MW01031345

RADICAL MEDICINE

"*Radical Medicine* is a thoughtful and comprehensive guide to everything I have learned and do daily. It really reminds us how difficult this work is, how subtle, how layered we are. Patients most often do not understand this and increasingly want the magic vitamin. I am going to post some things from the book on the office bulletin board, so that people can appreciate what is really involved in healing."

ROBERT ZIEVE, M.D., AUTHOR OF *BEYOND THE MEDICAL MELTDOWN,* FOUNDER AND DIRECTOR OF THE CENTER FOR HEALTHY MEDICINE

"I am impressed with the breadth and depth of *Radical Medicine.* In fact, just after reading this wonderful book I was able to help two of my most puzzling cases. Thank you, Dr. Williams."

BRETT JACQUES, N.D., CONTRIBUTOR TO THE *TEXTBOOK OF ANTI-AGING MEDICINE*

"*Radical Medicine* has set the standard in holistic medicine. Every important issue has been identified. What a magnificent book."

HARVEY BIGELSEN, M.D., AUTHOR OF *DOCTORS ARE MORE HARMFUL THAN GERMS,* FOUNDING MEMBER OF THE AMERICAN HOLISTIC MEDICAL ASSOCIATION

"This is the bible of true health. I have had so much joy reading it. Every dentist should be working with someone like Dr. Williams."

SANDOR HITES, D.D.S.

"As a patient, I found that the content of *Radical Medicine* directly reflected my own recognition of what my body/being needed for health and healing. I am now being treated at the Paracelsus Clinic in Switzerland, and their biological medical model mirrors some of the overall healthcare and wellness approaches explained in this revelatory and fascinating book. *Radical Medicine* contains a lifetime of wisdom."

JEANNINE WALSTON, COFOUNDER AND EXECUTIVE DIRECTOR OF EMBODIWORKS, A NONPROFIT PROVIDING INTEGRATIVE CANCER CARE RESOURCES

"*Radical Medicine* is an outstanding book, an important and useful contribution to natural medicine."

Pablo Bellavite, M.D., coauthor of *The Emerging Science of Homeopathy*

"*Radical Medicine* brings tremendous scope, wisdom, and experience to the table. I am looking forward to integrating its pearls into my practice."

Chris Jeong, L.Ac.

"*Radical Medicine* is truly amazing—a wonderful work with such depth that I didn't want to put it down. I thought I knew more than most doctors in certain areas but was surprised when I felt an eagerness to get back to working with holistic medicine while reading it. I didn't think there was any resource out there that would elicit that reaction. I am blown away at its depth."

James Johnson, holistic health advocate

"I'm amazed at Louisa L. Williams's knowledge in holistic dentistry—great book!"

Frances Chen, D.D.S.

"*Radical Medicine* is cutting-edge, comprehensive, and easy for my clients to read."

Robley Pryor, colonic therapist

"Very impressive—there are no competitors to this unique book."

John Iams, physical therapist, founder of the Primal Reflex Release Technique

"*Radical Medicine* is terrific. I appreciate the central role it has correctly ascribed to the harm being inflicted by traditional dentistry."

Charles G. Brown, Esq., National Counsel, Consumers for Dental Choice

"*Radical Medicine* is breathtaking. The coverage of all areas of health is amazing, including the accurate history of craniopathy. Louisa L. Williams is to be congratulated for creating a masterpiece."

Reid Rasmussen, D.C., chiropractic physician

RADICAL MEDICINE

Cutting-Edge Natural Therapies That Treat the Root Causes of Disease

Louisa L. Williams, M.S., D.C., N.D.

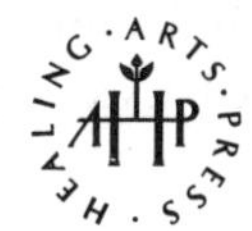

Healing Arts Press
Rochester, Vermont • Toronto, Canada

Healing Arts Press
One Park Street
Rochester, Vermont 05767
www.HealingArtsPress.com

Healing Arts Press is a division of Inner Traditions International

Originally published in 2007 by International Arts Publishing under the title *Radical Medicine: Profound Intervention in a Profoundly Toxic Age*

Note to the reader: *This book is intended as an informational guide. The remedies, approaches, and techniques described herein are meant to supplement, and not to be a substitute for, professional medical care or treatment. They should not be used to treat a serious ailment without prior consultation with a qualified health care professional.*

Library of Congress Cataloging-in-Publication Data

Williams, Louisa L.
Radical medicine : cutting-edge natural therapies that treat the root causes of disease / Louisa L. Williams.
p. ; cm.
Includes bibliographical references and index.
Summary: "A 'radical' approach to holistic healing that examines the root causes and cures for ailments such as Alzheimer's disease, breast cancer, and heart attacks"—Provided by publisher.
ISBN 978-1-59477-411-9 (hardcover)
1. Naturopathy. I. Title.
[DNLM: 1. Naturopathy—methods. 2. Diet Therapy. 3. Holistic Health. 4. Toxins, Biological. WB 935]
RZ440.W553 2011
615.5'35—dc22

2010051949

Printed and bound in India by Replika Press Pvt. Ltd.

10 9 8 7 6 5 4 3 2 1

Text design and layout by Priscilla Baker
This book was typeset in Garamond Premier Pro with Schneidler and Agenda used as display typefaces

To send correspondence to the author of this book, mail a first-class letter to the author c/o Inner Traditions • Bear & Company, One Park Street, Rochester, VT 05767, and we will forward the communication, or contact the author at **www.radicalmedicine.com**.

To my patients, who honor me with their trust and perseverance, and whose courage to live the principles embodied in Radical Medicine*—despite the pressure from an allopathically oriented media and often doubting family and friends—has inspired and shaped the contents of every aspect of this book.*

❧

NAVIGATING RADICAL MEDICINE

Radical Medicine was written for holistically oriented individuals who are not satisfied with simply "getting by" with marginal health and for those healthcare practitioners who are committed to supporting their patients in the pursuit of optimal health.

Reading chronologically from chapter 1 through chapter 18 will provide you with a good overview of the typical flow of treatment protocols for most individuals. In clinical practice the specific "trees" (the dental and tonsil focal infections or scar interference fields described in chapters 11, 12, and 13) are often treated after the larger "forest" (the systemic drainage and detoxification protocols detailed in chapters 2, 3, and 4) has been addressed.

However, for those who are already quite knowledgeable in holistic health, reading a chapter of interest out of the normal order should pose no challenge. Each part is comprehensive and complete enough on its own to be understood, especially if you refer to the glossary for the definition of any unfamiliar terms.

Helpful resources for obtaining recommended products and further information are provided throughout the book as well as in the resources section at the end.* All information is current and accurate as of the time of this printing. However, new and better products are constantly being developed. **For the author's most up-to-date recommendations, see www.radicalmedicine.com.**

Although this book is inteneded for both practitioners and patients alike, *Radical Medicine* is not your typical self-help book. While there are a few home treatments that you can do yourself—such as the elimination/challenge test for food allergies described in chapter 6—for the most part the treatments recommended in this book must be administered by well-trained and knowledgeable professionals.

It is always essential to remember that any therapeutic measure effective enough to significantly help can also hurt, especially if employed by an inexperienced individual. Therefore, potential patients should earnestly seek out holistic physicians, dentists, and other practitioners who are able to diagnose the underlying causes of their particular dysfunction or disease and prescribe the most effective treatments.

The information presented in this book is intended to provide insight and complement the advice of your physician, not replace it. **Please refer to appendix 1, "Description of Holistic Practitioners," for more information and to the resources section for help in locating appropriate professionals.**

---

*The author receives no financial remuneration from any of the companies whose products are recommended in this book.

CONTENTS

ACKNOWLEDGMENTS

A true accounting of all the holistic practitioners who should be acknowledged here would take up many more pages than this brief section allows. Let me just say, however, that I am truly indebted to all the very devoted and hardworking colleagues from whom I have learned so much, and who have been instrumental in the evolution of this book. It has been, and continues to be, a great privilege to be a part of this holistic community in which we all share the same dedication to healing without harm.

Specifically, my very genuine thanks and gratitude go to:

Mikhael Adams, N.D.; the late Gérard Guéniot, M.D.; and Etienne Vandekerkhove for their insight into the European field of drainage and their encyclopedic knowledge of the gemmotherapy remedies.

Dan Green, D.D.S.; Douglas Cook, D.D.S.; Oloph Granath, D.D.S.; Scott Loman, D.D.S.; and Robert Jarvis, D.D.S.; for their input into chapters 3 and 11, based on their invaluable experience in the forefront of the field of holistic dentistry.

Sally Fallon, for her courage in tirelessly propagating sound nutritional advice based on ancestral wisdom and valid scientific research that is so well conveyed in her book, *Nourishing Traditions,* and her journal, *Wise Traditions,* which are both greatly referenced throughout this book, and especially in chapter 5.

Marie Bishop and Christopher Cogswell, for their encouragement, editing support, extensive holistic knowledge, and insightful suggestions.

Jerry Bouquot, D.D.S., for the use of his clear and convincing photographs of a healthy jawbone as compared to a dead gangrenous one, which is typically seen in dental focal infection sites.

Joan Grinzi, R.N., executive director of the Price-Pottenger Nutrition Foundation, who facilitated the use of the before-and-after photos of native peoples seen in chapter 16 from the incomparable research of America's father of holistic dentistry, Weston A. Price, D.D.S.

Raymond Silkman, D.D.S., and Terrance Spahl, D.D.S., two orthopedically oriented holistic dentists who generously shared their valuable patient photographs that so graphically illustrate in chapter 16 the very serious structural malformations that can occur from deficient nutrition, the incorrect use of braces, and other factors.

Jerome Mittelman, D.D.S., and Beverly Mittelman, B.S., C.N.C., for their very demonstrative photos of dental malocclusion generated by prolonged thumb-sucking and pacifier use.

Carmen Marcadis, D.C., for her constructive criticism and exceptionally helpful editing suggestions in chapter 17.

Bryan Janssen; Perry Janssen, M.A.; Terry Saracino; and Mitch Visnick; for their editing and insights in chapter 18, based on their years of personal and professional experience undergoing as well as teaching psychospiritual approaches.

Robert Shane, for his input and suggestions in the energetic testing material in appendix 3, based on his numerous years of experience working with a multitude of various energetic testing methods.

And finally, I want to thank my colleague Dietrich Klinghardt, M.D., Ph.D., for the invaluable knowledge and extensive clinical expertise I have gained from his brilliant teaching and insight, which contributed tremendously to the writing of chapters 3, 4, 9, 10, 11, 12, and 13, as well as other parts of this book.

I further want to thank Sarah Scott, Jamaica Burns, Nancy Ringer, Mary Miller, and Jeanie Levitan for their skillful editorial work; Jennifer Taylor for her excellent illustrations; and Melanie Lamoureux for her creative and artistic vision.

Personally, I want to express my deep gratitude and appreciation for my Ridhwan teacher, Laurie Wattell, whose warmth and wisdom created a holding field that has tremendously furthered my own self-understanding and growth. I further want to thank my brilliant parents, Fred and Margaret Williams, whose love of knowledge and literature prompted my long educational odyssey as well as my interest in finally authoring a book.

AN INTRODUCTION TO RADICAL MEDICINE

Radical: 'ra-di-kəl (Latin: radix), *going to the root or origin; pertaining to what is fundamental, far-reaching, and thorough*

Radical medicine is a form of holistic medicine that is committed to curing disease, not simply suppressing or palliating symptoms. It has two central tenets. The first is that only through getting to the roots or underlying cause of the problem can true healing occur. For example, many holistic physicians give natural thyroid medication to their patients when blood test results indicate hypothyroidism. However, if these physicians fail to diagnose and treat an underlying common cause of hypothyroidism—mercury intoxication from amalgam fillings—they ultimately do their patients a great disservice.

> **physician/practitioner:** The term *physician* refers to all licensed doctors (N.D.s, M.D.s, D.C.s, D.O.s, and D.D.S.s). The term *practitioner* refers to licensed doctors as well as other holistic specialists such as acupuncturists, nutritionists, and physical therapists. See appendix 1, "Description of Holistic Practitioners," for more information.

The second tenet of radical medicine is that although drinking pure water, exercising regularly, and eating organic foods are all important—even essential—these general health guidelines are no longer sufficient to ensure the preservation of good health for most individuals. Unfortunately, in these modern toxic times, our immune systems have been subjected to poisons unparalleled in previous centuries and unimaginable by our earlier ancestors. The pervasive petrochemicals polluting our homes and environment, the injection of DNA-damaging childhood vaccinations, the placement of toxic mercury amalgam fillings in our mouths, and the excessive use of antibiotics and other prescription drugs are just a sample of the modern traumas that have rendered many individuals chronically ill—and perhaps, in some cases, essentially incapable of ever truly getting well. Until these and other "obstacles to cure" are adequately addressed, general guidelines—although important to maintaining a healthy lifestyle—are simply no longer adequate to fend off degenerative disease and help individuals regain their birthright of optimal health.[1] Indeed, in our current toxic environment, much more "radical" measures are required.

A TERMINAL DIAGNOSIS FOR MODERN MEDICINE

Many health-minded individuals have gone to great lengths to feel better. They purchase water filters, shop at health food stores, take nutritional supplements, and try to exercise regularly. Some have gone even further and avoid their primary food allergy, purchase herbal and homeopathic remedies when they get sick, and do ongoing personal growth work. And yet, for the majority of even these highly motivated individuals, the abundant energy, vitality, and feeling of well-being that define optimum health are rarely realized. Furthermore, many live in fear—often unconsciously—of succumbing later in life to cancer, heart disease, Alzheimer's, or any of the other devastating illnesses that have become so epidemic in our modern world. And sadly, the long-awaited cures that doctors, numerous charities and associations, and various telethons have been promising us for decades are "just around the corner" continue to remain elusive.

Cardiovascular Disease—Reputedly Our Number One Killer

In 1900, the number of deaths resulting from heart disease was 27,427; in 2002 it was 696,947.[2] These figures themselves dramatically depict the obvious failure of modern medicine to find an adequate treatment for heart disease. However, when another figure is added to the equation—the $3.2 billion (and counting) spent by the American Heart Association since 1949 to increase knowledge about the disease—this failure is all the more conspicuous.[3] In fact, cardiovascular disease—a more recently utilized category that encompasses all forms of heart disease including heart attack, congestive heart failure, and stroke—is considered to be the leading cause of death and disability in the United States.[4]

MORE U.S. DEATHS FROM HEART DISEASE OR CANCER?

Although it was recently reported that cancer had eclipsed heart disease as the number one disease killer, this statistic did not include Americans over the age of eighty-five. Furthermore, it accounted for only heart disease—myocardial infarction (heart attack) and angina pectoris (chest pain)—and excluded other heart ailments that make up the broader category of cardiovascular disease. However, when *all* ailments of the heart and circulatory system are included within this broader category, deaths from cardiovascular disease far outweigh deaths from cancer.[5]

Cancer—We're Not Winning the War

In 1900, *3 percent* of Americans were diagnosed with cancer during their lifetime.[6] In less than four decades, between 1907 and 1936, cancer rates rose by an astounding 90 percent.[7] Finally, in 1971, President Nixon declared a "War on Cancer" and Congress passed the National Cancer Act to try and quell this epidemic disease.

Based on numerous media reports over the next several decades, it did appear that allopathic medicine was making progress in treating this devastating disease with chemotherapy, radiation, and surgery. However, the National Cancer Institute recently reported that these previously optimistic reports on the decline of several types of cancer were actually false and simply reflected significant delays in the reporting of cancer cases. In fact, in 2002 the institute revealed that many cancer rates had, in reality, been on the *rise,* including breast and lung cancer rates in women and prostate cancer rates in men.[8] And although often-touted statistics point out that the incidence of lung cancer has declined in men, this has nothing to do with new medical treatments or advances in science but correlates directly with the decline in smoking that began with the Surgeon General's emphasis on quitting in 1964, and the subsequent widespread advertising and educational efforts launched to propagate the hazards inherent in this dangerous habit.[9]

U.S. SMOKING RATES

The incidence of smoking in men began to decline in 1964 after the Surgeon General's warning on the dangers of tobacco first became public. However, the number of female smokers continued to grow for another twenty years. Overall, though, the percentage of Americans of both sexes who smoke fell from 42 percent in 1965 to 22 percent in 2000. And due to this reduction, women's lung cancer rates are predicted to also decline.[10]

Despite this reduction in lung cancer rates due to a reduced incidence of smoking, cancer is reported to be our number two killer and was responsible for 557,271 deaths in 2002.[11] Indeed, overall cancer rates have risen, from the previous rate of affecting approximately one in three individuals (as reported in 1997) to the present percentages estimated by the American Cancer Society of striking approximately 50 percent of all men and 40 percent of all women.[12] And, as with cardiovascular disease, although for the last thirty years the medical establishment has been given over $40 *billion* in donations to find a cure, we are actually no closer to winning the war on cancer than we were a century ago.[13] In fact, the United Nations' cancer research agency recently postulated that by 2030 cancer will kill more than 13.2 million people a year—almost double the number who died from the disease in 2008.[14]

Allopathic Medical Treatment—"At Least" the Third Leading Killer

In the summer of 2000, the *Journal of the American Medical Association* (*JAMA*) reported that the annual death rate from *iatrogenic* causes—that is, deaths caused by doctors through the adverse effects of prescription drugs and surgery, errors in medical judgment, and nosocomial (hospital-induced) infections—was estimated at 225,000 annually, rendering it at least the third-leading cause of death in the United States, just behind cardiovascular disease and cancer.[15] This statistic would be shocking in and of itself if it weren't for the fact that this 225,000 figure included *only* deaths occurring in hospitals, and therefore excluded outpatient iatrogenic deaths, estimated to be 190,000 annually. Additionally, the author of this *JAMA* article, Barbara Starfield, a physician and researcher at the Johns Hopkins School of Hygiene and Public Health, further disclosed that this estimate of 225,000 was much lower than the figures arrived at by an Institute of Medicine (IOM) study the previous year, in which iatrogenic deaths were estimated to range from 230,000 to 284,000 annually.

allopathic: The term *allopathic* means "other than, or against, disease." It refers to the treatment of disease utilizing prescription drugs that are antagonistic to and suppressive of disease symptoms (e.g., antihistamines, antibiotics, and anti-inflammatories) and the surgical removal (-ectomy) of diseased tissue (e.g., appendectomy, hysterectomy, and tonsillectomy). Medical as well as osteopathic physicians are taught allopathic principles and practices in their respective medical colleges.

iatrogenic: The term *iatrogenic,* from the Greek *iatros* (physician) and *gennan* (to produce), refers to any adverse state or condition produced by a doctor due to poor treatment.

nosocomial: The term *nosocomial* derives from the Greek roots *nosos* (disease) and *komeion* (to take care of). It refers to any disease originating in a medical institution or hospital.

THE 225,000 IATROGENIC DEATHS REPORTED ANNUALLY

This figure of 225,000 is only the mortality, or death, rate. It does not include the effect of allopathic care on morbidity—that is, chronic illness or disability as a result of adverse reactions to prescription drugs, errors in medical judgment, or nosocomial infections.

The breakdown of each category within this estimated iatrogenic death rate of 225,000 is:

12,000 deaths per year from unnecessary surgery
7,000 deaths per year from medication errors in hospitals
20,000 deaths per year from other errors in hospitals
80,000 deaths per year from nosocomial infections
106,000 deaths per year from non-error, adverse effects of medications[16]

It is also essential to keep in mind one other crucial fact: typically, iatrogenic deaths are grossly underreported due to physicians' natural reluctance to admit fault. What percentage of doctors are going to risk losing their license and livelihood by admitting fault through honestly reporting deaths caused from extremely toxic chemotherapy (and other) drugs, excessive doses of radiation, unwise surgery in an already weakened patient, and so forth, in this highly litigious society? Further complicating the issue, many patients die nowadays while taking two, seven, or even more medications at the same time. This typical protocol of *polypharmacy* can baffle even the most knowledgeable toxicologist seeking the actual cause of death. And the possibility of funding by the allopathic medical-pharmaceutical industry to have more autopsies performed to shed light on this matter is not very likely. In this same *JAMA* article, Dr. Starfield disclosed that "most deaths resulting from these underlying [iatrogenic] causes are likely to be recorded according to the immediate cause of death (such as organ failure)."*

*Dr. Starfield asserts that "more consistent use of 'E' codes" (which represent injuries and other adverse effects that are caused by environmental or external events and are used in addition to the diagnostic code that characterizes the pathology), such as "Complications of Surgical and Medical Care" (ICD codes 960–979 and 996–999), "might improve the recognition of the magnitude of their effect." (Barbara Starfield, "Is US Health Really the Best in the World?" *JAMA* 284:4 [July 26, 2000], 483.)

Thus, *most* deaths that result primarily from the adverse effects of drugs, surgery, or nosocomial infections typically receive a diagnostic code of the *secondary* cause of death, such as heart failure or kidney failure.

Taking these three factors in mind—the exclusion of outpatient iatrogenic deaths (estimated at 190,000), *JAMA*'s conservative estimate of iatrogenic deaths as compared to the IOM's the year before (225,000 versus 230,000 to 284,000), and the natural inclination of physicians not to admit fault by recording deaths according to the immediate cause of mortality rather than the primary iatrogenic factor—leads to the even more startling possibility that this infamous doctor-induced third place in mortality may be dangerously conservative. That is, if all doctors—those practicing in hospitals, large clinics, and smaller offices—began to properly and completely code and report the real cause of their patients' death *honestly,* this iatrogenic death rate could very possibly eclipse our number two killer, cancer, and might even surpass the number one killer itself, cardiovascular disease.

These appalling statistics are such a frank indictment of the hazards of modern allopathic medicine that they are almost too unimaginable for the mind to comprehend. However, these figures emanate not from an angry counterculture publication that could be viewed with suspicion but from the highest bastions of medicine itself—Johns Hopkins University and the *Journal of the American Medical Association.*

"Death by Medicine"—Actually the Number One Killer

In 2004, Gary Null, Ph.D., a nutritionist and leader in the field of holistic medicine, decided to remedy the omission in Dr. Starfield's research and include outpatient deaths. He and a group of Ph.D., M.D., and N.D. researchers subsequently began to tabulate *all* the annual deaths in the United States caused by allopathic medicine—both inpatient and outpatient. What they discovered was nothing less than shocking. Null and his team found that conventional medicine had actually eclipsed both heart disease and cancer, achieving the ignominious position of number one in U.S. mortality rates.[17] Thus, the healthcare system that the vast majority of Americans subscribe to in this country is not only *not* delivering effective therapeutic intervention but actually causing more death than any disease it has ever purported to treat. Readers who want to read more about this astounding new study should google "Death by Medicine."

Not a New Phenomenon

It is important to point out that these iatrogenic deaths are not a new phenomenon—that is, they are not simply secondary to a recent spate of newly approved toxic drugs or current imprudent hospital procedures. As reported in a 1998 *JAMA* article, an extensive meta-analysis of the electronic databases of hospitals from 1966 to 1996 revealed that the incidence of fatal adverse drug reactions (ADRs) caused by prescription medications *alone* has remained quite stable over the last thirty years. In fact, the authors of this longitudinal study even chose to exclude deaths caused by errors in drug administration to show that "there are a large number of serious ADRs even when the drugs are properly prescribed and administered." However, even when these researchers excluded medical errors, unnecessary surgeries, and nosocomial infections, ADRs alone were still estimated to be between the fourth- and sixth-leading causes of death in the United States for the last three decades.[18*]

1.5 MILLION PEOPLE ANNUALLY HARMED BY ERRORS IN DRUG ADMINISTRATION

A July 2006 study found that 1.5 million people are harmed every year by medication errors, and that at least 7,000 of these individuals are killed annually by these iatrogenic mistakes. This study further revealed that hospitalized patients, on average, are subjected to one medication error *every single day.*[19]

---

*It is important to point out that the researchers counted deaths from heart disease and stroke separately, rather than grouping them in the broad category of cardiovascular disease, as Dr. Starfield's study did. This rendered ADRs ranking fourth, with an estimated 137,000 deaths per year, after heart disease, cancer, and stroke, rather than third, after cardiovascular disease and cancer. And when the researchers applied the more conservative estimate of 76,000 deaths, ADRs ranked as the sixth-leading cause of death, after pulmonary disease and accidents (and, again, ADRs would have moved up to fifth place if the researchers had used the broader category of cardiovascular disease).

Americans Spend the Most for the Worst Health Care

When another alarming statistic is factored in—that although the United States spends billions on health care, out of thirteen countries it ranks an average of twelfth in regard to sixteen health indicators (e.g., neonatal mortality, life expectancy, and so forth)—defending America's current system of health care becomes even more untenable.[20]

COUNTRIES RANKED ACCORDING TO QUALITY OF HEALTH CARE

The thirteen countries, in order of their average ranking (with first being the best), were Japan, Sweden, Canada, France, Australia, Spain, Finland, the Netherlands, the United Kingdom, Denmark, Belgium, the United States, and Germany.

In May 2006, "stunning new research" revealed that even though the United States spends twice as much as England on health care for its citizens, Americans still have higher rates of diabetes, stroke, lung disease, and cancer. Even when the researchers "crunched numbers" to remove the influence of lifestyle factors such as obesity, Americans were still found to be approximately twice as unhealthy as their British counterparts.[21] (And England's healthcare system is considered to be generally inferior to that of its neighbors.) Dr. Michael Marmot, an epidemiologist and coauthor of the study, found that even economic status was not a factor. In fact, the *richest* third of Americans were shockingly found to be in worse health than the *poorest* third of the English.[22] However, no researchers speculated on the most likely culprit of our spectacularly high morbidity and mortality rates: the United States' strong financial commitment to the allopathic medical and pharmaceutical industry, and this industry's very real and fatal "side effects." Thus, prescription drugs and surgery, the primary tools that modern medicine uses to purportedly heal disease, have actually reached the infamous position of being among its top killers—*rendering the cure often worse than the disease.*

M.D.s—"Bought and Paid For"

The initiation of real change and reform in this seriously flawed state of medical practice has a rather pessimistic prognosis due to the viselike grip pharmaceutical companies maintain over the majority of doctors. For example, in the January 26, 2006, edition of the *Journal of the American Medical Association* (*JAMA*), it was reported that the pharmaceutical industry spends approximately 90 percent of its $21 billion annual marketing budget on promotions for doctors (approximately $13,000 per practicing physician annually) in an effort to influence their prescribing behavior.[23] And in a related study published in the *New England Journal of Medicine* in 2004, the authors revealed that the pharmaceutical industry funds the majority of allopathic physicians' continuing medical education programs, accounting for $900 million of the $1 billion spent on this mandatory ongoing training.[24] Additionally, as reported in another *JAMA* study published in 2005, the pervasive influence pharmaceutical companies wield begins not simply when physicians receive their licenses to practice but in medical school, where drug companies spend an estimated $12 billion annually on weekly promotions and teaching materials. In fact, these researchers found that by their third year, medical students either receive a gift from or go to an event sponsored by a drug company approximately *once a week,* resulting in an "environment with progressively fewer boundaries between medicine and the pharmaceutical industry."[25]

And perhaps even more disturbing, when the American Medical Association attempted in 2002 to educate physicians about the ethical guidelines governing gifts from drug companies, $645,000 of their $695,000 education budget was funded by none other than the drug companies themselves.[26] Thus, not only has our present "bought and paid for" medical system failed to provide the promised cures for serious disease, but it has increasingly come under the pervasive influence of profit-motivated pharmaceutical drug companies.[27] And since prescription drug sales are the fastest-growing portion of healthcare costs—increasing at a rate of approximately 12 percent per year—the number of iatrogenic deaths can only be expected to rise.[28]*

*Twelve percent is an average figure; prescription drug sales grew at the highest rate ever recorded—18 percent—in 1999. (M. Angell, *The Truth About Drug Companies* [New York: Random House, 2004], xii.)

It should be noted that there are many allopathic physicians and scientists who are truly caring, dedicated, and working hard to find real answers behind this modern epidemic of chronic and degenerative disease. But it is time—in fact, it is past time—for these physicians and scientists, as well as the pharmaceutical industry, insurance companies, government agencies, and the general public, to stop and take a hard and unbiased look at these frightening statistics that reveal the very serious level of dysfunction in the United States' current healthcare practices.

HOLISTIC MEDICINE—PRESENTLY INSUFFICIENT

Clearly, allopathic Western medicine is an ailing system, and in light of its alarming iatrogenic statistics and dangerous treatments, it is hard to imagine how it could ever be a viable solution to our current healthcare crisis. But many may ask if holistic medicine is truly the answer, and if it is a viable alternative in the treatment of serious disease. It certainly seemed to be in former times.

From the 1700s through the early 1900s, famous natural healers, such as Vincenz Priessnitz and Sebastian Kneipp of Europe and Benedict Lust and Henry Lindlahr in America, claimed seemingly miraculous cures for asthma, rheumatism, tuberculosis, and even smallpox and syphilis.[29] Perhaps even more astonishing is how these men facilitated these cures purely through natural methods, such as hot and cold hydrotherapy (water treatments), heliotherapy (sunbathing), herbs, fresh air, rest, and simple whole foods.[30] These "nature cures" sound quite remarkable—and even highly improbable—today. And, in actuality, the doubt that arises in most readers' minds is not only understandable but, for the most part, quite valid in regard to this issue. In the majority of cases, these natural measures truly *are no longer* effective enough to treat modern-day diseases or dysfunction.

So what has changed? No one would argue against the fact that the world certainly has, but few are aware of the major effect modern toxins have wrought on our bodies. Although the modern industrialized world has afforded us good sanitation and freedom from much of the drudgery of the past, it has also brought with it air and water pollution, chemical preservatives in our foods, and toxic metals that poison the earth as well as our bodies. In addition to these external stressors, we suffer the liability of inherited genetic weakness that these pollutants caused in our forefathers and foremothers. Put simply, we're just no longer the sturdy stock that most of our grandparents (or great-grandparents, depending on your age) were. We currently suffer from the *double violation* of both a weakened genetic inheritance from our twentieth-century-born parents and the toxic medical, dental, and environmental assaults we are subjected to during our formative immune-system-building years. Ask any older chiropractor who used to heal a child's ear infection with only one cervical (neck) adjustment or any retired naturopath who remembers curing menstrual cramps through a few hydrotherapy sessions: patients simply do not respond as they used to.

Because of this modern-day double whammy of nature (genetic weakness) and nurture (environmental toxicity), general holistic health guidelines are simply no longer efficacious. Add to this the fact that too many patients present to the holistic physician's doorstep only after their immune systems have been ravaged by medications with two pages of side effects written in fine print, chemotherapy, radiation, or aggressive surgeries and the prognosis becomes exceptionally grave. Clearly, stronger intervention is needed.

RADICAL MEDICINE'S ANSWER

In addition to the natural therapies of diet, exercise, and rest that have been generally prescribed for the sick, both currently and in previous centuries, it is essential to further facilitate healing in modern-day patients, who typically present with complex issues and multiple toxic insults. To do this you must first be a good detective. In order to truly effect a cure, it is imperative that the holistic practitioner initially ascertains a correct *diagnosis,* and through that understanding then prescribes an appropriate *therapy.* That is, just as in quality psychological work, only when you know where you've been can you see a clear direction of where you need to go. It is the same way in medicine. The true cause of a patient's disease or dysfunction is always paramount, and when it is revealed through a thorough history, exam, and necessary laboratory work, this well-considered diagnosis both signals and shapes the appropriate treatment, or treatments, needed. Thus, a practitioner must always endeavor to go to the root of the problem to fully utilize the knowledge and master the methods of treatment that are conveyed in *Radical Medicine.* In fact, as described earlier, the term *radical* for this field of holistic medicine was chosen not for its common connotation of "unorthodox" or "extreme" but for its original denotation as that which goes "to the root or origin" and that which is "fundamental, far-reaching, and thorough."[31]

Holistic Diagnoses: Getting to the True Roots of Disease

The term *diagnosis* derives from a Greek word that literally means to "see through" in order to arrive at a "superior" level of knowledge or understanding.[32] Thus, a true diagnosis, according to the earliest Greek origins of the word, requires that the physician "see through" patients' various signs and symptoms to arrive at such a masterful level of understanding that the actual cause of the disease or dysfunction is clearly evident. For example, "irritable bowel syndrome" (IBS)—alternating constipation and diarrhea with intermittent pain—is not a valid "diagnosis" as Hippocrates and the early Greeks first defined it. However, "irritable bowel syndrome secondary to a gluten allergy and an appendix scar interference field"* *is,* in that it "sees through" the patient's overt bowel symptoms to the underlying deeper causative factors. Furthermore, this more descriptive and holistic diagnosis is much more clarifying and thus often relieving to patients, who in most cases have only received the standard allopathic approach to IBS—that is, "stress reduction" and suppressive prescription drugs. However, when the true cause of their chronic pain and suffering is known, this knowledge helps transform patients' despair into hope, and also into very real and tangible action to initiate healing. Thus, the more descriptive diagnosis "sees through" the overt symptoms to guide both the patient and the physician toward the most effective therapies, as well as the possibility of a real cure through treating the cause and not just the effects of disease.

*A *scar interference field* is any external or internal scar that creates chronic irritation and disturbance in the body. What is so insidious about interference fields is that they rarely cause disturbance locally. That is, the scars are usually quite asymptomatic (have no symptoms). However, they often create *disturbed fields* distally, in other parts of the body, such as a hysterectomy scar that can trigger intermittent migraine headaches, fatigue, and/or depression. (For more information about scar interference fields, see part 4.)

DANGEROUS DIAGNOSES

Karl Menninger, M.D., the innovative and brilliant psychiatrist who cofounded the Menninger Clinic in Topeka, Kansas, for the treatment of mental illness, noted that the very word *cancer* is enough to "kill some patients who would not have succumbed (as rapidly) to the malignancy from which they suffer."[33]

Effective Treatments

In many cases, a holistic diagnosis has the additional benefit of clearly indicating a specific treatment, consisting of simply the removal of what the founder of homeopathy, Samuel Hahnemann, referred to as the "obstacles to cure." In Hahnemann's day, in the late eighteenth and early nineteenth centuries, these obstacles included the excessive use of opium, "blood-letting in torrents," and the widespread use of mercury-containing calomel powder.[34] Sadly, two centuries later, this highly toxic metal is still in widespread use by conventional dentists, and it is even approved by the primary dental trade union, the American Dental Association (ADA). Thus, our modern-day "obstacles" *still* include mercury; the mercury amalgam fillings in our mouths must be replaced with less toxic alternatives. Another common obstacle to healing is the slow poisoning of our bodies by the toxic chemicals that are unfortunately so pervasive in every aspect of our lives. However, by simply removing these toxic personal care and cleaning products from our homes and workplaces and replacing them with nontoxic alternatives, this chemical load can be considerably lightened. Additionally, chronic dental focal infections such as failed root canals, abscessed teeth, and impacted or incorrectly extracted wisdom teeth can be a major block to healing and frequently the instigator of serious disease. Often these teeth must be "sacrificed" and removed through appropriate *cavitation surgery* methods to fully restore health.

Other efficacious treatments described in *Radical Medicine* originated in Europe and are still so esoteric that only a small minority of knowledgeable and holistically oriented practitioners utilize them in their practice. However, their long-lasting and curative effects are so significant that the use of these remedies and techniques in holistic medicine is truly indispensable. These include gemmotherapy remedies from Italy (developed in Belgium in the 1950s) to gently and effectively drain accumulated toxins from organs and tissues, as well as neural therapy from Germany and auriculotherapy from France to treat chronic foci (scar interference fields and dental, sinus, tonsil, and genital focal infections). Another essential therapy that originated from Europe, called constitutional homeopathy, is included in this book because it is the single most effective healing modality that specifically addresses a patient's miasmic, or inherited, susceptibility to disease. Recently updated by the revolutionary contributions of Indian physician Rajan Sankaran and his Mumbai colleagues, constitutional homeopathy is an essential component to every patient's healing protocol. Other important treatments detailed in *Radical Medicine* include the use of nutritional supplements and homeopathic nosodes (remedies made from diseased tissue that stimulate the body to mobilize its immune defenses against that disease) in the treatment of vaccinosis (disease and dysfunction caused by immunization); functional appliances prescribed by orthopedically oriented dentists in treating temporomandibular (jaw joint) dysfunction (TMD) and malocclusions (bad bites); and quality psychospiritual work to address the self-sabotaging mental and emotional issues inherent in many individuals' early childhood development that can most insidiously generate and continue to maintain chronic illness.

These "radical" treatments not only are of major importance in the cure of many degenerative diseases but also are essential for those individuals who aren't satisfied living with even the "minor" stress of chronic symptoms. Furthermore, these mild aches and pains, intermittent constipation or diarrhea, too frequent colds and bouts of flu, moderate fatigue, and other relatively functional (versus seriously pathological) health issues always signal some form of underlying disturbance that—without effective intervention—will only continue to escalate as you age. *Radical Medicine* is therefore written not just for the seriously ill but also for those who consider optimal health and freedom from chronic pain and dysfunction their birthright. It is also written for those who have done everything that each new bestselling diet book and every weekly magazine inserted in the Sunday paper recommends, but who still continue to suffer from chronic and sometimes debilitating symptoms, or even simply an overall lack of well-being.

Radical Medicine is also written to educate holistic practitioners so that they can more effectively serve the growing number of patients dissatisfied with conventional allopathic medical care. It is especially targeted toward the doctors and practitioners with integrity and a caring attitude who have been less than satisfied with their treatment results. Through providing the underlying reasons as to why such a great percentage of patients nowadays are so "therapy resistant" and difficult to heal, I hope that this book will resolve a great deal of confusion for many frustrated healthcare practitioners. Furthermore, *Radical Medicine*'s numerous scientific references should satisfy even the most skeptical physicians and, it is hoped, rekindle the original passion that first influenced their decision to study (holistic or allopathic) medicine.

Finally, it is important to point out that addressing and healing all the various chemical, physical, and emotional insults our bodies have suffered in these modern times may not be a quick process; in fact, based on the amount of toxins most of us have been subjected to, it rarely is. For example, the estimated naturopathic time frame for getting well is based on the general formula that it takes one month of treatment for every year an individual has felt unwell. Thus, for a thirty-five-year-old with a mouthful of amalgam fillings who has been tired ever since her first pregnancy at age twenty, it may take around one and a half years after beginning effective treatment to feel consistently energetic every day. For a fifty-year-old who for years was prescribed antibiotics for childhood acne, it may take up to two years to completely clear the resulting intestinal dysbiosis (overgrowth of pathogenic bacteria and fungus), repopulate the gut (intestines) with healthy flora, and restore normal immune system functioning.

A Journey of Greater Self-Understanding

There are benefits, however, to this more lengthy journey of real cure versus the often-advertised quick fixes. This journey can be best understood through the spiritual principle that we are here to learn and evolve, which is just as true for our physical bodies as it is for our souls. This truth was best expressed by the Lebanese poet

Kahlil Gibran in his masterpiece, *The Prophet,* as "Your pain is the breaking of the shell that encloses your understanding."[35] Thus, examining and clearing these physical obstacles that act as both blocks and passageways to our self-understanding and spiritual growth is an important (and some would argue even essential) aspect in our psychospiritual development. Furthermore, the wisdom and strength gained from suffering, as well as the experience of feeling the demonstrable changes that effective treatment makes in our bodies, can instill a profound level of sensitivity and awareness rarely appreciated by those seemingly lucky few who have always enjoyed robust health. In fact, in holistic medicine there is a rather well-known but unwritten law that patients who undergo this physical metamorphosis are much more motivated to seek out advanced emotional and spiritual growth work as their healing progresses. And, fortunately, in contrast to the very numerous aforementioned drawbacks of our modern toxic age, one of the major benefits of living now is that psychological and spiritual healing is more accepted today and much more readily accessible than it was for our parents (or grandparents, depending on your age). Furthermore, these effective psychological therapies and spiritual paths are not just helpful but essential for those evolved individuals who have healed their physical bodies sufficiently enough to clearly feel the pull and attraction of the truly ultimate healing of *self*-understanding and divine love. And that, of course, is always the most radical medicine of all.

self: The word *self* here refers to the realization of one's divine nature or "true" self, in contrast to the separate ego. This was expressed in the ancient Indian scriptures called the *Upanishads* (circa 3000 BCE) as the Atman:

There are two selves, the separate ego
And the indivisible Atman. When
One rises above I and me and mine,
The Atman is revealed as one's real Self.[36]

NOTES

1. S. Hahnemann, *Organon of the Medical Art,* ed. W. O'Reilly (Palo Alto, Calif.: Birdcage Books, 1996), 227.
2. K. Kochanek et al., "Deaths: Final Data for 2002," *National Vital Statistics Reports* 53, no. 5 (October 12, 2004): 5.
3. American Heart Association; www.americanheart.org/presenter.jhtml?identifier=10809.
4. American Heart Association, www.heart.org/HEARTORG.
5. T. Maugh II, "Cancer No. 1 Killer in US," *Press Democrat,* January 20, 2005, A5.
6. B. Goldberg, "Lies, Damn Lies and Statistics," *Alternative Medicine,* January 2002, 12.
7. A. Fonder, *The Dental Physician* (Rock Falls, Ill.: Medical-Dental Arts, 1985), 27.
8. S. Begle, "New Statistics Show Increase, Not Decline, in Cancer Rates," *Our Toxic Times,* December 2002, 19–20 (reprinted from the *Wall Street Journal,* October 16, 2002).
9. B. Goldberg, "Lies, Damn Lies and Statistics," *Alternative Medicine,* January 2002, 12; T. Maugh II, "Cancer No. 1 Killer in US," *Press Democrat,* January 20, 2005, A5.
10. T. Maugh II, "Cancer No. 1 Killer in US," *Press Democrat,* January 20, 2005, A5.
11. Centers for Disease Control, "Fast Stats A to Z," www.cdc.gov/fastats/cancer.htm.
12. R. Buckman, *What You Really Need to Know about Cancer* (Baltimore: Johns Hopkins University Press, 1997), xiii; B. Goldberg, "Lies, Damn Lies and Statistics," *Alternative Medicine,* January 2002, 12.
13. B. Goldberg, "Lies, Damn Lies and Statistics," *Alternative Medicine,* January 2002, 12.
14. Reuters, "Cancer Deaths to Double by the Year 2030," Cancer on msnbc.com, June 1, 2010, www.msnbc.com/id/37451524.
15. B. Starfield, "Is US Health Really the Best in the World?" *Journal of the American Medical Association* 284, no. 4 (July 26, 2000): 484.
16. Ibid., 483.
17. Gary Null et al., "Death by Medicine," *Life Extension Magazine* (March 2004) www.lef.org/magazine/mag2004/mar2004_awsi_death_02.htm.
18. J. Lazarou et al., "Incidence of Adverse Drug Reactions in Hospitalized Patients," *Journal of the American Medical Association* 279, no. 15 (April 15, 1998): 1200–1205.
19. T. Maugh, "Drug Mistakes Hurt or Kill 1.5 Million Each Year in US," *Press Democrat,* July 21, 2006.
20. B. Starfield, "Is US Health Really the Best in the World?" *Journal of the American Medical Association* 284, no. 4 (2000): 483.
21. C. Johnson and M. Stobbe, "Study Shows Americans Sicker Than English," *Washington Post,* May 2, 2006.

22. Krugman, "Sicker Than We Ought to Be," *Press Democrat,* May 7, 2006, G1.

23. "Medical Schools Should Ban Drug Company Gifts, Samples, Contributions to Continuing Education, *JAMA* paper states," *Medical News Today,* January 31, 2006, 1, www.medicalnewstoday.com/medicalnews.php?newsid=36608; "*Journal of the American Medical Association:* Medical Schools Should Ban Drug Company Gifts, Publish More Information Online," *Health Beat,* January 26, 2006, 1, www.ihealthbeat.org/index.cfm?action=mmediadanditemid=118308.

24. B. Coyne, "Drug Co. Marketing Threatens Medical Students' Independence," *The New Standard,* September 7, 2005, 1, http://newstandardnews.net/content/?action=show_itemanditemid=2328.

25. Ibid.

26. A. Paulin, "Of Junk and Junkets," *Mother Jones,* January/February, 2002, 20.

27. Dr. B. Koerner, "No Free Lunch," *Mother Jones,* March/April 2003, 24.

28. M. Angell, *The Truth About Drug Companies* (New York: Random House, 2004), xii.

29. F. Kirchfield and W. Boyle, *Nature Doctors* (Portland, Ore.: Medicina Biologica, 1994), 21; H. Lindlahr, *Natural Therapeutics,* vol. 2 (Essex, England: C. W. Daniel Company, 1981), 48–50.

30. H. Lindlahr, *Natural Therapeutics,* vol. 2 (Essex, England: C. W. Daniel Company, 1981), 48–50.

31. L. Brown, ed., *The New Shorter Oxford English Dictionary* (Oxford: Clarendon Press, 1993), 2462.

32. Ibid., 659, 1108.

33. J. Goldberg, *Deceits of the Mind and Their Effects on the Body* (New Brunswick, N.J.: Transaction Publishers, 1991), 87.

34. S. Hahnemann, *Organon of the Medical Art,* ed. W. O'Reilly (Palo Alto, Calif.: Birdcage Books, 1996), 120–22, 227.

35. K. Gibran, *The Prophet* (New York: Alfred A. Knopf, Inc., 1923), 52.

36. E. Easwaran, *The Upanishads* (Tomales, Calif.: Nilgiri Press, 1991), 96.

PART ONE

UNDERSTANDING DISEASE PATTERNS AND INITIATING TREATMENT

The four miasms, which detail the four levels of disease individuals can succumb to, are described in the first chapter of this book because they are a valuable aid in both diagnosis and treatment. Diagnostically, understanding these four levels helps practitioners determine the severity of dysfunction their patient is experiencing, which helps them estimate the length of treatment that may be needed in each case. Knowledge of the four miasms additionally helps practitioners more accurately prescribe the remedies that most specifically match the symptoms and the level of dysfunction of the patient's particular illness.

Incorporating this information into their practice helps practitioners determine an individual's therapeutic progress—or lack of it. Thus, the four-miasm theory serves as an excellent indicator of whether patients are truly getting well and moving in the direction of optimal health, or whether they are making no significant progress—or worse, regressing and exhibiting more serious signs of illness. This centuries-old miasmic knowledge is particularly valuable in exposing symptom suppression (e.g., through prescription drugs) versus true healing and cure (through nonsuppressive natural medicines).

Readers of *Radical Medicine* will benefit from keeping this paradigm in mind, as it will be referenced throughout the book. For example, when individuals are seriously poisoned by mercury amalgam fillings, as described in chapter 3, they can manifest symptoms of the fourth and most debilitating miasm (known as the *luetic*), ranging from severe insomnia to multiple sclerosis. On the other hand, individuals who have mild to moderate dairy or wheat allergies, as described in chapter 6, often experience symptoms from the second miasmic level (known as the *sycotic*). However, through simply avoiding this particular food group and taking supportive nutritional and herbal supplementation, this sycotic group can typically fully recover from the effects of this immune system weakness relatively rapidly.

Chapter 2 describes how essential it is to effectively excrete toxins from the body, which can be achieved through the European healing system of drainage—often the first step in many treatment plans. The recommended drainage remedies, termed *gemmotherapy,* are made from embryonic plant parts, typically young buds, rootlets, and seeds. The advantage of using fresh, embryonic plant parts to make herbal remedies full of detoxifying and regenerative phytochemicals (antimicrobials, essential oils, hormones, vitamins, minerals, antioxidants, amino acids, and so on) is intuitively obvious. It is even more apparently obvious when you compare these remedies to the typical herbal remedies that are derived from mature, older plants that may have absorbed significant amounts of toxic metals and chemicals during their lifetime and contain older, less vital, and less bioavailable phytoconstituents. In contrast, the use of young embryonic plants bursting with nutrients, growth hormones, and vital energy is clearly superior, and an ideal way to both detoxify and regenerate overburdened and weakened tissues and organs in the body.

The basic understanding of miasmic disease tendencies and the practice of drainage provided in part 1 lays the groundwork for the more specific detoxification needs that are discussed in part 2.

1

THE FOUR MIASMIC DISEASE TENDENCIES

Samuel Hahnemann, the founder of homeopathy, established the term *miasm* in homeopathic language in 1828, after twelve years of intensively searching for the underlying cause of chronic disease.[1] In his seminal text, *Organon of the Medical Arts,* Hahnemann stated:

> It will help the physician to bring about a cure if he can determine the most probable exciting cause in an acute disease and the most significant phases in the evolution of a chronic, longlasting disease, enabling him to discover its underlying cause, usually a chronic miasm.[2]

MIASM, DIATHESIS, AND REACTION MODE—ALL SYNONYMS

Miasm derives from the Greek word *miasma,* meaning "defilement," "pollution," or "emanations from swampy grounds."[3] Since the term *miasm* carried with it these obviously negative connotations, other more acceptable terms were later adopted.

For example, *diathesis,* a Greek word meaning "arrangement" or "disposition" (referring to an individual's particular constitution), was originated by Jacques Menetrier and is often used by European homeopaths in lieu of the term *miasm.*[4] *Diathesis* is also used in modern orthodox medical terminology, but in a slightly different context. *Dorland's Medical Dictionary* (twenty-sixth edition) defines the word *diathesis* as "a constitution or condition of the body which makes the tissues react in special ways to certain extrinsic stimuli and thus tends to make the person more than usually susceptible to certain diseases." Although this definition clearly shows *diathesis* to be synonymous with *miasm,* the term *diathesis* has become more diluted in everyday medical practice—for example, a *spasmodic* diathesis (tendency to have muscle spasms), a *cystic* diathesis (tendency to form cysts), a *bilious* diathesis (tendency to gallbladder dysfunction), and similar terms are commonly used. Medical dictionaries do not reference the four primary miasms, established in the 1800s, that actually encompass all these various tendencies. Therefore, few medical doctors are aware of this term's specific origins in homeopathic medicine.

Another common term employed by European homeopaths is *reaction mode,* which refers more specifically to how an individual responds to stress based on his or her particular disease susceptibility.

Whichever term you find more preferable, however, *miasm, diathesis,* and *reaction mode* all denote both the inner predisposition to chronic disease and the susceptibility to succumbing to that disease when under stress. This susceptibility can be inherited from your family or acquired during your lifetime.*

It should be noted that the term *constitution* is not an exact synonym to these three terms because it has both negative and positive connotations. For example, an individual who enjoys good health may be described as "having an excellent constitution." In contrast, *miasm, reaction mode,* and *diathesis* refer only to the negative predisposition toward illness, dysfunction, and disease.

*This susceptibility could perhaps even be *causally* or *karmically* transmitted—that is, the energetic disease imprint is received from an unresolved pattern of transgressions from a past life.

MIASMIC THEORY

Hahnemann observed that there were three primary miasms to which his patients could succumb—the *psoric, sycotic,* and *luetic*.[5]* These three miasms seemed to relate to diseases that were quite prevalent in Hahnemann's time. The psoric miasm was linked to the skin disease scabies (caused by the scabies itch mite, and characterized by intense itching and eczema), the sycotic miasm was linked to the sexually transmitted disease (STD) gonorrhea, and the luetic miasm was linked to the STD syphilis.

Inheriting Miasms

These diseases—scabies, gonorrhea, and syphilis—were all quite prevalent in the 1800s, which initially inspired Hahnemann to formulate his theory. Although these diseases are rarer nowadays, their influence in our genetic memory is not. That is, even if a man of the early 1800s eliminated his syphilitic chancre (infected sore) with the allopathic treatment of the day, such as a caustic ointment, his treatment did not deeply purge the disease from his system but simply suppressed the obvious visible signs of it on his skin. Even a century later, his great-grandchildren can still harbor a latent syphilitic tendency, or the luetic miasm, in their system. As a result, his weakened progeny can experience luetic-like symptoms, from mild to major insomnia or anxiety or even cancer.

It is important to point out that when an individual suffers from these and other symptoms of a particular miasm, he or she will not necessarily have directly inherited or acquired the actual causative microorganism of the disease. For example, the great-grandchildren of the preceding example will not necessarily have inherited or acquired the spirochete *Treponema pallidum,* which is the causative microorganism in syphilis. The individual simply has a genetic tendency that predisposes him or her to the "panoply of disorders that are common to the miasm."[6]† That is, this individual reacts to life's inevitable stressors—be they structural (e.g., a car accident), chemical (e.g., refined sugar), or psychological (e.g., a painful divorce)—with symptoms reflecting his or her particular miasmic tendency.

Acquiring Miasms

Although each miasm or reaction mode can be inherited genetically from your parents, it can also be acquired during your life. The most common environmental causes of miasms are intoxication (e.g., the injection of toxic metals and pathogenic microbes from a vaccine) and suppression through the action of pharmaceutical drugs (e.g., excessive antibiotics). Additionally, if you are directly exposed to syphilis or gonorrhea through a sexual partner, you can succumb to the effects of the particular miasm and may then, in the absence of appropriate holistic intervention, begin to manifest luetic-like or sycotic-like symptoms for the rest of your life. Furthermore, many homeopaths believe that any of the miasms can be transferred over time between sexual partners, even without any direct evidence of infection through the related causative microorganism.

Other Factors

Over time, miasmic theory has been added to and amended by other homeopaths, which has led to a broader and more descriptive paradigm. Thus, today, miasms have come to be used to describe a general category of inherited or acquired flaws or weaknesses in a person's constitution that can lead to symptoms similar to, but not always duplicating, the disease pattern upon which Hahnemann originally based his classification system. For example, the miasm of sycosis later came to be associated with symptoms not only due to exposure to gonorrhea but also secondary to the adverse effects of vaccinations.[7]

NEBEL IDENTIFIES A FOURTH MAJOR MIASM

In 1902 Antoine Nebel, the Swiss physician who originated the concept of drainage (which will be discussed

**Psoric* is pronounced *'soar-ick;* the *p* is silent. *Sycotic* is pronounced *sigh-'ko-tick*—not to be confused with the word *psychotic*! *Luetic* is pronounced *loo-'eh-tick.*

†However, note that some homeopaths argue that the causative microorganism—*Sarcoptes scabiei* in the psoric miasm, *Neisseria gonorrhoeae* in the sycotic miasm, *Mycobacterium tuberculosis* in the tuberculinic miasm, and *Treponema pallidum* in the luetic miasm—is directly transmitted through DNA from generation to generation. Others say that it is just the energetic signature or imprint of the microbe that is passed on to the next generation in a miasmic-type transference.

in chapter 2), further chiseled a place for himself in homeopathic history by adding a fourth miasm to Hahnemann's original three-miasm paradigm. Nebel discovered over years of clinical observation that the symptoms of tuberculosis reflected not only the disease state itself but also a specific flaw in a person's constitution causing a range of symptoms he termed *tuberculinism.*[8] This renowned Lausanne doctor felt that the existing three miasms described by Hahnemann did not encompass the unique aspects embodied in a tuberculinic constitution, and that this particular presentation of disease and dysfunction therefore required a separate diathesis. Over a century later, this fourth miasm is still quite valid in that it appropriately characterizes the profound exhaustion of individuals with depleted immune systems, as exemplified by the pandemic cases of AIDS, chronic fatigue, and autoimmune syndromes worldwide. The tuberculinic miasm has therefore withstood the test of time and is considered by many modern homeopaths as a valid and distinct reaction mode in its own right. With Nebel's final contribution, the four-miasm theory has become the most typical paradigm used to categorize medicines such as homeopathics and drainage remedies, as well as to assess patients' treatment progress over time.

HOW MANY MIASMS ARE THERE?

In homeopathic circles, whether there are really only three, four, or a multitude of miasms presently existing today is still a hotly debated question. One renowned homeopathic Mumbai school, led by Dr. Rajan Sankaran, teaches that there are at least ten major miasmic disease categories to which a patient may succumb (as described in Dr. Sankaran's *An Insight into Plants,* volumes 1 and 2). Other homeopathic practitioners argue that new miasms resulting from chronic exposure to and the resulting debilitating effects of X-rays, plutonium, the AIDS virus, excessive antibiotics, and other modern-day toxins should be recognized. However, a twenty- or thirty-miasm classification system makes for an unwieldy and difficult-to-interpret paradigm. Furthermore, the symptoms from these more modern toxins can still fit into the original broad and wide-ranging four-miasm paradigm, thus rendering the demand for a multitude of new categories relatively unnecessary. For example, the symptoms of AIDS correlate quite well with those of the tuberculinic miasm. Therefore, for the purposes of this book, as well as for the ease of tracking patients' progress—or lack of it—in treatment, the four-miasm paradigm is appropriate and quite functional. However, if you are a homeopathic practitioner planning on studying with Dr. Sankaran or one of his colleagues, you will come to realize very soon in his classes that the ten-miasm system is indispensable in this brilliant body of work, and quite essential in ascertaining a patient's correct remedy. (To learn more about the Sankaran system, visit the website of the California Center for Homeopathic Education at www.cchomeopathic.com or the Marin Naturopathic Medicine clinic at www.marinnaturopathicmedicine.com and click on "homeopathy.")

THE SUPPRESSIVE EFFECTS OF ALLOPATHIC DRUGS AND THE MANIFESTATION OF MIASMS

One of the major factors that trigger miasms—these latent flaws and weaknesses in our genetic code—is allopathic *suppression,* that is, the excessive use of drugs and surgery in conventional medicine to suppress the symptoms of illness or disease. The prescription of numerous toxic and synthetic medications, unnecessary surgery, invasive tests, and other iatrogenic procedures greatly weaken the body's defense mechanisms and can awaken or increase the potency of an individual's inherited miasmic traits. In fact, many homeopaths believe that the injection of live or attenuated (deadened) viruses in vaccinations may be strong enough to actually "engraft upon the organism [patient]" an acquired miasmic susceptibility that was not even previously part of his or her genetic potential.[9] (See chapter 15 for more about vaccinations.)

Suppression is causative in both the formation of environmentally caused miasmic weakness and the triggering of latent inherited miasms. However, it is also important to point out that inherited miasmic weaknesses and their resulting symptoms may never manifest if a person is blessed with a relatively stress-free life. This idyllic state is quite rare, though, especially in these modern times, when prescription drug use has come to be regarded as normal—over 50 percent of Americans are taking at least one medication—and organic foods and natural medicine have been relegated to the secondary status of "alternative."[10] Therefore, it is the relatively exceptional and robust human being nowadays who is *not* significantly affected by the suppressive effects of past or present drug use and other hazards of modern civilization. In fact, the expression of miasmic weakness and disease is currently so widespread that it is quite unusual to meet an adult who is not significantly affected by signs and symptoms of chronic dysfunction (e.g., acne, constipation, headaches, joint pain, frequent colds and bouts of flu, or fatigue) or more debilitating illnesses (e.g., chronic depression or anxiety, diabetes, heart disease, cancer, Alzheimer's, or Parkinson's).

Acute Illnesses Are Often Nature's "Safety Valve"

When the use of allopathic drugs suppresses the external expression of disease, natural drainage of the emunctories, or excretory organs, is blocked and the pathology is driven deeper. Although acute skin rashes, diarrhea, fever, coughing, sneezing, or nasal congestion may be mitigated, this short-term gain in symptom relief creates more serious dysfunction down the road, as toxins are internalized and sequestered more profoundly in the body. Thus, many of the external manifestations of illness are actually relief processes and considered by holistic physicians to be "nature's provisional safety valve"—as much a biological law and necessary process as the elimination of sweat and urine is a physiological process.[11] The temporary relief gained from the plethora of *anti*-type pharmaceutical drugs—antibiotics, antihistamines, anti-inflammatories, and so forth—unfortunately comes at the expense of our more weakened immune systems. Furthermore, these suppressive drugs have caused a great many individuals not only to manifest latent psoric or sycotic dysfunction but also to deteriorate to the level of the two most pathological reaction modes: tuberculinic and luetic. This is especially true when the real cause of the chronic symptoms—for example, mercury toxicity (chapter 3), a dairy allergy (chapters 5 and 6), a tonsil focus (chapter 12), or suppressed grief (chapter 18)—is never diagnosed and therefore never appropriately treated.

acute: An *acute* condition or disease is usually brief in duration and self-limiting, such as a cold, tonsillitis, flu, or bladder infection that comes on suddenly and lasts for a short period of time.

GERM THEORY
"The Curse of Louis Pasteur"

This title, from the compelling book written by holistic nutritionist Nancy Appleton, dramatically states the pernicious effect that this often-lauded nineteenth-century French physician had on the course of modern medicine. Like the first holistic physician Hippocrates' emphasis on the individual's terrain, miasmic theory asserts that it is the individual's degree of resistance or susceptibility that determines whether he or she will become sick, as well as what type of specific illness uniquely manifests. This is in contradistinction to Pasteur's belief that human blood is pure and sterile but can be contaminated by airborne microbes, such as bacteria and viruses, that precipitate illness.[12] This "germ theory of disease"—a theory very dear to the hearts of pharmaceutical company executives—became the prevalent belief system in medicine primarily due to Pasteur's widespread influence. The germ theory has flourished for three major reasons: it is simple to understand, it frees individuals from having to take responsibility for their health, and it boosted pharmaceutical companies into the multibillion-dollar industry they enjoy today. Dr. Appleton describes the ramifications of this theory in her book:

> Pasteur's influence with the germ theory was vast. There seemed to be no turning back, particularly during the first half of the twentieth century. Even today, the path seems "Pasteurian." We continue to look for magic pills and potions rather than to the individual's lifestyle.
>
> From the germ theory came pasteurization (killing the germs, along with many valuable enzymes), and now ultra-pasteurization (which kills all of the enzymes), antibiotics, antiseptics, and vaccines. These scientific advancements are all in pursuit of killing the germ or discovering the right cure for the common cold and other diseases.[13]

terrain: One's biological *terrain,* also referred to as *soil* or *earth,* is made up of connective tissue cells (fibroblasts), white blood cells (leukocytes), nerve endings, blood vessels, and colloidal substance (the extracellular matrix or ground substance). This matrix or connective tissue *mesh* or *sea* is a gel-like substance that surrounds every cell in the body and is the medium in which the external environment communicates with the cells in the body. The ubiquitous matrix system is considered by many holistic physicians to be the body's primary terrain, which reacts to external stimuli, communicates to the cells, and has the ability to adapt and change. (See chapter 9 for more information on the matrix connective tissue.)

In contrast to Pasteur's germ theory, two of Pasteur's colleagues, Claude Bernard and Antoine Béchamp, agreed with Hippocrates' original assertion that it is our bodies' internal milieu or terrain that is primarily responsible for the manifestation of chronic disease versus optimal health. Along with the famous American physiologist Walter Cannon, who coined the term *homeostasis* in the mid-1920s, these holistic pioneers were in agreement that the true initiators of disease were a toxic internal environment resulting from a person's lifestyle and inherited predisposition to disease (miasms)—and not invasive germs.[14] Unfortunately, due in part to Pasteur's "tireless self-promotion," ambition and genius for business, and even documented deception, plagiarism, and "scientific misconduct" in his laboratory research methods and reporting, the more simple-to-grasp presumption of the invading microbe became the prevailing popular theory.[15] Historical medical writer Alan Cantwell summarizes the profound effect that the germ theory of disease has had on the course of modern medicine:

> My study of Béchamp had shattered the icon of Pasteur. The chemist [Pasteur] made germs respectable and he was a genius at popularizing microbes as a cause of human disease. . . . [H]e also put science on the wrong track. Pasteur's dogma transformed the art and science of medicine into a multibillion dollar biotechnical business in search of a perfect pill and a perfect vaccine to cure man of all his ills. In the process the physicians were blinded.[16]

homeostasis: *Homeostasis* is defined by *Dorland's Medical Dictionary* (twenty-sixth edition) as "a tendency to stability in the normal body states (internal environment) of the organism, achieved by a system of control mechanisms" of the nervous, hormonal, metabolic, and other bodily systems. Thus, homeostasis is the state of healthy functioning that occurs when normal maintenance and regulation of the body is properly maintained.

It must be stated that germ theory is not completely invalid. If someone sneezes on you, microbes can spread into your system. However, if you have a healthy constitution, you either will not succumb to illness or will have a short-lived cold or flu. But if your immune resistance is lowered and latent miasmic tendencies have become active, then the cold or flu may linger and can even develop into a more serious disease. Thus, holistic practitioners understand that *although the microbe and the individual's miasmic susceptibility are both factors in the initiation of disease processes, it is the individual's miasmic susceptibility that has the greater influence.* Even Pasteur humbly acknowledged this on his deathbed, admitting, "Claude Bernard was right . . . the microbe is nothing, the terrain is everything."[17]

The health of your internal terrain can be assessed through a thorough history that should include any significant illness in your parents, grandparents, and other relatives; a review of your present symptoms; a physical examination; and relevant laboratory tests. This data can be used to initially determine your primary *active* miasm (or miasms) and help your health practitioner choose the appropriate drainage remedies (as well as other treatment) based on that miasmic level (or levels). Your individual and family history may indicate other *dormant* inherited miasms, but these should not be treated until they become active. For example, you may inherit various miasmic tendencies—some of which the public is well aware of, such as a family predisposition toward breast cancer—but these latent miasms may never manifest in your lifetime. If you have the good fortune not to experience any major life stressors that trigger these dormant tendencies, as well as a strong body as a result of good genes and a healthy lifestyle, then miasmic weaknesses may never become a significant factor in your life.

THE CORRELATION OF MIASMS TO THE STAGES OF DISEASE

Because of the widespread influence of Pasteur's germ theory, most individuals and even many holistic practitioners have never heard of miasms, diatheses, or reaction modes. The primary reason is that the theory of miasms is not only not espoused by modern orthodox medicine but even considered incorrect and passé. This present-day thinking is exemplified by the current definition of miasm in *Dorland's Medical Dictionary* (twenty-sixth edition): "[Miasm or miasma was] . . . alleged to be the cause of diseases . . . before the true cause became known."[18] (The true cause being a germ or microbe.)

However, despite the overwhelming influence of germ theory in modern-day medicine, the four-level miasmic paradigm has held up for three centuries in homeopathic circles because it is consistent with the truth—that is, how disease actually develops over time. The four miasms mirror the reality of how illness commonly manifests—from dysfunctional conditions to degenerative disease—in an individual's life.

The typical stages in the pathology of disease—that is, the signs and symptoms that arise as chronic illness progresses—were brilliantly outlined in 1952 by Dr. Hans-Heinrich Reckeweg of Germany.[19] His observations and research clearly established that chronic disease was caused by *homotoxins*—endogenous (produced within the body) or exogenous (externally derived) poisons that "impregnate the cells of the connective tissues, organs and brain, as well as the lymphatic and nervous system, causing them to function abnormally and degenerate." Dr. Reckeweg coined the term *homotoxicology* to describe this "gradual poisoning process" underlying the development of serious disease. And by careful observation in his clinical practice as well as through laboratory research testing that challenged different tissues with various toxic insults, he found that disease was simply a process that fell into six distinct and progressively more serious stages:[20]

> All those processes that we call diseases are an expression of biologically appropriate defense mechanisms against exogenous or endogenous homotoxins (excretion, reaction, and deposition phases) or of the attempt on the part of the body to compensate for the homotoxic damage sustained (impregnation, degeneration, and neoplastic phases) so as to stay alive as long as possible.[21]

endogenous: *Endogenous,* from the Greek, means "to produce or grow from within." Thus, endogenous toxins originate from within the body due to faulty metabolism, incomplete digestion, or long-term inflammation or chronic focal infections.

exogenous: *Exogenous* derives from the Greek word *exogennan,* meaning "to develop or originate outside the organism." Thus, *exogenous* refers to toxins such as mercury fillings, petroleum chemicals, microbes, and even excess cold, wind, or damp (Chinese medical terms) that affect and infect the body externally. The degree of these exogenous toxins' effects on the system is directly contingent on the particular miasmic level in which the individual is operating.

Thus, according to Reckeweg's clinical and laboratory research, the first three stages of disease, known as *excretion, reaction,* and *deposition,* are involved with defending against toxins; these stages are quite analogous to the first two reaction modes, in which the body attempts to throw off toxins (psoric) and then attempts to wall them off in deeper tissues (sycotic). Furthermore, Reckeweg's *impregnation, degeneration,* and *neoplastic* stages, in which the body valiantly tries to compensate for the noxious effects of the damaged and degenerated tissue, are quite parallel to the adaptive defense mechanisms seen in the tuberculinic and luetic reaction modes.

Functional Illness—The Psoric and Sycotic Miasmic Levels

To best illustrate the relationship between Reckeweg's six homotoxicology phases of disease and the four miasms, let's look at one typical scenario. After an initial toxic insult such as eating an allergenic (and devitalized through pasteurization) food like cow's milk, the defensive reaction of a child who has a dairy sensitivity is to try and throw off or purge the toxic effects as a psoric would, through coughing, sneezing, a runny nose, vomiting, or diarrhea.* If this excretion phase fails or is incomplete, or if the toxic stress is very strong—as would be the case if the child ingested lots of milk and ice cream—an inflammatory reaction phase occurs. The initial stages of inflammation in this phase also fall within the psoric reaction mode. However, more serious inflammatory reactions—chronic diarrhea, tonsillitis, appendicitis, and so forth—are more characteristic of the next level of defense, the sycotic miasm.

Over time, as the child continues to eat dairy products and has no adequate holistic intervention, and especially if he or she receives suppressive allopathic medications such as multiple courses of antibiotics, his or her system must next choose a new strategy, called the deposition phase. This is a classic defense mechanism of the sycotic miasm in which the body relocates toxins to tissues that are not vital to life—such as the deeper skin layer, the joints, and the genital organs. In this case of a dairy allergy, a child's diarrhea or gut pain may eventually diminish, only to be replaced by menstrual cramps or joint pain when he or she becomes a teenager. Or for a child who has reacted to dairy with numerous colds and tonsillitis, a more serious tonsil focus often becomes stably implanted in his or her system. Such a chronic tonsil focus rarely triggers specific throat symptoms but affects deeper tissues, such as the gut, and can cause symptoms such as gas, bloating, intermittent fatigue, and mild anxiety or depression. Other "rheumatic" manifestations secondary to a tonsil focus can include joint pain, heart palpitations, and frequent urination.† Additionally, other classic sycotic miasmic signs associated with this deposition phase include nasal polyps, lipomas, warts, obesity, gout, and swelling of the lymphatic nodes.

lipomas: *Lipomas* are benign fatty tumors under the skin. They are considered insignificant by allopathic physicians, but holistic practitioners recognize them as manifestations of disordered fat metabolism due to faulty liver, gallbladder, and pancreas metabolism.

Reckeweg categorized these three phases—excretion, reaction, and deposition—as humoral reactions, that is, those taking place primarily in the fluids of the body: the blood, lymph, phlegm, and bile. As is the case for the psoric and sycotic miasms, the symptoms in these three phases are typically intermittently quite unpleasant and difficult, but not seriously debilitating. That is, these three humoral phases are characterized by reversible illness and dysfunction, rather than the more challenging pathological changes seen in the tuberculinic and luetic miasmic levels.

Degenerative Disease—The Tuberculinic and Luetic Miasmic Levels

Over more time, as the exogenous (external) and endogenous (internal) toxins continue to insidiously and adversely affect normal function and damage tissues, the adaptive mechanisms of the system become depleted and start to move into what Dr. Reckeweg classified as the three cellular degeneration phases. Typical manifestations of the first of these phases, the impregnation phase, include asthma, chronic viral infections, rheumatism (chronic joint and muscle pain), and migraine headaches—all of which are also characteristic of the tuberculinic reaction mode. To further clarify this phase by using our initial dairy-allergy scenario, if a psoric or sycotic child is diagnosed with a sensitivity to cow's milk, it can be quite curative to have him or her simply avoid these foods as well as to prescribe drainage remedies for a relatively brief period of time. However, the dairy-allergic child, teen, or adult who is functioning (dysfunctioning) in the more serious tuberculinic/impregnation phase would require not only the avoidance of dairy and the prescription of drainage remedies but other holistic intervention such as supplemental digestive enzymes (see chapter 7), treatment of a possible tonsil focus (see chapter 12), and constitutional homeopathy (see chapter 14).

The next of these three more serious cellular stages of chronic or lingering diseases Reckeweg termed the degenerative, because abnormal matter actually deposits itself in the tissues, resulting in chemical changes in the body's terrain. This phase encompasses tuberculinic

*In this example, the child has an existing dairy allergy; therefore, the primary emunctories have already been somewhat compromised and the mucosae of the secondary emunctories are being utilized as the next line of defense. (See chapter 2.)

†The five rheumatic disturbed fields secondary to a tonsil focus are described in depth in chapter 12.

conditions such as lupus, scleroderma (in fact, all autoimmune diseases are characteristic of the tuberculinic reaction mode), rickets, pneumonia, and scoliosis, as well as luetic reaction mode diseases such as multiple sclerosis, muscular dystrophy, myocardial infarction (heart attack), and liver cirrhosis. Finally, without appropriate treatment and major lifestyle changes, the body, in a desperate attempt to survive, begins to make holes in itself (ulcerate) to drain toxic matter or to sclerose (create scar tissue) and wall off areas of chronic inflammation, infection, or other disturbance. Reckeweg called this the neoplastic phase, in which major tissue destruction takes place, such as in the case of malignant cancers and neurological degenerative diseases (Alzheimer's, Parkinson's, and so on). The neoplastic phase occurs solely within the fourth and most pathological miasmic level—the luetic reaction mode. Table 1.1 depicts the correlation between these two paradigms of how disease progresses.

An Invaluable Aid to Diagnosis, Treatment, and Prevention

As can be seen through the clear interrelationships of these two paradigms, Hahnemann's miasmic levels of disease, which were originally described in the nineteenth century, were later validated by Reckeweg's principles of homotoxicology, or disease pathogenesis, taught in the twentieth century. Through the use of this correlation, practitioners can more easily assess a patient's miasmic level and phase of dysfunction or disease to determine the appropriate extent of intervention and the particular type of treatment required. For example, an exhausted and weakened tuberculinic patient may

TABLE 1.1. THE CORRELATION BETWEEN THE FOUR MIASMS AND RECKEWEG'S SIX HOMOTOXICOLOGY PHASES

Functional Illness	Degenerative Conditions

THE SIX PHASES

Excretion	Reaction	Deposition	Impregnation	Degeneration	Neoplastic

THE FOUR MIASMS

Psoric	Sycotic	Tuberculinic	Luetic
skin issues (rashes, acne, eczema, psoriasis, and so on) overactive vital force—violent, brief eliminations (diarrhea, fever, sweating, vomiting, rashes, itching) good energy; quick to recover from illness active in evening, tired in morning mild joint pain allergy and hay fever symptoms parasites, hemorrhoids	deeper skin issues (warts, moles, lipomas, severe acne or eczema, and so on) intermittent fatigue and irritability chronic or intermittent joint pain intestinal dysbiosis/digestive dysfunction more frequent colds, sore throats, sinusitis bladder, prostate, menstrual dysfunction	slow to recover from illness (frequent but inefficient fevers) susceptible to viruses recurrent colds, bronchitis, asthma, earaches, et cetera depression, anxiety, severe fatigue insomnia, exhausted in morning painful arthritis, scoliosis, osteoporosis	disturbed and imbalanced energy premature aging, memory loss anxiety, severe insomnia muscle cramps and achiness, especially at night and especially in the legs destruction of tissue—ulcers, acne rosacea, cancer, multiple sclerosis (MS), amyotrophic lateral sclerosis (ALS), Alzheimer's, Parkinson's, et cetera

See plate 1 for a color rendition of this chart.

require many months of drainage and other remedies and treatment before mercury amalgam filling removal is appropriate. However, a patient functioning more in the sycotic diathesis may be strong enough to commence amalgam removal right away, in conjunction with drainage and specific heavy-metal detoxification treatments. Thus, when remedies and other holistic therapies are prescribed with a person's unique diathesis taken into account, not only are healing reactions milder but treatments are also more appropriate and therefore effective.

This paradigm also allows holistic practitioners, as well as their patients, to track *real* healing progress, rather than simply temporarily ameliorating symptoms through medications or other ultimately ineffective therapies. As patients are genuinely getting well, their improvement will be dramatically demonstrated by the movement of their symptoms in a *reverse* progression—from degenerative and luetic to more functional and psoric. Therefore, holistic practitioners can utilize these two paradigms as diagnostic indicators, along with physical examination and laboratory tests, to determine whether patients are truly moving in the direction of optimal health, versus making no progress, or worse, regressing and getting more ill.

Additionally, through the understanding these paradigms convey, more specific and personalized treatments can serve as preventive measures by helping to deter an individual's miasmic tendencies from ever manifesting. For example, when acute symptoms and ill health begin to arise, the holistic practitioner recognizes that the patient is not just "catching a bug that's going around" but mirroring his or her particular reaction mode. As these once-dormant diatheses are triggered and various related signs and symptoms start to manifest, drainage and detoxification remedies, as well as constitutional homeopathy and other treatments discussed in this book, have the capability not only to heal the outward presentations of dysfunction and disease but also to help resolve the underlying miasmic influence and end the cycle of susceptibility. Thus, when effective nonsuppressive remedies are prescribed to naturally drain and detoxify, they help prevent the manifestation of latent diseases such as cancer, Alzheimer's, and rheumatoid arthritis in the patient's lifetime. These holistic therapies are especially valuable before pregnancy to diminish the transference of miasms from parent to child. Drainage and detoxification therefore are extremely important forms of preventive medicine, for both patients and their progeny.

MIASMS AND THE FAMILY TREE

Hahnemann believed that it took three generations to clear miasmic disease patterning out of a family tree. However, this process can be speeded up and the intensity of the disease manifestations greatly mitigated with appropriate holistic treatment and a healthy lifestyle.

THE FOUR MIASMS IN DETAIL

In reading the following in-depth descriptions of the four primary miasms, you may find yourself caught in that medical school syndrome of believing that you are suffering from the effects of every single one of them. In this particular case, though, you are probably correct! With the increasing toxicity of this modern world and the increasing prevalence of the mixing of genes from different cultures and races in mobile populations, acquired and inherited miasmic tendencies have combined to result in almost everyone experiencing at least *some* symptoms from each of these four reaction modes. However, although many of the characteristics of each of these miasms may seem to fit your present health condition, one or two should predominate. This is your primary reaction mode, which can guide the choice of drainage remedies that will work for you, as well as serving as a means to measure your treatment progress.

The Psoric Miasm or First Reaction Mode

History

The psoric miasm was first elucidated by Hahnemann in 1827. Primarily due to lack of adequate hygiene, skin diseases were quite prevalent in the eighteenth and nineteenth centuries. In fact, in contradistinction to the daily bathing we take for granted nowadays, baths and showers were rare. It wasn't until the 1930s that sewer and water systems allowed most Americans the "luxury" of indoor plumbing and a level of hygiene—and health—never before experienced in previous generations. Hahnemann discovered that many of his patients who were not responding well to homeopathic remedies had a history of suppressing skin diseases.[22] The impulse to remove skin eruptions was almost as prevalent then as it is today. All kinds of corrosive ointments, toxic internal substances, surgery, and cauterization were utilized to relieve the itching and to clear unsightly blemishes, rashes, eczema, psoriasis, and other forms of "mange." Hahnemann noted, however, that when these suppressive procedures were used, patients later developed more serious and harder-to-treat illnesses such as gout, asthma, chronic digestive dysfunction, and more severe allergic and skin reactions.[23]

psoriasis: Psoriasis is a chronic autoimmune skin condition that causes psoriatic plaques—areas of chronic inflammation and excessive skin production—and affects the joints in 10 to 15 percent of cases. Psoriasis—a more severe skin condition than eczema—was a suitable appellation for Hahnemann's first miasm, psora.

mange: *Mange* was a catchall term in the eighteenth and nineteenth centuries to describe all the various types of dermatological illnesses.

Later in the nineteenth century, the famous American homeopath James Tyler Kent poetically compared the psoric miasm to original sin. He wrote that the symptoms of the psoric diathesis represented "the very first sickness of the human race, that is the spiritual sickness . . . which in turn laid the foundation for other disease."[24] The inheritance of a miasm can be characterized as a flaw or wound in the etheric blueprint that organizes and governs our vital force. Believers in reincarnation assert that this wound is why we incarnate—so that we can deal with and ultimately transcend our inherent imperfections and chronic egoic patterns that we manifest in each lifetime. Since the psoric level represents the initial stage of this weakened blueprint, this miasm signified for Kent the first "fall from grace" or separation from God. Allopathic medicine's attempt to cover the classic psoric skin eruptions is analogous to its present-day tendency to liberally prescribe antidepressant drugs, in an attempt to hide the external manifestations of disease without addressing the deeper internal causes. However, these suppressive and palliative treatments not only drive the physical toxins in deeper but also hinder an individual's psychological understanding and potential spiritual realization.

Robust Vital Force: "Bulldozers of Life"

The psoric miasm is primarily characterized by long periods of good health alternating with brief and strong reactions to infrequent illnesses. When psoric individuals do get sick, their robust vital force allows them to quickly excrete toxins through the emunctories. People functioning primarily in this first reaction mode eliminate their endogenous and exogenous poisons through short-term fever, diarrhea, sweating, rashes, vomiting, and other brief purges by the body. And while individuals in the tuberculinic or luetic miasm may suffer from influenza for weeks or even months, psorics often succumb to illness for only a few days and feel great relief afterward through the rapid elimination of these toxins.

Thus, patients who react primarily in a psoric manner have the good fortune to experience functional disorders that are reversible. Their immune systems are strong enough to eliminate toxins, and these eliminations do not exhaust them because they have an abundant store of reserve energy (unlike the tuberculinic). Therefore, psorics never become chronically ill because they do not hold on to things, and they excrete toxins rather than retaining and depositing them in their tissues. Because they are so constitutionally strong and resilient, Mikhael Adams, N.D., a world-renowned authority on this miasmic paradigm, refers to psoric patients as the "bulldozers of life."[25]

CONFLICTING OPINIONS ABOUT THE PSORIC MIASM

It should be noted that there is an opposite and conflicting opinion in the homeopathic literature in regard to the psoric reaction mode. Most South American and some European authors describe the psoric as a "constitutional state of deficiency or lack" (P. S. Ortega), with a tendency to be pessimistic and withdrawn (Jean Elmiger). However, it is the opinion of other homeopaths (Gérard Guéniot, Mikhael Adams, Vinton McCabe, and Michel Bouko Levy, among others) that these deficiency symptoms are seen in the more degenerated (sycotic and tuberculinic) miasms, after the psoric has exhausted his or her store of reserve energy. This controversy could be due to the fact that many of these same South American and European homeopaths have never recognized the tuberculinic miasm as a distinct and separate diathesis, seeing it instead as a subset of psora that they have termed *pseudopsora* (we'll discuss this subject further in the description of the tuberculinic miasm).

Hyperactive Defensive Reactions

When psorics do get sick, their symptoms are synonymous with the classic autonomic reaction to any first insult. That is, they typically initially react to stress in a hyperactive defensive manner, triggering the fight-or-flight response

HANS SELYE'S GENERAL ADAPTATION SYNDROME AND THE FOUR REACTION MODES

Reactions to Stress

Hans Selye, a professor of endocrinology at the University of Montreal, first established "stress" as a medical concept when he published a paper in 1936 titled "A Syndrome Produced by Diverse Nocuous Agents." In this paper, Selye recounted that when laboratory animals were placed under stress, they all exhibited the same signs and symptoms. Furthermore, these signs and symptoms were the same no matter what type of stressor the animals were subjected to, from extremes of temperature to overcrowded living conditions or infectious microbes. Among other reactions, the adrenal cortex would enlarge, the thymus involute (shrink), and the mucosa of the stomach bleed and eventually ulcerate. Selye therefore concluded that the body has a generalized set of reactions to literally *any* type of attack, and he termed this response the general adaptation syndrome (GAS).[26] Furthermore, Selye observed that within this generalized response of the body to adapt or compensate to stress, there was a specific order or level of bodily responses that could be classified into three general stages—*alarm*, *resistance*, and *exhaustion*.

Stages of Decompensation

In order to correlate Selye's GAS stages with the four reaction modes, we'll begin with a healthy psoric example. As long as psoric individuals are not unduly challenged in life, the manifestations of this diathesis remain dormant. However, when adverse life circumstances do arise, these individuals respond by exhibiting rare and brief active defensive responses in the form of acute illnesses or volatile but transitory emotional outbursts. These initial psoric responses of *overreaction* to stress closely parallel Selye's *alarm* response of sympathetic fight-or-flight reactions throughout the body, which he had consistently observed in his laboratory research.

However, after prolonged stress, or even after a single significant event such as the implantation of mercury amalgam fillings or the simultaneous injection of several vaccines,* a primary psoric individual can decompensate to one of the other three reaction modes. If the stress is chronic and strong enough, but not severely debilitating, the individual may begin to exhibit symptoms typical of the next level of pathology—the sycotic miasm. This second reaction mode, analogous to Selye's second adaptive stage, which he termed *resistance*, is characterized by hypofunctioning—that is, a generalized lowered level of energy and reduced metabolic functioning.[27] However, if the individual has a strong inherited tubercular genetic weakness and receives high doses of suppressive antibiotics, steroids, and so forth, this psoric patient may move directly into the more degenerative tuberculinic diathesis, correlating to Selye's exhaustion stage. Or in the case of the grandson of Indiana Congressman Daniel Burton, who was administered nine different vaccines with the mercury preservative thimerosal all in a single day, a psoric child can even move directly into the most pathological level, the degenerative luetic stage.[28] Burton's grandson, who was healthy before he received the shots, is now autistic. In figure 1.1, the miasmic levels are correlated with Dr. Selye's similar stages of stress.

It's important to point out that the decompensation from a less pathological to a more pathological reaction mode is not always linear. Psorics may decompensate to the next level of sycosis, characterized by reduced functioning but with no serious tissue destruction, or they can jump directly into the more degenerative tuberculinic or luetic reaction modes, particularly if they are exposed to an overwhelmingly toxic stress as well as having an underlying weak inherited predisposition.

*Vaccinations can be toxic to the body either through their mercury- and aluminum-laden preservatives or through the attenuated (deadened) viruses and bacteria used in them. (See chapter 15 for more information on the devastating effects of vaccines, or vaccinosis.)

characteristic of the sympathetic nervous system. This is signaled by excessive excretions or behavior—brief diarrhea, vomiting, a two-day flu, or an angry and confrontational response—in an attempt to throw off the toxin or reduce the stressful feeling.

The psoric hyperfunctioning and overreaction closely correlate with the excretion and reaction phases of Dr. Reckeweg's homotoxicology paradigm. They are also quite analogous to the first stage of defense, known as the alarm reaction, in Hans Selye's general adaptation syndrome.[29]

Targeted Organ: External and Internal Skin

Psoric reactions manifest primarily in the skin, gastrointestinal system, and respiratory system. As the late Dr. Guéniot, who was one of the leading European experts in drainage, pointed out in his lectures, the intestinal and respiratory mucosae can be thought of as simply the invagination of the skin, through the mouth and anus and through the nose and lungs, respectively.[30] Thus, the psoric miasm can be thought of as affecting *all* skin surfaces—both internal and external.

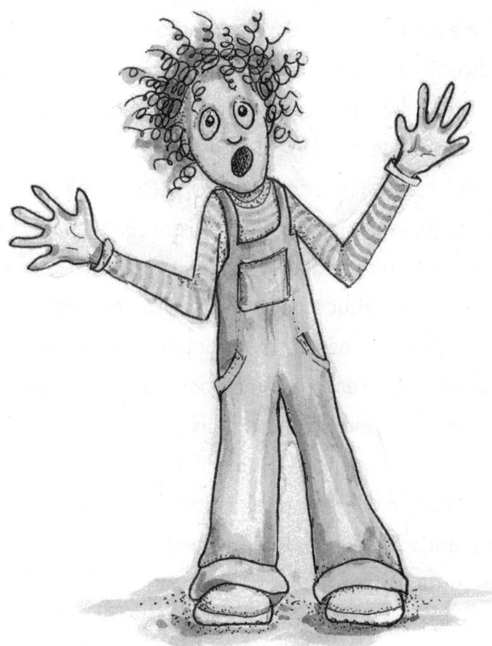

Selye's alarm stage ≈ psoric miasm

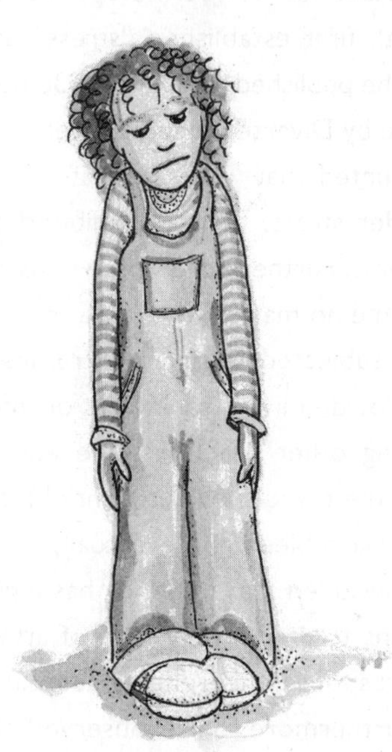

Selye's resistance stage ≈ sycotic miasm

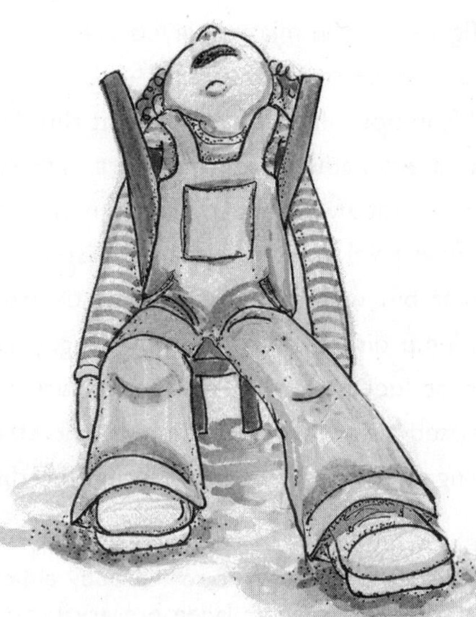

Selye's exhaustive stage ≈ tuberculinic miasm

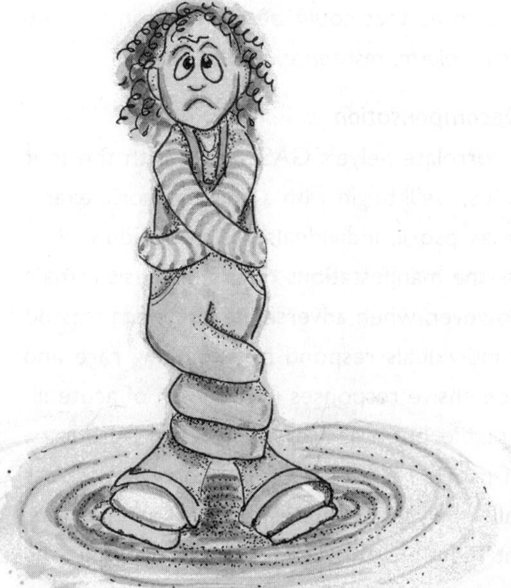

Selye's exhaustive/destructive stage ≈ luetic miasm

Figure 1.1. The four miasmic levels correlate to Dr. Hans Selye's three stages of adaptation to stress.

The psoric's complexion can have a general lackluster look, or it may be warm or flushed in appearance. People in this diathesis are prone to skin rashes, eczema, mild acne, urticaria (hives), boils, dandruff, and pruritus (itching). In fact, pruritus is pathognomonic, or extremely characteristic, of the psoric miasm. Psorics can also have rectal itching as well as foul-smelling stools. Other gastrointestinal symptoms include parasites, hemorrhoids, sugar cravings, constant hunger, and a nervous stomach. Brief and rather violent colds, bouts of flu, or sore throats and mild asthma are characteristic of a psoric's respiratory symptoms. Hay fever, mild sinusitis, and allergies may also occur in this reaction mode, but they are usually due to environmental factors such as pollen and dust, rather than foods.

pathognomonic: *Pathognomonic* means that a sign or symptom is so characteristic of a disease process that a diagnosis can be confidently made from this one aspect.

Other Symptoms

Other psoric symptoms include intermittent migraines, dysmenorrhea (menstrual cramps), menorrhagia (excessive menstrual flow), transient urinary dysfunction, muscle tension, hyperthyroid tendencies such as mild periodic tachycardia (fast heart rate), and nocturnal emissions (ejaculation during sleep). Psychologically, psorics can be nervous and quick-tempered, energetic, spontaneous, self-confident to the point of arrogance, irritable and angry, and overly active in the evening and tired in the morning. They can have difficulty completing tasks and may be inclined to have too many thoughts at one time, which tend to crowd each other out.

Levels of Functioning within the Miasm

Some of these symptoms may seem inconsistent with the previously described healthier picture of the psoric miasm, but each reaction mode can exhibit various levels of strength or weakness. For example, as a psoric woman's system becomes fatigued, disturbing symptoms may begin to appear in the form of hormonal disturbances such as dysmenorrhea and menorrhagia. However, as long as there is no major deposition of toxins in deeper tissues, such as the formation of uterine fibroids or endometriosis (a condition in which the uterine mucous membrane tissue is found outside the uterus, which can trigger menstrual cramps) in the case of the sycotic miasm, or the exhausting and severe dysmenorrhea and menorrhagia that occur in the tuberculinic miasm, then these menstrual symptoms still fall within the psoric diathesis picture. Thus, one female may experience an hour of mild menstrual cramps and another six hours of more intense pain, but both women may still be functioning within the psoric reaction mode.

However, a person in optimal health reacts to stress in the manner of the healthiest level of the psoric miasm—with brief and rare illnesses that eliminate toxins but do not exhaust the system. Most holistic health practitioners believe that occasional colds, for example, are actually good exercise for the immune system, and that those individuals who brag about never getting sick are the most susceptible to more severe illnesses such as cancer and heart disease.

Furthermore, it is important to keep in mind that there are many levels of clinical signs and symptoms. That is, the itchy anal symptoms classically experienced by children with pinworms are a psoric manifestation, whereas more severe and chronic intestinal parasitic infestation that causes gas, bloating, constipation, and intermittent bouts of fatigue would be typically classified under the dysfunctional sycotic diathesis.

Psoric Symptoms Can Indicate Progress

The holistic practitioner can use psoric symptoms to trace the success—or failure—of therapy. For example, if a former tuberculinic patient who has undergone extensive holistic care begins to break out in a rash around the liver and crave sweets, these symptoms may well be signs of progression, and not regression. A careful evaluation of the patient's present symptoms as well as energetic testing* can help confirm whether he or she is indeed showing marked improvement by exhibiting these—although new and somewhat disturbing—detoxifying and rebalancing psoric symptoms. In fact, sometimes the increased energy that is characteristic of a psoric diathesis can be rather disconcerting and feel too "speedy" to patients who have grown accustomed to a chronically fatigued

*Energetic testing can include kinesiology, electroacupuncture, and reflex arm length (RAL) testing. For more information, see appendix 3.

and enervated state.* However, as patients move from the psoric miasm's more active state to its more dormant one, over time they begin to enjoy more consistent emotional equilibrium, without the extreme "highs" and "lows," and to appreciate the uniqueness of their own emerging vital force.

Psoric Miasms Are Currently Uncommon

The pure psoric miasm is rarely seen nowadays. Because of our weakened genes and pervasive allopathic suppression, most individuals—and sadly even many children—typically present in holistic medical practices with dysfunction characteristic of the other three more disturbed reaction modes. However, many babies, some children, and the rare adult can sometimes begin treatment at the psoric level and in general return to optimal functioning within a relatively briefer time frame (e.g., three to six months) than is the usual case with the other reaction modes (e.g., one to three years).

The Sycotic Miasm or Second Reaction Mode

History

Hahnemann believed that the sycotic miasm originated from both active gonorrhea as well as the suppression of this venereal disease that was so widespread in the 1800s. The term *sycosis* derives from the Greek *sukosis,* which in turn derives from the Greek *sukon,* or "fig," a reference to the localized skin exudates, called *fics* or *figs,* that gonorrhea produces.[31] In 1892, the renowned British homeopath James Compton Burnett further described *vaccinosis,* a term originally coined in German literature to describe a syndrome contracted from the adverse effects of smallpox vaccinations.[32] Since both sycosis and vaccinosis produced similar symptoms, over time these two syndromes came to be grouped together under the umbrella term *sycosis.* Thus, individuals can experience the symptoms of the sycotic diathesis because they have genetically inherited this miasm, because they have acquired and/or suppressed gonorrhea in their lifetime, or because of the ill effects of smallpox vaccinations, as well as other vaccines. Additionally, individuals functioning primarily in the psoric miasm may begin to evidence symptoms characteristic of the sycotic diathesis as a result of major stress or chronic suppression through allopathic drugs.

*An agitated and hyperactive state can also indicate the release of aromatic hydrocarbons such as benzene, toluene, and xylene. See chapter 4 for more information on the detoxification of toxic chemicals.

MIASMS AND VACCINATIONS

Although Dr. Burnett first identified sycotic-type symptoms as adverse reactions to the smallpox vaccination, other homeopaths later found that ill effects from other vaccines were also characteristic of the sycotic reaction mode. Severe neurological reactions to vaccines, such as the current epidemic of autism, are characteristic of the luetic reaction mode.

Defensive Reactions: Underreaction and Adaptation

The sycotic *taint* or *contamination,* as it has been called, has been aptly referred to as the "pathology of adaptation," because instead of purging toxins it retains and adapts around them.[33] Thus, in contrast to a psoric's strong but overreactive system, the second reaction mode is characterized by underreaction and gradual but progressive weakening. Over time, as the sycotic's immune system and metabolic pathways become more impaired and compromised, the body grows less and less able to eliminate accumulated toxins. At this point, unable to efficiently purge metabolic wastes, toxic metals and chemicals, and pathological microbes, the congested internal terrain attempts to adapt by moving the toxins around and hiding them. Endogenous and exogenous wastes are relocated to less strategic tissues, such as the deeper skin layers, which can result in warts, lipomas, skin tags, cystic acne, psoriasis, and so forth, or the joints, manifesting in tendonitis, bursitis, or arthritis. Through the redistribution of toxic materials to these less vital tissues, the body is able to preserve the functioning of the organs that are more crucial to survival, such as the heart, kidneys, and liver.

Intestinal Dysbiosis Is Characteristic

As the pathology of this miasm progresses, more important tissues eventually become involved, including those of the respiratory, genitourinary, and gastrointestinal systems. In fact, the sycotic miasm is known as the primary diathesis of *dysbiosis*—the overgrowth of pathological intestinal flora.[34] For example, even a robust psoric can break down within just a matter of months and move into the initial stages of the more weakened sycotic reaction mode if he or she ingests excessive strong antibiotics over a period of time—especially if this individual has inherited latent weaknesses of this diathesis from sycotic parents. The ensuing dysbiosis from this depletion of friendly intestinal flora often manifests in the classic sycotic symptoms of chronic gas, bloating, constipation, diarrhea, liver congestion, enzyme deficiency, hypoglycemia, and even diabetes. The inevitable malabsorption of nutrients resulting from these various forms of digestive dysfunction greatly contributes to the fatigue, mild depression, and short-term memory loss that is also characteristic of this diathesis.

It should be noted that the sycotic's fatigue is nowhere near as incapacitating as the tuberculinic's exhaustion; it is characterized more by a chronic lack of reserve energy that is typically felt first thing in the morning or at the end of the day. A sycotic therefore usually requires more than eight hours of sleep, including frequent naps, and often "catches up on sleep" by staying home and resting on weekends and holidays. However, this mildly but chronically enervated state, as well as the associated emotional symptoms of low-level depression, fuel the sycotic's cravings for sugar's quick energy as well as creamy "comfort" foods, which, unfortunately, only strengthen the dysbiosis/malabsorption/craving cycle. Thus, the sycotic's state may be characterized as one of chronic frustration—rarely feeling sick enough to seek appropriate holistic care, and yet never feeling quite well enough to accomplish his or her life's goals and dreams.

Ear, Nose, and Throat Symptoms

The sycotic's chronic dysbiotic state has a profound effect on all the mucosae of the body. Consequently, other symptoms commonly seen in this diathesis include intermittent sinusitis, nasal congestion and frequent colds, postnasal drip, bronchitis, and other signs of chronic congestion such as edema, headaches, and weight gain. (Recurrent bouts of tonsillitis and other ear, nose, and throat symptoms that have been classified under the angina miasm by some homeopaths are actually subsumed under the broader umbrella of this sycotic diathesis.) The tonsil focus that can develop as a result of inadequate treatment and/or allopathic suppression (antibiotics or surgery) can greatly contribute to the sycotic's mild but chronic fatigue, brain fag, irritability, and intermittent back pain. The associated streptococcus-induced autoimmune syndrome PANDAS,* with its symptoms of hyperactivity, tics and twitches, and mild to moderate obsessive-compulsive behaviors, also falls primarily within this reaction mode. (However, when these Tourette's-like symptoms become extreme, they typically fall into the more degenerative luetic diathesis.)

> **brain fag:** *Brain fag* is a common homeopathic term, sometimes called *brain fog*, that describes significant exhaustion of the mental facilities and short-term memory loss.

Genitourinary Symptoms

The genitourinary mucosae can also be affected at this miasmic level, causing congestive symptoms such as cystitis (bladder infection), enuresis (bed-wetting), frequent urination, prostatitis, vaginal discharge, premenstrual syndrome (PMS) and dysmenorrhea, ovarian cysts, and uterine fibroids.

Psychological Manifestations

The sycotic also adapts behaviorally. Dr. Mikhael Adams vividly characterizes the sycotic state as one in which individuals hold on to things as much emotionally as physically. For example, sycotic individuals often ruminate for long periods before acting because they have difficulty concentrating and making decisions. And despite the fact that individuals affected by this miasm can be highly intelligent, performance at work or school is typically acceptable but never really outstanding because their sycotic condition robs them of much of their vital energy. In contrast to the more expressive psorics, sycotics typically appear calm and exhibit an attitude of passive indifference. This habitual suppression of feelings, however, may eventually give rise to chronically obsessive thoughts, irritability, and occasional violence.

---

*PANDAS is the acronym for pediatric autoimmune neuropsychiatric disorders associated with strep infections. PANDAS is covered in chapter 12.

Sycotic Pandemic: Pediatric Manifestations

Although many people think that a person is born in a healthy state and deteriorates over time, the fact is that homeopathic practitioners are now witnessing more and more infants who begin life in the already weakened sycotic state. One clear indication of potential sycosis can be observed in babies who are born with many moles or birthmarks. Other typical pediatric sycotic manifestations seen in the infant or child include colic, allergies, recurring colds, ear infections (otitis media), eczema, psoriasis, and warts. In fact, these childhood illnesses have become so widespread nowadays that they're actually considered by most allopathic pediatricians to be relatively normal childhood manifestations.

Conclusion

In contrast to the psoric's overreactive immune system, the sycotic's response is typically underreactive. An individual who is experiencing the effects of the sycotic reaction mode has chronic symptoms of congestion and a lack of vitality, but no significant tissue destruction. However, if the stresses in life—chemical, structural, or psychological—begin to cause significant tissue damage, the individual may then begin to demonstrate pathology characteristic of the more degenerative tuberculinic or luetic reaction modes.

The Tuberculinic Miasm or Third Reaction Mode

A Note on the Order of the Miasms: There is a conflict among drainage and homeopathic practitioners as to which miasm—the tuberculinic or the luetic—is the most debilitating. The French, who most often use the term *diathesis,* classify the tuberculinic as the fourth, or most pathological, diathesis. More commonly, however, and according to Dr. Mikhael Adams, the tuberculinic is labeled the third reaction mode, because it is not quite as serious or as difficult to treat as the luetic miasm. Furthermore, the French homeopaths also differ in that they recognize a fifth diathesis of *dysadaptation,* which affects primarily the digestive system. Many doctors, however, feel that the sycotic miasm is inclusive of this fifth diathesis.

History

As described earlier, the Swiss homeopath Antoine Nebel is credited with identifying and describing the tuberculinic miasm in 1902.[35] Through his research, Nebel found that the tubercular nosode prepared from the tuberculosis bacillus previously isolated by Koch would heal many of his patients who were previously unresponsive to treatment. However, he observed that it was often necessary to add drainage remedies to mitigate the mucosal aggravations of the respiratory system (nasal and sinus congestion, sore throat), musculoskeletal system (joint and muscle pain), and genitourinary system (kidney, bladder, vaginal, and prostate infections) that the tuberculosis bacillus often provoked.[36]

> **nosode:** A *nosode* is a potentized homeopathic remedy made from a diseased tissue or a product of the disease that, similar to a vaccine, stimulates the system to mobilize its immune defenses against the disease or miasmic tendency of the disease. Hahnemann was the first to conceive of nosodes through his homeopathic preparation of the psorinum remedy, made from the sero-purulent matter of a scabies vesicle. For more information on nosodes and vaccines, see part 5.

Among homeopaths, a hotly debated point of contention is whether tuberculinism is a *pseudopsora,* a combination of the psoric (scabietic) and luetic (syphilitic) miasms, or a unique and specific miasm in its own right. However, George Vithoulkas, one of the world's leading homeopaths, points out that the history of disease "clearly contradicts" this psoric-luetic pseudopsora theory. Tuberculosis, he contends, is one of the oldest disease entities on the planet and has been identified in the skeletons of the earliest primitive peoples.[37] Thus, it would seem logical that tuberculosis, which predates even the disease of syphilis that underlies the luetic miasm, should be considered a miasm in its own right. Furthermore, the current plethora of patients with environmental sensitivities and chronic fatigue confirms the very autonomous and specific nature of this diathesis, which has dramatically escalated in modern times due primarily to the devastating suppressive practices of allopathic dentistry and medicine.[38]

The Disease of Tuberculosis

Tuberculosis (TB), as an active disease state, is defined as an acute or chronic infection caused by the microbe *Mycobacterium tuberculosis,* in which pathological tubercles are formed, chiefly in the lungs, that can fibrose (form scar tissue) and caseate (degrade into a cheeselike tissue).[39] Infection occurs predominantly by inhalation but can also arise through the ingestion of infected cow's milk or contact with fomites (contaminated utensils, dishes, and bedclothes), especially in environments lacking in modern hygiene.[40] Symptoms of tuberculosis include coughing—which is usually productive, with sputum—as well as fever, night sweats, general malaise, weight loss, hemoptysis (spitting up blood), chest pain, and dyspnea (difficulty breathing). People with weakened immune systems such as infants, the elderly, alcoholics, those suffering from malnutrition, and individuals on prolonged courses of immunosuppressive drugs (corticosteroids) are most susceptible.

caseation: *Caseation* is a pathological process in certain diseases in which cells die and form a dry, amorphous-type tissue resembling cheese.

fomites: *Fomites* refers to objects, such as utensils, dishes, and bedclothes, that are not in themselves harmful but are able to harbor pathogenic microorganisms and thus serve as agents of transmission of infection.

Although TB most typically conjures up memories of the disease of consumption that swept across Europe in the nineteenth and twentieth centuries, researchers postulate that it first occurred eight thousand years ago in the Middle East.[41] Thus, TB and its wasting effects have been known in our genetic code since antiquity. And although tuberculosis is more rare today due primarily to modern hygiene standards and better heating, its miasmic effects are currently pandemic—predominantly because of the vitiating effects of suppressive allopathic drugs.

consumption/phthisis: *Consumption* and *phthisis* are both synonyms for *tuberculosis*.

"Mutant" Humans

As with the other miasms, a tuberculinic reaction mode can manifest in an individual because of an inherited genetic tendency, because that person succumbs to the disease of TB, or because that person has the effects of the diathesis "engrafted" upon him or her through the severely debilitating effects of suppressive medications or toxic vaccinations.[42] Thus, as is the case for the sycotic miasm, the damage from vaccinations alone is a major cause of the tuberculinic diathesis. In fact, Dr. Gérard Guéniot asserted that it is "criminal" to vaccinate a child under the age of seven, before the immune system has matured, or to give antibiotics to children (except in dire emergencies) under the age of three, before the liver has fully developed its detoxification pathways.* He further asserted that when children are not allowed to go through a fever or fight off a virus (with the support of natural, nonsuppressive remedies, hydrotherapy, rest, emotional support, and so forth), they are subsequently unable to structure their immune system properly to develop a fully functional "immunological self or identity." According to Guéniot, this practice produces "mutant human beings," whose impaired immune systems can have profound repercussions in every area of their lives.[43] His conclusion is in complete accordance with the holistic model of health, in which parts of the body are seen as not separate but synergistic. An impaired immune system impairs a child's potential to develop into a fully individuated and emotionally mature human being. Furthermore, when the "natural" or "nonspecific" immune system development that normally occurs between the ages of three months and seven years is interrupted or truncated by the use of suppressive vaccinations, antibiotics, and other synthetic medications, it lays the groundwork for future autoimmune diseases that are pathognomonic of the tuberculinic reaction mode.

"The Seat of All Autoimmune Diseases"

The tuberculinic diathesis is considered by Dr. Guéniot and other leading holistic practitioners to be the "seat of all autoimmune diseases."[44] Even allopathic physicians

*When the liver has not fully developed its detoxification pathways, the bacterial carcasses, bacterial mutations (cell-wall-deficient organisms), and inflammatory by-products left behind from antibiotic therapy cannot be adequately cleared from the system. Thus, the matrix or connective tissues and organs can become congested and more and more dysfunctional over time. Furthermore, antibiotics wipe out more than 90 percent of a child's bacterial intestinal flora—the good along with the bad. And although this intestinal flora can reflourish after a course of antibiotics, it is often incomplete, especially if the child ingests excessive sugar and other devitalized and toxic foods that feed the pathogenic flora or receives many courses of antibiotics due to frequent infections. (See chapter 7.)

recognize that many autoimmune diseases are clearly triggered by prescription drugs. And the most common chemical culprits of toxic reactions and autoimmune dysfunction identified in the bible of conventional medicine itself, *The Merck Manual,* are antibiotics. The side effects of these excessively prescribed medications include skin rashes, fever, anemia, liver damage, and such autoimmune syndromes as interstitial nephritis (inflammation of the kidneys), lupus (connective tissue disorder), and myasthenia gravis (intermittent muscle weakness, primarily in the face).[45] In fact, the effects of antibiotics and other suppressive medications are so great that Guéniot estimated that at least *80 percent* of all diseases have an underlying autoimmune causative mechanism, rendering the broad and insidious influence of the tuberculinic miasm even more dramatic.[46]

Physical Appearance

The classic picture of a person reacting primarily within the tuberculinic diathesis is similar to that of the "Camilles" of the nineteenth century who suffered the actual disease: an emaciated individual with a thin neck and hands, a narrow chest, and beautiful, shiny eyes with dilated pupils.[47] However, due to the widespread intestinal dysbiosis (which often begins in the sycotic diathesis) and the concomitant malabsorption with resulting hormonal dysfunction, tuberculinic patients nowadays can also present as overweight and even obese.

Sensitivity

A keynote (primary symptom) of tuberculinics is their extreme sensitivity, both emotionally and physically. Due to this propensity, tuberculinics often initially overreact to toxins or microbes by having a high fever, profuse sweating, and major muscle aches and pains. However, unlike psorics, tuberculinics use up all their reserve energy with this initial violent reaction.[48] Therefore, a cold, flu, tonsillitis, or other infection lingers for a prolonged period and may often move deeper into the system, with resulting bronchitis or pneumonia. Although the tuberculinic system may try valiantly to mount a fever to throw off the toxins, these efforts are typically ineffective in fully clearing the chronic infection. Thus, the violent eliminations of a two-day flu that make psorics feel better often exhaust tuberculinics, and the smoldering underlying infection and its debilitating effects subsequently last for weeks or even months.

> **keynote:** *Keynote* is a common homeopathic term that refers to a symptom that is so striking and predominant that on its own it strongly suggests a specific remedy or, in this case, a specific miasm. The keynote of psora is overreactivity, of sycosis is underreactivity, and of tuberculinism is both sensitivity and exhaustion.

Chronic Fatigue

There is fatigue, for example, that is experienced in the sycotic miasm, and then there's *fatigue.* It is this level of bone-weary, "brain-dead," sick fatigue that the tuberculinic knows most intimately. In fact, chronic fatigue syndrome is a common illness representative of the tuberculinic diathesis.

Miasms have been described as "the hook" for viruses and other toxins—meaning that the potential tendency toward a weakened terrain greatly magnifies the probability for opportunistic microbial invasion.[49] Nowhere is this more evident than in the tuberculinic miasm, in which individuals are most susceptible to the mononucleosis and Epstein-Barr viruses that often precipitate and underlie chronic fatigue and illness. And the tuberculinic's significantly weakened immune system is susceptible to *all* viruses, including hepatitis, meningitis, herpes, influenza, polio, diphtheria, pertussis, and AIDS. Cancers also occur in this reaction mode, typically leukemias, but they are often not as severe as those encountered in the luetic diathesis.

Targeted Organ: Lungs

As is the case for tuberculosis, the lungs are the primary targeted tissues in the tuberculinic miasm. Thus, as previously described, a tuberculinic individual characteristically experiences chronic intermittent ailments of the lungs and respiratory system such as recurrent colds, earaches, and sore throats. These typically "minor" illnesses that last for only a few days in psorics, however, can last for weeks in tuberculinics and often move into the chest, with ensuing bronchitis, pneumonia, and even tuberculosis itself. Other prevalent syndromes disturbing to the tuberculinic's respiratory system include allergies, especially to milk, as well as asthma. And quite understandably, the tuberculinic individual is especially sensitive to cold and drafts and can also be very short-winded and have shallow breathing.

Bone Abnormalities

The second most commonly targeted tissues of active tuberculosis, the spine and bones,* are also weakened in the tuberculinic reaction mode. Secondary to the tubercular bacillus's renal (kidney) affinity, which causes sodium, potassium, and calcium imbalance, mineralization deficiencies commonly occur in childhood and adolescence, with resulting softening and deformation of the bones. Therefore, rickets, scoliosis, osteomyelitis (bone infection), rheumatoid arthritis, and knot knees, bow legs, or hyperextension of the knees (genu valgum, genu varum, or genu recurvatum, respectively) are all classic signs of a child (dys-)functioning primarily in the tuberculinic diathesis. Older tuberculinic individuals are more prone to osteoporosis.

Emotional Lability

In this more serious and pathological reaction mode, it is understandable that the deeper endocrine and emotional levels of coping are affected. Adrenal exhaustion and hyperthyroid as well as hypothyroid conditions (e.g., Hashimoto's thyroiditis) are classically prevalent. Furthermore, individuals are often nervous and high-strung, restless, ungrounded, indecisive, and emotionally labile and can swing from elation to major apathy and depression. Thoughts of suicide are common but not as seriously considered as they are in the luetic reaction mode. More typically, individuals in the tuberculinic miasm often live with the "quiet desperation" of feeling tired of life and always at their limit.

Healing Takes Time

Using traditional Chinese medicine terminology, after psorics have continually drawn upon their *yang chi* and sycotics have further drained much of their remaining vital reserve energy, tuberculinics must depend on utilizing the deeper *yin chi*. The yin energy in the body is the nurturing and mothering energy represented by the blood and the most essential vital organs (the kidneys, liver, heart, pericardium,* lungs, and spleen). The typical exhaustion experienced in the tuberculinic reaction mode is characteristic of the progressive depletion of this deep yin vital essence. Therefore, treatment length for these most sensitive and very depleted individuals can take much longer than for sycotics or psorics. And although this news can be quite sobering to tuberculinic patients, being able to clearly correlate their chronic symptoms with this miasm and to therefore understand the underlying inherited and acquired causes that precipitated their exhausted state can be quite emotionally enlightening. Thus, the catharsis of an authentic diagnosis as well as the knowledge of the estimated time frame and treatment protocol required to get well can often be a rather empowering first step toward recovery.

> **chi:** *Chi* or *qi*, according to the ancient Chinese, is the fundamental substance constituting the universe. Chi movement initiates and maintains all the vital activities and functions of the body. *Yang* refers to the active masculine force or principle in the universe represented by fire and movement in the system. *Yin* refers to the passive feminine force that is represented by water and tranquility.

The Luetic Miasm or Fourth Reaction Mode

History

The term *luetic* comes from the Latin *lues,* meaning a plague, pestilence, or decay. And in Hahnemann's day in nineteenth-century Europe, syphilis was so widespread that it was indeed considered a plague. Hahnemann noticed, however, that as was the case for the corrosive ointments used in psoric-type skin diseases, the allopathic treatment of cauterizing ulcerated syphilitic chancres actually worsened the disease by blocking a valuable drainage route out of the body.[50] After observing numerous patients with suppressed syphilis, as well as their progeny, exhibiting a constellation of symptoms similar

*Pott's disease or tuberculosis spondylitis is characterized by inflammation, abscess, and lysis (destruction) of spinal vertebrae, which can result in a gibbous, or humpback, curvature.

*The pericardium is the serous and fibrous sac that surrounds the heart. In Chinese medicine, the pericardium meridian is considered to be the master of heart function and, therefore, the primary governing force regulating the entire circulatory system. (R. Low, *The Secondary Vessels of Acupuncture* [Wellingborough, Northamptonshire, England: Thorsons Publishers Limited, 1983, 60–61].)

to those of the actual disease, Hahnemann termed this miasmic tendency *luetic.*

As was noted in the preceding discussion of the tuberculinic miasm, practitioners often debate which is the most serious diathesis—the tuberculinic with significantly impaired immune defenses or the luetic with destructive immune reactions. Many holistic practitioners argue that the luetic reaction mode is the more pathological in light of the fact that the most challenging diseases—multiple sclerosis (MS), amyotrophic lateral sclerosis (ALS, also known as Lou Gehrig's disease), Parkinson's, and most cancers—are characteristic of this fourth reaction mode. Since this has also been the author's experience, the luetic miasm has been placed last, as the most pathological reaction mode in this four-miasm paradigm.

Tissue Destruction

Ulceration, sclerosis, metastasis, and other forms of tissue destruction are pathognomonic of the luetic miasm. Such destruction may occur in the blood vessels with arteriosclerosis, in the stomach or small intestine in the case of gastric or duodenal ulcers, in the nerve fibers and their surrounding myelin sheaths with ALS or MS, or anywhere in the body with the overgrowth and metastasis of malignant tumors. While the strategy of the psoric is to eliminate externally to the skin, and the strategy of the sycotic is to concentrate and hide toxins in benign tumors or growths, the luetic makes a hole for drainage in the form of ulcerations, necrosis (destruction of tissue), or sclerosis (scarring of tissue).

> **necrosis:** *Necrosis,* from the Greek word meaning deadness, is the progressive degradation and death of cells and tissues caused by the destructive action of enzymes. This eating away of tissue can occur in cancer, syphilis, gangrene, bony dislocations that cut off the blood supply, and some bacterial infections.

> **sclerosis:** *Sclerosis* refers to the induration, or hardening, of tissue. Sclerosis of the nerves in the brain occurs in Alzheimer's; sclerosis of the blood vessels occurs in arteriosclerosis. Although on the surface sclerosis seems to be a completely undermining process, it is actually another attempt—albeit a desperate one—at drainage and therefore survival, as the body increases the diameter of the blood vessels through hardening and shrinking the wall of the artery.

The degenerative tendency of sclerosing, or scarring, blood vessels in arteriosclerosis affects the entire cardiovascular system. Thus, chronic hypertension, mitral valve prolapse, heart disease, congestive heart failure, myocardial infarctions (heart attacks), and cerebrovascular accidents (strokes) are characteristic of the luetic reaction mode. The venous system is also affected, which typically manifests in varicose veins, phlebitis, or hemorrhoids.

Besides the aforementioned MS, ALS, and Parkinson's diseases, Alzheimer's and other forms of senile dementia are also classic signs of the luetic individual. Additionally, the neuropathy that can occur in diabetes (numbness, pain, and muscle wasting) as well as the seizures, tics, and chorea (involuntary movements) that are characteristic of neurological dysregulation are inherent in this miasm.

Premature Aging

The destructive tendencies just described are typical of the premature aging—both physically and mentally—that luetics commonly experience. Patients affected by this miasm therefore often appear older than their age, with excessive wrinkles and a blotchy, ruddy (acne rosacea), or grayish skin discoloration. The eyes are particularly affected, with astigmatism, corneal ulcerations, and severe photophobia commonly diagnosed.

> **astigmatism:** *Astigmatism* is an irregularity in the curvature of the lens of the eye that results in a distorted visual image.

> **photophobia:** *Photophobia* is an abnormal sensitivity to light.

Psychological Manifestations

Another keynote typical of the luetic reaction mode is anxiety. This can manifest in various ways, such as with chronic nervousness, "hurry sickness," restlessness, irritability, depression, manic depression, suicidal inclinations, psychoses, violent behavior, and even murderous tendencies. Like the tuberculinic, the luetic is deeply exhausted, but this is not as evident due to the chronic anxiety and the nervous—sometimes frenetic—activity that often overlays the fatigue.

Symptoms Are Worse at Night

Luetics are particularly aggravated at night. In fact, they usually experience some form of sleep disorder and often severe insomnia. Unfortunately, this only compounds the luetic's chronic anxiety. Another common luetic manifestation that typically occurs in the late afternoon or evening is achiness in the limbs, especially in the lower extremities. Chronic disturbance in this area, including cramping in the calves and other muscle spasms, numbness, paresthesias, and restless legs, can signal an individual's progression into this more degenerative diathesis.

> **paresthesia:** *Paresthesia* is defined as any "morbid or perverted or abnormal sensation" (*Dorland's Medical Dictionary,* twenty-sixth edition). Numbness, prickling, formication (a sensation of small insects crawling over the skin), and burning are all types of paresthesias.

DISEASES CAN SPAN SEVERAL MIASMS

A dysfunctional state or disease can extend across two miasms. For example, cancer can develop in both the tuberculinic and luetic miasms, but it is typically more severe and malignant in the luetic individual. Similarly, although susceptibility to the polio virus is a tuberculinic sign, the tissue destruction and paralysis seen in the more aggressive forms of polio fall within the luetic reaction mode. And although vulnerability to viruses such as herpes is a tuberculinic trait, the actual eruption of the skin lesions falls into the destructive luetic category.

Some illnesses can even span all four miasms. For example, several bouts of tonsillitis can occur in a psoric child. But a tendency toward chronic childhood tonsillitis falls squarely within the sycotic reaction mode. The formation of a serious and chronic tonsil focus—scarred but relatively silent tonsils that initiate disturbance elsewhere in the body—can be characteristic of an exhausted and depressed tuberculinic, or even an anxious and sleep-deprived luetic. (Sycotics can also have a tonsil focus, but it is milder than in the tuberculinic and luetic diatheses.)

Treating the Luetic

The primary underlying disturbance in the luetic reaction mode is a serious breakdown in homeostasis—that is, in normal metabolism and communication in the body, which is essential for a healthy and functional system. This tendency makes treatment problematic for two major reasons: it can be extremely difficult to judge therapeutic progress due to the luetic's unpredictable reaction to different therapies, and these unpredictable healing reactions can sometimes be quite serious. Therefore, practitioners must be quite circumspect with these patients and, when there is a choice of remedies or treatments, always err on the side of prescribing extremely gently.

As with the tuberculinic patient, clear communication about the patient's luetic miasmic level—in which this chapter can hopefully be useful—can forewarn the patient about possible healing aggravations as well as helping him or her recognize real therapeutic progress. The insight and deeper understanding gained from knowing the causes of the patient's illness and the estimated treatment time are invaluable both emotionally and financially by helping the doctor and patient concentrate on the truly useful therapies, while avoiding treatments that are not lasting or curative. Awareness of the seriousness of the luetic level can help motivate a patient to commit to a necessarily lengthier—often from two to three years—treatment plan. And the effectiveness of any treatment plan, and especially this longer and more complex one, depends as much on the individual patient's attitude and compliance as it does on the practitioner's skill and experience.

DETERMINING THE PRIMARY MIASM(S)

Determining your primary miasm is often rather depressing—even frightening, in some cases. However, knowing where you stand with your health can also be enlightening and freeing. From this position of understanding, individuals can make more knowledgeable decisions about their particular course of treatment.

Most Individuals Die from Luetic Diseases

It has been estimated that more than 80 percent of us devolve to the luetic reaction mode at some point in our lives. This is exemplified by the fact that it's rare to hear about people dying peacefully in their sleep from a natural death anymore, which has been said to most optimally occur around 120 years of age, or even later.[51] Lamentably, most individuals transition nowadays through the quick (heart attack) or slow (cancer, Alzheimer's, et cetera) effects of devastating degenerative diseases characteristic of the luetic diathesis, often quickened by the toxic effects of allopathic medication.

Treating the Weakest Link

On the strength of one link in the cable
Dependeth the might of the chain;
Who knows when thou mayest be tested?
So live that thou bearest the strain.

RONALD ARTHUR HOPWOOD (1868–1949),
THE LAWS OF THE NAVY

As can be seen from the foregoing lengthy and rather complex descriptions, determining the primary miasm or miasms in which an individual is reacting can be difficult. Further complicating this diagnosis is the fact that different tissues and organs in the same patient can be responding in different reaction modes simultaneously. For example, a patient may present with sycotic skin reactions (warts or lipomas), tuberculinic fatigue, and luetic insomnia. To further add to the confusion, nowadays a patient's chief complaints (major symptoms) can be daunting in number and quite challenging to categorize into one or two primary diatheses. However, the well-known maxim "a chain is only as strong as its weakest link" can be helpful when applied to the theory of miasms. Thus, even if a patient is predominantly presenting with sycotic-like symptoms but also has a few tuberculinic signs and symptoms, then treatment should include drainage remedies that can address the tissues in the more degenerated tuberculinic reaction mode.

MULTIPLE SYMPTOMS

Although medical schools typically teach that having five to ten chief complaints is a sign of malingering or hypochondria, currently most holistic practitioners realize that this is rarely the case. In fact, multiple symptoms have almost become the rule nowadays more than the exception. This is due primarily to the toxic effects of our modern world, such as chronically ingesting foods laden with pesticides and preservatives, exposure to toxic pharmaceutical drugs and heavy metals, and air and water pollution. Thus, in the case of a patient who grew up downwind of a nuclear power plant on a farm where the spraying of pesticides was as common as an afternoon rain shower, ten to twenty chief complaints when that patient presents as an adult is consistent with his history and appropriate to this level of serious exposure.

The Four-Miasm Paradigm Is an Approximate Guide

Finally, it is important not to become too dogmatic about this paradigm by assigning individuals a single rigid and strict miasmic label indefinitely.* Although the four reaction mode categories can be an invaluable aid in estimating a patient's treatment time frame as well as a means for judging therapeutic progress, the paradigm is only an *approximate* guide or instructive tool that can change over time. Individuals, through their own determination, will, positive attitude, and dedicated adherence to an effective treatment protocol, can accelerate their healing profoundly and therefore more quickly progress toward their optimal goal—functioning in a dormant psoric level, with rare and brief colds, bouts of diarrhea, or other minor illnesses. Infrequently experiencing these mild illnesses is actually a sign of a healthy and functioning body, which "exercises" the individual's immune system as well as intermittently detoxifying. In contrast, individuals who boast that they *never* get sick can actually be in a very adapted and defended luetic state and may more quickly succumb to a heart attack or other debilitating disease.

Ill Patients Are Often the Most Dedicated

Patients with major symptoms, or even those with minor ones who are simply sensitive enough to realize that something is not right with their physical or emotional health, can more fully appreciate the healing process

*This is especially true given the fact that, due to our forty-six chromosomes, the number of different variations occurring in fertilized eggs is in the *three hundred thousand billion* range. Thus, in light of the immense complexity of the human species, each individual is infinitely unique and the four-miasm paradigm can be used only as a very helpful, but very approximate, guide. (H. Cotton, *The Defective Delinquent and Insane* [New York: Arno Press, 1980 (orig. pub. 1921)], 20.)

than those who have never been ill. This is especially the case for those in the tuberculinic or luetic reaction modes, who are often the most dedicated and persistent toward the goal of reaching optimal health, in spite of their more challenging path to wellness. For making a prognosis for each particular patient, the following statement, made by Caleb Harry,* an eighteenth-century physician at Bath, rings as true today as it did then: "It is much more important to know what sort of patient has a disease than what sort of disease a patient has."[52]

*Dr. Caleb Harry (1755–1822) was an eminent physician at the health resort of Bath in southwest England. He was the first to observe, treat, and document exopthalmic goiter disease (enlargement of the thyroid gland with hyperthyroid symptoms). However, he has rarely been credited for this discovery, and the disease was subsequently named after an Irish physician, Robert Graves, a century later.

NOTES

1. G. Vithoulkas, *The Science of Homeopathy* (New York: Grove Press, 1980), 122–23.
2. S. Hahnemann, *Organon of Medicine* (Blaine, Wash.: Cooper Publishing, 1982), 11.
3. J. Yasgur, *Homeopathic Dictionary* (Greenville, Pa.: Van Hoy, 1998), 153.
4. D. Kenner and Y. Requena, *Botanical Medicine: A European Professional Perspective* (Brookline, Mass.: Paradigm Publications, 1996), 25, 84.
5. M. Wood, *The Magical Staff* (Berkeley, Calif.: North Atlantic Books, 1992), 67.
6. V. McCabe, *Homeopathy, Healing, and You* (New York: St. Martin's Griffin, 1997), 261.
7. J. C. Burnett, *Best of Burnett* (New Delhi: Jain, 1992), 147–49.
8. J. Elmiger, *Rediscovering Real Medicine* (Boston: Element Books, 1998), 211.
9. G. Vithoulkas, *The Science of Homeopathy* (New York: Grove Press, 1980), 129.
10. R. Navarrette, "Why Are Americans So Eager to Pop Pill after Pill after Pill?" *Press Democrat,* July 17, 2005, G1.
11. J. Allen, *The Chronic Miasms* (New Delhi: Jain Publishers, 1998), 112.
12. N. Appleton, *The Curse of Louis Pasteur* (Santa Monica, Calif.: Choice Publishing, 1999), 6.
13. Ibid., 41.
14. Ibid., 59, 61.
15. Ibid., 38–40, 58.
16. Alan Cantwell Jr., *The Cancer Microbe* (Los Angeles: Aries Rising Press, 1990), 151.
17. Ibid., 47.
18. J. Friel, ed., *Dorland's Illustrated Medical Dictionary,* 26th ed. (Philadelphia: W. B. Saunders Company, 1981), 818.
19. H. Reckeweg, *Homotoxicology* (Albuquerque, N.M.: Menaco, 1989), 13–14.
20. Gosch, *Vital Energy Medicine* (Provo, Utah: Chronicle Publishing Services, 2003), 59.
21. P. Bellavite and A. Signorini, *The Emerging Science of Homeopathy* (Berkeley, Calif.: North Atlantic Books, 2002), 29.
22. S. Hahnemann, *The Chronic Diseases, Their Peculiar Nature and Their Homeopathic Cure,* vol. 1 (New Delhi: Jain, 1998), 97–98.
23. J. Elmiger, *Rediscovering Real Medicine* (Boston: Element Books, 1998), 207.
24. V. McCabe, *Homeopathy, Healing and You* (New York: St. Martin's Griffin, 1997), 261.
25. M. Adams, "Biotherapeutic Drainage Course" (lecture, Scottsdale, Ariz., April 1998).
26. A. Fonder, *The Dental Physician* (Rock Falls, Ill.: Medical-Dental Arts, 1985), 7.
27. H. Selye, *The Stress of Life* (New York: McGraw-Hill, 1956), 31.
28. L. Reagan, "What about Mercury?" *Mothering,* March/April, 2001, 55.
29. H. Selye, *The Stress of Life* (New York: McGraw-Hill, 1956), 31.
30. G. Guéniot, *Transcript of Dr. Gérard Guéniot's Seminar* (Toronto: Seroyal, 1998).
31. J. Jouanny et al., *Homeopathic Therapeutics* (France: Boiron, 1994), 31.
32. J. C. Burnett, *Best of Burnett* (New Delhi: Jain, 1992), 147–49.
33. J. Jouanny et al., *Homeopathic Therapeutics* (France: Boiron, 1994), 31.
34. M. Adams, "Biotherapeutic Drainage Course," (Scottsdale, Ariz., April 1998): 13–14.
35. J. Elmiger, *Rediscovering Real Medicine* (Boston: Element Books, 1998), 211.
36. J. Jouanny et al., *Homeopathic Therapeutics* (France: Boiron, 1994), 25.
37. G. Vithoulkas, *The Science of Homeopathy* (New York: Grove Press, Inc., 1980), 126–27.
38. Ibid.

39. R. Berkow et al., eds., *The Merck Manual,* 15th ed. (Rahway, N.J.: Merck Sharp and Dohme Research Laboratories, 1987), 114.
40. H. Choudhury, *Indications of Miasm* (New Delhi: Jain, 1998), 7.
41. J. Yasgur, *Homeopathic Dictionary* (Greenville, Pa.: Van Hoy, 1998), 267.
42. G. Vithoulkas, *The Science of Homeopathy* (New York: Grove Press, Inc., 1980), 129.
43. G. Guéniot, *Transcript of Dr. Gérard Guéniot's Seminar* (Toronto: Seroyal, 1998), 9.
44. G. Guéniot, *Seminar Notes* (Toronto, June 1999), 7.
45. R. Berkow et al., eds., *The Merck Manual,* 15th ed. (Rahway, N.J.: Merck Sharp and Dohme Research Laboratories, 1987), 315–18.
46. G. Guéniot, *Seminar Notes* (Toronto, June 1999), 7.
47. V. McCabe, *Homeopathy, Healing and You* (New York: St. Martin's Griffin, 1997), 270–71.
48. M. Bouko Levy, *Homeopathic and Drainage Repertory* (France: Editions Similia, 1992), 15.
49. R. Jacobs (quoting Dr. Scott-Morley), *21st Century Medicine Seminar* (notebook) (San Francisco: BioResource, Inc., September 1999).
50. J. Elmiger, *Rediscovering Real Medicine* (Boston: Element Books, 1998), 210.
51. M. Fischer, *Death and Dentistry* (Springfield, Ill.: Charles C. Thomas, 1940), 2; G. Pitskhelauri, *The Long Living of Soviet Georgia* (New York: Human Sciences Press, 1982), 13, 37.
52. D. Kenner and Y. Requena, *Botanical Medicine: A European Professional Perspective* (Brookline, Mass.: Paradigm Publications, 1996), 21.

2

DRAINAGE FOR DETOXIFICATION AND REGENERATION

There is but one disease—deficient drainage.
Sir William Arbuthnot Lane

In some holistic circles, the terms *drainage* and *detoxification* are used interchangeably. However, although these two practices are closely related, they are not synonymous. *Detoxification* is a general term that usually refers to cleansing a particular area of the body, such as the liver or colon, or ridding the body of a specific toxin, such as mercury, a parasite, or candida (intestinal yeast overgrowth).* Unfortunately, many popular detoxification protocols fail to take into account the ability of a particular patient's excretory organs to discharge these accumulated poisons. And when detoxification measures are too rigorous for their constitutions, patients can experience a major *healing crisis*—that is, an increased intensity of their symptoms.

healing crisis: A *healing crisis* or, better, *healing reaction* occurs when a patient experiences an increased intensity of symptoms before he or she begins to feel better. It is a normal process that often occurs during treatment. The reoccurrence of symptoms that the patient has had before can indicate that he or she is retracing the path back to health, as his or her organs and tissues detoxify, ridding themselves of accumulated waste.

In contrast, the field of *drainage,* originating in Europe at the turn of the twentieth century, is a modality more focused on the individual. This holistic school of healing is based on the belief that true cleansing is accomplished only through stimulation of the body's organs and tissues to release toxins *at their own unique pace* and *within their own metabolic limits.* Drainage remedies are prescribed very carefully, according to the patient's particular illness and level of functioning, whereas detoxification protocols are more often simply generalized recipes touted as suitable for everyone.

DR. LANE'S "MIRACLE" CURE

Sir William Arbuthnot Lane (1856–1943), regarded as England's foremost abdominal surgeon in the first half of the twentieth century, was also a firm believer in homeopathy and alternative medicine and particularly in the importance of treating intestinal stasis and autointoxication (poisoning by toxins produced within the body). At one time while speaking to the staff of Johns Hopkins Hospital and Medical College he said, "Gentlemen, I will never die of cancer. I am taking measures to prevent it. . . . Drain the body of its poisons, feed it properly, and the miracle is done."

As discussed in chapter 1, a patient's symptoms reflect his or her miasm, or inherited (genetic) or acquired

**Candida albicans* is the most pathogenic and common opportunistic yeast to thrive in a toxic bowel. The overgrowth of candida, along with pathogenic bacteria, has become so prevalent nowadays that it has earned its own medical term: *dysbiosis.* (For more information about dysbiosis, see chapter 7.)

(environmentally caused) disease potential. For example, when under stress, whether it is a physical, biochemical, or psychological stress, one person may react with anxiety, another may get a blinding headache, while another may succumb to the flu. Each type of illness exemplifies the preexisting weakness in a specific tissue or organ system that is characteristic of the individual's miasmic tendency. Drainage remedies, as well as the constitutional homeopathic remedies described in chapter 14, are prescribed taking into account this miasmic tendency as well as the patient's particular disturbed and dysfunctioning organs and tissues.

NATURAL DRAINAGE IN THE BODY

In a healthy body, what might be termed *organic drainage* occurs automatically every day. Through the excretion of bile, feces, urine, and sweat, as well as the expulsion of carbon dioxide simply through breathing, the body is constantly in the process of draining and purifying itself. However, when defecation, urination, perspiration, or respiration is disturbed in any manner—perhaps, for example, because the body is overloaded from toxic stressors such as mercury amalgam fillings, inflamed from a dental or tonsil focal infection, or chronically congested from dysfunctioning metabolic pathways in the liver—drainage becomes less efficient, and over time illness ensues.

The Primary Emunctories

Natural organic drainage is realized through the body's emunctories. The term *emunctories* derives from the Latin *emungere,* meaning "to cleanse," and refers to the organs and tissues that excrete toxins in the body. The primary emunctories in the body are thus the major excretory organs: the liver and gallbladder (bile excre-

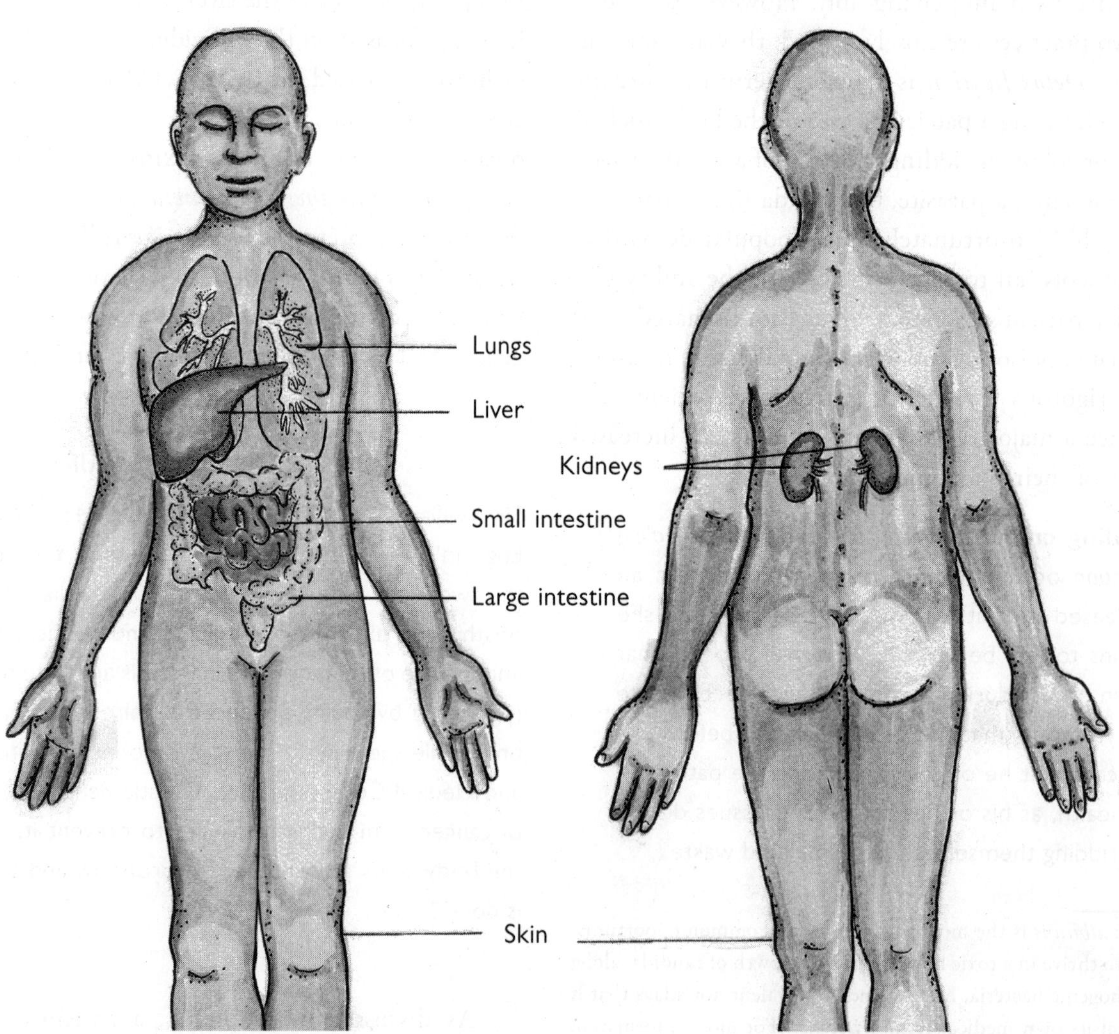

Figure 2.1. The primary emunctories in the body (see plate 2 for a color rendition of this figure)

tion), the kidneys (urination), and the intestines (defecation). Also included in this list are the lungs, which remove carbon dioxide through exhalation, and the skin, which removes waste through perspiration (see figure 2.1). In a healthy body, toxins are transported to these emunctories expediently through the blood and more slowly through the lymph fluid and the tissues (the extracellular matrix; see chapter 9). When these primary emunctories fail to function optimally, however, the body utilizes its next line of defense in draining toxins—the secondary emunctories.

The Secondary Emunctories

The secondary emunctories are all of the mucous membranes of the body. The mucous membranes, or mucosae, are the thin layers of tissue that line body cavities that open directly to the exterior. These membranes secrete mucus, which is a slimy, sticky substance that moistens and protects these body cavities. Their surface area is vast; in fact, the mucosae are estimated to be one hundred times greater in area than the external skin.[1]

The major secondary emunctories in the body are the mucous membranes of the eyes, nose, mouth, ears (Eustachian tubes), throat (pharynx and tonsils), and

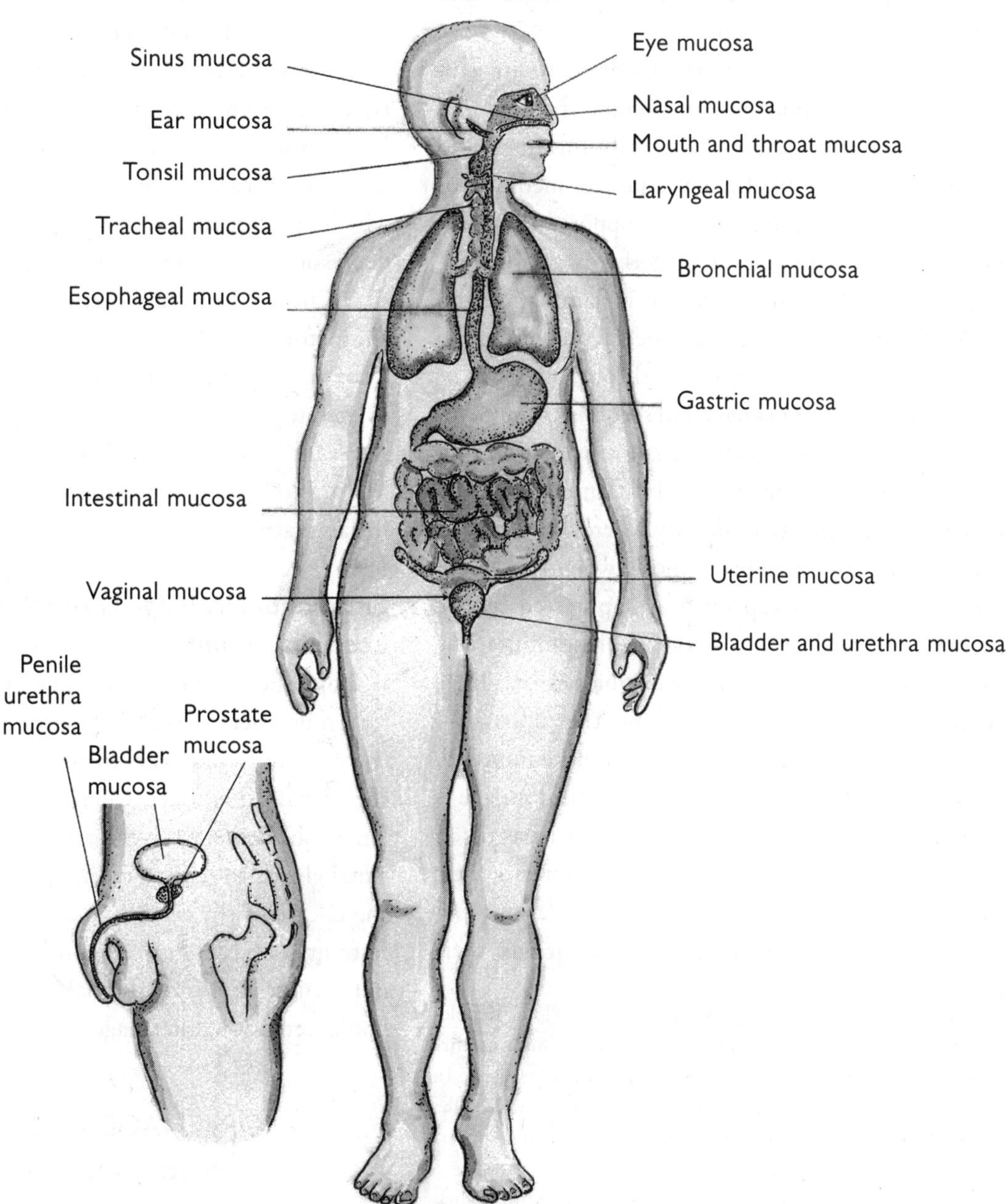

Figure 2.2 The secondary emunctories: the mucous membranes in the body (see plate 3 for a color rendition of this figure)

sinuses; those of the larynx, trachea, and bronchi; those of the esophagus, stomach, and intestines; those of the bladder and urethra; and those of the genital organs—in women the vagina and uterus, and in men the urethra (which travels through the prostate gland and penis).* (See figure 2.2.)

Although less efficient than the primary emunctories, the mucosae are an excellent backup drainage system for the body. When the primary emunctories fail, the body will try to drain toxins via these secondary pathways through such measures as frequent urination (bladder mucosa), sneezing (nasal mucosa), coughing (throat mucosa), loose stools (intestinal mucosa), and even vomiting (stomach mucosa).

However, if these outlets fail to drain toxins sufficiently, the body's mucosae can become irritated and inflamed. Over time, these chronically inflamed and very moist mucosal tissues become a perfect medium for infection through the proliferation of opportunistic bacteria, fungi, and viruses. In fact, all the diagnoses ending in the suffix *-itis,* which refers to inflammation and infection,† are really just medical labels representing the body's failed attempt to drain toxins through either of its first two defenses—the primary and secondary emunctories. Thus, *tonsillitis, bronchitis, sinusitis, cystitis* (bladder infection), *colitis* (chronic intestinal inflammation), and *prostatitis* are all terms that identify where drainage was inadequate in the body. Furthermore, when the mucosae's limited excretion capability is suppressed by the numerous "*anti*-medications"—the *anti*histamines, the *anti*-inflammatories, and even the *anti*biotics that leave bacterial carcasses littered throughout the mucosae—the body's ability to drain toxins is even more impeded. The enormity of this suppression of natural drainage is particularly magnified in individuals who have taken numerous medications for many years to curtail their symptoms. Although these allopathic medications can be necessary in certain life-threatening situations, their long-term use is a primary cause of chronic dysfunction and disease.

The Tertiary Emunctories

Broadly speaking, *any* organ or tissue that has the capability to excrete toxins may be considered an emunctory. However, since these tertiary emunctories do not excrete as well as the primary and secondary emunctories, they typically hold on to and store toxins, which invariably precipitates various levels of dysfunction and disease. For example, toxins accumulating in the synovial membranes that line the joints (and secrete lubricating synovial fluid) can lead to chronic arthritis. A buildup of inflammatory by-products in the serous membrane that surrounds the heart (and secretes a watery lubricating fluid) can eventually give rise to cardiovascular disease. Mercury amalgam fillings and bacterial focal infections in the head can so congest the meningeal membranes, which envelop the brain and spinal cord, that fatigue, depression, and memory loss often ensue.

When it fails to function normally as a primary emunctory, the skin can act as a tertiary emunctory. That is, when the skin's sweat (sudoriferous) glands fail to excrete waste, the body attempts to drain through the skin's oil (sebaceous) glands and deeper dermal tissues, leading to rashes, acne, and eczema (skin dryness and inflammation).

Emotional Drainage through the Lacrimal Glands

It should be mentioned that one of the smallest emunctory routes serves a dual function. The lacrimal glands continually secrete tears to clean, lubricate, and moisten the eyeballs. However, when grief and sadness accumulate in the heart, parasympathetic nerves trigger the lacrimal glands to secrete additional tears, which facilitates the release of the tension and pain these feelings manifest in the body. Thus, the tiny lacrimal glands serve one of the most vital and essential excretory functions in our bodies: emotional drainage.

DRAINAGE TECHNIQUES
History and Overview

In these toxic times, treatment must often begin with drainage remedies or therapies, which aid the body

*In men, the urethra, which is approximately 8 inches long, doubles as a passageway for both urine and sperm. Thus, the male urethra is part of the reproductive system as well as the urinary system. In women, these systems utilize separate tissues—the uterus and vagina are part of the reproductive system, and the urethra, which is approximately 1.5 inches long, is part of the urinary system.

†Although the suffix *–itis* by definition refers only to inflammation, many of the terms using this suffix, such as *cystitis,* also denote accompanying infection.

in effectively cleansing and purifying itself. Mikhael Adams, a leading naturopathic physician in the field of drainage, clearly illustrates this point by explaining that treatment must "open the door" and release toxins in the body before attempting any repair or regeneration of tissue. And in light of the fact that essentially *everyone* has been exposed to significant levels of toxic metals, petroleum chemicals, prescription drugs, devitalized foods, and other poisons of modern civilization, more and more holistic practitioners are prescribing unique drainage remedies at the beginning of each patient's treatment protocol. In addition, the use of drainage remedies and therapies ensures not only that toxins are effectively discharged from the body but also that they are released as gently as possible.

THESE TOXIC TIMES

The journal *Public Health Reports* has found that individuals nowadays are burdened with an astounding number of chemicals—an average of 167 per person. Of these chemicals, 76 have been found to cause cancer, 94 are toxic to the brain and nervous system, and 79 have been found to cause birth defects.[2]

This "body burden" of toxic chemicals has risen so precipitously in modern times that it can no longer be naturally eliminated without the assistance of external drainage and detoxification remedies and therapies.

The term *drainage* has been used in various contexts throughout its history. In this chapter, it is used primarily to describe remedies that gently and naturally discharge toxins from the body. Over the past two centuries, the most common drainage treatments have been homeopathic and herbal remedies. However, drainage treatments include some that do not utilize remedies at all, such as structural therapies like massage and hydrotherapies in the form of saunas, steam baths, douches, and wet sheet packs, which encourage the body to sweat toxins out through the skin. In fact, broadly speaking, *any* product or technique—from a massage to a vitamin or mineral supplement—can be considered a form of drainage if it effectively stimulates tissues and organs to discharge poisons from the body.

Massage

Manual lymphatic drainage (MLD), first employed by two physical therapists, Emil and Estrid Vodder in France, is an exceptionally effective massage technique that mechanically releases toxins and directs them out through the lymphatic channels of the body.[3] MLD is recognized as a superior therapeutic method for reducing edema and lymphatic congestion as well as for cleansing the tissues of metabolic wastes, excess water, large protein molecules, and toxic chemicals, metals, and microbes.

Other excellent massage methods that effectively detoxify the tissues are Tui-Na (Chinese medical massage), Rolfing, and Anatomy Trains (a Rolfing type of massage). All of these techniques are best employed in conjunction with homeopathic or herbal drainage remedies and after any "obstacles to cure" (such as mercury amalgam fillings or dental and tonsil foci) are cleared (or in conjunction with their clearing).

Hydrotherapy

Vincent Priessnitz (1799–1852), born in what is now the Czech Republic, is considered the founder of hydrotherapy; he used cold compresses, wet sheet packs, and douches (streams of water directed at specific areas of the body) in the treatment of disease. In 1840 his hydrotherapy clinic had over 1,600 patients, and his reputation was so great that he treated members of royalty, as well as Chopin and Napoleon. Based on Priessnitz's work and that of later practitioners, who employed hot water, steams, and saunas, hydrotherapy became an integral subject for the first naturopathic schools in Europe and America, and it is still taught today in all of the naturopathic medical schools.*

Homeopathic Remedies

Homeopathy, a system of medicine that uses minute quantities of specially prepared plant, animal, or mineral substances to stimulate healing in the body, originated in 1789 through the astute observations and careful research of German physician Samuel Hahnemann (1755–1843).[4] Chapter 14 describes in detail Dr. Hahnemann's specialty of constitutional homeopathy—

*For more information on Priessnitz, read *Nature Doctors,* by Friedhelm Kirchfeld and Wade Boyle.

the use of a single remedy to treat the overall mental, emotional, and physical makeup of an individual. Homeopathic remedies have been employed over the years not only in a constitutional manner but also for the specific purpose of draining toxins from the body.

Satellite Homeopathic Remedies

The use of homeopathic remedies for drainage was pioneered by Swiss physician Antoine Nebel (1870–1954).[5] Around 1910, Dr. Nebel noticed that after he gave patients a tubercular nosode—a strong homeopathic remedy made from diseased tissue that stimulates the body to mobilize its immune defenses against that disease—they often would have extreme reactions. Common responses included respiratory ailments such as nasal congestion, sore throat, and coughing; inflammatory reactions in the genitals such as bladder or prostate infection; and inflammation of the joints resulting in arthritic aches and pains. Although these bodily healing crises were quite disturbing and sometimes debilitating to the patients, to Nebel they were understandable, since tuberculosis bacteria have an affinity for producing disease in the lungs, genitals, and joints. Nebel reasoned that the body was simply responding to the homeopathic tubercular nosode by releasing its burden of accumulated microbes and toxic waste products in these tuberculosis-sensitive tissues. The problem was that the response could often be excessive.

After repeatedly witnessing these reactions in his practice and through years of clinical trial and error, Nebel concluded that patients' strong reactions to the potent homeopathic nosodes were a common—and actually appropriate—response. However, in order to address the discomforting and often painful symptoms, Nebel began to use other homeopathics as secondary remedies to augment the release of accumulated toxins in the tuberculosis-sensitive tissues. This use of a secondary, or satellite, homeopathic remedy to "channel" and purge the poisons residing in a patient's lung, genital, and joint tissues represented the formal birth of drainage remedies. Some examples of these satellite homeopathic remedies include Antimonium tartaricum to clear inflammation from the lungs, Cantharis vesicatoria to expel toxins from the bladder mucosa, Chimaphila umbellata to stimulate prostate drainage, and Rhus toxicodendron to discharge toxins from the joints. All of these homeopathic remedies are prescribed in a low potency (such as 6C)* so that they act at a very specific physical level on these particular tissues in the body. One of Nebel's most exceptional students, Leon Vannier, embraced Nebel's idea of channeling the toxins and actually coined the term *drainage* around 1920.[6]

Combination Homeopathic Remedies

A few years later, in 1927, a Belgian dowser† named George Discry and a Professor Reutter from the University of Geneva collaborated to formulate a line of remedies to stimulate drainage in the body. In contrast to Nebel's use of a single homeopathic remedy, Discry and Reutter combined several homeopathic remedies in one bottle. These formulas were innovative in that they were the first known to combine homeopathic plant and metal remedies. Furthermore, the metals in these remedies were potentized at a specific 12X‡ potency, allowing them to cross cell membranes to stimulate intracellular detoxification. In 1949, the UNDA company in Belgium began to manufacture these remedies, called the "numbered compounds"; they are still being produced today according to Discry and Reutter's original formulations.[7] Combination (or complex) remedies consisting of several homeopathic remedies mixed together in a single bottle are also available from other homeopathic companies. Although these combination remedies are not as effective in the long run as the use of accurately prescribed single homeopathic remedies, they are often helpful in the treatment of acute disease.

---

*The term *potency* refers to the power, vitality, or strength of a homeopathic remedy, based on the amount of dilution and succussion (shaking) the remedy undergoes. A low potency such as 6C has more of a physical effect in the body than a higher potency such as 1M, which acts more on the mental and emotional planes. (See chapter 14 for more detailed information on potency.)

†Dowsing is a paraphysical phenomenon in which information is divined through various instruments such as a dowsing rod (forked stick) or pendulum. In the hands of a true master, it is a dramatically accurate form of energetic testing.

‡It is generally agreed among homeopaths that the 12X to 15X potencies affect cell membranes most specifically, lesser potencies have more influence extracellularly, and greater potencies have an intracellular effect. Potencies in the M range and greater, however, have been observed to also affect the etheric body (that is, the mental and emotional level).

Herbal Remedies

In 1947, Belgian physician Pol Henry (1918–1988) made an innovative discovery.[8] Instead of utilizing mature adult plants to prepare herbal remedies, as herbalists had traditionally done in the past, Henry began to experiment with using very young parts of plants, such as the buds, sprouts, and rootlets. He found that the growth factors in these freshly harvested young parts, as well as the strong, active essence of life in them, rendered the remedies made from these very young herbs much more potent than botanical remedies extracted from the dried mature parts of plants.*

In his clinical practice, Henry found that these young, embryonic remedies were superior at activating congested organs and tissues to gently release and drain toxins from the body. At first, this new and unique form of drainage through phytotherapy (botanical medicine) was called blastotherapy or embryophytotherapy, but over the years it has come to be referred to primarily as gemmotherapy (the prefix *gemmo-* comes from the Latin *gemma-*, meaning bud) and more recently as plant stem cell therapy.[9]

GEMMOTHERAPY
Superior Drainage

Single satellite homeopathic remedies, combination homeopathic remedies, and gemmotherapy remedies all have drainage and cleansing effects in the body. However, in clinical practice I have found that gemmotherapy remedies are the most useful. The reasons for this are threefold. First, in the treatment of ill patients gemmotherapy remedies are the most effective in gently stimulating congested and depleted organs and tissues to release their accumulated toxins. Second, when subjected to energetic testing methods (such as kinesiology and reflex arm length testing; see appendix 3), gemmotherapy remedies consistently show superior results to single satellite or combination homeopathic drainage remedies. Finally, both forms of homeopathic drainage remedies have the potential to antidote, or cancel out, a patient's constitutional homeopathic remedy, in contrast to gemmotherapy remedies, which do not antidote homeopathics.* And as will be discussed in chapter 14, since it is my belief that constitutional homeopathy, according to the new Sankaran system, is one of the most—if not *the* most—curative forms of healing known, avoiding even the *possibility* of antidoting or interfering with the resonance of a patient's constitutional remedy is essential.

How Gemmotherapy Drainage Remedies Are Made

In order to preserve as much of their active constituents as possible, as soon as they are harvested the young plant parts (buds, sprouts, rootlets, et cetera) are tinctured, or mixed in a glycerin and alcohol solution. After three weeks of soaking, the plant parts are filtered out and the liquid extract is diluted with water, glycerin, and alcohol. Table 2.1 lists the commonly used gemmotherapy remedies, including their common and Latin names as well as the part of the tree, shrub, or plant that is used for making them.†

The Benefits of Using Embryonic Plants

Modern research has borne out what Dr. Henry found clinically—that the strong energetic and growth factors contained in the young parts of plants render these gemmotherapy remedies much more potent than traditional herbal remedies derived from mature plant parts. For example, in one French study, seven types of antioxidants (including vitamin C, anthocyanidins, and flavonoids) were isolated in the young buds of the black currant plant (*Ribes nigrum*) versus only three found in the more mature leaf portions of this plant.[10] Furthermore, the young buds

---

*Henry utilized both clinical and laboratory research in developing these remedies. His laboratory research was quite extensive and included the use of plasma protein electrophoresis, reticuloendothelial indexes, measurement of haptoglobin and ceruloplasmin levels, and flocculation tests of different globulins and other proteins. These blood test results allowed Henry to arrive at a blood protein profile, or investigative gemmogramme, that characterized a patient's terrain and indicated which gemmotherapy remedy was appropriate. For more in-depth information refer to *Botanical Medicine: A European Professional Perspective*, by Dan Kenner and Yves Requena, and *Gemmothérapie*, by Pol Henry (the latter is in French, however).

*Some would argue that single satellite and combination homeopathics have such a low potency—6C to 15C in most cases—that they won't disturb a constitutional remedy, which is typically given in a higher potency. However, in my experience they sometimes can, especially if the satellite or combination remedy is taken over time or if the patient is very sensitive.

†Pol Henry described only thirty-nine gemmotherapy remedies in his book. The other gemmotherapy remedies were developed by, among others, French physicians A. O. Julian and Max Tetau.

TABLE 2.1. THE GEMMOTHERAPY DRAINAGE REMEDIES

Remedy Common Name	Latin Plant Name	Plant Part Used
Ash	*Fraxinus excelsior*	buds
Beech	*Fagus sylvatica*	buds
Bilberry	*Vaccinium myrtillus*	young shoots
Black Currant	*Ribes nigrum*	buds
Black Elder	*Sambucus nigra*	buds
Black Poplar	*Populus nigra*	buds
Boxwood	*Buxus sempervirens*	young shoots
Bramble	*Rubus fructicosus*	young shoots
Cedar of Lebanon	*Cedrus libani*	young shoots
Chaste Tree	*Vitex agnus-castus*	young shoots
Cowberry	*Vaccinium vitis-idaea*	young shoots
Crab Apple	*Malus sylvestris*	buds
Dog Rose	*Rosa canina*	young shoots
Dogwood	*Cornus sanguinea*	buds
Elm	*Ulmus campestris*	buds
European Alder	*Alnus glutinosa*	buds
Fig	*Ficus carica*	buds
Giant Redwood	*Sequoia gigantea*	young shoots
Grape Vine	*Vitis vinifera*	buds
Grey Alder	*Alnus incana*	buds
Hawthorn	*Crataegus oxyacantha*	buds
Hazel	*Corylus avellana*	buds
Hedge Maple	*Acer campestre*	buds
Holly	*Ilex aquifolium*	young shoots
Hornbean	*Carpinus betulus*	buds
Horse Chestnut	*Aesculus hippocastanum*	buds
Horsetail	*Equisetum arvense*	young shoots
Judas Tree	*Cercis siliquastrum*	buds
Juniper	*Juniperus communis*	young shoots
Lemon Tree	*Citrus limonum*	bark
Lilac	*Syringa vulgaris*	buds
Linden Tree	*Tilia tomentosa*	buds
Maidenhair Tree	*Ginkgo biloba*	buds
Maize	*Zea mays*	rootlets
Mistletoe	*Viscum album*	young shoots
Mountain Pine	*Pinus montana*	buds
Oak	*Quercus pedonculata, Q. robur*	buds
Olive	*Olea europaea*	young shoots
Oriental Plane Tree	*Platanus orientalis*	buds
Raspberry	*Rubus idaeus*	young shoots
Rosemary	*Rosmarinus officinalis*	young shoots
Rye	*Secale cereale*	rootlets
Service Tree	*Sorbus domestica*	buds
Silver Birch	*Betula verrucosa*	buds, sap, seeds
Silver Fir	*Abies pectinata*	young shoots
Sweet Almond	*Prunus amygdalus*	buds
Sweet Chestnut	*Castanea vesca*	buds
Tamarisk	*Tamarix gallica*	young shoots
Virginia Creeper	*Ampelopsis veitchii*	young shoots
Walnut	*Juglans regia*	buds
Wayfaring Tree	*Viburnum lantana*	buds
White Birch	*Betula pubescens*	buds, bark of roots, rootlets, male catkins
White Willow	*Salix alba*	buds

were found to have substantially higher levels of amino acids (the building blocks of proteins) than the leaves. In fact, the vitality of black currant buds is most dramatically illustrated by their high content of arginine—5.7 milligrams in a bud as compared to 0.77 milligram in a mature leaf—since this amino acid stimulates the release of growth hormone, which is necessary for healthy plant (and human) maturation.[11] As a result of these constituents, black currant bud has potent anti-inflammatory properties through its action of draining toxins from arthritic joints and other inflamed tissues; it is also useful in the treatment of allergies and chronic fatigue because of its stimulating effects on the adrenal glands.

In table 2.2 the dramatic benefits of utilizing embryonic plant parts versus mature plant parts are further compared.

Specific Drainage of Organs and Tissues

Gemmotherapy remedies, as well as other botanical medicines, act on specific organs and tissues in the body through a mechanism called tropism. This term, from the Greek *tropos,* meaning "to turn," refers to the affinity certain plants have for certain tissues. For example, Juniper (*Juniperus communis*), the gemmotherapy remedy made from the young shoots of the evergreen juniper shrub, has a natural tropism for the

TABLE 2.2. EMBRYONIC VERSUS ADULT PLANT TISSUE

Embryonic plants contain all of the genetic information of the future plant.	Adult plants have *lost* most of the genetic information of the embryonic stage.
Embryonic plants contain all of the active phytochemicals of various parts of the plant.	Adult plants have a *low* concentration of phytochemicals, which differ from harvest to harvest.
Embryonic plants are nontoxic.	Many adult plants contain toxic metabolites, such as lead, arsenic, and so on, as a result of soil and/or air pollution.*

This table is based on information from PSC Distribution, www.epsce.com.

*In ingesting an extract from an adult herb—that is, by *not* using gemmotherapy remedies—individuals may indeed be ingesting toxins. In fact, a recent study published in the *Journal of the American Medical Association* found that some herbal remedies contain dangerous levels of mercury, arsenic, and lead. (R. Saper et al., "Heavy Metal Content of Ayurvedic Herbal Medicine Products," *JAMA* 292:23 [December 15, 2004], 2868–73.)

liver. Due to this affinity or tropic tendency, Juniper as well as Rosemary, Rye, and Hazel are the primary gemmotherapy remedies used in the treatment of hepatic congestion, impaired liver detoxification (phase 1 oxidation or phase 2 conjugation), faulty bile formation and excretion, cirrhosis, and any of the other host of liver-related maladies. Similarly, Walnut (*Juglans regia*), made from the bud of the walnut tree, has an affinity for the pancreas and is therefore indicated in the treatment of pancreatic enzyme deficiency, insulin dysfunction (syndrome X), intestinal bloating, and other digestive conditions. Hawthorn (*Crataegus oxyacantha*), extracted from the buds of the hawthorn shrub, has a strong affinity for the heart and its blood vessels and is an invaluable alterative—that is, it has a normalizing or balancing effect on the cardiovascular system and can therefore either stimulate activity (in the case of low blood pressure or heart failure) or sedate activity (in the case of hypertension or arrhythmia), depending on the individual's particular needs.

Because plants have this quality of tropic affinity for certain tissues and organs in the body, practitioners can prescribe gemmotherapy remedies according to exactly where drainage is required in a patient's system.

Personalized Remedies

Gemmotherapy preparations are superior drainage remedies in that they strengthen and tonify tissues while supporting them in releasing accumulated toxins. As a result, tissues release toxins gently and efficiently, within their own metabolic capability and limits, and the potential for strong healing reactions is greatly diminished.

A further distinctive characteristic of gemmotherapy remedies is that like homeopathic remedies, they are categorized according to a patient's level of health, or miasmic tendency. This additional personalizing factor renders these remedies even more effective in draining organs and tissues, since they can be appropriately prescribed to match the patient's degree of (weak or strong) functioning. When holistic practitioners prescribe gemmotherapy remedies taking into account their patient's miasmic tendencies as well as the specific organs and tissues that require drainage, these remedies are most efficacious, in that they are typically never too insignificant nor too overpowering to the patient.

Long-Lasting Effects

The potency and long-lasting effects of these remedies have been consistently witnessed by holistic practitioners for almost a century. In most cases, after the first several courses of drainage effected by gemmotherapy remedies, individuals' organs and tissues are rejuvenated and begin to excrete much more efficiently on their own. (Many other detoxification protocols often exhaust various metabolic pathways and tissues and achieve only short-term gain.) After the initial period of treatment with gemmotherapy remedies, further drainage remedies are usually required only intermittently—typically in response to acute intoxication (e.g., new paint at an individual's workplace) or to augment the drainage of toxins from a major focus, such as after the removal of a tooth that has had a failed root canal (dental focal infection).

PLANT STEM CELL THERAPY
Concentrated Gemmotherapy Remedies

Although the founder of gemmotherapy, Dr. Pol Henry, utilized only concentrated gemmotherapy remedies in his research, Dr. Max Tetau of France later diluted these herbal solutions. Tetau, who, along with Dr. A. O. Julian, greatly expanded this field of botanical medicine, chose to dilute gemmotherapy remedies at a 1X, or a 1:10, dilution level. He did this for two reasons: He found that these young embryonic extracts could be quite powerful, and by diluting them he could reduce strong healing reactions. Additionally, being diluted like homeopathics, these remedies more readily fit into the French pharmacopoeia, rendering them eligible for insurance reimbursement and therefore making them more affordable.*

More recently, however, companies in Belgium (HerbalGem, or Gemmos LLC in the United States) and Italy (Forza Vitale, or PSC Distribution in the United States) have reinstated the concentrated form of gemmotherapy according to Henry's original research. These undiluted remedies are often referred to as plant stem cells (PSCs) because these concentrated extracts contain "stem cells"—or *meristems*—that are capable of stimulating the growth of new cells and tissues in the body.

Effectiveness

A good example of the exceptional regenerative nature of plants is that a single cutting placed in water can grow into an entirely new plant.† In a similar way, embryonic plant cells can help grow and repair, as well as rejuvenate and regenerate, organs and tissues in the human body (without the negative side effects engendered from human stem cells). Thus, not only are these concentrated embryonic herbals more powerful drainage and detoxification remedies than the more diluted gemmotherapy remedies reformulated by Tetau and others, but they are also significantly more effective at regenerating tissues and organs.

Concentrated PSC remedies are loaded with nourishing phytochemicals, including vitamins, minerals, bioflavonoids and antioxidants, plant growth hormones (auxins, gibberellins), amino acids, nucleic acids, and anticancer and antimicrobial (antibacterial, antifungal, antiparasitic, antiviral) constituents, as well as important phytochelating agents (sap, enzymes, antioxidants, et cetera) essential for detoxification. Through the specific action of these potent phytochelating agents, these young herbal remedies are superior at removing both endogenous (made within the body) and exogenous (originating outside the body) toxins from the body.

Dosage

Since plant stem cell remedies are highly concentrated, patients can take small doses. For example, a typical adult PSC dosage ranges from one to six drops, three times a day.* In stark contrast, Tetau's more diluted gemmotherapy remedies often require prescriptions of twenty-five to seventy-five drops or more, three or four times a day, which necessitates the ingestion of large amounts of glycerin (which is too sweet for many and contraindicated in cases of intestinal dysbiosis) and alcohol (which is contraindicated in cases of liver dysfunction). In the same way, traditional herbal remedies made from older, mature plant parts also require higher daily doses to generate any curative effects in the body. The resulting higher amounts ingested—often from 50 to 150 drops per day—can be irritating and even toxic to some liver-compromised patients.

Treatment of Common Conditions

The following list gives a brief snapshot of the remarkable effectiveness of these herbal remedies in the treatment of many common symptoms and diseases.†

*Although since they weren't succussed, Tetau's gemmotherapy remedies were not strictly homeopathic.

†Such plant regeneration is accomplished through the apical meristems, or undifferentiated cells located in the growing tips of the buds and roots of all plants. Meristems have high levels of nucleic acids. Once undifferentiated meristem cells enter the body, they can become differentiated and selectively detoxify and regenerate the organs and tissues for which they have an affinity. (J. Rozencwajg, *Dynamic Gemmotherapy: Integrative Embryonic Phytotherapy* [New Zealand: Natura Medica Ltd., 2008], 3.)

*In fact, these remedies are so potent that they are best diluted in a half glass of water and sipped. Sensitive patients should consider diluting these remedies even more, such as one drop in an 8-ounce (or larger) glass of water, sipped throughout the day, as a daily dose. Over time, as patients improve, this very gentle dose can be increased.

†This information derives from PSC Distribution (www.epsce.com) and from their continuing education courses.

Allergies and Fatigue

Black Currant (*Ribes nigrum*) helps regenerate exhausted adrenal glands by stimulating corticosteroid production. This "natural DHEA" herbal reduces fatigue and is a major anti-inflammatory and antiallergenic remedy. Black Currant is loaded with vitamins, minerals, plant steroids, fatty acids, amino acids, and antioxidants. In fact, just 10 drops of Black Currant provides 1,000 milligrams of vitamin C.

BLACK CURRANT

Black currant buds contain abscisic acid, a naturally occurring hormone that allows the plant to adjust to outside stress, just like the adrenal cortisol hormone does in our bodies. They also have significant amounts of indoleacetic acid (IAA), a member of a group of phytohormones called auxins—the first plant hormone family identified by Darwin in 1880. The IAA in the extract Black Currant supports tissue regeneration in the adrenals and other tissues, acts as a natural anti-inflammatory in cases of allergies and painful arthritis (in place of harmful NSAID medications), and has been proven to destroy cancerous cells while leaving healthy cells intact. Black Currant contains high levels of flavonoids such as anthocyanins, catechins, epicatechins, quercetin, and rutin, which provide further potent anti-inflammatory, antioxidant, and antiallergenic effects. The extract is also loaded with vitamins B_1, B_2, B_3, and B_{12}, biotin, vitamins C and E, and calcium and contains trace amounts of minerals such as boron, copper, chromium, iron, magnesium, manganese, sodium, phosphorus, selenium, silica, and sulfur.

Caution: Black Currant should not be prescribed to those with high cortisol levels because it can raise these levels and further stress the already impaired adrenals in this particular patient population.

Asthma

Wayfaring Tree (*Viburnum lantana*) is indicated in cases of asthma, dyspnea (difficulty breathing), bronchial spasmodic coughs, and other lung-related symptoms. This extract, made from the buds of the wayfaring tree, contains significant amounts of amentoflavone, a phytochemical that reduces pro-inflammatory cytokine production, enhances natural killer-cell antibodies, and has been shown to reduce tumor nodule formation in induced lung metastasis in mice. Wayfaring Tree also contains phenylpropanoid glycosides and iridoid glucosides that inhibit harmful free radical production and are liver protective, acetic acid to combat bacterial and fungal infections, the natural antihistamine astragalin, and potent antioxidants such as citric acid, malic acid, and epicatechin.

More serious forms of asthma may require Hazel, Black Currant, or Black Poplar.

Eczema and Aging Skin

Cedar of Lebanon (*Cedrus libani*) reduces eczema outbreaks and itching and hydrates the skin and hair. It is indicated in the dry types of eczema characterized by skin flaking.

For wet or weeping types of eczema, Elm (*Ulmus campestris*) is indicated. Elm contains ulmic acid, which has an anti-inflammatory action much like that of oatmeal and is rich in calcium, magnesium, and vitamins A, B, C, and K.

CEDAR OF LEBANON

Cedar of Lebanon's antiseborrheic (normalizing and rehydrating) and sedative (anti-itch) phytoconstituents include cedarin, cedrol, thujopsene, and widdol. This remedy, made from the embryonic young shoots of the cedar of Lebanon tree, contains sesquiterpenes that can cross the blood-brain barrier and have been indicated as potentially effective in the treatment of Alzheimer's, multiple sclerosis, Parkinson's disease, and Lou Gehrig's disease. Cedar of Lebanon is also loaded with vitamins A, B_1, B_2, B_3, D, and E and fatty acids and contains trace amounts of copper, cobalt, iron, iodine, magnesium, manganese, phosphorus, sodium, silica, and zinc, as well as other minerals.

Herpes

Elm (*Ulmus campestris*) has anti-inflammatory and antiviral action that makes it an important remedy in treating herpes simplex lesions. Other plant stem cell remedies indicated for herpes include Grapevine (the polycrest antiviral remedy), Dog Rose, and Oak. (But note that Oak is contraindicated in individuals with hypertension, hyperthyroidism, or elevated levels of testosterone since this extract stimulates adrenal and pituitary function, which could already be excessive in this population of patients.)

> **polycrest:** A polycrest remedy is one that has a broad range of applications and is useful in both acute and chronic disorders. For example, Black Poplar is the polycrest remedy for heavy metal detoxification because it fits—and treats—so many symptoms of heavy metal poisoning.

Hormone Balancing for Men

Giant Redwood (*Sequoia gigantea*) is indicated in cases of male infertility to increase sperm count and to help reduce any associated sexual asthenia (weakness) and memory loss during andropause (male menopause). Giant Redwood has significant concentrations of amino acids (methionine, aspartic acid, glutamic acid, proline, and phenylalanine), vitamin D, and essential oils. It has been shown to be effective in reducing benign prostatic hypertrophy (BPH) and improving urinary function.

Maidenhair (*Ginkgo biloba*) can be added to the prescription in cases of male infertility and impotency secondary to impaired penile blood flow. Maidenhair contains antioxidant flavonoids (such as quercetin) and terpenoids (such as ginkgolides) that improve blood flow by dilating blood vessels and reducing the stickiness of platelets. (Caution: Maidenhair is contraindicated for those who are taking blood-thinning prescription medications, such as Coumadin or Plavix, and for those with idiopathic thrombocytic purpura [ITP]).

Oak (*Quercus pedonculata*) is a general hormonal tonic that stimulates the production of testosterone, reduces benign prostatic hypertrophy (BPH), and can lessen the incidence of premature ejaculation. Oak contains beta-sitosterol, a natural plant sterol that can lower cholesterol and ease symptoms of BPH. (Caution: Oak is contraindicated in cases of hypertension or hyperthyroidism.)

Hormone Balancing for Women

Raspberry (*Rubus idaeus*) helps balance estrogen and progesterone production and is indicated in cases of amenorrhea (absence or cessation of menstrual periods), dysmenorrhea (painful periods), menorrhagia (excessive menstrual bleeding), and premenstrual syndrome (PMS), as well as for menopausal symptoms. Raspberry contains fragarine, a uterine tonic. It also contains ellagic acid, a phenolic compound that has been shown to inhibit cancer in mice, and quercetin, which has demonstrated anticarcinogenic activity in skin, colon, and mammary cancers.

Cowberry (*Vaccinium vitis-idaea*) also helps balance estrogen and progesterone production, but it is indicated more often in the treatment of adverse menopausal symptoms such as hot flashes and female senescence (aging). Cowberry contains potent antioxidants such as catechin, citric acid, and lycopene, as well as proanthocyanidin A-1, which contains small amounts of estrogen.

Insomnia and Anxiety

Linden Tree (*Tilia tomentosa*) increases serotonin levels in the body, which can help patients fall asleep as well as increase the duration of their sleep. It is also an excellent antianxiety remedy and has been used successfully as a natural tranquilizer for adults as well as hyperactive children. Linden Tree contains farnesol, flavonoid glycosides, and essential oils that have been shown to reduce anxiety and hypertension, lower triglyceride levels, and induce lipogenesis (weight loss). (Caution: Linden Tree is contraindicated for those who are taking selective serotonin reuptake inhibitor [SSRI] medications such as Prozac, Paxil, Celexa, or Zoloft.)

Fig (*Ficus carica*) is often prescribed in conjunction with Linden Tree as a mild antidepressant and antianxiety remedy and to further induce more restful sleep. Fig is also indicated in gut-related dysfunction and therefore can be an excellent choice for patients who suffer from both mental and emotional symptoms and gastrointestinal dysfunction. Fig contains the protease ficin, which is twenty times more powerful than papain (an enzyme found in papaya) in stimulating protein digestion. Ficin's anti-inflammatory action supports the healing of gastric and peptic ulcers, and it acts as a vermifuge in the treatment of intestinal worms. Fig contains significant amounts of vitamins B_1, B_2, B_3, and B_5 and calcium, as well as trace amounts of boron, copper, iron, magnesium, manganese, phosphorus, potassium, and zinc.

Memory Loss

European Alder (*Alnus glutinosa*) improves cognition by increasing cerebral circulation and tonifying arterial walls. Grey Alder (*Alnus incana*) is indicated in cases of more serious dementia and Alzheimer's, as well as in cases of other degenerative neurological diseases such as Parkinson's and multiple sclerosis. European Alder and Grey Alder both contain beta-sitosterol and brassinolide, which have anticancer and immune-modulating effects.

However, Grey Alder also contains betulinic acid, which has very potent anticancer activity.

Optimal Preparation

The Italian company Forza Vitale has the highest-quality concentrated plant stem cell extracts in the world, according to my personal testing. Forza Vitale carefully harvests its buds and young shoots at the most optimal times from the Italian Apennines, ensuring that they are 100 percent embryonic. In contrast, other companies' products may contain some nonembryonic plant material such as cataphylls (scales around the buds) and branches, whose high tannin content can significantly reduce the absorption of vitamins, minerals, and numerous other phytochemicals into the remedy. Forza Vitale's buds and young shoots are certified organic, and the company uses allergen-free certified organic grape alcohol, as opposed to the more allergenic grain alcohol from corn. Finally, Forza Vitale's light brown bottles have a nontoxic natural organic latex rubber dropper that ensures the correct dosage in drops and eliminates leakage. Each bottle has a shelf life of five years.

▶ Plant stem cell remedies are available to healthcare professionals from two companies in the United States: PSC Distribution at (631) 477-6696 or www.epsce.com and Gemmos LLC at (877) 417-6298 or www.gemmos-usa.com.

Prescription

I *highly* encourage practitioners to attend educational seminars on the use of plant stem cell remedies before prescribing them to their patients. Each remedy has many indications (as well as some contraindications) and numerous phytochemicals that should be understood both scientifically and clinically. Furthermore, for optimal results, plant stem cell remedies should be correlated to the findings of blood, urine, and other appropriate laboratory tests.

Both Gemmos LLC and PSC Distribution offer excellent continuing education seminars.

USING DRAINAGE REMEDIES

Compatibility with Other Remedies

The gemmotherapy drainage remedies discussed in this chapter are quite compatible with other treatment protocols. They not only can be given simultaneously with constitutional homeopathic remedies (with no fear of antidoting), other herbal remedies, nutritional supplements, and even prescription medications but are often greatly synergistic, augmenting the action of other treatments through their draining and tonifying effects. (However, caution should always be used with patients who are taking prescription drugs, especially in the case of tuberculinic or luetic patients.)

USING DRAINAGE REMEDIES WITH PRESCRIPTION MEDICATIONS

Drainage remedies can reduce the side effects of prescription medications by facilitating the release of toxins through the liver, kidneys, and other emunctories. Many holistic practitioners have had great success using drainage remedies with patients who are taking strong doses of chemotherapy to treat cancer. However, practitioners must be skilled and experienced in such treatments, as results can be very unpredictable with these more compromised luetic patients.

Achieving Organic Drainage

Toward the middle and end of the typical patient's treatment protocol—whether it has been under way for six months or five years—very little to no intermittent drainage is required, as the patient's body has begun to be able to cleanse and organically drain itself. Thus, after several treatment periods, practitioners will often note progress through observing that their patients more and more rarely require drainage support, which is indicative of the healthier dormant psoric level of functioning.

The Unlayering Effect or "Peeling the Onion"

As drainage remedies begin to detoxify the body, a clearer picture of an individual's true pathology and "obstacles to healing" arises. As these major obstacles to healing become clear and are treated, drainage remedies are often needed again to facilitate the release of the accumulated toxins that have been coaxed out from intracellular and tissue stores. This unlayering effect, often referred to as "peeling the onion," is an essential aspect of the unwinding process that characterizes holistic healing.

It is critical at this stage that manifestations of healing are not misidentified as symptoms of an acute (suddenly occurring) illness and treated in an inappropriate suppressive manner. For example, applying cortisone cream on an abdominal rash that is a transient manifestation of liver drainage, or taking an antihistamine during drainage of a chronic sinus focus, can set back a patient's progress considerably.* Practitioners may find energetic testing to be helpful in identifying and measuring these healing vicissitudes as they naturally arise.

CLEARING "PSYCHOSOMATIC" EFFECTS

Drainage can help arrest mental and emotional toxic patterns as effectively as it clears chronic metabolic stagnation. In other words, as drainage encourages the release of toxins (heavy metals, chemicals, food-allergy antigens, and so on) from the system, it often concurrently mitigates many so-called psychosomatic disturbances. There is nothing new (or "New-Agey") about this psychophysical clearing process; in fact, it was recognized millennia ago by ancient Chinese acupuncturists who correlated anger to liver congestion, fear to kidney dysfunction, and lack of—or inappropriately excessive—joy to heart disturbances.[12] Thus, by encouraging drainage through the liver, kidneys, and other emunctories, drainage remedies have the potential to improve short-term memory, increase concentration, stimulate creativity, deepen spiritual awareness, and over time create a greater capacity for happiness. As a result, drainage not only helps facilitate the optimization and regeneration of our physical bodies but also furthers the evolution of our psychological and spiritual growth.

Lifestyle Recommendations during Drainage Protocols

During treatment with a drainage protocol, drinking lots of pure water will augment drainage and hydrate detoxifying tissues. For those taking gemmotherapy or plant stem cell remedies, mineral-free water is optimal, as it will not interfere with the minerals contained in the remedies and will further draw toxic material from the body. Water filtered by reverse osmosis is the preferred type of mineral-free water, but distilled water is also sufficient.

- ▶ Long-term use of mineral-free water is a controversial and much-debated issue in the holistic health community. Dennis Higgins, M.D., who has studied this subject for over twenty years, developed a product that avoids the issue. Higgins's water filter gives individuals the option of mineral-free reverse osmosis water to drink during drainage protocols, as well as clean springlike water that is filtered through a coral calcium filter at other times. For more information, contact the Radiant Life Company at (888) 593-8333 or www.radiantlifecatalog.com or contact Mary Cordaro at (818) 766-1787 or through www.marycordaro.com.

Additionally, exercise and massage greatly augment the mechanical release of toxins stored in the tissues. Adequate sleep—from eight to even ten hours per night—is also highly recommended during this period to facilitate the physical discharge of these toxins, as well as the release of any accumulated dark thoughts and feelings associated with these life-negative poisons. A dream diary and effective psychospiritual work (see chapter 18) can also be extremely important during this time.

It is also essential to greatly decrease, if not altogether avoid, the consumption of alcohol and refined sugar. In its early phases, drainage can increase cell membrane and tissue porosity, which can make a single glass of wine drunk the night before feel like it was an entire bottle the next day! Reducing or avoiding caffeine is also important, as its contracting and stimulating effects are at cross-purposes with the relaxing and releasing effects of drainage remedies and can therefore significantly reduce the discharge of toxins and lengthen treatment time. Patients might consider transitioning from coffee to black tea to green tea or, better, herbal tea. (See chapter 5 for more information on the toxic effects of sugar and caffeine.)

CONCLUSION

Currently, the vast majority of individuals on this planet are deeply intoxicated from modern refined foods, prescription (and street) drugs, and exposure to toxic metals and chemicals. Furthermore, most have inherited weak

*Of course, extremely uncomfortable symptoms may be managed with allopathic medications if patients are unable to consult with their holistic practitioner.

constitutions from parents (and grandparents, for those who are of Generation X or younger) who grew up under the influence of the increasingly pervasive toxins of the twentieth century. The goal of therapeutic drainage is to reduce the limiting influence of these inherited and acquired miasmic weaknesses so that individuals can enjoy the robust and energetic state of the healthy dormant psoric individual, who experiences rare dysfunction or illness. The plant stem cell remedies described in this chapter are a key element in this healing process, as they are the most potent and effective of all the drainage remedies.

When patients begin to heal and are able to move away from the "survival mode" existence of the tuberculinic and luetic diatheses, they can begin to focus more on their own personal growth and spiritual well-being. Thus, by removing the toxic wastes that not only obstruct the healthy functioning of the physical body but also obscure the vision of an individual's sense of self and own unique life path, drainage remedies can have beneficial repercussions over time in literally every aspect of life—physical, mental, emotional, *and* spiritual.

NOTES

1. K. Slagel, "Dental and Systemic Therapy with Innate Microbial Isopathic Homeopathic PleoSANUM Remedies," International Academy of Biological Dentistry and Medicine: 20th Anniversary Meeting, Carmel, Calif. (March 31–April 2, 2006), 8.
2. Thornton et al., *Public Health Reports,* 2002.
3. "Manual Lymph Drainage," www.vodderschool.com/manual_lymph_drainage_overview.
4. S. Hahnemann, *Organon of the Medical Art,* ed. W. O'Reilly (Palo Alto, Calif.: Birdcage Books, 1996), xv.
5. J. Jouanny et al., *Homeopathic Therapeutics: Possibilities in Chronic Pathology* (France: Boiron S.A., 1994), 24.
6. Ibid., 25.
7. H. Fagard, *UNDA Numbered Compounds Guide* (Wood Dale, Ill.: Seroyal, n.d.), 4–9.
8. M. Tetau, *Gemmotherapy: A Clinical Guide* (Paris: Editions du Detail, Inc., 1987), 9, 12–13.
9. Ibid., 9.
10. Ibid., 25.
11. Ibid.
12. D. Connelly, *Traditional Acupuncture: The Law of the Five Elements* (Columbia, Md.: Traditional Acupuncture Institute, 1994), 26, 41, 56, 67, 80.

PART TWO

DETOXIFICATION OF TOXIC METALS AND CHEMICALS

❧

Woo ah Mercy, mercy me
Ah, things ain't what they used to be.
No, no, where did all the blue skies go,
Poison is the wind that blows
from the north and south and east
Woo mercy, mercy me

Ah things ain't what they used to be, no, no
Oil wasted on the oceans and upon
Our seas, fish full of mercury, Ah. Oh

Ah things ain't what they used to be
What about this overcrowded land
How much more abuse from man can she stand?

Oh mercy, mercy me.
Ah things ain't what they used to be.
No, no, no, radiation underground and in the sky;
animals and birds who live nearby are dying oh,

Oh mercy, mercy me.
Ah things ain't what they used to be.
No, no, no, radiation underground and in the sky;
animals and land how much more abuse from man can she stand?

"MERCY MERCY ME (THE ECOLOGY),"
BY MARVIN GAYE*

As described in chapter 2, as drainage remedies help the body's tissues heal and excrete accumulated toxins, disturbing symptoms of detoxification often arise, including headaches, fatigue, and achy muscles and joints. Such symptoms are a normal manifestation of healing, and often they are mistaken for transient illnesses or "normal" emotional ups and downs. However, knowledgeable holistic practitioners—especially those who use energetic testing methods (see appendix 3)—can help patients determine when these symptoms signal something deeper: the presence of *xenobiotics*, or toxic metals or chemicals foreign to the body.

A healthy body will not tolerate xenobiotic poisons. As drainage initiates a more functional metabolism and improved excretion, the body starts to recognize and reject what is not "self," that is, any stores of these toxic metals and foreign chemicals. The symptoms of malaise

*Thanks to Dr. Alan Miller, who reintroduced me to this quite prophetic song, which was written over thirty years ago but, unfortunately, is still as relevant today as it was then. Words and music by Marvin Gaye, copyright 1971 (renewed 1999) Jobete Music Co., Inc. All rights controlled and administered by EMI April Music Inc. All rights reserved. International copyright secured. Used by permission.

that commonly result, sometimes referred to as a healing crisis, should be thought of, therefore, as a natural progression—*not* a regression—in an individual's health. They alert the body to the presence of these unwanted toxins.

Although the drainage remedies described in chapter 2 have a profound effect in helping to expel these toxins, no remedy can ever effect a complete cure in a body in which toxic metals have actually been *implanted*, as is the case with dental amalgam fillings. The same holds true for a body in which the toxic load of xenobiotics is continually *re-dosed*, as is the case for someone who uses petroleum-laden soaps and cosmetics every day.

Thus, often the initial—and certainly the most significant—detoxification treatment is the removal of toxic metals and chemicals from the body. Such treatment includes replacing dental mercury amalgam fillings and nickel- or palladium-gold crowns with less toxic alternatives, as well as exchanging conventional personal care and cleaning products for petroleum-free choices. Supplementation with antioxidants, algae, and other nutrients is also often required, as is an additional course of drainage remedies, to reduce the impact of removing these poisons from the body. When carefully selected and appropriately prescribed, these drainage and detoxification supplements can greatly mitigate the destruction xenobiotics wreak in the body's cells and tissues over time.

Chapter 3 describes the devastating effects of toxic metals in the body as well as treatments for the damage they cause, including removing the offending substances and appropriate supplements. Chapter 4 details the pandemic problem of toxic chemicals in everyday products and suggests alternative petroleum-free options, as well as an effective supplementation protocol to help repair the damage such toxins have in the body.*

*While metals are themselves chemical elements, their properties differ from those of petroleum-based chemical compounds. Therefore, the discussions of metals and chemicals are divided into separate chapters.

3

TOXIC METALS

The term *metal* derives from the Latin *metallum* and the Greek *metallon,* meaning "mine,"[1] suggestive of metals' origin in the earth. Metals can be classified into three major categories:

1. *Macrominerals.* These minerals, some of which are classified as metals, are essential to life and are present in relatively high quantities in the body and in our food. They include calcium, magnesium, and potassium.
2. *Microminerals.* These minerals, some of which are classified as metals, are also essential for life but are present in relatively small amounts in the body and in our food. They include copper, iron, zinc, and chromium.
3. *Toxic metals.* These metals are poisonous to the body and include mercury, lead, and cadmium.

A CLOSER LOOK AT MINERALS AND TOXIC METALS

Macrominerals

There are seven macrominerals in the body: calcium, chloride, magnesium, phosphorus, potassium, sodium, and sulfur. Of these seven, four are classified as metals: calcium, potassium, magnesium, and sodium.

Microminerals

There are fourteen primary microminerals, also known as trace minerals: chromium, cobalt, copper, fluoride, iodine, iron, manganese, molybdenum, nickel, selenium, silicon, tin, vanadium, and zinc. All but fluoride, iodine, selenium, and silicon are classified as metals. The body also contains trace amounts of aluminum, arsenic, barium, bismuth, bromine, cadmium, gallium, gold, silver, strontium, and other metals, but whether they are essential to the health of the body or simply toxic residues is still a debatable point among scientists and researchers.

Toxic Metals

The term *heavy metals* is often used as a synonym for *toxic metals*, but these two terms do not have exactly the same meaning. A toxic metal is any metal that poisons the body. A heavy metal is any metallic mineral with a specific gravity of five or more times that of water. As an example, aluminum in its acidic form (see page 77) is one of the most poisonous toxic metals, but it is not by definition a heavy metal because its specific gravity is 2.7. And heavy metals are not always toxic. For example, chromium, copper, iron, manganese, and zinc are heavy metals, but they are also microminerals necessary for the health of the body; they are toxic only if taken in the wrong form or in too high a concentration.

Toxic metals are the subject of this chapter. Mercury will be the primary focus due to the unconscionable use of this heavy metal in dental fillings. (Chapter 15 will cover the debilitating effects of the mercury-containing preservative used in vaccines called thimerosal.) We'll also investigate other toxic metals used in dentistry, such as so-called porcelain crowns, which contain high concentrations of aluminum, as well as gold crowns, which are often made up of a mixture of carcinogenic nickel and toxic palladium.

GOVERNMENT RESPONSE TO ENVIRONMENTAL TOXICITY

There is no longer any question that toxic metals in our air, water, soil, and food supply have a deleterious effect on our health and immune systems. In fact, in the late 1960s and early 1970s, when the words *ecology* and *environment* first began to become part of our everyday lexicon, the U.S. government instituted numerous pollution controls to limit citizens' exposure to toxic metals. Since then, air-polluting carbon monoxide and lead emissions from automobiles have been reduced by 80 percent.[2] Toxic industrial emissions have also greatly decreased.[3] Furthermore, in 1970 the government enacted the Occupational Safety and Health Act (OSHA) to help protect U.S. workers (particularly those who worked in industrial settings) from exposure to toxins in the workplace.[4] Other federal antipollution measures followed in great number.

ecology: Although it didn't become part of everyday speech until the late 1960s and early 1970s, the word *ecology* was first coined by Ernst Haeckel all the way back in 1866, in reference to Darwin's description of the mutual relations of organisms to their physical environment as well as to each other. (Theron Randolph, *Human Ecology and Susceptibility to the Chemical Environment* [Springfield, Ill.: Thomas, 1962], 5.)

Although Greenpeace, the Sierra Club, and other environmental groups would correctly argue that U.S. regulations and programs have been inadequate and implemented only after intense lobbying and political pressure, the government's vast response to environmental pollution measured simply in sheer numbers—agencies, employees, and funding—cannot be denied.

MERCURY AMALGAM FILLINGS

No Government Response to Dental Amalgam Toxicity

In *dramatic* contrast to the government's response to environmental pollution, however, is its extraordinary lack of response in regard to an even more insidious and quite personal toxic insult: the placement of mercury amalgam fillings directly in our mouths. Mercury amalgam fillings are approximately 50 percent mercury, a heavy metal that is second only to plutonium in its toxicity. These dental fillings are significantly more damaging to human health than mercury emissions in the environment. In fact, studies have found that the amount of mercury amalgam in our mouths—not mercury pollution of food, air, or water—is the most significant factor determining the level of mercury stored in our bodies.[5]

Approximately 85 percent of the U.S. population has received one or more of these mercury amalgam fillings.[6] In total, an estimated 144 million adult U.S. citizens, and 2 billion people worldwide, have mercury amalgam fillings.[7] Yet the government's silence on this subject—probably the greatest health controversy since thalidomide and DES*—continues to be deafening. Despite the glaring scientific evidence that has mounted over the past few decades as to the clearly poisonous nature of this toxic metal, the U.S. Food and Drug Administration (FDA) continued until recently to not categorize dental mercury as a classified medical device (as are, for example, elastic bandages and examination gloves).[8]

MERCURY AMALGAM AND THE FDA

After a ten-year legal battle waged by attorney Charles G. Brown (known to most as Charlie Brown) and holistic advocates, the FDA finally agreed in July 2009 to classify dental mercury amalgam as a class II device, meaning that it would not require proof of safety but would be subject to certain controls. Although this was indeed a victory, consumer activists and holistic dentists and physicians contend that mercury amalgam should actually be classified as a class III device—that is, a potentially dangerous device that would need to be proven safe to be sold and used in dentistry. Since scientific research has incontrovertibly proven that mercury amalgam fillings are not safe, classifying them as a class III device would lead to these toxic fillings being banned in dentistry.[9]

*Thalidomide, a prescription drug commonly used in England and Germany in the 1950s and 1960s as a sedative, hypnotic, and pain reliever, was pulled off the market in 1962 because it causes severe birth defects in infants born to mothers who use it during pregnancy. DES (diethylstilbestrol), a synthetic estrogen formerly prescribed to prevent miscarriage and premature labor, was banned in the United States in 1971 after many daughters of women who had taken it during pregnancy later developed vaginal cancer.

ADA Says That Mercury Amalgam Is Safe

The American Dental Association (ADA), a trade organization composed primarily of nonholistic dentists, has continued to deny that mercury amalgam is harmful.[10] In fact, the ADA (and ADA-influenced state dental boards) considers replacing amalgam fillings out of concern about mercury toxicity "unethical"—a fact well known by hundreds of holistic dentists who have been harassed, been taken to court, and even lost their license because of this practice.[11] This pro-amalgam position was well exemplified in a 1998 report by the ADA's Council on Scientific Affairs:

> The Council concludes that, based on available scientific information, amalgam continues to be a safe and effective restorative material. . . . There currently appears to be no justification for discontinuing the use of dental amalgam.[12]

On the other hand, the ADA has been very careful to extricate itself from any potential for liability, demonstrated in the following quote from a tort liability suit argued in Santa Clara County in October 1992:

> The ADA owes no legal duty of care to protect the public from allegedly dangerous products used by dentists. The ADA did not manufacture, design, supply, or install the mercury-containing amalgams.[13]

Nonetheless, the ADA continues to assert its pro-amalgam position, as anyone who visits its website (www.ADA.org) can ascertain:

> Dental amalgam is considered a safe, affordable, and durable material that has been used to restore the teeth of more than 100 million Americans.[14]

Why do the ADA, the FDA, and amalgam manufacturers continue to deny the toxic effects of mercury fillings? At this point, they probably fear class action lawsuits, much like what happened to the tobacco companies. Amalgam-based lawsuits, however, have already been initiated in Canada and in several states in the United States.[15] In fact, many holistic practitioners believe that only through the courts will a ban on mercury amalgam finally be enacted. Although the ADA has been trying for years to sidestep its untenable position by suggesting the alternative use of white fillings (plastic composite and glass ceramic) *simply* because they are more pleasing cosmetically, this stance is probably not sufficient to stem the tide of future lawsuits. It seems that in our sadly failing system of irresponsible capitalism-at-any-cost, only the threat of litigation and political pressure—and not ethics or consciousness—can really drive the system to eventually institute needed reforms.

Fortunately, in June 2008 the Consumers for Dental Choice (CDC), tirelessly led by attorney Charlie Brown, won an important lawsuit against the FDA and its thirty-year policy of protecting mercury amalgam fillings. Based on this legal settlement, the FDA changed its website in June 2008 from supporting the use of amalgams to now warning about the potential toxicity of mercury fillings for children, pregnant women, nursing mothers, and heavily mercury-burdened individuals. The ADA was understandably stung by the FDA's new stance and continues to advocate the safety of mercury amalgam fillings, despite overwhelming scientific evidence to the contrary.

- ▶ To read more about the ADA's continued defensive stance regarding mercury amalgam fillings and the FDA's changing stance, visit the Consumers for Dental Choice website at www.toxicteeth.org.

THE SUPPRESSION OF THE TRUTH

The holistic dentist who strongly suspects mercury (or nickel, palladium, or any other toxic metal) as the primary cause of a patient's symptoms risks losing his or her license in vocalizing this diagnosis in the face of the ADA's position on the "safety" of amalgam fillings.[16] This prevailing false dogma even forces a doctor or dentist to hesitate about—or even decide against—telling a patient the diagnosis. Most strikingly and sadly paradoxically, the most intimidating and hostile government in the world to holistic intervention and honest communication about the toxicity of mercury amalgam is that of the United States—the land of the free and the First Amendment. Fortunately, though, more and more holistic dentists as well as physicians have been speaking out about this subject over the past few decades, as the evidence mounts—through research published in peer-reviewed journals—that mercury amalgam fillings are incontrovertibly poisonous and damaging to every part of the human body.

European Countries and Canada Are More Progressive

Sweden, Norway, Germany, Austria, France, Belgium, and England have all instituted various curbs on dental amalgam, from banning the transport of hazardous liquid mercury (in France) to disallowing any coverage for amalgam fillings through state-run health insurance.[17] Sweden attempted to ban the use of mercury amalgam fillings by 1997 after research showed that the fillings were linked to immune system and other health disorders. However, after pressure from the Swedish dental establishment, the government softened its stance and presently limits the use of mercury amalgam for environmental concerns.[18] In Norway, 90 percent of the fillings done over the past few years have been mercury-free alternatives;[19] in fact, in January 2008, Norway became the first nation to legislate an outright ban on the use of amalgam fillings in dental work. Norway's minister of environment and development stated, "Mercury is among the most dangerous environmental toxins. Satisfactory alternatives to mercury in products are available, and it is therefore fitting to introduce a ban."[20] And in none of these European countries can mercury amalgams be placed in children, pregnant women, or people with kidney problems.[21] Similarly, in North America Canada bans the use of mercury fillings in pregnant women and children under the age of seven.[22]

In contrast, despite the efforts of two courageous U.S. representatives, Congressman Dan Burton of Indiana and Congresswoman Diane Watson of California, the United States has enacted no laws in regard to informed consent for or restricting the use of mercury amalgams. Although in each session over the past few years, Burton and Watson have introduced a bill that would ban the placement of amalgam fillings in pregnant women and in children under the age of eighteen and that also would require a warning to all consumers that amalgam fillings contain approximately 50 percent mercury, "a highly toxic element," this bill has still not received its first hearing.

HALF OF U.S. DENTISTS CHOOSE NOT TO USE MERCURY AMALGAM

Although the FDA continues to allow unregulated use of mercury amalgam in the military and other institutions, a national dental poll recently found that over 50 percent of dentists are mercury-free. Although the majority don't advertise themselves as "holistic," the damning findings on the toxicity of mercury amalgam fillings are so clear that over half of U.S. dentists have wisely decided to stop using this dangerous, archaic, and controversial filling material.

Informed Consent Law Enacted in California

A few progressive states such as California have passed "informed consent" laws to warn patients about the toxicity of mercury amalgam fillings. In December 1993, the California Environmental Law Foundation was one of the first to successfully sue amalgam companies for failing to warn dental patients of the dangers of amalgam fillings.[23] Subsequently, Jeneric Pentron, one of the nation's largest amalgam manufacturers and the first to comply among almost three dozen other amalgam-producing companies, began to provide warning signs that were to be prominently displayed in dentists' offices. Unfortunately, a federal court later overturned the ruling, not because the ruling wasn't valid, but because federal guidelines supersede state law, and since the FDA does not require such a warning, a state cannot make the warning mandatory.[24] Nevertheless, amalgam manufacturers now include warnings and contraindications to the use of amalgam in their "Directions for Use" inserts.[25] Regrettably, patients never see this information.

Fortunately, a later victory for opponents to the use of mercury in dentistry occurred in 2003, when the final language for warnings on dental amalgams was approved by the San Francisco Superior Court:

> Dental amalgam, used in many dental fillings, causes exposure to mercury, a chemical known to the state of California to cause birth defects or other reproductive harm. Root canal treatments and restorations including fillings, crowns, and bridges use chemicals known to the state of California to cause cancer. The U.S.

Food and Drug Administration has studied the situation and approved for use all dental restorative materials. Consult your dentist to determine which materials are appropriate for your treatment.[26]

California's Proposition 65, the Safe Drinking Water and Toxic Enforcement Act, now mandates that dental offices with more than nine employees must give patients this warning and receive their informed consent before giving them amalgam fillings. And though it applies only to larger dental offices, this precedent-setting informed consent law is having an effect on smaller dental practices throughout the state as well, many of which voluntarily follow its guidelines.[27]

Old News for Holistic Patients

The practice of removing amalgam fillings is so widespread in holistic circles that it has almost become cliché. In fact, in many holistic practitioners' offices nowadays, a majority of patients who present for their initial history and exam have already replaced their mercury fillings and done a certain amount of mercury detoxification. However, the vast majority of these individuals still feel that mercury has not been completely cleared from their system, and physical exam, laboratory work, and energetic testing often prove them right. The information in this chapter will hopefully prove valuable not only for those individuals who still have mercury amalgam fillings but also for those who have replaced their fillings with nontoxic alternatives but still haven't adequately detoxified their bodies from this most insidious poison.

FACTS ABOUT MERCURY AMALGAM FILLINGS

The "Silver Filling"

Using the popular term *silver filling* to describe dental amalgam not only is confusing and misleading to the consumer but borders on malpractice. Dr. Hal Huggins, a pioneering U.S. dentist who has worked to expose the toxicity of mercury in dental amalgam fillings, has referred to this euphemistic terminology as "uninformed consent."[28] In fact, silver makes up only approximately 35 percent of the filling. Mercury itself is the major component, ranging from 49 to 54 percent of the amalgam filling.[29] The rest of the amalgam is made up of tin at approximately 12 percent, copper at 0.5 to 3 percent, and zinc at around 1 percent.[30]

Amalgam *Means Mixture*

The term *amalgam* derives from the Greek word *malagma*, meaning "soft mass," and is used to define any mixture or alloy of two or more metals. In the past, dentists used an extremely toxic "wet" method of preparing the dental amalgam, manually mixing in their offices one part of a metallic powder composed of silver, tin, copper, and zinc with one part of liquid mercury. Fortunately, nonholistic dentists and their assistants currently use a less hazardous (but still quite toxic) "dry" or "no-touch" form of amalgam prepackaged in capsules.

THE HISTORY OF MERCURY USE IN DENTISTRY

The use of mercury mixed or "amalgamated" with silver and other metals in dental fillings originated with the English chemist Benjamin Bell around 1819. Several years later, in 1826, a French dentist named Auguste Traveau began using mercury amalgam fillings,[31] and in 1835, Edward and Moses Crawcour, two entrepreneurs with no professional training, brought mercury amalgam to the United States and advertised it widely as a cheap new filling.[32] Reputable dentists were so enraged by the use of this toxic metal that in 1840 they banded together and formed the first organization of dentists in the United States, the American Society of Dental Surgeons. This professional organization considered the use of mercury amalgam fillings to be malpractice, and their use could result in automatic expulsion from the society.[33]

ADA Amalgam-Using Dentists Referred to as "Quacks"

Despite disapproval from professionals, the use of mercury amalgam continued to grow, for both economic and technical reasons. For one, in the nineteenth century the main dental filling material was gold, which was quite expensive and required considerable skill to use. Mercury amalgam, on the other hand, was cheap and could be used without much training or expertise, as it molded easily into a cavity and hardened quickly. Over time, dentists who were attracted to using the easier-to-place amalgam quit the American Society of Dental Surgeons, and in 1859 a group of them formed the American Dental Association (ADA). (As described earlier in this chapter, the ADA has maintained to this day that mercury amalgams are safe.) Incensed, dentists in the American Society of Dental Surgeons began to refer to these ADA amalgam-using dentists as *quacks,* from the German word *quecksilber,* or *quicksilver,* which is another name for mercury.[34]* (Ironically, the term *quack* today is often used by conventional mercury-amalgam-using dentists to slander their holistic, nontoxic-alternative-using colleagues, as well as by allopathic physicians to denigrate holistic practitioners.)

Research Capabilities Were Limited

How could ADA dentists utilize amalgam as a filling material when the toxicity of mercury was generally well known at the time? For one thing, research capacities in the nineteenth and early twentieth centuries were still quite primitive.[35] Therefore, the initial harmful effects of mercury in the human body—much less the long-term effects—could not be easily identified or propagated through published research studies. And although in the 1920s and 1930s scientists in Germany—notably the great chemist Alfred Stock, who actually sacrificed his life studying the toxic effects of mercury—began reporting that amalgam fillings were indeed quite harmful, the anti-German sentiment growing prior to World War II caused many American dentists and scientists to dismiss this mounting evidence.[36]

The Mid-Twentieth-Century "Golden Age of Dentistry"

During World War II, the use of amalgam fillings boomed. Many GIs' teeth were in bad condition, most often because of dietary deficiencies (this was, after all, just after the Great Depression), the rise of modern toxic commercial foods such as hydrogenated margarine and refined sugar (see chapter 5), or simply a lack of money for dental care. Because it was affordable and easy to use, amalgam seemed the perfect choice for dental fillings in the cost-cutting military. As soon as they were drafted or enlisted, as well as throughout their military career, millions of U.S. servicemen and women received mercury amalgam fillings from military dentists. This mercury amalgam boom, along with the now common use of novocaine to control pain, led to what has been called the "golden age of dentistry" from the late 1940s to the late 1960s.[37] Lamentably for the consumer, the "golden" aspect referred not to the dental material used, but to the fact that the demand for dental services exceeded the supply. As a result, without much effort (or skill in some cases), more and more dentists were trained in the quicker, easier, and financially lucrative placement of mercury amalgam fillings.

Unfortunately, those of us born during this period, known as the baby-boom generation, were the primary youthful recipients of the brunt of this blatantly toxic yet popular practice. Making matters worse, the now controversial Dr. Spock even recommended in his *Baby and Child Care* book that cavities should begin to be filled as early as age three—an age when immature immune systems are particularly susceptible to the damaging effects of mercury.[38]

The Copper Amalgam

Another type of mercury amalgam known as the copper amalgam, consisting of 66 percent mercury and a whopping 33 percent copper, is particularly toxic due to its extremely unstable galvanic nature and was widely denounced as early as the 1920s.[39] In spite of this, copper amalgams were very popular in pediatric dentistry and were placed in children's teeth until the late 1960s in Sweden and through the 1980s in the United States.[40] Even more astonishing, the copper amalgam has recently received the approval of a CE marking—the form of certification used by the European Union to signify that a product has been approved for sale in all the European Union countries, similar to FDA approval in the United States.

Dr. Hal Huggins has monitored more than 1,000 multiple sclerosis patients and found that mercury amalgams, and *particularly* high-copper amalgams, are instrumental in the causation of this neurological disease. Through his years of research, Dr. Huggins has found that the high-copper amalgam filling releases *fifty times* more mercury than regular amalgam fillings.[41]

---

*Aristotle was the first to call mercury "quicksilver" or "living silver." In fact, the scientific symbol for mercury, Hg, stands for the Greek word *hydrargyrum,* meaning "water silver."

MERCURY LEACHES INTO THE BODY

In no way is mercury "locked into" the amalgam filling, as the ADA and many nonholistic dentists have claimed. Even the National Institutes of Dental Research (and, at times, the ADA) has publicly acknowledged this fact. Mercury *readily* escapes from amalgam fillings in the form of vapor created by chewing, brushing the teeth, or grinding the teeth.[42] This vapor, made up of metallic or elemental mercury, is absorbed into the lungs when a person breathes through the mouth and into the brain when a person breathes through the nose. Some mercury is also dissolved in the saliva in the mouth and swallowed into the gastrointestinal tract.

The Lungs' Pathway to the Body

Approximately 80 percent of the metallic mercury released by amalgam fillings is absorbed into the lungs when a person breathes through the mouth. It then diffuses rapidly across the alveolar membranes into the rest of the body. In comparison to other forms of mercury, such as those ingested through eating fish, metallic mercury is lipid soluble and freely passes through cell membranes. Once within the cell, metallic mercury is oxidized by the catalase enzyme into the highly reactive inorganic or ionic mercury. This inorganic mercury binds to sulfur-containing enzymes in the cell, thereby inactivating their cellular function and causing "cellular suffocation": blocking intracellular respiration, obstructing the cell's ability to scavenge harmful free radicals, and impairing important detoxification pathways. Once bound, mercury leaves the cell, circulates in the blood or lymph, and is deposited in an organ or tissue.[43]

The Nasal Pathway to the Brain

When a person breathes through the nose, mercury vapor from amalgam fillings passes through the two nasal cavities and travels directly into the brain and spinal cord. Through his brilliant and innovative research, Alfred Stock found that because of this direct route to the brain, nose-breathing of mercury vapor is ten times more toxic than mouth-breathing.[44]* In addition, the metallic mercury absorbed into the brain from the upper nasal cavity is in a significantly stronger concentration than that which the body receives through mouth-breathing, since it has completely bypassed the general blood circulation and its various detoxifying processes.

*The same is true for other toxic vapors. Thus, in a toxic environment—for example, a room with a new carpet or new paint—breathe through your mouth rather than your nose, and exit as soon as possible.

The Saliva Pathway to the Gut

One to two liters of saliva is secreted into the mouth every day, where it moistens the mucous membranes and rinses the teeth before being swallowed.[45] In addition to amylase, the enzyme that is best known of its components, saliva contains sodium and chloride, or salt, as well as potassium and bicarbonate ions. The sodium, chloride, potassium, and bicarbonate ions act as electrolytes, and when saliva washes over amalgam fillings, electrolytic action corrodes the amalgam, increasing the release of mercury.[46]*

The instability of mercury in amalgam fillings in the presence of saliva is not a new discovery but was documented as far back as 1878 by Dr. H. S. Chase. Chase found that mercury amalgam fillings act like miniature batteries in the mouth not only because they are made up of five different metals (causing galvanic corrosion; see page 63), but because the electrolytes in saliva have current-generating properties. In his research, Chase proved that this low-level but ongoing electrical current corrodes the metals in the filling, causing metallic mercury to be continuously leached from the amalgam filling.[47]

After dissolving in saliva and being swallowed, mercury travels along with food through the esophagus and down to the stomach and small intestine. From there, the digestive system passes nutrients from the food into the liver through the blood (portal veins), and the rest passes into the large intestine and is excreted through the feces. However, due to mercury's enervating effects on the digestive tract, as well as most individuals' limited ability for effective digestion and excretion as a result of antibiotic use and an unhealthy diet, much of this mer-

*Ions are atoms that have a positive or negative charge due to the loss or gain of one or more electrons. Ions can be dissolved in solution and are then referred to as electrolytes. Electrolyte solutions are capable of conducting electricity. Examples of ions are the hydroxyl ion (OH-), the hydrogen ion (H+), and the potassium ion (K+). The primary ions of electrolyte solutions in the body are sodium, potassium, calcium, magnesium, chloride, phosphate, and bicarbonate.

cury ends up stored in the stomach, intestines, and liver. In fact, one study found that approximately 80 percent of the body burden of mercury is stored in the gut (small and large intestines).[48]

The Neural, Venous, and Pharyngeal Pathways to the Brain

In addition to the nasal pathway, metallic mercury can enter the brain via two other pathways: by axonal transport (passage along a nerve fiber) and by venous circulation (passage through blood vessels). As we'll discuss later in this chapter (see pages 67–68), studies have shown that mercury can travel from the mouth through cranial veins or along the trigeminal nerve to the primary hormone-regulating centers of the brain—the hypothalamus and the pituitary gland. This direct passage to these important hormonal glands is well illustrated through autopsy studies that have found that the pituitary gland can contain *twenty* times more mercury than the neighboring cerebral cortex tissue.[49]

Another possible transit route for metallic mercury to enter the pituitary is through the pharynx (the upper soft palate in the very back of the throat). In a human embryo, the anterior pituitary develops from a pouch (Rathke's pouch) in the upper palate. After birth, a vestigial portion of the pituitary remains in the pharynx, termed the *pharyngeal pituitary.* It is very possible that metallic mercury from amalgam fillings diffuses directly through this pharyngeal pituitary tissue into the pituitary in the brain.

METHYLATION
How Toxic Mercury Becomes Even More Toxic in the Mouth

In the presence of bacteria, metallic or inorganic mercury is *methylated*—that is, it receives a methyl group and is chemically changed into a new compound, called *organic mercury* or *methylmercury.* Unfortunately for the individual with a mouthful of amalgam fillings, numerous studies have found that methylmercury is ten times more toxic, and hence exceedingly more difficult to detoxify in the body, than the original inorganic mercury.[50] Since dysbiosis, or the existence of pathogenic bacteria in the intestine, is pandemic nowadays, it is not hard to understand why this more toxic form of mercury is so widespread. Often, however, mercury arrives in the gut already methylated, having been exposed in the mouth to bacteria-laden dental focal infections (chronic abscesses and failed root canals), gingivitis, periodontitis,* and tooth decay—or even the various nonpathogenic bacteria that normally reside in the mouth.[51] (See chapter 7 for more on dysbiosis and chapter 11 for more on dental focal infections.) In fact, bacteria in the mouth, gut, or anywhere else in the body where mercury has metastasized greatly potentiate the toxicity of this metal by converting it to the more pathogenic compound of methylmercury.

FACTORS THAT AUGMENT MERCURY RELEASE
From Galvanism to Gum-Chewing

Dental Galvanism

Dorland's Medical Dictionary defines the term *dental galvanism* as "a physicochemical phenomenon in which two or more dissimilar metals that have been used to restore or replace missing teeth produce the flow of an electric current."[52] This electrical current occurs between dental restorations—fillings, inlays, onlays, or crowns—that contain dissimilar metals. Most commonly, dental galvanism occurs between a gold crown and a mercury filling or an aluminum-containing porcelain crown. A galvanic current can also exist within a single tooth containing dissimilar metals, such as an amalgam filling that has five different metals in it, or a gold crown placed on top of an amalgam filling.

Dental galvanism is not a new phenomenon. In fact, every standard dental textbook states that mercury amalgam fillings can generate electricity in the mouth and are therefore unstable.[53] Despite this, dental-school professors still train students to use mercury amalgam fillings, and new dental graduates overwhelmingly use them in their practices—and many continue to use

---

*Gingivitis is simply inflammation of the gums, whereas periodontitis, or periodontal disease, is a collective term describing inflammation and degeneration of the gingivae (the gums), alveoli (the sockets in the jaw where the teeth insert), periodontal ligament (the ligament attaching teeth to the jaw), and cementum (the bonelike connective tissue that covers the root of a tooth).

them throughout their career. (Only approximately 15 percent of U.S. dentists are currently not using mercury amalgam.[54] However, as research proving the toxicity of mercury amalgam becomes more widespread, more dentists—although they may not advertise themselves as holistic—are choosing less toxic alternatives for their patients.) Additionally, dental schools give very little to no training on the inadvisability of placing restorations of dissimilar metals near each other, such as a gold crown next to an amalgam filling.

Galvanic Corrosion Increases Mercury Off-Gassing

Mercury amalgam fillings are made up of mercury, silver, copper, tin, and zinc; with all these dissimilar metals, even a single filling can create an electric current in the mouth. This dental galvanism, or *electrogalvanism,* of an amalgam filling was proven to off-gas mercury in a 1994 study conducted by Professor James Masi of the University of Southern Maine. Dr. Masi found that electrogalvanism causes corrosion of amalgam, resulting in some degree of micro-cracking in the material—regardless of the age of the filling—that allows mercury to readily migrate out into the mouth and the rest of the body.[55]

Gold and Mercury Produce "Dental Batteries"

Electrogalvanism is dramatically increased when gold, nickel, palladium, aluminum, and other metal fillings, inlays, onlays, crowns, or bridges are placed near an amalgam filling. Gold in particular, having a high positive charge, greatly augments the rate of corrosion of the negatively charged mercury in amalgam fillings, and thus it especially potentiates the release of this toxic metal into the body.[56] When mercury amalgam makes contact with gold in the mouth, they form a galvanic cell or "dental battery," with the mercury functioning as an anode and the gold as a cathode, and current running between them. The *anodic corrosion* of mercury resulting from its interaction with gold in a galvanic cell has been measured at ten to twenty times higher than corrosion in the amalgam filling alone. Furthermore, the galvanic currents from these gold-mercury dental batteries have been reported at a hundred to several hundred millivolts, and sometimes even exceeding a thousand millivolts.[57]

corrosion: *Corrosion* derives from the Latin root *rodere,* meaning "to gnaw" like a rodent. In the case of a gold crown on top of or next to an amalgam filling, *anodic corrosion* occurs when the gold "gnaws away" at the mercury.

Often No Obvious Symptoms in the Tooth or Body

Surprisingly, these strong electrical currents in the mouth are often completely asymptomatic (causing no pain) or relatively asymptomatic (causing, as an example, only mild irritation in the tooth or gums). Sometimes, however, they are quite painful; the *galvanic pain,* as it's called in the dental profession, can be felt in the tooth itself and in surrounding tissues.[58] Unfortunately, many dentists misdiagnose galvanic pain and refer patients to endodontists for a root canal, thus destroying a healthy tooth that simply needed a new nonmetallic restoration.

These dental batteries can also produce pain elsewhere in the body. In these cases, the gold crown or amalgam filling is referred to as a *dominant focus,* and the painful or otherwise disturbed area in the body that results from the dental galvanism is referred to as a *disturbed field.* A dental focus and disturbed field can be identified through a patient's history (When did you receive the gold crown, and when did the pain first begin?), as well as through energetic testing methods such as kinesiology and arm length testing (Matrix Reflex Testing). When the amalgam filling or gold crown is replaced with a less toxic alternative, a decrease in symptoms and negative energetic testing often substantiate the enormity of the effects of the dental galvanism. (For a more in-depth discussion of dental foci, see chapter 11.)

A Major Cause of Nervous Disorders

When we compare the artificially induced galvanic currents in the mouth with the electrical currents naturally produced in the human body, it becomes clear that the allopathic (nonholistic) dental profession could be contributing to the plethora of mental, nervous, and hypersensitivity symptoms that exist today. To illustrate this connection, it's helpful to look at a few examples. Brain waves range between 50 and 100 microvolts (a microvolt is 0.001 of a millivolt), and the heartbeat averages 300 microvolts.[59] Nerve transmissions are around 60 millivolts or less, and cell membranes have a potential energy ranging from 90 to 100 millivolts. In contrast, galvanic currents in a mixed-metal mouth can range from 100 to 1,000 millivolts, far outpowering the normal physiological currents. This dental galvanism, as well as the increased levels of mercury and other toxic metals that result from the constant galvanic corrosion, could be linked to chronic irritability, anxiety, agitation, and other nervous and emotional symptoms. In fact, the consensus among leading holistic dentists is that the sickest patients they see are usually the ones who have or had mixed metals in their mouths.[60]

"Astronomical" Amounts of Mercury Released

To find out just how strong the mercury-releasing effects of dental galvanism can be, Austrian researchers examined a patient's tooth containing a twenty-five-year-old amalgam filling covered with a gold crown. Using atomic absorption spectrometry, they measured the mercury content in the root of that tooth and found it to be 1,200 parts per million (ppm)—that is, 1,200 micrograms of mercury per gram of dental tissue.[61] In their published results, these researchers point out that even 50 ppm of mercury measured in a hair is strong enough to cause toxic symptoms, whereas 1,200 ppm, especially in the root of a tooth, where it can be transported to all parts of the body through the blood, is an *astronomical* amount.

Nickel, Aluminum, and Other Toxic Metals Also Induce Oral Galvanism

Unfortunately, despite this and other published studies, the placement of a gold crown next to or opposing a tooth with an amalgam filling, or on top of a tooth without thoroughly removing the mercury filling underneath, is still quite common even today.* And although these gold-amalgam pairings are the most typical galvanic cells, galvanic corrosion also occurs between other metals used for dental restoration, such as the aluminum in porcelain crowns or the nickel used in stainless-steel braces.[62] In fact, when children with preexisting amalgam fillings receive nickel-containing braces, Dr. Hal Huggins warns their parents to be on the lookout for personality changes in them within even just a few days, due to the increased electrical and toxic load in their mouth.[63]

Stimulation and Temperature

Chewing

In the 1980s, researchers clearly established that the rate of mercury release from amalgam fillings is dramatically increased during and after chewing.[64] M. Vimy and F. Lorscheider, two cutting-edge Canadian researchers on amalgam safety, found that eating three meals a day released enough mercury from amalgam fillings to give subjects an average dose of 20 micrograms of this toxic metal. They concluded that the doses released from amalgams were as much as eighteen times the allowable daily limit established by some countries for mercury exposure from all sources in the environment.[65]

A German study measuring the mercury content in saliva of 430 subjects after they had chewed sugar-free gum found the following:

1. Subjects with amalgam fillings had a significant elevation in the mercury content of their saliva during chewing. In fact, the mercury level of their saliva exceeded the World Health Organization's limit for drinking water by more than a thousand (ug/L).
2. Subjects who had undergone amalgam replacement had significantly lower mercury levels during chewing than subjects who still had amalgams, but these figures were still seven times higher than the levels of those who had never had any amalgam fillings (indicating possible mercury stores still in the gums and jawbone).[66]

A classic kinesiology test for mercury toxicity is to have patients with amalgam fillings chew gum for a few seconds. The resulting release of mercury invariably elicits an autonomic muscle weakening response (in which a previously strong indicator muscle goes weak) with typical therapy localizations positive over the frontal

*For patients with financial constraints, well-meaning dentists sometimes replace mixed-metal amalgams over time. However, a replacement gold crown next to or opposing mercury amalgam can create strong galvanic currents that are even more harmful than the original mouthful of amalgams, especially when the two are allowed to coexist in the mouth for years. It is better for patients to save up the money, or for the dentist to extend credit, so that the mercury amalgam fillings can be replaced expeditiously, typically at a pace of one quadrant a month. (See "Detoxification from Mercury," beginning on page 87, for more information.)

cortex, sinuses, tonsils, liver, and various cranial ganglia. Analogous to the German study, even patients who have had amalgam fillings removed and have detoxified considerably can sometimes elicit positive mercury tests in these areas by chewing gum.

Tooth Brushing, Smoking, Hot Drinks, Bruxism, Acids, and EMFs

The rate of mercury release is significantly increased after tooth brushing, smoking, or drinking hot fluids (elevating the air temperature in the mouth intensifies mercury vaporization), bruxism (grinding the teeth), ingesting weak acids (such as vinegar or citrus), sitting in front of a computer's electromagnetic field or using a cell phone, and working under fluorescent lights.[67]*

Dental Cleanings

Quite understandably, since all forms of stimulation in the mouth increase the rate of mercury release from amalgam fillings, a teeth cleaning at a dentist's office, which causes very strong vibrations in the mouth, can be one of the most serious offenders. Many patients with amalgam fillings report that they feel unwell after this presumably healthy procedure, and scientific studies have shown that teeth cleanings release dangerously high levels of mercury vapor.[68] Patients with amalgams, therefore, would be well advised to delay teeth cleanings if possible until after their amalgams have been replaced, or at least not to have their amalgam surfaces polished during this annual or semiannual procedure.

MERCURY CONTINUOUSLY LEACHES OUT OF EVEN "OLDER" AMALGAM FILLINGS

Most allopathic dentists contend that older amalgam fillings no longer leak significant amounts of mercury. But anyone can see that "all mercury/silver fillings leak out substantial amounts of mercury constantly" simply by viewing *Smoking Tooth,* an excellent 8½-minute video (found on the website of the International Academy of Oral Medicine and Toxicology) that shows mercury vapor leaking from a twenty-five-year-old amalgam filling.[69] In fact, not only do older amalgams leak mercury vapor continuously, but that vapor contains 1,000 times more mercury than the EPA allows in the air we breathe.[70] These "toxic time-bombs," as Sam Ziff, a leading dental researcher, characterized them, should be carefully removed by a knowledgeable holistic dentist or physician who has determined that the patient is healthy enough to effectively detoxify afterward.

It is also important to keep in mind that the continued presence of amalgam fillings disallows the release of mercury from the rest of the body. The fillings in the mouth resonate energetically with stores of mercury in the cells and tissues, maintaining a perpetual chronic toxic equilibrium level throughout the body. Thus, even patients with just one or two amalgam fillings will never enjoy the level of health that they potentially could with a mercury-free mouth. As these cases illustrate, mercury amalgam fillings are one of our most significant modern-day obstacles to cure.

*Although no study has yet been done, for individuals with amalgam fillings, surely those with temporomandibular disorders, malocclusions (bad bites), and/or traumatic bites (teeth don't fit together well) have more mercury chronically released than those with normal occlusions (see chapter 16).

MERCURY DEPOSITS IN THE BODY

It has been said that the placement of even just one amalgam filling leads to mercury "micrometastasis" to every cell in the body.[71] Over the past few decades, various animal and human studies have proved that mercury released from amalgam fillings has a particular affinity for several specific organs and tissues. These include the brain and central nervous system, spinal ganglia, kidneys, liver, gastrointestinal tract, adrenals, lungs, and jawbone.[72] However, the brain—as the mercury-poisoned Mad Hatter in *Alice in Wonderland* so dramatically illustrates—is by far the primary target organ.

Mercury Deposits Primarily in the Brain

The neurotoxic effects of mercury are lethal to brain tissue, as the video *How Mercury Causes Brain Neuron Degeneration* (on the International Academy of Oral Medicine and Toxicology website) graphically depicts. In this video documentation of Dr. Fritz Lorscheider's research from the University of Calgary in Canada, even a small amount of mercury—comparable to the amount leaching from amalgam fillings—strips the sheathing (covering) from nerves within minutes and causes the formation of the neurofibrillary tangles that typically occur in the neurodegenerative disease Alzheimer's.[73] Mercury is deposited in the brain through three primary routes: the bloodstream (through failure of the blood-brain barrier and via the valveless cranial veins), transport along nerves, and direct inhalation through the nose.

Failure of the Blood-Brain Barrier

As discussed earlier in this chapter, when mercury is inhaled into the lungs, it can pass into the blood and circulate to every organ in the body. Through the cerebral arteries, mercury and other toxic substances are able to pass directly into the brain cells.[74] Normally the tightly packed capillaries in the brain form a barrier, known as the *blood-brain barrier*, to guard against the passage of toxic materials into brain tissue. However, the blood-brain barrier can be bypassed after trauma and in cases of acute or chronic inflammation.[75] Additionally, the blood-brain barrier is much less effective in the hypothalamus region, which communicates directly with the pituitary gland—a region where many postmortem studies have found the highest amounts of mercury deposition. And not surprisingly, the population with the highest postmortem content of mercury in their pituitary gland is dentists.[76]

> **blood-brain barrier:** The term *blood-brain barrier* describes the normally protective effect of capillaries in the brain, which are more tightly packed than capillaries in the body and are surrounded by large numbers of neuroglial cells (brain cells). This more dense anatomical arrangement forms a barrier to the passage of certain materials. In a healthy person (whose body does not contain amalgams, petroleum chemicals, toxic foci, et cetera), glucose, oxygen, and certain ions (e.g., potassium, sodium, and magnesium) pass through the blood into the brain, but proteins and *most* antibiotics do not.

Although the brain makes up only about 2 percent of the body's total weight, it utilizes approximately 20 percent of the oxygen the body as a whole needs, making it the most metabolically active organ in the body. However, a brain with a high concentration of mercury rarely receives this high level of oxygen. Thus, mercury amalgam fillings are one of the major causes of brain fatigue and memory loss, both common complaints nowadays. This fact is not anecdotal but has been proven and published in numerous peer-reviewed scientific journals. Such reports have linked Alzheimer's *incontrovertibly* to mercury toxicity.[77] (We'll discuss this subject at length in "Mercury-Related Diseases," beginning on page 72.)

The Valveless Cranial Veins

The cranial venous system has a unique feature: it has no valves. Many veins in the body, especially those in the limbs, contain valves that prevent the backflow of blood. In the cranium, valves are not possible due to the need to maintain intra-cranial pressure at every moment. Forceful acts such as sneezing, crying passionately, or running short sprints, for example, force a tremendous amount of arterial blood through the carotid arteries into the brain. If the cranial veins had valves, these normal actions could build up excessive pressure and potentially cause a stroke.

Because it lacks valves, the cranial venous system presents a much more open pathway than the rest of the body's veins for the transport of mercury from the jaws and teeth, as well as for the transport of oral microbial toxins such as pathogenic bacteria. Störtebecker, the brilliant Swedish doctor who dedicated much of his life to the research of mercury toxicity, asserted that this free flow of mercury and microbes was a major contributor to the development of multiple sclerosis (MS) and other neurological diseases such as epilepsy and schizophrenia, as well as brain cancer. He based this belief on two research findings. First, radiographic cranial contrast studies* demonstrated this direct venous access to the brain for mercury in the teeth and jaws. Second, postmortem studies of MS patients revealed that the cranial and spinal plaques (sclerosed or scarred tissue) that characterize this disease were always located around the walls of the veins. Dr. Störtebecker noted that these veins were always surrounded at least initially by white blood cells, indicating an inflammatory process resulting from infection (caused by bacteria transported from the mouth), and "enhanced" by the co-transport of mercury and other toxic metals.[78]

*Contrast studies involve injecting some type of radiopaque substance, such as barium, into the veins of the face and brain so that they can be visualized more clearly on an X-ray. Störtebecker conducted these radiographic studies on postmortem human skulls, with the contrast dye injected directly into the teeth and jaws.

As discussed earlier in this chapter, microbial action in the case of abscessed or even just inflamed teeth and gums converts metallic mercury to methylmercury, which is from ten to one hundred times more toxic than metallic mercury and one of the most poisonous substances known to humankind.[79] Considering that the valveless cranial venous system provides open transport for both mercury and microbes, an amalgam filling in conjunction with a dental focus such as an abscessed tooth or failed root canal is a potentially lethal combination, which over the years can lead to serious neurological disease and brain cancer.

Since this valveless system extends throughout the central nervous system—that is, not only in the brain but along the entire spinal cord—the transport of microbes and metals can "take place freely in every direction."[80] Thus, microbes from genital infections can readily migrate to the brain, and in turn, oral mercury and bacteria can be transported to the genital region. This "venous highway" between the head and the pelvis helps explain the presence of mercury in the pelvic tissues and nerves (Frankenhäuser's and the sacral ganglia) commonly found through energetic testing methods. (We'll discuss the fascinating but little-known craniovertebral venous pathway further in chapter 13.)

Axonal Transport along Nerves

In 1923, animal studies published simultaneously in France and the United States proved that nerves not only conduct electrical signals but also transport nutrients and toxins. Both studies proved that herpes, when inoculated into the eye of an animal (in these studies, a rabbit or guinea pig), would spread through the ophthalmic branch of the fifth cranial nerve into the brain stem.* Since then, axonal transport, as passage of a sub-

*The fifth cranial nerve, or trigeminal nerve, supplies sensory and motor nerve fibers to the face, including the teeth, mouth, and nasal cavity. It has three branches: the ophthalmic (eye) in the upper face, the maxillary in the middle face and upper jaw, and the mandibular in the lower face and lower jaw.

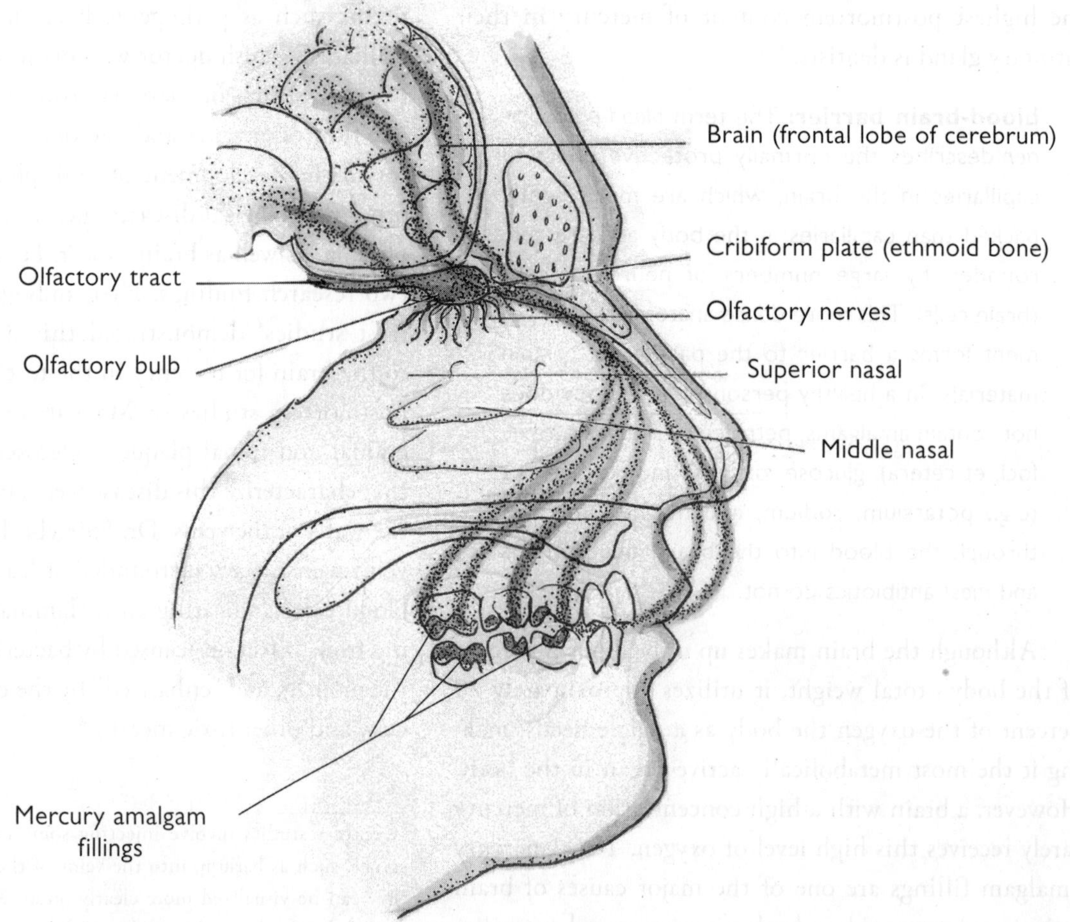

Figure 3.1. The neurological pathway of smell (and mercury transport)

stance along a nerve fiber is called, has been well documented in the cases of viruses (rabies, polio, and herpes) and bacteria (tetanus, leprosy, and diphtheria). Through his extensive research beginning in the early 1960s, Störtebecker discovered that heavy metals, like mercury and lead, and bacterial toxins are taken by axonal transport through the maxillary and mandibular branches of the fifth cranial nerve to the brain.[81] Other studies have demonstrated mercury transport along the hypoglossal nerve (of the tongue) and its ganglion into the brain.[82]

Inhalation through the Nose

As described earlier in this chapter, in the 1930s at the University of Berlin, Dr. Alfred Stock, originally from Poland, proved conclusively that inhaled mercury vapor spreads from the mucosa of the upper nasal cavity directly into the brain.[83] This pathway is the same route by which oils, gases, and other scent factors are received by the brain. Tiny nerve fibers project from the epithelium (skin) of the upper part of the nasal cavity. These olfactory (scent) nerves travel directly through the ethmoid bone (which forms the walls of the nasal cavity) to the olfactory bulb, the olfactory area of the cerebral cortex. The olfactory nerves transmit gases such as mercury vapor in the same way that they transmit scents, through specific neural signals that directly enter the cortex of the brain.[84] The olfactory transport of toxins has been found to occur within a range of a few hours to two days from the time of exposure.[85]

In this way, mercury vapor from corroded amalgams that is inhaled through the nose travels a direct pathway to the brain and adversely affects the olfactory bulb of the cortex, as well as the rest of the brain. It is indeed no wonder so many dentists have an impaired, or in some cases completely nonfunctional, sense of smell.

Mercury Deposits in the Kidneys

The kidneys, along with the aforementioned brain, spine, lungs, liver, gut (small and large intestines), and jawbone, are also an area of significant mercury deposition in the body. In numerous studies of monkeys, sheep, rabbits, rats, and humans, the kidneys have been found to show greatly increased concentrations of mercury after placement of dental amalgam fillings.[86] In one animal study, for example, after the placement of amalgam dental fillings, subjects experienced a 54 percent reduction in kidney function within thirty days, and a 60 percent reduction within sixty days.[87] Even more alarming, these findings were both subclinical *and* subhistological—that is, the animal subjects had no overt symptoms of illness, nor did their kidneys show any adverse tissue changes postmortem. Despite causing a 60 percent reduction in kidney function within just two months, the mercury poisoning was demonstrated to be insidiously silent.

Mercury Transferred from Mother to Fetus

Mercury from amalgam fillings is readily transferred from mother to fetus during pregnancy.[88]* The transplacental migration of mercury from amalgam fillings—crossing the placenta and depositing in the fetus—has been positively correlated to the number of amalgam fillings in the mouth of the mother.[89] The potential toxic effects to the fetus from this mercury include "neurotoxicity, kidney dysfunction, reduced immunocompetence, effects on the oral and intestinal bacterial flora, fetal and birth effects, and effects on general health."[90]

Mercury can also pass from mother to infant during breast-feeding. As is the case for transplacental migration, the concentration of mercury in breast milk collected immediately after birth has a "significant association with the number of amalgam fillings" in the mother.[91] (However, mercury poisoning through placental transfer has been demonstrated to be more harmful than mercury poisoning through breast-feeding.)[92]

SIGNS AND SYMPTOMS OF MERCURY POISONING

Neurological and Psychological Symptoms: Erethism

> Erethism (Greek—*erethisma* = "stimulation")—A psychic disturbance marked by irritability, emotional instability, depression, shyness, and fatigue, as in chronic mercury poisoning.
>
> DORLAND'S MEDICAL DICTIONARY, TWENTY-SIXTH EDITION

*When a patient has high levels of mercury and yet has never had an amalgam filling, it is often due to this maternal-transfer factor and thimerosal-laced vaccinations (see chapter 15), as well as mercury (and other toxic metals) absorbed from the environment (i.e., the diet, air, and water).

> Erethism—This physical or emotional disturbance is characterized by self-consciousness, timidity, embarrassment with insufficient reason, anxiety, indecision, lack of concentration, depression or despondency, resentment of criticism, irritability or excitability; these appear sometimes to cause a complete change of personality. Headache, fatigue, weakness, and either drowsiness or insomnia are frequent complaints; in advanced cases there may be hallucinations, loss of memory, and intellectual deterioration.
>
> E. Browning,
> *Toxicity of Industrial Metals*

Erethism, a neuropsychological syndrome characterized by mental and emotional instability, was first recognized at the end of the eighteenth century as a specific effect of mercury intoxication.[93] Mercury had long been—and still is—heavily used in industry before it became popular in the use of dental fillings. The expression "mad as a hatter" comes from the hat industry, from the time when hatters (hat makers) used mercuric salts in the manufacture of fur and felt hats. These workers would absorb the mercury through their skin and eventually begin to display various neuropsychological symptoms, sometimes to the point of insanity. (The use of mercuric salts was eliminated in the early 1940s, after several studies were published on the severely toxic effects of this hat-making manufacturing practice.[94])

Pandemic Erethism?

Erethism, or micro-mercurialism, as it was called by the brilliant chemist Alfred Stock in the 1920s, can result from exposure to even relatively low concentrations of vapor leaching from mercury amalgam fillings.[95] The resulting symptoms—emotional instability, irritability, anxiety, and depression—certainly call into question the increasing diagnoses of mental disorders that accompanied the maturation of the baby boomers, the generation of children most affected by mercury amalgam fillings. Seven new antidepressants were introduced between 1987 and 1997 (Prozac, Zoloft, Paxil, Effexor, Serzone, Remeron, and Wellbutrin).[96] With little awareness of the impact of mercury amalgam fillings and other possible causes of neuropsychological disturbances, such as exposure to toxic chemicals, food allergies, and poor diet, physicians prescribed these new antidepressants to the estimated 20 million people in the United States who suffer from depression, to the approximately 16 million purportedly afflicted with "social anxiety disorder," and to millions of others with any manifestation of mental and emotional disease.[97] How much have mercury amalgam fillings—or exposure to mercury in the womb from the mother's amalgams—contributed to both major and minor psychological symptoms? According to the scientific research, plenty.

MERCURY INTERFERES WITH NEUROTRANSMITTER UPTAKE IN THE BRAIN

One neurological explanation for the mental and emotional symptoms associated with exposure to mercury is that mercury damages astrocytes, star-shaped cells found in the central nervous system that play an important role in providing nutrients to the nerves and in the repair and functioning of the brain and spinal cord. Mercury also interferes with the uptake of neurotransmitters such as dopamine, serotonin, acetylcholine, and norepinephrine, which play a pivotal role in mood regulation, sleep, and behavior.[98]

Neuropsychological disorders such as anxiety, tension, depression, manic depression, memory loss, and even hallucinations have been linked in numerous studies to mercury exposure.[99] For example, in one study, twenty-five women with amalgams had significantly higher scores on two psychological scales measuring depression, fatigue, insomnia, excessive anger, and anxiety, in contrast to twenty-three female controls without amalgams.[100] Other studies have found manifestations of *erethismus mercurialis* such as irritability, excitability, outbursts of temper, aggression, and quarreling to be significantly increased in dentists and personnel working in dental offices that utilize amalgam.[101] Mental symptoms resulting from mercury exposure also include loss of memory, dementia, intellectual impairment (difficulty in receiving and understanding information), difficulty reading, inability to concentrate, and disturbed consciousness and speech.[102] And although the term *erethism* is little known, millions suffer silently from the mild to major mercury-induced symptoms of it every day of their lives.

Other Mercury-Induced Symptoms

Beyond neuropsychological symptoms, mercury intoxication resulting from amalgam fillings results in numerous and quite varied conditions. They include:

abdominal bloating
allergies
asthma
chronic fatigue
colitis
constipation or diarrhea
eczema
electrical sensitivity
hair loss (alopecia)
hearing loss
hypothyroidism
infertility
muscle and joint weakness and pain
narrowing of the field of vision
numbness and tingling in the fingers, toes, nose, and lips
painful menstruation
persistent coughs
premature aging
tremors
urination disorders[103]

In fact, these chronic symptoms are so numerous that it is often quite challenging to distinguish between mercury toxicity and other conditions that also cause a plethora of symptoms in the body, such as candidiasis (infection with candida, usually *Candida albicans*), exposure to toxic petroleum chemicals, and food allergies. Distinguishing among these various etiologies—as well as understanding the interaction between them—requires considerable clinical experience. This experience, in combination with quality energetic testing, is essential to an accurate diagnosis and a successful treatment plan. Knowledge of the harm mercury amalgams do can also save patients considerable time and money that they might otherwise have spent on ineffective therapies.

Secondary Candidiasis

Candidiasis, or infection with parasitic candida fungi, especially *Candida albicans,* often accompanies mercury poisoning. In the early 1990s, Dr. Dietrich Klinghardt posited that the body allows *Candida albicans* to proliferate specifically because it binds with mercury.[104] He explains:

> Mercury suffocates the intracellular respiratory mechanism and can cause cell death. So, the immune system makes a deal: it cultivates fungi and bacteria that can bind large amounts of toxic metals. The gain: the cells can breathe. The cost: the system has to provide nutrition for the microorganisms and has to deal with their metabolic products ("toxins").[105]

As a parallel, Klinghardt asserted that the effects of chlorella, an algae proven to attenuate and clear microbes such as viruses from the body, could be due just as much to its mercury-binding ability as to any specific antimicrobial aspect.[106] Direct evidence of such a mercury/microbe synergy has been seen in industry, where "biomasses" of bacteria (streptococci and staphylococci), fungi (candida), and parasites (amoebas) are utilized in mining because of their ability to accumulate and bind metals in their cell walls.[107]

Through clinical experience, many holistic practitioners have affirmed the Klinghardt axiom, as the theory is now known, finding that after patients have had their amalgam fillings removed and have appropriately detoxified, their candidiasis-like symptoms of fatigue, intestinal gas and bloating, and general malaise are significantly reduced or even clear up completely. In contrast, when patients do not have their amalgam fillings replaced, their "fight" against candida, intestinal parasites, or bacterial focal infections is typically a frustrating uphill battle that is never completely resolved.

Oral Pathology

One particular pathology associated with chronic mercury poisoning calls into further question the practice of placing mercury in the mouth. Since the early 1900s, research has identified mercury as specifically toxic to the oral mucosa and teeth, causing recession and inflammation of the gums, or gingivitis; recession and infection of the gums, or periodontitis; and loose and decaying teeth (the upper and lower molars and sometimes the upper incisors and canines).[108] In light of this characteristic toxicology, not to mention the systemic poisoning of the rest of the body, the placement of mercury amalgam in the teeth and sensitive oral mucosa should be considered, if not frank malpractice, at the very least bordering on it.

Mercury-Related Diseases

As is the case for the symptoms of mercury poisoning, studies have linked numerous diseases to mercury exposure. The following pages list only a brief selection of the most severe of them. The "Recommended Reading" section, beginning on page 672, includes a number of books on the subject of mercury amalgam poisoning that explore this subject in greater depth.

Alzheimer's Disease

> No one knows yet what causes Alzheimer's disease, believed to affect as many as 4 million people in this country. Experts believe that by the year 2050, the number may reach 14 million.[109]
>
> *Marin Independent Journal*, December 17, 2001

On the contrary, many people who keep up with the scientific literature *do know* that one of the major causative factors underlying the onset of Alzheimer's is mercury toxicity.[110] Dr. Boyd Haley's and his colleagues' animal studies at the University of Kentucky were so clearly definitive in proving that mercury produces the same brain aberrations and dysfunctional behavior that are seen in Alzheimer's patients, in fact, that he stated: "The results of this experiment are terrifying. I'm getting the rest of my mercury fillings taken out right now, and I've asked my wife to have hers replaced too."[111]

Dr. Sam Ziff, one of the leading holistic dental researchers writing about mercury toxicity, states: "How long can this blatant and contrived ignorance of peer-reviewed research demonstrating conclusively that mercury, regardless of source, is a major factor of Alzheimer's disease, continue?"[112]

Aluminum has also been correlated to the causation of Alzheimer's.[113] However, postmortem studies have revealed that mercury is even more culpable than aluminum in the onset of Alzheimer's and other forms of dementia and memory loss.[114]

Amyotrophic Lateral Sclerosis (ALS)

ALS, also known as Lou Gehrig's disease, is characterized by destruction of the motor nerves in the spinal cord with resulting progressive loss of muscular function. It has no medical treatment and is considered 100 percent fatal by conventional medicine.[115] Although ALS has not been as conclusively linked to mercury toxicity as Alzheimer's, several research studies point to a positive correlation. One Japanese study, for example, found mercury toxicity to be associated with ALS as well as other neurodegenerative diseases such as multiple sclerosis and Parkinson's.[116] Another study proved that mercury can travel along nerves from the peripheral muscles to the spinal cord and brain stem motor neurons,* demonstrating a possible "oral amalgam to brain" mechanism in the development of ALS.[117] Scientists have also found that mercury accumulation in the motor neurons of the spinal tract degenerates these nerve cells, and that ALS can develop either by excessive mercury accumulation or through inadequate mercury detoxification.[118]

In a recently published book, one ALS patient describes his remarkable improvement from this "terminal illness," primarily through the removal of his amalgam fillings and mercury detoxification. In his informal survey of over one hundred PALS (that is, people with ALS), all but six had—or had a history of—amalgam fillings. The group of six without amalgams included a former dentist, a dental technician, a practicing dentist, an insecticide sprayer, and an avid golfer—all occupations with exposure to mercury and toxic chemicals.[119] Although his observations can only be classified as anecdotal, the implications of mercury poisoning in the etiology of ALS cannot be ignored and deserve more research analysis.

Cancer

There is no longer any question that exposure to petroleum chemicals is a major cause of many cancers.[120] However, more and more research now strongly implicates heavy metals' role in the causation of cancer as well. Mercury amalgam fillings themselves have been

*This movement along nerves is termed *axonal transport*. For more information on axonal transport, see chapter 9.

highly implicated as a primary causative factor in cancer, and especially in leukemias.[121] In fact, *all* components of amalgam filling are found to trigger adverse immune system responses that predispose the body to cancerous cellular invasion and other disease. For example, tin causes a reduction of weight in the thymus gland and decreases the survival rate of thymocytes (thymus cells); zinc inflames brain lymphocytes (white blood cells); copper inhibits T-cell and B-cell responses (they amplify antibody production against microbes); and mercury causes abnormal levels of white blood cells, as well as the development of antinuclear antibodies (signaling inflammatory processes) and chromosomal damage.[122]

Several studies have demonstrated a positive correlation between the number of amalgam fillings and mercury levels in the brain.[123] In one dramatic study of postmortem analyses of human cadavers, Dr. Magnus Nylander of Sweden and his colleagues found a statistically significant correlation between the content of mercury in each subject's brain (the cerebral cortex and occipital lobe) and the amount of amalgam (the size and number of fillings) in their mouths.[124]

Animal studies have shown that infection, by means of intracerebral inoculation (injecting directly into the brain), can trigger the formation of malignant gliomas (brain cancer).[125] Störtebecker of Sweden has asserted for decades that malignant gliomas of the brain often result from the direct spread of microbial carcinogens from the peri-apical (root) area of the teeth—that is, from dental focal infections (as discussed in chapter 11).[126] Furthermore, the pathogenicity and spread of these toxic microbes are often potentiated by the electrogalvanic corrosion of a gold crown on or near a mercury filling, as well as by the methylation of this mercury through bacteria.[127] As described earlier in this chapter, methylmercury, derived from the complexing of oral bacteria with inflamed or abscessed teeth (dental foci), is highly toxic and has been shown to be able to travel directly through the blood, lymph, and nerves into the brain. Unfortunately, the great majority of scientists and physicians seem to still be unaware of the "principle of the shortest pathway," first pointed out by Dr. Störtebecker in 1961, which describes the movement of mercury from its source to the nearest organ; in the case of mercury-filled and infected teeth, that "shortest pathway" is the few inches separating them from the brain.[128*]

Cardiovascular Disease

The occurrence of heart disease did not become statistically significant until the early twentieth century, beginning in the 1920s.[129] Over the next forty years, the incidence of coronary heart disease rose dramatically, and it became the leading cause of death in the United States. During this period not only did the use of margarine and refined oils increase approximately 400 percent (as opposed to dietary cholesterol, which increased only 1 percent),[†] but the implantation of mercury amalgam fillings also rose exponentially.[130] Although many are aware of the dietary correlation, few know about the correlation between mercury amalgam fillings and heart disease.

One study published in 1990 found that individuals with amalgam fillings had significantly higher blood pressure and a greater incidence of chest pain (angina), rapid heartbeat (tachycardia), and anemia than those who were dentally mercury-free.[131] Another study used EKGs to find that mercury causes arrhythmias (abnormal heartbeat) and other cardiac irregularities.[132] As pointed out by the Ziff brothers, two noted dental researchers, the existing scientific evidence firmly establishes that exposure to mercury amalgams (along with smoking, stress, and refined oils and foods) damages the tissues of the cardiovascular system; the Ziffs theorize that mercury poisoning could be the "missing link" in the etiology of the prevalence of heart disease.[133]

---

*The principle of the shortest pathway has been verified through Dr. Magnus Nylander's research, which found through postmortem analysis of dentists that their pituitary gland had excessively high mercury content as compared to other parts of their brain. This pattern of deposition indicates that the mercury was inhaled through the nose. That is, when dentists worked on patients' amalgam fillings, they inhaled the resulting mercury vapor through their nose, and the mercury deposited most highly in the part of the brain that was just a few inches away from the source of nasal exposure. Perhaps most disturbing is that these high concentrations were found even in dentists who had been practicing only a few years. (P. Störtebecker, *Mercury Poisoning from Dental Amalgam* [Orlando, FL: Bio-Probe, 1985], 207–212.)

†See chapter 5 for more information on the harmful effects of margarine and other refined fats and oils.

MORE RESEARCH NEEDED: ARRHYTHMIAS AND DENTAL GALVANISM

A topic begging for more research would be the correlation between heart arrhythmias and dental galvanism. The sinoatrial node, the pacemaker of the heart, produces the impulse that stimulates the heart to beat. This node has been shown to be greatly affected by mercury but is probably even more influenced by the combination of mercury and gold (or any other dissimilar metal) that creates the toxic and electrical double whammy known as dental galvanism.

Infertility, Miscarriage, and SIDS

The role of petroleum chemicals in the disruption of the lock-and-key mechanism between hormones and their receptor sites is well known.[134] Less widely propagated are the hormonal disorders associated with mercury toxicity. In studies, however, the body burden of heavy metals—lead, cadmium, and mercury—has been clearly and positively correlated with pregnancy complications and menstrual disorders.[135] Additionally, mercury exposure has been shown to prevent ovulation, generate miscarriages, and cause fetal malformations.[136]

Multiple studies have documented that mercury crosses the placenta and deposits in the fetus, and that this deposition correlates to the number of amalgam fillings in the mother.[137] Researchers in Munich autopsied 108 SIDS babies and 46 aborted fetuses and found that mercury concentrations in the tissue correlated positively with the number of mercury amalgam fillings in the mother.[138] The subjects in this study were nursed not at all or for only a few weeks, so mercury absorption took place in utero, not through breast-feeding. Based on these findings, the relationship between mercury amalgam fillings and infertility, miscarriage, and SIDS clearly needs further scientific investigation.

Multiple Sclerosis

Several studies have found that mercury amalgam fillings are significantly correlated with the pathology underlying multiple sclerosis (MS).[139] As discussed earlier in this chapter (see page 67), Dr. Störtebecker has found that the plaques scattered in the brain that are characteristic of MS are identical to those caused by mercury toxicity in combination with oral infection.[140] Dr. Weston Price, the father of holistic dentistry in America, also found a relationship between infected root-canalled teeth and neurological disease in his research.[141] Using MRI (magnetic resonance imaging), Huggins and Levy found objective biochemical changes (photolabeling of cerebrospinal fluid proteins) in their MS patients following the removal of their amalgam fillings and root-canalled teeth.[142] In his book *Solving the MS Mystery: Help, Hope and Recovery*, Dr. Huggins blames much of the etiology of this disease on the high-copper amalgam (see page 61), which releases fifty times more mercury than other amalgam fillings.[143]

Parkinson's Disease

Parkinson's disease is the second most common neurodegenerative disorder after Alzheimer's, affecting 1 percent of the population over age fifty.[144] The *New York Times* and NBC's *Nightline* reported in November 2000 that chemicals in the environment could be a major contributing factor in the development of Parkinson's, based on a study reported at that time at the Society for Neuroscience.[145] Actually, scientists have suspected environmental toxins as a cause of Parkinson's for over a century, based on the finding that people who live or work in rural or farm areas (with pesticides) have a significantly increased risk for developing this disease.[146]

Mercury's demonstrated ability to cross the blood-brain barrier into the substantia nigra and basal ganglia, where movement disorders like Parkinson's arise, implicates amalgam fillings as a strong etiological factor in this disease.[147] In one recent study, exposure to mercury vapor caused in subjects a tremor consistent with the essential tremor that is diagnostic of Parkinson's.[148] It should be noted, however, that this correlation is not new. It has been well established for centuries that heavy metals such as copper and mercury produce lesions in the basal ganglia that result in tremors (tremor mercurialis or shaking palsy).[149] And in clinical experience, holistic physicians who employ energetic testing have found that Parkinson's patients typically test positive for both chemical and metal toxins as well as dental and tonsil focal infections.

OTHER SOURCES OF MERCURY

Unfortunately, even those of us who make every effort to avoid toxins—buying exclusively organic products, filtering our water, using nontoxic cleaning products, and so on—can still have significant exposure to toxic chemicals and metals in our everyday life. Mercury, as an example, is found in many personal care products (mascara, hair dyes, and bleaching creams, to name a few),* in medicines (such as some vaccines), in the food we eat (especially certain types of fish), and in the environment (especially in industrial areas). As a result, even if we do not have amalgam fillings, we still face mercury poisoning as a simple fact of living in modern-day life.

The Abominable Practice of Mercury-Laden Vaccines

One way in which both children and adults are exposed to mercury is through injection with vaccines containing the widely used mercury-containing thimerosal preservative. The practices of giving children numerous vaccines as well as amalgam fillings are particularly tragic, since according to the Centers for Disease Control (CDC) the two groups that are most vulnerable to methylmercury are children under the age of fifteen and fetuses.[150] In fact, the FDA recently acknowledged that in the first six months of life, children get more mercury than is considered safe by the EPA.[151]

The other group most at risk—fetuses—may now also receive mercury-containing thimerosal due to the CDC's recent recommendation that pregnant women receive the flu vaccine before the start of flu season. The Advisory Committee on Immunization Practices (ACIP), which advises the CDC on vaccination practices, has recommended that the flu vaccine be given only after fourteen weeks of pregnancy to avoid the *coincidental* association of the vaccine with miscarriage. Unfortunately, both the CDC and the ACIP seem to be quite unaware of a recent study, published in the *American Journal of Epidemiology,* showing that "the greatest susceptibility to methylmercury neurotoxicity occurs during late gestation, while early postnatal vulnerability is less."[152]

On June 8, 1999, the FDA "recommended" that vaccine makers phase out vaccines that contain thimerosal.[153] However, since the FDA did not enact a ban on this mercury-containing preservative, it remains in use, even if considerably reduced. It is still contained, for example, in some DTP, DT, tetanus, meningococcal, and flu shots.[154] And many thimerosal-containing vaccines have been shipped off to other countries in the world, putting those nations' infants and children at risk of *vaccinosis* (vaccine-caused illnesses).

For more information on thimerosal, as well as other toxic metals and chemicals in vaccines, see chapter 15, which discusses this subject in detail.

Thermometers, Antiseptics, and Calomel

Mercury used to be common in first-aid supplies such as thermometers, antiseptics, and calomel. Many of us remember playing with mercury thermometers as children, and even the mercury itself if a thermometer was dropped and broke open. Thankfully, many localities as well as drugstores have banned the sale of mercury thermometers, and they are now being replaced by digital thermometers.[155]

Many of us will also remember the pale reddish orange antiseptics Mercurochrome and Merthiolate (Eli Lilly's trade name for thimerosal), which burned as they were applied to our skinned knees. Since mercury does have a mild bacteriostatic* effect, it was a staple in every medicine cabinet until just recently (1998), when it was banned in most regions along with thermometers.[156]

Calomel, or mercurous chloride, is a form of inorganic mercury that has been used for centuries in skin creams and other products. As recently as 1996, it was linked to cases of mercury poisoning in Arizona, California, New Mexico, and Texas.[157] (The FDA still allows the use of mercury in cosmetics to 0.0065 percent by weight.) Calomel was also used to treat ailments including yellow fever, typhus, and syphilis.

Pink disease—also known as acrodynia, erythoedema, Feer's disease, or Swift's disease—was once a common

*See the "Best Bets" list (page 137) for sources of nontoxic cosmetics and other personal care products.

*Mercury is more *bacteriostatic* than *bactericidal*. That is, it slows the growth of bacteria but does not kill them altogether. In fact, mercury-containing thimerosal has been found to be "no better than water in protecting mice from fatal streptococcal infection." Furthermore, it has been found to be more deadly to healthy cells than it is harmful to bacteria. (D. Kirby, *Evidence of Harm* [New York: St. Martin's Press, 2005], 83.)

syndrome caused by inorganic mercury poisoning in infants and children from calomel-containing teething powders and Mercurochrome. The disease was purportedly eliminated in the 1950s when these child-care products were banned, but many adults still suffer from the effects of this form of mercury poisoning from their childhood.[158] Pink disease is characterized by severe leg cramps, weight loss, palpitations, weak and flabby muscles, irritability, severe photophobia (eye sensitivity to light), a prickling sensation on the skin, and peeling, painful fingernails. Additionally, as David Kirby points out in his book on the use of mercury-containing thimerosal in vaccines, *Evidence of Harm,* susceptible children demonstrate neurological symptoms "instantly recognizable to parents of an autistic child":

> The first sign is a loss of joyfulness. The children stop playing and laughing, and may go weeks or months without smiling. Their faces reflect sadness; the forehead is wrinkled, the look melancholy or even desperate. The children appear to suffer physically and morally. At the same time, the children stop talking. Some cry constantly. Most are cranky, complain, and moan. Affectivity is modified. Most often it is diminished or disappears completely. Some children appear unaware of their parents, don't respond to their kisses, do not seem to notice them when they come close or leave. In most children, there is some irritability, sometimes hostility.[159]

Industrial Exposure

Numerous industries expose workers to mercury, among other toxins. These include battery manufacturing, drug manufacturing, fungicide and insecticide production, fluorescent and neon light manufacturing, mining, mirror production, paint manufacturing, papermaking, and photography.[160]

Mercury in Fish

There has been much debate over the amount of mercury exposure that results from eating fish. The media's warnings to avoid consumption of certain types of fish, although worthwhile, create the illusion that this is the most important step in avoiding mercury exposure—which it isn't. A 1991 WHO study looking at the average amount of mercury that was being absorbed daily from known sources found that seafood intake resulted in an average of 2.34 micrograms of mercury absorption per day, as compared to dental amalgams, which cause from 3.0 to 17.0 micrograms of mercury absorption per day.[161] In fact, fish have been described as only a "distant second" to dental amalgam as a source of mercury toxicity.[162] This hierarchy has been borne out by scientists at the Institute of Forensic Medicine at the University of Munich, who found that for mercury contained in the liver, kidneys, and brain, the percentage that is organic mercury derived from food is actually quite low (5 to 8 percent), as compared to the percentage that is inorganic mercury released from dental amalgam fillings (95 percent).[163]

Of course, fish do ingest and concentrate pollutants in their bodies, and mercury is particularly common in lake fish. Therefore, it is best to avoid fish from contaminated waters—that is, polluted rivers or lakes and waters close to the shore. These include scavenger fish like catfish and carp, as well as shoreline feeders such as sole and flounder. Swordfish, tuna, and salmon have been found at various times to have high levels of mercury. However, other researchers contend that these deep-sea fish increase their selenium content to compensate and protect themselves from the effects of mercury, which protects the consumer as well.[164]

A growing number of clean and environmentally friendly farms are producing fish. However, farm-raised fish are often raised with antibiotics and pesticides, and the trout and salmon dyed with red food dyes.[165] Therefore, the safest choice is to eat only deep-sea fish or fish from clean waters, and limit your intake if you have had difficulty detoxing from amalgam fillings or are pregnant or nursing.

- ▶ For more information on eating fish, visit the Monterey Bay Aquarium's website at www.seafoodwatch.org to access the aquarium's excellent fish-eating pocket guides, which give information on sustainable seafood choices for different parts of the country.

- ▶ If you suspect the fish you have just ingested contained mercury, take 2 to 4 capsules of Pure Radiance C or another powerful antioxidant to help detoxify it from your system. Pure Radiance C is available from the Synergy Company at (800) 723-0277 or www.thesynergycompany.com; it is one of the core vitamin C supplements not chemically synthesized or derived from genetically modified compounds. This natural antioxidant is made from organic and wild berries and provides strong immune system support that helps the body detoxify more efficiently. Additionally, vitamin C helps elevate red blood cell glutathione levels. Glutathione is the most important antioxidant amino acid in the body.

OTHER TOXIC METALS AND THEIR SOURCES

In light of the strong evidence of dental galvanism's culpability in the etiology of serious pathology, it is extremely important to your health and longevity to be an informed consumer at the dentist's office. The number one rule is not to mix metals in your mouth. Mercury amalgams are themselves composed of mixed metals and by themselves alone create galvanic currents. Even without amalgam fillings, mixing other metals in your mouth, such as gold, palladium, nickel, or aluminum in crowns, inlays, or onlays, can also create disturbing galvanic currents. A completely metal-free mouth is the safest way to go. (Though in some difficult dental cases that require a number of extractions, metal crowns and bridges may be required, in which case they should be made of a high-quality gold.)

The following section gives a brief summary of the effects of toxic metals.* It's important to note that some heavy metals—cobalt, copper, chromium, iron, manganese, and zinc—are essential for healthy functioning at trace amounts but toxic in large concentrations. I've included mercury here so that the list is complete and can be photocopied for quick reference or to show to a dentist or physician.

*The primary sources for this information about toxic metals are the *Handbook on Metals in Clinical and Analytical Chemistry* by Seiler, Sigel, and Sigel; *Hazardous Materials Toxicology* by Sullivan and Krieger; *Mercury Poisoning from Dental Amalgam* by Störtebecker; *Toxic Metal Syndrome* by Casdorph and Walker; *How to Stay Young and Healthy in a Toxic World* by Gittleman; and Russell Jaffe's handout *Chelation Therapy for Acute and Chronic Metal Intoxication* from his 1994 presentation to the American Academy of Biological Dentistry.

Aluminum

Aluminum is the third most abundant element in the earth's crust. Although it's a common misconception that aluminum is always toxic, in actuality there are two forms—water soluble and acid soluble—and the first is thought to be *not* toxic.

The water-soluble form of aluminum is an organically bound colloid found in plants and has no known negative effects. Its role in the human body is not conclusively known, but many scientists believe that the water-soluble form is an essential element in human nutrition. According to Professor Gerhardt Schrauzer, head of the chemistry department at the University of California at San Diego, organic aluminum's "known biological function is to activate the enzyme succinic dehydrogenase and increase the survival rate of newborns, and it is probably an essential mineral for human nutrition."[166]

There is strong evidence that the acid-soluble form of aluminum is a causative factor in Alzheimer's, amyotrophic lateral sclerosis (ALS), Parkinson's, and some brain cancers. Other neurotoxic effects of this form of aluminum include severe fatigue, depression, ataxia (shaky movements and unsteady gait), short-term memory loss, and difficulty performing mental functions such as arithmetic. Aluminum also negatively affects the body's metabolism of calcium and phosphorus and can therefore contribute to osteomalacia (abnormal softening of the bones) and osteoporosis (demineralization of the bones). It has also been associated with heart disease, headache, and frequent colds. Aluminum can compromise digestion by neutralizing pepsin, an enzyme that digests protein in the stomach, contributing to symptoms of colic, flatulence, heartburn, and ulcers. Aluminum, like mercury, can be absorbed in the gut and permeate the blood-brain barrier.

Potential sources of aluminum: Dental porcelain* and ceramic crowns and bridges; deodorants and antiperspirants; antacids; buffered aspirins; anti-diarrhea drugs; some baby formulas (both cow and soy-based); food additives; aluminum cans; aluminum foil; some baking powders; some pickles and processed cheeses; self-rising

*Most porcelain crowns are actually porcelain fused to metal (PFM). These crowns create galvanic currents through the interaction of the aluminum in the porcelain with the gold, nickel, or other metal in the underlying metal "sleeve" or "shoulder" of the crown.

flour; feminine hygiene products (douches); aluminum pots, pans, and other cookware; tap water; leather; glues; paints; and cosmetics (e.g., powders).

ALUMINUM COOKWARE

Many holistically minded individuals choose to use nontoxic glass and ceramic cookware* to avoid the leaching of toxic aluminum into food from aluminum pots and pans. The sale of aluminum-lined cookware is prohibited in Germany, France, Belgium, Great Britain, Switzerland, Hungary, and Brazil, but it is still permitted in the United States. However, most aluminum cookware nowadays is anodized, or dipped into a hot acid bath, which seals it by changing its molecular structure so the aluminum won't leach into food.[167]

*Stainless steel is not a good material for cookware due to its nickel content. See the "Nickel in Cookware" sidebar on page 81.

Arsenic

Arsenic is ubiquitous in the earth. We still don't know whether it is essential for human nutrition as a trace element. Arsenic toxicity affects the heart, gastrointestinal tract (nausea, colic, diarrhea), skin (cancer), kidneys, and nervous system (e.g., dizziness, seizures, tingling and burning of the hands and feet, visual impairment, deafness, muscular weakness, loss of coordination, and peripheral neuropathy). Other symptoms include loss of hair, dermatitis, headaches, fatigue, and cirrhosis of the liver. Breathing in arsenic from dust or cigarette smoke causes coughing, difficulty breathing, and restlessness.

Potential sources of arsenic: Cigarette smoke; air, water, and soil pollution from insecticides, herbicides, and copper-smelting factories; well water; bottom-feeding sea creatures like shrimp and lobster; pigments and dyes; wallpaper; ceramics; glass; some paints; and wood preservatives and treatments.

Barium

Barium is moderately prevalent in the earth's crust. It has been well established as a neurotoxin and has not been demonstrated to be essential to animals or plants. Long-term retention is rare but has been reported after contrast studies (X-rays) in the colon and lung.

Potential sources of barium: Contrast studies in radiology; some dental composites; paints; rubber; ceramics and plastics; paper fillers; explosives; jet fuel; pesticides; photography supplies; and, formerly, medications for tuberculosis, skin diseases, and heart disease.

Cadmium

Cadmium has no known biological function within the body. It accumulates primarily in the kidneys and liver, with signs of resulting kidney dysfunction being the most common, including recurrent stones, polyuria (frequent urination), and impairment of calcium metabolism contributing to osteoporosis and osteomalacia. Symptoms of cadmium poisoning from cigarette smoke include chronic fatigue, forgetfulness, various mental aberrations, emphysema and lung cancer, chronic lower back and kidney-area pain, and kidney stones. Cadmium crosses the placenta and concentrates in amniotic fluid, and it is highly toxic to the developing fetus. High cadmium levels have been associated with learning disabilities and lowered achievement and intelligence scores.

Other symptoms of cadmium poisoning include decreased appetite, sore joints, mouth sores, dry and scaly skin, loss of hair, weight loss, decreased growth (due to cadmium's direct antagonism to zinc), decreased body temperature, impotence, and anosmia (loss of the sense of smell). Signs of cadmium poisoning include lung cancer; rheumatoid arthritis; benign prostatic hypertrophy (enlargement of the prostrate) and prostate cancer; vitamin D, zinc, and iron deficiencies; excess protein, glucose, amino acids, and enzymes in the urine; and hypertension (high blood pressure) and heart disease.

Potential sources of cadmium: Cigarette smoke; air pollution from the manufacture of coal, oil, cement, batteries, paint, and rustproofing materials; soldering; car exhaust; dust; fungicides typically sprayed on apples, tobacco, and potatoes; pesticides; superphosphate fertilizers; drinking water (especially soft); oysters and other seafoods; dairy products, including evaporated milk; organ meats, such as kidney and liver; refined wheat flour (which increases the cadmium-to-zinc ratio); silver polish; some dental prosthetics; antiseptics and medications for dandruff and oily skin; some refined foods; motor oil; car seat covers; plastics; electroplated ice-cube trays; synthetic dyes in clothing and some art pigments; fireworks; and furniture and floor coverings.

Chromium

Chromium functions biologically as part of an organic complex known as glucose tolerance factor (GTF), which acts synergistically with insulin to increase cellular uptake of glucose. Inorganic or metallic chromium is used along with nickel to strengthen stainless steel, as well as to brighten and protect it from corrosion. However, this hexavalent form of chromium can cause DNA damage and is considered carcinogenic. In industry, dermal (skin), gastrointestinal, renal (kidney), and pulmonary (lung) disorders have been documented in cases of large doses of or chronic exposure to chromium.

Potential sources of chromium: Dental crowns, bridges, and braces; surgical implants; some detergents and bleaches; air pollution; dyes and pigments; copy machine toner; glues; photography supplies; silverware; cookware; jewelry; fireworks; and blue jean snaps and belt buckles that touch the skin.

Cobalt

In the body, cobalt is found within vitamin B_{12} in the form of adenosylcobalamin, cyanocobalamin, or methylcobalamin. B_{12} is essential in the production of hemoglobin and red blood cells, the synthesis of DNA, and the formation of creatine, choline, and methionine. In industry, metallic cobalt is used to maintain the melting point in steel alloys. The toxicity of cobalt is considered to be fairly low.

Potential sources of cobalt: Dental crowns, bridges, and braces; surgical implants; jewelry; paints and varnishes; colored pottery; cement; some medicines for treating hypertension; radiation therapy to stimulate bone marrow; and, in the past, brewing beer.

Copper

This essential trace mineral is found in all body tissues but is most concentrated in the brain, heart, kidneys, and liver. Though copper toxicity is generally considered to be rare, Dr. Carlton Fredericks reported in the 1970s that high copper levels from copper water pipes laid down primarily after World War II contribute greatly to mental illness, especially schizophrenia. Dr. Paul Eck of Analytical Research Labs has asserted that copper today is what lead was to the ancient Romans—an unsuspected toxin that greatly contributes to a society's debility and aging.

Acute copper toxicity can cause nausea, vomiting, abdominal pain, diarrhea, diffuse muscle pain, and abnormal mental states. Clinically, excess levels of copper have been linked to ulcerative colitis and neurobehavioral impairment including anxiety, hyperactivity, irritability, anorexia nervosa, compulsive and addictive behavior, depression, and schizophrenia. Chronic copper toxicity has been documented to induce a "shaking palsy," similar to the "tremor mercurialis" of mercury intoxication. Excessive copper intake can reduce iron and zinc levels in the body. Sexual hormone disorders such as premenstrual syndrome, endometriosis, fibroid tumors, and menstrual dysfunction in women and impotence, overaggressiveness, and hair loss in men have been linked to copper toxicity.

Potential sources of copper: Dental amalgam (especially high-copper amalgam) and gold crowns and bridges; inorganic copper supplements; copper plumbing (especially in combination with soft water); IUDs (intrauterine devices for birth control); copper cookware; insecticides and fungicides; fireworks; photography supplies; pigments; jewelry; some cough and decongestant medications; birth control pills; leather; and fabric preservatives.

Gold

Although found in extremely low levels of concentration in the body, gold has not yet been identified as an essential trace element. Acute gold toxicity can cause disorders in the digestive tract and skin. Chronic exposure has been noted to sometimes cause neurobehavioral effects of confusion or dementia. In one major MELISA Medica study measuring the lymphocyte sensitivity of 617 subjects, gold actually tested as the *fourth* most allergenic metal, after the well-known toxic metals nickel, mercury, and cadmium.[168] Another study found gold concentrations in saliva, blood, serum, urine, and feces samples to correlate to the number of gold crowns or inlays in subjects. The amount of gold in the saliva, measured both before and after chewing gum, reached the range of oral gold therapy for rheumatoid arthritis, from which frequent and severe side effects have been reported.[169]

Potential sources of gold: Dental crowns, inlays, onlays, and bridges; chrysotherapy (gold injection or oral gold therapy for arthritis); angiocardiography and nuclear medicine; jewelry; and some coins.

Iron

Iron is the fourth most abundant element in the earth's crust. Ferrous iron is an essential trace element and the oxygen-carrying component bound to hemoglobin in red blood cells. Iron deficiency is the most prevalent deficiency in humans. However, iron excess, or hemosiderosis, is also common, occurring most often in white males. This iron overload is most often due to hemochromatosis, a hereditary disorder that affects 5 to 10 percent of the U.S. population. However, symptoms of iron overload such as fatigue and lack of mental clarity can unfortunately mirror those of iron deficiency. Thus, blood tests are essential for an accurate diagnosis. Other signs and symptoms of iron excess can include arthritis, diabetes, impotence, sterility, premature menopause, and cirrhosis. Iron accumulation in the body can eventually cause brain damage and dementia, cancer, and heart disease.

Potential sources of iron: Mineral supplements (furthermore, vitamin C enhances the uptake of iron); stainless-steel and iron cookware (cast-iron frying pans); enriched flour (as is used in the manufacture of commercial breads, crackers, cereals, pasta, cakes, and cookies); and dyes, inks, paints, and pigments.

Lead

Lead, widely distributed in the earth's crust, has long been known as a toxin. In 1972, the United States finally banned tetraethyl lead as a gasoline additive, after fifty years of millions of tailpipes spewing out lead into the air, soil, and water. The use of lead additives in residential paint was banned in the United States in 1977, due to the widespread danger of lead poisoning in children. However, many older homes and buildings still contain lead paint, and lead pigments are still used in outdoor paints. Lead is easily absorbed through the lungs, and children absorb as much as 50 percent of dietary lead found in vegetables, meat, and milk (in contrast, adults absorb only 20 to 30 percent). Each year in the United States lead exposure leads to about 200 children dying from encephalopathy (degenerative brain disease); another 800 are diagnosed with permanent brain damage and 3,200 with temporary mental impairment.

Common symptoms of lead poisoning in children are hyperactivity, long-term learning disorders, lowered I.Q., and impaired growth. Other symptoms include colic and abdominal cramping, irritability, fatigue, hearing loss, general malaise, muscle pain, fatigue, insomnia, paralysis, peripheral neuritis (inflammation of the peripheral nerves), anemia, seizures, mania, dementia, delirium, stupor, and coma. Lead may slowly and insidiously accumulate in children through storage in the bones, causing irreversible deficient cognitive development or the later onset of Alzheimer's.

Potential sources of lead: Car exhaust from leaded gasolines, which are still in use in some countries (such as India); paint chips and dust in older homes and buildings; lead-based paint; industrial smoke and fumes from lead smelters, coal-burning refineries, and processing plants; waste incineration; landfills; manufacture and incineration of batteries; air, water, soil, and food pollution; lead pipes and solder in water systems; glass and lead crystal; fireworks; newsprint; inks; pesticides; some pottery and ceramics; cigarettes; and some mascaras and hair dyes.

LEAD CRYSTAL

After the British journal *Lancet* (one of the most respected medical journals in the world) reported that wine and other alcohols greatly increase the leaching of lead from crystal, the FDA recommended that food and beverages not be stored in lead crystal and that children and women of child-bearing age not drink from it.[170]

Manganese

Manganese, the tenth most abundant metal in the earth's crust, is an essential trace element for human health and catalyzes over fifty biochemical reactions. In fact, it is second only to zinc in activating enzyme systems. However, industrial exposure to or excessive consumption of manganese can lead to "manganism" or "manganese madness," with resulting neurotoxic effects such as emotional lability, irrationality, hallucinations, impulsivity, and violent behavior. Chronic exposure produces Parkinson's-like symptoms, including muscular weakness, a slow shuffling gait, a "flat" or masklike facial expression, "pill-rolling" movements of the fingers, and impaired speech.

Potential sources of manganese: Soy-based infant formulas; stainless-steel utensils, cookware, buckles, and snaps; pharmaceutical products and antiseptics; gasoline exhaust; pesticides and fertilizers; leather tanning; ceramics; and dyes and varnishes.

Mercury

Mercury is the only metal that is liquid at room temperature. Traces of mercury are ubiquitous in the earth's crust, and often found near gold. Mercury is a general protoplasmic (cell) poison. Its toxicological action occurs primarily through the manner in which it binds to sulfur groups in enzymes, thereby inactivating them. The most common route of exposure is through inhalation of mercury vapor, whether through the nose, from which it passes into the brain, or through the lungs, where it quickly penetrates the alveolar membranes and is absorbed into the general circulation.

Mercury is absorbed into the red blood cells, tissues, and organs and readily passes the blood-brain barrier, where it accumulates in the central nervous system (CNS). Chronic exposure to mercury from dental fillings can cause a classic triad of gum and CNS symptoms: gingivitis, tremors, and erethism (insomnia, shyness, memory loss, emotional lability, nervousness, and anorexia). Mercury also adversely affects the kidneys, liver, lungs, eyes, skin, gastrointestinal tract, heart, pituitary, thyroid, pancreas, spleen, and reproductive organs.

Bacteria, such as may be present in cases of intestinal dysbiosis, gingivitis, or abscess, can methylate mercury, causing it to take the much more toxic and dangerous methylmercury form.

Potential sources of mercury: Dental amalgam; some fungicides and insecticides; some adhesives; latex paints; polluted water and seafood; air pollution from volcano emissions, mining, combustion of fossil fuel, smelting of iron, and production of cement and plastics; sewage sludge; broken mercury thermometers; leaking batteries; mercurial diuretics, ointments, and antiseptics; cinnabar (used in jewelry); some fabric softeners; some felt; film; tattooing; floor waxes and polishers; wood preservatives; and some hair dyes, mascaras, and bleaching creams.

Nickel

Nickel, widely distributed in the earth's crust, is thought to be essential to human health in trace amounts and may help activate certain enzymes. Excess nickel accumulates in the kidneys and interferes with hormone production. It also suppresses natural killer cells and interferon production and can cause chromosomal changes. The National Institute of Occupational Safety and Health classifies nickel as a carcinogen at any exposure level.

Nickel is also highly allergenic. Dermatitis (skin rashes) and urticaria (itching and hives), as well as other symptoms from contact sensitivity, have been documented in 10 to 20 percent of females and 1 percent of males.

Nickel exposure affects the brain and nervous system and can cause frontal headaches, vertigo, insomnia, lethargy, nausea, and irritability. Diseases associated with significant nickel exposure include cancer (especially lung, nasal, colon, kidney, gastric, liver, pancreas, brain, and muscle and bone cancers); heart attack; thyroid dysfunction; autoimmune disorders; infectious diseases; and psoriasis and eczema. Many cases of chronic rhinitis, sinusitis, and asthma have been linked to the nickel content of the stainless steel contained in dental crowns, bridges, and braces. Nickel toxicity, like that of mercury and many other heavy metals, is quite insidious because of the often gradual onset of symptoms and the presence of symptoms distant from the site of sensitization (e.g., nickel-containing stainless-steel braces causing urticaria on the arms and hands).

Potential sources of nickel: Dental crowns, bridges, and braces; hydrogenated fats and oils; surgical implants; cigarettes; nickel-cadmium batteries; stainless-steel utensils and cookware; jewelry; thimbles, scissors, and needles; coins; pigments and dyes; asphalt; air and water pollution from smelting, refining, and processing stainless steel and other nickel alloys; certain foods (cocoa, chocolate, soy products); and zippers, snaps, and buckles on blue jeans and other clothing.

NICKEL IN COOKWARE

Nickel began to be added to stainless steel after World War II to increase the strength of this alloy. Stainless steel is 50 to 88 percent iron, 11 to 30 percent chromium, and up to 31 percent nickel. For cookware, a more preferable option to stainless steel is enamel-covered cast iron or enamel-covered steel (such as the cookware manufactured by Le Creuset), stoneware (such as that manufactured by Corningware), or glass.* Of course, all nonstick cookware should be avoided as much as possible, since when it is overheated the nonstick coating (such as Teflon) emits a toxic gas. A class-action lawsuit on this issue was filed against Du Pont in April 2006.[171]

*Corning glassware is no longer in production, but eBay is a good source.

Palladium

Palladium is a platinoid element, along with platinum, ruthenium, rhodium, osmium, and iridium. Platinoids are found in trace amounts in the earth but are not essential elements in the body. Platinoids can cause hypersensitivity and allergic reactions: cough, wheezing, dyspnea (difficulty breathing), chronic bronchitis, irritation of the eyes and nose, dermatitis, and itching. Little research exists on palladium, but clinically many holistic practitioners have observed chronic toxic effects resulting from the placement of palladium alloy crowns and bridges. Dental palladium alloys are associated with environmental sensitivity, depression, passivity, nervousness, weight gain, migrating pains in the body, hair loss, and hyperthyroidism. Furthermore, palladium toxicity has been reported to be even more therapy-resistant than mercury toxicity, and therefore more difficult to chelate out of the body.

Potential sources of palladium: Alloys in dental crowns and bridges; industrial pollution; air pollution from catalytic converters in cars; and copy toner.

Platinum

Like palladium, platinum is a platinoid element that is not essential for human health. The platinum-based compound cisplatin is used chemotherapeutically to treat testicular, ovarian, bladder, prostate, thyroid, head, and neck tumors. Cisplatin has caused renal (kidney), gastrointestinal, hematologic (blood), and otologic (ear) toxicity, so its use is limited. Platinum is widely used as an alloy with gold in dental crowns, inlays, onlays, and bridges.

Potential sources of platinum: Dental crowns, inlays, onlays, and bridges; jewelry; chemotherapy (in cisplatin); and industrial pollution.

Silver

Silver, a relatively rare element, occurs only in trace quantities in the earth's crust. It is not an essential constituent of the human body. Silver poisoning, although rare, can cause gastroenteritis, diarrhea, hypotension (low blood pressure), paralysis, and respiratory failure. Chronic exposure can cause liver and kidney fatty-tissue degeneration. Major exposure causes deposition of silver in the skin or eyes (argyria), which appears as a blue/black/gray discoloration.

Potential sources of silver: Dental amalgam and, formerly, silver-point root canals; industrial exposure; colloidal silver* as an antibacterial treatment for burns, opthalmia neonatorum (conjunctivitis) in newborns,† osteomyelitis (bone inflammation), and urinary tract infections from catheters; formaldehyde; some water purification systems; photographic film; jewelry; and silver tableware and flatware.

Thallium

Thallium is ubiquitous in the earth's crust at low levels. It is not an essential element in the body and is quite toxic. Thallium compounds are tasteless and odorless. Most thallium is easily absorbed through the lungs, gastrointestinal tract, and skin. Thallium poisoning can cause acute symptoms of constipation, pain or paresthesia (a prickling or tingling) in the extremities, insomnia, and excessive thirst. Chronic neurologic signs include restlessness, ataxia (incoordination), tremors, stupor, psychotic

*Although colloidal silver has significant antibacterial action and can be effective for short-term use, if used excessively over time it can wipe out the body's intestinal flora (the good as well as the bad) and cause argyria, an irreversible condition in which silver salts deposit in the skin (giving it an ashen gray color), eyes, and internal organs. Those who wish to use colloidal silver products should research them and choose wisely, as well as not take them excessively.

†Silver nitrate eyedrops are still used prophylactically in the treatment of opthalmia neonatorum (conjunctivitis in newborns) if gonorrhea infection is suspected in the mother. However, these eyedrops themselves can cause a chemical conjunctivitis that exudes a purulent (pus) discharge. More recently, they have been replaced by erythromycin ointment. *Mothering* magazine notes that blindness from gonorrhea does not happen instantaneously, and no tests have determined if preventive eye drops are more effective than watching your baby for signs of trouble. The ointment blurs the baby's vision so "if you decide to go ahead with the eye treatments (and in some states you have no choice), be sure to delay it for one hour," taking some time to bond together first. If you choose to skip the antibiotics, be sure to report any signs of irritation or infection, explaining to your baby's healthcare provider that she was not given the drops at birth. (Newborn Decisions," *Mothering,* www.mothering.com/pregnancy-birth/newborn-decisions?pag=0,1.)

changes, and convulsions. Alopecia (balding) is considered a classic sign of thallium poisoning. Thallium has been used in mercury thermometers and reputedly has been added to some amalgam fillings, which may have contributed to the paralysis and ataxia that occurred in some cases of major mercury poisoning.

Potential sources of thallium: Silver alloys; some fungicides and insecticides (which are banned in much of the world now); cigarettes; cement making; myocardial imaging; imitation jewelry; dye pigments; optical lenses; and air pollution from plants, mines, and smelters.

Tin

In 1970 tin was reported to be an essential element in animals, but its specific biological actions remain unknown. Although a 1990 Kyoto study points to tin deficiency as a factor in male pattern baldness as well as impaired hearing in older men,[172] tin compounds produce irritation of the eyes, mucous membranes, throat, and skin, and some are hepatotoxic (toxic to the liver). Neurotoxic effects from tin include severe anxiety, neurasthenia (severe weakness), and signs of encephalopathy (degenerative brain disease) including severe headaches, alterations in consciousness, seizures, and delirium.

Potential sources of tin: Amalgam fillings and some crown and bridge alloys; bactericides and other pharmaceuticals; fingernail polish; perfumes; silverware; paints; tin cans; soaps; soft plastics; pesticides; and wood preservatives.

Titanium

Titanium is the ninth most common component of the earth's crust. There is no evidence to indicate that it is an essential element needed by the human body, and it is generally thought to be nontoxic, although the National Institute of Occupational Safety and Health considers it a carcinogen.

Excessive exposure to titanium dioxide, which occurs primarily in industry, can result in pulmonary irritation and fibrosis, bronchitis, contact dermatitis, and allergy symptoms. The organs primarily targeted by titanium intoxication, however, are the lungs. It is recommended that people with titanium implants have no other metals in their body, because titanium increases the rate of corrosion in the less precious (less inert) metal. That is, in the presence of titanium and mercury amalgam, the mercury in the amalgam will corrode much faster than is usual, and in the presence of titanium and gold, titanium will corrode faster than is usual.

Potential sources of titanium: Dental and surgical implants; enamels, paints, lacquers, and inks (white pigment); pharmaceuticals (including antibiotics and antidepressants); toothpastes; sunscreens; cosmetics; ointments and lotions; white cheese (e.g., mozzarella); food additives; and pesticides.

Zinc

Zinc is widely distributed in the earth's crust. It is an essential trace element in the body and catalyzes more biochemical enzymatic reactions than any other mineral. Acute symptoms of oral zinc poisoning are primarily gastrointestinal, including nausea, stomach pain, and vomiting. Other organs targeted by chronic toxic zinc exposure include the skin, eyes, respiratory tract, kidneys, blood (anemia), and brain (fatigue). Toxic doses or chronic exposure to zinc can cause copper and iron deficiency, decrease white blood cells, and lower HDL cholesterol, increasing the risk for heart disease.

Potential sources of zinc: Amalgam fillings and dental cements; pharmaceuticals such as vaginal douches, bactericides, and skin and sunblock creams; deodorants; chemosurgery for skin cancers; astringents and eye drops; paints; inorganic or excessive mineral supplementation; food additives; and brass, bronze, steel, and iron alloys.

Conclusion

More research needs to be conducted on the toxic effects of many of these metals. It is especially needed in the case of nonindustrial settings, where the effect of chronic exposure to aluminum-filled "porcelain" crowns, palladium-containing crowns and bridges, and even nickel-containing stainless-steel cookware is still relatively unknown. Such research should include the interactions of these metals, such as the galvanic and corrosive effects of titanium implants placed next to gold crowns and bridges. Suffice it to say that a mouth filled with mixed metals must always be a primary consideration by all holistic practitioners when ill patients present in their offices.

"THE DAMAGE DONE"

Neil Young's famous song about heroin addiction could just as well be written for the effects of dental amalgams and other toxic metals. In other words, there is a reason that only a minority of individuals feel symptomatic relief after their amalgam fillings have been removed: *the damage has already been done.* That is, mercury and other toxic metals have already infiltrated their organs, cells, and connective tissue and, without treatment, will adversely affect their functioning for years, or even decades.

Damage within Days of Amalgam Placement

The placement of amalgam fillings in the mouth causes biological damage almost immediately. Degenerative changes in the brain are initiated within *days* of an amalgam filling.[173] White blood cells that have been ruptured by mercury, known as "shadow cells," release their enzyme packets into the bloodstream and set up a multitude of chronic allergic and immune responses.[174] And the glomeruli and tubules in the kidneys and the grapelike alveoli in the lungs are significantly damaged very early—within *months* after amalgam fillings are put in the mouth.[175]

Mercury Poisoning Can Cause Irreversible Effects

Depending on the dose (the amount of amalgam filling, plus the galvanic effect of any other metals in the mouth), the duration (the length of time amalgam has been in the mouth), and the patient's primary miasmic tendency (psoric, sycotic, tuberculinic, or luetic), mercury can have either reversible or irreversible toxic effects.[176] Even the best of holistic practitioners have reported very little reversal of symptoms for patients in wheelchairs from the effects of MS (multiple sclerosis) or ALS (amyotrophic lateral sclerosis) and for patients suffering severe dementia from Alzheimer's. However, over time, appropriate therapy has been shown to slow or stop the progress of the insidious effects of these diseases.

Mercury Poisoning Can Be Reversible

For those with less severe symptoms, much can be done. However, to truly rid the body of mercury and other toxic metals requires a wide range of treatments and considerable perseverance on the part of the patient and practitioner. It is important that appropriate detoxifying drainage remedies (such as plant stem cell remedies) and supplements be prescribed. Other important factors include clearing toxic focal infections in the teeth, tonsils, sinuses, and genitals (see part 4); eating a clean diet and treating chronic intestinal dysbiosis (see chapter 7); and mitigating one's miasmic tendency through the correct constitutional homeopathic remedy (see chapter 14). In most cases, clearing the damaging effects of mercury amalgams that have been implanted in the mouth for years and even decades requires much determination and commitment on the part of the individual as well as the holistic practitioner, but optimal health and well-being are always worth the journey.

PROBLEMS WITH LABORATORY DIAGNOSIS

The Catch-22 of Testing for Mercury and Other Toxic Metals

Unfortunately, proof of mercury intoxication can be difficult to obtain. Blood, urine, stool, hair, and skin analysis tests for mercury and other toxic metals can be misleading. The major problem underlying accurate testing is the fact that the tests are primarily measures of excretion, and *failure to excrete toxins is the primary causative factor in the development of mercury poisoning.* In other words, tests on patients who excrete mercury relatively efficiently often show them to have high levels of this poison, while tests on subjects who don't excrete mercury well and exhibit marked evidence of micromercurialism often show them to have low levels.[177] In fact, the relationship between the body's excretion of mercury and its mercury levels may be contingent on not just the amount of mercury exposure but also the severity of damage and area of deposition. For example, patients may have a falsely negative urine test for mercury if the mercury in their body has damaged their kidneys or deposited primarily in the brain and thyroid. This catch-22 scenario—that is, the sicker patients are, the more likely they are to have a negative test—makes laboratory testing for mercury and other toxic metals particularly challenging.

Porphyrin Tests Are Nonspecific

Dr. Hal Huggins has recommended testing for porphyrins, chemicals excreted in the urine due to mercury's inactivation of hemoglobin formation. However, this test is nonspecific, because other toxic metals as well as root canal toxins also affect porphyrin levels. In addition, the porphyrin test can be expensive, and it is difficult to find a lab that will run it.[178]

Blood Tests Are Nonspecific (but Can Reveal a "Toxic Footprint")

Analyzing the mercury content in the blood is not helpful either. Mercury remains in the blood for only a few minutes before it is sequestered in other tissues. In studies using adult sheep, after placement of amalgams, mercury levels in the blood remained relatively low, while the surrounding body tissues had high concentrations.[179] In addition, in humans, blood tests for other compounds (such as glucose, liver enzymes, iron, and cholesterol) and blood cell counts (red blood cell count, white blood cell count, platelets, hemoglobin, and so on) can determine how mercury may be affecting parts of the body, but they are not specific to systemic intoxication and can often be within normal limits even in patients with obvious symptoms of mercury toxicity.

However, Sam Queen, a leading medical researcher and clinical nutritionist who has studied the issue of amalgam toxicity for decades, has found that the following positive signs can reveal a "toxic footprint" of mercury intoxication:[180]

Elevated: IgA, IgM, B2M (beta-2-microglobulin), total bilirubin, MCV (mean corpuscular volume)

Elevated or Low: BUN (blood urea nitrogen), total cholesterol

Low: cortisol, G-6-PD (glucose-6-phosphate dehydrogenase)

- ► For more information on the effect of toxic metals on blood, and how to interpret these findings, contact Queen's Institute for Health Realities in Colorado. To contact the Institute for Health Realities, call (719) 598-4968 or visit www.healthrealities.org.

Skin Patch Test Not Conclusive and Too Toxic

Some physicians have recommended the use of a mercury skin patch test, which would detect hypersensitivity to mercury as evidence of systemic poisoning, but again a negative test would not be necessarily conclusive. Also, rubbing even a highly diluted amount of mercury on the skin is obviously toxic to the patient, and it should not be tested on pregnant women or those who are severely toxic from amalgams, such as patients with multiple sclerosis.[181]

Hair Analysis Can Be Unreliable

Hair analysis has the advantage of measuring long-term exposure to toxins and can differentiate between different metals, but it has been shown to be unreliable in the past. Results have varied dramatically between split samples (samples of the same hairs sent to two different laboratories), and hair samples can be contaminated by hair sprays, shampoos, dyes, and permanent and straightening products. However, more recent standardization of laboratory analysis as well as better sampling methods have improved the accuracy of the results.[182]

- ► Quality hair analysis laboratories include Analytical Research Labs at (800) 528-4067 or www.arltma.com and Doctor's Data at (800) 323-2784 or www.doctorsdata.com.

Neuropsychological Tests Are Prohibitively Expensive

A neuropsychological test to assess signs of micromercurialism (as well as poisoning from lead, aluminum, nickel, and other toxic metals) is excellent and completely noninvasive for detecting potential Alzheimer's and other dementias. However, no research exists on the value of this testing for the more subtle signs of suboptimal functioning—poor attention span, inability to concentrate, or memory deficit—because the cost of the test is so high that no physician ever orders it without frank signs of significant mental deficit already present.

Scans, Biopsies, and Spinal Taps: Expensive, Invasive, and Rarely Positive

Like a neuropsychological test, an MRI (magnetic resonance imaging) or CAT (computerized axial tomography) scan to test for neurological dysfunction is very

THE USE OF DMPS AND DMSA CHELATION THERAPY

Because of the many unsatisfying results from the testing methods described thus far, provocation (in which a patient takes relatively high doses of the chelating drug or supplement to draw out higher amounts of toxic metals prior to testing) has gained popularity. The most popular of these drugs are DMPS (sodium 2,3-dimercaptopropane-1-sulfonate) and DMSA (meso-2,3-dimercaptosuccinic acid). Even in the case of these two strongly provocative chelators, however, false negative results continue to occur in urinary testing. And there are two further problems with these drugs.

Should Not Be Used When Amalgams Are Still Present

The first problem is that these drugs can sometimes cause severe toxic reactions if they are given—DMPS is usually injected and DMSA is given orally—before all of an individual's amalgams have been removed.[183] Unfortunately, to make a diagnosis based on laboratory testing—especially to receive insurance coverage—this is precisely the time when this challenge test should be run.[184]

DMPS and DMSA Are Mildly to Moderately Toxic Drugs

The second problem is that these two chelators are drugs, and both clinical experience and energetic testing (see appendix 3) have shown that they are mildly to moderately toxic. Although current research (by Daunderer in Germany, Klimnet in Russia, and Aposhian in the United States) has shown both DMPS and DMSA to have no side effects, the clinical experience of holistic practitioners has shown this not to be the case.[185] Among other side effects, these chelation drugs can cause severe aggravation of symptoms, including increased ataxia (muscular incoordination), paralysis, and disturbed mental functioning. In fact, Dr. Hal Huggins now advises patients not to take DMPS because of "the high risk of adverse side effects."[186]* DMPS and DMSA also chelate beneficial minerals along with the toxic ones, leaving many patients exhausted and nutritionally depleted afterward. Boyd Haley, a chemistry professor and leading expert on the toxicity of mercury amalgams, suggests that natural vitamin and mineral supplements should be used first, since DMSA and DMPS do not "effectively enter the cells or cross the brain-blood barrier as do natural compunds."[187]

Because of these issues, DMSA and DMPS are probably best reserved for the treatment of acute and immediately life-threatening exposure to high levels of mercury, such as can occur in industrial settings, or, as Dr. Haley suggests, "only after the use of natural compounds has failed."[188]

*Dr. Huggins does currently use low doses of DMSA, however—typically 25 mg, Monday, Wednesday, and Friday, depending on the patient's particular biochemical profile.

expensive. In addition, these scans detect brain dysfunction only after major pathology has occurred, such as brain injury from a stroke or tumor or general brain atrophy in the case of dementia. Although the newer PET (positron-emission tomography) scans that measure cerebral blood flow are more precise at detecting abnormal brain dysfunction in earlier stages, they are also expensive, and the "mostly harmless" radioactive tracer the scan uses is not usually acceptable to holistically oriented individuals.[189] The most definitive information can be gained from biopsy of brain, kidney, or gut tissue, but no one wants this dangerous procedure performed. Several experts believe that biopsies can actually spread dormant cancer cells in the breast, prostate, and other glands, as well as cause inflammation and even infection in the site. A lumbar puncture, or spinal tap, for the examination of cerebrospinal fluid for abnormalities associated with dementia, multiple sclerosis, or other neurological pathologies is also invasive, expensive, painful, and not without side effects.

Stool Analysis Requires Provocation

Stool analysis for mercury content has become available in the past few years. The body excretes as much as twenty times more mercury through the intestine than the kidneys.[190] Unfortunately, in most cases, in order to be significant stool analysis also requires chelation therapy. As previously discussed, chelation drugs can cause adverse effects such as severe fatigue, mineral depletion, and severe aggravation of symptoms.

Liver Function Tests: An Indirect Method

The liver works to remove toxic metals and chemicals from the body. The efficiency of this process can be measured through the urine. Thus, an individual's ability to excrete foreign toxins, or xenobiotics, can be measured through a urine test. This test, although it doesn't directly measure the amount of mercury existing in the body, is a good indirect test of the body's burden of xenobiotics. It is an excellent measurement of liver function to run on all patients with moderate to major health disturbances, before they commence the amalgam removal process.

- Doctor's Data in Chicago offers a Hepatic Detox Profile that patients can take home, process themselves, and mail in for analysis. To contact the company, health professionals should call (800) 323-2784.

The MELISA Test

The MELISA test is one of the safest and most sensitive measures of mercury toxicity. Since it measures the reaction of the white blood cells (or lymphocytes) to mercury and other heavy metals, it does not require any provocation by toxic chemicals such as DMPS, DMSA, or EDTA. It is also more specific than other tests and can differentiate between an allergic reaction to inorganic or metallic mercury from dental amalgams and ethyl mercury used in thimerosal (the controversial toxic preservative used in vaccines). For more information on the MELISA test, healthcare professionals can call (888) 342-7272 or go to www.neuroscienceinc.com.

THE BEST SOLUTION Correlation of Signs and Symptoms with Laboratory Findings

No perfect objective test for the detection of heavy metal toxicity presently exists. And it's important to remember that no laboratory test ever stands alone. Laboratory tests should always be compared and correlated with a thorough history (e.g., determining the presence and type of fillings and other dental work and the patient's risk of exposure to toxins through occupation or lifestyle); a physical exam (looking for hyperreflexia, a strong clonus response,* finger tremors in the extended hand, and other signs of dysfunction), including inspection of the teeth and mouth; and energetic testing to help determine the specific toxicity and which areas of the body have had the most accumulation and damage. At the present time, the correlation of these tests with a regular blood panel and fecal stool analysis with provocation by nontoxic chelators (such as the drainage remedies described in chapter 2) can give the least stressful and most complete picture of whether heavy metal toxicity is present.

- Doctor's Data laboratory in Chicago is one of the best and most experienced labs in testing for heavy metals. To order a fecal metal test kit, health professionals should call (800) 323-2784.

DETOXIFICATION FROM MERCURY

Clinical Readiness

The sad fact is that those who *most need* to have their mercury amalgam fillings or other toxic dental work removed are often those who *can't handle* the ensuing symptoms of detoxification. For example, neither the luetic individual with chronic anxiety, insomnia, and hand tremors nor the exhausted and achy tuberculinic patient has enough functional liver detoxification pathways, kidney filtration, or efficient intestinal transit to effectively release toxic metals from his or her body during and after removal of amalgam fillings. In fact, if they don't have the capability of detoxifying adequately, many people find that their health worsens after having their amalgams or other toxic metals drilled out.

Systemic Release of Mercury after Amalgam Removal

The toxic effects of having mercury and other metals removed from the mouth are twofold. First, despite the efforts of even the best holistic dentist, inhalation and ingestion of mercury vapor always occurs at some level while the metal is being drilled out. Second, as soon as this "antenna" of large amounts of metal in the head has been removed, the body can begin to more readily sense

*Ankle clonus is a series of abnormal reflex movements induced by sudden foot dorsiflexion (jerking the ball of the foot toward the head). Dr. Dietrich Klinghardt has correlated a strong ankle clonus response with upper motor neuron dysfunction usually secondary to dental amalgams.

and release its stores of toxic metals from other areas in the body. Thus, when the dense amounts of mercury in the mouth have been removed, the body wisely begins to get busy expelling this toxin from elsewhere in the body—from the organs, tissues, and cells in which it has been chronically held.

We might consider this process a form of systemic osmosis—that is, the movement of molecules in the body from areas of greater concentration to areas of lesser concentration. As described earlier in this chapter, mercury in dental amalgam leaches into the body and circulates widely. When this store of mercury is removed, the body begins to release other stores, and gradually deeper and more concentrated stores begin to drain and detoxify. Unfortunately, though, as many holistic practitioners have painfully observed, in individuals with chronic illness (those functioning primarily in the tuberculinic and luetic reaction modes) this innate body wisdom is often seriously limited, and disturbing and sometimes quite debilitating detoxification symptoms can ensue. In contrast, healthier patients (those functioning more in the sycotic and psoric levels) may experience only mild symptoms or none at all.

Clinical Experience and Energetic Testing Most Valuable

A knowledgeable and experienced holistic practitioner can use energetic testing (see appendix 3) to determine exactly when a patient is ready to handle the effects of amalgam removal. In many cases, patients with a multitude of debilitating symptoms require drainage remedies, avoidance of their primary food allergy, treatment of one or more chronic foci, a constitutional homeopathic remedy, and/or quality nutritional supplementation before they are strong enough to effectively detoxify mercury after amalgam filling removal. These treatments can range from a period of weeks to months, and even years.

Energetic testing allows practitioners to assess individuals "in vivo." As practitioners work with patients to strengthen their detoxification systems, energetic testing allows them to measure patients' progress, even when clinical progress is unclear. The testing will inevitably point more directly to the toxic metal as the body becomes clearer and more aware of what is self versus what is *not* self. At the point at which it is evident clinically as well as energetically that toxic metals are impeding a patient's therapeutic progress, the practitioner can then test the patient to determine which remedies will best help him or her during and after amalgam removal and refer the patient to a holistic dentist. For a patient with a strong detoxification system, amalgam removal proceeds quite well and detoxification symptoms are minimal.

Finding a Holistic Dentist

"The Jury's In!"

One phrase that holistic practitioners have heard countless times is that "the jury's still out" in regard to the amalgam toxicity issue. When patients query nonholistic dentists about the safety of amalgam fillings, this response is usually what they hear. This response is so prevalent, in fact, that we might conclude that these allopathically oriented dentists must have read it in an ADA newsletter or heard it at one of their conventions. In point of fact, it's quite a good line. It has the ring of impartiality and awareness of both sides of the issue, and it implies that the dentist has kept up with the scientific literature on amalgam. Unfortunately this is rarely the case. As the great preponderance of scientific research published in peer-reviewed journals attests, not only is the jury *in,* but it's reached a verdict and it's unanimous: mercury amalgam fillings are incontrovertibly guilty of causing chronic debilitating symptoms and serious disease. Thus, it's best to steer clear of the ADA-misinformed dentists who rely on this catchphrase. They're either not reading the current scientific literature or are too immersed in (and toxic from) their habitual pattern of placing amalgam fillings to have the courage to admit their past mistakes and make positive changes.

Referral through Physicians or Holistic Dental Organizations

The best way to find a qualified holistic dentist is through a referral from your holistic doctor or practitioner, who will have dealt with many dentists and seen the results of their work in their mutual patients, including how clearly (or not) those patients test energetically after amalgam removal. Receiving a referral from a friend is another avenue, but it may not be as reliable as that from a doctor who has seen the work of many dentists. Another great source of information is the Dental Amalgam Mercury Solutions (DAMS) organization. It keeps an ongoing list of quality holistic dentists in the United States and elsewhere. DAMS can provide you with a list of amalgam-free holistic dentists in your area as well as a packet of information to help you screen these prospective dentists.

Additional good referrals can come from the three main holistic dental organizations in the United States: the International Academy of Biological Dentistry and Medicine (IABDM), the International Academy of Oral Medicine and Toxicology (IAOMT), and the Holistic Dental Association (HDA). All three of these organizations post on their websites lists of holistic dentists and physicians knowledgeable in the removal and detoxification of mercury. And the Consumers for Dental Choice organization maintains a list of dentists who support amalgam-free dentistry on its website.

▶ To find a local holistic dentist, contact one of the following organizations:

- Consumers for Dental Choice: (202) 822-6307 or www.toxicteeth.org
- DAMS: (651) 644-4572, dams@usfamily.net, or www.amalgam.org
- HDA: (619) 923-3120 or www.holisticdental.org
- IABDM: (281) 651-1745 or www.iabdm.org
- IAOMT: (863) 420-6373 or www.iaomt.org

Interview Questions

When interviewing a potential dentist, always ask first about the mercury amalgam issue, and reject any dentist who is still using this toxic material, especially if you want to have amalgam fillings removed. It is difficult to trust a dentist to *completely and thoroughly* drill out all the amalgam material if he or she is still placing it into some patients' mouths. Furthermore, if the dentist is still using mercury amalgam, it's likely that he or she has not had all the education necessary to learn how to remove amalgam safely.

Another important question is how often the dentist uses inlays and onlays. Many dentists as a matter of routine jump from a filling to a crown and in the process remove substantial amounts of healthy tooth material. In contrast, although it requires more time and skill, the best holistic physicians move from a filling to a bigger filling, or if necessary an inlay (an even larger filling made in a laboratory), if the decay is extensive enough to call for this larger restoration. If an inlay is not sufficient, the practitioner may place an onlay, which covers the top of the tooth like a "mini crown." If the decay or fracture area is very extensive, only then is the placement of a crown warranted. By going through this step-by-step conservative process, holistic dentists remove as little healthy tooth material as possible, leaving more of their patients' natural tooth intact.

You should also ask a potential dentist about the tools and procedures he or she uses during amalgam removal; we'll discuss these next.

Important Procedures in a Holistic Dental Office

A dentist should observe the following precautions to help ensure safe and effective removal of toxic metals:

Rubber dam. The tooth should be isolated with a thin piece of latex, known as a rubber dam, so that particles of the toxic metals that are drilled out of the tooth do not mix with saliva and become absorbed in the gums or swallowed. A rubber dam can have certain drawbacks, however. The clamps used to hold it may stress weak teeth unduly, for example. Other barrier methods are sometimes employed, and in rare cases, if the dentist is very fast and diligent, she or he may work without one. For patients with latex sensitivity, dams made with other materials are available.

Oxygen. Patients should have a nose mask so they can breathe clean compressed air during the procedure and not inhale mercury vapor directly. Some holistic offices don't consider this to be essential, but others do and offer it to all patients.

Section versus drill. The dentist should begin by sectioning out (removing in chunks) the filling as much as possible. This decreases the amount of drilling that is necessary, which grinds down the metal to dust and vapor and therefore releases more toxic material into the gums, saliva, and air.

Low- and high-speed drills. After the filling has been sectioned out, the dentist will use a drill to remove the last bits of amalgam. High-speed drills engender excessive heat and vibration, which can damage a tooth's pulp and dentin. Many holistic dentists utilize a high-speed drill with a new burr, a *very* light touch, and lots of water to drill out the remaining amalgam. But for the very last remaining deep stores of amalgam in the tooth, the dentist should use a low-speed drill (with a maximum of 20,000 rpm) to minimize the risk of killing the tooth. (Low-speed drills should also be employed with shallow cavities and in children, if possible.)

Water. The dental drill and the dental assistant should continue to spray water on the tooth throughout the procedure to keep it cool, since heat directly increases the release of mercury vapor.

Suction. The dental assistant should use a high-speed suction to vacuum up toxic metal particles and vapor released during drilling.

Masks. The dentist and the assistant should both wear mercury vapor masks to protect them from mercury vapor (research has shown that the pituitary glands of dental personnel can have a thousand times more mercury than those of the average person).[191] This is important not only for the health of the dentist and staff, but also for the patient. No one wants to have dental procedures performed by a dentist or staff with significant cerebral deficit secondary to mercury toxicity.*

Glasses. The dentist, assistant, and patient should all wear protective goggles or glasses. The dentist may want magnifying lenses in his or her eyewear so that he or she can see very clearly in order to remove every bit of toxic metal, glue or cement, and decay from the tooth.

Air quality. The dental office should be well ventilated. A powerful vacuum hose should draw the mercury vapor and particles away from the patient and dental staff and deposit it in another part of the building where it can be trapped and filtered. The office should employ negative ion generators to help charge the mercury vapor ions so they can then be collected away from the patient on a positive plate.

Disposal. After mercury amalgam is removed from the mouth, it should be handled like toxic waste (even the ADA insists on this, although it continues to declare that mercury amalgam is perfectly safe). The amalgam must be stored in a tightly closed container and sent to a recycling company that is legally responsible for disposing of it as toxic waste.[192] (Unfortunately, much of the scrap amalgam is illegally going to landfills, to hazardous trash pickup services that may burn it and increase the off-gassing, or down sewer lines.)[193]

*Some patients make it a habit to request morning appointments so that the dentist is fresher and his or her accumulation of toxic metal isn't as great as it will be in the afternoon.

Scheduling and Removal Protocols

No matter how diligently dentists and practitioners endeavor to prepare and detox patients before and after, amalgam removal is always stressful. The release of toxic mercury vapors, the discomfort of drilling, and (for some) the emotions surrounding an invasive dental procedure combine to make the day relatively unpleasant for most patients. However, many holistic patients have successfully reframed this scenario—focusing on the fact that a substantial amount of toxicity is being skillfully removed is quite exciting. These individuals also realize that when they follow the correct detoxification protocols their overall health will greatly benefit. Thus, many knowledgeable patients actually look forward to their holistic dentist appointments.

Scheduling Depends on the Patient's Detoxification Capabilities

For properly prepared healthy individuals functioning primarily at the psoric level, amalgam quadrants may be removed as rapidly as every two to three weeks. In contrast, for ill individuals functioning more in the tuberculinic or luetic reaction modes, removals should be scheduled for no more than once every month to three months, depending on the level of impairment of their excretion pathways. Everyone's particular history and constitution are unique, however, and therefore each patient must be evaluated individually by an experienced holistic practitioner to determine the best schedule for removing amalgam fillings.

quadrant: There are four quadrants in the mouth that divide the mouth into four equal parts. Teeth are described as being located in one of the four quadrants: the right maxillary, left maxillary, right mandibular, or left mandibular.

BEWARE OF REMOVING ALL FILLINGS IN A SINGLE SESSION

A leading holistic dentist has recently claimed that it's best to remove all four amalgam quadrants under light sedation in a single treatment session. In my experience, this is not a wise decision. Patients who have all their amalgam fillings removed in a single session often complain afterward of fatigue, insomnia, and joint pain and present with positive signs of acute mercury intoxication.

CYCLES OF SEVEN

It's sometimes said that the immune system runs on a cycle of seven days. However, the basis underlying this belief is difficult to ascertain. The life span of the red blood cell is about 120 days, white blood cells' life span ranges from several months in a healthy body to only a few days in a toxic environment, and platelets live from 5 to 9 days. Although none of these variations exactly involve the number 7, clinical experience shows that stressing the immune system exactly 14 to 28 days after it has initially been stressed from amalgam removal can be disturbing to some patients. Therefore, patients would be well advised not to schedule an appointment for another amalgam removal on the seventh, fourteenth, twenty-first, or twenty-eighth day after a removal.

Remove the Quadrant with the Highest Galvanic Effect First

The general protocol is to first remove the quadrant that has the highest galvanic current, and thus is the most disturbing to the body. A dentist can determine the strength of galvanic currents with a galvanic meter and through energetic testing. Often, it is obvious which quadrant is most disturbing. For example, if a patient has only one gold crown and it sits between two amalgam fillings, then its quadrant is clearly producing high galvanic currents and should most likely be removed first.

Some holistic practitioners espouse the sequential removal method, though I have not found it to be critical. This method involves testing the galvanic current of each tooth and removing first the amalgam filling that has the highest current, then the next highest, and so forth. However, removing a filling from one quadrant and then from another quadrant is slow, and rather traumatic to the patient in the long run. It also increases the amount of anesthesia that is used overall, since the dentist does not numb and remove dental work from an entire quadrant at a time. Since anesthesia has its own toxic effects (we'll discuss these shortly), quadrant removal, which minimizes the use of anesthesia, is the most efficient.[194]

In General, Remove Visible Mercury First

The most common protocol is to remove all visible amalgam fillings first. Next crowns and amalgam-filled root canals are evaluated; if any mercury exists underneath them—unfortunately, a very common occurrence for work done by nonholistic dentists—it is removed. Nickel, palladium, aluminum, and other toxic metal restorations—crowns, onlays, inlays, and fillings—are then evaluated and, if they are toxic, removed. Finally, any dental foci that need to be treated surgically are addressed.

This sequence can vary, however, according to the individual situation. Sometimes a patient presents with such a toxic dental focus—that is, an infected root canal or abscessed tooth—that it must be addressed immediately. Even in this situation, though, it is best to remove any visible mercury amalgam from this affected tooth first. In fact, sometimes removing the mercury from these dental foci will so dramatically decrease the toxic load at the site that extraction of the tooth may not be necessary. However, when cavitation surgery of the dental focus is clearly necessary, removal of the neighboring amalgam fillings beforehand ensures better healing of the future extraction site. In the case of patients with complex situations—that is, amalgam fillings, gold and porcelain-metal crowns, and several root canals—it is imperative that they be in the hands of an experienced holistic physician and dentist in order to arrive at a comprehensive and effective treatment plan.

Avoiding the "Frying Pan into the Fire" Syndrome

Dr. Hal Huggins's use of this famous phrase refers to the fact that when patients have their amalgam fillings replaced with other toxic materials, their immune system is doubly challenged. That is, they are now stressed by the mercury that is released when fillings are removed and also by the new toxic metals placed in their mouth. Thus, when unknowledgeable dentists remove fillings, crowns, or other dental work and replace them with ones made of gold, porcelain, aluminum, nickel, palladium, or noninert composite materials, in the process using highly toxic glues and cements, patients often become more ill than they were originally—they've jumped "from the frying pan into the fire."

Following the Five Dental Detox Days Protocol (see page 95) and taking appropriate supplements for a few months following amalgam removal will help the body drain, detoxify, and heal as quickly as possible. This is important for detoxifying the body from the effects of not only the metals that were removed but also the glues and cements that were used in the replacement restorations, which by their very nature are always toxic to some degree.

Specific Dental Materials

Metal-Free Considered Best

Unfortunately, there is no perfect material to replace teeth. We want our teeth back—but of course this is not possible. So we must compromise with the least reactive and most inert materials available. Regrettably, there are no easy answers to the question of which materials are the most suitable, because every material has its downside. In the experience of many holistic practitioners, though, using composite materials and keeping the mouth metal-free is the best solution. However, dental realities—such as trying to find a suitable material for a large bridge (spanning two or more tooth extractions)—must also be considered, and sometimes a high-quality gold or porcelain material is necessary.

High-Quality Composite Materials Test as the Most Inert

In 1996, a Spanish study reported that dental plastic composites were potential sources of estrogenic xenobiotics (hormone-altering, and thus possibly cancer-inducing, chemicals).[195] However, this study subjected these dental composites to extreme heat (100°C or 212°F) followed by immersion in the strongest of acid (pH 1) and then alkaline (pH 13) media.[196] More reasonable studies, such as one from Canada, have found that composites release carcinogenic compounds such as bisphenol A at a level 140 times lower than the acceptable levels established by the government. Furthermore, such studies show that the BIS-GMA (bisphenol A glycidyl methacrylate) breakdown products of formaldehyde and methacrylic acid are 10,000 and 1,6000,000 times lower, respectively, than relevant reference doses (the EPA's maximum acceptable oral dose of a toxic substance).[197] Other studies have indicated that composites have a high degree of biocompatibility (are relatively inert and nontoxic in the body) when properly placed by a knowledgeable and well-trained holistic dentist.[198] And researchers at the University of Zurich who tested two popular materials, Tetric Ceram and Herculite, found that these composites, when placed properly, had excellent durability.[199]

Energetic testing has shown that composites are the most inert dental materials presently available. However, the durability of these composite restorations is highly dependent on the technical expertise of the dentist placing them, and patients should therefore search for an experienced holistic dentist who is knowledgeable and skilled in working with these materials. (For help in finding a holistic dentist, consult with the resources listed on page 89.)

Many dentists use glass ceramic and porcelain for restorations even though these materials contain aluminum oxide. They claim that ceramic and porcelain do not leach any aluminum into the body because the aluminum oxide is strongly bound, and some research studies support these claims.[200] However, energetic testing continues to show that these materials are toxic for some patients. It could be that although the aluminum oxide doesn't leach out into the mouth, the metal content is still high enough to have a disturbing electromagnetic field effect. Although even high-quality (inert) composites have minute amounts of metal in them, the levels are so low that they do not engender a significant galvanic effect in the body.

Dental Material Testing

Ideally, all patients will be tested to determine which dental restoration materials are least stressful to their bodies, but testing is especially important for very sensitive individuals. Blood serum compatibility tests are available to help identify existing sensitivity problems to various chemical groups and compounds, or prospective dental materials can be tested energetically on each patient. Some practitioners use both methods to help ensure the patient receives the most compatible material possible. However, neither method is foolproof, and the results of these tests should always be weighed against the findings from the patient's history and exam.

► The two major companies specializing in blood serum compatibility testing for dental materials are Scientific

Health Solutions, Inc., at (800) 331-2303 and Clifford Consulting and Research at (719) 550-0008.

Both blood tests and energetic testing have one thing in common: for the most part, the same relatively inert and nontoxic materials tend to test over and over again as the best. Therefore, patients who don't choose to be tested individually or who are relatively strong and healthy often decide to let their dentist choose the most suitable material out of the "90 percenters"—that is, the materials that consistently tend to test as relatively neutral and nondisturbing. For over a decade, I've kept a list of these "clean" dental materials for just this purpose. This list (see below) can help you and your holistic dentist choose the most suitable material to use.

"Clean" Dental Materials

Note: Manufacturers change the names and compounds in their dental materials often. Therefore, this list should be used *only* as a general guide to assist patients, doctors, and dentists in the selection of the most compatible dental materials. Conferring with a holistic physician or dentist is the best guarantee that you will receive the most suitable material available.

▶ The list of "clean" dental materials requires updates from time to time. For the most up-to-date version, visit www.radicalmedicine.com.

1. *Fillings:* Estelite Palfique, Fuji 7, Heliomolar, Holistore, Point 4, Tetric Ceram
2. *Crowns, Inlays, Onlays, and Bridges:* Eris (Empress II), Paradigm Mz-100 86, Premise Indirect (formerly Belle Glass), Procad, Vita,* RXG Gold (if necessary for a big bridge; otherwise, metal-free materials are best)
3. *Anesthetic:* The Hubbell technique or bupivacaine (Marcaine)
4. *Bonding for Fillings, Inlays, Onlays, and Crowns:* All Bond A and B; Bistite II DC; Clearfil Photo Bond; Estelite Palfique; Holistore Light; Opti Bond I, II, FI, 3A, and 3B; Prelude 1 and 2; Prime and Bond; SE Bond
5. *Cements for Inlays, Onlays, and Crowns:* Dual Cement, Durelon (ESPE) Carboxylate Cement, Pro Tec Cement, Rely X-Luting, Temp Bond, Variolink II
6. *Temporary Cements for Temporary Inlays, Onlays, and Crowns:* Durelon (ESPE) Carboxylate Cement, Temp Bond Clear, Temp Bond NE
7. *For Sealing Composite Fillings after Adjustments:* Permaseal
8. *Dentures:* Flexite Supreme, Vitalon 1060*

*Paradigm Mz-100, Procad, and Vita are used with the Cerec 3D instrument for inlays, onlays, or crowns made in the office.

HOLISTORE AND PREMISE INDIRECT

For over a decade Dr. Douglas Cook, one of the leading holistic dentists in the United States, has found Holistore (from the Den-Mat company) and Premise Indirect (formerly Belle Glass) "with no shade" to be the most compatible and inert dental restoration materials. The "shade" in Belle Glass is an iron oxide. Because the "no shade" version doesn't have this metal tint, it appears colorless and can look a little strange in the mouth. Therefore, if the dental work is in a visible front tooth, the patient might choose the "shade" option for this particular restoration.

The Use of Local Anesthetics in Dentistry

"Clearly Carcinogenic"

In 1994, *Scientific American* published an article questioning the safety of lidocaine, the world's most popular local anesthetic, widely used in dentistry and medicine. In the body, lidocaine breaks down into aniline, a coal tar product that has been known for centuries to be "clearly carcinogenic."[201] In fact, almost *all* local anesthetics approved for use in the United States—lidocaine, mepivacaine, prilocaine, bupivacaine, procaine (novocaine),† and so forth—break down in the body to toxic anilines. In animal studies, aniline (2,6-xylidine) has been linked to the onset of breast cancer (99.999 percent causative), prostate cancer, brain cancer, leukemia, sarcomas, and carcinomas. Anilines have also been identified as causing cardiac arrest, neuromuscular disease, asthma, central or

*Note to holistic dentists: tissue tone 99, no cadmium, heat-cure 20 hours at 167°F.

†Novocaine is known to be quite allergenic, and many dentists have stopped using it simply on that account. (P. Lazarus, "Multiple Sclerosis and Amyotrophic Lateral Sclerosis: More Hope Than We Think?" *Let's Live,* April 1980, 72.)

peripheral nerve injury, dementia, severe depression, and possibly even suicide and criminal behavior.[202]

Why Does Southern California Have Less Cancer than Northern California?

In 1994, after examining numerous epidemiological studies of cancer in California, a California oral surgeon, Dr. Alfred Nickel, noted that northern California had a significantly higher rate of breast cancer than southern California. He proposed that this difference could be due to the different types of dental anesthetics used in each region. Nickel cited the fact that for more than fifty years dentists and oral surgeons in southern California had been commonly using the Hubbell technique, an alternative aniline-free anesthesia system that incorporates oxygen, Demerol, and barbiturates like Brevital and Pentothal. In contrast, patients in northern California typically received only various types of local anesthetics during their dental visits. Dr. Nickel stated in a 1997 interview that this link between cancer and local anesthetics, especially in the case of the high-socioeconomic-status Bay Area population, which often utilizes regular and cosmetic dentistry, "may be the most significant factor in U.S. cancer mortality since 1930."[203]*

The Hubbell Technique and Bupivacaine Are Currently the Safest Options

Dr. Nickel developed an aniline-free anesthetic called Septocaine (articaine) and had it approved by the FDA in April 2000. Unfortunately, it contains both a synthetic preservative and epinephrine—a compound that can stimulate the sympathetic nervous system and cause adverse heart and neurological reactions in many sensitive patients. Therefore, until another alternative is available, the Hubbell technique is a safer option.

Another alternative is the preservative-free, epinephrine-free local anesthetic bupivacaine, also known as Marcaine. Studies have shown that in the body bupivacaine breaks down into aniline at a greatly decreased rate, as much as 85 percent less than other anesthetics.[204] The liver and kidneys can effectively purge this smaller residual of aniline from the body, particularly if supported by nutritional supplements and drainage remedies after the dental visit. One uncomfortable drawback of bupivacaine is that it is longer acting than other local anesthetics; however, still being numb at dinnertime after receiving a filling in the morning is a small price to pay for less exposure to aniline.

▶ To order bupivacaine, contact the ApothéCure pharmacy in Dallas, Texas, at (800) 969-6601. Unfortunately, until it is available in dental carpules, dentists must order the anesthetic in vials and transfer it into carpules in their offices.

Other anesthesia alternatives include acupuncture, auriculotherapy (ear acupuncture), hypnosis, or even no anesthetic at all if the filling is shallow and the patient is not very sensitive to pain. Music during the procedure is also beneficial; the journal *Anesthesia and Analgesia* recently reported that when patients can hear music they enjoy during their treatment they require significantly lower levels of anesthetic sedation.[205]

More Research Is Needed

Clearly, much more research needs to be conducted on anesthetics, and once again, the FDA has much to answer for in regard to its lack of response in informing the public of this clear carcinogen. In the meantime, avoiding anesthetics as much as possible is the safest option. When anesthetics are necessary, patients should request preservative-free, epinephrine-free bupivacaine or the Hubbell technique. They also should consider supplementing with extra antioxidants, using drainage remedies, and re-dosing with the appropriate constitutional homeopathic remedy after dental treatments.

The Acute Detoxification Period

There is no one perfect detoxification protocol for cleansing the body of toxic metals. Many holistic practitioners have their own particular detoxification "recipe" that has proved successful over time. For detoxification following the removal of amalgam fillings, the Five Dental Detox Days Protocol (see page 95) has proved effective for me for many years.

Mercury is excreted from the body primarily through the bowels; studies have shown that the fecal excretion of heavy metals is generally five times that of urinary excretion.[206] In 1991, researchers in Sweden placed one

*Lung cancer became a major hazard in the 1930s, which is attributed to an increase in smoking during World War I. (D. W. Kufe et al., eds., *Holland Frei Cancer Medicine,* 6th edition [Hamilton, ON: BC Decker, 2003], section 27.)

small amalgam filling in an eleven-year-old girl who had no previous history of cavities or fillings. They then measured the mercury content of her stool for the next three days. The researchers were quite surprised to find that in comparison to a control group, the fecal excretion of mercury in this child was *enormous* the third day after the dental visit, measured at an astronomical level of 400 micrograms in a twenty-four-hour period. To put this number into perspective, the WHO standard for the maximum acceptable total intake of mercury from food is 45 micrograms in a twenty-four-hour period.[207]

Through the information gleaned from this and other research studies, it is clear that mercury excretion peaks approximately three days or so after the placement of amalgam fillings. With this cycle in mind, the five-day period following the *removal* of amalgam (or other toxic metals) is the most essential time period to actively encourage the effective detoxification and release of toxic metals. The Five Dental Detox Days Protocol is an acute detoxification process designed to maximize the body's ability to detoxify during these five days—the day of removal and the four days afterward—when high levels of toxic metal are released.

Even under normal systemic metabolic conditions, and even more so when the body is processing toxic metals, intermediary metabolites such as urea, pyruvic acid, lactic acid, and so forth are produced. Thus, during the five crucial days following a dental procedure, the patient's system is burdened not only with toxic metals but also with these endotoxins, as well as the exotoxins produced by the anesthetic, cement, and glue used during the procedure. However, in my experience, when patients adhere to the protocol guidelines during these five days—and they have been adequately prepared beforehand—they rarely experience any negative symptoms or toxic sequellae (aftereffects) following amalgam removal.

OUTLINE: THE FIVE DENTAL DETOX DAYS PROTOCOL

Here is a quick "big picture" look at the Five Dental Detox Days Protocol. The key point in this protocol is to treat *chronic* mercury amalgam toxicity *acutely* just after removal of fillings, for the most optimal excretion of heavy metals.

- **Don't Get Constipated!** It is important to have good bowel movements during these five detox days; a colonic or home enema may be indicated.
- **Double (or Triple or More) Dosages.** Doubling or tripling up (or more) on dosages of supplements and herbal remedies can greatly enhance the mobilization and excretion of toxic metals out of the body.
- **Mineral Supplementation.** Sulfur crystals, Quinton marine plasma, Schuessler's cell salts, or other quality mineral supplements are essential in chelating toxic metals out of the body and replenishing needed minerals.
- **Re-dose Homeopathic Remedy.** After dental drilling, re-dose your constitutional homeopathic remedy or Arnica 30C and/or Hypericum 30C, if you are not on your constitutional remedy.
- **Nutrient-Dense Diet.** Avoid toxic refined foods and allergenic foods as well as high-oxalate foods such as spinach, soy, peanuts, and chocolate. Eat a nutrient-dense diet to further ensure efficient bowel transit time and heal leaky gut.
- **Oral Cleansing.** Once a day, do Dr. Karach's oil pulling treatment.
- **Lifestyle.** Drink pure water, get extra sleep, and don't plan any major events during these five days. Infrared or low-temperature saunas can also be very helpful in detoxification. Be sure to call your holistic doctor and dentist if you are not feeling well.

The Five Dental Detox Days Protocol In Depth

The following detoxification recommendations help stimulate the most efficient release of heavy metals from the body during these five crucial days of *acute* detoxification. After this period of intense detoxification, doses are reduced for longer-term chelation over the next three to six months, which is the average amount of time it takes the majority of patients to effectively detox mercury from their system.*

*Three to six months is *generally* the period of time that the body needs to detoxify from mercury amalgam poisoning. However, mercury and other metals can still be concentrated and stored in focal areas, such as the tonsils, teeth, and genitals, and in scar tissue. As these foci are treated and cleared, often patients will need to re-dose with Black Poplar and other chelating and antioxidant products to effectively remove these deeper stores of heavy metals. In the same manner, when patients are prescribed their constitutional homeopathic remedy—the deepest treatment anyone can receive—toxic metals and chemicals may arise once again (as noted clinically as well as through energetic testing) in their more knowledgeable and wiser bodily terrains.

Don't Get Constipated

Eighty percent of toxic metals are excreted through the colon, so it is very important to have good bowel movements during these five detox days, and a colonic or home enema may well be indicated. Note that the highest excretion is on the third day, so you may want to schedule a colonic for that day in advance to ensure optimal intestinal detoxification.

Colon Cleansing

A colonic or a home enema during the Five Dental Detox Days Protocol can help ensure a more complete release of mercury and other toxins. Additionally, a colon cleansing supplement, such as bentonite clay, charcoal, or slippery elm, can help the body more effectively bind the toxic metals and evacuate them through the bowels. Herbal Laxative from Thorne is a good product. Quality acidophilus and bifidobacterium also greatly support the colon in regenerating healthy flora, which assists in more efficiently clearing toxic metals. Original Synbiotic Formula and High ORAC Synbiotic Formula from BioImmersion are recommended before, during, and after the five detox days. (For more information about BioImmersion products, see chapter 7.)

- Herbal Laxative is available from Thorne at (800) 228-1966. Original Synbiotic Formula and High ORAC Synbiotic Formula are available from BioImmersion at www.bioimmersion.com or (425) 451-3112.

Double (or Triple or More) Dosages

Doubling up on the chelation remedies you are taking (e.g. Black Poplar, Mountain Pine, Rosemary, White Willow, Pure Radiance C, enzymes, etc.) during these five days is completely appropriate as you encourage the movement of heavy metals out of the body.

Plant Stem Cell Remedies

The plant stem cell (PSC) remedies described in detail in chapter 2 help heal and strengthen the body's excretion capabilities. Black Poplar is the primary chelating remedy prescribed before and after amalgam removal, but Mountain Pine, European Alder, White Willow, Rosemary, Juniper, and other gemmotherapy botanicals can also be an essential part of the detoxification protocol.

Made from the embryonic parts of plants, plant stem cell remedies have demonstrated a remarkable ability to significantly reduce the body's stores of toxic metals. Research studies and clinical experience have shown the following plant stem cell remedies to be especially effective chelation agents.*

Black Poplar (*Populus nigra*): This herbal extract made from the buds of the black poplar tree is considered to be the polycrest detoxifier—that is, the detoxification remedy that is most effective at removing toxic metals and chemicals from the body. This number one position would make perfect sense to environmentalists who already use poplar trees in *phytoremediation*—the use of plants to clean up toxins in the environment. In fact, poplar trees have been described as being able to "suck up" toxic waste "like soda straws" from the ground and safely metabolize these toxic compounds in their woody tissue.[208] In the same way, these young buds help remove heavy metals and toxic chemicals from our bodies, primarily through the action of the enzyme phytochelatin synthase. This enzyme polymerizes sulfur-rich glutathione into phytochelatins, which bind strongly to such heavy metals as cadmium, mercury, and arsenic.[209] This exceptionally superior form of chelation is specific and selective for toxic metals, and therefore it does not deplete the body of essential minerals, as do chelation protocols using synthetic pharmaceutical drugs (such as EDTA, DMPS, and DMSA).

Mountain Pine (*Pinus montana*): This remedy contains the powerful flavonoid antioxidant pycnogenol, well known to naturopaths in the treatment of osteoarthritis. Mountain Pine is known as the primary plant stem cell remedy for arthritis. Lesser known, however, is its effectiveness as a chelator of heavy metals from the body.† It is

*The following information derives from PSC Distribution (www.epsce.com). As discussed in chapter 2, these highly potent remedies should be prescribed carefully; like all natural medications, they have contraindications for certain patients.

†Pycnogenol has been shown in research studies to be effective in treating a variety of disorders including ADHD, adverse menopausal symptoms, asthma, and diabetic leg ulcers (G. Belcaro et al., "Diabetic Ulcers: Microcirculatory Improvement and Faster Healing with Pycnogenol," *Clinical and Applied Thrombosis/Hemostasis* 12 (July 2006): 318–23). Other potent antioxidant constituents in Mountain Pine include ascorbic acid, catechin, cysteine, and pinocembrin. This plant stem cell remedy also contains adenine, also known as vitamin B_4, which is important for energy production and the induction of apoptosis ("programmed cell death," which is essential in the treatment of cancer). Mountain Pine also contains significant amounts of vitamins B_1, B_2, B_3, and B_5 and calcium, as well as trace amounts of easy-to-assimilate copper, iron, magnesium, manganese, phosphorus, potassium, and zinc.

often prescribed for patients burdened with toxic metals who also suffer from arthritis, soft-tissue destruction (in the cartilage, tendons, and ligaments), and other musculoskeletal pain and dysfunction.

White Willow (*Salix alba*): Since aspirin medications originally derived from white willow, it makes sense that this remedy, known as a "natural NSAID,"* is well known for relieving joint and muscle pain and inflammation (as in cases of rheumatoid arthritis, osteoarthritis, bursitis, tendonitis, fibromyalgia, and so on). White Willow has also been shown to be an effective chelator for mercury and other heavy metals.† Therefore, it is an excellent choice for patients who both need to detoxify from their mercury amalgam fillings and have musculoskeletal pain and dysfunction.

Evidence shows that at a standard dose, White Willow is the equivalent of 50 mg of aspirin—that is, a very small dose (the recommended dose of aspirin as a painkiller being 325 mg every six to eight hours). Furthermore, White Willow doesn't impair blood coagulation to the same extent that aspirin does, nor does it significantly irritate the stomach lining. Nevertheless, to be safe, the risks of aspirin therapy should be considered to apply to White Willow. Thus, this remedy should not be given to children (to avoid the risk of Reye's syndrome); to patients with aspirin allergies, bleeding disorders, kidney disease, or idiopathic thrombocytic purpura; or to individuals who are taking blood thinners (such as Coumadin or Plavix) or other anti-inflammatory medications.

European Alder (*Alnus glutinosa*): This major remedy for both heart disease and gastrointestinal dysfunction additionally helps clear toxic metals and pesticides from the body.‡ Because it increases cerebral blood flow, European Alder is also indicated for the most common syndrome resulting from heavy metal poisoning: memory loss and senile dementia.

- Plant stem cell remedies, as well as educational seminars on their use, are available to healthcare practitioners from two companies in the United States: PSC Distribution at (631) 477-6696 or www.epsce.com and Gemmos LLC at (877) 417-6298 or www.gemmos-usa.com. Plant stem cell remedies should be prescribed by a knowledgeable practitioner, as they are contraindicated for some patients.

Vitamins and Enzymes

Because the potent plant stem cell remedies are loaded with bioavailable vitamins, minerals, amino acids, and other nutrients, patients who take them do not need to take large quantities of other nutritional supplements. However, natural vitamin C and enzymes are almost always indicated.

Pure Radiance C: Pure Radiance C is derived from organic and wild berries; tests show it to be far superior to conventional vitamin C supplements that are chemically synthesized and are often derived from genetically modified compounds that most often originate from China.

Take approximately 2 capsules per day before amalgam removal. After the removal, double the dose to 4 capsules or more per day for five days. Then return to the normal dose of 2 capsules per day for the next three to six months.

This natural vitamin C has powerful antioxidant activity. It contains camu camu berries wildcrafted in the Amazon (one of the richest sources of vitamin C), amla berries wildcrafted in the Himalayan valleys (the most revered and regenerative herb in Ayurvedic medicine), and a blend of organic blueberries, raspberries, cranberries, cherries, rose hips, and lemon peel, which provide beneficial cofactors such as bioflavonoids, quercetin, hesperidin, anthocyanins, and proanthocyanins to further activate antioxidant activity. Many other types of vitamin C supplements contain ascorbic acid, only a fractionated part of the vitamin C complex, which can hyperacidify the body and may cause excessive bleeding and diarrhea. In contrast, Pure Radiance C is alkalinizing and does not cause excessive bleeding or stimulate diarrhea.

**NSAID* is the acronym for nonsteroidal anti-inflammatory drug, examples of which include aspirin and ibuprofen.

†The naturally occurring salicylic acid in White Willow can stimulate antibiotic, anti-inflammatory, and immune system responses. This remedy also contains antioxidants including apigenin, ascorbic acid, beta-carotene, catechin, cyanidin, and rutin; vitamins A, B_1, B_2, and B_3 and calcium; and trace amounts of easy-to-assimilate chromium, iron, magnesium, manganese, phosphorus, potassium, selenium, silica, and zinc.

‡European Alder contains brassinolide, a plant sterol that can reduce and detoxify fermentation in the gastrointestinal tract, and lupeol, a triterpene that has shown promise in the treatment of pancreatic cancer. This plant stem cell remedy also contains L-serine, which plays a central role in the production of myelin for nerve regeneration.

▶ Pure Radiance C is available from the Synergy Company at (800) 723-0277 or www.thesynergycompany.com.

Digestive Enzymes: Digestive enzymes are often required to enhance the breakdown of toxins and help the body more efficiently eliminate waste. Over the decades I have found that BioGest and Dipan-9 from Thorne test best, as well as Gastric Comfort (#601) for those who have a history of ulcers or gastritis. Dipan-9 and Gastric Comfort can also double as metabolic enzymes, if additional catalytic energy is needed to break down toxic metals and chemicals.

Dipan-9 is a proteolytic formula—the protease (protein-digesting) enzyme in it helps break down protein waste products and destroy the protein coats of harmful organisms in the gastrointestinal tract and blood. Proteolytic enzymes further help eliminate incompletely digested food particles, which allows the immune system a rest, and thus, more efficient surveillance of the entire body. This increased surveillance translates into an increased capacity to recognize and defend against toxins such as mercury and other heavy metals through the release of macrophages and natural killer cells. Finally, through this more rapid and efficient cleansing of undigested food particles, proteolytic enzymes support more complete gastrointestinal functioning and therefore more effective excretion of toxic metals.

Although Gastric Comfort does not contain protease, the other enzymes in this formula—amylase, lipase, cellulase, etc.—have a similar detoxifying effect in patients with ulcers, gastroesophageal reflux disease (GERD), and a sensitivity to the stronger protease action on the gastric and intestinal mucosa.

▶ Dipan-9 is available from Thorne at www.thorne.com and Gastric Comfort is available from Enzymes, Inc., at www.enzymesinc.com.

Mineral Supplementation

On each of the five detox days, take 1 or 2 vials of Quinton marine plasma (isotonic or hypertonic) to replace minerals displaced by the mercury fillings. Additionally, take 1 teaspoon to 1 tablespoon of sulfur crystals (MSM) two, three, or four times a day to help support liver detoxification and activate glutathione. Finally, Dr. Schuessler's cell salts (2 to 4 tablets, two to three times a day) can be indicated to further support and strengthen the teeth and jawbone after the drilling.

Quinton Marine Plasma

The very assimilable Quinton marine sea plasma is a new addition to my five detox days recommendations. French physiologist René Quinton (1897–1925) discovered that the nutrient-rich environment of enormous oceanic plankton blooms creates an excellent supplement for our internal biological terrain, almost perfectly matching the 7.4 to 7.6 alkaline pH of blood and extracellular fluid. For over a century, Quinton and other scientists and physicians have clinically demonstrated that this "marine plasma" assists in healing a diverse number of conditions.

Drinking the vials is the most typical method of application, at a recommended dose of 1 or 2 vials daily during the dental detox protocol. Furthermore, holding the contents of each vial in the mouth for two to five minutes before swallowing enhances the absorption of minerals into traumatized tooth, gum, and jawbone tissues after drilling. These vials are also indicated after cavitation surgery to help remineralize the tissues and normalize bleeding at the surgery site. Quinton's marine plasma has additionally been successfully implanted rectally and vaginally, sprayed into the nasal sinuses, inhaled with a nebulizer, and used as a dental rinse.

This supplement is extremely effective, yet in the great majority of cases it can be used by even the most sensitive patient without fear of strong reactions. However, two possible contraindications should be noted. Quinton hypertonic plasma (with three times the mineral concentration of human blood) has the potential to increase blood pressure and anxiety in some cases. Therefore, in patients with hypertension or significant anxiety, the isotonic form should be used.

▶ For more information on Original Quinton products, go to www.originalquinton.com.

Sulfur

Sulfur is the third most abundant mineral found in our bodies, surpassed only by calcium and phosphorus. All body cells contain sulfur compounds. We receive sulfur primarily through the ingestion of protein, from the two major sulfur-containing amino acids: cysteine and methionine.* Any dietary excess of these amino acids is oxidized to sulfate and either excreted in the urine or stored in the form of glutathione in the liver. Glutathione is a key antioxidant, essential in detoxifying pharmaceutical drugs and other toxic compounds, free radicals, reactive oxygen species, and other signs of oxidative stress.

Sulfur is necessary for the production of cartilage, heparin (a blood anticoagulant), fibrinogen (which is essential for blood clotting), thiamine (vitamin B_1), biotin, lipoic acid, and coenzyme A (which is involved in the metabolism of carbohydrates, proteins, and lipids and in the production of energy). It is also essential for the production of insulin in the pancreas, for the phase II detoxification sulfation pathway in the liver, for creation of the protective mucosal barrier in our intestines, for balanced hormone metabolism and excretion, and for the production of collagen (for joint support) and keratin (for healthy hair, nails, and skin).

In the 1970s, Stanley Jacob, M.D., at the University of Oregon, was researching the effects of dimethyl sulfoxide (DMSO). He found phenomenal success utilizing this organic sulfur compound in pain reduction and wound healing. However, since DMSO had a bitter taste and disturbingly pungent odor and sometimes caused skin irritation when applied topically, Jacob began to experiment with a DMSO metabolite, dimethyl sulfone or methylsulfonylmethane (MSM). He found MSM to be more beneficial since it was odorless, did not cause any skin irritation, and was retained in the body for significantly longer periods than DMSO. Researchers believe that this longer retention—DMSO is held for 120 hours, versus MSM at 480 hours—was due to the "extensive tissue building" that MSM accomplishes in the body. Furthermore, Dr. Jacob reported astounding healing benefits with MSM, including significant pain relief, anti-inflammatory effects, muscle spasm reduction, antiparasitic properties (particularly against giardia), immune normalizing effects (which are helpful in cases of rheumatoid arthritis, lupus, and scleroderma), and the reduction of constipation through restoration of normal intestinal peristalsis.[210]

MSM quickly became a popular nutritional supplement and was soon a major multilevel-marketing favorite. Although many benefited from the wide distribution of MSM, the negative aspects of multilevel marketing—the pressure to sign up as many people as possible to make more money—somewhat tarnished the reputation of this important sulfur compound. Furthermore, many companies added other nutrients and even chemical preservatives to their MSM products, which often disturbed or diluted its effectiveness in the body. Other companies pulverized MSM crystals and added anticaking ingredients so they could encapsulate it in pill form, which, as Patrick McGean, an independent researcher, has found, disrupted the sulfur crystal matrix, resulting in a less potent and less effective product.

After years of lesser-quality MSM products that do not produce adequate results in patients, one product, Lignisul MSM Granular Crystals, has finally tested consistently. This MSM product is made up of natural unpulverized sulfur crystals, with no additives. These sulfur crystals have become an important component of my amalgam detoxification protocol, as well as an important mineral supplement for almost every patient.

▶ Lignisul MSM Granular Crystals are available from PC NetwoRx, Inc., at www.msm-msm.com or (800) 453-7516.

Sulfur can greatly enhance the mercury detoxification process. It has a major antioxidant action in the body, being a major sulfur donor for the amino acids methionine and cysteine, enabling formation of glutathione (the most powerful antioxidant in our bodies), and potentiating nutritional antioxidants such as vitamin C, vitamin E, coenzyme Q10, and selenium. When sulfur combines with mercury it forms mercuric sulfate, a compound that can be expelled from cells, processed by the liver, and excreted through the gut. Sulfur further enhances the permeability of cell membranes, which makes it easier for cells to receive nutrition and excrete waste products and toxins. Furthermore, the sulfur compound MSM is one of the few antioxidants that can easily pass the blood-brain barrier, allowing it to stimulate nerve cells to start excreting waste products, restore cell

*A small percentage of sulfur comes in the form of nonprotein foods such as garlic, onions, and broccoli. Methionine is an essential amino acid, meaning that it cannot be synthesized by the body and we must receive it in our diets. Cysteine can be synthesized by our bodies, but the process requires a steady supply of sulfur. Taurine and cystine, the other two sulfur-containing amino acids, are synthesized from cysteine. (M. Nimni et al., "Are We Getting Enough Sulfur in Our Diet?" *Nutrition and Metabolism* 4:24 [2007], www.nutritionandmetabolism.com/content/4/1/24.)

membrane elasticity and permeability, and repair oxidative damage to these sensitive brain cells and tissues.

Lignisul MSM Granular Crystals, and even MSM in general, has shown no evidence of toxicity. Some patients have reported detoxification effects—primarily gastrointestinal distress in the form of diarrhea—but they seem to recover quickly upon stopping this supplementation. Another common side effect is a skin rash, but this psoric sign is almost always a signal of successful detoxification and moving in the *correct* direction of health. Thus, in most cases doctors and patients celebrate this sign of the elimination of toxins through the skin. However, if the rash becomes too disturbing, nonsuppressive herbal creams may be helpful, and the patient should stop taking sulfur until the intensity of the rash subsides.

Often patients confuse MSM with sulfa drugs or sulfites in wine; if they have a bad reaction to the latter, they think they are allergic to sulfur. Such an allergy is impossible, however, since sulfur is an essential element and is in every cell in our bodies. In fact, sulfa drugs do not contain sulfur; they are sulfonamides—that is, synthetically made antibiotics.

Paradoxically, although MSM often relieves muscle cramps, a small percentage of patients experience increased muscle cramping, especially in the calves at night, when taking this product. Supplementation with calcium and magnesium usually resolves this issue.

▶ Thorne's Magnesium Citramate and Calcium Magnesium Citramate are excellent nutritional supplements for relieving muscle cramping. Contact Thorne Research, Inc., at (800) 228-1966.

MSM also has topical applications. Patients with gingivitis, or even the more severe periodontitis, report exceptional healing of their gum pockets and reduced bleeding when they brush with sulfur crystals two times a day.

Cell Salts

Even with the use of a high-quality drill expertly managed by a knowledgeable holistic dentist, drilling is still very stressful to the teeth and surrounding tissues. Cell salts, also known as tissue salts, can be extremely helpful in strengthening the teeth, gums, and jawbone after amalgam removal. These remedies can also be miraculous in saving a weakened tooth threatened with root canal treatment, as may be the case when a patient continually feels pain and swelling for weeks or months after a new dental restoration has been placed. When gentle equilibration of the filling, inlay, onlay, or crown (drilling away any high spots that interfere with occlusion) doesn't alleviate the symptoms, the use of cell salts can often strengthen the tissues and reduce the swelling enough to obviate a root canal or extraction of the tooth. As is the case for all remedies, it is most helpful to have a knowledgeable practitioner use energetic testing to best determine which of these cell salts the patient requires, as well as the particular dosage and the estimated duration of treatment.

▶ Cell salts can be found at most health food stores. They also can be ordered from Seroyal at (800) 263-5861.

Cell salts were developed by Dr. William Schuessler in 1872. He believed that illness was often related to a deficiency of one of twelve mineral substances. The salts are triturated (ground) together with lactose and formed into soft tablets. When the tablets dissolve sublingually (under the tongue), the salts pass into the bloodstream and then act in a homeopathic manner as catalytic agents (stimulating chemical reactions or processes) in the body. (For more extensive information on cell salts, see page 338.)

***Calcarea fluorica* 6X:** Calc fluor, as this salt is known, is found in all the bones in the body as well as in tooth enamel. As a supplement, it can strengthen loose teeth and support the remineralization of enamel. The typical dose is two tablets taken one to three times a day for at least a few weeks before and after dental drilling. Calc fluor is also a good alternative to the toxic sodium fluoride used as an anti-cavity supplement; children can take two tablets one to three times a week.

***Calcarea phosphorica* 6X:** Calc phos, as this salt is known, is the most widespread mineral salt in the body and is found in literally every tissue. It is a reinforcing and remineralizing remedy that gives solidity to bones and tissues and can also help heal gums after dental drilling. The typical adult dosage is two tablets taken one to three times a day for at least a few weeks before and after dental drilling. Like Calc fluor, Calc phos is an effective anti-cavity agent, and it also can encourage tooth growth in cases of delayed eruption or otherwise abnormal bone or tooth development; children can take two tablets one to three times a week.

***Magnesium phosphoricum* 6X:** This mineral salt, familiarly known as Mag phos, is found in the blood, bones, teeth, nerves, and brain. It is most well known for its antispasmodic function, and it is often prescribed for the treatment of muscle spasms and menstrual cramps. For the same reason, since much of pain sensitivity is due to cramping and tension, Mag phos is often indicated for all types of pain reduction, including teething and after the trauma of dental drilling. The typical adult dosage is two tablets taken one to three times a day for at least a few weeks after dental drilling. Mag phos is also beneficial for hardening tooth enamel and in cases of deficient bone and tooth mineralization, and it is often prescribed along with Calc phos to both the young (infants and children) and the old (to reduce or prevent osteoporosis).

***Silicea* 6X:** Silica is found in connective tissues, bones, hair, nerves, teeth, the pancreas, and the heart. Silicea cell salt is beneficial after dental drilling because it helps restore silica, giving stability to the connective tissue, gums, teeth, and jawbone. The typical adult dosage is two tablets taken one to three times a day for at least a few weeks after dental drilling. Silicea is often given in conjunction with Calc fluor, Calc phos, or Mag phos to children with delayed development of the teeth and bones. Caution: This remedy can have the additional action of discharging foreign materials from the body. Therefore, homeopathic Silicea should *cautiously* be prescribed to individuals who have implants (hip, breast, dental, organs, pins, or screws) and *never* during pregnancy.

Re-dose Homeopathic Remedy

Since dental drilling can potentially antidote a constitutional remedy, you should re-dose yours at least once upon returning from the dental office. Those who are not on a constitutional remedy should re-dose with Arnica montana 30C to reduce swelling and inflammation. If the drilling was particularly deep, Hypericum 30C, the "arnica of the nerves," should be taken at a different time during the day. (For instance, take Arnica 30C in the morning and Hypericum 30C in the evening.)

With significant swelling, bleeding, and inflammation, Arnica 200C may be indicated. Similarly, if there are signs of nerve damage—most specifically numbness along the cheek and jaw lasting longer than a day—Hypericum 200C or even the 1M potency may be needed. Contact a certified homeopath or naturopathic physician for guidance on how to use these higher potencies.

- ▶ Arnica and Hypericum are available at most health food stores in the 30C potency.

Nutrient-Dense Diet

To further ensure efficient bowel transit time, it is important to avoid your major food allergy. For most of us, this is either dairy or wheat/gluten foods. Of course, avoiding sugar, trans fats, and other toxic refined foods will also support healthy digestion and more efficient detoxification. Organic bone broths (high in glycine to heal leaky gut), fermented vegetables and juices, and eating according to the wise traditions of our foremothers and forefathers will further help eliminate mercury and is essential for optimal intestinal elimination during these five days.*

Reducing our intake of foods high in oxalates is also important, since these toxic salts bind with mercury, lead, and other heavy metals and deposit them in tissues where they can't be easily chelated out of the system. A high-oxalate diet can also cause kidney stones and vulvodynia (pain in and outside of the vagina) and has been implicated in autism and chronic fatigue. Foods especially high in oxalates include:

Spinach	Soy protein
Peanuts	Pecans
Lemon peel	Lime peel
Rhubarb	Swiss chard
Parsley	Sweet potatoes
Pokeweed	Black pepper
Chocolate	Instant coffee
Leeks	Tea
Okra	Wheat germ

William Shaw, Director of the Great Plains Laboratory for Health, Nutrition and Metabolism, reports that

*Also see the Weston A. Price diet recommendations at www.westonaprice.org/environmental-toxins/1447-mad-as-a-hatter.html.

calcium and magnesium citrate are effective binders of oxalates, allowing this salt form of oxalic acid to be precipitated out through the stool. Therefore, supplements such as Calcium Magnesium Citramate or Magnesium Citramate by Thorne are beneficial to take with meals during this detox period.[211]

Oral Cleansing

The age-old Ayurvedic method of "oil pulling," as described by Dr. Karach, is especially helpful in drawing out the toxins (mercury, anesthetics, bacteria, etc.) in the mouth and surrounding tissues after dental drilling. After returning home from the dental office, and for each of the five detox days, hold a few tablespoons of organic unrefined sesame oil in your mouth for as long as you can (anywhere from three to ten minutes), intermittently swishing it around, "chewing" it, and gargling. When you can't hold it any longer (without serious drooling), spit it out. Then gargle and rinse with salt and baking soda, and brush your teeth.

As the oil absorbs lipophilic (fat-loving) toxic chemicals, metals, and microbes from the oral mucosa, it changes color from golden to white and becomes thinner in consistency. The degree of these changes indicates the level of toxins in the mouth as well as throughout the entire body, since the blood circulates through the oral mucosa. Environmentally sensitive patients may particularly benefit from the chemical-clearing effects of this treatment.

Although the use of coconut oil is becoming increasingly popular, I have not found it to be as effective as sesame oil, which has stood the test of time for millennia in Ayurvedic medicine. Additionally, the natural lecithin content and high levels of oleic, linoleic, and linolenic oils in sesame oil render it particularly nutritive to nearby brain cells and nerves.

- ▶ Unrefined sesame oil can be found at any health food store; of course, organic is preferred. Organic virgin sesame seed oil is also available from Biotics (www.bioticsresearch.com); healthcare practitioners may want to stock it in their offices.

Lifestyle

Drink plenty of pure water, get extra sleep (eight to even ten hours per night would not be excessive while your body is healing), eat as pure a diet as possible, and don't plan any major events or strenuous activities during these five detox days.

Low-temperature, particularly infrared, saunas can also be appropriate during the detox days, though caution must be used. The use of saunas for detoxification has a long history. In Almaden, Spain, where mercury in the form of cinnabar (a yellowish red mercuric sulfide) has been mined for centuries, miners with clinical signs of mercurialism are placed in a saunalike environment where they can sweat it out.[212] During this treatment, the concentration of mercury in their sweat is considerably greater than that of their urine.[213] Thus, sauna or sweat therapy for *acute poisoning* from recent heavy metal exposure can be quite effective, especially for individuals who are relatively robust and strong.

In contrast, in the treatment of *chronic* mercury poisoning from years of exposure to amalgam fillings, many holistic practitioners are in agreement with Dr. Mats Hanson, the scientific director of the Swedish Association of Dental Mercury Patients, who has found that "saunas can . . . be useful in connection with amalgam replacement, but not before that and not on a long-term basis."[214] As further noted by Dr. Michael Lebowitz, a leading U.S. kinesiologist, long-term sauna use is often exhausting for sensitive patients, and its use can weaken patients' functioning in the more depleted tuberculinic or luetic miasm.[215]

TOWEL OFF THE TOXINS

Be sure to wipe off your sweat with a towel intermittently during a sauna. Your sweat will contain heavy metals as well as petrochemicals and other toxins that you don't want to reabsorb. Wiping off frequently is an easy and effective means of enhancing the benefits of a sauna.

The infrared sauna is at a lower temperature and is therefore safer than high-temperature saunas, which can put a strain on the heart. Furthermore, because infrared saunas can penetrate the body more deeply (up to 2 inches compared to traditional saunas that reach ⅛ inch), you can get a good sweat going at only about 120°F. Thus, infrared saunas excrete toxins more efficiently through the skin without depleting individuals as much as traditional saunas.

As a general rule of thumb, individuals should simply monitor their response and adjust the heat, duration, and frequency of sauna use according to their own particular constitution. In general, individuals functioning at the healthy psoric level (and some at the sycotic level) benefit much more from saunas than those functioning at the more depleted tuberculinic and luetic levels.

If you are adequately prepared and follow these directions, you should experience only mild and intermittent symptoms during this period of detoxification. If you do experience any significant symptoms beyond the mild fatigue and malaise that is common after dental drilling, do not hesitate to contact your holistic practitioner and dentist.

Comments on the Five Dental Detox Days

As we've learned from allopathic drugs, hitting the body with a hammer—that is, with strong products and excessively large dosages—may be called for in a life-threatening emergency but does not benefit anyone in the long run. Seemingly short-term gains never last in living systems. Thus, although many potent heavy metal detoxification protocols exist and make great promises, in my experience they are rarely curative over time. The holistic physician's primary purpose is always to encourage the patient's *own* organs and tissues to cleanse and purify at his or her body's own rate and physiological and metabolic limits.

Excessive faith in megadosages or an external product to cure all of one's ills is almost always ultimately defeating. The body cannot detoxify more than it has the metabolic capacity for at any one time, no matter how powerful the drug. Strong drugs and medications are our well-meaning Western response to the horror of amalgam fillings and other toxins; however, they're always excessively "yang"—that is, too strong and unbalancing for our bodies. Drugs (and even synthetic, fractionated vitamin and mineral supplements) *force* processes upon the body; natural remedies such as herbs, homeopathics, and natural nutritional supplements *support* the body's own processes and its innate wisdom. Through the use of these natural remedies the body becomes more aware of the "500-pound gorilla" of toxic metal stores and begins to recognize them as "nonself." As it becomes more functional, the body begins to process and clear these toxins at its own pace, within its own limits.

That said, the Five Dental Detox Days Protocol should be considered not a cure-all but simply a guide to reasonable supplementation that has "held up" for years clinically and energetically in the treatment of heavy metal poisoning. Every individual is unique, however, and therefore patients are best served when they consult with a holistic practitioner who can use energetic testing to determine exactly which products and remedies will best help them detoxify in the days and months following amalgam removal.

CONCLUSION

Removing toxic metals from the body is an essential step in the detoxification protocol of every holistically oriented individual. However, this removal must be done at an appropriate time, when the patient is strong enough to detoxify these heavy metals from his or her body, with the help of appropriate nutritional supplements and remedies.

The fact that the practice of placing the second-most-toxic metal in the mouth in the form of amalgam fillings is not only still legal in the United States but righteously defended by the ADA should be incredulous not only to holistically oriented patients but also to any rational and thoughtful individual. This incredulity only grows upon review of the scientific literature on this subject, in which the toxicity of mercury amalgam fillings is not only evident but conclusively proven. A quote from *Discover* magazine most succinctly illustrates the "unimaginably toxic and dangerous" nature of this heavy metal:

> Let's start with a straightforward fact: Mercury is unimaginably toxic and dangerous. A single drop on a human hand can be irreversibly fatal. A single drop in a large lake can make all the fish in it unsafe to eat.[216]

In fact, the past and ongoing practice of placing amalgam fillings in the mouth is such a travesty to public health that I can't help but be reminded of earlier "more primitive" times when other quite lethal practices were perpetrated on innocent patients. The following historical account of another example of such gross malpractice seems a fitting conclusion to this chapter:

> In the mid 1800s, a young Hungarian-born physician by the name of Ignaz Philipp Semmelweis was working in the obstetrical ward of a famous Viennese hospital. After some time, he noticed that death from puerperal (childbirth) fever for women in the doctor's ward where obstetricians delivered babies and medical students were trained was more than four times higher than for women being treated in another section of the hospital by midwives. Although Dr. Semmelweis did not know then that germs can cause disease in susceptible patients in this pre-Pasteur, pre-Lister period, he suspected that medical students who handled (gloveless) deliveries on his ward in between their examination of cadavers could be the cause. So he instituted a highly innovative concept for that time—the washing of the hands.
>
> Semmelweis proceeded to introduce a chlorine hand-washing technique to the medical ward and had washbasins placed between the rows of beds. He instructed all medical students to wash their hands after dissecting corpses, as well as after examining women on the ward. The results were nothing short of miraculous. Before the hand-washing practice, approximately one out of every eight women would die giving birth. However, after instituting this simple hygienic practice, the death rate dropped almost immediately to less than one in one hundred.
>
> Surprisingly, however, this discovery that saved hundreds of women's lives was not well received. In fact, the opposite occurred. Orthodox obstetricians, incensed that they could possibly be at fault, insulted and hounded Semmelweis at every opportunity. These harsh attacks by his colleagues finally drove him out of Vienna and eventually caused his mental breakdown. In fact, this originally happy, open-minded, and brilliant individual slowly became morose, moody, and psychologically unstable. Quite sadly, Dr. Semmelweis died alone at age forty-seven from "paralysis of the brain" in a mental institution.[217]

This analogy may seem extreme to those not in holistic circles. But for those holistic dentists and practitioners who have been, and continue to be, persecuted by the modern-day method of professional censure—the loss of their hard-earned licenses by ADA-influenced dental boards, the stress of lawsuits for simply removing amalgam fillings, and the loss of their income and often sense of self-worth—the similarities are clear. I hope that holistic dentists, holistic practitioners, and their loyal and knowledgeable patients will keep this story in mind every time they are ridiculed by the establishment over the mercury amalgam controversy. Someday, the use of mercury amalgam fillings will be seen to be as ludicrous as a doctor not washing his or her hands before delivering a baby.

NOTES

1. *Webster's New Universal Unabridged Dictionary,* deluxe 2nd edition (New York: Simon and Schuster, 1983), 1131.
2. J. Sullivan and G. Krieger, *Hazardous Materials Toxicology* (Baltimore: Williams and Wilkins, 1992), 2.
3. Ibid.
4. Ibid.
5. M. Kauppi, "Mercury Exposure from Amalgam Fillings in German Children," *Heavy Metal Bulletin* 1, no. 1 (1997): "extra pages," 1; J. Robbins, *Reclaiming Our Health* (Tiburon, Calif.: H. J. Kramer, 1998), 3.
6. S. Ziff, *Silver Dental Fillings: The Toxic Time Bomb* (New York: Aurora Press, 1984), vi.
7. M. Kauppi, "Brave 'New' Metal World!" *Heavy Metal Bulletin* 1, no. 1 (April 1994): 3.
8. Editors, "Dentists Left Twisting in the Wind on Amalgam!" *Bio-Probe Newsletter* 18, no. 2 (March 2002): 3, 4.
9. FDA News Release, "FDA Issues Final Regulation on Dental Amalgam," July 28, 2009, www.fda.gov/NewsEvents/Newsroom/Pressannouncements/ucm173992.htm.
10. Quicksilver Associates, *The Mercury in Your Mouth* (New York: Quicksilver Press, 1996), 3.
11. L. Cashman, "Kerger Lawsuit Gains Traction," *International DAMS Newsletter,* Summer 2005, 4.
12. ADA Council on Scientific Affairs, *Journal of the American Dental Association* 129 (April 1998): 494, 501.
13. Editors, "Dentists Left Twisting in the Wind on Amalgam!" *Bio-Probe Newsletter* 18, no. 2 (March 2002): 3.

14. American Dental Association, "Statement on Dental Amalgam," August 2009, www.ADA.org/1741.aspx.

15. M. Kauppi, "Class Action Suit in Canada," *Heavy Metal Bulletin* 1, no. 1 (1997): "extra pages," 2; DAMS, Inc. Information Packet from DAMS (Dental Amalgam Mercury Solutions), Minneapolis, 5; L. Cashman, "Kerger Lawsuit Gains Traction," *International DAMS Newsletter,* Summer 2005, 4.

16. ADA Council on Scientific Affairs, *Journal of the American Dental Association* 129 (April 1998): 494, 501.

17. A. Gittleman, *How to Stay Young and Healthy in a Toxic World* (Los Angeles: Keats Publishing, 1999), 73.

18. David Howard, "Swedish Government Announces Total Ban of Amalgam Dental Fillings," www.davidhoward.com.au/resources/article15.html.

19. "Summary of Amalgam Use in Norway," www.bioprobe.com?ReadNews.asp?article=78.

20. What Doctors Don't Tell You, "Amalgam Fillings: Norway Is First to Ban Mercury in Teeth," March 27, 2008, www.wddty.com.

21. A. Martin, "Many Countries Have Curbs on Dental Mercury," *International DAMS Newsletter* 2 and 3 (October 2001): 26.

22. C. Brown, "FDA Panels Repudiate Staff Position," www.toxicteeth.org.

23. J. Wheaton, "Prop 65 Warnings for Mercury in Dental Fillings," Environmental Law Foundation (Oakland, Calif.), news release, December 14, 1993.

24. F. Jerome, *Tooth Truth* (San Diego: ProMotion Publishing, 1995), 95.

25. Editors, "Dentists Left Twisting in the Wind on Amalgam!" *Bio-Probe Newsletter* 18, no. 2 (March 2002): 2.

26. Editors, "California Court Enforces Propositon 65," *Bio-Probe Newsletter* 19, no. 2 (March 2003): 4.

27. Ibid.

28. H. Huggins, *It's All in Your Head* (New York: Avery, 1993), 15.

29. M. Kauppi, "Brave New Metal World!" *Heavy Metal Bulletin* 1, no. 1 (April 1994): 1; K. Sehnert et al., "Is Mercury Toxicity an Autoimmune Disorder?" *International DAMS Newsletter,* Winter 1996, 4.

30. M. Kauppi, "Brave New Metal World!" *Heavy Metal Bulletin* 1, no. 1 (April 1994): 1.

31. H. Huggins, *It's All in Your Head* (New York: Avery, 1993), 59.

32. S. Ziff, *Silver Dental Fillings: The Toxic Time Bomb* (New York: Aurora Press, 1984), 9.

33. Ibid., 10

34. Quicksilver Associates, *The Mercury in Your Mouth* (New York: Quicksilver Press, 1996), 26.

35. M . Ziff and S. Ziff, *The Missing Link?* (Orlando: Bio-Probe, 1991), 45.

36. F. Jerome, *Tooth Truth* (San Diego: ProMotion Publishing, 1995), 88.

37. Ibid.

38. T. W. Clarkson, "Mercury—An Element of Mystery," *New England Journal of Medicine* 323, no. 16 (October 18, 1990): 1138.

39. M. Kauppi, "CE-Marking of Dental Materials Is a Joke!" *Heavy Metal Bulletin* 6, no. 2 (October 2000): 3.

40. L. Friberg, "Inorganic Mercury," *World Health Organization Environmental Health Criteria* 118 (Geneva, 1991): 32.

41. L. Cashman, "Solving the MS Mystery: Help, Hope and Recovery, by Hal A. Huggins, D.D.S., M.S. [2002]," *Dental Truth,* December 2003, 8.

42. Bioactive Services, *Mercury Amalgam Toxicity,* 1, no. 7: 1.

43. F. Lorscheider et al., "Mercury Exposure from 'Silver' Tooth Fillings: Emerging Evidence Questions a Traditional Dental Paradigm," *The FASEB Journal* 9 (April 1995): 505–6; R. Jaffe, "Chelation Therapy for Acute and Chronic Metal Intoxication," AABD lecture notes, Carmel, Calif. (1994): 7.

44. P. Störtebecker, *Mercury Poisoning from Dental Amalgam—A Hazard to the Human Brain* (Orlando: Bio-Probe, 1985), 19, 28.

45. G. Tortora and N. Anagnostakos, *Principles of Anatomy and Physiology,* 5th ed. (New York: Harper and Row, 1987), 597, 598.

46. P. Störtebecker, *Mercury Poisoning from Dental Amalgam—A Hazard to the Human Brain* (Orlando: Bio-Probe, 1985), 54.

47. M. Ziff and S. Ziff, *The Missing Link?* (Orlando: Bio-Probe, 1991), 46, 47.

48. P. Borinski, "Die Herkunft des Quecksilbers in des menschlichen Ausschridungen," *Zahnaerzt. Rundschau* 40 (1931): 223–30.

49. P. Störtebecker, *Mercury Poisoning from Dental Amalgam—A Hazard to the Human Brain* (Orlando: Bio-Probe, 1985), 172.

50. U. Heintze et al., "Methylation of Mercury from Dental Amalgam Mercuric Chloride by Oral Streptococci In Vitro," *Scandinavian Journal of Dental Research* 91 (1983): 150–52; C. U. Eccles and Z. Annua, eds., *The Toxicity of*

Methyl Mercury (Baltimore: Johns Hopkins University Press, 1987), 117; I. Rowland et al., "The Methylation of Mercuric Chloride by Human Intestinal Bacteria," *Experientia* (Basel) 31 (1975): 1064–65.

51. P. Störtebecker, *Mercury Poisoning from Dental Amalgam—A Hazard to the Human Brain* (Orlando: Bio-Probe, 1985), 29.
52. J. Friel, ed., *Dorland's Illustrated Medical Dictionary,* 26th ed. (Philadelphia: W. B. Saunders Company, 1981), 535.
53. M. Ziff and S. Ziff, *The Missing Link?* (Orlando: Bio-Probe, 1991), 47.
54. L. Cashman, "Victory in California and Arizona," *International DAMS Newsletter* 10, nos. 3 and 4 (February 2000): 1.
55. Quicksilver Associates, *The Mercury in Your Mouth* (New York: Quicksilver Press, 1996), 24–25.
56. Ibid., 24.
57. P. Störtebecker, *Mercury Poisoning from Dental Amalgam—A Hazard to the Human Brain* (Orlando: Bio-Probe, 1985), 131–32; Y. Momoi et al., "A Measurement of Galvanic Current and Electrical Potential in Extracted Human Teeth," *Dental Research* 65, no. 12 (1986): 1441–44.
58. Y. Momoi et al., "A Measurement of Galvanic Current and Electrical Potential in Extracted Human Teeth," *Dental Research* 65, no. 12 (1986): 1441–44.
59. P. Störtebecker, *Mercury Poisoning from Dental Amalgam—A Hazard to the Human Brain* (Orlando: Bio-Probe, 1985), 132.
60. S. Ziff and M. Ziff, *Dentistry without Mercury* (Orlando: Bio-Probe, Inc., 1995), 7; J. Pleva, "Mercury from Dental Amalgams: Exposure and Effects," *International Journal of Risk and Safety in Medicine* 3 (1992): 11.
61. J. Pleva, "Mercury from Dental Amalgams: Exposure and Effects," *International Journal of Risk and Safety in Medicine* 3 (1992): 1–22.
62. J. Pleva, "Corrosion and Mercury Release from Dental Amalgam," *Journal of Orthomolecular Medicine* 4, no. 3 (1989): 155.
63. L. Cashman and M. Brake, "Seeing the Physical Causes of Behavioral Problems," *International DAMS Newsletter* 9, no. 2 (Spring 1999): 3.
64. M. Vimy and F. Lorscheider, "The Effects of Dental Amalgams on Mercury Levels in Expired Air," *Journal of Dental Research* 60 (1985): 1668–71; A. Aronsson et al., "Dental Amalgam and Mercury," *Biological Metals* 2 (1989): 25–30; C. Svare et al., "The Effects of Dental Amalgams on Mercury Levels in Expired Air," *Journal of Dental Research* 60 (1981): 1668–71.
65. M. Vimy and F. Lorscheider, "Serial Measurements of Intraoral Air Mercury: Estimation of Daily Dose from Amalgam," *Journal of Dental Research* 64 (1985): 1072–75.
66. M. Kauppi, "Mercury in Saliva," *Heavy Metal Bulletin* 3, no. 1 (April 1996): 23.
67. J. Patterson et al., "Mercury in the Human Breath from Dental Amalgam," *Bulletin of Environmental Contamination and Toxicology* 34 (1985): 459–68; C. Enwonwu, "Potential Health Hazard of Use of Mercury in Dentistry: Critical Review of the Literature," *Environmental Research* 42 (1987): 264; P. Störtebecker, *Mercury Poisoning from Dental Amalgam—A Hazard to the Human Brain* (Orlando: Bio-Probe, 1985), 151–52; M. Kauppi, "Live and Love in a Metal-clad Room," *Heavy Metal Bulletin* 6, no. 2 (October 2000): 7; M. Kauppi, "Electromagnetic Fields Increase Mercury Excretion," *Heavy Metal Bulletin* 4, no. 1 (May 1997): 17; Swedish Association of Dental Mercury Patients, *ABC on Mercury-Poisoning from Dental Amalgam Fillings* (Orlando: Bio-Probe, 1997), 8.
68. D. Kennedy, "Smoking Tooth," www.IAOMT.org.
69. Ibid.; W. Clifford, "Minute Amounts of Metals Wreak Havoc, Particularly in Nerves and Brain," *Well Mind Association Newsletter,* January 1994, 2.
70. D. Kennedy, "Smoking Tooth," www.IAOMT.org.
71. L. Williams, "From Bechamp's Microzyma to Naessen's Somatid," *Raum und Zeit* 3, no. 1 (1991): 55.
72. L. Hahn, "Whole-body Imaging of the Distribution of Mercury Released from Dental Fillings into Monkey Tissues," *The FASEB Journal* 4 (November 1990): 3256–59; G. Danscher et al., "Traces of Mercury in Organs from Primates with Amalgam Fillings," *Experimental and Molecular Pathology* 52 (1990): 291–99.
73. F. Lorscheider, "How Mercury Causes Brain Neuron Degeneration," from the video library of the International Academy of Oral Medicine & Toxicology, www.IAOMT.org.
74. P. Störtebecker, *Mercury Poisoning from Dental Amalgam—A Hazard to the Human Brain* (Orlando: Bio-Probe, 1985), 33–34.
75. G. Tortora and N. Anagnostakos, *Principles of Anatomy and Physiology,* 5th ed. (New York: Harper and Row, 1987), 310.
76. P. Störtebecker, *Mercury Poisoning from Dental Amalgam—A Hazard to the Human Brain* (Orlando: Bio-Probe, 1985), 207–12.
77. S. R. Saxe et al., "Alzheimer's Disease, Dental Amalgam and Mercury," *Journal of the American Dental Association* 130, no. 2 (February 1999): 191–99; W. Ehmann et al.,

"Brain Trace Elements in Alzheimer's Disease," *Neurotoxicology* 7, no. 1 (Spring 1986): 195–206; C. Cornett, "Imbalances of Trace Elements Related to Oxidative Damage in Alzheimer's Disease Brain," *Neurotoxicology* 19, no. 3 (June 1998): 339–45.

78. P. Störtebecker, *Mercury Poisoning from Dental Amalgam—A Hazard to the Human Brain* (Orlando: Bio-Probe, 1985), 34–43, 118–21.
79. H. Casdorph and M. Walker, *Toxic Metal Syndrome* (Garden City Park, N.Y.: Avery Publishing Group, 1995), 151.
80. P. Störtebecker, *Mercury Poisoning from Dental Amalgam—A Hazard to the Human Brain* (Orlando: Bio-Probe, 1985), 34.
81. Ibid., 38–48, 149; P. Störtebecker, *Dental Caries as a Cause of Nervous Disorders* (Orlando: Bio-Probe, 1982), 38.
82. B. Arvidson, "Retrograde Axonal Transport of Mercury," *Experimental Neurology* 98 (1987): 198.
83. P. Störtebecker, *Mercury Poisoning from Dental Amalgam—A Hazard to the Human Brain* (Orlando: Bio-Probe, 1985), 50.
84. D. Guembel, *Principles of Holistic Therapy with Herbal Essences,* 2nd ed. (Brussels: Haug International, 1993), 34.
85. P. Störtebecker, *Dental Caries as a Cause of Nervous Disorders* (Orlando: Bio-Probe, 1982), 40–41.
86. F. Lorscheider et al., "Mercury Exposure from 'Silver' Tooth Fillings: Emerging Evidence Questions a Traditional Dental Paradigm," *FASEB Journal* 9 (April 1995): 506.
87. Quicksilver Associates, *The Mercury in Your Mouth* (New York: Quicksilver Press, 1996), 51.
88. F. Lorscheider, "Mercury Amalgams and Health," *Clinical Pearls News* 6, no. 6 (June 1996): 67.
89. M. Wolff, "Occupationally Derived Chemicals in Breast Milk," *American Journal of Industrial Medicine* 4, no. 12 (1983): 259–81; M. Vimy, "Mercury from Maternal 'Silver' Tooth Fillings in Sheep and Human Breast Milk. A Source of Neonatal Exposure," *Biological Trace Element Research* 56, no. 2 (February 1997): 143–52; F. Lorscheider, "Mercury Amalgams and Health," *Clinical Pearls News* 6, no. 6 (June 1996): 67.
90. B. Eley, "The Future of Dental Amalgam: A Review of the Literature. Part 6: Possible Harmful Effects of Mercury from Dental Amalgam," *British Dental Journal* 182, no. 12 (1997): 455–59.
91. H. Drexler and K. Schaller, "The Mercury Concentration in Breast Milk Resulting from Amalgam Fillings and Dietary Habits," *Environmental Research* 77, no. 2 (May 1998): 124–29.
92. J. Dorea and A. Barbosa, "Maternal Mercury Transfer," *Environmental Research* 93 (2003): 113.
93. U.S. Department of Health, Education, and Welfare, Review Committee, Criteria for a Recommended Standard: *Occupational Exposure to Inorganic Mercury* (1973), www.cdc.gov/niosh/73-11024.html: 16–17.
94. Ibid.
95. I. Trakhtenberg, "Chronic Effects of Mercury on Organisms," U.S. Department of Health, Education, and Welfare publication no. (NIH) 74-473 (translated from the Russian, 1974): 134.
96. J. Abramson, *Overdosed America* (New York: HarperCollins, 2004), 115–17.
97. Ibid., 232–33.
98. R. Siblerud, "The Relationship between Mercury from Dental Amalgam and Mental Health," *American Journal of Psychotherapy* 43, no. 4 (October 1989).
99. Ibid.
100. R. Siblerud et al., "Psychometric Evidence That Mercury from Silver Dental Fillings May Be an Etiological Factor in Depression, Excessive Anger and Anxiety," *Psychological Reports* 74 (1994): 67–80.
101. W. Ross and M. Sholiton, "Specificity of Psychiatric Manifestations in Relation to Neurotoxic Chemicals," *Acta Psychiatrica Scandinavica Supplementum* 303 (1983): 100–104.
102. J. Pleva, "Are Promoters of Dental Amalgam Poisoned by Mercury?" *Journal of Orthomolecular Medicine* 9, no. 2 (1994): 76.
103. D. Kennedy, *How to Save Your Teeth* (Delaware, Ohio: Health Action Press, 1996), 97.
104. D. Klinghardt, "Amalgam/Mercury Detox as a Treatment for Chronic Viral, Bacterial and Fungal Illnesses," lecture at the annual meeting of the International and American Academy of Clinical Nutrition, San Diego (September 1996): 1.
105. Ibid., 2.
106. Ibid.
107. B. Volesky, *Biosorption of Heavy Metals* (Boca Raton, Fla.: CRC Press, 1990), 101–3.
108. E. Browning, *Toxicity of Industrial Metals* (London: Butterworths, 1961), 204.
109. B. Ashley, "Facing Alzheimer's Together," *Marin Independent Journal,* December 17, 2001, E1.
110. S. Khatoon et al., "Aberrant Guanosine Triphosphate-Beta-Tubulin Interaction in Alzheimer's Disease," *Annals*

of Neurology 26, no. 2 (August 1989): 210–15; S. R. Saxe et al., "Alzheimer's Disease, Dental Amalgam and Mercury," *Journal of the American Dental Association* 130, no. 2 (February 1999): 191–99; W. Ehmann et al., "Brain Trace Elements in Alzheimer's Disease," *Neurotoxicology* 7, no. 1 (Spring 1986): 195–206; C. Cornett, "Imbalances of Trace Elements Related to Oxidative Damage in Alzheimer's Disease Brain," *Neurotoxicology* 19, no. 3 (June 1998): 339–45.

111. Quicksilver Associates, *The Mercury in Your Mouth* (New York: Quicksilver Press, 1996), 59–60.

112. S. Ziff, "Editorial on the Alzheimer's/Mercury Connection," editorial flyer (March 2001).

113. H. Casdorph and M. Walker, *Toxic Metal Syndrome* (Garden City Park, N.Y.: Avery Publishing Group, 1995), 118–27.

114. H. Huggins, "Medical and Legal Implications of Components of Dental Materials" (master's thesis, University of Colorado, 1989), 25.

115. R. Berkow et al., eds., *The Merck Manual,* 15th ed. (Rahway, N.J.: Merck Sharp and Dohme Research Laboratories, 1987), 1438–39.

116. Y. Mano et al., "Amyotrophic Lateral Sclerosis and Mercury—Preliminary Report," *Rinsho Shinkeigaku* 30, no. 11 (November 1990): 1275–77.

117. B. Arvidson, "Inorganic Mercury Is Transported from Muscular Nerve Terminals to Spinal and Brainstem Motoneurons," *Muscle and Nerve,* October 1992, 1089–94.

118. Editor, "'Lou Gehrig's Disease and Mercury," *International DAMS Newsletter* 4, no. 1 (Winter 1994): 3.

119. L. Cashman, "Eric Is Winning," *International DAMS Newsletter,* Summer 2005, 14.

120. A. Kimbrell, ed., *Fatal Harvest: The Tragedy of Industrial Agriculture* (San Rafael, Calif.: Palace Press International, 2000), 43, 52–53.

121. H. Huggins, "Proposed Role of Dental Amalgam Toxicity in Leukemia and Hematopoietic Dyscrasias," *International Journal of Biosocial and Medical Research* 11, no. 1 (1989): 84–93.

122. Ibid.

123. E. Duhr et al., "HgEDTA Complex Inhibits GTP Interactions with the E-site of Brain Beta-tubulin," *Toxicology and Applied Pharmacology* 122 (1993): 273–80; N. Brookes, "In Vitro Evidence for the Role of Glutamate in the CNS Toxicity of Mercury," *Toxicology* 76 (1992): 245–56; D. Eggleston et al., "Correlation of Dental Amalgam with Mercury in Brain Tissue," *The Journal of Prosthetic Dentistry* 58, no. 6 (December 1987): 705–6.

124. P. Störtebecker, *Mercury Poisoning from Dental Amalgam—A Hazard to the Human Brain* (Orlando: Bio-Probe, 1985), 161–63.

125. P. Störtebecker, *Dental Caries as a Cause of Nervous Disorders* (Orlando: Bio-Probe, 1982), 160–63.

126. Ibid., 167.

127. P. Störtebecker, *Mercury Poisoning from Dental Amalgam—A Hazard to the Human Brain* (Orlando: Bio-Probe, 1985), 131–33.

128. Ibid., 6.

129. M. Ziff and S. Ziff, *The Missing Link?* (Orlando: Bio-Probe, Inc., 1991), 21.

130. S. Fallon, *Nourishing Traditions* (San Diego: ProMotion Publishing, 1995), 5.

131. R. Siblerud, "The Relationship between Mercury from Dental Amalgam and the Cardiovascular System," *Science of the Total Environment* 99 (1990): 23–25.

132. S. Dahhan and H. Orfaly, "Electrocardiographic Changes in Mercury Poisoning," *American Journal of Cardiology* 14 (August 1994): 178–83.

133. M. Ziff and S. Ziff, *The Missing Link?* (Orlando: Bio-Probe, Inc., 1991), 90.

134. T. Colborn et al., *Our Stolen Future* (New York: Penguin Books, 1996), 68–75.

135. I. Gerhard and B. Runnebaum, "Toxic Factors and Infertility, Heavy Metals and Minerals," *Geburtshilfe und Frauenheilkunde* 52 (1992): 383.

136. I. Gerhard and B. Runnebaum, "Fertility Disorders May Result from Heavy Metal and Pesticide Contamination Which Limits Effectiveness of Hormone Therapy," *Zentralblatt fuer Gynaekologie* 114 (1992): 593.

137. M. Vimy, "Mercury from Maternal 'Silver' Tooth Fillings in Sheep and Human Breast Milk. A Source of Neonatal Exposure," *Biological Trace Element Research* 56, no. 2 (February 1997): 143–52; F. Lorscheider, "Mercury Amalgams and Health," *Clinical Pearls News* 6, no. 6 (June 1996): 67.

138. G. Crowther, letter to the editor, *International DAMS Newsletter* 4, no. 3 (Summer 1998): 9.

139. R. Siblerud and E. Kienholz, "Evidence That Mercury from Silver Dental Fillings May Be an Etiological Factor in Multiple Sclerosis," *Science of the Total Environment* 142 (1994): 191–205; P. Le Quesne, "Metal-induced Diseases of the Nervous System," *British Journal of Hospital Medicine* 28 (1982): 534–38; J. Clausen, "Mercury and Multiple Sclerosis," *Acta Neurologica Scandinavica* 87, no. 6 (1993): 461–64.

140. P. Störtebecker, *Mercury Poisoning from Dental Amalgam—*

A Hazard to the Human Brain (Orlando: Bio-Probe, 1985), 118–21.

141. H. Huggins and T. Levy, "Cerebrospinal Fluid Protein Changes in Multiple Sclerosis after Dental Amalgam Removal," *Alternative Medicine Review* 3, no. 4 (1998): 295.

142. Ibid., 295–300.

143. L. Cashman, "Solving the MS Mystery: Help, Hope and Recovery," *International DAMS Newsletter,* Summer 2005, 8.

144. P. Kidd, "Parkinson's Disease as Multifactorial Oxidative Neurodegeneration: Implications for Integrative Management," *Alternative Medicine Review* 5, no. 6 (2000): 502.

145. K. Head, "Parkinson's: Better Living through Chemicals?" *Alternative Medicine Review* 5, no. 6 (2000): 501.

146. Ibid.

147. Chun-Han Ngim and G. Devathasan, "Epidemiologic Study on the Association between Body Burden Mercury Level and Idiopathic Parkinson's Disease," *Neuroepidemiology* 8 (1989): 128–41; V. Uverrsky et al., "Metal-triggered Structural Transformations, Aggregation and Fibrillation of Human Alpha-syneclein. A Possible Molecular NK between Parkinson's Disease and Heavy Metal Exposure," *Journal of Biological Chemistry* 276, no. 47 (September 11, 2001): 44284–96.

148. H. Biernat et al., "Tremor Frequency Patterns in Mercury Vapor Exposure, Compared with Early Parkinson's Disease and Essential Tremor," *Neurotoxicology* 20, no. 6 (December 1999): 945–52.

149. P. Störtebecker, *Mercury Poisoning from Dental Amalgam—A Hazard to the Human Brain* (Orlando: Bio-Probe, 1985), 86.

150. D. Richardson, "Flu Vaccine: Stay Out of My Womb!" *International DAMS Newsletter* 11, no. 1 (October 8, 1999): 5.

151. L. Reagan, "What about Mercury?" *Mothering* 105 (March/April 2001): 54.

152. D. Richardson, "Flu Vaccine: Stay Out of My Womb!" *International DAMS Newsletter* 11, no. 1 (October 8, 1999): 7.

153. M. Tucker, "Vaccines under Fire," *Pediatric News* 8, no. 33 (1999): 1, 7.

154. Institute for Vaccine Safety at the Johns Hopkins Bloomberg School of Public Health, "Thimerosal Content in Some U.S. Licensed Vaccines" (updated September 28, 2010), www.vaccinesafety.edu/thi-table.htm.

155. S. Williams, "No More Mercury," *Newsweek,* August 14, 2000, 67.

156. A. Fuentes, "Eli Lilly and Thimerosal," *In These Times,* November 11, 2003, www.InTheseTimes.com/article=649.

157. Washington State Department of Health, "Mercury Poisoning Cases Traced to Face Cream," *EPI Trends* 1, no. 2 (August 1996): 4.

158. M. Kauppi, "Pink Disease Victims Organize," *Heavy Metal Bulletin* 5, no. 3 (August 1999): 4, 5; D. Kirby, *Evidence of Harm* (New York: St. Martin's Press, 2005), 62, 63.

159. D. Kirby, *Evidence of Harm* (New York: St. Martin's Press, 2005), 62, 63.

160. T. Levy, "Teeth—The Root of Most Disease?" *Extraordinary Science,* April/May/June 1994, 10.

161. D. Klinghardt and L. Williams, *Amalgam Toxicity Handbook* (Seattle: AANK, 1994), 4.

162. L. Cashman and M. Brake, "Seeing the Physical Causes of Behavioral Problems," *International DAMS Newsletter* 9, no. 2 (Spring 1999): 2.

163. B. Strittmatter, *Identifying and Treating Blockages to Healing* (New York: Thieme, 2004), 37.

164. S. Fallon, *Nourishing Traditions* (San Diego: ProMotion Publishing, 1995), 238.

165. L. Forristal, "Is Something Fishy Going On?" *Wise Traditions* 1, no. 3 (Fall 2000): 43–46.

166. J. D. Wallach and Ma Lan, *Rare Earths Forbidden Cures* (n.p.: Wellness Publications, 1994).

167. Debra Lynn Dadd, *Natural Home* (July/August 2000): 16.

168. V. Stejskal et al., "MELISA: An In Vitro Tool for the Study of Metal Allergy," *Toxicology In Vitro* 8 (1994): 991–1000.

169. M. Kauppi, "Gold and Palladium in Body Fluids," *Heavy Metal Bulletin* 6, no. 2 (October 2000): 15.

170. Lynn Lawson, *Staying Well in a Toxic World: Understanding Environmental Illness, Multiple Chemical Sensitivities, and Sick Building Syndrome* (Chicago: Noble Press, 1994), 144.

171. M. Pennybacker, "Chemicals That Stick Around," *Natural Home,* September/October 2006, 80.

172. J. Wallach, *Dead Doctors Don't Lie,* audiotape.

173. P. Störtebecker, *Mercury Poisoning from Dental Amalgam—A Hazard to the Human Brain* (Orlando: Bio-Probe, 1985), 125.

174. R. Kupsinel, "Mercury Amalgam Toxicity: A Major Common Denominator of Degenerative Disease," *Journal of Orthomolecular Psychiatry* 13, no. 4 (1984): 8, 240.

175. Ibid.

176. World Health Organization, "Mercury," *World Health Organization and UN Environment Program* (1976): 22.

177. S. Denton, "The Mercury Cover-up," *Health Consciousness Magazine,* June 1989, 3.

178. H. Huggins, *It's All in Your Head* (New York: Avery, 1993), 93–95.
179. F. Lorscheider and M. Vimy, "Mercury Exposure from 'Silver' Fillings," *Lancet* 337 (May 4, 1991): 1103.
180. S. Queen, "Toxic Footprints in Chemistry and Biotransformation," IABDM 20th Anniversary Conference, March 31–April 2, 2006, 7.
181. R. Kupsinel, "Mercury Amalgam Toxicity," *Journal of Orthomolecular Psychiatry* 13, no. 4 (1984): 1.
182. D. Bass et al., "Trace Element Analysis in Hair: Factors Determining Accuracy, Precision, and Reliability," *Alternative Medicine Review* 6, no. 5 (2001): 472–81.
183. D. Klinghardt and L. Williams, *Amalgam Toxicity Handbook* (Seattle: AANK, 1994), 1.
184. I. Trakhtenberg, "Chronic Effects of Mercury on Organisms," U.S. Department of Health, Education, and Welfare publication no. (NIH) 74–473 (translated from the Russian, 1974): 123.
185. H. Aposhian, "Human Studies with the Chelating Agents, DMPS and DMSA," *Clinical Toxicology* 30, no. 4: 505–28; H. Aposhian, "DMSA and DMPS—Water Soluble Antidotes for Heavy Metal Poisoning," *Annual Review of Pharmacology and Toxicology* 23 (1983): 193–215.
186. L. Cashman, "Solving the MS Mystery: Help, Hope and Recovery," *Dental Truth,* December 2003, 8.
187. B. Haley, "A Biochemist's Views on Detoxification," *Dental Truth,* March 2005, 5.
188. Ibid.
189. R. Casdorph and M. Walker, *Toxic Metal Syndrome* (New York: Avery, 1995), 68.
190. F. Lorscheider, "Mercury Amalgams and Health," *Clinical Pearls News* 6, no. 6 (June 1996): 67.
191. M. Breiner, *Whole Body Dentistry* (Fairfield, Conn.: Quantum Health Press, 1999), 77.
192. ADA Council on Scientific Affairs, "Dental Mercury Hygiene Recommendations," *Journal of the American Dental Association* 130 (July 1999): 1125–26.
193. F. Jerome, *Tooth Truth* (San Diego: ProMotion Publishing, 1995), 93.
194. S. Ziff et al., *Dental Mercury Detox* (Orlando: Bio-Probe, 1988), 49.
195. N. Olea et al., "Estrogenicity of Resin-based Composites and Sealants Used in Dentistry," *Environmental Health Perspectives* 104, no. 3 (March 1996): 298.
196. Editors, "Are Dental Composites Safe?" *Bio-Probe Newsletter* 16, no. 1 (January 2000): 1.
197. Ibid.
198. S. Ziff and M. Ziff, *Dentistry without Mercury* (Orlando, Fla.: Bio-Probe, 1995), 39–40.
199. M. Kauppi, "New Dental Materials and Techniques," *Heavy Metal Bulletin* 1, no. 2 (October 1994), 13–14.
200. Ibid., 14–15.
201. T. Beardsley, "Take the Pain? Lidocaine Comes under Suspicion as a Carcinogen," *Scientific American* 270, no. 5 (1994): 28–29.
202. A. Nickel, "Update on Heart Attacks and Cancer" (2000): 1.
203. R. Francis, "The Alarming Local Anesthetics," *Beyond Health News,* May/June 1997, 3.
204. A. Nickel, "Update on Heart Attacks and Cancer" (2000), 2.
205. "Power of Music," *The Press Democrat,* June 14, 2005, D1.
206. P. Borinski, "Die Herkunft des Quecksilbers in des menschlichen Ausschridungen," Zahnärztliche Rundschau 40 (1931): 223–30.
207. C. Malmstroem et al., "Amalgam-derived Mercury in Feces," ISTERH Third International Conference and NTES Fourth Nordic Conference, Stockholm (May 25–29, 1992): 1–8.
208. "Poplar Trees Popular among Pig Farmers?" American Forests Forest Bytes, www.americanforests.org/ForestBytes/122003.php.
209. P. Rea, O. Vatamaniuk, and D. Rigden, "Weeds, Worms, and More: Papain's Long-Lost Cousin, Phytochelatin Synthase," *Plant Physiology* 136 (September 2004): 2463–74.
210. S. Jacob, *The Miracle of MSM: The Natural Solution for Pain* (New York: G. Putnam's Sons, 1999), 22–23.
211. William Shaw, "The Role of Oxalates in Autism and Chronic Disorders," www.westonaprice.org/food-features/1894-the-role-of-oxalates-in-autism-and-chronic-disorders.html.
212. P. Störtebecker, *Mercury Poisoning from Dental Amalgam—A Hazard to the Human Brain* (Orlando: Bio-Probe, 1985), 9, 64.
213. M. Kauppi, "Sweating Out Mercury," *Heavy Metal Bulletin* 6, no. 2 (October 2000): 14.
214. Ibid.
215. M. Lebowitz, notes from an Applied Kinesiology seminar (September 1992).
216. K. Wright, "Our Preferred Poison," *Discover,* March 2005, 58.
217. J. Robbins, *Reclaiming Our Health* (Tiburon, Calif.: H. J. Kramer, 1998), 15–16.

4

TOXIC CHEMICALS

In the late 1940s, when the use of amalgam fillings began to boom, the chemical age also took off, fueled by technology developed during World War II. Before the war, virtually no petroleum-based pesticides and few petroleum-based household products had been in use. Environmentalist Lynn Lawson reminisces about this less toxic era in her book, *Staying Well in a Toxic World:*

> Farmers fertilized fields with manure, not chemicals . . . flyswatters or sticky pest strips caught flies. Housewives washed clothes with soap, not detergents. Synthetic fabrics, except for rayon, did not exist; there was no "need" for fabric softeners. Women wore cotton or, rarely, silk stockings. Perfumes were made from flowers, medications mostly from plants.[1]

In contrast, from the 1940s to the end of the century an astonishing 87,000 new chemicals were synthesized in the United States alone. This trend has continued, with new chemicals now being invented at a rate of at least 2,000 per year.[2]

> **toxic chemical:** By broad definition, the term *toxic chemical* can refer to *any* chemical substance that can induce morbidity (illness) or mortality (death)—whether it is an inorganic compound such as lead or mercury, an organic compound such as methyl alcohol or DDT, or a naturally occurring poison such as snake venom. However, this chapter will focus on synthetic organic compounds (and a few inorganic compounds) derived primarily from petrochemicals.

"NEXT TO NOTHING" KNOWN ABOUT MOST OF THESE CHEMICALS

Today, more than 5 million chemicals are known worldwide, with 65,000 in commercial use and 10,000 produced at a rate greater than a million pounds per year.[3] But what is particularly alarming is that we know next to nothing about the toxic effects of the great majority of these chemicals. In fact, a National Research Council study found that complete information on the hazards to human health were available for only 10 percent of pesticides and for only 18 percent of chemically derived medications. Furthermore, almost no tests have been conducted to determine the synergistic effects of chemicals when they are combined in the air we breathe, the food we eat, and the shampoos, shaving creams, and lotions we absorb daily through our skin.[4] As a 2004 report by the Pesticide Action Network North America (PANNA) stated, "Almost nothing is known about the long-term impacts of multiple chemicals in the body over long periods."[5]

PESTICIDES LINKED TO CANCER

The statistics on pesticides are especially dramatic. In 1950, less than 10 percent of cornfields were sprayed with pesticides; in 1993, 99 percent were chemically treated.[6] In 1996, an estimated 98 percent of all U.S. families used a pesticide at least once a year.[7] One of the most commonly used pesticides, atrazine, is strongly suspected of causing breast and ovarian cancer in humans.[8] Furthermore, at least twenty peer-reviewed studies have linked the use of pesticides to cancer in children.[9] Even the conservative

National Cancer Institute has estimated that as many as 98 percent of all cancers may be correlated to chemical exposure.[10] Pesticides and other modern industrial chemicals have also been connected with an increased incidence of other illnesses, including neurological diseases such as Parkinson's and amyotrophic lateral sclerosis (ALS), hormone disruptions including infertility and impotency, emotional and sociopathic disorders,* and autoimmune syndromes such as thyroiditis and lupus.[11]

The Toxic Hazards of Modern-Day Farming

Farmers, whom you might logically consider to be a healthier population than city-dwellers, have been found in at least seven studies to have higher rates of leukemia, Hodgkin's disease, non-Hodgkin's lymphoma, multiple myeloma, and cancers of the bone, brain, connective tissue, eye, kidney, lip, pancreas, prostate, skin, stomach, and thyroid. This litany of degenerative and toxicity-induced diseases concentrated in those who enjoy "clean" country air is more understandable, however, if you take into account the fact that of the billion pounds of pesticides used in the United States every year, more than three-quarters is used on farms.[12]

PCBs Resist Natural Decay

Chemicals do not confine themselves to isolated farming areas. Polychlorinated biphenyls (PCBs), by-products of the production of pesticides, paints, varnishes, wood, rubber, and plastics, are found everywhere—in soil, air, and water; in the mud of lakes and rivers; in the ocean; and in fish, birds, and other animals. In 1929, the Swann Chemical Company (which became part of Monsanto in 1935) first manufactured PCBs. They were finally banned in the United States in 1976 as much for their toxicity as for their "persistence"—that is, their resistance to natural decay for years, decades, or even centuries. Today, PCBs are found all over the globe, even in the remote and once pristine Arctic.[13]

*Here's a heart-stopping statistic: "In World War II, . . . the military found that 80 percent of its riflemen would not fire at an exposed enemy soldier, and as a result they had to devise ways to make killing more acceptable and reflexive (one method was to use cutouts of the human figure). By the Vietnam War, as many as 90 percent of GIs had overcome their reticence and could automatically shoot to kill," according to Lt. Col. Dave Grossman, a retired West Point psychology professor specializing in child violence, in a 2002 article in the *Marin Independent Journal.*

Dioxins and Other Potent Carcinogens

Dioxins, a family of seventy-five chlorinated chemicals, are so extremely toxic that an amount the size of a fist is enough to kill every person on earth. "TCDD, the most lethal form of the dioxin family, is a known human carcinogen and hormone disrupter and is recognized as the most toxic synthetic compound ever produced. All humans and animals now carry body burdens of TCDD and other dioxins."[14] As a by-product of twentieth-century life from the manufacture of chlorine-containing chemicals such as pesticides and wood preservatives, as well as from bleaching paper with chlorine, incinerating trash, and burning fossil fuels, dioxins have been detected virtually everywhere—in air, water, soil, and food. Dioxins accumulate in the fat stores of the human body.[15] In fact, in 1982 the EPA National Human Adipose Tissue Survey found that dioxin was present in *100 percent* of adipose (fat) tissue specimens sampled from across the United States.[16] (The other four chemicals to also enjoy this privilege were the solvents styrene, 1,4-dichlorobenzene, xylene, and ethylphenol.)[17]Although studies have clearly confirmed that dioxin-exposed workers show a statistically significant increase in lung cancer, the EPA's reluctance to regulate dioxin as a clear carcinogen has allowed this chemical to continue to be a major pollutant.[18]

Fortunately, a November 2005 ruling by a Michigan judge has allowed a class-action lawsuit to go forward against Dow Chemical for exposing residents around Lake Huron to dioxin-contaminated soil and dust and a variety of illnesses including cancer.[19] (Dow Chemical is also currently under attack for its pesticide chlorpyrifos, a known nerve toxin and endocrine disruptor that was recently banned from almost all household use but is still being widely used in agriculture.[20])

THE BODY BURDEN
Toxic Chemicals Pandemic

Chemical exposure is so inherent to modern-day life that no person is free from a body burden of toxins, as several studies have conclusively shown.

For example, a 2002 study led by scientists at the Mount Sinai School of Medicine and the Environmental Working Group tested the blood and urine of nine subjects for 210 toxic chemicals. (The reason they studied only nine subjects is that testing for 210 chemicals is prohibitively expensive.)[21] Although these nine volunteers did not work with chemicals on the job or live near chemical or industrial plants, the study found on average 91 industrial toxic compounds in each subject, with a total of 167 different compounds in the group as a whole. These 167 chemicals included:

76 chemicals linked to cancer in humans or animals
77 chemicals toxic to the immune system
94 chemicals toxic to the brain and nervous system
86 chemicals that interfere with hormone regulation
79 chemicals associated with birth defects or abnormal development[22]

These startling results were corroborated by a November 2005 report from the Canadian organization Environmental Defense, titled *Toxic Nation: A Report on Pollution in Canadians*. The report gave results of blood and urine tests for a broad range of Canadians; the tests detected in each subject an average of forty-four chemicals, including forty-one carcinogens, twenty-seven hormone disruptors, twenty-one respiratory toxins, and fifty-three reproductive-system toxins.[23] The authors of the report concluded, "Toxic chemicals contaminate people no matter where they live, how old they are or what they do for a living."[24] A similar study in the United States in 2003 tested 9,282 Americans for 116 chemicals; over half tested positive for twenty-nine pesticides, with an average of thirteen pesticides in each subject.[25]

A 2005 study by the Environmental Working Group (EWG) provides the most damning evidence of our out-of-control toxic environment. These researchers tested cord blood—the blood that is pumped back and forth between the nutrient- and oxygen-rich placenta and a developing fetus—for chemical contamination. Scientists had once thought that the placenta shields cord blood; however, the EWG researchers reported that the cord blood of the average baby at birth now contains at least two hundred chemicals. Of the 287 chemicals they detected, they found the following:

180 cause cancer in humans or animals
217 are toxic to the brain and nervous system
208 cause birth defects or abnormal development in animal tests

As this study clearly demonstrates, from the beginning modern-day infants face an enormous toxic hurdle. And most disturbing of all, as the EWG researchers conclude, "the dangers of pre- or post-natal exposure to this complex mixture of carcinogens, developmental toxins, and neurotoxins have never been studied."[26]

CHEMICAL REGULATION

Profit-Driven Chemical Companies Tend to Oppose Regulation

In light of the overwhelming evidence linking cancer and other diseases to toxic chemicals, you might think that we would take major steps to help transform nonorganic farms to organic ones and to regulate industries that continue to produce obvious toxic chemicals. However, in the present capitalism-at-any-cost climate, making changes that could possibly inhibit profits for large corporations is always a daunting uphill battle. This economic obstacle to regulation and reform is especially challenging in light of such statistics as the fact that in 1995 alone, the one hundred largest U.S. chemical companies made over $35 billion in profits.[27]

Intentions Can Be Genuine

The rationale supporting the production of toxic chemicals has not always been economic. On many World War II front lines, diseases carried by insects killed more American GIs than the enemy. Therefore, when the Swiss firm J. R. Geigy invented dichlorodiphenyltrichloroethane (DDT) in 1943, the U.S. government, elated with this new "miracle white powder," dusted millions of soldiers and refugees with it in order to prevent malaria and typhus.[28] By the end of the war, sales of DDT had escalated as farmers, public health officials, and the rest of America used this "atomic bomb of the insect world."[29] By 1951, the company now known as Ciba-Geigy and its licensees, including DuPont and General Chemical Company, were selling a staggering $110 million of DDT per year.[30] However, by as early as the late 1950s evidence of the darker side of this pesticide—its very deadly effects—came into light, including the revelations of Rachel Carson's widely read book *Silent Spring*. Despite this clear toxic link, DDT's registration wasn't revoked until more than two decades later, in 1972.[31]

Ramifications of the Lengthy Regulation Process

Unfortunately, the snail-like pace at which toxic chemicals are regulated has still not been remedied. Even now, it takes an average of five to ten years to remove a hazardous pesticide from the market once it has been recognized as dangerous.[32] The lengthy regulation process can have dire ramifications. In fact, a 2003 CDC study found DDE, a breakdown product of DDT, in 99 percent of the 9,282 American subjects tested.[33] This startling statistic results from subjects being exposed to DDT residues in soil (in soil DDT has a half-life of two to fifteen years, meaning in that time half of the residues will break down and half will remain), eating foods imported from countries that have still not banned DDT, breathing air or drinking water near waste sites or landfills, and ingesting breast milk from mothers who have been exposed.[34]

THE RESPONSIBLE USE OF PETROCHEMICALS

To many holistically minded individuals, the modern use of petrochemicals evokes images of shortened lives destroyed by cancer and other degenerative diseases, environmental abominations such as a plastic six-pack holder wrapped tightly around a pelican's neck, and garish fast-food signs littering once-pristine small towns. However, few of us would choose to give up the convenience of our automobiles (with approximately 360 pounds of plastic parts*), the luxury of airplanes, which allow us to travel to a vacation destination in a matter of hours rather than days or weeks (airplanes have approximately 2 tons of plastic components), or the fuel it takes to power them.[35] Nor would we willingly part with our computers, telephones, or Gore-Tex rain gear.

The solution to this double-edged sword of great benefit as well as vast destruction is the responsible use of modern-day chemicals and plastics. Unfortunately, a cursory review of the government's abysmal track record in protecting its citizens strongly suggests that relying on regulatory agencies to inform or shield us from toxic chemicals is not a prudent choice. However, by limiting our exposure to chemical toxins in our immediate environment, that is, our workplace, our home, and our body, we can substantially decrease our toxic burden over time. When we combine this measure with effective nutritional, homeopathic, hydrotherapy, and lifestyle protocols, we can effect significant change in our present health and well-being, as well as greatly reducing our risk of future degenerative disease.

The following sections discuss the pervasive chemicals found in the workplace, in schools, in cars, and in our homes. We'll cover in depth the toxic chemicals found in personal care and cleaning products, since the effective protocol for exposure to these products is so simple: identify them and then replace them with petroleum-free alternatives.

*Plastics are made from large molecules called polymers that consist of long repeating chains of smaller molecules, called monomers. Monomers are extracted from petrochemicals such as crude oil and natural gas.

THE WORK ENVIRONMENT

The Overworked American Workers

U.S. workers currently have less time off than workers in any other developed nation in the world. With an average of only thirteen vacation days per year, U.S. workers have even surpassed cultures with a reputation for a stronger work ethic, such as the Japanese, who have twenty-five vacation days, and the Germans, who have thirty-five.[36] Furthermore, the United States is the only developed country in the world without mandatory vacation time.[37] Considering the "24-7" work ethic fostered in thousands of corporations and dot-coms over the past few decades, this often translates into very little to no time off. Therefore, many Americans spend much of their lives at work. Look around you: what kind of environment are you living in eight to ten (or more) hours per day for five (or six or seven) days a week?

Sick Building Syndrome

Few, if any, could have predicted the devastating effect that the energy crisis of the late 1970s would indirectly have on thousands of people's health through the building trade. But after the crisis, in an attempt to conserve energy as much as possible, airtight windows and doors, concrete floors, insulation foam, impermeable layers of plastic paints and adhesives, and plastic vapor barriers were all employed to render buildings airtight and more energy efficient.[38] This trend spawned modern offices and homes in which trapped chemical vapors, molds, bacteria, dust, and stale air continuously circulate.

The popular UFFI (urea foam formaldehyde insulation), which was sprayed into thousands of homes and buildings, sickened many literally overnight when it off-gassed formaldehyde, a proven carcinogen.[39] Further concentrating the toxic vapors in energy-efficient sealed structures, strong formaldehyde resins and glues were mixed with particleboard, plywood, and fiberboard in the cabinets, flooring, walls, and furniture put into virtually every American home and office built or renovated since World War II. When we also consider the popular use of formaldehyde-laden prefabricated cubicle walls, off-gassing from wall-to-wall carpeting and its glues, and toxic fumes from felt pens, inks, copy machines, perfumes, and car exhaust in parking garages, it's no wonder that many sickened and exhausted workers have little energy for anything other than hitting the couch as soon as they get home. In fact, after conducting a five-year study of the twenty most common toxic chemicals, the EPA reported that indoor air was three to seventy times more toxic than outdoor air, even in heavily polluted areas such as Los Angeles and Bayonne, New Jersey.[40]

According to the World Health Organization, this "chemical soup" that many people subject themselves to for forty or more hours per week can be the source of sick building syndrome (SBS), causing such vague and numerous symptoms as sore throats, headaches, sore eyes, joint pains, nausea, and chest tightness.[41] SBS has many synonyms—tight building syndrome, environmental illness, multiple chemical sensitivity syndrome (MCSS)—and has even been referred to as "twentieth-century disease," since many people become sensitized in a new or newly remodeled workplace (or home). The great majority of these people are unaware that their symptoms are associated with the toxicity of their workplace. Dr. Sherry Rogers, a leading physician in environmental medicine, calls these people the "walking wounded," because their various and quite diverse symptoms are rarely recognized by allopathic physicians as possible chemical sensitivity.[42] In fact, many of the most typical symptoms—mood swings, inability to concentrate, "spaciness," anxiety, and depression—are often disparaged as simply psychosomatic when patients' standard laboratory tests and X-rays come back negative.[43]

Furthermore, many of these workers' mild, vague, and intermittent symptoms are not considered severe enough even to warrant a doctor's visit. The fatigue, headaches, irritability, and sneezing, coughing, and congestion associated with chronic allergic reactions—indicative of the body's struggle to drain and detoxify chemical irritants—are so common and ubiquitous nowadays that chemical intoxication is rarely considered. Even more alarming than the diminished quality of life toxic chemicals induce, however, is the warning these symptoms sound for future serious disease. Dr. Samuel Epstein, professor of occupational and environmental medicine at the University of Illinois Medical Center in Chicago, cautions that most cancer diagnoses represent events and exposures that occurred often decades before.[44]* Because these major health problems may not manifest until years after a worker has been exposed, proving a direct cause-and-effect relationship is difficult and often obstructs employees from receiving compensation from their employer.[45]

Factory and Trade Occupations and Farming

Because of their more obvious direct chemical exposure, people working in factories and in trades are studied more than office workers and therefore are more often cited in the literature to be at risk for developing occupationally induced cancer and neurological disease. Significantly elevated cancer rates have been found among painters, asbestos workers, welders, plastics manufacturers, dye and fabric makers, firefighters, miners, printers, and radiation workers.[46] Other hazardous occupations include artists (who work with paints, solvents, dyes, and so on), gas station and refinery workers, cosmetologists, copy shop employees, housecleaners and janitors, dry-cleaning workers, photo processors, chemists, nurses and medical doctors (who are exposed to anesthesia, chemotherapy, drugs, antiseptics, et cetera),

*The long-term cause-and-effect scenario is further illustrated by the cases of "status thymicolymphaticus" diagnosed in the first half of the twentieth century, when infants' "bulging thymus glands" were irradiated by doctors who didn't understand that this gland is normally enlarged during the early maturation years of the immune system. Those who underwent irradiation as infants typically developed tumors later, when they were in their late twenties—almost three decades after their initial X-ray exposure. (Marc Lappe, *Chemical Deception* [San Francisco: Sierra Club Books, 1991], 90.)

dentists and their assistants (who work with anesthesia, glues, cements, et cetera), microchip manufacturing workers, and, of course, farmers and field workers.[47]

The U.S. Bureau of Labor Statistics rates the mining, agricultural, construction, and manufacturing industries as the most dangerous occupations in respect to exposure to chemical and hazardous substances.[48] However, as discussed earlier, farming exceeds even these occupations, with farmers and field workers exhibiting much higher rates of cancer than the general population and dying more often from these cancers. Children of workers in these toxic occupations also have higher rates of cancer. In fact, childhood brain cancers and leukemias have been consistently correlated with parental exposure to paint, petroleum products, solvents, and pesticides.[49] And these statistics don't take into account the fact that many cases of pesticide poisoning go unreported because of field workers' fear of losing a job, doctors' failure to recognize and/or report pesticide-related illnesses, and the failure of insurance companies to submit doctors' reports to the proper authorities.[50] Even more alarming, not only for farm workers but also for people living near farms, is that 51 percent of pesticide poisoning cases reported between 1998 and 2000 occurred when pesticides *drifted* from a site.[51]

Government Agencies Fail to Protect Workers

Unfortunately for the health of its citizens, the U.S. government's two occupational safety agencies—the Occupational Safety and Health Administration (OSHA) and the National Institute for Occupational Safety and Health (NIOSH)—which are charged with protecting both workers and the environment, are both understaffed and underfunded. What's more, lengthy lawsuits from industries and chemical companies often block research into chemical safety as well as the health and safety regulations the two agencies try to impose. By 1988, for example, eighteen years after its founding, OSHA had managed to set limits on only twenty-four of the thousands of chemicals in the American workplace. In 1991, when OSHA tried to set standards for 200 other chemicals based on well-established research, the courts ruled against the agency.[52] Unfortunately, this lack of government oversight continues today. In testimony from 2010, Public Employees for Environmental Responsibility (PEER) stated that OSHA has been "missing in action" in regulating the more than 70,000 chemicals that kill tens of thousands of workers each year.[53]

Even when companies' or industries' violations of chemical safety regulations are cited, the fines are often so small that leading safety expert John Moran has referred to them as "a goddamn joke. In construction nobody worries about OSHA anymore. They don't take it seriously."[54] Similarly, although the EPA by law is required to publish complete information on chemicals used in farming, industry, and the American home, only two reviews of the more than 19,000 pesticides on the market were completed by 1992.[55]

More recently, however, chemical toxicity issues have come to be of greater concern for regulators, perhaps because of greater concern about toxicity in the public. For example, in 2005 the Florida Department of Agriculture fined the company Ag-Mart $111,200 for eighty-eight pesticide violations that probably resulted in severe birth defects (and infant deaths) in the children of three female workers.[56] Although the fine was not a large amount of money for a major agribusiness, the impact of the decision has broader reach. For example, the sixth-largest supermarket chain, Publix Super Markets, stopped selling Ag-Mart's tomatoes in the fall of 2005 based on these reports, and Ag-Mart also came under fire in North Carolina for 369 violations of pesticide regulations.[57]

THE SCHOOL ENVIRONMENT

Sick School Syndrome

Schools are not immune to SBS and in fact have generated their own acronym—SSS, or sick school syndrome. In 1989 the EPA reported "in public buildings such as offices, schools, and nursing homes, eight common chemicals were increased [over outdoor air levels] by factors of about a hundred." Thus, students, teachers, and other school employees often suffer from respiratory illnesses, headaches, skin rashes, dizziness, and other chronic symptoms from the fumes released by carpet glue, cockroach and termite sprays, floor polish, particleboard shelving, and other modern building materials.[58]

At the elementary level, classrooms are less likely to contain some of the toxins—perfumes, aftershaves, hair spray, and cosmetics—that abound in higher school levels. However, many extremely toxic chemicals are used in nearly every elementary school's arts and crafts curriculum, such as rubber cement, permanent felt-tip markers, pottery glazes, enamels, spray fixatives, and wallpaper paste.[59] Additionally, pesticide spraying is still quite routine in most school districts.[60] Numerous chemicals used in these pesticides have been correlated to abnormalities in children's behavior, perception, cognition, and motor skills.[61] For example, in a 2002 study reported in the *Journal of the American Medical Association,* researchers found that children are increasingly being poisoned by forty-eight commonly used pesticides in schools, of which twenty-four are probable or possible carcinogens and twenty-five are linked with reproductive defects, thirty-three with liver or kidney damage, and thirty-three with neurotoxicity.[62] Commenting on this study, Jay Feldman, the executive director of Beyond Pesticides, a national environmental group, noted, "It makes no sense to send children back to school with inhalers and then spray pesticides that cause respiratory problems in the school buildings and grounds."[63]

Electromagnetic Field Pollution

Strong electromagnetic fields (EMFs) in and around schoolyards can compound the toxic stressors enervating young immune systems. Studies have shown that EMFs are responsible for a two- to threefold increase in the cancer rate of children exposed to them, particularly in terms of leukemia, lymphoma, and brain tumors.[64] Learning disabilities have also been linked to EMFs, as have lowered levels of the neurotransmitters dopamine and serotonin, which correlate to behavioral disorders, depression, and suicide.[65] EMF exposure comes from high-tension wires and power transformers, fluorescent lighting and computers, and common electronics such as cell phones and portable music players.

Playing Hooky or Avoiding a Toxic Environment?

It is important for parents to consider these chemical and EMF toxins when their children complain of being sick of school. In truth, their children may simply be sick *at* school. Many children with attention deficit disorder (ADD) or attention-deficit-hyperactivity disorder (ADHD) improve dramatically when schools reduce their use of chemical toxins, open windows to let in fresh air, limit or ban cell phone and music-player usage, and exchange fluorescents for full-spectrum lights.

Mixed News for Children

Fortunately, school environments have recently seen some changes for the better. In New York, for example, the state senate voted in 2005 to require schools to begin using "green" cleaning products.[66] And seventeen states have currently enacted laws that require or recommend the use of integrated pest management (IPM), which focuses on pest prevention and the use of only the least toxic pesticides, in their schools. Schools in Seattle, Washington, as well as twenty-one school districts in North Carolina have adopted IPM successfully over the last few years and implemented "creative, cost-effective programs that ensure clean, safe learning environments for children."[67]

But the news is not all good. Although thirty-three states have passed some type of legislation to address pesticide use in and around schools, no federal legislation exists to fully protect schoolchildren around the country. On the national front, the School Environment Protection Act (SEPA), written to reduce the use of pesticides in schools and also to prevent pesticide drift from farmland to schools, has still not become law, despite numerous attempts to pass the bill since 1999.[68]

THE POWER OF DIET

In an uplifting study conducted in 2005 at Emory University, researchers were astonished at the significant "plunge" in children's pesticide levels after their diet was converted from conventional to organic foods.[69] The "dramatic and immediate protective effect" of converting to an organic diet is particularly heartening given that, compared to adults, children's developing organ and immune systems are more vulnerable to pesticides, and they consistently take in more toxic chemicals relative to their body weight. For example, a 2003 CDC study showed that young children carry the highest body burden—almost twice that of adults—of the insecticide and nerve toxin chlorpyrifos.[70]

► For information on advocating for toxin-free schools, go to www.beyondpesticides.org and www.panna.org.

THE AUTOMOBILE ENVIRONMENT

Toxic Chemical Off-Gassing in Cars

New cars off-gas so many toxic vapors that some models display warning labels on the inside of their windshield. From the formaldehyde-laden carpet and foam seat cushions to the vinyl or leather-treated interiors, new automobiles generate noxious fumes that are obvious to the environmentally sensitive and insidiously intoxicating even to those oblivious to these odors. Unfortunately, in areas of heavy traffic or industry, rolling down the windows only slightly reduces the internal toxicity, as the passengers are then barraged with exhaust fumes and air pollution.

Even the environmentally friendly hybrids subject passengers to the toxic "new car smell." In fact, a recent study by the Michigan-based Ecology Center found that cars from Toyota—the producer of the popular Prius—along with those from Chrysler, Subaru, Volkswagen, and Mercedes had some of the highest concentrations of polybrominated diphenyl ethers (PBDEs).* In regard to toxic phthalates (plasticizers),† Toyota cars once again tested with some of the highest levels, along with automobiles from Hyundai, Ford, and Chrysler.

In contrast, cars from the Swedish manufacturer Volvo (now owned by Ford) had the lowest levels of toxic chemicals in both categories, due to the fact that the company has been "working for many years on creating a clean interior climate, which is also suitable for people who are particularly sensitive, such as those suffering from asthma and allergies."[71] And in 2009 an American car (the Chevrolet Cobalt) tested as the least toxic vehicle for the first time, proving that "GM has the innovation and know-how to make healthy vehicles."[72]

► See www.healthystuff.org for the Ecology Center's consumer guide to toxic chemicals in cars and children's car seats. The group tests over 700 new and used vehicles for chemicals that off-gas from the steering wheel, dashboard, seats, and carpets.

*PBDEs are toxic flame retardants added to plastic widely used in household products and electronic devices.

†Phthalate esters are esters of phthalic acid mainly used as plasticizers to increase the flexibility and durability of plastic.

Electromagnetic Field Stress in Hybrids

At the end of *Thank You for Smoking,* the dark comedy about an executive working for Big Tobacco, the protagonist meets with new clients from the cell phone industry. Mirroring his strategy with tobacco, he offers them this advice: "Look into the mirror and repeat: 'There is no conclusive scientific evidence linking cell phone usage and brain cancer.'" Unfortunately, this statement is not just reserved for black comedies but continues to be the primary defense for the cell phone industry, as well as other industries that generate powerful electromagnetic fields (EMFs). Many holistically oriented individuals are shocked to find that hybrid cars can also fall into this category.

As early as 1990, after amassing one hundred studies, the EPA recommended that EMFs be classified as a class B carcinogen—that is, a probable human carcinogen. However, after significant pressure from electronics and military lobbyists, the EPA decided to rescind its decision, concluding in its final report simply that studies had shown a "causal link" between EMFs and leukemia, lymphoma, and cancer in children.[73] EMF radiation from cell phones has been studied extensively, and even many mainstream scientists have begun to admit its link with cancer. However, the EMFs generated by the huge batteries in hybrid cars such as the best-selling Toyota Prius and the Honda Civic Hybrid have received little attention. Although a small number of drivers have become ill after beginning use of a hybrid car (experiencing excessive drowsiness, headaches, anxiety, heart palpitations and increased blood pressure, tinnitus, brain fog, memory loss, and other symptoms), most drivers remain oblivious to the EMFs produced by hybrid car batteries.[74]

Evidence for EMF stress in hybrid cars remains contradictory and inconclusive primarily because many gauss meters used to measure EMF strength are unreliable and inaccurate. And there has been little professional research conducted on the EMFs that hybrid batteries—not to mention all the other automotive gadgetry that has become popular, such as GPS systems and onboard cell phones—generate. Until this issue is addressed more thoroughly, individuals should consider testing hybrids themselves with a reliable gauss meter before purchasing them.* I've used the Trifield Meter (model 100XE) to measure EMFs from hybrid batteries as well as automotive GPS navigation systems, and I've found that both generate significantly disturbing magnetic fields. Disturbingly, the backseat of the hybrid, which is closest to the battery, tests especially high, and this is where infants and children—our most susceptible passengers—sit.

- The TriField (model 100XE) gauss meter is relatively inexpensive and reasonably accurate. To order, call (800) 658-7030.
- To most accurately measure EMFs it is best to consult with an expert. Please contact Mary Cordaro through her website www.marycordaro.com when you need to make important decisions about your car, home, workplace, or other potentially electromagnetically stressful environments.

CELL PHONE SAFEGUARDS

To protect against ipsilateral brain cancer (tumors found on the side of the head on which cell phones are used), take the following steps:

1. Reserve your cell phone for emergencies and use a landline at home and work.
2. Turn your phone off when carrying it in your purse or pocket to reduce radiation exposure.
3. Do not allow your children to use cell phones; they are significantly more vulnerable to radiation than adults due to their thinner cranial bones.
4. Use a speaker phone or headset. When using the speaker phone option, hold the phone at least 6 inches away from your head when making a call. Another option is to use a well-shielded headset with an air tube so that there is no wire going up to your head.
5. Use a Pong cell phone holder (www.pongresearch.com), which reduces overall radiation by 60 perecnt and reduces cell phone "hot spot" radiation by 85 percent while still maintaining full signal strength.

Together, these precautions can drastically reduce your exposure to this damaging and ultimately carcinogenic radiation.

---

*A gauss meter can be used to measure EMFs not only in cars but also at home and at work (see "Measuring EMF Stress at Home" on page 121). The EPA has set a safety level of no greater than 1 mG (milligauss). However, Dr. Joseph Mercola, an osteopath and creator of the most frequently visited natural health website today, has recommended that for optimal wellness EMFs should not exceed 0.5 mG. (J. Mercola, "Are EMFs Hazardous to Our Health?" www.loveforlife.com.au/node/5064 [July 7, 2008], 1–7.)

THE HOME ENVIRONMENT

Sick House Syndrome

The heavily chemical-laden building materials used in "tight" new house construction or newly remodeled homes has generated yet another acronym—SHS, or sick house syndrome. The one place that should be sacrosanct, where an individual should be able to rest and relax, can be just as—or more—devastating to a person's health as a toxic work environment. While houses share many of the toxic aspects of new buildings, such as carpet, insulation, paint, and particleboard or plywood cabinets or furniture, they also carry an additional burden from the synthetic chemicals emanating from couches and mattresses, kitchen cleaners and disinfectants, refrigerant gas leaks, gas ovens, bathroom chemicals and perfumes, and fireplace smoke.

COMPACT FLUORESCENT LIGHT BULBS

The new compact fluorescent light (CFL) bulbs, like their predecesors, regular fluorescent bulbs, contain mercury. Although a CFL contains less mercury—4 to 15 mg compared to approximately 20 mg in a regular fluorescent—when either bulb breaks, mercury is released into the environment.[75] This potent neurotoxin can severely harm the nervous system in unsuspecting people and animals in the home as well as sanitation workers handling these broken bulbs in the garbage and landfills. When these bulbs break they are supposed to be taken to hazardous waste collection sites, but few people know this and few states, counties, and cities have outlawed disposing of these potentially dangerous bulbs in the trash.

For light-sensitive individuals, CFL and regular fluorescent bulbs have both been shown in numerous scientific studies to worsen skin conditions such as eczema, dermatitis, and rashes and to trigger migraine headaches and seizures.[76]

For these thousands of light-sensitive individuals, as well as for all health-minded people, avoiding fluorescent lighting is the safest bet for now. Stick with Edison's original incandescent light bulb until the Environmental Protection Agency realizes the colossal mistake it is making and provides the public with a safer, environmentally friendly alternative.

Children Are Most Vulnerable to Toxic New Homes

Chemicals embedded in new carpets and building materials are particularly hazardous to infants and children because their newly developing immune systems make them more vulnerable to toxins. In fact, studies of infants exposed to the "mere 'background' environmental levels of such pollutants" prenatally—that is, even before birth—have consistently shown delays and disturbances in neurological development.[77] Sensitive adults are similarly affected. In fact, holistic practitioners who specialize in environmental medicine often note that many new patients' symptoms began just after they remodeled their home, or after they moved into a newly constructed house.

Toxic Lawns

The internal house environment is not the only issue because a majority of homeowners use herbicides, insecticides, and pesticides both inside and outside of the house. However, an increasing amount of research clearly demonstrates that these chemicals are dangerous to children and pets. (Pesticides kill more than 30,000 pets each year and increase the risk of illnesses such as cancer in children.) In addition to polluting the air and water, these chemicals cause depression, vision problems, breathing difficulties, and cancer in the people that apply them.[78] Despite the advertising efforts of Monsanto (a $7.5 billion company), the active ingredient glyphosate in Roundup, the world's most widely used herbicide, was recently reported in a study by Swedish oncologists to have *clear links* with the onset of lymphoma, a form of cancer.[79] Fortunately, organic alternatives for lawn care are quite successful and many communities are currently endeavoring to go pesticide-free.

- ▶ For more information on alternatives to toxic lawn care products, visit www.beyondpesticides.org/lawn and www.panna.org.

DIAGNOSIS OF TOXIC CHEMICAL POISONING

Insidious, Invisible, and Pervasive

Toxic chemicals are often referred to as "the great masqueraders" because they produce such a wide spectrum of symptoms that can range from those of the severely impaired environmentally ill individual to the sneezing a new employee has every morning in his cubicle at work. In fact, these invisible and even often odorless chemicals are so ubiquitous that they can be difficult to diagnose.[80] Because many typical symptoms such as headaches, joint pain, mild intermittent short-term memory loss, and fatigue are completely subjective, they cannot be validated by standard laboratory tests.

Feeling Relief away from a Toxic Home or Office

One simple way to pinpoint the source of toxicity is to notice how you feel at work, at home, or in the car. Many sensitive individuals readily smell or just even "sense" toxic chemicals as soon as they walk into a new building. Others may not immediately perceive the toxic environment, but when questioned by an alert practitioner they may realize that they don't generally feel well at work (e.g., at the hospital, tight office building, or beauty salon), or on the weekends even while relaxing in their newly constructed home. Experiencing the relief of their symptoms during business trips or vacations may point to a toxic home or office, especially when headaches, allergies, fatigue, and other symptoms manifest once again when they return to their regular routine.

Testing Methods and Personal Histories

Individuals who are very ill or those considering a workers' compensation claim may want to invest in specialized testing at laboratories that focus on toxic chemicals. Blood and urine sample testing have been found to be more valid than hair analysis. Sam Queen, director of the Institute for Health Realities and a leading authority on the effects of toxic metals and chemicals, has found the following "toxic footprints" of blood that often indicate the presence of toxic chemicals:[81]*

*For more information on the effect of toxic chemicals on blood and how to interpret these findings, contact the Institute for Health Realities in Colorado at (719) 598-4968, or go to www.healthrealities.org.

Solvents: Elevated triglycerides
Pesticides: Elevated HDL; low cholesterol/HDL ratio
Petrochemicals: Elevated IGE, eosinophils, and basophils

► One of the best labs for chemical testing is Pacific Toxicology Laboratories in Los Angeles: (800) 538-6942 or www.pactox.com.

Holistic practitioners trained in environmental illness can also identify the effects of toxic chemicals by simply listening to a thorough history. If an individual's decline in health began just after he or she moved into a new house or started work in a "tight" building, the cause-and-effect relationship of toxic chemicals is often relatively obvious. Furthermore, when a patient lists a present or past toxic profession such as a painter, artist, chemist, nurse, farmer, and so forth on the history form, this should serve as a red flag to question the patient further during the history.

Finally, since so many symptoms are rarely severe enough to evoke positive neurological findings during standard physical exams, energetic testing can be valuable in helping to estimate the extent of toxic insult and the organs and tissues most affected.

MEASURING EMF STRESS AT HOME

As described earlier in "The Automobile Environment," gauss meters can help identify EMF stressors at home, including computers, microwave ovens (these should not be used at all, however; see chapter 5) and other kitchen appliances, telephones (landlines and cells), hair dryers, and even the electrical wiring in walls (especially those that have the electricity coming into the house on the wall outside a particular room). The EPA has set a safety level of no greater than 1 mG (milligauss). However, Dr. Joseph Mercola has recommended that for optimal wellness, EMFs should not exceed 0.5 mG.[82]

Do as much remedial action and rearranging as you can to reduce EMFs in your home, including keeping all electrical equipment as far away from your bed as possible. EMFs reduce with distance, so if you can't change your bedroom to another room, for example, at least move your bed six feet or more away from a wall that tests positive for high electromagnetic field levels from electrical wiring. Many individuals have made their bedroom an EMF-free haven and report sleeping much more soundly at night as a result.

DEALING WITH A TOXIC ENVIRONMENT

Toxic chemicals have become so pervasive in our society that trying to decide exactly where to begin and what treatments to undertake for these *xenobiotics*—that is, chemicals foreign to the body—can feel rather overwhelming. However, several significant measures can considerably reduce a person's xenobiotic load and initiate effective drainage and detoxification in the body. These holistic steps can help reduce or eliminate current symptoms, as well as reduce the risk for future degenerative disease.

Avoidance

If an individual is very ill and works in a toxic environment, transferring to another job site or even quitting may be options to consider. Some employers offer work-at-home opportunities that can both reduce the financial burden of possible workers' compensation payments and provide the employee with a safe means of earning income. Likewise, if someone lives in a new, remodeled, or mobile home that is extremely toxic, moving out is invariably cheaper than trying to replace most of the building materials with nontoxic alternatives, not to mention the savings on medical bills. An excellent solution is to find an older home, built prior to the 1950s or 1960s—but make sure that it is free of asbestos.[83]

Similarly, parents of a child in a toxic school building may want to consider transferring their child to a different school if they meet resistance in talking to teachers and administrators about nontoxic chemicals and installing windows that open.

In regard to new cars, the answer is easy—don't buy one. In fact, the Tappet Brothers (Tom and Ray Magliozzi) of National Public Radio's *Car Talk* would wholeheartedly agree based on the great financial loss that occurs simply after driving off the dealer's lot! Furthermore, individuals can still enjoy a late-model car by buying one that is six months to one year old, after it has off-gassed enough to be reasonably nontoxic. If individuals are very ill or extremely sensitive, however, they often choose to purchase a much older car with a cloth (not vinyl or treated leather) interior and with more metal than plastic surfaces.

Ventilation and Protection

Open windows, fans, and air filters can be helpful in clearing out chemical vapors, molds, dust, and other contaminants. After the installation of a new carpet or building a new addition on a house, one to two weeks of keeping windows open and twenty-four-hour air filtration can greatly mitigate chemical off-gassing. In a new car, using an air filter that plugs into the cigarette lighter and driving with the windows down (in nonpolluted areas) for several weeks can help dispel toxic fumes considerably.

Ventilation measures are considerably more difficult in the workplace, however, especially if other workers don't experience any stress from—or at least don't equate their symptoms with—the toxic work environment. Conservative relief options include placing an air filter next to your desk, working near an open window (if there is one), and taking more frequent breaks outside in lieu of a longer lunch period. A more drastic measure such as wearing a mask in an office environment can make a person the object of ridicule and is considered inappropriate in front of clients or customers, so it is not a viable choice.

In contrast, masks, protective suits, safety goggles, and other protective gear are often required in industry, mining, construction, laboratories, and other occupations that are recognized as exceptionally toxic and hazardous. However, when you are employed at these toxic or potentially toxic sites, it is important to conduct your own research and not simply trust the company's safety requirements or recommendations. Many of the industry guidelines are based on risk assessments—that is, the *probability* of harm from poisonous chemicals on the job site. Furthermore, these guidelines originate from governmental regulatory agencies where bureaucratic and political influences greatly affect the final published safety recommendations. Additionally, the company considers the financial impact of cleanup and its healthcare costs, and not simply the well-being of the workers. Thus, often many of the safety requirements for workers are based on standards of toxicity far below those recommended through independent laboratory evaluations. In fact, James Huff, a senior researcher at the National Institute of Environmental Health Sciences, has commented:

> This whole risk-assessment process is not science, it's voodoo stuff. . . . Just look at the standard-setting for various countries. Europe and Canada and the United States are miles apart as to what we think is the safe level for dioxin, and we're all supposed to be using risk assessment.[84]

Therefore, painters, chemists, miners, factory workers, manicurists, and other workers who labor in seriously toxic environments should research and acquire the most effective masks, goggles, and protective clothing possible to ensure that their health is not seriously compromised while at work. The savings in money spent on medical bills and the possible loss of income from taking too many sick days—or worse, disability—as well as the improved quality of life (and hopefully a longer life) are well worth the money expended for top-quality equipment.

Prevention

Fortunately there are currently numerous resources for nontoxic construction materials and furnishings for individuals who are planning to build a new house or addition. Although these cleaner materials can add an estimated 10 to 20 percent or more to the overall building costs, the enhanced quality of life in a nontoxic environment and mitigating the possibility of future healthcare costs from chemically induced illnesses are well worth the investment. The magazine *Natural Home* is one of the best resources for locating the most current environmentally friendly and nontoxic products and materials needed to remodel or build. Additionally, Mary Cordaro, a healthy home consultant and certified Bau-biologist,* is an excellent guide and teacher in helping individuals transform their home into a less toxic environment. For more than twenty years, she has specialized in the diagnosis of sick building syndrome and in building and remodeling healthy, green homes. Mary often keeps it simple for her clients by starting with the most essential room in the house—the bedroom. For example, she advocates first simply unplugging as much as possible, replacing the

*Originating in Germany, Bau-Biologie is the study of how homes and workplaces affect the health of both humans and the planet.

bedding with organic, hypoallergenic materials, and then, as you can afford it, replacing the mattress and remodeling as needed. She also has excellent advice on reducing indoor air pollution in your home, tips for traveling in airplanes and hotels, and information about the dangers of cell phones and cell towers on her website, www.marycordaro.com.

▶ To order *Natural Home* call (800) 340-5846, or go to www.naturalhomeandgarden.com.

PERSONAL CARE PRODUCTS

Although shampoos, soaps, and deodorants are certainly part of the home, the toxic influence of these personal care products is so widespread and complex it necessitates its own section. Additionally, it is the one area over which we have significant control, and we can therefore make many life-affirming changes here, right away, with relatively little expenditure. One of the most effective methods to treat current symptoms as well as to greatly reduce the chance of future degenerative disease is to simply replace toxic cosmetics and soaps in the bathroom and kitchen with nontoxic alternatives.

"The Harmless Aspect of the Familiar"

When she commented on "the harmless aspect of the familiar," wildlife biologist Rachel Carson was referring to the fact that hazards that are universally common or used repetitively, such as insecticides, can assume a rather ordinary and harmless reputation over time.[85] This astute observation is perhaps even more fitting for the use of personal care products. That is, the repetitive and seemingly harmless application of mascara, shampoo, shaving cream, and nail polish can feel so familiar and "normal" that the thought of these everyday products being carcinogenic can sound rather absurd at first. However, although many individuals tend to equate poisonous chemicals only with major offenders such as pesticides, exhaust fumes, and new paint fumes, newer research disputes this belief.

Phthalate Plasticizers: Linked to Cancer and Infertility

In a 1999 study of 3,800 Americans, government researchers at the CDC's National Center for Environmental Health found a "surprisingly high" amount of diethyl phthalate, a chemical used in soaps and cosmetics, in the subjects' blood and urine. This chemical was one of twenty-four toxins tested for in this first landmark nationwide study of environmental toxins in the body.[86] Phthalates (pronounced "THAY-lates") belongs to a class of compounds known as plasticizers, which are found in insect repellents, paints, adhesives, plastic bottles, and cellophane, and also quite abundantly in nail polish, hair spray, perfumes, and cosmetics.[87] Many phthalates are known to be overtly carcinogenic, while some have been identified as estrogenic hormone disruptors that have caused birth defects in animal studies.[88] The adverse endocrine effects of these plasticizers were further revealed in a study published in *Epidemiology* in 2003 that showed a clear link between the urinary excretion of phthalates and depressed sperm counts—and therefore infertility.[89] Infertility has become a major twenty-first-century issue, as has the opposite situation of multiple births that fertility drugs heavy-handedly generate in couples who may not be able to afford the cost of raising twins, triplets, or even quintuplets. In fact, almost 10 percent of U.S. couples have reported fertility problems according to the U.S. Department of Health and Human Services; on average, a man born in the 1970s has only three-quarters the sperm of a man born in the 1950s.[90]

Regulation of Personal Care Pollutants

Health Hazards Are Relatively Unknown

What is more frightening is that very few of the ingredients used in personal care products have been evaluated for their toxic effects. For example, in the 1990s, when the U.S. Congress investigated the potential health hazards of cosmetic products, it was found that out of approximately 3,000 chemicals used by the cosmetics industry, 884 had been reported to NIOSH as toxic substances.[91] A related investigation, based on the 1985 congressional hearings on neurotoxins and titled "Neurotoxins: At Home and the Workplace," concluded that "countless . . . substances applied daily to the skin of consumers in the form of soaps, perfumes, aftershaves, and detergents have yet to be tested for their chronic neurotoxic effects."[92] Furthermore, in a 2005 report, the Environmental Working Group (EWG) found that a full 89 percent of the 10,500 ingredients used in personal care products have not been evaluated by the FDA or by the self-regulating panel of the cosmetics industry, the Cosmetic Ingredient Review (CIR).[93] In fact, these chemical compounds sold on supermarket and drugstore shelves and found in almost everyone's medicine cabinet have emerged as such a major class of contaminants that they have spawned their own acronym—PPCPs, or pharmaceutical and personal care pollutants.[94]

Lax Regulations

Another major problem is the lack of government regulation over personal care products containing suspected or known toxins. With the exception of color ingredients that need to be authorized for use, it is not necessary to get FDA approval for a new cosmetic. In fact, the FDA is not even legally required to test cosmetics ingredients for safety.[95] The FDA can—and will—take action only after a cosmetic has been on the market and enough evidence has accumulated over time to prove in a court of law that the product is hazardous.[96] However, after nearly seventy years of monitoring cosmetics, the FDA has banned or restricted only *nine* personal care ingredients. In contrast, the European Union has banned 450 ingredients for use in cosmetics.[97] Furthermore, as these statistics reflect, the FDA spends less than 1 percent of its budget on cosmetics safety surveillance.[98]

Thus, safety issues have fallen primarily on the industry's self-regulating panel, the Cosmetic Ingredient Review (CIR), which is billed by the FDA as the organization that "thoroughly reviews and assesses the safety of ingredients used in cosmetics."[99] However, in 2005, a report by the Environmental Working Group (EWG) revealed that the CIR, which is funded by the cosmetics industry's trade association, has not examined 99.6 percent of the ingredients in cosmetics for potential health impacts.[100] These lax guidelines by both the U.S. government and the cosmetics industry have resulted in practically no toxicity regulations being implemented on personal care products. In fact, the admonition "Buyer Beware!" is probably more fitting for the purchase of cosmetics, shampoos, and soaps than for any other product sold in the United States.

Lack of Research on the Effects of Personal Care Products

Many questions remain unanswered about the direct effects of personal care products. For example, no tests have been conducted to ascertain the degree of absorption into the body when a moisturizing lotion containing toxic solvents and preservatives is spread all over the body, or when phthalate-laden hair spray is used daily. It is also entirely unknown whether an adult's diagnosis of cancer or a senior's dementia can be due to—or at least greatly compounded by—a lifetime of using cosmetics, colognes, shampoos, aftershaves, and deodorants. Furthermore, it is rarely suspected or acknowledged how much these daily toxic insults act as promoting factors, or tumor-accelerating factors, which are often suspected as the trigger for cancer and other degenerative diseases when combined with other more well-known environmental toxins. For example, some medications (such as an antimalarial drug called praziquantel) interact with benzene, a chemical found in nail polish remover, and dramatically increase its chromosome-breaking ability and leukemogenicity (tendency to cause leukemia).[101]

Virtually No Long-Term Studies

Unfortunately, the small amount of research conducted has been primarily *short term*—that is, focused on the often acute allergic reactions to cosmetics and perfumes. These symptoms typically include skin rashes, photosensitivity, dizziness, nausea, and respiratory illnesses. In contrast, longitudinal studies of chronic systemic toxicity from a lifetime of contact with these chemicals are almost nonexistent. Furthermore, since studies have shown that typical tumor-latency periods can be decades long—for example, over eleven years in the case of a large study of 28,460 benzene-exposed workers in China—the odds of the government footing the bill for a complex study of profit-driven makeup and personal care companies is probably next to nil.[102]

However, when the rate of multiple myeloma (malignant tumor of the bone marrow) is found to be *four* times the rate of the general population in a study of 58,000 cosmetologists, hairdressers, and manicurists, it certainly suggests a profound long-term impact.[103] Or furthermore, when women who use hair dye have been shown to have a *50 percent* higher risk of developing non-Hodgkin's lymphoma (another form of cancer, the incidence of which has risen 250 percent since 1950),[104] and that there is an almost doubled risk of multiple myeloma in men who use hair dye, the carcinogenicity and mutagenicity of these products sold in every drugstore come greatly into question.[105] Other studies have revealed that women who use permanent hair dyes once a month are twice as likely to develop bladder cancer as nonusers, and hairdressers who work daily around these chemicals have a fivefold increase in risk.[106] Currently in North America, Europe, and Japan, more than one in three women, and one in ten men over the age of forty, use some form of hair coloring, with 75 percent of both men and women using the more toxic permanent hair dyes.[107]

Chemical Absorption

Skin Absorption

All chemicals penetrate the skin to some extent, and many do so significantly. In fact, medications to prevent seasickness, treat angina (chest pains), and deliver estrogen and other hormones are manufactured in adhesive disks that ensure dermal absorption by being placed on the skin. Based on this, noted environmental physician Sherry Rogers cautions that individuals should be as cognizant about their makeup as their food:

> Skin absorption is so good that more and more prescription medicines are being manufactured in a patch form. . . . People who slather creams, colognes, and oils on their skin do not realize that it is just like *eating them,* for they reach the bloodstream as though they had eaten them.[108]

Thus, women who consider themselves holistically oriented and buy their groceries only at Whole Foods are unknowingly sabotaging themselves when they purchase their makeup at department stores that carry cosmetics loaded with petrochemicals. In fact, common petroleum solvents such as propylene glycol and xylene are used routinely in lotions, creams, and fragrances for their very soluble nature—that is, their ability to permeate through the skin. A recent report by the Environmental Working Group (EWG) revealed that 55 percent of all personal care products contain these "penetration enhancers."[109] Dermal penetration is further enhanced by dampness and heat that open the pores of the skin. Therefore, slapping on cologne or aftershave after a shave or spreading moisturizing lotion all over the body after a warm bath or shower greatly potentiates the dermal absorption of the toxic chemical ingredients into systemic circulation. Additionally, the ingestion of phthalate plasticizers and silicone from a lifetime of wearing (and licking off) lipstick alone is estimated at four pounds.[110] Because girls are using cosmetics at much younger ages now, they are increasing their lifetime exposure to the toxic chemicals in these products. In fact, by age thirteen, 84.9 percent of female children use lip gloss and 71.6 percent use blush.[111] In the adult population, a survey of 2,300 people revealed that adults generally use at least nine personal care products per day, with an average of 126 unique chemical ingredients received daily.[112]

Inhalation

Secondhand or "sidestream" exposure to perfumes and scented cosmetics, as with cigarette smoke, can be even more aggressive than skin applications. Perfume or cologne molecules travel directly to the brain from the nostrils via the olfactory bulb, the "nose brain" of the frontal cortex. Once in the frontal cortex, the molecules connect with—and disrupt—the master regulating centers of the hypothalamus and the pituitary glands.* The symptoms of dysfunction in the body's neurological (brain and nervous system) and hormonal centers are as prevalent as the damaged immune system signs of allergies, asthma, and cancer that are also associated with toxic chemicals. In fact, one study found perfume exposure caused dizziness, inability to concentrate, spaciness, mood changes, depression, sleepiness, and short-term memory lapses in over half of the 427 subjects surveyed.[113]

Neurological Damage Can Be Permanent

Symptoms of neurological damage are all the more disturbing because a nerve cell doesn't divide and regenerate like a liver or blood cell; therefore, nerve damage can be irreversible. As one neurotoxicologist testified before the U.S. Congress, "As one depletes these nerve cells, it is suspected [that] throughout a lifetime of chemical exposure eventually the result . . . is expressed either by subtle behavioral changes . . . or more frank neurological deficits."[114]

*The hypothalamus regulates emotions (limbic system) and the body's autonomic nervous system functions (temperature, food intake, digestion, thirst, urination, heart rate, respiration, et cetera), while the pituitary is the primary hormonal control gland.

Although cigarette smoke has become greatly regulated, individuals are still bombarded with fragrances from other people's perfumes and colognes, scented shampoos, soaps, or cosmetics and air fresheners and "skunk mail" (scented inserts in magazines). In fact, escaping toxic environments is almost impossible if you have to do any shopping. The air in department stores and shopping malls, for example, was found to have more chemicals than the air in auto parts and tire shops, carpet stores, rooms with chemical air "fresheners," and, surprisingly, even more than in the nauseatingly aromatic detergent sections of grocery stores.[115]

Perfumes Are Always Toxic

The chemical toluene, which is carcinogenic and damaging to the liver, has been found most abundantly in both auto parts stores and the perfume sections of department stores. Toluene is so pervasive in perfumes that a study conducted by the EPA in 1991 found the chemical in every fragrance sample collected.[116] Additionally, the National Academy of Sciences found that 95 percent of the chemicals used in fragrances were synthetic compounds derived from petroleum.[117] The other notoriously toxic solvents used in the multi-billion-dollar fragrance industry include acetone (causes dizziness, nausea, and incoordination), benzaldehyde (causes eye irritation and possible kidney damage), benzyl alcohol (causes headache, nausea, and vomiting), and trichloroethane (causes vomiting and severe eye irritation), combined with over 5,000 other "aroma chemicals."[118] These toxic ingredients are not just confined to perfumes, colognes, and aftershaves. Fragrance is also added to many toiletries, household products, and pesticides, and its use has increased *tenfold* since the 1950s.[119]

Brain Scan Reveals Damage from Perfume

One of the most dramatic—and hopefully most convincing—images to help both women and men steer clear of perfume, cologne, and aftershave is a SPECT (single photon emission computerized tomography) scan taken of a patient's brain before and after being exposed to perfume. After the patient inhaled perfume, a UCLA radiologist took a scan immediately afterward and again thirty minutes later. Both scans showed that there was significant diminished cerebral blood flow and inflammation of the blood vessels consistent with "exposure to neurotoxic substances."[120] To view this scan, visit www.ourlittleplace.com/spect.html.

Six-Dollar Ingredients Priced at $230

One important reason for the widespread use of these synthetic aromatics is that they are cheap—usually less than $10 a pound. When this price is compared with the price of natural scents like jasmine or tuberose that cost more than $10,000 a pound, it is understandable why profit-driven cosmetic and perfume companies use synthetic scents.[121] Surprisingly, the expensive perfumes are often just as guilty as the cheap ones of averaging hundreds of ingredients per scent with only a small minority containing natural oils. In fact, when one French perfumer was asked how much the ingredients really cost in a perfume selling for $230 in a department store, he answered, "Four to six dollars."[122]

Death by Perfume?

In 1991, the Environmental Protection Agency (EPA) investigated thirty-one fragrance products that could contribute to indoor air pollution and pose a risk to human health.[123] In her book *Drop-Dead Gorgeous,* Kim Erickson lists the ingredients of a popular designer perfume that were revealed through this study:

beta-pinene	toluene
benzaldehyde	camphene
benzyl alcohol	2-ethyl-1-hexanol
linalool	3,7-dimethyl-1,3,7-octatriene
benzyl acetate	$C_{15}H_{24}$
alpha-terpinol	crotonaldehyde
beta-citronellol	2-furaldehyde
ethanol	gamma-terpinolene
limonene	alpha-terpinolene
beta-phenethyl alcohol	phenyl acetaldehyde
beta-myrcene	o-allytoluene
alpha-cedrene	acetophenone
t-butanol	allocimene
ethyl acetate	2-methyl-4-phenyl-1-butene
carvone	

Erickson notes that many of these fragrance ingredients—such as allocimene, benzyl acetate, camphene, carvone, ethyl acetate, 2-ethyl-1-hexanol, 2-furaldehyde, limonene, and linalool—are also named under the EPA's Toxic Substance Control Act. And some—including benzaldehyde, benzyl alcohol, benzyl acetate, 2-furaldehyde, and acetophenone—are listed as possible carcinogens by the EPA, the National Toxicology Program, or the state of California. Furthermore, t-butanol and toluene can cause harm to a developing fetus, while benzaldehyde, ethyl acetate, and t-butanol have narcotic effects in humans that may result in disorientation, loss of coordination, and coma. Finally, in a section of her book titled "Death by Perfume," Erickson describes the violent and even near-death reactions some individuals have experienced after major exposures to toxic fragrances. In fact, these exposures have rendered an estimated 15 percent of the population highly sensitive to all fragrances, where even casual exposure can bring on symptoms of nausea, difficulty breathing, dizziness, muscle weakness, loss of concentration, and disorientation.[124]

Treatment

Avoidance

Whether individuals have noticeable symptoms or not, toxic chemicals are continually accumulating in their body if they use personal care products purchased from department stores, drugstores, or grocery stores. Because petroleum-free products are now available from alternative sources, individuals who are still buying and using petrochemical-laden products have the option to begin replacing these toxic products. As one woman who got well primarily through the elimination of toxic chemicals explained, "After spending thousands of dollars on doctors and tests, what would it hurt to buy new soaps and deodorants?"[125] By simply buying natural products for the bathroom and kitchen to replace old chemical-laden supplies, individuals can make a major first step in detoxifying their bodies and reduce or even possibly eliminate the onset of future degenerative diseases generated by the constant use of toxic chemicals.

In her bestselling book, *The Cure for All Cancers,* the late Hulda Clark, Ph.D., addressed the elimination of personal care and other products containing toxic petroleum derivatives.[126]* Since the publication of her book in 1993, many ill patients have benefited from Clark's detoxification program of removing all personal care products containing propylene glycol, benzene, and other known toxic chemicals. Unfortunately, many of Clark's alternative suggestions containing borax, cornstarch, and beet root performed poorly, frustrating patients so much that they would often return to their toxic and easier-to-use products. To combat this problem, I have tested cosmetics, soaps, and shampoos for over fifteen years and have compiled the results in a "Best Bets" list format to guide patients toward the cleanest, most nontoxic products, which additionally *perform well* on the skin and hair. (The "Best Bets" list is provided later in this chapter, beginning on page 137.)

It's also important to realize that the expense during this transition is really not an obstacle, because nontoxic cosmetics and shampoos are usually comparably priced to drugstore products, and are often much cheaper than the department store's pricier brand names. Furthermore, because many of the nontoxic cosmetics come from the health food store or by mail order, you're less likely to make as many rash purchases as when shopping at the local drugstore or at expensive department stores (like that $35 eye cream with the free gift!). Therefore, through shopping carefully for nontoxic items, individuals don't accumulate as many cosmetics as they did before that often languish in the back of a bathroom cabinet. In contrast, the natural products that are purchased are more well-considered choices in most cases, and therefore more highly prized and more fully utilized.

Thus, intoxication through conventional personal care products is one form of pollution that we can control very easily—simply stop buying them.

Detox Symptoms

If individuals are only mildly toxic, that is, they do not work—or have not worked in the past—in a toxic

*Dr. Clark asserted that the cause of cancer was primarily due to parasites that thrive unimpeded in individuals whose immune systems have been compromised by toxic chemicals. In the author's experience, parasites—similar to *Candida albicans* yeast—are simply opportunistic to more lethal invaders and insults to the body. These include mercury amalgam fillings, petroleum chemicals, highly pathogenic bacteria generated in dental and tonsil focal infections (foci are covered in part 4), and chronic negative mental and emotional patterns (addressed through constitutional homeopathy in chapter 14 and psychospiritual work in chapter 18).

profession, have worn very little makeup throughout their life, haven't dyed their hair for a number of years, and so forth, the detoxification period triggered by changing from toxic to nontoxic products may go relatively unnoticed. However, if they have been moderately to severely intoxicated from a past or present toxic profession, worn lots of makeup and used hair coloring for many years, grew up in a polluted city or farm (pesticide-filled) environment, and so forth, there can be significant withdrawal symptoms. In fact, in these latter cases where individuals' liver and kidney functioning is already compromised, the extra burden of stored toxic chemicals that begin to be released through simply the cessation of their daily dermal and nasal "hit" can be rather overwhelming to the body. Thus, individuals with a heavy body burden of chemicals can react quite similarly to addicts who go through withdrawal after giving up heroin cold turkey. For example, women who are detoxifying from the past or present use of nail polish, hair spray, and hair dyes that contain benzene, styrene, toluene, and other aromatic hydrocarbons that have a benzene-ring structure similar to the structure of Dexedrine-like compounds have often reported experiencing symptoms similar to withdrawal from "speed," such as agitation, hurriedness, and anxiety. In contrast, those who are clearing greater stores of alcohol solvents such as methylene glycol or propylene glycol, found in numerous cosmetics and creams, often experience fatigue, depression, and other "downer" types of withdrawal symptoms. Regardless of whether a person is able to identify the effects of aromatic "speedy" hydrocarbons or "downerlike" alcohol solvents withdrawal, the overall detoxification process itself can generate excessive free radicals and intermediary metabolites in the body that can contribute to a generalized sense of malaise and just feeling "sick" in many individuals.

Nutritional Support

Therefore, regardless of a patient's level of chemical intoxication with personal care products, at the minimum he or she should, as part of any detoxification protocol, be taking a good antioxidant supplement, as well as an algae product that binds not only toxic metals, as discussed earlier, but also toxic chemicals. The antioxidants Pure Radiance C and High ORAC Synbiotic Formula, generally at a dose of 2 capsules each per day with meals, are almost always included in a detoxification protocol.

- Pure Radiance C can be ordered from the Synergy Company (www.thesynergycompany.com) at (800) 723-0277.

- High ORAC Synbiotic Formula can be ordered from BioImmersion (www.bioimmersion.com) at (425) 451-3112. (Triple Berry is a similar formulation but comes as a powder for those who prefer this form over capsules.)

Drainage Remedies

Besides the aforementioned nutritional supplements, drainage remedies are often needed to support the release of xenobiotics from the body. Individuals who have had a significant history of chemical intoxication should seek guidance from a holistic practitioner who is knowledgeable not only in nutrition but also in drainage and homeopathy.* This is especially true for artists, hairdressers, nurses, painters, and others employed long-term in toxic professions, who are likely functioning in the more degenerated tuberculinic and luetic reaction modes. These more seriously poisoned individuals especially need to be in the hands of a skilled and experienced practitioner who can handle the difficulties of healing reactions that often arise as layers of toxicity and chronic metabolic dysfunctioning are cleared from the body.

Many plant stem cell drainage remedies have demonstrated a remarkable ability at significantly reducing the body's stores of chemical pollutants. The following remedies have been shown to be highly effective at chelating toxic chemicals, as proven both in scientific research studies and clinically through laboratory testing in patients.†

Black Poplar (*Populus nigra*): This herbal extract made from the buds of the black poplar tree is considered to be the *polycrest detoxifier*—that is, the detoxification remedy that is most effective at removing both toxic metals and chemicals from the body. As discussed in chapter 3, this makes perfect sense

*During this detoxification period, it is beneficial to have the patient on a constitutional remedy, which is discussed in detail in chapter 14.

†The following information derives from PSC Distribution (www.epsce.com).

because poplar trees have been described as actually being able to "suck up" toxic waste and chemicals from the ground and then safely metabolize them. In fact, studies have shown that black poplar trees can absorb nearly 3,000 gallons of ground effluent (ammonia, nitrogen, et cetera) per acre per day.[127] In the same way, these young buds help remove heavy metals and toxic chemicals from our bodies, primarily through the action of the enzyme phytochelatin synthase. Black Poplar has also been shown to be effective in removing chlorinated solvents, 1, 4-dioxane (a suspected carcinogen widely used in paints, varnishes, and cosmetics), and other toxic petrochemicals.

European Alder (*Alnus glutinosa*): This major remedy for both heart disease and gastrointestinal dysfunction additionally helps clear both toxic metals and pesticides from the body. European Alder can significantly improve cerebral and systemic blood circulation, which helps reduce and heal the neurological symptoms (memory loss, cognitive dysfunction, and depression) that commonly occur after exposure to toxic chemicals.

Hazel (*Corylus avellana*): This polycrest remedy for detoxification of the liver and lungs also restores elasticity in these and other organs and tissues by reducing scar tissue in the body. In the same way that it breaks down scar tissue, it is currently showing promise as an important remedy for breaking down stores of phthlates (plasticizers) and other toxic chemicals in the body. Doctors and practitioners should correlate history and blood findings with energetic testing to determine if this remedy is indicated in their patients' protocols.*

Juniper (*Juniperus communis*): This polycrest remedy for all liver and kidney disorders is also effective in detoxifying petrochemicals from the body. The young shoots of juniper are loaded with antioxidants; essential oils; vitamins B_1, B_2, and B_3 and calcium; and small but easily assimilable amounts of chromium, iron, magnesium, manganese, phosphorus, potassium, selenium, silica, and zinc.

Rye (*Secale cereale*): This major liver remedy also detoxifies stores of polyaromatic hydrocarbons such as benzene, toluene, and xylene from the body. Rye contains squalene, an isoprenoid compound that has been shown to aid in the elimination of xenobiotics in animal studies.

For the most effective results, the patient's symptoms and laboratory test findings should be carefully correlated with the most appropriate plant stem cell remedies. Furthermore, many of these potent remedies have significant contraindications with which practitioners should become well versed. When prescribed incorrectly or without knowledge of their contraindications, even natural medications can potentially cause harm. It is essential for all professionals who want to utilize these remedies in their practice to take continuing education courses from knowledgeable instructors to become adept at prescribing the most curative treatment plans possible.

▶ For educational seminars about and to order plant stem cell remedies, contact PSC Distribution at (631) 477-6696 or www.epsce.com, or Gemmos LLC at (877) 417-6298 or www.gemmos-usa.com.

Colon Detoxification

Finally, since many toxic chemicals such as PCBs are stored in adipose (fat) tissues, supplements that help the body produce as well as excrete bile (bile emulsifies or breaks down fat) are also important. The director of the Environmental Medicine Center at Southwest College of Naturopathic Medicine in Arizona, Dr. Walter Crinnion, utilizes psyllium, which he notes is still the only known fiber that can increase the fecal bile content and thus promote the release of toxic chemicals stored in fat tissues.[128] Herbal Laxative from Thorne is an excellent combination product that has a bulking action on the stool, which allows a fuller release of these petrochemicals. Dr. Crinnion also combines low-temperature saunas (see "Hydrotherapy," page 130) and colonic irrigations with psyllium supplementation to further help reduce the toxic chemical load.[129]

▶ Herbal Bulk is available from Thorne at (800) 228-1966.

*Please note that Hazel is contraindicated in cases of lung cancer or tuberculosis and should not be prescribed to patients on SSRI antidepressants such as Prozac, Paxil, or Celexa because it might excessively increase serotonin levels.

Tonifying Chi

Additionally, to help mitigate the often mind-numbing exhaustion that detoxification from both heavy metals and petrochemicals can intermittently generate, it may be necessary to tonify chi (bolster energy) with a Chinese medicinal herb compound, a supplement to suppost the adrenal glands, or a drainage remedy.

The balanced Chinese herbal called Jing can support both kidney yin deficiency (exhaustion, dryness, lower back ache, vague anxiety, or depression) and kidney yang deficiency (fatigue, chill, or lack of drive and enthusiasm). This herbal can be taken first thing in the morning as well as in the late afternoon during the bladder/kidney time (3 p.m. to 7 p.m.),* in which many people feel the highest level of fatigue.

For more severe exhaustion states and chronic hypoadrenalism, Cortrex provides excellent support to the adrenal glands, taken in combination with vitamin C, the B vitamins, zinc, and licorice root. Also, many people benefit from taking the gemmotherapy remedy Black Currant (*Ribes nigrum*), which is indicated for kidney and adrenal exhaustion and is also antiallergenic and anti-inflammatory.[130] Black Currant is often added to plant stem cell protocols, which typically combine four to eight remedies, because it is considered a *polycrest adjuvant,* which means that it supports and strengthens the effects of the other remedies in the mix.

- ▶ Jing is available from Dragon Herbs at (888) 558-6642. Generally, individuals take from 1 to 3 capsules in the morning and from 1 to 3 capsules in the afternoon, or as dictated by their particular fatigue pattern. However, it's always helpful to take kidney chi remedies during the bladder/kidney period between 3 p.m. and 7 p.m. It's important to keep in mind that although Jing is a relatively gentle and balanced tonification remedy, no herb—Chinese or Western—should be taken for extended periods of time without practitioner supervision. Thus, after a couple of months, if the fatigue is still significant, you should confer with an acupuncturist or Chinese herbal specialist.
- ▶ Cortrex is available from Thorne at (800) 228-1966. Dosages can range from 1 to 3 capsules per day, but Cortrex should not be taken in the evening because it could disturb sleep. Individuals should be under the guidance of a holistic practitioner if they feel the need to take this product for more than one or two months. Additionally, since the licorice in this combination product is not "deglycyrrhizinated," it could cause an increase in blood pressure if taken over an extended period of time.
- ▶ To order Black Currant and other plant stem cell remedies, see the contact information on page 129.

Hydrotherapy

Sweating out xenobiotics is even more effective than with heavy metals, because the majority of chemicals in the body are stored in the fat and therefore are more easily released from the skin through sweating. However, the same admonitions apply as with mercury detoxification. As a general rule, saunas are usually too strong for patients who are already ill and weak and primarily functioning in the more debilitated tuberculinic and luetic reaction modes. However, for patients who are more advanced in their detoxification protocol and have the kidney chi and liver metabolic ability to excrete these xenobiotics relatively efficiently, saunas can be quite valuable. Traditionally, slow and steady sweating—from thirty to sixty minutes three to five times a week in low-temperature saunas (dry saunas between 110° and 120°F and steam baths at around 110°)—most effectively encourages the release of fat-soluble pesticides, solvents, and pharmaceutical drugs through the skin from their cellular and tissue stores.[131] Additionally, Dr. Joseph Kees of Germany has found that slightly more aggressive forms of hydrotherapy—such as the use of homeopathic ointments and a "mummy wrap" of damp elastic bandages before the patient exercises—can effectively discharge stored xenobiotics from the body. Independent laboratories have confirmed that significantly elevated levels of pesticides and mercury are found in sweat samples from Dr. Kees's patients.[132]

*In traditional Chinese medicine (TCM) five-element theory, the flow of each meridian reaches its highest energy at a certain time during the day. For example, the bladder meridian is most active between 3 p.m. and 5 p.m., and its paired meridian, the kidney, reaches its peak between 5 p.m. and 7 p.m. When the *chi,* or energy, is impaired in the kidney meridian—a common cause of fatigue—individuals often experience a "4 p.m. droop," or feeling of significant fatigue, almost daily.

Dr. Karach's Oil Therapy

This method of natural chelation is one of the treatments recommended for the Five Dental Detox Days Protocol (see page 102). This method is also highly recommended for longer periods during the detoxification of toxic chemicals.

Toxic chemicals are fat-soluble and therefore *lipophilic*—that is, "fat-loving." Thus, this Ayurvedic oil technique—popularized by a Russian doctor named Karach—is a helpful chelation method for these chemicals. In this treatment, a big mouthful of organic unrefined sesame oil is held in the mouth for as long as possible (three to ten minutes, or until serious drooling begins!) and then spit out. During this time, lipophilic chemicals in the oral mucosa, as well as those circulating in the blood vessels traveling through the oral mucosa, are absorbed into this sesame oil. Since the average circulating time—or time required for the blood to completely circulate from the head to the toes—is approximately one minute, this oral therapy also helps absorb toxic chemicals traveling in the blood from other parts of the body. After spitting out the oil, gargle with salt and baking soda, and then brush your teeth. Environmentally ill patients suffering from multiple chemical sensitivities find this treatment quite valuable and often employ it once or even twice a day.

> **Ayurvedic:** Ayurvedic medicine originated around 2000 B.C. in India with Hindu brahmins (priests or wise men) who wrote scriptures, known as the Vedas, to reveal knowledge about life—spiritually, psychologically, and physically.

Identifying Xenobiotics

Labels Can Be Misleading

The foreign chemicals known as xenobiotics, which our bodies don't recognize and therefore can't easily detoxify, are not always easy to identify. For example, the word *nontoxic* on a label should not be trusted at face value. Rather than meaning "not at all toxic," as the word implies, it can actually mean that only "less than half" of the laboratory animals exposed to the product died within two weeks, or that no "serious" (i.e., extreme) damage occurred through eye or skin contact. Not exactly a glowing endorsement! Additionally, the term *natural* is not regulated, so it can simply mean that there are some natural-sounding ingredients included, such as herbs or essential oils, rather than that a product is completely clear of all artificial colors, fragrances, and preservatives. Finally, the term *hypoallergenic* can be placed on a label simply if *some* of the most common allergens have been removed, such as fragrances, cornstarch, cottonseed oil, lanolin, and cocoa butter.[133] However, the product can still contain many other allergenic ingredients, including various toxic chemicals that often induce a multitude of sensitivity reactions.

Many Products Do Not List Their Ingredients on the Label

Furthermore, reading labels is sometimes not an option. Some hygiene items such as deodorant soaps, antiperspirants, sunscreens, fluoridated toothpastes, and antidandruff shampoos are classified by the FDA as over-the-counter drugs rather than cosmetics because they claim to affect the body's structure or function—"fight" tooth decay or dandruff, for example—and therefore aren't required to list their ingredients. Even when cosmetic products do list their ingredients, trade secrets and proprietary ingredients such as "fragrances" and "flavors" are not required to be divulged on the label.[134]

When in Doubt, Don't Buy It

If the ingredients are listed but the label reads like a chemistry textbook, then obviously that product is toxic and the choice to purchase it or not is clear. However, many manufacturers who are trying to cash in on the current holistic health movement include plenty of natural ingredients on the label, with just one or two strange chemical-sounding names at the end of the list. In these cases, referring to the list beginning on page 132 of the most typical toxic chemicals used in the personal hygiene and cosmetics industries can help consumers identify which terms refer to toxic additives and which refer to "clean" or harmless ingredients. However, if you are still in doubt, either don't buy the product or have your holistic doctor or a practitioner who utilizes energetic testing test it for you.*

Toxic Chemicals Seen—and Not Seen—on Personal Care Product Labels

The following section lists common toxic chemicals used in personal care products, along with some reported adverse reactions. However, because thousands of solvents, emulsifiers, preservatives, and fragrances are in use currently, as well as thousands of new compounds being produced yearly, you should refer to trustworthy Internet sites for the most up-to-date information. The Environmental Working Group maintains the Skin Deep cosmetic safety database at www.cosmetics-database.com, which lists information on almost 15,000 personal care products and the approximately 7,000 ingredients that make up these products. The website www.health-report.co.uk/ingredients-directory.htm is also a good resource. For even more in-depth information, readers may want to consult *A Consumer's Dictionary of Cosmetic Ingredients* by Ruth Winter, *Drop-Dead Gorgeous* by Kim Erickson, and *Natural Detoxification* by Jacqueline Krohne and Frances Taylor. All of these sources were used to create the following two lists of the most common toxic chemicals contained in personal care products.

Chemicals Often Seen on Cosmetic and Hygiene Product Labels

Because no research studies have yet been conducted on the long-term effects of using products that contain even low levels of known carcinogens and hormone disruptors, the adverse symptoms and illnesses listed here have been reported from both small and large dosages of these toxic chemicals. These adverse reactions are sometimes dismissed as resulting only from a "large dosage," but that term can be difficult to define—is it giving rats megadoses in a single study or is it a woman using cosmetics laced with toxic chemicals daily for decades? Unfortunately, no one will know until some longitudinal studies are conducted.

Acetone: A solvent found in nail polish and nail polish removers, colognes, and cosmetics (as well as in glues, dishwashing detergents, paints, lacquer removers, and lubricating oils). It can cause skin rashes, nail splitting and peeling, and irritation of the lungs and eyes. In large doses, it has a narcotic action and can cause drunkenness, tremors, and loss of consciousness. In 1992, the FDA banned the use of acetone in astringents.

Acrylate or acrylate copolymer: Found in thickening agents, binders, and fixatives and widely used in nail polish, artificial nails, blushes, mascara, eye shadows, deodorants, and hair sprays. It is considered to be a strong irritant and allergen. Research studies have shown that inhalation is lethal to rats.

Alcohols or aliphatic hydrocarbons:

Butyl

- *BHA or butylated hydroxyanisole.* Used as a preservative and antioxidant in cosmetics. May cause allergic contact dermatitis (skin rash) and is a suspected human carcinogen.
- *BHT or butylated hydroxytoluene.* Used as a preservative and antioxidant in cosmetics. May cause allergic contact dermatitis and is a suspected human carcinogen. It is prohibited as a food additive in England.
- *Butyl acetate (aka acetic acid, butyl ester).* Used in perfumes, nail polish, and nail polish remover. May cause conjunctivitis (eye irritation) and acts as a narcotic in high doses.
- *Butyl alcohol or butanol.* Used in fats, waxes, and shellac and as a clarifying agent in shampoos. May cause mucous membrane irritation, dermatitis, headache, dizziness, drowsiness, and pulmonary (lung) problems.
- *Butylene glycol.* A humectant in hair sprays and setting lotions. May cause transient stimulation of the central nervous system (brain and spinal cord), depression, vomiting, drowsiness, coma, respiratory failure, and convulsions. Renal damage may proceed to kidney failure and death.
- *Butyl myristate.* A fatty alcohol used in nail polish and nail polish removers, lipsticks, and creams. May cause skin irritation.
- *Butylparaben.* Used as an antifungal preservative. Parabens are hormone-disrupting chemicals that

*For more information about energetic testing, refer to appendix 3. It should be noted here, however, that personal care products, as well as dental materials, should test neutral on the body—that is, cause no change in the muscle strength, arm length, leg length, or energy field measurements. Thus, as opposed to supplements and remedies, we don't want to *eat* or *drink* these products—we simply want them to be as neutral as possible. Therefore, the body need not respond with a "yes" signal, as it does to vitamin and mineral supplements, for example. There is one exception to this rule: when a personal care product is very clean and contains exceedingly fresh and beneficial ingredients, sometimes it will actually test positive (that is, as *very* healthy for the skin and the entire body), rather than just neutral.

can mimic estrogen. Parabens may be listed on the label under the term "fragrance."

Ethyl

- *EDC or ethylene dichloride.* A wetting and penetrating ingredient in cosmetics. May cause mucous membrane irritation and, in large doses, breast, stomach, and skin cancer.
- *EDTA or ethylenediamine tetraacetic acid.* A sequestering agent in shampoos. May cause skin and mucous membrane irritation, asthma, skin rashes, and kidney damage.
- *Ethyl acetate.* A solvent used in nail enamels and nail polish removers and perfumes. May cause local skin irritation and is a central nervous system (brain and spinal cord) depressant. Prolonged inhalation may cause kidney and liver damage.
- *Ethyl alcohol or ethanol or grain alcohol.* Just like any alcohol—wine, vodka, or gin—ethanol is not toxic in small amounts. However, before it can be used in cosmetics legally, it must be denatured. The acetone, turpentine, benzene, and denatonium benzoate that are used to denature ethanol renders the resulting product unpalatable and toxic. (Many holistic companies simply ignore this FDA ruling, which is a holdover from Prohibition days, and utilize grain or pure ethanol in their products.) See also *SD alcohol.*
- *Ethylene glycol.* A solvent and humectant in many cosmetics. When ingested may cause central nervous system (brain and spinal cord) depression, drowsiness and coma, vomiting, respiratory failure, kidney damage, and death. Adverse reproductive and developmental effects have also been reported.
- *PEG or polyethylene glycol.* A binder, plasticizing agent, solvent, and emollient widely used in hair straighteners, baby products, pharmaceutical creams, fragrances, and lipsticks. May cause allergic reactions. The ingestion of large doses has produced kidney and liver damage and cancer in rats.
- *SD alcohol.* Stands for "specially denatured" ethyl alcohol. Denatured alcohol is ethanol that has additives that make it unpalatable and toxic. SD alcohol is very common in cosmetics as an astringent, solvent, and antimicrobial. Environmental Working Group rates it as a moderate hazard, as it has been associated with cancer and endocrine disruption.[135]

Methyl

- *Methyl alcohol or methanol or wood alcohol.* A solvent, fuel, and denaturant from the distillation of wood that converts to the even more toxic formaldehyde and formic acid in the liver. The primary use of methyl alcohol is in making other chemicals. May cause headaches, vertigo, nausea, vomiting, abdominal cramps, mild central nervous system depression, sweating, weakness, delirium, blurred vision, and blindness.
- *Methyl paraben or methyl p-hydroxybenzoate.* A preservative widely used in cosmetics. May cause allergic reactions. Parabens are hormone-disrupting chemicals that can mimic estrogen. Beginning in 1998, studies have revealed that parabens had estrogenic activity in mice, rats, and human breast cancer cells.[136] Measurable concentrations of six different parabens (methylparaben, ethylparaben, p-propylparaben, isobutylparaben, n-butylparaben, and benzylparaben) were found by British researchers in 2004 in biopsy samples from breast tumors.[137] Parabens may also be listed on the label under the term "fragrance."

Propyl

- *Propyl alcohol or propanol.* A solvent and denaturant derived from propane and used in the manufacture of cosmetics and in lotions and mouthwashes. Hulda Clark first alerted the public to the danger of propyl alcohol in her book *The Cure for All Cancers.* Next to benzene, she found it to be the most toxic solvent used.[138] Propyl alcohol has similar effects to isopropyl alcohol including dry and cracking skin, brown spots and premature aging of the skin, central nervous system depression, and possibly cancer.
- *Propylene glycol.* A moisture-carrying and skin-penetration ingredient widely used in cosmetics. Propylene glycol, also used as an antifreeze and in hydraulic brake fluid, is considered by the FDA to be "safe" as a cosmetic ingredient up to a 50 percent concentration. However, when drums of propylene glycol are delivered to cosmetic manufacturers, the Material Safety Data Sheet warns workers to "avoid skin contact."[139] May cause allergic reactions, respiratory and throat irritation, liver abnormalities, blood and

kidney disorders, and central nervous system depression.

- *Propylparaben.* Preservative and antimicrobial used widely in cosmetics and hygiene products. May cause contact dermatitis. Studies have shown that parabens are hormone-disrupting chemicals that can mimic estrogen and therefore be carcinogenic. Parabens may also be listed on the label under the term "fragrance."

Benzoic acid: An antifungal derived from barks and berries or from benzene and used in many cosmetics and personal lubricants. A mild skin irritant and may cause allergenic reactions.

Colors: *D & C Green No. 6 or FD& C Red or Yellow No. 6, et cetera.* There are approximately seventy-five D and C and twenty F, D, and C artificial color pigments used in cosmetics.[140] May be allergenic, irritating to the skin and eyes, and asthma inducing, and are also believed to be carcinogenic.

Formaldehyde: A common preservative, disinfectant, and defoamer widely used in cosmetics, nail hardeners, nail polish, soap, hair-growing products, and so forth. Vapors are intensely irritating to mucous membranes. Ingestion may cause severe abdominal pain, internal bleeding, headaches, chronic fatigue, vertigo, coma, and death; allergenic and irritating to the skin; a known carcinogen. Cosmetic use of formaldehyde has been banned in Japan and Sweden. *Formaldehyde* may be listed on the label under the trade name Formalin or Formal, or it may not be listed on the label at all (for instance, if the product is classified as an over-the-counter drug).

Fragrance or perfume: These include both natural and synthetic aroma additives and can indicate the presence of up to 4,000 ingredients, including parabens. May cause headache, dizziness, rashes, skin hyperpigmentation, violent coughing, and vomiting. Many fragrance ingredients are suspected or known carcinogens and hormone disruptors.

Imidazolidinyl urea or diazolidinyl urea: The second most common synthetic preservative (after the parabens) used in cosmetics. May cause contact dermatitis, and can release formaldehyde at certain temperatures. Some research scientists consider it dangerous to use around the eyes.

Lanolin: A natural emulsifier from the oil glands of sheep that is used in many cosmetics. It is a common allergen and may cause skin rashes, but it is not a toxic chemical.

Mineral oil: A lubricant, binder, and protective ingredient made from petroleum chemicals that is also known as *liquidum paraffinum, paraffin oil, paraffin jelly, paraffin wax,* and *petrolatum.* It is used in creams, hair conditioners, suntan lotions, shaving creams, and powders. Baby oil is 100 percent mineral oil. Mineral oil may cause allergic reactions and photosensitivity, promote acne and premature aging by coating the skin like plastic and interfering with the skin's ability to eliminate toxins, and may be contaminated with cancer-causing polycyclic aromatic hydrocarbons (PAHs).

PPD (4-paraphenylenediamine): Used since 1909 and still present in over two-thirds of permanent hair dyes, PPD replaces the melanin pigment in hair after it has been broken down by peroxide. PPD is also found in some dark-colored cosmetics and temporary tattoos. It can cause allergic symptoms, including contact dermatitis, contact urticaria syndrome (rash, itching, wheezing, difficulty swallowing, and vomiting), and in rare cases anaphylactic shock.[141] The state of Maine recently included PPD on its list of "chemicals of high concern" and categorized it as "persistent, bioaccumulative, and inherently toxic."[142]

PVC or polyvinyl chloride: Has moisture-resistant properties and is used in cosmetics, nail enamels, and creams, as well as in plumbing fixtures and raincoats. PVC causes cancerous tumors when injected into rats.

PVP or polyvinylpyrrolidone: An emollient and softener in shampoos, hair sprays, rouges, and creams. Ingestion may cause gas and fecal impaction or damage to lungs and kidney. Strong circumstantial evidence indicates that foreign bodies in the lungs may be caused by the use of hair spray. Also has caused tumors in rats.

Propellant: A compressed gas that is used to expel the contents in shaving cream and cosmetic preparations. Since chlorofluorocarbons were banned due to their depletion of the ozone layer, butane, propane, carbon dioxide, and nitrous oxide are now utilized. May cause heart problems, birth defects, lung cancer, nausea, dizziness, lung damage, and other disorders.

Quaternium 7, 15, 31, 60, et cetera: Used as a preservative, surfactant, and germicide in many cosmetics including aftershaves, shampoos, antiperspirants, hair color, hand creams, and mouthwashes. May irritate the eyes, skin, and mucous membranes, and ingestion can be fatal. Can also break down into nitrosamine compounds that can cause cancer. *Benzalkonium chloride,* one of the most popular of these quaternium compounds, may cause muscular paralysis, low blood pressure, and central nervous system depression and weakness.

Salicyclic acid or methyl salicylate: A naturally occurring substance that is prepared synthetically for use as a preservative and antimicrobial in skin softeners, deodorants, dandruff preparations, face masks, hair dye removers, suntan lotions, and creams. Absorption of large amounts may cause vomiting, abdominal pain, respiratory disturbances, mental disturbances, and skin rashes. It is also used in making aspirin, topical acne drug creams, and some "anti-aging" beta- or alpha-hydroxide products.

Sodium benzoate: A preservative and antiseptic used in eye creams, vanishing creams, and toothpastes. May cause allergenic reactions.

Sodium lauryl (or laurel or laureth) sulfate or ammonium laureth sulfate (SLS): A detergent (foaming agent), surfactant, and emulsifier derived from the reaction of sulfuric acid on coconut or other oils and found in 90 percent of all shampoos and bubble baths; also found in toothpastes, hand lotions, and cream depilatories. It is a known skin irritant. With prolonged skin contact, concentrations should not exceed 1 percent of the ingredients. Also may cause eye irritation (can irreversibly affect eye and vision development in children), gum disease, tooth and hair loss, diarrhea, liver toxicity, central nervous system depression, and death. Can also break down into nitrosamine chemicals that can cause cancer. SLS is absorbed through the skin and scalp and is an estrogen mimic; it has been implicated in contributing to PMS and menopausal symptoms, reducing male fertility, and increasing female cancers such as breast cancer.[143]

Talc and talcum powder: Used for that slippery sensation felt in baby and adult powders, eye shadows, dry rouges, masks, cake foundations, and creams. It is a possible lung irritant and carcinogen. Talc-based powders have been linked to ovarian cancer because of the genital and sanitary napkin use of talcum powder. Also has caused coughing, vomiting, and pneumonia from prolonged inhalation in babies.

Triethanolamine or TEA: A dispersing agent and detergent (foaming agent) in lotions, shaving creams, soaps, and shampoos. With prolonged skin contact, concentrations should not exceed 5 percent. May cause allergenic reactions and eye and skin irritations. TEA, as well as *DEA* or *diethanolamine,* and *MEA* or *monoethanolamine,* can break down into carcinogenic nitrosamines and be absorbed through the skin. These chemicals are restricted in Europe due to their link with an increased incidence of liver and kidney cancer.

Chemicals Often Not *Seen on Cosmetic and Hygiene Product Labels*

The following list includes toxic chemicals that are rarely listed on product labels, often because they are disguised under the term "fragrance," they are considered proprietary and therefore don't have to be disclosed, they were used only in the distillation or extraction process of other ingredients and not directly added to the product, or the FDA considers the products they are contained in over-the-counter drugs, which aren't required to reveal all ingredients on the label.

Aromatic Hydrocarbons:

- *Benzene* (and its derivatives *naphthalene, aniline, phenol,* and *hydroquinone*). A solvent from coal and petroleum used in nail polish remover and in the manufacture of many cosmetics, personal lubricants, dyes, waxes, oils, and detergents. Benzene is a powerful bone-marrow poison (aplastic anemia), and cases of leukemia have been linked to it since 1897. It was banned in 1978 as a household solvent, and safety standards for cosmetics manufacturing workers has been set at ten parts per million during an eight-hour day. (We inhale benzene primarily through car exhaust and cigarette smoke.) May cause nausea, vomiting, fatigue, skin and mucous membrane irritation, and narcotic behavior including lightheadedness, disorientation, loss of consciousness, and coma. Benzene exposure has been linked with leukemia, aplastic anemia, and uterine and breast cancer.

- *Styrene.* A solvent used in the manufacture of cosmetics and added directly to such cosmetics as liquid eyeliners and perfumes. (The most common exposure is through takeout Styrofoam cups and plastic food wrap.) May cause eye and mucous membrane irritation, neurotoxic effects in the central (memory dysfunction, headache, dizziness) and peripheral (incoordination, motor dysfunction, nerve damage in hands and feet) nervous systems, loss of consciousness, and death.
- *Toluene.* A solvent used in nail polish,* nail hardeners, dyes, perfumes, and cosmetics (and typewriter correction fluid, glues, markers, paints, and inks). May cause symptoms of neurotoxicity including ataxia (muscular incoordination), tremors, hearing loss, dizziness, vertigo, emotional instability and delusions, liver and kidney damage, and anemia, and can harm developing fetuses.
- *Xylene.* Solvent in the manufacture of some cosmetic ingredients (and in cleaners, air fresheners, glues, marking pens, and paints). More toxic than benzene and toluene, xylene can have carcinogenic and neurotoxic effects and can cause reproductive abnormalities and death through respiratory or cardiac arrest.

Formaldehyde: See page 134.

Methylene chloride: A solvent found in perfumes, nail enamels, cleansing creams, aftershave lotion, and some shampoos. May cause cancer, liver and kidney damage, central nervous system disorders (delusions, hallucinations, tremors), headaches, insomnia, unconsciousness, and death. In 1988, it was determined to be safe in cosmetics only for brief use by the Cosmetic Ingredient Review board.

Phthalates: A family of plasticizers and solvents used in perfume, deodorants, nail polish, hair spray, hair gels, and cosmetics. Are known hormone disruptors and implicated in causing low sperm counts and infertility, as well as sexual abnormalities and deformities. Many are known carcinogens.

Why Do Companies Continue to Use These Obvious Toxins?

Antimicrobial and Solvent Effects

After reading about all of the hazards associated with these chemicals, you may wonder why companies would even use petrochemicals. One reason is that these chemical compounds *have* demonstrated mild to moderate antiseptic, antibacterial, and antifungal properties in laboratory tests, and therefore function well as preservatives in products. Furthermore, many of these chemicals also have strong solvent properties that help mix the ingredients together as well as allowing them to penetrate the skin better. However, these benefits can never offset the greater harm toxic chemicals potentially have to your health. For example, mercury has antimicrobial properties. So, beginning in 1928, Eli Lilly began to sell mercury as a topical antiseptic named Merthiolate, also known by the name of thimerosal when it was used in the injectable form.[144] In 1982, the FDA finally banned Merthiolate for over-the-counter topical use; but it wasn't until 1999 that thimerosal was "recommended" to be phased out in vaccines due to this compound's proven toxicity to the human cell.[145]*

Familiar, and Therefore Harmless?

Much like swabbing a little reddish orange Merthiolate or Mercurochrome on a skinned knee in the 1950s, the extensive use of petrochemicals that are suspected or even known carcinogens in personal care products today has also become the norm. Cited earlier in this book, Rachel Carson's timeless quote about "the harmless aspect of the familiar" is appropriate here as well.[146] That is, there is a universal tendency to believe that if everyone uses these products—and if drugstores, supermarkets, and department stores stock and sell them—then they must be okay. Fortunately, freethinking individuals realize that this is not the case, and that trusting the purported good intentions of corporations or governmental organizations can be a recipe for disaster—and possibly chronic illnesses.

*Depending on the brand, toluene may comprise up to 50 percent of the ingredients.

*See chapter 15 for more information on the use of thimerosal in vaccines, and resulting autism in susceptible infants and children.

The Oil Industry's Influence in Promoting the Use of Petrochemicals

Another reason that these chemicals are used is for profit. In fact, a full 10 percent of the billions of barrels of crude oil produced annually goes to cosmetics, medicines, polyester, pesticides, carpets, paints, rubber, and plastic products.[147] The use of these petrochemicals in cosmetics, mouthwashes, and oral and nasal medications started in the early 1900s due in no small part to the influence and research of Rockefeller's Standard Oil Company.[148] During the period of Prohibition in the United States (1920–1933), the search was on to find a nontoxic, nonpotable (unfit to drink) substitute for ethanol, or ethyl alcohol, found in wine, beer, and liquors, so that destitutes and chronic alcoholics did not try to ingest hair tonic, paint thinner, or mouthwashes to get their alcohol "fix." Due to its unpalatable taste and the oil industry's influence, isopropyl alcohol seemed to be the perfect solution.[149] Although it was found to be twice as toxic as ethanol, it caused questionable symptoms in early studies (e.g., narcosis, ataxia and unsteady gait, and heart irregularities), and no long-term studies were conducted, isopropyl alcohol was declared safe enough by governmental health agencies for external and some internal ("a few cubic centimeters") use.[150]

THE DANGEROUS NATURE OF RUBBING ALCOHOL

Today, isopropyl alcohol is still used in many cosmetics and sold in every drugstore as "rubbing alcohol." However, few people are aware that this seemingly harmless chemical was the cause of the fifth most common call to U.S. poison control centers in 1990, with 80 percent of the 17,000 cases reported to be in the pediatric age group.[151] In fact, the scientific literature is rife with reports of comas, near-death accidents, and even some fatalities of infants and children in which the common practice of a rubbing alcohol sponge bath to reduce fever was employed.[152] In a 1986 study, researchers noted that the studies conducted in the early 1900s did not measure the dangers of *prolonged* dermal exposure of isopropyl alcohol that can occur for four or more hours with sponge bathing with isopropyl alcohol and then wrapping up the body afterward.[153] During this exposure, the liver converts isopropyl alcohol into the more toxic chemical acetone, and the kidneys then attempt to excrete it out of the body. Coma and death can occur, however, by the delayed metabolism and slower excretion rates that occur in younger and more immature systems.[154] Isopropyl alcohol is also used widely as an antiseptic before injections, which is inhaled by countless doctors, nurses, and patients daily in clinics and hospitals.

Alternatives to Toxic Chemical Preservatives Exist

Even more amazing is that existing alternatives to isopropyl alcohol and other known toxic petrochemicals in our cosmetics and hygiene products are often overlooked. Companies can choose to use natural preservatives such as vitamin A, C (ascorbic acid), or E; grapefruit seed extract (citric acid); and tea tree or other strongly antimicrobial essential oils.[155] Additionally, if people truly realized that when they apply their cosmetics and lotions, they are actually "ingesting" them through their skin and into their bloodstream, they would begin to demand fresher products with a shorter shelf life, just as they do with their food.

The "Best Bets" List of Nontoxic Personal Care Products

Unfortunately, just buying your personal care products at the health food store does not ensure that they are completely nontoxic, although it is a giant leap forward from purchasing these items at drugstores, groceries, or department stores.* However, many cosmetics, shampoos, and moisturizing lotions—even at the best health food stores—still contain toxic chemical preservatives, or ingredients that were distilled or manufactured with the use of these petroleum solvents.

This "Best Bets" list contains my recommendations for the best nontoxic cosmetic and hygiene products currently available. Please note that this list was current at the time of publication of this book and will be updated regularly on my website, www.radicalmedicine.com. However, it's important to remember that companies can—and often do—change product ingredients from time to time and sometimes sell out to larger corporations. Therefore,

*In fact, if this all feels too overwhelming, just skip this list for now and simply start buying your shampoo, shaving cream, and kitchen cleansers at the health food store. This, in itself, will greatly mitigate your toxic chemical exposure and body burden over time.

it is not possible to guarantee the continued nontoxicity of every product. Always read labels, test borderline products with your holistic doctor or practitioner, and don't buy anything from companies that won't fully discuss with you the sources of their ingredients.

The suggested products on the list are from holistic companies endeavoring to use truly natural ingredients. Furthermore, they have been energetically tested on numerous patients for many years and are shown to be the most inert and clean products available. The product(s) in **bold** type are the ones that have performed best on the skin or hair and are therefore the most popular among holistic patients.

▶ Readers are encouraged to go to the Environmental Working Group's website, www.cosmeticsdatabase.com, to find out more about products not listed on the Best Bets list. However, remember that the Best Bets list includes not only products that have tested as "clean" but also products that have performed well on my patients' hair and skin.

TESTING PRODUCTS ENERGETICALLY

It is possible that some of the products on the Best Bets list might have traces of petrochemicals, but the amount of good ingredients in them—herbs, essential oils, and so forth—greatly outweigh the small amount of bad. Testing products for purity at a lab is very expensive and not always definitive, so this option is not always feasible.* However, for the most part, when a product's label has no toxic ingredients and the company that makes it is on this list, you can trust that it's a clean product.

Through energetic testing, holistic doctors and practitioners can determine which products don't cause stress on the body. Generally, a nontoxic product tests clear on an average patient as well as on a sensitive patient. However, sometimes extremely sensitive patients need to forgo wearing any makeup and use only the hygiene products that pass their personal "sniff test" or skin and nervous system sensitivity until their health is stabilized.

*One of the challenges with lab testing is that you have to specify the ingredients you are looking for—so if you don't name it, they won't look for it. A product may also test in a lab as "nontoxic" but be revealed to be subtly disturbing through energetic testing.

Some of these products are readily available at most health food stores; however, those that are not can be ordered by mail. The companies that manufacture these mail-order products are listed in *italics* after the product name. A resource list of these "clean" recommended companies is included at the end of the Best Bets list, with each company's phone number and website.

Deodorant

Strong: **MiEssence Deodorant** (*Annie's Organics*)
Strong: **Real Purity Deodorant** (*Real Purity*)
Mild: Sea Breeze Body Freshener (*Vital Image*)
Very mild: Crystal rock, stick, or spray (health food stores or *F/T Ltd.*)

Soap

Face and Body Wash (*Vital Image*)
Liquid or bar soaps (Dr. Bronner's and many others at health food stores)*

Shaving Cream

Shaving Cream (*Real Purity*)
Shaving Miracle (*Vital Image*)

Toothpaste

Calendula Toothpaste (health food stores or *Weleda*)†
MiEssence Anise Toothpaste (*Annie's Organics*)‡
Doctor Burt's (health food stores or *Burt's Bees*)
Plant Gel or Salt Toothpaste with Baking Soda (health food stores or *Weleda*)

*However, Dr. Bronner's soap often contains a significant amount of peppermint or other essential oils that can potentially antidote constitutional homeopathic remedies. Other good soaps commonly found at health food stores include those made by Adra Natural Soap, Bee and Flower, French Milled, River Soap Company, Sappo Hill, Simmons Special, and Suisun Bay. In addition, many health food stores carry locally produced soaps that may not be on this (California-derived) list.

†The Calendula Toothpaste is mint-free and therefore appropriate for those on a homeopathic remedy.

‡The best of both worlds: this anise toothpaste has a gentle essential oil aroma with antiseptic/antibacterial properties but is not strong enough to antidote a homeopathic remedy.

Mouthwash

IPSAB or Ipsadent (health food stores or *Heritage Store*)*

Shampoo and Conditioner

John Masters Shampoo and Créme Rinse (health food stores or *John Masters Organics*)

MiEssence Desert Flower Shampoo and Shine Herbal Hair Conditioner (*Annie's Organics*)

All Paul Penders products (*Paul Penders*)

Mangrove Foaming Shampoo & Hair Conditioner (*Keys*)

Pure Abundance (*Aveda*)†

Hair Gel

B-5 Design Gel (health food stores or *Aubrey Organics*)

John Masters Styling Gel or Hair Texturizer (health food stores or *John Masters Organics*)

Shine On (health food stores or *John Masters Organics*)

Hair Spray

None (mix a little of one of the above gels with water in a spray bottle)‡

Hair Color

Aveda Color Conditioners (*Aveda*)§

Light Mountain Henna or Color the Gray Henna (health food stores or *Light Mountain*)

Logona Henna (health food stores or *Logona*)**

Sunglitz Crème Lightening System (*Farouk*)

*Put a little Ipsadent in water and gargle, or better, put a few drops in a Panasonic Oral Irrigator and spray onto gums and teeth. The Oral Irrigator is available from the Sharper Image at (800) 344-4444. The essential oils in this mouthwash can antidote a homeopathic remedy, however. If you are in optimal health you don't need a mouthwash.

†This product is not entirely chemical free but is among the best available products at this time.

‡Through years of energetically testing products as well as detoxing patients from petroleum chemical exposure, it has been my experience that the four most toxic products a woman can use are hair dye, hair spray, nail polish, and perfume.

§This product is not entirely chemical free but is among the best available products at this time.

**This product is not entirely chemical free but is among the best available products at this time.

Facial Cleansing Creams, Moisturizing Lotions, Masks, and Toners

All Éminence Organics products (*Éminence Organics*)*

All EvanHealy products (*EvanHealy*)

All Grateful Body products (*Grateful Body*)

All MyChelle products (health food stores or *MyChelle Dermaceuticals*)

All Royal Labs products (*Royal Labs*)

All Vital Image products (*Vital Image*)

Pure Organic Shea Butter (health food stores or *Organic Essence*)†

All Paul Penders products (*Paul Penders*)

All Super Salve products (*Super Salve*)

Apitherapy Goldenrod Honey Facial Masque (*Honey Gardens*)

Hand and Body Lotion (health food stores or *Avalon Organics*)

Radiance Day Cream (health food stores or *Burt's Bees*)

Lip Balm

Honey House Propolis Salve (*Honey Gardens*)

John Masters Organic Lip Calm (health food stores or *John Masters Organics*)

Suntan Lotion

Reflect Outdoor Balm (*Annie's Organics*)

Jason Sunbrellas Sun Care (PABA-free; health food store or order from *Jason Natural Cosmetics*)

Real Purity Suntan Lotion (if no PABA skin sensitivity; *Real Purity*)

Sunblock Lotion (SPF 15) (*Super Salve*)

Nail Polish

None (use a buffer for a natural shine)‡

*Éminence has superlative products. However, their paprika-containing products, such as Eight Greens Phyto Masque (in the AntiAging Kit) and the Almond Mineral Treatment, can be a little too stimulating for sensitive skin.

†This excellent moisturizer has light sun protection too, approximately 5–6 SPF.

‡Conventional nail polish can consist of greater than 50 percent toluene (a known carcinogen), as well as other toxic chemicals including sulfonimide, formaldehyde (a known carcinogen), and phthalate (endocrine disruptor) resins. (M. Kennedy, "The Green Corner," *Naturopathic Doctor News & Review* [May 2006]: 17.) Even the formaldehyde-free, toluene-free, and phthalate-free alternative brands contain toxic isopropyl alcohol and other synthetic chemicals.

Perfume, Cologne, and Aftershave

None (Use natural essential oils in moderation for special occasions. They can be diluted with neutral-smelling almond oil; the Aura Cacia company extracts its oils cleanly and can be found in many health food stores.)

Lipstick

Hemp Organics Hempcolors (health food stores or *Hemp Organics*)

Peacekeeper Lipsticks and Lip Gloss (health food stores or *PeaceKeeper Cause-Metics*)

Lavera Lipsticks (health food stores or *Lavera*)

Paul Penders Lipsticks (*Paul Penders*)

Real Purity Lipsticks (*Real Purity*)

Super Salve Lipsticks (*Super Salve*)

Un-Petroleum Terra Tints (health food stores or *Un-Petroleum*)

Blush, Concealer, Base, Eyeliner, Eyeshadow, Mascara, and Powder

All Lavera products (health food stores or *Lavera*)

All Paul Penders products (*Paul Penders*)

All Real Purity products (*Real Purity*)

All Super Salve products (*Super Salve*)

Body Powder

Body Powder (health food stores or *Jason Natural Cosmetics*)

Herbal Baby Powder (*Super Salve*)

Best Bets Resources

- Annie's Organics: www.anniesorganics.com
- Aubrey Organics (800) 282-7394: www.aubrey-organics.com
- Avalon Organics (888) 659-7730: www.avalonorganics.com
- Aveda (800) 328-0849: www.aveda.com (you can't order Aveda products by mail, but you can ask for the location of a hair salon near you that uses Aveda products, as well as one that has been approved to do hair coloring)
- Burt's Bees (919) 998-5200: www.burtsbees.com
- Éminence Organics (888) 747-6342: www.eminenceorganics.com
- EvanHealy (858) 513-7559: www.evanhealy.com
- Farouk (800) 237-9175: www.farouk.com (sold only to professionals)
- F/T Ltd. (800) 829-7625: www.thecrystal.com
- Grateful Body (800) 600-6806: www.gratefulbody.com
- Hemp Organics (877) 524-4367: www.colorganics.com
- Heritage Store (800) 862-2923: www.caycecures.com
- Honey Gardens (802) 985-5852: www.honeygardens.com
- Jason Natural Cosmetics (877) 527-6601: www.jasonnatural.com
- John Masters Organics (800) 599-2450: www.johnmasters.com
- Keys (877) 878-4082: www.keys-soap.com
- Lavera (877) 528-3727: www.lavera-usa.com
- Light Mountain (262) 889-8561: www.lightmountain-hair-color.com
- Logona (828) 252-1420: www.logona.com
- MyChelle Dermaceuticals (800) 447-2076: www.mychelle.com
- Organic Essence (707) 465-8955: www.orgess.com
- Paul Penders: www.paulpenders.com
- PeaceKeeper Cause-Metics (866) 732-2336: www.iamapeacekeeper.com
- Real Purity (800) 253-1694: www.realpurity.com
- Royal Labs (800) 760-7779: www.royallabs.com
- Super Salve (505) 539-2768: www.supersalve.com
- Un-Petroleum (877) 263-9456: www.unpetroleum.com
- The Vital Image (800) 414-4624: www.thevitalimage.com
- Weleda (800) 241-1030: www.weleda.com

Other "Best Bets" Guidelines

Cleaning Supplies and Paper Goods

Debra Lynn Dadd, the author of *Nontoxic, Natural, and Earthwise* and a columnist for *Natural Home* magazine, does much of her cleaning with a squirt bottle of a fifty-fifty mix of vinegar (distilled white) and water, a bottle of liquid soap (like Dr. Bronner's), and a can of Bon Ami cleaning powder.[156] However, you can also trust your health food store to provide reasonably clean and non-toxic cleaning products. So in this section we'll forgo a long list of itemized detergents, cleaners, and paper products and just recommend high-quality and dependable companies that are environmentally aware.

Bio Kleen
Bon Ami
Country Save
Earth Friendly
Ecover
KD Gold (not found at health food stores; call (888) 759-7256 or go to www.kdgold.com)
Life Tree
Method
Seventh Generation
Whole Foods

► The Seventh Generation company has authored the book *Naturally Clean: The Seventh Generation Guide to Safe and Healthy, Non-Toxic Cleaning,* which is an excellent resource that explains the dangers of traditional household cleaners.

PAPER GOODS AND FEMININE PRODUCTS

It's just as important to use clean paper goods as it is to use nontoxic cleaners. Bleaching paper with chlorine creates dangerous toxins such as dioxin, furans, and other organochlorines. Traces of chlorine, dioxin, and other toxic chemicals can be easily transferred to moist and warm mucosal tissues such as the nose and eyes, as well as the vagina. In fact, these toxic organochlorines in sanitary napkins and tampons, often worn for hours at a time, can be readily absorbed into the vaginal mucosa and then into the systemic circulation. Therefore, it's essential to buy these feminine items at the health food store and make sure they are labeled "non-chlorinated." The same goes for the baby wipes used on infants' sensitive skin, which can affect their immune systems.

Clothing

Since World War II, synthetic fibers such as polyester, acrylic, and nylon have been developed almost as rapidly as pesticides.[157] Although the relief from ironing is gratifying, our moist skin readily absorbs the organic solvents (toluene and xylene), chlorine, formaldehyde, silicon, synthetic dyes (cadmium, mercury, and benzidine), pesticides, and other substances used in the manufacture of these fabrics.[158] These chemicals are also inhaled through the air we breathe—as many sensitive individuals will attest to when walking through a department store's clothing sections. Therefore, except for that long beaded dress for special occasions, it's a good idea to try to wear as much natural-fiber clothing as possible, primarily the following.

Organically grown and dyed cotton
Organic linen
Ramie
Silk
Wool (unmothproofed)
Leather (often comes with toxic tanning agents or dyes, however)

► Organically grown and dyed cotton should also be used in the place where we spend one-third of our lives—bed. Possibly the most economical place to buy certified organic cotton sheets and bedding, as well as natural latex mattresses (considered the best for their purity, durability, and sustainability), is the Organic Company, at (605) 593-5650 or www.theorganiccompany.com.

Additionally, Mary Cordaro, an expert in the field of natural homes and home furnishings, specializes in researching and stocking the highest-quality organic bedding currently available (she's like the "Good Housekeeping Seal of Approval" for organic and nontoxic products and building materials). Contact her at (818) 766-1787 or through www.marycordaro.com.

Dry Cleaning

Perchloroethylene, or "perc," is a degreaser and the major chemical used to dry-clean clothes. It is a known thyroid-hormone disruptor and has been linked to infertility in both men and women, and menstrual disorders in women.[159] Studies conducted since the 1970s have correlated perc with cancer and several kidney, liver, neurological, and hormonal problems.[160] However, the American Council on Science and Health (ACSH) asserts that the "teeny" doses of perc to which consumers are exposed are not dangerous.[161]* Nevertheless, when you need to dry-clean certain necessary items, keep in mind the following:

- Remove the plastic and air the clothes outside or in a separate well-ventilated room before wearing them. (It can take a week to substantially reduce perc residues, but even a day or so decreases your exposure by about 20 percent.)
- Some cleaners are now offering professional multi-process wet cleaning without perc. Look in the yellow pages or google "perc-free dry cleaners" to locate an eco-friendly wet cleaner near you.
- Many clothes that are labeled "dry clean only" can actually be hand-washed or washed on the delicate cycle with cold water.

Plastic Bottles and Tin Can Liners

Phthalates, bisphenol A, and other components of plastic can leach into foods, especially those with a high fat content,† such as peanut butter, milk, cheese, and margarine, as well as into juices, carbonated drinks, and water.[162] Many of these plasticizers have been identified as hormone disruptors, and some are overtly carcinogenic.[163] Plastic is not only used to package everything from spring water to seafood, it also lines tin cans, where it can leach bisphenol A and other estrogen mimickers into such products as canned fruits and vegetables.[164] Here are some solutions for this disturbing and growing toxic phenomenon:

- Don't buy soft water bottles. If the bottle easily dents in when squeezed, it will readily leach plastic. These plastic bottles are usually imprinted with a #1 on the bottom, indicating that they are meant for one-time usage only. Those imprinted with a #7 should be avoided too, as they leach toxic bisphenol A. Try to buy water in strong and rigid polycarbonate plastics. Check the recycling symbol on the bottom of your bottle. For plastics that leach less, look for bottles marked #2 HDPE (high-density polyethylene, such as Nalgene), #4 LDPE (low-density polyethylene), or #5 PP (polypropylene). Furthermore, don't leave these bottles in the sun, where even these sturdier plastics can leach chemicals. Even better, buy or carry your own water (filtered at home) in glass.
- Only use BPA-free baby bottles. In 2006, Europe banned all products containing bisphenol A made for children under age three; in December 2006, San Francisco banned these products as well.
- Don't use stainless steel water bottles that contain nickel as an alternative to plastic. Nickel is both a major allergenic (an estimated 10 to 20 percent of the population is sensitive to nickel; women are more susceptible) and a carcinogenic heavy metal. The other metals contained in stainless steel—molybdenum, chromium, iron—can also leach into water and are toxic.
- Avoid canned foods.
- Use glass whenever possible.

BEST BET WATER BOTTLE

The crème de la crème of water bottles is the "Violiv" violet glass. First used by the ancient Egyptians for long-term storage, violet glass was later rediscovered in the 1800s by Jacob Lorber, an Austrian naturalist, who noted the preserving and enhancing effects of the glass on olive oil. More recently, in the 1980s, Dutch biologist Yves Kraushaar perfected the violet glass formula. Violet glass blocks harmful visible light rays while enhancing transmission of UV(a) and infrared frequencies, which regulate intercellular communication. Through this biophoton process, foods stored in violet glass stay fresher and contain nutrients much longer, and water is optimized for more

*The ACSH receives some funding from Dow Chemical, a manufacturer of perc, but the director says that all money is "no-strings-attached" and that the group's work is independently peer-reviewed.

†Most toxic chemicals are lipophilic, or fat-loving.

efficient hydration. Violiv violet glass products are available in the United States from Vitality Glassware at www.naturalhomesource.com, or (800) 373-4548.

Supplements: Tablets and Capsules

That red, green, or yellow vitamin tablet you may be ingesting daily is shiny and easy to swallow for a reason. In order for tablet ingredients to stick together, manufacturers use glues, binders, and even *shellac*—euphemistically described on the label as "pharmaceutical glaze," "confectioner's glaze," or "natural glaze."[165] Other coatings include corn protein, which many people are sensitive or allergic to, and which may be described on the label as "natural vegetable," "natural protein," "vegetable," or "maize protein."[166] Tablets also contain flowing agents (talc), lubricants (magnesium stearate, calcium stearate, ascorbyl palmitate, castor oil, hydrogenated vegetable oil, and fractionated vegetable oil), binders (corn starch, dextrose sugar, polyethylene glycol, and wax), solubilizing agents (sodium lauryl sulfate), and plasticizers (propylene glycol and phthalates).[167] Furthermore, tablets require up to 20,000 pounds of pressure per square inch to make—which can degrade the nutrients up to 25 percent.[168]

Although encapsulated products are a better bet most of the time, they too might contain added sugars and lubricants. These common lubricants—magnesium and calcium stearate primarily—can inhibit the absorption of nutrients and reduce dissolution of the tablet.[169] Therefore, so you don't waste money on your nutritional supplements, use the following suggestions:

- Don't buy nutritional supplements at a drugstore, department store, or discount store. These commercial products usually are substandard.
- With rare exceptions, do not buy tablets.
- Buy nutritional supplements in capsule form from a health food store or from your holistic physician or practitioner.

THE USE OF BEEF IN CAPSULES

Many nutritional companies have stopped using gelatin capsules made from beef because of the bovine spongiform encephalopathy (BSE) or "mad cow disease" scare. Although many high-quality nutritional supplement companies such as Thorne still don't believe that there has been any BSE contamination from the use of their gelatin capsules made from American—not British—beef, just to be safe they switched in 2001 to plant-derived (from the southern pine tree) capsules.

TOXIC CHEMICALS AND TOXIC METALS
Partners in Poison

Similar to the mercury-microbe synergistic relationship described in chapter 3, I have found in clinical practice an opportunistic relationship between the presence of toxic chemicals and toxic metals in the body. For example, it is exceedingly difficult if not impossible for artists, anesthesiologists, house painters, women who wear lots of cosmetics, or other patients who are continually exposed to petrochemicals daily to fully detoxify from mercury amalgam fillings and other toxic metals. One reason for this synergistic effect is that these "partners in poison" both cause devastating effects in the body—impairing organ functioning, immune system defenses, intracellular respiration, and nerve transmission. However, toxic chemical solvents also have a specific effect on the protective membrane that surrounds each of the 75 trillion cells existing in our body, which allows for a deeper and more destructive cellular ingress of toxic metals.

Toxic Chemicals Destroy Cell Membranes

Although many toxins attack cell membranes, lipophilic (fat-loving) toxic chemicals are especially injurious to these membranes, which are composed of 70 to 90 percent phospholipids. In fact, organic petroleum solvents and toxic detergents are known necrotizers, or destroyers, of cell membranes.[170] Not only do these fatty cell membranes serve as a protective boundary around each of our cells, but they also mediate the entrance of nutrients, hormones, enzymes, antibodies, and neurotransmitters, as well as the exit of waste from the cell. However, chronic exposure to these solvents (butyl-, methyl- or propyl- alcohols) and detergents, as well as to aromatic hydrocarbons (e.g., benzene, toluene, styrene), can render the cell membrane too fluid and slippery, which causes neurotransmitters to miss their binding site on the protein receptors that are normally stably sandwiched between these fatty phospholipids.[171] When neurotransmitter transmission is disrupted, messages that are normally communicated to the cell can become scrambled, resulting in memory loss, difficulty concentrating, and "brain fog." Motor commands to the limbs may also become garbled, causing muscle incoordination and difficulty walking. Additionally, this systemic cell membrane dysregulation triggers increased adrenaline production, which can cause agitation and anxiety.

"Drunk" Cells Decompensate Further

These symptoms are also typical in individuals who have imbibed excessive amounts of the chemical ethanol from alcoholic drinks. Thus, the same mechanism in the body occurs for alcoholics as it does for environmentally sensitive individuals who are exposed to too much perfume or have walked into a freshly painted house. In both instances, the membrane-disrupting effects of an excessive load of toxic chemicals cause brain cells to become more and more dysfunctional. Over time, these "drunken" cells further decompensate by absorbing cholesterol and mineral-based fat compounds in a desperate attempt to become more stable and functional.[172] However, at this point neurotransmitter signaling, as well as ionic transport into and out of the cell (the sodium-potassium pump and calcium channel functioning), become even more impaired.

Toxic Metals Infiltrate "Leaky" Cells

The membrane-disrupting effects of chemical solvents can dissolve parts of the cell membrane and render a cell more vulnerable (and "leaky") to external toxins, similar to leaky gut syndrome. In damaged and leaky cells, mercury, cadmium, and other heavy metals can easily combine with the cell membrane's damaged phospholipids. This infiltration of foreign toxic metals has the most devastating effect of all on cells by further reducing their fluidity, flexibility, and function, and when the destruction is too great, resulting in their death.[173] Thus, by damaging membranes and allowing the deeper penetration of toxic metals into each cell, petroleum chemicals have a direct adverse effect on the detoxification of amalgam fillings and other toxic metals out of the body. This has been seen clinically in cases of patients with a significant history of exposure to toxic chemicals who have a more difficult time detoxifying mercury, even after the removal of their amalgam fillings.

Pathogenic Microbes Proliferate

Additionally, in this pathological state, the cells that haven't died function in a chronic state of malnutrition that leaves them significantly more vulnerable to pathogenic bacteria, viruses, and fungi. In fact, trying to clear chronic intestinal dysbiosis—the pathogenic overgrowth of bacteria and candida yeast—is futile when patients have a mouthful of fillings and crowns made up of heavy metals and continue to expose themselves to toxic chemicals in their personal care products. In the majority of cases, it is necessary that patients replace their amalgam fillings and petrochemical-laden cosmetics and soaps with nontoxic alternatives before treatment can have any significant beneficial effect on their dental or tonsil bacterial focal infections. Thus, many candida symptoms, viral fatigue syndromes, and chronic intestinal parasites are often opportunistic to the bigger toxic threat to survival—chronic exposure to toxic metals and chemicals. Fortunately, as this toxic load is reduced, damaged cell membranes are able to regenerate, and healthy regulation and normal metabolism can be restored.*

DEFINING "HEALTHY" SENSITIVITY

Just What Is Normal and Healthy Nowadays?

Before concluding this chapter, it is important to define exactly what is normal and healthy currently in regard to etiquette as well as the degree of reactivity we experience from exposure to toxic chemicals. For example, is it appropriate to sit for three hours on an airplane next to a man reeking of aftershave, or can we get up and request another seat? Should we stay and eat with friends in a new restaurant with strong odors from new carpet and paint, or can we leave immediately and try to get another reservation on a Friday night? Finally, if we

*Furthermore, sensitive patients who were previously allergic to almost everything become stronger and have a more functional immune system after detoxifying these toxic chemicals and metals. They then typically only have to avoid a more reasonable amount of food allergens, such as only one or two primary food groups, instead of their previous twenty or thirty foods.

decide to endure these chemical assaults, is it "normal" to feel nothing, or to have symptoms? These issues are not only grappled with daily by environmentally ill individuals but also deliberated by those who perhaps don't feel the immediate symptomatic effects quite as strongly, yet are very conscious of the toxic consequences that these xenobiotics have on the body.

Is Anyone Impervious to Toxic Chemicals?

Many people in the West seem to strive for that "superman" or "superwoman" image that lies in our collective consciousness, able to handle any stress with perfect equanimity. However, are these excessively vital people who seem to live obliviously in a newly painted and carpeted home or who spray perfume on themselves daily truly healthy? Furthermore, are these superhumans impervious to the future possibility of cancer, heart disease, Parkinson's, or Alzheimer's? That is, can truly robust individuals adapt to modern supertoxins such as PCBs (polychlorinated biphenyls), dioxin, formaldehyde, and phthalates? Based simply on the rising rates of cancer and other degenerative diseases, this does not appear to be the case. A renowned San Francisco allergist and immunologist, Alvin S. Levin, remarked on this issue:

> Over many centuries, our bodies have miraculously evolved to tolerate or require most of the naturally occurring substances that surround us. Yet there are many synthetic substances in our environment to which our bodies have not had sufficient time to adapt. At the present moment, we're being exposed to concentrations of these chemicals that . . . tax our adaptive mechanisms to their maximum.[174]

"Lay Off That 'Sensitive' Crap!"

Thus, if no one's immune system is strong enough to combat significant doses of these foreign and highly toxic chemicals, we may ask, what is appropriate sensitivity and behavior nowadays? One reader of *The Wary Canary,* a newsletter for the environmentally ill (who see themselves as canaries in coal mines warning others of dangerous fumes), expresses her disgust with the typically pejorative use of the word *sensitive:*

> Lay off that "sensitive" crap! If your kid plays in the streets and is run over by a truck, do you say, "Poor thing, he's sensitive to Fords"? We're basically dealing with poisons, not frail health.[175]

Thus, the term *sensitive* does not always equate with *sick.* In fact, the opposite of sensitive—*insensitive*—is not exactly a state to strive for either. Perhaps the ideal mirrors more of a balance in life, similar to the Tao in Taoism or the Middle Path in Buddhism. That is, healthy individuals could be defined as those who have detoxified enough to be quite sensitive and aware of toxic chemicals in their environment, but who have also received enough effective therapies to not become unreasonably ill from the typical exposures of everyday life. For example, a few minutes of smelling obnoxiously strong aftershave or perfume may trigger in the healthy and sensitive individual only transient symptoms such as a mild headache, fatigue, or irritability for a few minutes to hours—as opposed to being debilitated for weeks in the case of an environmentally ill individual. Thus, symptoms are like a warning bell, and when heard clearly by an advanced and "clean" patient, they signal appropriate action. In life, appropriate actions made now can often help prevent future misfortune—such as the onset of degenerative disease.

The Healthy and Sensitive Individual

In fact, awareness and sensitivity to our symptoms, although they can make our life more challenging at times, can also enrich and prolong our lives. They motivate us to seek needed holistic help, clean up our diet, replace our kitchen and bathroom products, examine our psychological conflicts, and become more aware of our bodies. Therefore, a working definition of a truly balanced and healthy individual living appropriately in this toxic twenty-first century might be the following:

> A "healthy sensitive" individual is one who is aware of toxic fumes and chemicals, avoids or mitigates his/her exposure, and is able to fully recover from typical toxic stressors in a reasonable period of time with no significant physiological, neurological, or psychological deficits.

The New Etiquette among Sensitive and Conscious Individuals

As this new consciousness pervades more and more of the planet, let's hope that people become more sensitive to toxic stressors, including the wearing of strong perfumes in public. Already this newer social etiquette is becoming more common, as growing numbers of holistically oriented individuals refrain from wearing scents or even strong essential oils in public. As this type of behavior increasingly becomes the norm, perhaps the pejorative connotation associated with the term *sensitive* will also change, and the word will be used appropriately as the dictionary originally has defined it: "connected with the senses" and "responsive to emotional, artistic, etc., impressions."[176]

CONCLUSION
Humans Have Lived with Poisons for Millennia

> We shall never completely master nature; and our bodily organism, itself a part of that nature, will always remain a transient structure with a limited capacity for adaptation and achievement. This recognition does not have a paralyzing effect. On the contrary, it points the direction for our activity. If we cannot remove all suffering, we can remove some, and we can mitigate some: the experience of many thousands of years has convinced us of that.[177]
>
> SIGMUND FREUD

Freud's quote magnifies the fact that human beings have lived with toxins for centuries. In fact, the decline of the Roman Empire has been blamed by many well-respected historians at least in part on the "sweet poison" of wine simmered in lead pots, which may have caused infertility, among other conditions.[178] In the early 1800s, Alfred Nobel was said to have suffered from dynamite-induced headaches, as did many of his factory workers.[179] At the turn of the twentieth century, Marcel Proust, who was asthmatic and quite sensitive to environmental toxins, often had to isolate himself in a cork-filled room and set perfumed visitors' chairs outside to air afterward.[180]* In World War I, troops were poisoned by mustard gas, and many survivors later developed chemical sensitivity.[181] In World War II, millions of soldiers and refugees were dusted with DDT. In Vietnam, military personnel were sprayed with defoliant, later resulting in the diagnosis of Agent Orange syndrome for many suffering GIs.[182] And chemicals used in the 1991 Gulf War caused such a host of chronic symptoms that this war received its own disease appellation—Gulf War syndrome. Finally, no one can deny that presently in our everyday world we are confronted daily with an onslaught of toxic chemicals in the air and water, in our homes and offices, and in our personal care products.

Lighten Your Chemical Burden over Time

Although the sheer amount of chemicals produced annually—in the *trillions* of pounds—and their poisonous nature can be staggering even to comprehend, as Freud stated in the 1800s, we do have the power to mitigate these toxins and remove some of the suffering that they cause. The choice is yours. Do you want to passively undergo the slow genocide chemicals cause, or will you choose the path of knowledge and resist conventional ignorance? Replacing your kitchen and bathroom products with nontoxic ones is a relatively painless and important first step. Changing your home, school, or office surroundings is a more complicated endeavor, but doing so can be well worth the effort if these environments are adversely affecting the health of you and your children. Finding a competent holistic practitioner to guide your detoxification protocol and suggest supportive supplements is also important, especially if you are ill. Making small steps daily will significantly lighten your toxic load within a few short months and also reduce the likelihood of future degenerative disease.

A Final Note for Skeptics

Skeptics may wonder why this information is not more widespread. Although the green movement is growing and is more popular than ever before, information and guidance about toxic chemicals in the house, cosmetics, work, school, car, and so forth are still rare in the mainstream news. And when the more disturbing truths about toxic chemicals and the industries that produce them are sometimes revealed in the news,

*Cork is an effective insulator against both temperature and noise.

there always seems to be a quote from some scientist that "pooh-poohs" the danger. This dearth of impartial news reporting is primarily due to the influence of multi-billion-dollar chemical companies on governmental organizations and the media. In fact, the extensive and pervasive control the chemical industry has on the media is illustrated in the following story reprinted from *Toxic Deception,* by Dan Fagin, Marianne Lavelle, and the Center for Public Integrity.

▶ For more information on the decline of independent investigative reporting and the growing influence of the government and corporations on our slowly eroding "free" press, go to www.projectcensored.org.

> On March 31, 1993, *Frontline,* a Public Broadcasting System television program, aired a provocative documentary called *In Our Children's Food* about the harmful effects of pesticides and the general inability of the federal government to regulate the widespread use of cancer-causing farm chemicals. The documentary, narrated by Bill Moyers and produced by Martin Koughan, later received an Emmy award from the National Academy of Television Arts and Sciences. The Investigative Reporters and Editors also honored the program as the best TV documentary in the United States in 1993.
>
> The morning after the program aired in most U.S. cities, however, a remarkable editorial appeared in the *Wall Street Journal* titled "Frontline Perpetuates Pesticide Myths." It was written by Dennis T. Avery, who was identified as a "fellow at the Hudson Institute" and "director of Hudson's Center on Global Food Issues." The author, an agricultural economist whose work is funded by agribusiness interests, charged in his opening paragraph that the Frontline documentary had "made recommendations that would increase our cancer and heart disease rates, increase the risk of world hunger, and plow down millions of square miles of wildlife habitat." Avery wrote about the "ignorance" of Rachel Carson, the respected author of the classic 1962 book *Silent Spring,* and also lamented the government's banning of the pesticide DDT, which, he said, was not "dangerous to people or birds."
>
> What was most intriguing was not the vitriol of Avery's editorial but its curious timing. No one places an op-ed article in a major newspaper the night before its publication; indeed, the Frontline program ended at 10 P.M., Eastern time. How did Avery do it?
>
> The question gnawed away at producer Koughan so much that he telephoned Avery directly. Koughan discovered to his dismay that the editorial actually had been submitted to the *Wall Street Journal* a full *week* before the Frontline program was broadcast. He later ascertained that the pesticide industry had somehow obtained a copy of *In Our Children's Food* a month before the airdate. An entire public-relations campaign had been waged against the show; individual PBS stations had been contacted, and the American Cancer Society had been persuaded to send out a nationwide bulletin to its members, advising them to disregard the information in the program. As Sheila Kaplan reported in *Legal Times,* the American Cancer Society instructed its branch offices on how to respond to public inquiries, asserting that "the program makes unfounded suggestions . . . that pesticide residues in food may be at hazardous levels."
>
> How did all this happen? Porter/Novelli, a public relations and lobbying firm based in New York City—representing major chemical companies such as Rhone-Poulenc Ag Company, DuPont, and Hoechst-Roussel, in addition to the pesticide industry-financed Center for Produce Quality—had quietly been doing pro bono PR work for the American Cancer Society. When word became known that a major, critical documentary was about to be telecast, the firm quickly sprang into damage-control action, orchestrating the American Cancer Society's "reaction" to the program. It was a public relations coup.[183]

Bill Moyers learned his lesson. Nine years later on March 26, 2001, he narrated a PBS documentary named

Trade Secrets, on the chemical industry and its suspected role in the increased incidences of learning disorders, breast and brain cancer in children, testicular cancer in teenage boys, and infertility in adults. However, this time, he didn't distribute the tapes in advance to journalists or reviewers. Moyers concluded his program by saying:

> We are flying blind, except the laboratory mice in this vast chemical experiment are the children. They have no idea what's happening to them. Neither do we.[184]

NOTES

1. L. Lawson, *Staying Well in a Toxic World* (Chicago: The Noble Press, 1993), 19.
2. D. Berkson, *Hormone Deception* (Chicago: Contemporary Books, 2000), 21.
3. R. Freeze, *The Environmental Pendulum* (Berkeley: University of California Press, 2000), 8.
4. D. Dadd, *Nontoxic, Natural and Earthwise* (New York: G. Putnam's Sons, 1990), 7.
5. K. Schafer et al., *Chemical Trespass: Pesticides in Our Bodies and Corporate Accountability* (Pesticide Action Network, May 2004), 3, www. panna.org/issues/publication/chemical-trespass-english.
6. S. Steingraber, *Living Downstream* (Reading, Mass.: Addison-Wesley Publishing Company, 1997), 5.
7. D. Fagin et al., *Toxic Deception* (Secaucus, N.J.: Carol Publishing Group, 1996), xvii.
8. S. Steingraber, *Living Downstream* (Reading, Mass.: Addison-Wesley Publishing Company, 1997), 5.
9. D. Fagin et al., *Toxic Deception* (Secaucus, N.J.: Carol Publishing Group, 1996), xvi.
10. C. Wilson, *Chemical Exposure and Human Health* (Jefferson, N.C.: McFarland and Company, Inc., 1993), 2.
11. L. Lawson, *Staying Well in a Toxic World* (Chicago: The Noble Press, 1993), 52–53; D. Berkson, *Hormone Deception* (Chicago: Contemporary Books, 2000), 143, 206–8, 209–10; Z. Gard, "Why Is Irritability, Anger and Viciousness Increasing?" *Explore!* 6, no. 4 (1995).
12. D. Fagin et al., *Toxic Deception* (Secaucus, N.J.: Carol Publishing Group, 1996), xvi, xvii.
13. T. Colborn, *Our Stolen Future* (New York: Dutton, 1996), 89–91.
14. "PVC—The Poison Plastic," http://archive.greenpeace.org/toxics/html/content/pvc1.html.
15. K. Schafer et al., *Chemical Trespass: Pesticides in Our Bodies and Corporate Accountability* (Pesticide Action Network, May 2004), 2, 3, www. panna.org/issues/publication/chemical-trespass-english.
16. "Body Burden: The Pollution in Newborns," July 14, 2005, 1–5, http://archive.ewg.org/reports/bodyburden2/execsumm.php.
17. K. Erickson, *Drop-Dead Gorgeous* (Chicago: Contemporary Books, 2002), 19.
18. T. Colborn, *Our Stolen Future* (New York: Dutton, 1996), 113.
19. Ibid., 113–17.
20. W. Crinnion, "Environmental Medicine: Excerpts from Articles on Current Toxicity, Solvents, Pesticides and Heavy Metals," *Townsend Letter for Doctors and Patients,* January 2001, 64.
21. "Body Burden: The Pollution in People," 2002, 1–5, http://archive.ewg/reports/bodyburden1/methodology.php.
22. "Executive Summary: What We Found," www.ewg.org/sites/bodyburden1/es.php.
23. T. Colborn, *Our Stolen Future* (New York: Dutton, 1996), 89–91.
24. "New Canadian Report Reveals Toxic Pollution in Humans," *Beyond Pesticides,* November 16, 2005, 1, www.beyondpesticides.org/news/daily.htm.
25. K. Schafer et al., *Chemical Trespass: Pesticides in Our Bodies and Corporate Accountability* (Pesticide Action Network, May 2004), 2, 3, www. panna.org/issues/publication/chemical-trespass-english.
26. "Body Burden: The Pollution in Newborns," July 14, 2005, 1–5, http://archive.ewg.org/reports/bodyburden2/execsumm.php.
27. M. Reeves et al., *Fields of Poison 2002* (Californians for Pesticide Reform, 2002), 1, www.panna.org/issues/publication/fields-poison-2002-english.
28. D. Berkson, *Hormone Deception* (Chicago: Contemporary Books, 2000), 23.
29. Ibid.
30. D. Fagin et al., *Toxic Deception* (Secaucus, N.J.: Carol Publishing Group, 1996), 1–2.
31. S. Steingraber, *Living Downstream* (Reading, Mass.: Addison-Wesley Publishing Company, 1997), 8.
32. R. Carson, *Silent Spring* (Boston: Houghton Mifflin Company, 1962), xxi.

33. K. Schafer et al., *Chemical Trespass: Pesticides in Our Bodies and Corporate Accountability* (Pesticide Action Network, May 2004), 5, www. panna.org/issues/publication/chemical-trespass-english.
34. "Toxic FAQs for DDT, DDE, and DDD," www.atsdr.cdc.gov/tfacts35.html.
35. Associated Press, "Try to Imagine No Plastic Anything," *Marin Independent Journal,* October 30, 1999, D1.
36. USA Today Snapshots, "Fewer Vacation Days in the USA," *USA Today,* December 27, 2001, 1.
37. C. Adams, "The Straight Dope: Vacation Daze," *Pacific Sun,* February 28–March 6, 2001, 10.
38. D. Pearson, *The New Natural House Book* (New York: Fireside, 1989), 42–43.
39. S. Rogers, *Chemical Sensitivity* (New Canaan, Conn.: Keats Publishing, Inc., 1995), 7.
40. L. Lawson, *Staying Well in a Toxic World* (Chicago: The Noble Press, 1993), 59.
41. Ibid., 51.
42. S. Rogers, *Chemical Sensitivity* (New Canaan, Conn.: Keats Publishing, Inc., 1995), 7.
43. B. Matthews, *Chemical Sensitivity* (Jefferson, N.C.: McFarland and Company, Inc., 1992), 18.
44. L. Lawson, *Staying Well in a Toxic World* (Chicago: The Noble Press, 1993), 39.
45. S. Stranahan, "The Clean Room's Dirty Secret," *Mother Jones,* March/April, 2002, 49.
46. S. Steingraber, *Living Downstream* (Reading, Mass.: Addison-Wesley Publishing Company, 1997), 65.
47. S. Stranahan, "The Clean Room's Dirty Secret," *Mother Jones,* March/April, 2002, 44–49.
48. J. Sullivan and G. Krieger, *Hazardous Materials Toxicology* (Baltimore: Williams and Wilkins, 1992), 2.
49. S. Steingraber, *Living Downstream* (Reading, Mass.: Addison-Wesley Publishing Company, 1997), 65.
50. M. Reeves et al., *Fields of Poison 2002* (Californians for Pesticide Reform, 2002), 1, www.panna.org/issues/publication/fields-poison-2002-english.
51. Ibid.
52. D. Fagin et al., *Toxic Deception* (Secaucus, N.J.: Carol Publishing Group, 1996), 81.
53. Environmental Resource Center, "How to Put the H Back into OSHA," April 5, 2010, www.ercweb.com/resources/viewtip.aspx?id=7562.
54. L. Lawson, *Staying Well in a Toxic World* (Chicago: The Noble Press, 1993), 124.
55. D. Fagin et al., *Toxic Deception* (Secaucus, N.J.: Carol Publishing Group, 1996), 81.
56. "Supermarket Rejects Ag-Mart Tomatoes Over Birth Defects in Florida," *Beyond Pesticides,* November 16, 2005, 8, www.beyondpesticides.org/news/daily.htm.
57. Ibid.
58. L. Lawson, *Staying Well in a Toxic World* (Chicago: The Noble Press, 1993), 308–10.
59. B. Matthews, *Chemical Sensitivity* (Jefferson, N.C.: McFarland and Company, 1992), 81.
60. L. Lawson, *Staying Well in a Toxic World* (Chicago: The Noble Press, 1993), 312.
61. P. M. Kidd, "Autism, an Extreme Challenge to Integrative Medicine. Part I: The Knowledge Base," *Alternative Medicine Review* 7, no. 4 (2002): 302.
62. Ibid.
63. "Parents Urge Schools to Start Year Without Toxic Pesticides; US Senator Introduces Bill to Protect Children from School Pesticide Poisoning," *Beyond Pesticides,* November 16, 2005, 1, 2, www.beyondpesticides.org/schools/alerts/asthma.htm.
64. Ibid., 2; B. Levitt, *Electromagnetic Fields* (San Diego: Harcourt Brace and Co., 1995), 176–77.
65. L. Lawson, *Staying Well in a Toxic World* (Chicago: The Noble Press, 1993), 313.
66. B. Levitt, *Electromagnetic Fields* (San Diego: Harcourt Brace and Co., 1995), 177–78.
67. "Parents Urge Schools to Start Year Without Toxic Pesticides; US Senator Introduces Bill to Protect Children from School Pesticide Poisoning," *Beyond Pesticides,* November 16, 2005, 1, 2, 9–10, www.beyondpesticides.org/schools/alerts/asthma.htm.
68. "Children, Pesticides and Schools: School Environment Protections ACE (SEPA)," *Beyond Pesticides,* November 16, 2005, 1–3, www.beyond pesticides.org/schools/sepa.
69. C. Lu et al., "Organic Diets Significantly Lower Children's Dietary Exposure to Organophosphorus Pesticides," *Environmental Health Perspectives* 114 (2006): 260–63.
70. K. Schafer et al., *Chemical Trespass: Pesticides in Our Bodies and Corporate Accountability* (Pesticide Action Network, May 2004), 4, www. panna.org/issues/publication/chemical-trespass-english.
71. J. Motavalli, "New Car Smell: It's Not So Sweet, " *E The Environmental Magazine,* January/February 2006, 2, www.emagazine.com/view/?3062.

72. "GM Chevy Cobalt Receives Top Honor in 3rd Annual Guide to Toxic Chemicals in Cars and Children's Car Seats," September 16, 2009, press release at www.healthystuff.org/departments/cars/press.releases.php.
73. J. Mercola, "Are EMFs Hazardous to Our Health?" July 3, 2008, 1–7, www.loveforlife.com.au/node/5064.
74. "Hybrid EMF Risk Still Uncertain," April 27, 2008, 1, www.hybridcars.com/safety/hybrid-emf-risk-still-uncertain.html; C. McKusick, "Car Radiation," www.emfblues.com/CarRadiation.html.
75. M. Adams, "Fluorescent Lights Release Toxic Mercury Directly into the Environment," February 11, 2008, www.naturalnews.com.
76. D. Gutierrez, "Fluorescent Light Bulbs Linked with Eczema, Seizures, Migraines, Skin Rashes," August 8, 2008, www.naturalnews.com.
77. P. M. Kidd, "Autism, an Extreme Challenge to Integrative Medicine. Part I: The Knowledge Base," *Alternative Medicine Review* 7, no. 4 (2002): 302.
78. "New Canadian Report Reveals Toxic Pollution in Humans," *Beyond Pesticides,* November 16, 2005, 3, www.beyondpesticides.org/news/daily.htm.
79. L. Hardell and M. Eriksson, "A Case-Control Study of Non-Hodgkin Lymphoma and Exposure to Pesticides," *Cancer* 85, no. 6 (March 15, 1999).
80. S. Rogers, *Chemical Sensitivity* (New Canaan, Conn.: Keats Publishing, Inc., 1995), 7, 14.
81. S. Queen, "Toxic Footprints in Chemistry and Bio Transformation," IABDM 20th Anniversary Conference (March 31–April 2, 2006), 7.
82. J. Mercola, "Are EMFs Hazardous to Our Health?" July 3, 2008, 1–7, www.loveforlife.com.au/node/5064.
83. B. Matthews, *Chemical Sensitivity* (Jefferson, N.C.: McFarland and Company, 1992), 80, 82.
84. D. Fagin et al., *Toxic Deception* (Secaucus, N.J.: Carol Publishing Group, 1996), 228.
85. S. Steingraber *Living Downstream* (Reading, Mass.: Addison-Wesley Publishing Company, 1997), 7.
86. Associated Press, "Study Finds Unexpectedly High Levels of Toxic Chemicals Inside Americans," *Marin Independent Journal,* March 22, 2001.
87. D. Berkson, *Hormone Deception* (Chicago: Contemporary Books, 2000), 299–301.
88. S. Steingraber, *Living Downstream* (Reading, Mass.: Addison-Wesley Publishing Company, 1997), 112.
89. CBC, "Environmental Toxins and Infertility in Men," *CellMate Reporter* 3 (First Quarter 2004): 1.
90. D. Fischer, "The Body Burden," *Lake County Record-Bee,* March 30, 2005, B1.
91. L. Lawson, *Staying Well in a Toxic World* (Chicago: The Noble Press, 1993), 279.
92. Ibid., 281.
93. Environmental Working Group, "Skin Deep: A Safety Assessment of Ingredients in Personal Care Products," 1, www.ewg.org/reports/skindeep/report/executive_summary.php.
94. Associated Press, "Personal Products Polluting Water," *Marin Independent Journal,* March 13, 2002.
95. R. Winter, *Cosmetic Ingredients* (New York: Crown, 1994), 7.
96. D. Dadd, *Nontoxic, Natural and Earthwise* (New York: G. Putnam's Sons, 1990), 174.
97. Environmental Working Group, "Skin Deep: A Safety Assessment of Ingredients in Personal Care Products," 4, www.ewg.org/reports/skindeep/report/executive_summary.php.
98. R. Winter, *Cosmetic Ingredients* (New York: Crown, 1994), 7.
99. Environmental Working Group, "Skin Deep: A Safety Assessment of Ingredients in Personal Care Products," 2, www.ewg.org/reports/skindeep/report/executive_summary.php.
100. Ibid.
101. Marc Lappe, *Chemical Deception* (San Francisco: Sierra Club Books, 1991), 94.
102. Ibid.
103. R. Winter, *Cosmetic Ingredients* (New York: Crown, 1994), 14–15.
104. D. Fischer, "The Body Burden," *Lake County Record-Bee,* March 30, 2005, B1.
105. Ibid., 15.
106. Ibid.
107. R. Williams, "Health Risks and Environmental Issues," *Townsend Letter for Doctors and Patients,* February/March 2004, 32.
108. L. Lawson, *Staying Well in a Toxic World* (Chicago: The Noble Press, 1993), 282.
109. Environmental Working Group, "Skin Deep: A Safety Assessment of Ingredients in Personal Care Products," 3, www.ewg.org/reports/skindeep/report/executive_summary.php.
110. Anna Soref, "Make Up Your Mind to Go Natural," *The Natural Foods Merchandiser,* January 2001, 50.
111. R. Winter, *Cosmetic Ingredients* (New York: Three Rivers Press, 1999), 9.

112. Environmental Working Group, "Skin Deep: A Safety Assessment of Ingredients in Personal Care Products," 2, www.ewg.org/reports/skindeep/report/executive_summary .php.
113. L. Lawson, *Staying Well in a Toxic World* (Chicago: The Noble Press, 1993), 282.
114. Ibid., 279–80.
115. Ibid., 281.
116. Lance A. Wallace et al., "Identification of Polar Volatile Organic Compounds in Consumer Products and Common Microenvironments," paper #A312 for presentation at the 1991 annual meeting of the Air & Waste Management Association, March 1, 1991.
117. U.S. Congress House Committee on Science and Technology, *Neurotoxins: At Home and in the Workplace* (Report 99–827), September 16, 1986.
118. R. Winter, *Cosmetic Ingredients* (New York: Three Rivers Press, 1999), 281–82, 287.
119. R. Williams, "Health Risks and Environmental Issues," *Townsend Letter for Doctors and Patients,* February/March 2004, 33.
120. "(SPECT) Scan of MCS Patient's Brain Before and After Challenge with Perfume Inhalation," www.ourlittleplace .com/spect.html.
121. U.S. Congress House Committee on Science and Technology, *Neurotoxins: At Home and in the Workplace* (Report 99–827), September 16, 1986, 287.
122. R. Winter, *Cosmetic Ingredients* (New York: Crown, 1994), 18.
123. K. Erickson, *Drop-Dead Gorgeous* (Chicago: Contemporary Books, 2002), 190–92.
124. Ibid., 191–94.
125. L. Lawson, *Staying Well in a Toxic World* (Chicago: The Noble Press, 1993), 286.
126. H. Clark, *The Cure for All Cancers* (San Diego: ProMotion Publishing, 1993), 8, 38–39.
127. "Poplar Trees Popular among Pig Farmers?" American Forests Bytes, www.americanforests.org/forestbytes/122003 .php.
128. Seroyal, *Gemmotherapy* (Richmond Hills, Ontario: Seroyal International, Inc., n.d.), 36.
129. W. Crinnion, "For the Sake of Your Children, Don't Eat Farmed Salmon," *Naturopathic Doctor News and Review,* April 2006, 14.
130. Ibid.
131. E. Lipski, *Digestive Wellness* (New Canaan, Conn.: Keats Publishing, Inc., 1996), 149.
132. M. Kauppi, "Sweating Out Mercury," *Heavy Metal Bulletin* 6, no. 2 (October 2000): 14.
133. D. Dadd, *Nontoxic, Natural and Earthwise* (New York: G. Putnam's Sons, 1990), 8, 175.
134. Ibid.
135. Environmental Working Group, "Alcohol Denatured," www.cosmeticsdatabase.com/ingredient .php?ingred06=700215.
136. R. Arditti, "Cosmetics, Parabens, and Breast Cancer," September 6, 2004, www.organicconsumers.org/bodycare/ breastcancer090604.cfm.
137. "Parabens," www.breastcancerfund/org/site.
138. H. Clark, *The Cure for All Diseases* (San Diego: ProMotion Publishing, 1995), 36.
139. K. Erickson, *Drop-Dead Gorgeous* (Chicago: Contemporary Books, 2002), 28.
140. R. Williams, "Health Risks and Environmental Issues," *Townsend Letter for Doctors and Patients,* February/March 2004, 33.
141. Jan Modric, "Hair Dye Allergies," May 18, 2007, www .healthhype.com/hair-dye-allergies.html.
142. Department of Environmental Protection, State of Maine, "Chemicals of High Concern List," www.maine.gov/dep/ oc/safechem/highconcern/acronyms.htm.
143. "Sodium Laureth Sulfate: What It Is, Where to Find It, and How to Avoid It," www.natural-health-information-centre.com/sodium-laureth-sulfate.html.
144. S. Tracey, "Plaintiffs' Response to Eli Lilly and Company's Supplemental Motion for Summary Judgment," 5, www .redflagsweekly.com/legal/2002_nov18.html.
145. Ibid., 11, 12.
146. S. Steingraber, *Living Downstream* (Reading, Mass.: Addison-Wesley Publishing Company, 1997), 7.
147. L. Lawson, *Staying Well in a Toxic World* (Chicago: The Noble Press, 1993), 38.
148. D. Grant, "The Pharmacology of Isopropyl Alcohol," *Journal of Laboratory and Clinical Medicine* 8 (October/ September 1922): 382–86; A. Lehman and M. Chase, "The Acute and Chronic Toxicity of Isopropyl Alcohol," *The Journal of Laboratory and Clinical Medicine* 29, no. 6 (June 1944): 561–67.
149. D. Grant, "The Pharmacology of Isopropyl Alcohol," *Journal of Laboratory and Clinical Medicine* 8 (October/September 1922): 382–86.
150. Ibid., 386; D. Macht, "A Toxicological Study of Some Alcohols, with Especial Reference to Isomers," *The Journal of Pharmacology and Experimental Therapies* 16, no. 1

(May 25, 1920): 1–10; W. von Oettingen, "The Aliphatic Alcohols: Their Toxicity and Potential Dangers in Relation to Their Chemical Constitution and Their Fate in Metabolism," U.S. Public Health Service Bulletin 281, (Washington, D.C.: Government Printing Office, 1943), 1–181.

151. L. Williams and D. Klinghardt, *Isopropyl Alcohol and Other Toxic Solvents* (AANK self-publlished, 1995): 24.

152. S. McFadden and J. Haddow, "Coma Produced by Topical Application of Isopropanol," *Pediatrics* 43 (January–June 1969): 622–23; P. Visudhiphan and H. Kaufman, "Increased Cerebrospinal Fluid Protein Following Isopropyl Alcohol Intoxication," *New York State Journal of Medicine,* April 15, 1971, 887–88; I. Vicas and R. Beck, "Fatal Inhalational Isopropyl Alcohol Poisoning in a Neonate," *Clinical Toxicology* 31, no. 3 (1993): 473–81; T. Mydler et al., "Two-Week Old Infant with Isopropanol Intoxication," *Pediatric Emergency Care* 9, no. 3 (1993): 146–48.

153. T. Martinez et al., "A Comparison of the Absorption and Metabolism of Isopropyl Alcohol by Oral, Dermal, and Inhalation Routes," *Veterinary Human Toxicology* 3, no. 28 (June 1986): 233–36.

154. I. Vicas and R. Beck, "Fatal Inhalational Isopropyl Alcohol Poisoning in a Neonate," *Clinical Toxicology* 3, no. 31 (1993): 473–81.

155. Anna Soref, "Make Up Your Mind to Go Natural," *The Natural Foods Merchandiser,* January 2001, 50.

156. D. Dadd, *Nontoxic, Natural and Earthwise* (New York: G. Putnam's Sons, 1990), 151.

157. Ibid., 219.

158. M. Kauppi, "Cadmium, Mercury, Formaldehyde and Benzidine in Your T-Shirt!" *Heavy Metal Bulletin* 3, no. 2 (September 1996): 10.

159. D. Berkson, *Hormone Deception* (Chicago: Contemporary Books, 2000), 269.

160. D. Fagin et al., *Toxic Deception* (Secaucus, N.J.: Carol Publishing Group, 1996), xxii.

161. E. McCarthy, "Clothes Call: Health Newsletter," *Elle,* 2001, 214.

162. S. Steingraber, *Living Downstream* (Reading, Mass.: Addison-Wesley Publishing Company, 1997), 112.

163. T. Colborn, *Our Stolen Future* (New York: Dutton, 1996), 223–24.

164. Ibid., 135.

165. A. Czap, "Supplement Facts ≠ All the Facts: What the New Label Does—and Doesn't—Disclose," *The Townsend Letter for Doctors and Patients,* July 1999, 117–19.

166. Ibid.

167. Ibid.

168. R. Marshall, "Just Say 'No' to Tablets," Pacific Research Laboratories product information guide, 2006.

169. A. Czap, "Supplement Facts ≠ All the Facts: What the New Label Does—and Doesn't—Disclose," *The Townsend Letter for Doctors and Patients,* July 1999, 117–19.

170. W. Rea, *Chemical Sensitivity,* vol. 1 (Boca Raton, Fla.: Lewis Publishers, 1992), 67.

171. R. Erdmann, *The Amino Revolution* (New York: Simon and Schuster, 1987), 226–27.

172. Ibid.

173. W. Rea, *Chemical Sensitivity,* vol. 1 (Boca Raton, Fla.: Lewis Publishers, 1992), 58, 67.

174. L. Lawson, *Staying Well in a Toxic World* (Chicago: The Noble Press, 1993), 35.

175. Ibid.

176. L. Brown, ed., *The New Shorter Oxford English Dictionary* (Oxford: Clarendon Press, 1993), 2776.

177. S. Freud, *Civilization and Its Discontents* (New York: W. W. Norton and Company, 1961), 37.

178. A. Gittleman, *How to Stay Young and Healthy in a Toxic World* (Los Angeles: Keats Publishing, 1999), 64.

179. C. Wilson, *Chemical Exposure and Human Health* (Jefferson, N.C.: McFarland and Company, Inc., 1993), 2–3.

180. Ibid., 3.

181. W. Rea, *Chemical Sensitivity,* vol. 1 (Boca Raton, Fla.: Lewis Publishers, 1992), 9.

182. Ibid.

183. D. Fagin et al., *Toxic Deception* (Secaucus, N.J.: Carol Publishing Group, 1996), vii–viii.

184. D. Bauder, "Bill Moyers Documentary Exposes Chemical Industry," *Marin Independent Journal,* March 26, 2001, E2.

PART THREE

NUTRITION AND DIGESTION

Throughout history, many profound cures effected through dietary changes have been recorded. However, for the majority of individuals today, diet *alone* is simply no longer an effective healing method. The harm inflicted on our bodies from modern-day toxic stressors is just too great. For example, even the purest diet possible cannot completely mitigate the systemic poisoning and immune system impairment caused by mercury amalgam fillings. Nor can it fully eliminate the damaging effects of long-term inhalation of toxic chemicals at work or in a new home, a chronic dental or tonsil focal infection (covered in part 4), or vaccinosis caused by DNA-altering vaccinations (see chapter 15). This is especially true for those depleted individuals who respond to treatment not from a healthier dormant psoric miasmic level, but instead from the more degenerated tuberculinic or luetic reaction mode. As Jane G. Goldberg, Ph.D., comments in her book *Deceits of the Mind and Their Effects on the Body,* although "whole foods must replace those fragmentalized, partial nonfood foods . . . food, however, often fails to have sufficient potency to reverse the kinds of serious nutritive dysfunctions that are present in most serious illnesses."[1]

On the other hand, it's also important to point out that *without* a clean diet, individuals can never truly reach and sustain an optimal level of health. The analogy of a fire can help explain this point. That is, if you are trying to put out a fire, it is extremely counterproductive to keep adding kindling to it. In the same way, if you are trying to detoxify your body through the use of nutritional supplements and various remedies, you will become frustrated and eventually fail if you keep eating the same toxic foods that continually fan the flames of pathogenic intestinal flora overgrowth, persistent systemic inflammation, and chronic metabolic, immune, and digestive system dysfunctioning.

The foods described in chapter 5, "Diet: Healthy and Harmful Foods," are an important component of the healing protocol for those who are ill and depleted, as well as for healthier individuals who enjoy the benefits of most fully metabolizing the nutrients contained within whole grains, organic fruits and vegetables, grass-fed meats, and fresh fish. Indeed, for those "advanced" patients who have removed their mercury amalgam fillings, replaced their petroleum chemical-laden personal care products, had their focal infections and scar interference fields treated, are on their deepest homeopathic constitutional remedy, and have done a significant amount of psychospiritual work (chapter 18), the energy and sense of well-being received from eating a clean and healthy diet can be most fully appreciated. This sense of well-being is so strong that these individuals rarely desire toxic foods but more and more crave the nutrient-dense foods in which they so readily enjoy beneficial effects. Therefore, chapter 5 is included in this book because of this major tenet of holistic radical medicine: although diet *alone* can no longer heal the majority of individuals suffering from chronic dysfunction and disease, *without a clean diet, individuals can never fully heal.*

Chapter 6, "Food Allergies: A Hidden Epidemic," covers another form of food toxicity. Like eating a healthy diet, avoiding wheat, milk, or other allergenic foods is often an essential component in a holistic patient's healing protocol. The chapter covers how to identify your primary food allergy, suggests other foods to substitute while avoiding your allergenic food(s), and explains how to treat the immune system and digestive weaknesses that first spawned the allergy during infancy and childhood.

The final chapter of part 3, "Dysbiosis," describes bowel toxicity from the overgrowth of opportunistic and pathogenic bacteria and fungi. The two biggest contributors to this pandemic intestinal disorder are the excessive use of antibiotics and the ingestion of refined sugar. The problems of refined sugar are described in detail in chapter 5, while chapter 7 covers the history, use, and abuse of antibiotics. This chapter also suggests nutritional supplements that can help restore normal flora (healthy bacteria) in the gut.

NOTES

1. J. Goldberg, *Deceits of the Mind and Their Effects on the Body* (New Brunswick, N.J.: Transaction, 1991), 230.

5

DIET: HEALTHY AND HARMFUL FOODS

Let thy food be thy medicine and thy medicine be thy food.
HIPPOCRATES, FATHER OF MEDICINE (460–370 BCE)

BIOCHEMICAL INDIVIDUALITY
Our Uniqueness

There is no single diet with a strict list of foods to eat that is espoused for everyone. Because of each individual's unique level of health and varied geographic, cultural, and genetic makeup, the pronouncement of a single ideal diet is impossible. For example, patients who are functioning more in the tuberculinic (exhaustion, depression, frequent headaches, colds, and respiratory congestion) or luetic (anxiety, insomnia, and neuropathy) miasms often require the more easily assimilable protein found in stews and broths made with organic beef, lamb, turkey, or chicken. However, when individuals are functioning in the healthier psoric reaction mode, they are able to include more salads and other raw fruits and vegetables in their diet.

The validity of the theory of miasms described in chapter 1, and therefore the uniqueness of each individual in response to life's stressors, has been confirmed by other physicians and scientists since Hahnemann's time in the eighteenth and nineteenth centuries. One of the most brilliant was the world-renowned biochemist Roger Williams from the University of Texas, who pioneered the concepts of *genetic polymorphism* and *biochemical individuality* in the 1950s.[1] Dr. Williams, who was the first to isolate pantothenic acid (vitamin B_5), discovered significant biochemical differences among individuals. These differences include *wide* variations in the composition of blood, saliva, gastric juice, bone, and skin; far-ranging physiological differences in organ and glandular functioning; and even major variations in the morphology of individuals' organs such as the stomach, brain, heart, intestines, and liver.[2] In fact, Dr. Williams asserted that the individual differences in these body fluids, tissues, and organs were just as unique to each person as their external characteristics such as height, weight, facial shape, size of feet, eye color, and so forth.[3]

For example, Dr. Williams noted that wide varieties exist not only in the location of the stomach in the abdomen but also in the size and shape of this digestive organ—with some stomachs in "normal" individuals able to hold six to eight times as much as others (see figure 5.1).[4] Coupling this information with individual differences in dentition and therefore chewing function, as well as variations in the emptying time of the stomach (which Williams also found significant), sheds considerable light on people's varied eating habits as well as their ability to lose or gain weight. Therefore, the information about various foods in this chapter is to inform, rather than to dictate a specific dietary one-size-fits-all regimen.

NUTRIENT-DENSE FOODS
Our Biochemical Common Denominator

However, in this modern world inundated with processed foods, there are obviously healthy foods (e.g., organic vegetables) and unhealthy foods (e.g., refined

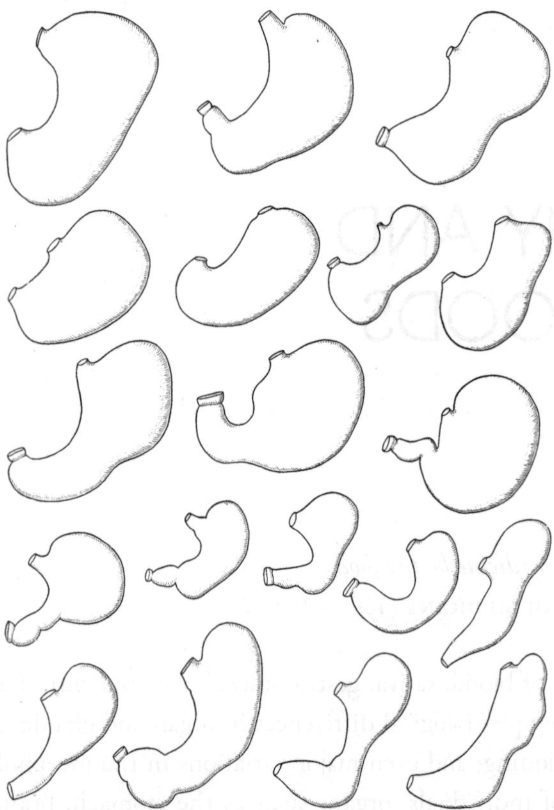

Figure 5.1. Human stomachs vary greatly in size and shape. These diagrams were derived from a study of 425 cadavers. (Reprinted from An Atlas of Human Anatomy, *by Barry J. Anson, published by W. B. Saunders Company, 1950, page 287, with permission from Elsevier.)*

sugar). In fact, Weston Price, D.D.S., who, with his wife, studied fourteen primitive cultures all over the world, found that despite the wide variety of foods eaten by different indigenous tribes—from the primitive Swiss and Gaels to the Eskimos, Native Americans, and South Sea Islanders—the intake of their nutrients was remarkably similar.[5] He found consistently that these healthy indigenous people all thrived on diets consisting of nutrient-dense foods such as wild game and seafood, raw and fermented dairy products, whole grains, and fresh vegetables and legumes, which provided them with readily assimilable proteins, fats, and carbohydrates. Therefore, this chapter will discuss the benefits and detriments of the obviously healthy and harmful foods, addressing them in alphabetical order.

food: If you refer to the definition of *food* in *Dorland's Medical Dictionary*—"anything which, when taken into the body, serves to nourish or build up the tissues or to supply body heat"—then refined sugar, margarine, and refined flours really don't even fall into the definition of food at all.

SALLY FALLON AND THE WESTON A. PRICE FOUNDATION

Much of the following information in this chapter is referenced from Sally Fallon's landmark book, *Nourishing Traditions.* This combination nutrition and recipe book is loaded with valuable and unique information—the majority of it rarely found in other conventional or even alternative books on food and nutrition. Everyone serious about food science and healthy eating should incorporate this essential nutritional reference guide into his or her library. The journal of the Weston A. Price Foundation (WAPF), the nonprofit charity organization founded by Sally Fallon in 1999 to disseminate the nutritional research and work of Dr. Price, is also highly recommended reading. This quarterly journal, *Wise Traditions,* is always packed with pertinent information on how to obtain and correctly prepare the most nutrient-dense foods, backed up by historical accounts of tried-and-true dietary methods our ancestors intuitively used to maintain optimal health, as well as modern research studies from peer-reviewed scientific journals.

▶ To order *Nourishing Traditions* or the *Wise Traditions* journal, or to join the WAPF, contact the Weston A. Price Foundation at (202) 363-4394, or go to www.westonaprice.org.

THE HEALTHY FOODS

The first half of the chapter will be devoted to information about the most nutritive foods essential to include in a restorative and healing diet.

Dairy

Dairy Sensitivities and Cautions

Unfortunately, a significant percentage of the population is allergic to milk and other dairy products. How to identify and treat a dairy sensitivity is discussed at length in chapter 6. For adults who are not sensitive, however, as well as for the percentage of dairy-allergic individuals who can eat small amounts of cow's milk products or can substitute goat, sheep, or buffalo milk products, it's important to find a source for raw dairy products. Furthermore, infants and children who did not inherit a genetic dairy-sensitivity predilection (primarily in the tuberculinic miasmic level) do exceptionally better when raised on raw dairy products.*

"Dead" Pasteurized Milk

Pasteurization (the heating of milk at 161°F or above for fifteen seconds) and ultra-pasteurization (the heating of milk at 280°F for at least two seconds) destroys helpful bacteria, makes proteins less available by altering the amino acids lysine and tyrosine, promotes rancidity of unsaturated fatty acids, and causes vitamin loss. Even worse, pasteurization alters the composition of calcium and magnesium and destroys the enzymes that help the body assimilate these minerals—rendering even the most dedicated milk drinkers susceptible to osteoporosis. Another common process, homogenization—the emulsification of fat globules in milk so that the cream doesn't rise to the top—makes the fat and cholesterol more prone to rancidity and is a suspected contributor to heart disease.[6] Unfortunately, the source of most commercial milk sold today is the modern Holstein cow, bred to produce huge quantities of milk—as much as three times more than the old-fashioned cow. She is often a genetically manipulated "pituitary freak," needing special feed and antibiotics to keep her well, which makes her produce milk that contains high levels of growth hormones.[7]

GROWTH HORMONES

Growth hormones in milk come from abnormal pituitary production in genetically manipulated cows, as well as through the injection of growth hormone to increase cows' milk production by 20 to 30 percent. Recombinant bovine growth hormone (rBGH), made by Monsanto, also known as recombinant bovine somatotropin (rBST), is injected into approximately 30 percent of U.S. dairy cows, and the resulting hormone-laden milk is added to cream, cheese, yogurt, and baked goods with no labels identifying the rBGH milk addition.[8] For more information, see "BGH Milk Implicated in Cancer" on page 178.

---

*These children have better immune system development, fewer colds and flus, less anxiety, and better growth.

The Benefits of Raw Milk

Due to intense harassment by state authorities, about half of U.S. states either ban or severely limit the sale of raw milk.[9] This ban is based on the false belief that raw milk is dangerous. In actuality, the bacterial count allowed for certified raw dairies is much lower than the bacterial count allowed even *after* pasteurization in conventional dairies. For example, raw milk must contain no more than 10,000 bacteria per milliliter, as compared to the allowance of 30,000 bacteria per milliliter after pasteurization in Georgia and New York's conventional dairy farms, and 15,000 per milliliter in California.[10] Furthermore, the measurement for anaerobic bacteria in raw milk must be performed once a week in all states, whereas for dairies that pasteurize there is no requirement for measuring anaerobic bacteria in any state.[11] Finally, all outbreaks of salmonella bacteria in contaminated milk in the past few decades (and there have been many) have occurred in *pasteurized* milk.[12]

Raw milk may be legally purchased directly from farms in many states. Farmers who have Jersey or Guernsey cows that feed on organic grass (not sprayed with pesticides) produce the most nutrient-rich milk. Raw goat's milk is also a good option. This too may need to be purchased through an arrangement with a farmer, since it is as strictly regulated as cow's milk by state authorities.

- ▶ The Weston A. Price Foundation's website, www.realmilk.com, lists farms with raw milk products. Aajonus Vonderplanitz also maintains a website, www.rawmilk.org.

Because goat's milk is slightly less allergenic than cow's milk, often it can be tolerated by individuals who are sensitive to cow's milk. Goat's milk differs from cow's milk in that it has smaller protein molecules, and its fat molecules have thinner, more fragile membranes and are half the size of those found in cow's milk (therefore, there is no cream line). Dr. Bernard Jensen has shown that goat's milk will digest in a baby's stomach in twenty minutes, whereas pasteurized cow's milk takes eight hours. Dr. Jensen found that he was able to heal severely ill patients—with constipation, ulcers, or juvenile arthritis, as well as severely malnourished and underweight individuals, to name a few—by having them drink seven to eight glasses of raw goat's milk a day within three hours after milking, while the life energy is high and the milk is still alkaline and can neutralize acids in the body. (After three hours, the lactose breaks down into lactic acid and the milk becomes too acidic.)[13]

Furthermore, goats graze freely and enjoy a large variety of leaves, grasses, and herbs. Therefore, their milk contains a rich amount of nutrients and more utilizable vitamin A and calcium than cow's milk—although it is deficient in vitamin B_{12} and folic acid (which must be supplemented in infants if this is their only source of nourishment).[14]

Raw Butter Is a Health Food

Butter (as well as cream) contains little allergenic lactose (the sugar in milk) or casein (the major protein in milk), so it can be tolerated even by many individuals who are sensitive to milk products. This is especially true if the individual has studiously avoided dairy for a period of time (at least two to three months) and taken supplements to support digestion and promote healthy intestinal flora.

Weston Price, D.D.S., was also a brilliant nutritionist. Through his extensive anthropological research, as documented in his groundbreaking book, *Nutrition and Physical Degeneration,* Dr. Price realized the great benefits of raw dairy products in the health and well-being of the primitive tribes and cultures that he visited and studied. Furthermore, through his extensive research and experience in the field, Dr. Price isolated a previously unknown and unique factor in butter that he termed the "X factor." This "vitamin-like activator,"[15] which helps the body absorb and utilize minerals (and is not completely destroyed by pasteurization), is highest in butter from dairy cows that graze on green grass primarily in the spring and fall.[16]

Russian scientists later described this X factor as a form of vitamin K and termed it *vitamin* K_2. Vitamin K_2 is produced by animal tissues, including the mammary glands, from vitamin K_1, which occurs in rapidly growing green plants eaten by the animals. Modern research has confirmed Dr. Price's observations that vitamin K_2 is an important nutrient that helps the body utilize minerals, protects against tooth decay, and supports normal reproduction as well as children's growth and development. It can also protect against arteriosclerosis (calcification of the arteries in heart disease) and is an important component of the brain.[17]

Dr. Price also found that vitamin K_2 works synergistically with vitamins A and D, activating certain proteins that these vitamins tell the cells to make, and therefore he recommended that raw butter be combined with cod liver oil (the best source of vitamins A and D). Both forms of cod liver oil and butter recommended here are essential for individuals at any age, but the essential nutrients they contain are critical for fetal development and thus are particularly crucial for women *and* their male partners to take at least several months before conception, as well as for women to ingest during pregnancy and breast-feeding. Growing children especially need the beneficial nutrients in these superfoods to support optimal growth and development of their teeth, bones, brain, and nervous system. Dr. Price found that our primitive ancestors who enjoyed excellent health consumed *ten times* the amount of these fat-soluble vitamins than the typical American does today.[18]

- ▶ To order raw butter (if you don't live in Arizona, California, Connecticut, Idaho, Maine, New Hampshire, New Mexico, Pennsylvania, South Carolina, or Washington, where it's legally sold in stores), refer to the classified section, "The Shop Heard 'Round the World," in the Weston A. Price Foundation's *Wise Traditions* journal, or go to www.realmilk.com for an update on the current situation in your state.

- ▶ Butter oil, produced from Guernsey and Devon cows that graze on grass, is the most concentrated source of vitamin K_2 and is exceptionally high in butyric acid. Butter oil is currently available as X-Factor Gold High Vitamin Butter Oil from Green Pasture at (402) 858-4818 or www.greenpasture.org, or from the Radiant Life Company at (888) 593-9595 or www.radiantlifecatalog.com. Blue Ice Fermented Skate Liver Oil and Cod Liver Oil are also highly recommended and can be ordered from either company.

GHEE

Since so many of us are sensitive to dairy, ghee is often a better choice than butter oil as an ongoing daily supplement. Ghee contains no lactase or casein. In fact, ghee sourced from cows that graze on grass in organic pastures has been shown through laboratory assays to have higher X factor content than butter oil.

Order organic ghee from Pure Indian Foods: (877) 588-4433 or www.pureindianfoods.com.

Another substance found in raw butter, cream, and whole milk, called the "Wulzen factor," *is* destroyed by pasteurization. In the early 1940s, the researcher Rosalind Wulzen of Oregon State College determined that this factor, also known as the anti-stiffness factor, protects against all kinds of calcification abnormalities such as degenerative arthritis, cataracts, and calcification of the pineal gland.[19]

Raw butter also contains a perfect ratio of omega-3 and omega-6 fatty acids, antitumor and antimicrobial short- and medium-chain fatty acids, conjugated linoleic acid (CLA), lecithin, cholesterol, and trace minerals. Furthermore, the short-chain fatty acid butyric acid, which is unique to butter, is the primary fuel colon cells need to function properly and produce normal levels of bifidus bacteria.[20]* Low butyric acid levels have been associated with ulcerative colitis, colon cancer, and inflammatory bowel disease. This four-carbon fatty acid also helps heal inflamed bowel tissue and has stopped the growth of colon cancer cells in vitro.[21]

Cheese: The Wine of Milk Products

Unlike raw butter and milk, raw cheese is available in most health food stores and even specialty grocery stores. Look for the words "milk," "fresh milk," or "raw milk" on the label to indicate that these cheeses were not made from pasteurized milk. Past claims linking raw cheese with pathogenic bacterial contamination have been completely rebuked in scientific literature.[22] Cheesemaking is a highly sophisticated science, and cheese has been called the "wine of milk products."[23] The full complement of enzymes found in cheese made from raw milk makes it much more digestible than processed cheeses containing emulsifiers, extenders, phosphates, and hydrogenated oils.[24] Raw goat and sheep's milk cheese is often preferable to cow's milk cheese, since many dairy-sensitive people can tolerate them somewhat better than cow's milk products.

*Butter oil is exceptionally high in butyric acid. In fact, rectal insertion of butter oil for relatively short periods (e.g., a protocol of two times a week for one month) can stimulate healthy levels of bifidus bacteria in the large intestine. This butyric acid protocol is most often indicated in patients who have taken probiotics for some time but still need to support the repopulation of the descending colon, sigmoid, and rectum.

- ► For more information on the safety of raw cheese, see the websites www.realmilk.com and www.rawmilk.org. Furthermore, the Weston A. Price Foundation at (202) 363-4394 or info@westonaprice.org and the Price-Pottenger Nutrition Foundation at (800) FOODS-4-U or info@price-pottenger.org are both excellent resources for information on nutrient-dense raw foods.

GENETICALLY ENGINEERED RENNET

Some 60 percent of all hard cheese products in the United States are made with a genetically engineered form of rennet called "chymosin" or "chymax," as well as "animal rennet."* Shopping at health food stores or buying from local dairy farmers can reduce the risk of eating this genetically engineered food.[25]

*Traditionally, rennet is an enzyme complex typically derived from the inner mucosa of animal stomachs, often from calves. These enzymes coagulate milk and cause it to separate into solids (curds) and liquid (whey) in the production of cheese.

Cultured Dairy Is Exceptionally Beneficial

Yogurt and kefir,* cottage and cream cheese, some sour butters in France and Germany, and crème fraîche are cultured, a process in which lactic-acid-producing bacteria digest and inactivate the milk sugar (lactose) and the milk protein (casein), or milk is heated and live cultures (*Lactobacillus bulgaricus* and *Streptococcus thermophilus*) are added.[26] Fermented milk products are less allergenic and easier to digest, have higher vitamin B and C contents, and contain friendly bacteria and lactic acid to aid the digestive tract, and the culturing process restores many of the enzymes destroyed during pasteurization.[27] Similar to the case with milk, yogurt and kefir made

*Kefir is a fermented milk product that is in a more liquid state than yogurt.

from the milk of goats,* sheep, and water buffalo (where available)† are often more easily tolerated than cow's milk yogurt. Eat yogurt plain or with only a little added maple syrup or fruit; avoid sugary yogurts or ones with artificial colors or flavors. If you are ill, practice stricter food combining; otherwise, your body can usually handle and digest the combination of (quality) protein and sugar.

- G.E.M. Cultures sells active live cultures to make kefir and other cultured dairy products; call (707) 964-2922.
- Piima is an excellent culture from Finland derived from the milk of cows that feed on the butterwort plant, which clabbers better and therefore makes a thicker yogurt or other cultured product. To order, go to www.culturesforhealth.com/Piima-Yogurt-Starter.html.

Eggs

Eggs and the Cholesterol "Myth"

A whole egg has 6 grams of protein, 5.6 grams of fat, and about 270 milligrams of cholesterol.[28] Because eggs have the highest amount of cholesterol of all common foods (liver and brains have more), they have been targeted for decades as one of the major causative factors in heart disease, primarily due to a multibillion-dollar advertising campaign waged by the margarine and vegetable oil industries.[29]

The Framingham Heart Study, which began in 1948 and involved about 6,000 people from the town of Framingham, Massachusetts, is often cited as proof of the cholesterol/animal fat theory. In actuality, this study proved nothing about the relationship between cholesterol and heart disease; in fact, the inverse relationship occurred, as the director of the study disclosed forty years later:

> In Framingham, Massachusetts, the more saturated fat one ate, the *more cholesterol* one ate, the more calories one ate, the *lower the person's serum cholesterol* . . . we found that the people who ate the most cholesterol, ate the most saturated fat, ate the most calories, weighed the least and were the most physically active.[30]

Other studies, including a survey of 1,700 patients with hardening of the arteries conducted by the famous heart surgeon Michael DeBakey, have found *no relationship* between the level of cholesterol in the blood and the incidence of atherosclerosis.[31] In fact, 80 percent of cholesterol is produced in the liver, and excess amounts are excreted in the bile and out through the feces. Therefore, abnormal lipid (fat) profiles are primarily due to the modern-day pandemic liver dysfunction occurring from toxic refined foods, and not the ingestion of whole natural foods such as eggs. (For more information on the cholesterol "myth," see the discussion on the cholesterol-lowering drugs called statins in appendix 4, "How Scientific Is Allopathic Medicine?")

The Benefits of Organic Free-Range Eggs

Any holistic practitioner who uses energetic testing will confirm what your own taste buds will tell you—there is a huge difference between eggs from organic free-range chickens and eggs from chickens housed in cramped cages and fed rations with antibiotics (to decrease the spread of disease in such close living quarters), preservatives, and mold inhibitors.[32] The eggs from organic free-range chickens have not been irradiated; rather, they come from chickens that move around freely, eat bugs and worms along with their pesticide-free feed, and are raised without antibiotics, growth hormones, or genetic modification.[33] Organically raised free-range eggs have more vitamins (200 percent more vitamin E and 600 percent more beta-carotene, or vitamin A), more lecithin, twice as much unsaturated fatty acids (400 percent more omega-3 fatty acids), and half the cholesterol as those produced in modern "egg factories."[34] Furthermore, these eggs contain a beneficial one-to-one omega-3 to omega-6 fatty acid ratio, whereas commercial eggs have been measured as having as much as nineteen times more omega-6 than omega-3—a very abnormal and harmful ratio.[35] Additionally, eating organic, free-range eggs is not only more nutritious but less dangerous, because more than 80 percent of commercial supermarket eggs have been reported to be contaminated with *Helicobacter pylori,* a

*Because the fat globules in goat's milk are smaller than in cow's milk, tapioca is often added to goat's milk yogurt to thicken it.

†Although water buffalo yogurt sounds like an excellent idea, some brands are unfortunately homogenized and therefore should be avoided.

bacterial species that can cause acute fever, diarrhea, and abdominal pain and is also the primary agent implicated in causing chronic ulcers.[36]

Both the late dietary expert Paavo Airola and a modern leading nutritionist, Aajonus Vonderplanitz, recommend that eggs be fertile—that is, that the hens have fraternized with roosters.[37] One benefit to fertilized eggs is that there is a higher ratio—approximately eight to one—of lecithin to cholesterol, which translates to approximately 1,700 milligrams of lecithin to 194 to 200 milligrams of cholesterol per egg.[38] Lecithin contains both choline and inositol, which help emulsify cholesterol and keep it moving in the bloodstream. A fertilized egg with its superior lecithin–cholesterol ratio helps naturally protect arteries from plaque buildup and future atherosclerosis.

The Raw versus Cooked Egg Controversy

Vonderplanitz and other nutritionists have recommended that eggs be eaten raw, although some have reported reactions to this practice possibly due to food allergies, sensitivity to egg whites, or salmonella contamination. Salmonella bacteria, when they are present, are found on the shells of eggs and can be cleaned off with soap and water. However, some evidence now suggests that a small percentage of eggs may contain salmonella inside their shells, which necessitates cooking for a minimum of three minutes.[39] On the other hand, three minutes of cooking can destroy a "protein G" in eggs that actually helps guide cholesterol to appropriately damaged areas of the intima, where it can repair this innermost layer of the blood vessel wall.

Eating raw eggs also brings up the controversial issue of the protein avidin in raw egg white that is said to bind to and interfere with biotin (a B vitamin) absorption. In one study in which cancer patients were fed thirty-six to forty-two raw egg whites daily for an entire year, however, no biotin deficiency occurred.[40] Others contend that the egg yolk contains plenty of biotin and that as long as the whole raw egg is eaten, no nutritional deficits can occur.[41] Additionally, unless the albumin in egg white is denatured to a certain degree by cooking, sensitive individuals may react more often to this allergenic substance in its raw state.

Finally, to add to the confusing decision making, it's important to remember that eggs (and fish) are one of the best sources of the important omega-3 essential fatty acid DHA, and overcooking can destroy much of this important "brain food."[42]* In the midst of all these conflicting opinions, many health-minded individuals tread the middle ground between raw and cooked eggs and eat them soft-boiled or lightly poached, which keeps the yolks runny and the whites as little cooked as possible.[43] For the highest nutritional content, the yolks should be a deep orange color.

Consumer Tips

Another important but little-known point is that free-range chickens lay fewer eggs in the winter because it is their time of rest. The custom of pickling eggs traditionally was undertaken in order to make eggs available during this fallow time, lasting approximately from November until February. For those of us trying to stay more in tune with nature, it may be wise to eat fewer eggs during the winter to support farmers in allowing chickens their natural cycle.

Additionally, although brown foods look more natural than white, the shell color of an egg depends on the breed of the hen that laid it and is not a marker of nutritional differences. And size—medium, large, or jumbo eggs—doesn't seem to matter in regard to nutritional content.[44] Finally, although there is a very minor difference, Grade AA is the highest-quality egg possible and Grade A is slightly less so (the yolk and white are less firm). In contrast, eggs given the Grade B rating are significantly lower in quality, are not sold in grocery stores, and are generally used only by commercial bakers and companies that produce egg products.

Fish

Mercury Contamination

Like the raw or cooked egg question, whether to eat fish and shellfish in light of their potential mercury content also remains controversial. Unfortunately, fish can pick up and concentrate heavy metals and other contaminants in two ways: first through direct contact with the gills and skin, and second through the food chain ingestion

*Consumers may want to be cautious in purchasing the new eggs being advertised as high in DHA because they are primarily the product of big agribusinesses and may not be as healthful as they purport.

of smaller fish, plants, and algae. The microorganisms in the water that smaller fish feed on—and they themselves are then eaten by larger fish—convert inorganic mercury into the more toxic organic methylmercury, which no amount of cleaning or cooking can protect us from absorbing into our systems.[45] Thus, it's best to avoid big predator fish such as shark, marlin, swordfish, and tuna. However, it is important to remember that these fish also contain substances such as omega-3 fatty acids that bind with mercury and help eliminate it from the body, and thus the benefits from occasional ingestion of these larger fish can outweigh the negative heavy metal aspects.[46] Because children under the age of eight do not have fully developed and functioning immune systems, they—as well as women who are pregnant or nursing—have been recently cautioned through government guidelines to eat no more than twelve ounces of fish per week.[47]

To help mitigate the effects of any mercury in the fish, two Pure Radiance C capsules or another natural antioxidant can be taken with a meal. Additionally, the gemmotherapy (or plant stem cell) remedy Black Poplar, which is a major heavy metal detoxifier, can be taken after a fish meal to help reduce mercury levels in the body.

- ▶ For more information on fish-eating guidelines for pregnant or nursing women or young children, go to www.americanpregnancy.org/pregnancyhealth/fishmercury.htm.
- ▶ Pure Radiance C is available from the Synergy Company at (800) 723-0277.
- ▶ For educational seminars and ordering information on gemmotherapy remedies, contact PSC Distribution at www.epsce.com or (631) 477-6696, or Gemmos LLC at www.gemmos-usa.com or (877) 417-6298.

Furthermore, as discussed in chapter 3, fish from contaminated waters such as toxic rivers (notably the Hudson in New York), lakes (e.g., the Great Lakes), and waters close to the shore (especially near heavily populated coastal areas or industrial facilities) should always be avoided. This would include scavenging fish such as catfish and carp, as well as shoreline feeders such as sole and flounder. Coal-burning plants and waste incinerators are the largest polluters of mercury into the atmosphere, from where this toxic metal later rains down into oceans, lakes, and streams. There bacteria convert it into the more toxic and absorbable methylmercury, which is collected in the tissues of marine mammals, waterfowl, and fish.[48]

Fish Is Brain Food

If the fish comes from deep, clean natural waters, however, it is one of the healthiest flesh foods we can eat. Fish is an excellent source of protein, minerals (notably iron, zinc, magnesium, and phosphorus), vitamins (especially A and D), and omega-3 essential fatty acids (EPA and DHA)—particularly in the oilier cold-water species such as bluefish, salmon, mackerel, sardines, tuna, halibut, lake trout, and sablefish.[49] The omega-3 essential fatty acids hold oxygen in cell membranes, where they not only act as a barrier to viruses, fungi, and bacteria but also greatly assist in the movement of toxic substances out of the interior of the cell to the skin, kidneys, lungs, or intestines, where they can be eliminated.[50] The long-chain omega-3 fatty acids EPA (eicosapentaenoic acid) and DHA (docosahexaenoic acid) are termed "essential" because humans must obtain them in their diet; the human body cannot synthesize them.

DHA is *critical* for optimal brain functioning as well as for good visual acuity. In fact, individuals with symptoms of dementia, as well as Alzheimer's, have as much as 30 percent lower DHA content in their brains. DHA is found in abundance only in salmon, mackerel, herring, sardines, anchovies, and bluefin, and in lesser amounts in eggs from free-range hens and some marine algae. Although the body can make its own DHA from the omega-3 fatty acids found in flaxseed oils (ALA or alpha-linolenic acid), this can be a difficult process because so many people lack the adequate vitamin (B_3, B_6, and C) and mineral (zinc and magnesium) cofactors to activate the enzymes required for conversion.* For example, studies of long-term vegetarians show that their DHA levels are very low. Furthermore, DHA levels of breast-fed infants of vegetarian mothers have been measured to be only one-third the level of infants whose mothers consumed meat, fish, and vegetables.[51] Based on these findings, as well as the fact that

*The enzymes elongase and delta-6-desaturase are required to convert the ALA to EPA and DHA. Furthermore, certain health conditions such as diabetes and autoimmune disease can inhibit this conversion.

plant-based DHA supplements are now available, vegetarian pregnant and nursing mothers should strongly consider supplementation to support the growth and development of their babies' brains and nervous systems.*

Cod Liver Oil

Modern Research Validates Traditional Wisdom

For centuries, cod liver oil has been a dietary staple in cultures around the world. Culled from articles in the *Wise Traditions* journal, here is a brief list of the uses of this superfood throughout history:[52]

~400 BCE: Hippocrates records the medicinal uses of fish oils.

1776: Used in a Manchester, England, infirmary for rheumatism.

Early 1800s: Widespread use in Germany and the Netherlands to treat the vitamin D deficiency disease of rickets, as well as eye diseases and tuberculosis.

1848: British physician John Hughes writes that the fishing villages in Scotland, Sweden, and Norway have used cod liver oil for centuries as a health and strengthening medicinal agent.

Early 1900s: Research expands the oil's use to include preventing and treating measles (reducing mortality by more than half), industrial absenteeism (reducing by two-thirds), and puerperal fever (reducing by up to two-thirds).

2000–2009: Research studies published in peer-reviewed journals demonstrate that cod liver oil supplementation is effective in treating numerous disorders and diseases, including rheumatoid arthritis, bone loss, multiple sclerosis, breast cancer, depression, wounds, hip fractures, upper respiratory tract infections and earaches in children, and diabetes, and, furthermore, that mothers who take cod liver oil during pregnancy have children with higher birth weights and intelligence.

Conventional Medicine and Megadoses of Vitamin D

Cod liver oil supplementation has become a hotly debated issue since doctors have recently become aware of a rather widespread vitamin D deficiency (based on laboratory testing) and have been prescribing megadoses of this vitamin to their patients. In fact, flying in the face of traditional wisdom for centuries, as well as modern scientific nutritional research, Dr. John Cannell and other allopathic practitioners associated with the Vitamin D Council have further concluded that vitamin A supplementation actually antagonizes the beneficial effects of vitamin D; therefore, they have recommended against the use of cod liver oil. The fallacy of this deduction was addressed in the Summer 2009 *Wise Traditions* journal by Sally Fallon and Chris Masterjohn,* who noted that quite the opposite is true. That is, the fat-soluble vitamin A and vitamin D are not antagonists at all but actually cooperate with each other, and that supplementing one without the other has caused harm. For example, in 1998, it was shown that even moderate amounts of vitamin D reduces stores of vitamin A in both the blood and the liver of chickens.[53] In contrast, receiving one's daily vitamin A requirement through diet and cod liver oil intake is an exceptionally safer route than the typical supplementation in pill form. Since vitamin A is fat-soluble, disposing of excesses is more difficult than with water-soluble vitamins, and vitamin A toxicity is a concern. However, recent studies have shown that vitamin A taken in water-soluble and solid forms was actually ten times more toxic than when it is ingested in oil.[54] This helps explain why Eskimos and other primitive peoples that Dr. Price studied consumed such high amounts of vitamin A in their diets and yet enjoyed superlative health.

The Source of Cod Liver Oil Is Key

For many years, I could not understand why every brand of cod liver oil that I ordered would energetically test so inconsistently. Dave Wetzel, owner of Green Pasture, solved this mystery a couple of years ago when he visited Iceland and Norway, where cod liver oil is not just a health food store supplement but a dietary staple.† Much like Weston A. Price did in his early-twentieth-century travels around the world, Wetzel found that

*One note of caution: the essential fatty acids EPA and DHA are natural blood thinners and not recommended if individuals are consuming high doses of aspirin or are on blood-thinning medication. Furthermore, supplementation should be reduced or ceased altogether before undergoing surgery.

*Readers are encouraged to read these articles at the www.westonaprice.org website.

†After eighteen months of research and interviews with manufacturers, laboratories, fisheries, fish meal plants, fish farms, and fish oil mills throughout the world, Wetzel culminated his studies by visiting six different mills in Iceland and Norway, as well as a cod fish farm, fishing boats, and a slaughterhouse.

the traditional method of cod liver oil preparation yielded the most superior product. This unheated extraction method includes the fermentation of codfish livers, which allows the nutrients to concentrate in the oil that rises to the top. Wetzel further found one fish oil mill that took the time to collect the vitamins from the oil, clean the oil of contaminants, and then return these naturally occurring vitamins to the final product. This yielded an oil with the most assimilable and nutrient-rich levels of vitamins A, D, E, and K; valuable omega-3 essential fatty acids EPA and DHA; and many known and unknown quinones, such as coenzyme Q10.[55]

In contrast, some of the other mills Wetzel observed fully cleaned and deodorized their oils and added nothing back, thus leaving a reduced vitamin A content and virtually no vitamin D. This is a major problem because, as described earlier, vitamins A and D work synergistically, so reduced vitamin D levels render the remaining vitamin A either ineffective or even toxic.[56] Other mills made the mistake of adding to the final product *synthetic* vitamins A and D after the high-heat deodorization methods.[57] Unfortunately, the majority of cod liver oil products on the market today contain the addition of these fat-soluble synthetic vitamins that have a great potential for harm. Today this is especially important because many patients are being prescribed megadoses of synthetic vitamin D, which can suppress immune system functioning and actually *hinder* the absorption of this important nutrient.

Through his pioneering research, Dave Wetzel has been able to provide a superior quality of cod liver oil with naturally occurring fat-soluble vitamins in the United States. This product, Blue Ice Fermented Cod Liver Oil, is now available to both physicians and the general public. His Blue Ice Fermented Skate Liver Oil, made from the skate fish, also tests well both energetically and clinically on patients, especially on individuals who have joint pain.

- ▶ Blue Ice Fermented Cod and Skate Liver Oil are available from Green Pasture at (402) 858-4818 or www.greenpasture.org or from the Radiant Life Company at (888) 593-9595 or www.radiantlifecatalog.com.

- ▶ X-Factor Gold High Vitamin Butter Oil, previously described under the "Dairy" section, is also available from Green Pasture. Dr. Weston Price advocated taking cod liver oil and butter from cows who grazed on green grass together, because the "X factor" (vitamin K_2) in butter and the vitamins A and D in cod liver oil have a synergistic effect, and therefore these fat-soluble vitamins are better utilized in the body when eaten together. Ghee is an excellent butter oil substitute for those sensitive to dairy.

- ▶ Pro DHA is a highly concentrated DHA formula available to practitioners from Nordic Naturals, (800) 662-2544 or www.nordicnaturals.com.

Wild versus Farm-Raised Salmon

When buying salmon, purchase fresh wild salmon from Alaska and the Pacific Northwest. Another good choice is canned Alaskan salmon that is fully cooked, shelf-stable, and not treated with preservatives. The majority of Atlantic salmon is farm raised and typically artificially colored with red food dyes (canthaxanthin or astaxanthin). (See plate 4 in the color insert.) Farmed rainbow trout also receives dyes in its feed and is often marketed as "salmon trout." Although these dyes have been categorized as "generally recognized as safe" (GRAS) by the FDA, allergenic responses after ingestion have been reported. In fact, England banned tanning pills containing the dye canthaxanthin in 1987.[58]

KRILL

In the wild, salmon feed on the crustacean krill, which turns their flesh red. Antarctic krill is high in omega-3 fatty acids. Unfortunately, when krill oil is manufactured for use as a supplement, the krill are crushed, and the lipids and proteins are extracted using (toxic) acetone and further heated (damaging the omega-3 EFAs) during industrial processing. Therefore, krill oil supplements are not recommended. Rather, use cod liver oil, which has a more balanced essential fatty acid (omega-3, omega-6, and omega-9) content.[59]

Most smoked salmon comes from farmed salmon unless the label specifically denotes that it is from Alaska. Alaskan wild salmon can be purchased fresh during May through October and all year round when individually quick-frozen (IQF).[60] The commercial feeds (fish or poultry by-products with corn, soy, or wheat filler—some with genetic modifications) that farmed fish feed on, as opposed to the smaller fish, algae, or seaweed consumed in the wild, significantly reduce salmon's normally high omega-3 fatty acid content and lowers its vitamin A and D levels. According to many authorities, salmon is the primary animal source of omega-3 fatty acid. Therefore, it is crucial to protect this important health food by supporting family-owned, independent Alaskan fisheries and other fishermen who fish from deep, clean waters elsewhere.[61]

FINFISH FARMING

"Finfish farming" (the term *finfish* refers to fish and is used to distinguish between fish with fins and shellfish) has polluted coastal waters with nitrogenous fish waste, antibiotics, hormones, and pesticides and endangers wild salmon and other fish when farmed fish escape and compete for food and weaken the genetic pool. Further, in the crowded ocean net pens, pathogens and parasites such as sea lice proliferate and can induce disease in wild fish populations. To learn more about this serious issue, read "Scientist Statement on the Aquaculture Industry's Impact on Marine Ecology and Human Health" at www.puresalmon.org/pdfs/scientist_letter.pdf.

Because intense crowding stresses fish immune systems, fish farms use antibiotics (e.g., erythromycin, amoxicillin) as well as hormones (e.g., human chorionic gonadotropin, 17-methyltestosterone) and pesticides. For example, the pesticide formalin (which contains formaldehyde) is used to control fungi on fish eggs, while pyrethroid is used to control sea lice.[62] In fact, farmed salmon receive *more antibiotics* per body weight than any other type of livestock. Even when fish are caught in the wild, catch techniques such as trawling (which scrapes the sea floor) destroy fish habitats, and the use of long lines that can stretch eighty miles or more kill an estimated 200,000 endangered wandering albatrosses and other sea birds annually. In addition to overfishing, these practices have severely depleted fish species, notably the Chilean sea bass that became wildly popular over a decade ago for its mild, succulent flavor.[63]

Fortunately, there are organizations promoting responsible fishing practices as well as informing consumers about the safest fish to purchase. The Monterey Bay Aquarium's Seafood Watch program offers information and a consumer's guide to safe, sustainably caught seafood. Even more heartening, Whole Foods markets have partnered with the aquarium and are selling only those fish on the approved list—a great relief for the many holistically oriented consumers who shop there. Furthermore, organic fish farms that utilize stringent standards to produce healthier fish without the use of toxic fertilizers, pesticides, antibiotics, and genetically engineered (GE) organisms are growing in number.

- ▶ Visit www.seafoodwatch.org for information on which seafood to buy or avoid, and to obtain a "Pocket Guide" of the best choices (green), the good choices (yellow), and the fish (finfish and shellfish) to avoid (red) in your particular area.

Caution with Shellfish

Parasites, viruses, and bacteria from sewage contamination can pollute fish and shellfish. However, freezing or cooking fish to an internal temperature of 140°F can destroy these parasites. Undercooked or raw fecal-contaminated shellfish can cause gastroenteritis, hepatitis, cholera, or typhoid, especially in a weakened immune system.[64] As with finfish, always inquire where the shellfish came from, and be especially careful of the water source when eating sushi, sashimi, or other raw seafood. It is indeed a travesty that the earth's waters have been so thoroughly polluted and have contaminated both finfish and shellfish. Like salmon and other cold-water fish, shellfish is considered to be a superior "brain food" with its high levels of omega-3 fatty acids and rich tyrosine amino acid content, which converts into the energizing neurotransmitters dopamine and norepinephrine.[65] However, due to this possible pollution threat, shellfish is one of the two foods (the other being pork) that Sally Fallon and other holistic nutritionists caution about eating too often, especially without knowing the water source of the crab, shrimp, mussel, or lobster.[66]

Fruits and Vegetables

Hold the Pesticides, Please!

Certified organically grown produce is not just ideal but essential based on the plethora of information now known about the harmful carcinogenic effects of pesticides, insecticides, and herbicides (previously detailed in chapter 4). "Transitionally grown" produce from land that hasn't received chemical applications for three years is a good second choice when organic isn't available.[67]

Protective against Degenerative Disease

Fruits and vegetables contain more vitamins and minerals than any other food group, as well as abundant amounts of indigestible cellulose that enhances intestinal regularity. The numerous phytochemicals found in fruits and vegetables such as the carotenoid and flavonoid antioxidants, the antiviral polyphenols, the antibiotic sulfur compounds, and the tissue-regenerating chlorophyll (a.k.a "plant blood") protect us against heart disease, cancer, and a host of other chronic degenerative diseases. Furthermore, although the majority of fruits and vegetables contain relatively few enzymes, some are exceptionally rich in them, including grapes, figs, and many tropical fruits such as avocados, papayas, dates, bananas, pineapples, kiwis, and mangoes.[68]

Caution with Fruit for Those with Severe Dysbiosis

For someone with major dysbiosis—overgrowth of pathogenic flora (fungus and bacteria) intra- and extra-intestinally—even the naturally occurring fructose in fruit can stimulate toxic microbial growth and should be avoided until the individual can better tolerate it. This is especially true in the case of highly sweet fruits such as bananas, mangoes, cherries, and figs, and all dried fruits (e.g., raisins, prunes, dates). Additionally, lab cultures have revealed species of the yeast *Candida albicans* in many processed juices—including apple, pineapple, orange, tomato, grape, apricot, and lemonade—primarily due to the aluminum from foil wrap packaging, so they should be avoided.[69] However, for those with mild dysbiosis and/or those who have done a significant amount of drainage and detoxification, organically grown fruit can serve as a healthy snack or dessert and an excellent alternative to the occasional (or not so occasional) emotional or physical sugar cravings.

Limiting Fruit Juices

Undiluted fruit juices are too sweet. In fact, there is as much sugar in a glass of orange juice as there is in a candy bar.[70] Furthermore, even freshly squeezed orange juice yields only about 114 milligrams of vitamin C and 200 milligrams of bioflavonoids, as compared with peeling and eating the whole orange, which yields significantly more vitamin C (~200 milligrams) and bioflavonoids (~2,000 milligrams).[71] Citrus fruits are also included in most lists as one of the top ten typical food allergens. This is especially true of oranges, probably due to their overconsumption in the U.S.[72] Fruit juice, if consumed at all, should be reserved as an occasional treat and is best freshly juiced or at least bought organic and in a glass bottle. Juices should always be diluted with water or San Pellegrino (or another quality sparkling water that can help wean individuals off soft drinks), and it should be limited in amount to only one or two ounces at a time—that is, no more fructose than you would consume in one piece of fruit.[73]

Fermented Fruits and Vegetables Are Optimal

Traditionally, fruit and vegetable beverages have been fermented with lactic acid to yield a nutritious drink rich in dilute natural sugars, mineral electrolytes, and beneficial lactobacillus flora. Since ancient times, healthful fermented beverages such as ginger ale, beet kvass, apple cider, and kombucha tea have been revered not only for their deliciously sweet, slightly acidic, and naturally fizzy taste, but also for their amazing healing properties, including being highly protective against cancer and other degenerative diseases.[74]* Thankfully, these predecessors to the present-day cancer-causing imitators—soft drinks—are making their way back into the homes of health-conscious individuals who ferment these drinks at room temperature for two to three days, or buy them directly from the health food store. Recipes for all these nutritious drinks can be found in Sally Fallon's *Nourishing Traditions*.

► Sally Fallon's *Nourishing Traditions* provides fermented drink recipes on pages 586 through 596 of the second edition. The beet kvass recipe is found on page 608 in the "Tonics and Superfoods" section. At home, use a large (1.5 liter) French canning jar with a rubber washer and hinges that snap on tightly to get the best (fizzy!) results. (Google "French canning jars" to view a selection of these jars if they are not available at your local health food store.)

*Sadly, most modern-day ginger ale is loaded with high fructose corn syrup or other refined sugars.

Lacto-fermented fruits and vegetables such as sauerkraut and pickles in Europe, kimchi (cabbage) in Korea, and umeboshi plums in Japan have also been prized by traditional cultures for centuries. The process of fermentation greatly enhances the digestive process by increasing enzyme levels, and the lactic acid that is produced promotes the growth of beneficial intestinal flora. These foods also provide high vitamin levels as well as antibiotic and anticarcinogenic factors.[75] It is important to remember that fermented fruits and vegetables, as well as fermented chutneys, are primarily used as condiments, so that even the most finicky child needs to ingest only a small amount served with meat, fish, or grains to receive the benefit of these true health foods. *Nourishing Traditions* has a great selection of recipes for making fermented foods at home, or individuals can buy them refrigerated at the health food store. Note that those products sitting on the shelf are pasteurized and/or often have added vinegar, which can encourage dysbiosis.

▶ Fermenting crocks are excellent for making these fermented vegetables and fruits at home. Contact the Radiant Life Company at (888) 593-8333 or go to www.radiantlifecatalog.com.

Caution with Juice Fasting

Fresh organic vegetable and fruit juices have been used in place of harmful drugs in healing protocols for cancer and other toxicity diseases for centuries. Juice fasting has been well documented in both Europe and the United States not only as being curative in healing disease but also as having rejuvenating and revitalizing effects. In fact, the great sixteenth-century physician Paracelsus called fasting "the greatest remedy; the physician within."[76] However, in this present period of more severe physical degeneration and disease typical of the tuberculinic and luetic miasms, fasting should be supervised by an experienced holistic practitioner and accompanied by intermittent colonics or enemas, gentle exercise, and most of all rest. Too many people nowadays try to fast while maintaining a full work schedule, while also overburdened with family responsibilities at home.

Eat Salads *First*

In many instances, the "old world" food traditions of Europe greatly surpass the eating habits in the more fast-paced "new world" of the United States. However, one custom Americans have that greatly benefits them in comparison to those living abroad is the custom of eating salads *first*. According to the Swiss medical researcher Kouchakoff, eating raw food before cooked food greatly reduces the immune system stress that can occur from simply eating (over)cooked food alone.[77] This "digestive leukocytosis" immune response (elevated white blood cell count) can be further reduced by not cooking foods at high temperatures.[78] This includes pasteurization, deep-frying, and barbecuing. Therefore—whether cooking meat or vegetables—lower-temperature steaming, stewing, or slow cooking are the best cooking methods.

THOROUGH CHEWING

Very thorough chewing also reduces digestive leukocytosis. This practice of effective mastication, known as "Fletcherism" after the U.S. author and holistic health advocate Horace Fletcher (1849–1919), had many followers, or "Fletcherites," in health spas and sanatoriums at the turn of the twentieth century.

Combining Flaxseed Oil and Cheese in Salads

Another exceptionally healthy habit is to use salad dressing composed of flaxseed oil mixed with balsamic or red wine vinegar. It will not be difficult to make using this dressing a habit because this combination tastes much more delicious than most bottled dressings. Be sure to buy organic and expeller- or cold-pressed ultra-high-lignan flaxseed oil to receive the highest amount of omega-3 fatty acid possible. The balsamic vinegar should be produced from organic grapes. However, individuals with severe dysbiosis should avoid the sweet-tasting balsamic vinegar until their symptoms and pathogenic intestinal bacteria and fungus (*Candida albicans*) are reduced (see chapter 7).

When flaxseed oil with its abundant omega-3 fatty acids is combined with the sulfur-containing proteins in raw cheeses such as Roquefort (especially sheep's milk Roquefort, due to its high content of antimicrobial lauric acid), Parmesan, or cottage cheese, a synergistic effect occurs that greatly enhances many essential metabolic processes.[79] In fact, the European biochemist Johanna

Budwig has used this combination successfully in the treatment of cancer and other degenerative diseases (see the upcoming section "Oils and Fats").[80]

Cooking Reduces Plant Toxins in Some Vegetables

Although the inclusion of raw food like frequent salads in the diet is important and well tolerated by most individuals, many vegetables are better when cooked. These vegetables include cabbage, broccoli, brussels sprouts, and kale, whose goitrogen content in the raw plant can block the production of thyroid hormone. Other vegetables in this category are beets, spinach, and chard (with oxalate raphides) and potatoes (with hemagglutinins).[81] Although spinach and cabbage are popular salad foods, they should be eaten raw only occasionally (unless the cabbage is fermented). In fact, Dr. Weston Price specifically recommended that *most* vegetables be cooked "since raw vegetables are usually too bulky to allow very much mineral to be obtained from them."[82] Steaming or light sautéing is the best way to cook most vegetables.

LEARNING MORE ABOUT PLANT TOXINS

In a recent *Wise Traditions* issue titled "Plants Bite Back: Plant Toxin Issue," many types of *phytotoxins* (plant toxins) are detailed. Covering evrything from the inflammatory alkaloids in nightshade plants (tomatoes, potatoes, eggplant, etc.), which can induce muscle and joint pain, to the toxic phytates (anti-nutrients) in grains, nuts, seeds, and beans, this issue is an essential read for all those who want to prepare their food appropriately with optimum nutritive value.

Also included is research on the salt form of oxalic acid, or oxalates, in foods (spinach, soy, peanuts, coffee, etc.). These cause pain when deposited in the body—for instance, 80 percent of kidney stones are caused by oxalates. Less well known is the role of oxalates in contributing to vulvodynia, chronic fatigue, and fibromyalgia, and even in aggravating the symptoms of autism. Finally, oxalates can bind and trap heavy metals, rendering mercury amalgam detoxification much more challenging. Thus, avoiding foods high in oxalates during the Five Dental Detox Days Proptocol (page 95) is optimum in order to allow as much release of heavy metals as possible.

See the Weston A. Price Foundation's *Wise Traditions* journal volume 11, number 1 (Spring 2010), pages 28–54, for more information.

Variety Is the Spice . . .

One mistake that many individuals make is not to vary the vegetables and fruits they consistently consume. In fact, our hunter-gatherer ancestors regularly ate more than a hundred different kinds of fruits and vegetables during a one-year period.[83] In contrast, too many of us get stuck in a pattern of eating only the familiar day after day—that is, broccoli, carrots, or potatoes. Individuals should try varying their diet with uncommon fruits and vegetables that can supply new and different ratios of nutrients. Make it a habit to purchase a new fruit (e.g., Asian pear, cherimoya, kumquat, mango, or plantain) or vegetable (e.g., burdock root, bok choy, daikon, fennel, or jicama) each time you shop. A good mnemonic to remember is "V & R"—that is, variety and rotation. With variety, individuals receive the varied nutrients they need, and through rotation they reduce the tendency to become allergic to one particular food or food group when it is overeaten.

Grains

Like dairy, grains are notoriously allergenic, especially wheat, corn, and soy. This reaction most likely occurs because our culture overconsumes grains in their refined state and ignores the traditional methods our ancestors used to render them digestible and nutritious. In fact, one of the quintessential aspects of traditional wisdom concerning grains that has been almost totally forgotten is the practice of soaking and fermenting them before cooking. Sally Fallon points out this major modern-day omission in preparing grains in her book *Nourishing Traditions:*

> Our ancestors, and virtually all pre-industrialized peoples, soaked or fermented their grains before making them into porridge, breads, cakes, and casseroles. . . . (Many of our senior citizens may remember that in earlier times the instructions on the oatmeal box called for an overnight soaking.)[84]

Today, grocery stores stock their shelves with sugary dry cereals that have been subjected to an extrusion process of extremely high heat and pressure. These boxed breakfast cereals contain toxic and denatured proteins as well as rancid oils, and they are not suitable for consumption by anyone, *especially* not by their most popular consumers—our children.

Soaking grains overnight and mixing them with a little whey (the "juice" from yogurt is also whey and works well) or buttermilk allows lactobacilli and other helpful microorganisms to break down and neutralize the phytic acid contained in the outer layer (or bran) of the grain. Untreated phytic acid combines with calcium, phosphorus, iron, and zinc and blocks the intestinal absorption of these minerals, leading to bone loss and serious mineral deficiencies, and may have a role in causing some forms of cancer. Although the modern practice of sprinkling bran on foods improves colon transit time at first, in the long run the possible adverse effects from this dose of unprocessed phytic acid outweigh the short-term gain.[85]

Grains that make a delicious morning porridge include quinoa (which has the highest protein content), teff, amaranth, buckwheat, oat groats, millet, triticale, barley, spelt, kamut, and brown rice. When making breads, the same whey soaking principles apply. Furthermore, because grains go rancid so quickly, eating freshly ground grain is optimum. Grain grinders should be the slow-speed variety as opposed to high-speed mills that can heat the grain to too high a temperature, causing much of the oil to go rancid.

► Slow-speed mills for grinding grains are available from the Radiant Life Company at (888) 593-8333 or www.radiantlifecatalog.com.

LITTLE-KNOWN GRAIN FACTS

- In 3000 BCE, the Incas valued quinoa so highly that they paid their taxes with this grain.[86]
- Teff, the smallest grain in the world, originated in Ethiopia. Teff seeds were discovered in a pyramid estimated to date back to 3359 BCE.
- Quinoa and buckwheat are technically not grains, but a fruit from the chenopodium family and the seeds of an herb related to rhubarb, respectively.[87]

Eating a variety of grains instead of the same old bowl of (refined) oatmeal every morning helps prevent individuals from becoming sensitive to the protein gluten—primarily in wheat, oats, rye, and barley—which is one of the most common allergens. Furthermore, similar to a varied fruit and vegetable intake, eating a diet full of diverse and properly prepared grains exposes individuals to many various healthful and assimilable nutrients not enjoyed by those who eat the same refined cereal daily.

Meat

Dietary Choices Are Unique to Each Individual

The question of whether or not to eat meat, or any animal products, ranks up there with other major controversial topics such as politics and religion. Unfortunately, our government and universities often spend the vast amount of their funding trying to find the best drug to suppress disease rather than studying which foods are truly the most nutritious and restorative—resulting in a dearth of research in this polemical subject. However, as previously described under the "Dairy" section, in the 1930s and 1940s Dr. Weston Price and his wife conducted their own anthropological research by traveling to various remote areas of the world and comparing the health of the inhabitants with what they ate. In his book *Nutrition and Physical Degeneration,* Price reported that out of the fourteen groups of people around the world that he found in superb health, none were vegetarian.[88] All of these native peoples consumed some form of flesh-derived food in their diet, including meat, organ meats, fish, shellfish, eggs, cheese, and butter.[89] Dr. Price noted the following from his worldwide experience:

> As yet, I have not found a single group of primitive racial stock which was building and maintaining excellent bodies by living entirely on plant foods. I have found in many parts of the world most devout representatives of modern ethical systems advocating restriction of foods to the vegetable products. In every instance where the groups involved had been long under this teaching, I found evidence of degeneration in the form of dental caries, and in the new generation in the form of abnormal dental arches to an extent very much higher than in the primitive groups who were not under this influence.[90]

Despite this evidence, many leading vegetarians and vegans such as Paul Pitchford have pointed out that large numbers of Taoists in China in previous generations lived exceptionally healthy lives without any animal products.[91] Although in India vegetarianism has been a dietary tradition among Hindus, Buddhists, and Taoists for twenty-five centuries, dairy products were also extensively used, so veganism cannot be validated by the health of these populations. Others argue that because of the lack of strict hygiene standards typical in many of these third-world countries, grubs and insects that adhered to plant leaves were often consumed, and therefore these diets were not strictly vegetarian or vegan.[92]

Many individuals who eat no meat, fish, fowl, dairy, or eggs choose veganism for moral reasons, believing that the eating of animal foods is cruel and unnecessary. In her book *Nourishing Traditions* Sally Fallon discusses one aspect of the spiritual issues underlying this deeply divisive issue:

> The desire to abstain from animal products, found so often in those of a spiritual nature, may in fact be a longing for a return to a former, more perfect state of consciousness that was ours before our souls took embodiment in physical bodies on the material plane. This longing attracts many to the belief that our bodies and souls can be purified, or that we can achieve spiritual enlightenment, through a meatless diet. Saintly individuals are often drawn to strict vegetarian habits, and some have been able to sustain themselves on a diet free of animal products for fairly long periods of time. Even so, it is a mistake to think that meat eaters lack spirituality—many highly spiritual people eat meat regularly. Perhaps they instinctively realize that when we eat animal products we are accepting, reverently and humbly, the requirements of the earthly body temple in which the soul is temporarily housed. . . . Seen in this light, strict vegetarianism can be likened to a kind of spiritual pride that seeks to "take heaven by force," and to shirk the earthly duties for which the physical body was created.[93]

On a purely clinical basis, many holistic practitioners have found that their weaker patients—primarily those individuals functioning in the tuberculinic or luetic reaction modes—cannot get well without frequent ingestion of the utilizable B_{12}, protein, and fat found in meat, fowl, eggs, and fish. This is especially the case during intense growth periods for pregnant and nursing mothers and growing children, as well as for those who lead a relatively busy life. This latter point—matching your dietary needs according to your energy output—was dramatically exemplified during part of the Vedic period (circa 3000 BCE) in India, when traditionally vegetarian Hindu Brahmins ate meat. The American followers of one of the greatest Indian spiritual teachers, Swami Vivekananda, recounted his story about these ancient Hindu priests who normally abhorred the eating of animal food:

> One day, asked about what he considered the most glorious period of Indian history, the Swami [Vivekananda] mentioned the Vedic period, when "five Brahmins used to polish off one cow." He advocated animal food for the Hindus if they were to cope at all with the rest of the world in the present reign of power and find a place among the other great nations, whether within or outside the British Empire.[94]

Thus, even for religious groups, diet is not always set in stone but a consideration that needs to be judiciously weighed and based on the changes and circumstances that are occurring in your life. These factors include consideration of your lifestyle, your particular job or profession and your level of activity at home and at work; your spiritual beliefs; your miasmic level of functioning (psoric, sycotic, tuberculinic, or luetic); and your unique biochemical individuality. Deciding on which animal products to ingest is always a personal decision, one that is up to each individual alone to make.

Organically Raised and Appropriately Prepared Meat

Whatever your choice—whether vegetarian or meat-eating—it is important to learn from the traditional wisdom of food preparation of native peoples who thrived in former times. Today, conventionally farm-raised animals such as cattle, sheep, pigs, and poultry are fed antibiotics, steroid hormones, and pesticide-laden feed.[95] In fact, the use of antibiotics in animal feed today accounts for *half* of the 35 million pounds of these drugs produced each year.[96] Despite this excessive use of antibiotic drugs to kill germs, diseased animals routinely pass inspection. In fact, the United States Department of Agriculture in 2000 implemented new rules reclassifying as safe for human consumption animals with cancer, lymphomas, sores, and diseases caused by intestinal worms, advising processors to "remove localized lesion(s) and pass unaffected carcass portions."[97] However, an animal whose cancerous tumor has been cut off is a far cry from the traditional food of hunter-gatherer societies that thrived on wild game.[98]

Fortunately, organically raised grass-fed meat and poultry are becoming more widely available, even in some conventional grocery stores. Additionally, large health food stores such as Whole Foods often stock buffalo and venison raised on the open range, as well as game birds such as duck, geese, pheasant, and wild turkey that are rich in nutrients and have a superior fatty acid profile to farm animals.[99] Eating a variety of organic meats, fowl, and fish is just as important and nourishing as varying your vegetable, fruit, and grain choices.

Another forgotten tradition from our ancestors is the use of every part of the animal. The primitive peoples Dr. Price studied prized the organ meats for their regenerating qualities as well as the muscle parts commonly sold today. In many cases they used the whole animal to make stocks and broths. Meat, chicken, and fish stocks contained the minerals of bone, cartilage, and marrow, and the vegetables that were included supplied electrolytes.[100] Bone broths are one of the two best sources of calcium (the other being milk products), as well as other minerals that protect against osteoporosis.[101]

Equally valuable is the gelatin that accumulates in these broths, which, through its hydrophilic colloidal nature, allows the body to more fully utilize proteins and other nutrients.[102] The great nutritionist Dr. Francis Pottenger first expounded on the importance of eating hydrophilic, or water-loving (and therefore gastric-juice-loving), raw foods versus overcooked foods. The "colloids," or organic molecules, in foods that have been overheated are hydrophobic and repel digestive juices, which makes cooked food more difficult to digest.[103]* However, the proteinaceous gelatin in meat broths, although cooked, is hydrophilic, so it attracts gastric and intestinal digestive juices and supports more complete digestion. Even most nutritionists and holistic practitioners are unaware of the exceptionally beneficial effects of gelatin in the treatment of many chronic digestive disorders, as well as other diseases including anemia, diabetes, muscular dystrophy, and cancer.[104]† In *Nourishing Traditions,* recipes for stock are described extensively, and information on how to freeze and store these broths to later serve in soups or add to a meat, chicken, or fish course is also included. Other sources of gelatin include cactus and beet juice, edible seaweeds, agar, okra, or even unflavored gelatin purchased at the health food store.[105]

▶ The Radiant Life Company (888-593-8333 or go to www.radiantlifecatalog.com) carries gelatin from grass-fed cows. Knox gelatin, which is not made from organic beef and contains MSG, is not recommended.

Raw Meat in Moderation

Dr. Pottenger concluded from his exhaustive nutritional research on cats that raw meat was superior to cooked.[106] Although our intestines are different physiologically and morphologically from cats', the value of raw meat has been espoused by other researchers as well, including Dr. Pottenger's colleague Weston Price. In his worldwide studies of primitive peoples, Dr. Price was struck by the fact that every one of the healthy cultures he observed ate a certain amount of raw animal protein.‡ Even today, almost every traditional culture includes some raw animal protein in its diet—steak tartare from France, carpaccio from Italy, kibbeh from the Middle East, and raw marinated fish from Scandinavia, Hawaii, Latin America, and Asia. In regard to the problem of possible parasites, Sally Fallon suggests that beef or lamb be frozen for fourteen days, and that fish be marinated or

---

*Again, more evidence that eating a salad or other raw food before the main cooked course stimulates digestive juices and improves the assimilation of nutrients.

†Of course, gelatin-rich broth made from the bones of grass-fed, organically raised animals is a far cry from the modern-day ugly twin Jell-O, which is loaded with sugar, additives, and artificial flavorings and colorings.

‡For more information on Dr. Price's findings, see the chapter 16 section on inadequate nutrition (page 507).

fermented in a parasite-reducing acid solution of lemon juice, lime juice, or whey, which supports more effective digestion as well.[107]

Low-Temperature Cooking of Meat

Fallon further recommends that meat should never be deep-fried or cooked at high temperatures where the internal temperature is raised above 212°F. Meat is best cooked rare or braised in water or stock to preserve many essential nutrients.[108] For example, vitamin B_{12} is resistant to temperatures below 250°C (482°F) and therefore remains intact in rare and medium-rare cooked meats.[109] Additionally, some traditional cultures reduce cooking time and temperature by marinating meat for twenty-four to forty-eight hours in wine, yogurt, or buttermilk, which tenderizes and predigests it.[110]

Excessive Amounts of Protein Not Recommended

Contrary to popular thinking among several of his detractors, Dr. Price did not advocate a high-protein diet. In fact, during the Depression, Price stated that a person's protein requirement could be fulfilled by as little as one egg (or a piece of meat equivalent to the bulk of one egg) per day, as well as one quart of whole milk daily per child. Price recommended that the most nutrient-dense protein be consumed, such as organic meats, bone broths, shellfish, anchovies, and sardines (eaten with the bones).[111]

Don't Forget the Fat!

All animal protein foods—meat, eggs, and milk—come with fat, and in this natural state that is how they should be eaten. The modern trend of consuming lean cuts of meat, egg whites without the yolk, and low-fat or skim milk products can cause serious deficiencies of essential fat-soluble vitamins (A, D, E, and K) and also renders the protein difficult to digest.[112] Even combining protein and fat—scrambled eggs and avocados, butter melting on rare filet mignon, and so forth—can help further supplement the fat-soluble vitamins A and D that are needed to fully assimilate the protein.

Nuts and Seeds

Nuts and seeds are concentrated foods rich in vitamins, minerals, and essential fatty acids.

Soaking and Dehydrating Nuts Augments Digestion

Nuts have numerous enzyme inhibitors and are best soaked or partially sprouted to make their nutrients most nontoxic and assimilable before eating. Therefore, raw nuts are significantly easier to digest if they are first soaked in salt water (a little tamari and Celtic or Himalayan salt adds to the taste) and then dried in a warm oven or dehydrator—and they make a great snack. The dry-roasted nuts from your local supermarket are not a good option; most are rancid by the time you buy them. Walnuts have large amounts of triple unsaturated linolenic acid and should be stored in the refrigerator, whereas almonds, pecans, cashews, macadamia nuts, and peanuts can be stored for many months at room temperature after soaking and dehydrating.[113]

The Benefits of Sprouting Seeds

The value of sprouting seeds has been known for centuries, beginning with the ancient Chinese, who on their oceangoing ships took along mung beans to sprout, which produced vitamin C, thus preventing scurvy on board. Sprouting also increases seeds' vitamin B and carotene levels, activates enzymes, inactivates carcinogenic aflatoxins, and neutralizes phytic acid and enzyme inhibitors.[114] One popular seed that should never be sprouted or eaten in any form is alfalfa. Alfalfa seeds contain an amino acid called canavanine that can be toxic, and research has shown that alfalfa sprouts can inhibit immune system functioning and contribute to inflammatory arthritis and lupus.[115] Nutritious seeds that can be sprouted include sunflower, pumpkin, sesame, chia, and radish. Chia seeds are second only to flax in their content of omega-3 fatty acids, and they are commonly used in baking in Mexico to promote endurance and energy.[116] Grains (wheat, rye, barley, and buckwheat) and beans (mung, adzuki, kidney, lima, and lentils) also germinate well.[117]

TAHINI AND FLAXSEED OIL

Sesame seeds contain a high amount of methionine and tryptophan, two important amino acids usually lacking in vegetables. Flaxseed oil can be added to tahini, which is made from hulled sesame seeds, to supply omega-3 fatty acids. The synergistic action of the omega-3 fatty acids in flaxseed oil and the sulfur-containing methionine in tahini is very beneficial.

Oils and Fats

Dietary fats and oils supply the body with energy; carry the fat-soluble vitamins A, D, E, and K; satisfy hunger four to five times more than carbohydrates do; provide building blocks for cell membranes, hormones, and prostaglandins; and function as a layer of insulation and shock absorption under the skin.[118] Furthermore, the much-maligned saturated fats—coconut oil, butter, and fat on meat—are not the cause of heart disease but actually protect against it. The fact is that rates of coronary heart disease, rare before 1920, have risen dramatically in the United States; since the mid-1950s, it has been the leading cause of all U.S. deaths.[119] If saturated fats were the primary culprit, you would expect that there would be a corresponding increase in their use. However, as Sally Fallon points out, the statistics just don't bear this out, and in actuality, just the reverse is true.

> During the sixty-year period from 1910 to 1970, the proportion of traditional animal fat in the American diet declined from 83 percent to 62 percent, and butter consumption plummeted from eighteen pounds per person per year to four. During the past eighty years, dietary cholesterol intake had increased only 1 percent. During the same period, the percentage of dietary vegetable oils in the form of margarine, shortening, and refined oils increased about *400 percent* while the consumption of sugar and processed foods increased about *60 percent*.[120]

Perhaps the most famous example of the failure of low-fat diets is in the case of the Pritikin diet. Many who stayed on this regimen for an extended period of time developed a variety of health problems including low energy, difficulty concentrating, depression, weight gain, and mineral deficiencies. In fact, Pritikin himself committed suicide after "he realized that his Spartan regime was not curing his leukemia."[121]

fats/oils: Lipids (or fats) that are solid at room temperature are called fats, and those that are liquid at room temperature are called oils.

The Health Benefits of Coconut Oil

The heart-protective factor of coconut oil is borne out by the fact that Asian and Polynesian people who have relied on this oil for centuries have the lowest heart disease rates in the world.[122] Saturated fats such as coconut oil also play other essential and beneficial roles in the body including immune system support, liver protection from alcohol and other toxins, and absorption of calcium by the bones. Furthermore, because coconut oil doesn't require pancreatic enzymes for digestion, it is more quickly absorbed into the liver, where its high concentration of medium-chain fatty acids are used as fuel to produce quick energy. Coconut oil also stimulates thyroid metabolism, and several studies have shown that its use is quite thermogenic (increasing heat in the body through metabolic stimulation), and it has been used to facilitate significant weight loss in overweight and obese individuals.[123]

Additionally, coconut oil is the largest and most assimilable source of lauric acid—an important antifungal, antiviral, antibacterial, and antiprotozoal monoglyceride.[124] In vitro, lauric acid has been shown to inactivate the HIV, measles, and herpes simplex viruses, as well as the cytomegalovirus.[125] Coconut oil is therefore currently included in some AIDS and anti-candida protocols because of its potent microcidal (microbe-killing) effects.

Because coconut oil is 92 percent saturated fat, it is extremely stable and doesn't break down into dangerous free radicals when heated. It is therefore the oil of choice for cooking and baking.[126] When shopping for coconut oil, look for a product that is nonhydrogenated, "food-grade," and a white semisolid in cool weather (below 76°F) and a creamy-colored oil in hot weather (above 76°F). It needs no refrigeration and has an exceptionally long shelf life without becoming rancid (after one year of storage at room temperature, no rancidity has been detected).

Olive oil, being a monounsaturated fat, is almost as stable and can be used for cooking and sautéing at mild to moderate temperatures.* Additionally, extra virgin olive oil is rich in antioxidants, but its longer-chain fatty acids can contribute to body fat more than the short- to

*As discussed in the "Dairy" section previously, raw butter should also be used liberally in your kitchen, but it should be only lightly heated and not subjected to moderate or high heat.

medium-chain fatty acids found in butter or the tropical coconut and palm oils.[127] Furthermore, research published in the *Arteriosclerosis, Thrombosis and Vascular Biology* journal in 1998 reported that the monounsaturated fatty acids found in olive and canola oils may actually contribute to the development of atherosclerosis, and therefore heart disease, more so than saturated fat.[128] However, olive oil, a major component in the health-oriented Mediterranean diet, does contain a beneficial anti-inflammatory substance called *oleocanthal,* which can inhibit the harmful effects of inflammatory cox-1 and cox-2 enzymes in arthritic syndromes—without the side effects (ulcers, diarrhea, and bloating) of NSAIDs and cox-2 inhibitors such as Vioxx (heart attacks and strokes).[129]*

► Two of the most unrefined and purest grades of coconut oil presently available are from Jungle Products (organic and "extra virgin") and Wilderness Family Naturals (800-945-3801). Both are available in health food stores or can be ordered from the Radiant Life Company at (888) 593-8333 or www.radiantlifecatalog.com.

Flaxseed Oil Advantages

Flaxseed oil—also called food-grade linseed oil—should also be considered a premium health food due to its high omega-3 content (57 percent). Americans generally consume far too many omega-6 essential fatty acids (found in most polyunsaturated vegetable oils) and not enough omega-3 essential fatty acids (found in flax and chia seeds, fish, eggs from free-range chickens, dark green vegetables, and walnuts).† As described previously under "Fruits and Vegetables," flaxseed oil makes a delicious salad dressing, and the oil or seeds are excellent freshly ground and sprinkled on cottage cheese, fruit, and cooked whole grains in the morning to promote healthy bowel functioning. Furthermore, flaxseeds are low in phytic acid and do not require soaking first if eaten in small amounts.[130]

In Europe, biochemist Johanna Budwig has researched the beneficial synergy between the essential fatty acids in flaxseed oil and the sulfur-based proteins in cottage cheese or in sesame seeds used in tahini. Dr. Budwig has used this antitumor and detoxifying combination extensively in the treatment of cancer and other degenerative diseases.[131] Because flaxseed oil can easily go rancid, it's essential to buy only refrigerated, low-heat expeller-pressed organic flaxseed oil in opaque bottles.

Salt

Essential for Our Blood, Sweat, and Tears

Our bodies require salt, or sodium chloride, in order to function. In fact, all our cells are bathed in water and salt to help maintain a normal electrolyte balance in order for cells to communicate and function properly. Furthermore, salt helps balance blood sugar levels, maintain energy levels, absorb nutrients, and support the functioning of the liver, kidneys, adrenals, and brain. Additionally, all our body fluids—blood, sweat, tears, lymph, and bile—require salt in order to maintain normal physiological functioning.[132] Salt, a strong alkalinizer for overly acidic tissues, is highly regarded in macrobiotic cooking to promote energy through strengthening the kidneys, counteracting toxins in the body, helping to emulsify oils, and clearing plaque in the blood vessels and for its integral and essential role in digestion, since it is used to make up the oral saliva and the hydrochloric acid in the stomach.[133]

Celtic and Himalayan Salts Are Superior

One of the purest salts available is Celtic salt, which is harvested from the ocean off the coast of Brittany, France. This natural sea salt is not heated, refined, or adulterated with aluminum and other compounds like conventional salt, and even many other so-called sea salts. Celtic salt provides the body primarily with organic sodium and chloride, as well as eighty-two other elements including organic iodine, magnesium, calcium, phosphorus, selenium, and manganese.[134] Furthermore, the balanced mixture of essential minerals in Celtic salt is almost identical to that of the salty amniotic fluid that surrounded us as

*NSAID stands for "nonsteroidal anti-inflammatory drugs" and includes aspirin, indomethacin (Indocin), ibuprofen (Motrin), naproxen (Naprosyn), piroxicam (Feldene), and nabumetone (Relafen). For more information on Vioxx, see appendix 4, "How Scientific Is Allopathic Medicine?"

†As previously discussed under "Fish," the body can manufacture DHA (found naturally in fish) from the omega-3 fatty acids found in flaxseed oil, though many individuals lack the adequate vitamin and mineral cofactors to activate the enzyme necessary for this conversion. Thus, to ensure receiving both the DHA and EPA from omega-3 fatty acids, most individuals should include both fish and flax in their diets.

fetuses. This coarse and moist light gray salt should be dried at a low heat in an oven (~150°F) or dehydrator and then ground in a salt mill over your food.

- ▶ Buy Celtic sea salt from your local health food store or from www.celticseasalt.com.
- ▶ Sur La Table has good salt and pepper grinders; the brand name is Unicorn.

Another excellent natural salt, commonly referred to as "pink salt" (because of its content of iron and other minerals), is derived from the foothills of the Himalayas. This 200-million-year-old fossil marine salt originating from the Mesozoic era contains calcium, magnesium, potassium, copper, iron, and other minerals and mirrors our bodies in its ratios of trace minerals.[135] Dr. Joseph Mercola, a prominent holistic practitioner, recommends the Himalayan salt over Celtic sea salt due to the chemical dumping and toxic oil spills that are unfortunately polluting the oceans and the stores of sea salt today. Himalayan salt is available in a range of crystal sizes, from coarse rock salt to a finer, more granular form. The Himalania company sells its salt with excellent custom graters and grinders. Unfortunately, health food stores do not always carry this salt, but it can be ordered online.

- ▶ Himalania-brand pink salt is available at health food stores or go to www.himalania.com.

Table Salt Toxicity

Unlike Celtic and Himalayan natural salts, table salt is highly refined to remove essentially all of its minerals except sodium chloride. Furthermore, although the addition of iodine to table salt was seemingly appropriate in the 1920s when thyroid goiters were more prevalent, today there are actually more problems with the excessive ingestion of iodine through table salt and salted foods, as exemplified by the increasing incidence of hyperthyroidism.* Additionally, table salt can typically contain added aluminum silicate, fluoride dextrose (sugar), bleaching chemicals, and preservatives, and it is dried at over 1,200°F, which changes its crystalline structure—and thus its ability to be readily absorbed and utilized in the body.[136†]

*Iodine occurs naturally in seafood and Celtic and Himalayan salt.

†To view a 400X magnification comparing the crystals of common table salt, sea salt, and Himalayan salt go to www.alohabay.com/products/saltinfo/salt_info_faq.html.

The Blood Pressure Controversy

The effect of salt on high blood pressure, or hypertension, is extremely complex. According to cardiologist Richard N. Fogoros, "After decades of research [and] over 20,000 scientific studies published on the relationship between salt and hypertension, conflict and contradiction [still] result."[137] Furthermore, based on the clear differences between natural sea salts and refined table salt, an important question for consumers as well as researchers to consider is, out of the 20,000 or so studies on salt, how many utilized Celtic or Himalayan salt? Likely very few, if any.

Additionally, many well-conducted longitudinal studies have found no connection between low-sodium diets and the reduction of hypertension and other forms of heart disease. For example, in one eight-year study in New York City of hypertensive individuals, the population on low-salt diets had more than *four* times the number of heart attacks (a significant risk of hypertension) than those on normal-sodium diets. In another massive study analyzing health outcomes for over twenty years by the U.S. National Health and Nutrition Examination Survey, a 20 percent *greater* incidence of heart attacks occurred in the population of individuals on a low-salt diet than in those on a normal dietary regimen.[138]

Until a long-term study is conducted on hypertensive individuals comparing the use of natural sea salts to refined table salt as well as a general low-sodium diet, it is up to educated consumers and their practitioners to make these dietary decisions. Dr. Joseph Mercola recommends that if your blood tests reveal a sodium level higher than 142 or a chloride level over 105, you may want to consider restricting your salt intake.[139] Additionally, a 2001 study in the *Hypertension* journal suggests that a small number of people are salt sensitive and thus more prone to hypertension and other forms of cardiovascular disease when they ingest high amounts of salt.[140] If you think you fall into this category, you may want to eat a low-sodium diet. (Unfortunately, once again, the researchers at Indiana University School of Medicine who conducted this study were not measuring the dietary effects of natural and unrefined sea salts on cardiovascular disease.)

Seaweed

Seaweeds or sea vegetables such as kelp, arame, wakame, kombu, and hijiki contain the greatest amount and broadest range of minerals of any organism—ten to twenty times the minerals found in land plants.[141] Because they contain hydrophilic mucilaginous gels such as algin, carrageenan, and agar, which attract digestive juices to the food bolus (the rounded mass of food that is swallowed and passes through the esophagus to the stomach), they also assist in digestion. Furthermore, the sodium alginate found in sea vegetables binds and chelates out many radioactive contaminants—such as the ubiquitous strontium 90 (found in nuclear waste and fallout), as well as lead, cadmium, mercury, excess iron, and other heavy metals that can accumulate in the body.[142]

Because of their high mineral and mucilaginous content, sea vegetables don't need to be consumed in large amounts to impart their nutritional benefits. This is fortuitous, since sea vegetables also contain long-chain complex sugars that can be difficult to digest. Furthermore, overconsumption of even the organic form of iodine found in these seaweeds can contribute to iodine poisoning and harm thyroid function.[143] Sea vegetables should therefore be eaten more as condiments in small amounts, and should be simmered a long time to begin the breakdown of their complex sugars. As always, their source is also important. Seaweeds should be purchased at health food stores or they should be from holistic sources to ensure that they were harvested from a clean water source.

If you are unfamiliar with cooking seaweed, begin by simply including it in brown rice. Make your brown rice as usual but include some arame in the cooking water that you bring to a boil and then simmer until the rice is cooked. You may need to add a little extra water to compensate for the water absorbed by the arame while cooking.

Soy, Fermented

Soy is another nutritious food that should be consumed more like a condiment. Contrary to common belief, traditionally in Asia the average consumption of soy foods is only 10 grams or about 2 teaspoons per day. Soy was first used as a food as early as 1134 BCE, but only after the Chinese learned to ferment soybeans.[144] Miso, tempeh, and tamari (soy sauce) are all fermented, which removes the harmful enzyme inhibitors and phytic acid found in soybeans. The soaking and processing of tofu removes some of these plant toxins, so it can be eaten safely in small amounts, or better, combined with miso or fish stock.[145] It's especially important to buy organically grown soy products, because the majority of the soybean crop has been genetically altered in this country.

THE HARMFUL "FOODS"

The second half of this chapter will be devoted to information about harmful substances that are commonly ingested.

Coffee

In hot, sunny fields liberally sprayed with pesticides, green coffee beans are picked and then roasted up to sixteen times. This processing yields both pesticide residues and harmful hydrocarbons that have been linked to pancreatic and colon cancers.[146] Furthermore, coffee contains more caffeine than any other popular beverage,* and caffeine is one of the most potent alkaloids in the methylxanthine family (which includes theophylline found in black and green teas and theobromine found in chocolate). Indeed, caffeine is highly addictive, and prolonged use depletes the adrenals (and the epinephrine and norepinephrine neurotransmitters); initially raises and then in a rebound fashion greatly lowers blood sugar (hypoglycemia); increases the heart rate, arrythmias, and blood pressure;† exhausts gastric juices (hydrochloric acid); decreases thymus gland size and circulating antibodies; promotes fibrocystic breast changes; depletes minerals and interferes with the calcium/phosphorus ratio; induces vitamin B_1 deficiency; and crosses both the placenta (to the fetus) and the breasts (to the nursing infant) virtually unchanged.[147]

CAFFEINE COMPARISONS

A 12-ounce cup of brewed coffee contains 200 milligrams of caffeine. In comparison, a 6-ounce Hershey's milk choc-

*With the exception of some "energy drinks," widely known to be health hazards.

†Sometimes it decreases blood pressure.

olate bar contains 25 milligrams, an 8-ounce cup of brewed tea contains 50 milligrams, a 20-ounce bottle of Coca-Cola contains 57 milligrams, and 2 tablets of Excedrin pain reliever contain 130 milligrams.[148]

Individuals who are still drinking coffee can use the following behavior-modifying steps to gradually detoxify this drug from their bodies and lifestyle. First, buy only organic coffee. Second, switch to decaffeinated organic coffee. Next, try switching to organic black or green tea. Finally, switch to herbal tea or grain beverages (if you're not sensitive to the roasted chicory, barley, and cardamom), or start your day with warm water and lemon juice.

The morning fatigue that triggers the desire for caffeine can be greatly mitigated by taking the steps outlined in this book—drainage, detoxification of heavy metals and toxic chemicals, treatment of dominant foci, and the correct homeopathic constitutional remedy. Furthermore, with quality psychospiritual work and increased self-understanding (see chapter 18), the underlying emotional craving for that morning fix of something warm and comforting (e.g., "mother's milk"), disguised as a cappuccino or latté, will begin to dissipate over time.

Genetically Engineered Food

Genetically engineered (GE) foods are also known as genetically modified (GM) foods, genetically modified organisms (GMO), biotech foods, gene-foods, bioengineered food, gene-altered foods, transgenic foods and "Frankenfoods."[149]

What Is It?

The process of genetically engineering foods involves the enzyme extraction of selected genes from a donor (e.g., an animal, plant, insect, bacterium, virus, and so forth) so that the genes can be copied and then inserted into a *completely different* host, such as a soybean, a tomato, a cow, or a pig. For example, genetic engineering or modification projects have included combining tomatoes with flounder genes, pigs with human genes, and GE cows that produce human breast milk.[150]

The GE process differs dramatically from traditional crop breeding, in which selected plants of the same or closely related species are combined through natural propagation methods such as pollination. This long-term practice only emphasizes certain characteristics in a plant or animal, but it *does not* involve interbreeding between widely different species. For example, corn can pollinate only with other strains of corn or with plants that are closely related to the corn family.[151]

The Dangerous Consequences of Genetic Engineering

One of the primary concerns with genetically modified foods is that the process is, in the words of Ronnie Cummins and Ben Lilliston, authors of *Genetically Engineered Food,* "unstable, inexact, and prone to mistakes with potentially fatal consequences."[152] For example, the August 9, 1990, *New England Journal of Medicine* reported that the toxicity of the dietary supplement L-tryptophan that caused 37 deaths, 1,500 cases of permanent disability, and over 5,000 cases of illness (eosinophilia myalgia syndrome or EMS) in the United States in 1989 was caused by genetic engineering. The Japanese manufacturer of the supplement, Showa Denko, had recently begun using genetically engineered bacteria to increase the efficiency of L-tryptophan production.[153] The FDA was aware of this practice but did not require safety tests of this new imported product because the agency mistakenly believed that "GE and non-GE L-tryptophan were 'substantially equivalent.'"[154] Furthermore, after this tragedy, instead of rigorously investigating the tryptophan from this Japanese company and its brand-new production methods, the FDA reacted simply by pulling all L-tryptophan off the market, depriving many people for several years of this previously (non-GE) safe nutrient that readily converts in the body to the neurotransmitter serotonin, and has been effective in treating some forms of depression, premenstrual tension, and insomnia.[155]

Danger Echoed in Scientific Research

Although independent scientific research on GE foods is rare, a prestigious biotech lab in Scotland, the Rowett Institute, won a highly competitive multimillion-dollar grant to study the impact of GE potatoes on the health of animals and humans in the late 1990s. The institute's findings were quite disturbing, however—both to the scientists themselves and for the biotech industry. The GE potatoes studied, spliced with the DNA from a plant and a commonly used virus (cauliflower mosaic virus [CaMV] promoter), were found to be poisonous to the lab rats on which they were tested.[156] Perhaps most alarming of all, these Scottish researchers found that it was the CaMV virus—spliced into *almost all* GE foods and crops—that was primarily culpable for causing the proliferation of cancerlike cells in the rats' intestines and stomachs, as well as underdeveloped brains, livers, and testicles and damaged immune systems.[157] Researchers in England and Canada have made similar discoveries, asserting that the "transgenic instability" of the CaMV virus can promote the "inappropriate overexpression of genes," which can very possibly be a major causative factor in cancer.[158]

Unfortunately, information gleaned from independent scientific studies about the real dangers of eating GE foods has not been widely propagated. After the Scottish scientists at the Rowett Institute published their findings in the U.K. *Sunday Herald* and the prestigious *Lancet* journal (October 1999), government funding was abruptly cut off and the team's leader, Dr. Arpad Pusztai, was promptly fired from the job he had held for thirty years, locked out of his lab, and "vilified by the pro-biotech establishment."[159]

BGH Milk Implicated in Cancer

The world's first genetically modified food product introduced in the United States was milk from cows injected with genetically engineered bovine growth hormone (rBGH). Also known as recombinant bovine somatotropin (rBST), this hormone stimulates the pituitary gland in cows to increase their milk production.[160] Created by the Monsanto Corporation, rBGH milk was approved by the FDA in 1994, although scientists from the Consumers Union and the Cancer Prevention Coalition warned that the significantly higher levels of insulin-like growth factor (IGF-1) in this milk and other dairy products was a powerful cancer promoter and had been linked to an increased risk of breast, prostate, and colon cancer, as well as glucose intolerance, hypertension, and swollen limbs in humans.[161] Furthermore, cows injected with rBGH are prone to many diseases and frequently secrete pus in their milk, requiring even more doses than normal of antibiotics.[162] The FDA was also warned by the Government Accounting Office in 1993 that the expected increased residues of antibiotics in the milk of rBGH-injected cows would add to the growing resistance to antibiotics. Although the FDA did not heed this and the other aforementioned warnings, other countries have, including many European countries, Canada, and Japan.[163]

Genetic Expression Unpredictable in "Frankenfoods"

The grains and vegetables produced with genetically modified organisms have been referred to as "Frankenfoods," since they are created in labs and are based on the simplistic premise that certain genes cause certain traits. In reality, however, heredity has been described as a remarkably "plastic potential expressing itself fluidly within particular environments."[164]

For example, when the gene for cystic fibrosis was discovered, the initial euphoria at possibly eradicating this disease was later dampened by the discovery that 350 different genetic mutations may occur on this gene, with many perfectly healthy people displaying a cystic fibrosis genetic profile.[165] Or, for example, when tomatoes were first engineered for increased carotene production, unexpected dwarfism occurred.[166] (That is, the more carotene a plant produced, the smaller it became.) Or when corn was genetically engineered to target pests, beneficial insect predators also suffered high mortality rates. Therefore, this transgenic corn was actually defeating its purpose of "integrated pest management," and further increasing the likelihood of the rapid development of resistance among pests.[167] In fact, nearly 60 percent of biotechnology research is aimed at developing plants that can tolerate more chemicals, resulting in an estimated *tripling* of the herbicides used on crops.[168]

Instead of this myopic and mechanistic approach to genetic coupling, an organism needs to be understood as a whole, in all of its complexities, to understand and predict the outcome of genetic inheritance. Indeed, it is the *interaction* of foreign DNA in a host, with the resulting multiplicity of reactions, that causes so many unknowable and unforeseeable hazards—and often disastrous consequences.[169]

More Frightening than Toxic Chemicals

Genetically altered crops easily contaminate other crops when pollen from GE plants is carried by wind, rain, birds, or insects and then pollinates other plants in adjacent fields or environments. For example, in one study of thirty-six batches of conventionally grown corn, soy, and canola seed, more than two-thirds had been contaminated through the "genetic drift" of GE crops.[170] These and other findings led a Washington-based advocacy group, the Union of Concerned Scientists, to conclude in 2004 that if federal rules and farming practices are not tightened soon, "the United States may soon find it impossible to guarantee that any portion of its food supply is free of genetically altered elements, which could seriously disrupt the export of foods, seeds, and oils . . . [and] gravely harm the domestic market for organic food."[171]

The implications of the far-reaching contamination by these GE foods prompted Stephanie Mills of the Sierra Club to assert that genetically engineered farming is even more frightening than the use of toxic chemicals:

> Here you are creating millions of novel organisms, organisms that the earth has never seen, and then releasing them into the environment. . . . Many of us have spent much of our working lives addressing the terrible ecological problems created by chemical pollution. [But] chemical pollution, however horrible, does dilute over time, and it often can be contained. However, once you release an organism into the environment it cannot be recalled or contained. It will not dilute but rather reproduce, disseminate, and mutate. It is unstoppable.[172]

Shop Organic!

An estimated 70 percent of all packaged goods found on supermarket shelves include some genetically modified ingredients. Even more alarming, the consumer has no way of identifying these products since there are no laws requiring labeling of GE products. Furthermore, although numerous polls have shown that 80 to 95 percent of Americans want these GE foods to be labeled, the large pharmaceutical firms that dominate genetic engineering—Monsanto, Aventis, DuPont, Dow Chemical, and others—continue to fight regulatory legislation.[173]

Fortunately, some of the major U.S. food industries, including Gerber, Heinz, and Frito-Lay, have become concerned enough by the preponderance of alarming scientific evidence that they have become GE-free.[174] Furthermore, other countries around the world that are not as influenced by large pharmaceutical firms and agribusinesses are strongly rejecting genetically modified foods. Japan and Europe are strongly opposed to GE foods, and African nations will not even accept GE seeds when they are given as food aid.[175] Meanwhile, in the United States, until GE foods are labeled, their prevalence in so many foods is just one more reason to shop at health food stores and to patronize farmers who grow organic, non-GMO crops.

An excellent educational tool about the hazards of GE foods is the film *The Future of Food.* Written, directed, and coproduced by Deborah Koons Garcia (the widow of Jerry Garcia of the Grateful Dead), this film investigates not only the health and environmental issues surrounding GE foods but also the harm that GE seeds and crops can do to small family-owned farms.[176] This ninety-minute film has been used widely throughout California in the movement to ban GE crops, which has been successful most recently in Marin and Mendocino counties.

▶ To watch the film *The Future of Food,* go to www.thefutureoffood.com.

THE AAEM CALLS FOR MORATORIUM ON GE FOODS

Recently, the American Academy of Environmental Medicine (AAEM) called for a moratorium on GE foods, stating that they "pose a serious health risk in the areas of toxicology, allergy and immune function, reproductive health, and metabolic, physiologic and genetic health." The academy further concluded that "there is more than a casual association between GM [GE] foods and adverse health effects."[177]

Irradiated Food

"Turning Garbage into Gold"

In the Spring 2002 *Wise Traditions* journal, Sally Fallon and Mary Enig announced that once again—as with the use of fluoride—"the Food Processing-Industrial Complex has turned garbage into gold."* That is, by using

*In the mid-1940s, fluoride began to be added to the water in various U.S. cities, allowing Alcoa a market for its toxic fluoride wastes that had accumulated in the process of its production of aluminum. Fluoride has been linked to bone fractures, dental fluorosis (damage to the enamel of the teeth), arthritis, hypothyroidism, and osteosarcomas (bone cancer) in young men. (S. Gibson, "Water Fluoridation—Therapy or Fallacy?" www.positivehealth.com/articles/dentistry/503.)

nuclear waste material to irradiate food, the Department of Energy's Byproducts Utilization Program greatly benefits by reducing disposal costs for military and civilian nuclear fuel wastes. Although the nuclear industry claims that there is no difference between irradiated food and nonirradiated food, the damaging effects of irradiated food have been studied and documented since the 1960s. For example, the massive doses of radiation used in irradiating meat (200 million times greater than in a chest X-ray) produce elevated levels of benzene, cyclobutanones, formaldehyde, and other carcinogenic "radiolytic" compounds.[178] Irradiating food also reduces its nutritional content, particularly A, C, E, and B-complex vitamins, and kills friendly bacteria and enzymes, rendering it a relatively "dead" food. In a short-term study testing the effects of irradiated food on children in India, blood tests taken after six weeks showed chromosomal damage. In another short-term study that used dogs as research subjects, enlarged spleens and swollen lymph nodes were noted in these animals after they had eaten irradiated beef for a few weeks.[179]

Another Reason to Shop at Health Food Stores

Food irradiation is popular among food manufacturers because it greatly extends shelf life. It is currently approved for use in meats, grains, some produce, herbs, and spices. Irradiated foods must be labeled, but products containing irradiated ingredients do not have to be labeled.[180] Labeling can include the use of the "radura" symbol:

It may also include the words "Irradiated to destroy harmful microbes," or even the ambiguous and confusing term "pasteurized."[181] Food irradiation is just another reason to shop at health food stores—your life and health depend on it.

Microwaved Food

Like irradiation, microwaving also creates carcinogenic "radiolytic" compounds. These ovens use an alternating current that agitates the molecules in foods, breaking the natural membranes as well as affecting the chemical structure of the nutrients. One study conducted by eight Swiss biochemists found that eating microwaved food consistently decreased hemoglobin levels, lymphocytes (white blood cells), and HDL (good cholesterol) in the blood of the research participants.[182]* German and Russian scientists who studied the biological effects of microwave cooking concluded that these ovens decreased the bioavailability of B-complex vitamins, vitamins C and E, essential minerals, and lipotropics (fatty acids, cholesterol, et cetera) and created carcinogenic free radicals.[183] In a Stanford study published in the *Journal of Pediatrics,* researchers found that human breast milk microwaved just enough to warm it resulted in destruction of 98 percent of its immunoglobulin A antibodies and 96 percent of its liposomal activity, which inhibits bacterial infections.[184] Even water should not be heated in a microwave, because microwave heat deforms the water molecules just the same as it denatures protein and other nutrients in food.

MSG

Glutamic acid is an amino acid that occurs naturally in many foods and is a component in folic acid and the chromium compound glucose tolerance factor (GTF).† It is a major excitatory neurotransmitter and is often referred to as a "brain fuel." This amino acid is also a necessary precursor to the inhibitory neurotransmitter GABA, as well as glutathione—a major deactivator of harmful free radicals and toxic metals in the body.[185]

However, free glutamic acid, or monosodium glutamate (MSG), which was originally synthesized in Japan in 1908, is quite a different matter. Introduced into the United States after World War II as a flavoring agent in foods and packaged as the product "Accent," MSG is a powerful neurotoxin. MSG has no flavor of its own, but it neurologically stimulates the brain in a way that causes individuals to experience a more intense flavor from their foods. In the estimated tens of millions of Americans who are affected by it, MSG causes a multitude of toxic and allergic reactions, collectively known

*The results of this 1989 research study were not well propagated because it was banned from publication by the Swiss courts. However, in 1998, the European Court of Human Rights finally allowed its publication. (G. Lazenby, *The Healing Home* [Guilford, Conn.: Lyons Press, 2001], 77.)

†When glutamic acid combines with ammonia, it becomes the amino acid glutamine. Glutamine is the only amino acid that easily passes through the blood-brain barrier.

as "Chinese restaurant syndrome" from a letter published in 1968 in the *New England Journal of Medicine.* These symptoms can encompass every aspect of the body, such as the skin (flushing and rashes), muscles (joint pain, stiffness, and flulike achiness), cardiovascular system (arrythmia, tachycardia, angina, and shortness of breath), gastrointestinal system (diarrhea, nausea and vomiting, and bloating), and the brain and nervous system (dizziness, depression, disorientation, mental confusion, anxiety, insomnia, shakiness, and seizures).* (See table 5.1.)[186]

Although the FDA requires that the ingredient "monosodium glutamate" be written on the labels of the foods in which it is contained, in some foods free glutamic acid is not added but is formed during the processing of the product, and is therefore not required to be listed. Furthermore, free glutamic acid is often included in numerous other foods and packaged goods under different names such as "textured protein," "gelatin" and "soy protein isolate."[187] Thus, simply reading labels to avoid this serious neurotoxin can be daunting even for the most learned consumer. As always, however, the best defense is to shop at health food stores, and even there, to avoid packaged goods with suspicious labels that list numerous ingredients such as those listed in table 5.2.

*Scientists and neurologists who have studied the effects of MSG-fed mice generally agree that free glutamic acid kills brain cells by exciting them to death. (J. Samuels, "MSG Dangers and Deceptions," *Health and Healing Wisdom* 22, no. 2 [Summer 1998], 4.)

Oils and Fats, Damaged

Caution with Seed and Vegetable Oils

None of the seed and vegetable oils—corn, sunflower, safflower, sesame, canola, and so forth—existed before the modern hydraulic press and petroleum-solvent extraction processes were invented after World War I.[188] Today, most polyunsaturated oils are processed commercially at very high temperatures with these extraction methods, where their natural "cis" configuration

TABLE 5.1. COLLECTED REPORTS OF ADVERSE REACTIONS TO MSG

Cardiac	**Neurological**	**Respiratory**
Arrythmia	Depression	Asthma
Extreme rise or drop in blood pressure	Dizziness	Shortness of breath
Rapid heartbeat (tachycardia)	Light-headedness	Chest pain or tightness
Angina	Loss of balance	Runny nose
Circulatory	Disorientation	Sneezing
Swelling	Mental confusion	**Skin**
Gastrointestinal	Anxiety	Hives or rash
Diarrhea	Panic attacks	Mouth lesions
Nausea/vomiting	Hyperactivity	Tingling
Stomach cramps	Behavioral problems in children	Flushing
Irritable bowel	Lethargy	Extreme dryness of the mouth
Bloating	Sleepiness	**Urological**
Muscular	Insomnia	Swelling of prostate
Flulike aches	Migraine headache	Nocturia
Joint pain	Numbness or paralysis	**Visual**
Stiffness	Seizures	Blurred vision
	Sciatica	Difficulty focusing
	Slurred speech	
	Shaking	
	Trembling	

Reprinted with permission from the Price-Pottenger Nutrition Foundation from its *Health and Healing Wisdom* journal, vol. 22, no. 2, Summer 1998.

(the hydrogen and carbon atom arrangement) is altered to an unhealthy "trans" configuration (when hydrogen molecules move to the opposite sides of the chemical structure).[189] When these polyunsaturated oils are unrefined and "expeller-pressed" with low heat, they are a healthier source of fatty acids but are still highly reactive and can go rancid quite easily when exposed to heat and oxygen. Thus, even when polyunsaturated vegetable oils are purchased from reliable companies that use low-heat processes, they must be refrigerated after opening or they can go stale or rancid. Ingesting old and rancid safflower, sunflower, or canola oils can cause free radical damage in the body, which has been linked to numerous health conditions and illnesses. For example, free radical damage to the skin can cause wrinkles, age spots, and other signs of premature aging, while in the blood vessels free radicals damage the intima (inner) walls, which allows for the buildup of plaque and cardiovascular disease. Free radicals have also been associated with cancer, autoimmune diseases (rheumatoid arthritis, thyroid dysfunction, and various anemias), Parkinson's disease, Lou Gehrig's disease (ALS), Alzheimer's, and cataracts.[190]

Furthermore, the dearth of omega-3 fatty acids in corn, safflower, sesame, and sunflower oils can create too great an imbalance of omega-6 fatty acids,

TABLE 5.2. HIDDEN SOURCES OF MSG

***Always* Contain MSG**	***Often* Contain MSG (or create MSG during processing)**	**Unexpected Sources of MSG**
Glutamate	Flavors and flavorings	Salad dressings
Glutamic acid	Seasonings	Frozen meals
Monosodium glutamate	Natural flavors and flavorings	Packaged and restaurant soups
Textured protein	Natural pork flavoring	Cheese
Hydrolyzed protein	Natural beef flavoring	Reduced-fat milk
Monopotassium glutamate	Natural chicken flavoring	Chewing gum
Calcium caseinate	Soy sauce	Ice cream
Sodium caseinate	Soy protein isolate	Cookies
Gelatin (commercial)	Soy protein	Vitamin-enriched foods
Yeast extract	Bouillon	Beverages
Yeast food	Stock	Candy
Autolyzed yeast	Broth	Cigarettes
	Malt extract	Medications
	Malt flavoring	I.V. materials
	Barley malt	Supplements, particularly minerals
	Whey protein	
	Carrageenan	
	Maltodextrin	
	Pectin	
	Enzymes	
	Protease	
	Corn starch	
	Citric acid	
	Powdered milk	
	Anything protein fortified	
	Anything enzyme modified	
	Anything ultrapasteurized	

Reprinted with permission from the Price-Pottenger Nutrition Foundation from its *Health and Healing Wisdom* journal, vol. 22, no. 2, Summer 1998.

which interferes with the production of important hormonelike messengers in the body called *prostaglandins*.[191] Over the past seventy-five years, the omega-6 to omega-3 fatty acid balance in the U.S. diet has become quite imbalanced, moving from the beneficial one-to-one ratio found in raw butter, for example, to an estimated thirty-to-one imbalanced ratio. Before these modern extraction methods were invented, traditional cultures received their dietary omega-6 fatty acids, as well as omega-3 and omega-9 fatty acids, the natural way: from whole and unprocessed foods such as legumes, grains, nuts, seeds, green vegetables, fish, olive oil, and animal fats.[192]

Caution with Canola Oil

Although canola oil contains a significant amount of omega-3 fatty acid (10–15 percent), traces (~2 percent) of toxic erucic acid, which is inherent in the rapeseed plant from which the oil is derived, still remain despite many hybridization attempts to eliminate it.[193] Additionally, rapeseed has been associated with fibrotic heart lesions, and canola oil is not allowed in infant formula in the United States or Canada.[194]

Caution with Soybean Oil

Soybean oil has over 50 percent omega-6 fatty acids and only a small amount of omega-3. Furthermore, soybean oil is the most commercially abundant food fat in the United States, and greater than three-fourths of it is partially hydrogenated.[195]*

Sesame and Peanut Oils Are Relatively Stable

Sesame oil contains 42 percent oleic acid, the stable monounsaturated fat found in olive oil, and a unique antioxidant (sesamol) that together render it useful for low- to moderate-temperature cooking.[196] Peanut oil, with a 48 percent oleic acid content, is also relatively stable and can be used occasionally for stir-frying. However, due to their high percentage of omega-6 linoleic acid, the use of peanut and sesame oils should be limited.[197]

*For more information on hydrogenation and soy, see the upcoming sections "The Toxic Process of Hydrogenation" and "Soy, Nonfermented."

Dangerous Trans-Fatty Acids

As mentioned previously, most of the commercial polyunsaturated vegetable oils are extracted at high heat (230°F) and then subjected to toxic solvents that destroy the fat-soluble antioxidant vitamin E and disrupt the natural "cis" pattern of the fatty acids into the indigestible "trans" configuration.

Cooking with these oils can compound the damage by converting even more "cis" to "trans" configurations. Trans-fatty acids have been correlated to heart disease (lowering the "good" HDL and raising the "bad" LDL), diabetes, cancer, low birth weight, obesity, and immune system dysfunction. In fact, scientific evaluation of the fat in arteries (plaque) reveals that only about 26 percent is saturated (from meat, butter, or coconut oil), while the majority of it is polyunsaturated (from margarine, vegetable oils, French fries, and junk foods).[198] Other studies have shown that trans fats increase cardiac risk twice as much as saturated fat in the diet.[199]

Another toxic chemical resulting from the high-heat methods used in making corn and potato chips, crackers, and other processed foods is acrylamide. This odorless neurotoxin has a long list of various names (including Acrylagel, acrylic acid monomer (AAM), propenamide, and vinyl amide) and has been classified by the National Institute for Occupational Safety and Health (NIOSH) as a carcinogen *at any* exposure level. Acrylamide has been associated with numerous neurological symptoms including numbness in the limbs, staggering gait, headaches, insomnia, and depression.[200]

CANCER RISK

A study conducted by researchers at the Harvard School of Public Health found that each weekly serving of French fries that girls consumed between the ages of three and five increased their risk of developing breast cancer as adults by 27 percent.[201]

The Toxic Process of Hydrogenation

Another process that creates trans fats is hydrogenation. This method turns liquid polyunsaturated oils to a solid state, such as with margarine and shortening. Manufacturers who hydrogenate begin with the cheapest oils such as soy, corn, cottonseed, or canola that are already rancid from the extraction process, mix them with nickel particles that act as a catalyst, subject them to high temperatures, and then steam-clean and bleach them (margarine's natural color is an unappetizing gray and it has a "horrendous" odor).[202] Hydrogenated fats or "partially hydrogenated" fats inhibit enzymes necessary for the body's normal metabolism of fats. In fact, the body needs *fifty-one* days to metabolize half of these trans fats, versus eighteen days for the natural cis fat.[203] Thus, it is frightening to imagine, but very possible, that your body can still be struggling to metabolize the partially hydrogenated pretzels eaten mindlessly on an airplane flight taken over a month ago! Equally disconcerting is the fact that trans-fatty acids readily enter the brain (as well as cross the placenta) and there can lodge in cell membranes and displace the important essential fatty acid DHA.[204]

Another problem with these trans fats is that they block "good" prostaglandin production and promote more of the inflammatory circulating hormones that lead to tissue destruction with resulting symptoms ranging from chronic joint pain and headaches to chronic autoimmune and heart disease.[205]

Read Labels Carefully

Hydrogenated and partially hydrogenated fats, as well as rancid vegetable oils, are prevalent in margarines, vegetable shortenings, salad dressings, most chips, popcorn, French fries, cookies, candy, cakes, doughnuts, pastries, most crackers, and many other products sold in fast-food chains and commercial grocery stores. For example, in one 1999 survey, the FDA found that partially hydrogenated oils were in 95 percent of the cookies, 100 percent of the crackers, and 80 percent of the frozen breakfast foods on supermarket shelves.[206] Thus, you should read labels carefully while shopping and avoid fast foods with hydrogenated oils or those subjected to high heat.

One positive note: Due to the preponderance of research—especially from a 1999 Harvard study reporting that an estimated 30,000 to 100,000 cardiac deaths could be prevented annually if people replaced their trans fat oils with healthier alternatives—the FDA ordered that food companies must disclose the amount of trans fats contained in their products as of January 2006. There is one loophole, however; the FDA is allowing products with less than a half gram of trans fat per serving not to disclose the amount of trans fats on the label. However, this allowance goes against the 2002 declaration of the Institute of Medicine at the National Academy of Sciences that they could not determine *any* level of healthy trans fat usage.[207]

A final piece of good news for consumers: Whole Foods and other conscientious health food stores have removed from their shelves the few products they had previously stocked (e.g., frozen whole-wheat pie or pizza crust) that contain trans fats.

Soy, Nonfermented

Plant Toxins in Soy

As mentioned in the previous "Soy, Fermented" section, the soybean did not serve as a food for the Chinese until sometime during the Chou dynasty (1134–246 BCE), when fermentation methods were discovered. Unfermented soybeans contain large quantities of natural toxins or "antinutrients," including enzyme inhibitors that block protein digestion and have been linked to the onset of pancreatic cancer in animals. They also contain hemagglutinin, which causes red blood cells to clump together; goitrogens, which depress thyroid function; and phytic acid, which can block the uptake of essential minerals such as calcium, magnesium, copper, iron, and especially zinc, which is essential for optimal brain and nervous system development.[208]

Estrogen-Mimicking Effects

Soy protein isolate (SPI), which is the key ingredient in most soy foods that imitate meat and cheese, baby formulas, and some brands of soy milk, contains aluminum (from the acid washing tanks), carcinogenic nitrites, artificial flavorings including MSG, and denatured proteins that are impossible to digest. Despite these risks, soy formula that contains the phytoestrogens (or isoflavones) genistein and daidzein is presently given to approximately 25 percent of formula-fed infants in the United States (15 percent od all infants). Furthermore, it has been estimated by one source that an infant fed exclusively soy-based formula receives the estrogenic equivalent of five or more birth control pills per day. This huge dosage of female hormones is cited as one of the causes—along with the increase of the environmental estrogen-mimickers such as PCBs and DDT breakdown products—of the earlier sexual maturation in girls as well as learning disabilities and lack of sexual development in boys.[209]

Currently Most Soy Is Genetically Engineered

Another reason to avoid nonfermented, nonorganic soy is that along with corn, rice, and wheat, it is one of the top genetically engineered crops. Based on the preponderance of alarming research discussed under the previous "Genetically Engineered Food" section, it's wise to avoid these "Frankenfoods" completely. In an October 2005 animal study conducted by the Russian Academy of Sciences, researchers found that rats fed GE soy were significantly smaller two weeks after birth than control rats. And within three weeks after birth more than half of the GE-fed rats died—55.6 percent as compared to 9 percent and 6.8 percent from the control groups.[210]

Linked to Immune System Dysfunction

Newer concerns about the use of soy infant formula were raised in a May 2002 article published in the *Proceedings of the National Academy of Science* in regard to the thymus—the gland where immune system cells grow and mature. When researchers injected mice with the soy isoflavones genistein and daidzein, they found that the weight of the thymus gland was reduced up to 80 percent and that thymus cells decreased in number by as much as 86 percent.[211] These dramatic indicators of the direct damage to the thymus from soy help explain the frequent infections, high fevers, and autoimmune problems (e.g., thyroid disease and diabetes) that are often linked to soy-fed infants and children. Additionally, soy isoflavones have been linked to thyroid cancer.[212]

Other Countries React

Fortunately, other countries have not been deaf to these warnings about the toxicity of soy. In Israel, the government has advised that *no* infants should receive soy formula, children up to 18 years should not eat or drink soy products more than three times per week, and adults should use caution eating soy because of its adverse effects on fertility and the potential increased breast cancer risk. The French government is also in the process of implementing new regulations, including reducing the isoflavone content in soy infant formula (one part per million) and requiring warning labels stating that soy foods are unsafe for children under age three, children treated for hypothyroidism, and women at risk for breast cancer.[213] In the United States, the Weston A. Price Foundation is considering arranging possible legal assistance for investigations by individuals who feel they or their children might have suffered serious medical consequences as a result of ingesting soy.

- ▶ If you feel that you or your children have suffered serious medical consequences as a result of ingesting soy, you may contact the Weston A. Price Foundation at westonaprice_soy@verizon.net, or (202) 363-4394. Serious conditions may include asthma, chronic fatigue, depression, diabetes, heart arrthymia, heart or liver disease, infertility and reproductive problems, irritable bowel syndrome, pancreatic disorders, premature or delayed puberty, rheumatoid arthritis, thyroid conditions, uterine conditions, and weight gain.

Read Labels Carefully—Even in the Health Food Store

Besides soy-based infant formula, nonfermented soy can be found in soy milk, ice cream, cheese, protein powders, "power" bars, granola, edamame, vegetarian chili, pasta, a new "woman's bread," and many meat-imitation products such as burgers, hot dogs, and sausage.[214] Sally Fallon and Mary Enig, who have spearheaded the drive to make individuals aware of the toxicity of non-fermented soy, have suggested that the widespread sale of soy infant formula as well as other soy foods may someday rival the use of asbestos in terms of public outrage and lawsuits. Unfortunately, you have to be perhaps even more careful of this product in health food stores than in commercial supermarkets. Therefore, once again, read labels carefully before purchasing any packaged goods.

- ▶ To order a *Soy Alert!* brochure or for more information, contact the Weston A. Price Foundation at (202) 363-4394 or www.westonaprice.org. Additionally, the Summer 2004 edition of *Wise Traditions* journal contains an excellent article, titled "Soy Alert! Not Milk and Uncheese: The Udder Alternatives," that details the disturbing manufacturing practices and toxic effects of soy milk, cheese, and ice cream.

Sugar

Everyone is born with an innate taste for sweets. In fact, our bodies are fueled by the sugar glucose, which is maintained at a constant level in our blood. Sugar is a carbohydrate—one of the three macronutrients that are essential in our diet, along with protein and fat. Eating complex carbohydrates—whole grains, vegetables, legumes, and fruit—supplies our bodies with the natural sugar that supports energy and healthy glucose metabolism.

TYPES OF SUGAR

There are six types of sugar: fructose, galactose, glucose, lactose, maltose, and sucrose. White or table sugar is made from the sucrose found in sugarcane and sugar beets.

Sugar Craving

Knowledgeable and holistically oriented individuals have experienced for themselves that they can derive this energy-supplying glucose from the naturally occurring sugar in whole foods, as well as from small portions of organic raw honey and maple syrup. The primary reason for overconsumption of sugar is not a lack of knowledge—it's sugar *craving*. Whether it is bingeing on cookies and ice cream or grabbing a seemingly innocuous muffin or "breakfast bar," much of the baby boom and subsequent generations have been hooked on sweets since their first introduction to formula or sweetened baby food. This sugar craving is further fueled through the barrage of advertising employed by Madison Avenue to persuade individuals that "drinking soda is fun!" or that eating plastic containers of pudding is comforting. These constant visual and auditory media cues interjected into our unconscious minds further strengthen the positive associations with sugar that we first developed during our most vulnerable years in infancy and early childhood.

Although food companies try to peddle their products as innocuously as possible, there is little difference between the consolation enjoyed from an addictive and toxic substance like sugar and that resulting from other drugs such as alcohol or tobacco. Furthermore, the physical ailments in which sugar has been implicated, from behavioral disorders, diabetes, and hypertension to degenerative diseases such as Alzheimer's, multiple sclerosis, heart disease, and cancer, can often be just as debilitating as the lung cancer from tobacco use or the dementia caused by alcoholism.[215] Consider the following devastating facts about diabetes: type 2 diabetes has increased tenfold among children in the past twenty years; a ten-year-old who has diabetes loses nineteen years of life expectancy; and presently *one-third* of five-year-olds are projected to get diabetes at some point in their lives.[216]

Real Conviction of Sugar's Harmful Effects

The answer to our overconsumption of sugar is not strict regulation—whether individually through short-lived diets or collectively as during the Prohibition years. What is required is a *real conviction* that sugar truly does harm to the body. This understanding is best gained through reading about the effects of refined sugar in books and other sources, including the preponderance of evidence attesting to the serious disorders and diseases that inevitably arise as a consequence of ingesting this non-nutrient.

Even more dramatically, individuals who personally commit to the radical steps required to truly heal their bodies—mercury amalgam removal, removal of toxic soaps and shampoos, avoiding their primary food allergy, clearing foci, and receiving their correct constitutional homeopathic remedy—can witness for themselves their progressively reduced sugar cravings in a clearer body and mind. Finally, through the remarkable process of quality psychospiritual work and inquiry into why we seek consolation from food, individuals can more fully observe their earliest feelings of deficiency, anxiety, or deprivation that most deeply drive their subconscious addiction to "fill the void" with toxic foods. Through their commitment and courage to free themselves from these unresolved feelings and habit patterns, individuals gain the strength, the willpower, and the real maturity over time to forgo refined sugar as well as other toxic substances in their lives.*

History of Refined Sugar

The abundant supply of sugar in processed foods is a very recent historical phenomenon. Sugar was an expensive luxury in colonial America, and a cube of sugar in your Christmas stocking was considered a

*For more information on "growing up as well as waking up," see chapter 18 on psychospiritual healing.

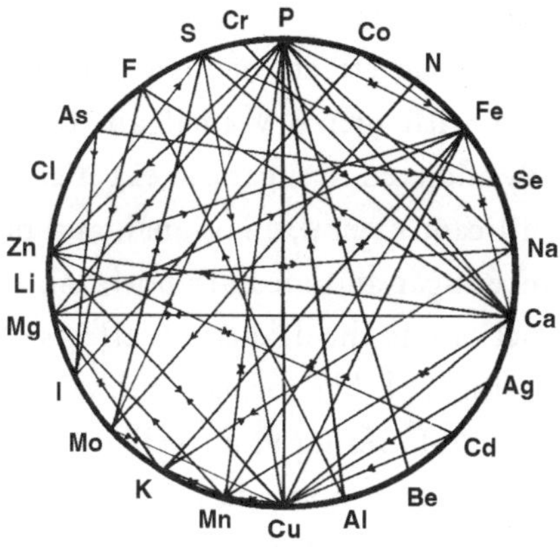

Figure 5.2. The mineral relationship wheel (reprinted with permission from Ken Eck of Analytical Research Labs in Phoenix, Arizona)

real treat.[217] Even before this period, the main source of sweets—since antiquity—has been primarily honey and fruit. When we compare this with the modern-day consumption of sugar in soft drinks (approximately 10 teaspoons per 12-ounce can or bottle) or even the so-called healthy fruit yogurts (approximately 6 teaspoons of sugar per 8-ounce cup), the explosion of sugar ingestion in the past century is clearly unequalled in history. In fact, the average intake of sugar in the 1800s was an estimated 12 pounds per year, whereas the average U.S. consumption currently is an alarming 150 pounds per year.[218] Perhaps most problematic of all, humankind has still not evolved in these brief two hundred years—and probably never will—the metabolic ability to utilize this refined food without significant harm. Sugar is the major culprit behind the rising obesity epidemic in this country. According to Robert Lustig, a pediatric neuroendocrinologist, sugar consumption is the key to obesity, by both stimulating fat storage and making the brain think it is hungry, setting up a "vicious cycle."[219] According to the Centers for Disease Control and Prevention, obesity alone is linked to 112,000 deaths per year in the United States.[220] Even more dramatic, almost one-third (30 percent) of all Americans are presently obese, and a whopping two-thirds (64 percent) are overweight, according to data collected between 1999 and 2002.[221]

Mineral Depletion

Sucrose, or white sugar, is difficult to define as a food because it is completely devoid of any nutrients.[222] During the refining process, the minerals we need to digest sugar—chromium, manganese, cobalt, copper, zinc, and magnesium—are stripped away, which forces the body to deplete its own mineral reserves to process and digest it. Depleting minerals is serious enough, but refined sugar ingestion does even worse—it imbalances them. Correct mineral ratios are very delicate and very essential in the body. If there is a shortage (or excess) of even just one of the seventeen essential minerals (out of eighty-four known minerals), the entire mineral balance is thrown off.[223] As demonstrated in the intricate mineral wheel in figure 5.2, minerals are synergistic and can function properly only in relationship to each other.

Dr. Melvin Page, a holistic dentist and nutritional giant like Weston Price, noted sugar's mineral imbalancing effect through his research on his dental patients. Page found that ingesting refined sugar causes phosphorus levels to drop and calcium levels to rise.[224] However, this excess calcium, stolen from the bones and teeth, was unable to be absorbed properly because the crucial calcium-phosphorus ratio (10:4) was out of balance. Dr. Page further observed that even though patients' blood calcium levels could look *perfectly normal* on laboratory tests, the "functional calcium," or usable calcium, was often quite deficient in the body. However, as soon as Dr. Page convinced his patients to stop eating sugar and replace it with whole foods, their calcium-phosphorus ratio would return to normal and their tooth decay, bone loss, and other nutritional problems began to diminish.[225]

Minerals not only are highly dependent on one another, so that an excess or deficiency in any one of them causes an imbalance in all the rest, but also affect directly or indirectly *all* the other nutrients in the body. Thus, a mineral imbalance from sugar ingestion also affects vitamins, proteins, enzymes, amino acids, and even fats and carbohydrates, which all require minerals to function. Normally, all of these nutrients are always fluctuating in the body due to internal and external changes in order to maintain homeostasis. However, when the fluctuations become too great and last for too long, our bodies lose their homeostatic balancing mechanism and nutritional deficiencies that can eventually lead to serious degeneration and disease creep in.[226]

Furthermore, when we consider the additional mineral-displacing effects of toxic metals, it is clear why a child with mercury amalgam fillings who is additionally addicted to sugar can experience any number of significant mental, emotional, and physical disorders. Since sugar and mercury both inhibit immune system functioning, the deleterious effects of these two poisons during a child's formative developmental and immune-system-building years will inevitably stretch into his or her teen and adult years, unless there is effective holistic intervention.

Disease and Dysfunction

The role of refined sugar in the epidemic of immune dysfunction and associated degenerative diseases today is perhaps most dramatically exemplified by the fact that the amount of sugar in two cans of soda can suppress immune system functioning for as much as five hours.[227] Thus, children or teens who drink on average four to five cans of soda a day would have little, if any, time during a twenty-four-hour period when their immune systems were fully functioning. Unfortunately, drinking soda is still popular among teens, even with the progress holistic medicine has made in the past few decades. One study has found that teenage boys in the United States ingest an average of 34 teaspoons of sugar daily, and teenage girls get an average of 24 teaspoons, with 40 percent of these empty calories coming from this "liquid candy," or soft drinks.[228]

Sugar's "unbalancing act" has been further implicated in depression, hypoglycemia, premenstrual syndrome (PMS), irritable bowel syndrome, headaches, psoriasis, osteoporosis, diabetes, Alzheimer's, heart disease, and cancer.[229]* In her book *Lick the Sugar Habit* Nancy Appleton has compiled a comprehensive list of all the damaging health effects of refined sugar, based on research from prestigious medical journals such as the *British Medical Journal, Lancet, Neurology,* and the *Journal of Clinical Nutrition.* Her list, expanded and updated, is reprinted on the following pages to convince even the most staunchly addicted readers that refined sugar causes *serious* dysfunction and disease, and that this fact is backed up by solid scientific research.

The excessive ingestion of sugar and other refined carbohydrates (e.g., breads, pasta, and white rice) has become so prevalent that it has recently spawned its own unique name—Syndrome X, coined by Stanford endocrinologist Gerald Reaven. The diagnosis of Syndrome X is confirmed in patients who have two of the following signs: insulin resistance,* elevated cholesterol or triglycerides, abdominal obesity, and high blood pressure.[230] This disorder results when excessive insulin is chronically secreted by the pancreas (hyperinsulemia) in response to the habitual ingestion of refined sugar and starches. The resulting high blood insulin levels eventually cause insulin resistance—a condition in which the receptors in the cells are no longer able to respond properly. Insulin resistance dominoes into more sugar cravings as well as chronic fatigue, which results from the glucose-starved cells, and over time into diabetes. Having Syndrome X greatly increases an individual's odds of getting diabetes, heart disease, and stroke, as well as some cancers.[231]

Politics

The sugar industry was second only to tobacco in campaign contributions to the Bush administration. These financial contributions paid off in 2003 when a global strategy proposed by the World Health Organization (WHO) to reduce obesity and curb the marketing of junk food to children was opposed by the Bush administration, which, along with Coca-Cola and General Mills, submitted a thirty-page document in an attempt to bury the WHO report. When this document, which stated in part that science did not support "linking . . . fruit and vegetable consumption to decreased risk of obesity and diabetes" and that "the assertion that heavy marketing . . . of fast food outlets increases the risk of obesity is supported by almost no data," was leaked to the press, it was strongly criticized in editorials around the world.[232] Fortunately, other countries have taken the advice of the WHO report more seriously, and several countries in Europe have already banned junk food marketing to children.[233]

---

*Whichever particular syndrome or disease individuals eventually succumb to is influenced by their genetic blueprint, or miasmic tendency, as discussed in chapter 1.

*Insulin resistance, when the cellular absorption of blood glucose is impaired, can be diagnosed by a glucose tolerance test.

145 REASONS WHY SUGAR IS RUINING YOUR HEALTH

(Reprinted with permission by Nancy Appleton, Ph.D., from www.nancyappleton.com.)

1. Sugar can suppress the immune system.
2. Sugar upsets the mineral relationships in the body.
3. Sugar can cause hyperactivity, anxiety, difficulty concentrating, and crankiness in children.
4. Sugar can produce a significant rise in triglycerides.
5. Sugar contributes to the reduction in defense against bacterial infection (infectious diseases).
6. Sugar causes a loss of tissue elasticity and function, so the more sugar you eat, the more elasticity and function you lose.
7. Sugar reduces high-density lipoproteins.
8. Sugar leads to chromium deficiency.
9. Sugar leads to cancer of the ovaries.
10. Sugar can increase fasting levels of glucose.
11. Sugar causes copper deficiency.
12. Sugar interferes with absorption of calcium and magnesium.
13. Sugar can weaken eyesight.
14. Sugar raises the level of neurotransmitters: dopamine, serotonin, and norepinephrine.
15. Sugar can cause hypoglycemia.
16. Sugar can produce an acidic digestive tract.
17. Sugar can cause a rapid rise of adrenaline levels in children.
18. Sugar malabsorption is frequent in patients with functional bowel disease.
19. Sugar can cause premature aging.
20. Sugar can lead to alcoholism.
21. Sugar can cause tooth decay.
22. Sugar contributes to obesity.
23. High intake of sugar increases the risk of Crohn's disease and ulcerative colitis.
24. Sugar can cause changes [stomach and intestinal ulcerations and inflammation] frequently found in persons with gastric or duodenal ulcers.
25. Sugar can cause arthritis.
26. Sugar can cause asthma.
27. Sugar greatly assists the uncontrolled growth of *Candida albicans* (yeast infections).
28. Sugar can cause gallstones.
29. Sugar can cause heart disease.
30. Sugar can cause appendicitis.
31. Sugar can cause multiple sclerosis.
32. Sugar can cause hemorrhoids.
33. Sugar can cause varicose veins.
34. Sugar can elevate glucose and insulin responses in oral contraceptive users.
35. Sugar can lead to periodontal disease.
36. Sugar can contribute to osteoporosis.
37. Sugar contributes to saliva acidity.
38. Sugar can cause a decrease in insulin sensitivity.
39. Sugar can lower the amount of vitamin E (alpha-tocopherol) in the blood.
40. Sugar can decrease growth hormone.
41. Sugar can increase cholesterol.
42. Sugar can increase systolic blood pressure.
43. Sugar can cause drowsiness and decreased activity in children.
44. A high sugar intake increases advanced glycation end products (AGEs), which is sugar bound non-enzymatically to protein.
45. Sugar can interfere with the absorption of protein.
46. Sugar causes food allergies.
47. Sugar can contribute to diabetes.
48. Sugar can cause toxemia during pregnancy.
49. Sugar can contribute to eczema in children.
50. Sugar can cause cardiovascular disease.
51. Sugar can impair the structure of DNA.
52. Sugar can change the structure of protein.
53. Sugar can make our skin age by changing the structure of collagen.
54. Sugar can cause cataracts.
55. Sugar can cause emphysema.
56. Sugar can cause atherosclerosis.
57. Sugar can promote an elevation of low-density lipoproteins (LDL).
58. A high sugar intake can impair the physiological homeostasis of many systems in the body.
59. Sugar lowers enzymes' ability to function.
60. Sugar intake is higher in people with Parkinson's disease.

61. Sugar can cause a permanent altering of the way proteins act in the body.
62. Sugar can increase the size of the liver by making the liver cells divide.
63. Sugar can increase the amount of liver fat.
64. Sugar can increase kidney size and produce pathological changes in the kidney.
65. Sugar can damage the pancreas.
66. Sugar can increase the body's fluid retention.
67. Sugar is enemy #1 of the bowel movement.
68. Sugar can cause myopia (nearsightedness).
69. Sugar can compromise the lining of the capillaries.
70. Sugar can make the tendons more brittle.
71. Sugar can cause headaches, including migraine.
72. Sugar plays a role in pancreatic cancer in women.
73. Sugar can adversely affect schoolchildren's grades and cause learning disorders.
74. Sugar can cause an increase in delta, alpha, and theta brain waves.
75. Sugar can cause depression.
76. Sugar increases the risk of gastric cancer.
77. Sugar can cause dyspepsia (indigestion).
78. Sugar can increase your risk of getting gout.
79. Sugar can increase the levels of glucose in an oral glucose tolerance test over the ingestion of complex carbohydrates.
80. Sugar can increase the insulin responses in humans consuming high-sugar diets compared with low-sugar diets.
81. A high-refined-sugar diet reduces learning capacity.
82. Sugar can cause less effective functioning of two blood proteins (albumin and lipoprotein), which may reduce the body's ability to handle fat and cholesterol.
83. Sugar can contribute to Alzheimer's disease.
84. Sugar can cause platelet adhesiveness.
85. Sugar can cause hormonal imbalance; some hormones become underactive and others become overactive.
86. Sugar can lead to the formation of kidney stones.
87. Sugar can cause the hypothalamus to become highly sensitive to a large variety of stimuli.
88. Sugar can lead to dizziness.
89. Diets high in sugar can cause free radicals and oxidative stress.
90. High-sucrose diets of subjects with peripheral vascular disease significantly increase platelet adhesion.
91. A high-sugar diet can lead to biliary tract cancer.
92. Sugar feeds cancer.
93. High sugar consumption of pregnant adolescents is associated with a twofold increased risk for delivering a small-for-gestational-age (SGA) infant.
94. High sugar consumption can lead to substantial decrease in gestation duration among adolescents.
95. Sugar slows food's travel time through the gastrointestinal tract.
96. Sugar increases the concentration of bile acids in stools and bacterial enzymes in the colon. This can modify bile to produce cancer-causing compounds and colon cancer.
97. Sugar increases estradiol (the most potent form of naturally occurring estrogen) in men.
98. Sugar combines with and destroys phosphatase, an enzyme, which makes the process of digestion more difficult.
99. Sugar can be a risk factor of gallbladder cancer.
100. Sugar is an addictive substance.
101. Sugar can be intoxicating, similar to alcohol.
102. Sugar can exacerbate PMS.
103. Sugar given to premature babies can affect the amount of carbon dioxide they produce.
104. A decrease in sugar intake can increase emotional stability.
105. The body changes sugar into two to five times more fat in the bloodstream than it does starch.
106. The rapid absorption of sugar promotes excessive food intake in obese subjects.
107. Sugar can worsen the symptoms of children with attention-deficit/hyperactivity disorder (ADHD).
108. Sugar adversely affects urinary electrolyte composition.
109. Sugar can slow down the ability of the adrenal glands to function.
110. Sugar has the potential of inducing abnormal

metabolic processes in a normal healthy individual and promoting chronic degenerative diseases.

111. Intravenous feedings (IVs) of sugar water can cut off oxygen to the brain.
112. A high sucrose intake could be an important risk factor in lung cancer.
113. Sugar increases the risk of polio.
114. A high sugar intake can cause epileptic seizures.
115. Sugar causes high blood pressure in obese people.
116. In intensive care units, limiting sugar saves lives.
117. Sugar may induce cell death.
118. Sugar can fool the brain into thinking you're always hungry.
119. In juvenile rehabilitation camps, when children were put on a low-sugar diet, there was a 44 percent drop in antisocial behavior.
120. Sugar can lead to prostate cancer.
121. Sugar dehydrates newborns.
122. Sugar can cause low-birth-weight babies.
123. Greater consumption of refined sugar is associated with a worse outcome of schizophrenia.
124. Sugar can raise homocysteine levels in the bloodstream.
125. Sweet food items increase the risk of breast cancer.
126. Sugar is a risk factor in cancer of the small intestine.
127. Sugar may cause laryngeal cancer.
128. Sugar induces salt and water retention.
129. Sugar may contribute to mild memory loss.
130. As sugar increases in the diet of ten-year-olds, there is a linear decrease in the intake of many essential nutrients.
131. Sugar can increase the total amount of food consumed.
132. Exposing a newborn to sugar results in a heightened preference for sucrose relative to water at six months and two years of age.
133. Sugar causes constipation.
134. Sugar causes varicose veins.
135. Sugar can cause brain decay in pre-diabetic and diabetic women.
136. Sugar can increase the risk of stomach cancer.
137. Sugar can cause metabolic syndrome.
138. Sugar ingestion by pregnant women increases neural tube defects in embryos.
139. Sugar can be a factor in asthma.
140. The higher the sugar consumption, the greater the chance of getting irritable bowel syndrome.
141. Sugar could affect the brain's central reward system.
142. Sugar can cause cancer of the rectum.
143. Sugar can cause endometrial cancer.
144. Sugar can cause renal (kidney) cell carcinoma.
145. Sugar can cause liver tumors.

SOURCES

1. A. Sanchez et al., "Role of Sugars in Human Neutrophilic Phagocytosis," *American Journal of Clinical Nutrition* 261 (Nov 1973): 1180–84; J. Bernstein et al., "Depression of Lymphocyte Transformation Following Oral Glucose Ingestion," *American Journal of Clinical Nutrition* 30 (1997): 613.
2. F. Couzy et al., "Nutritional Implications of the Interaction Minerals," *Progressive Food and Nutrition Science* 17 (1933): 65–87.
3. J. Goldman et al., "Behavioral Effects of Sucrose on Preschool Children," *Journal of Abnormal Child Psychology* 14, no. 4 (1986): 565–77.
4. S. Scanto and J. Yudkin, "The Effect of Dietary Sucrose on Blood Lipids, Serum Insulin, Platelet Adhesiveness and Body Weight in Human Volunteers," *Postgraduate Medicine Journal* 45 (1969): 602–7.
5. W. Ringsdorf, E. Cheraskin, and R. Ramsay, "Sucrose, Neutrophilic Phagocytosis and Resistance to Disease," *Dental Survey* 52, no. 12 (1976): 46–48.
6. A. Cerami, H. Vlassara, and M. Brownlee, "Glucose and Aging," *Scientific American,* May 1987, 90; A. T. Lee and A. Cerami, "The Role of Glycation in Aging," *Annals of the New York Academy of Science* 663: 63–67.
7. M. Albrink and I. H. Ullrich, "Interaction of Dietary Sucrose and Fiber on Serum Lipids in Healthy Young Men Fed High Carbohydrate Diets," *American Journal of Clinical Nutrition* 43 (1986): 419–28; R. Pamplona et al., "Mechanisms of Glycation in Atherogenesis," *Medical Hypotheses* 40, no. 3 (March 1993): 174–81.

8. A. Kozlovsky et al., "Effects of Diets High in Simple Sugars on Urinary Chromium Losses," *Metabolism* 35 (June 1986): 515–18.
9. E. Takahashi, Tohoku University School of Medicine, *Wholistic Health Digest,* October 1982, 41.
10. J. Kelsay et al., "Diets High in Glucose or Sucrose and Young Women," *American Journal of Clinical Nutrition* 27 (1974): 926–36; B. J. Thomas et al., "Relation of Habitual Diet to Fasting Plasma Insulin Concentration and the Insulin Response to Oral Glucose," *Human Nutrition Clinical Nutrition* 36C, no. 1 (1983): 49–51.
11. M. Fields et al., "Effect of Copper Deficiency on Metabolism and Mortality in Rats Fed Sucrose or Starch Diets," *Journal of Clinical Nutrition* 113 (1983): 1335–45.
12. J. Lemann, "Evidence That Glucose Ingestion Inhibits Net Renal Tubular Reabsorption of Calcium and Magnesium," *Journal of Clinical Nutrition* 70 (1976): 236–45.
13. *Acta Ophthalmologica Scandinavica* 48 (March 2002): 25; H. Taub, ed., "Sugar Weakens Eyesight," *VM Newsletter,* May 1986, 6.
14. "Sugar, White Flour Withdrawal Produces Chemical Response," *The Addiction Letter,* July 199, 4.
15. William Dufty, *Sugar Blues* (New York: Warner Books, 1975).
16. Ibid.
17. T. W. Jones et al., "Enhanced Adrenomedullary Response and Increased Susceptibility to Neuroglygopenia: Mechanisms Underlying the Adverse Effect of Sugar Ingestion in Children," *Journal of Pediatrics* 126 (February 1995): 171–77.
18. Ibid.
19. A. T. Lee and A. Cerami, "The Role of Glycation in Aging," *Annals of the New York Academy of Science* 663 (1992): 63–70.
20. E. Abrahamson and A. Peget, *Body, Mind and Sugar* (New York: Avon, 1977).
21. W. Glinsmann, H. Irausquin, and K. Youngmee, "Evaluation of Health Aspects of Sugar Contained in Carbohydrate Sweeteners. F. D. A. Report of Sugars Task Force" (1986), 39; K. K. Makinen et al., "A Descriptive Report of the Effects of a 16-Month Xylitol Chewing-Gum Programme Subsequent to a 40-Month Sucrose Gum Programme," *Caries Research* 32, no. 2 (1998): 107–12; Riva Touger-Decker and Cor van Loveren, "Sugars and Dental Caries," *American Journal of Clinical Nutrition* 78 (October 2003): 881–92.
22. H. Keen et al., "Nutrient Intake, Adiposity, and Diabetes," *British Medical Journal* 1 (1989): 655–58.
23. A. Tragnone et al., "Dietary Habits as Risk Factors for Inflammatory Bowel Disease," *European Journal of Gastroenterology & Hepatology* 7, no. 1 (January 1995): 47–51.
24. J. Yudkin, *Sweet and Dangerous* (New York: Bantam Books, 1974), 129.
25. L. Darlington, N. W. Ramsey, and J. R. Mansfield, "Placebo-Controlled, Blind Study of Dietary Manipulation Therapy in Rheumatoid Arthritis," *Lancet* 8475, no. 1 (February 1986): 236–38.
26. L. Powers, "Sensitivity: You React to What You Eat," *Los Angeles Times,* February 12, 1985; J. Cheng et al., "Preliminary Clinical Study on the Correlation Between Allergic Rhinitis and Food Factors," *Lin Chuang Er Bi Yan Hou Ke Za Zhi* 16, no. 8 (August 2002): 393–96.
27. W. J. Crook, *The Yeast Connection.* (Tenn.: Professional Books, 1984).
28. K. Heaton, "The Sweet Road to Gallstones," *British Medical Journal* 288 (April 14, 1984): 1103–4; G. Misciagna et al., "Diet, Physical Activity, and Gallstones," *American Journal of Clinical Nutrition* 69, no. 1 (1999): 120–26.
29. J. Yudkin, "Sugar Consumption and Myocardial Infarction," *Lancet* 1, no. 7693 (February 6, 1971): 296–97; S. Reiser, "Effects of Dietary Sugars on Metabolic Risk Factors Associated with Heart Disease," *Nutritional Health* (1985): 203–16.
30. T. Cleave, *The Saccharine Disease* (New Canaan, Conn.: Keats Publishing, 1974).
31. S. Erlander, "The Cause and Cure of Multiple Sclerosis, the Disease to End Disease," 1, no. 3 (March 3, 1979): 59–63.
32. T. Cleave, *The Saccharine Disease.* (New Canaan, Conn.: Keats Publishing, 1974).
33. T. Cleave and G. Campbell, *Diabetes, Coronary Thrombosis and the Saccharine Disease* (Bristol, England: John Wright and Sons, 1960).
34. K. Behall, "Influence of Estrogen Content of Oral Contraceptives and Consumption of Sucrose on Blood Parameters," *Disease Abstracts International* (1982): 431–37.
35. W. Glinsmann, H. Irausquin, and K. Youngmee, "Evaluation of Health Aspects of Sugar Contained in Carbohydrate Sweeteners. F. D. A. Report of Sugars Task Force" (1986), 36–38.

36. L. Tjäderhane and M. Larmas, "A High Sucrose Diet Decreases the Mechanical Strength of Bones in Growing Rats," *Journal of Nutrition* 128 (1998): 1807–10.

37. N. Appleton, *Healthy Bones* (New York: Avery Penguin Putnam, 1989).

38. H. Beck-Nielsen, O. Pedersen, and S. Schwartz, "Effects of Diet on the Cellular Insulin Binding and the Insulin Sensitivity in Young Healthy Subjects," *Diabetes* 15 (1978): 289–96.

39. P. Mohanty et al., "Glucose Challenge Stimulates Reactive Oxygen Species (ROS) Generation by Leucocytes," *Journal of Clinical Endocrinology and Metabolism* 85, no. 8 (August 2000): 2970–73.

40. L. Gardner and S. Reiser, "Effects of Dietary Carbohydrate on Fasting Levels of Human Growth Hormone and Cortisol," *Proceedings of the Society for Experimental Biology and Medicine* 169 (1982): 36–40.

41. S. Reiser, "Effects of Dietary Sugars on Metabolic Risk Factors Associated with Heart Disease," *Nutritional Health* 203 (1985): 216.

42. H. G. Preuss, "Sugar-Induced Blood Pressure Elevations Over the Lifespan of Three Substrains of Wistar Rats," *Journal of the American College of Nutrition* 17, no. 1 (1998): 36–37.

43. D. Behar et al., "Sugar Challenge Testing with Children Considered Behaviorally Sugar Reactive," *Nutritional Behavior* 1 (1984): 277–88.

44. A. Furth and J. Harding, "Why Sugar Is Bad For You," *New Scientist,* September 23, 1989, 44.

45. A. T. Lee and A. Cerami, "Role of Glycation in Aging," *Annals of the New York Academy of Sciences* 663 (November 21, 1992): 63–70.

46. N. Appleton, *Lick the Sugar Habit* (New York: Avery Penguin Putnam, 1988).

47. "Sucrose Induces Diabetes in Cat," *Federal Protocol* 6, no. 97 (1974).

48. T. Cleave, *The Saccharine Disease* (New Canaan, Conn.: Keats Publishing, 1974), 131.

49. Ibid., 132.

50. O. Vaccaro, K. J. Ruth, and J. Stamler, "Relationship of Postload Plasma Glucose to Mortality with 19 Year Follow-up," *Diabetes Care* 10 (October 15, 1992): 328–34; M. Tominaga et al., "Impaired Glucose Tolerance Is a Risk Factor for Cardiovascular Disease, but Not Fasting Glucose," *Diabetes Care* 2, no. 6 (1999): 920–24.

51. A. T. Lee and A. Cerami, "Modifications of Proteins and Nucleic Acids by Reducing Sugars: Possible Role in Aging," in *Handbook of the Biology of Aging* (New York: Academic Press, 1990).

52. V. M. Monnier, "Nonenzymatic Glycosylation, the Maillard Reaction and the Aging Process," *Journal of Gerontology* 45, no. 4 (1990): 105–110.

53. D. G. Dyer et al., "Accumulation of Maillard Reaction Products in Skin Collagen in Diabetes and Aging," *Journal of Clinical Investigation* 93, no. 6 (1993): 421–22.

54. S. Veromann et al., "Dietary Sugar and Salt Represent Real Risk Factors for Cataract Development," *Ophthalmologica* 217, no. 4 (July–August 2003): 302–7.

55. V. M. Monnier, "Nonenzymatic Glycosylation, the Maillard Reaction and the Aging Process," *Journal of Gerontology* 45, no. 4 (1990): 105–10.

56. A. M. Schmidt et al., "Activation of Receptor for Advanced Glycation End Products: A Mechanism for Chronic Vascular Dysfunction in Diabetic Vasculopathy and Atherosclerosis," *Circulation Research* 84, no. 5 (1999): 489–97.

57. G. F. Lewis and G. Steiner, "Acute Effects of Insulin in the Control of VLDL Production in Humans. Implications for the Insulin-resistant State," *Diabetes Care* 19, no. 4 (April 1996): 390–93; R. Pamplona et al., "Mechanisms of Glycation in Atherogenesis," *Medical Hypotheses* 40 (1990): 174–81.

58. A. Ceriello, "Oxidative Stress and Glycemic Regulation," *Metabolism* 49, no. 2, suppl. 1 (February 2000): 27–29.

59. N. Appleton, *Lick the Sugar Habit* (New York: Avery Penguin Putnam, 1988).

60. W. Hellenbrand, "Diet and Parkinson's Disease. A Possible Role for the Past Intake of Specific Nutrients. Results from a Self-administered Food-frequency Questionnaire in a Case-control Study," *Neurology* 47, no. 3 (September 1996): 644–50.

61. A. Cerami, H. Vlassara, and M. Brownlee, "Glucose and Aging," *Scientific American,* May 1987, 90.

62. F. S. Goulart, "Are You Sugar Smart?" *American Fitness,* March–April 1991, 34–38.

63. Ibid.

64. J. Yudkin, S. Kang, and K. Bruckdorfer, "Effects of High Dietary Sugar," *British Journal of Medicine* 281, no. 6252 (November 22, 1980): 1396.

65. F. S. Goulart, "Are You Sugar Smart?" *American Fitness,* March–April 1991, 34–38.

66. Ibid.
67. Ibid.
68. Ibid.
69. Ibid.
70. J. Nash, "Health Contenders," *Essence* 23 (January 1992): 79–81.
71. E. Grand, "Food Allergies and Migraine" *Lancet* 1 (1979): 955–59.
72. D. Michaud, "Dietary Sugar, Glycemic Load, and Pancreatic Cancer Risk in a Prospective Study," *Journal of the National Cancer Institute* 94, no. 17 (September 4, 2002): 1293–1300.
73. A. Schauss, *Diet, Crime and Delinquency* (Berkeley, Calif.: Parker House, 1981).
74. L. Christensen, "The Role of Caffeine and Sugar in Depression," *Nutrition Report* 9, no. 3 (March 1991): 17–24.
75. Ibid.
76. J. Cornee et al., "A Case-control Study of Gastric Cancer and Nutritional Factors in Marseille, France," *European Journal of Epidemiology* 11 (1995): 55–65.
77. J. Yudkin, *Sweet and Dangerous* (New York: Bantam Books, 1974), 129.
78. Ibid., 44.
79. S. Reiser et al., "Effects of Sugars on Indices on Glucose Tolerance in Humans," *American Journal of Clinical Nutrition* 43 (1986): 151–59.
80. Ibid.
81. R. Molteni et al., "A High-fat, Refined Sugar Diet Reduces Hippocampal Brain-derived Neurotrophic Factor, Neuronal Plasticity, and Learning." *NeuroScience* 112, no. 4 (2002): 803–14.
82. V. Monnier, "Nonenzymatic Glycosylation, the Maillard Reaction and the Aging Process," *Journal of Gerontology* 45 (1990): 105–11.
83. J. Frey, "Is There Sugar in the Alzheimer's Disease?" *Annales De Biologie Clinique* 59, no. 3 (2001): 253–57.
84. J. Yudkin, "Metabolic Changes Induced by Sugar in Relation to Coronary Heart Disease and Diabetes," *Nutrition and Health* 5, nos. 1–2 (1987): 5–8.
85. Ibid.
86. N. J. Blacklock, "Sucrose and Idiopathic Renal Stone," *Nutrition and Health* 5, nos. 1–2 (1987): 9–12; G. Curhan et al., "Beverage Use and Risk for Kidney Stones in Women," *Annals of Internal Medicine* 28 (1998): 534–40.
87. *Journal of Advanced Medicine* 7, no. 1 (1994): 51–58.
88. Ibid.
89. A. Ceriello, "Oxidative Stress and Glycemic Regulation," *Metabolism* 49, no. 2, suppl. 1 (February 2000): 27–29.
90. *Postgraduate Medicine* 45 (September 1969): 602–7.
91. C. J. Moerman et al., "Dietary Sugar Intake in the Etiology of Biliary Tract Cancer," *International Journal of Epidemiology* 2, no. 2 (April 1993): 207–14.
92. Patrick Quillin, "Cancer's Sweet Tooth," *Nutrition Science News* 6, no. 4 (April 2000); M. Rothkopf, *Nutrition* 6, no. 4 (July/August 1990).
93. C. M. Lenders, "Gestational Age and Infant Size at Birth Are Associated with Dietary Sugar Intake among Pregnant Adolescents" *Journal of Nutrition* 127, no. 6 (June 1997): 1113–17.
94. Ibid.
95. R. M. Bostick et al., "Sugar, Meat, and Fat Intake and Non-dietary Risk Factors for Colon Cancer Incidence in Iowa Women," *Cancer Causes and Control* 5 (1994): 38–53.
96. Ibid.; W. Kruis et al., "Effects of Diets Low and High in Refined Sugars on Gut Transit, Bile Acid Metabolism and Bacterial Fermentation," *Gut* 32 (1991): 367–70; D. S. Ludwig et al., "High Glycemic Index Foods, Overeating, and Obesity" *Pediatrics* 103, no. 3 (March 1999): 26–32.
97. J. Yudkin and O. Eisa, "Dietary Sucrose and Oestradiol Concentration in Young Men," *Annals of Nutrition and Metabolism* 32, no. 2 (1988): 53–55.
98. A. T. Lee and A. Cerami, "The Role of Glycation in Aging," *Annals of the New York Academy of Science* 663 (1992): 63–70.
99. C. Moerman et al., "Dietary Sugar Intake in the Etiology of Gallbladder Tract Cancer," *International Journal of Epidemiology* 22, no. 2 (April 1993): 207–14.
100. "Sugar, White Flour Withdrawal Produces Chemical Response," *The Addiction Letter,* July 1992, 4; C. Colantuoni et al., "Evidence That Intermittent, Excessive Sugar Intake Causes Endogenous Opioid Dependence," *Obesity Research* 10, no. 6 (June 2002): 478–88.
101. Ibid.
102. *The Edell Health Letter* 7 (September 1991): 1.
103. A. L. Sunehag et al., "Gluconeogenesis in Very Low Birth Weight Infants Receiving Total Parenteral Nutrition," *Diabetes* 48, no. 4 (April 1999): 791–800.
104. L. Christensen et al., "Impact of a Dietary Change on Emotional Distress," *Journal of Abnormal Psychology* 94, no. 4 (1985): 565–79.
105. "Sugar Changes into Fat Faster than Fat," *Nutrition Health Review,* Fall 1985.

106. D. S. Ludwig et al., "High Glycemic Index Foods, Overeating and Obesity," *Pediatrics* 103, no. 3 (March 1999): 26–32.
107. N. L. Girardi, "Blunted Catecholamine Responses after Glucose Ingestion in Children with Attention Deficit Disorder," *Pediatrics Research* 38 (1995): 539–42; J. L. Berdonces, "Attention Deficit and Infantile Hyperactivity," *Revista de Enfermería* 24, no. 1 (January 2001): 11–14.
108. N. J. Blacklock, "Sucrose and Idiopathic Renal Stone," *Nutrition Health* 5, nos. 1 and 2 (1987): 9–17.
109. F. Lechin et al., "Effects of an Oral Glucose Load on Plasma Neurotransmitters in Humans," *Neurophychobiology* 26, nos. 1–2 (1992): 4–11.
110. M. Fields, *Journal of the American College of Nutrition* 17, no. 4 (August 1998): 317–21.
111. A. I. Arieff, Veterans Administration Medical Center in San Francisco, "IVs of Sugar Water Can Cut Off Oxygen to the Brain," *San Jose Mercury,* June 12, 1986.
112. E. De Stefani, "Dietary Sugar and Lung Cancer: A Case Control Study in Uruguay," *Nutrition and Cancer* 31, no. 2 (1998): 132–37.
113. Benjamin P. Sandler, *Diet Prevents Polio* (Milwakuee, Wis.: The Lee Foundation for Nutritional Research, 1951).
114. Patricia Murphy, "The Role of Sugar in Epileptic Seizures," *Townsend Letter for Doctors and Patients,* May 2001.
115. N. Stern and M. Tuck, "Pathogenesis of Hypertension in Diabetes Mellitus," in *Diabetes Mellitus, a Fundamental and Clinical Test,* 2nd edition (Philadelphia: Lippincott Williams and Wilkins, 2000): 943–57.
116. D. Christansen, "Critical Care: Sugar Limit Saves Lives," *Science News* 159 (June 30, 2001): 404.
117. D. Donnini et al., "Glucose May Induce Cell Death through a Free Radical-mediated Mechanism," *Biochemical and Biophysical Research Communications* 219, no. 2 (February 15, 1996): 412–17.
118. Allen S. Levine, Catherine M. Kotz, and Blake A. Gosnell, "Sugars and Fats: The Neurobiology of Preference," *Journal of Nutrition* 133, no. 3 (2003): 831S–34S.
119. S. Schoenthaler, "The Los Angeles Probation Department Diet-Behavior Program: An Empirical Analysis of Six Institutional Settings," *International Journal of Biosocial Research* 5, no. 2 (1983): 88–89.
120. H. Deneo-Pellegrini et al., "Foods, Nutrients and Prostate Cancer: A Case-control Study in Uruguay," *British Journal of Cancer* 80, nos. 3–4 (May 1999): 591–97.
121. A. L. Sunehag et al., "Gluconeogenesis in Very Low Birth Weight Infants Receiving Total Parenteral Nutrition," *Diabetes* 48, no. 4 (April 1999): 791–800.
122. C. M. Lenders, "Gestational Age and Infant Size at Birth Are Associated with Dietary Intake Among Pregnant Adolescents," *Journal of Nutrition* 128 (1998): 1807–10.
123. M. Peet, "International Variations in the Outcome of Schizophrenia and the Prevalence of Depression in Relation to National Dietary Practices: An Ecological Analysis," *British Journal of Psychiatry* 184 (2004): 404–8.
124. V. Fonseca et al., "Effects of a High-fat-sucrose Diet on Enzymes in Homocysteine Metabolism in the Rat," *Metabolism* 49, no. 6 (2000): 736–41.
125. N. Potischman et al., "Increased Risk of Early-stage Breast Cancer Related to Consumption of Sweet Foods among Women Less than Age 45 in the United States," *Cancer Causes Control* 10 (December 2002): 937–46.
126. E. Negri et al., "Risk Factors for Adenocarcinoma of the Small Intestine," *International Journal of Cancer* 2, no. 2 (1999): 171–74.
127. C. Bosetti et al., "Food Groups and Laryngeal Cancer Risk: A Case-control Study from Italy and Switzerland," *International Journal of Cancer* 100, no. 3 (2002): 355–58.
128. M. Shannon, "An Empathetic Look at Overweight," *CCL Family Found* 20, no. 3 (November–December 1993): 3–5.
129. Harry G. Preuss, M.D., of Georgetown University Medical School.
130. *Johns Hopkins Medical Letter: Health After 50,* May 1994.
131. Allen S. Levine, Catherine M. Kotz, and Blake A. Gosnell, "Sugars and Fats: The Neurobiology of Preference," *Journal of Nutrition* 133, no. 3 (2003): 831S–34S.
132. D. A. M. Booth et al., "Sweetness and Food Selection: Measurement of Sweeteners' Effects on Acceptance," in *Sweetness,* edited by J. Dobbing (London: Springer-Verlag, 1987).
133. T. L. Cleve, *On the Causation of Varicose Veins* (Bristol, England: John Wright, 1960).
134. Ibid.
135. Yaffe Ket et al., "Diabetes, Impaired Fasting Glucose and Development of Cognitive Impairment in Older Women," *Neurology* 63 (2004): 658–63.
136. Liliane Chatenoud et al., "Refined-cereal Intake and

Risk of Selected Cancers in Italy," *American Journal of Clinical Nutrition* 70 (December 1999): 1107–10.

137. Sunmi Yoo et al., "Comparison of Dietary Intakes Associated with Metabolic Syndrome Risk Factors in Young Adults: The Bogalusa Heart Study," *American Journal of Clinical Nutrition* 80, no. 4 (2004): 841–48.

138. Gary M. Shaw et al., "Neural Tube Defects Associated with Maternal Periconceptional Dietary Intake of Simple Sugars and Glycemic Index," *American Journal of Clinical Nutrition* 78 (November 2003): 972–78.

139. Nicholas J. Krilanovich, "Fructose Misuse, the Obesity Epidemic, the Special Problems of the Child, and a Call to Action," *American Journal of Clinical Nutrition* 80 (November 2004): 1446–47.

140. G. Jarnerot, "Consumption of Refined Sugar by Patients with Crohn's Disease, Ulcerative Colitis, or Irritable Bowel Syndrome," *Scandinavian Journal of Gastroenterology* 18, no. 8 (November 1983): 999–1002.

141. Allen S. Levine, Catherine M. Kotz, and Blake A. Gosnell, "Sugars and Fats: The Neurobiology of Preference," *Journal of Nutrition* 133, no. 3 (2003): 831S–34S.

142. E. De Stefani, M. Mendilaharsu, and H. Deneo-Pellegrini, "Sucrose as a Risk Factor for Cancer of the Colon and Rectum: A Case-control Study in Uruguay," *International Journal of Cancer* 75, no. 1 (1998): 40–44.

143. F. Levi, S. Franceschi, E. Negri, and C. La Vecchia, "Dietary Factors and the Risk of Endometrial Cancer," *Cancer* 71, no. 11 (June 1993): 3575–81.

144. A. Mellemgaard et al., "Dietary Risk Factors for Renal Cell Carcinoma in Denmark," *European Journal of Cancer* 32A, no. 4 (April 1996): 673–82.

145. A. E. Rogers, H. M. Nields, and P. M. Newberne, "Nutritional and Dietary Influences on Liver Tumorigenesis in Mice and Rats," *Archives of Toxicology Supplement* 10 (1987): 231–43.

Sugar's Different Guises

The $8 billion multinational sweetener industry has many names for sugar, which can be quite confusing when reading labels.[234] Additionally, although manufacturers have to list ingredients by weight, they often include different types of sugar in a product. These various names for sweeteners may be either not recognized (e.g., dextrin, pentose, or inversol) or unnoticed, since they are buried in the middle of a lengthy product ingredient list.[235] Once again, when shopping, it is imperative to read labels. In the case of sugar, we must be diligent in learning to recognize the many names for sweeteners on the product ingredient labels, even at the health food store (e.g., dehydrated cane juice, raw sugar, Sucanat, et cetera). This section details the most typical terms used to define sweeteners—both acceptable and unacceptable—and their various effects on the body.

Acesulfame-K

This artificial sweetener, whose chemical name is 5,6-dimethyl-1,2,3-oxathiazine-4(3H)-one-2,2-dioxide, is also known as ace-K, ACK, Sunett, Sweet One, Swiss Sweet, Sweet and Safe, and Twinsweet. It is the sweetener used in Pepsi One.[236] In 1998, acesulfame-K was fully approved by the FDA for all sweetening purposes, despite previously raised objections by the Center for Science in the Public Interest (CSPI). After reviewing the data from the safety tests, the CSPI found that the studies were of "mediocre quality" and that two rat studies suggested that acesulfame-K might cause cancer. Furthermore, other studies have shown that the breakdown products in this artificial sweetener adversely affect thyroid function in animals and that it can stimulate insulin secretion and aggravate hypoglycemia (low blood sugar). Despite the FDA's approval, CSPI and other independent scientists maintain their objections to acesulfame-K due to the inadequate safety testing and the possible link to carcinogenicity.[237]

Agave Syrup (also known as Agave Nectar or Chicory Syrup)

As a recent *Wise Traditions* journal has reported, agave's "big dirty secret" is that it is neither "raw" nor made from the sap of the yucca (agave) plant.[238] In fact, agave is extracted from the large starchy agave root bulb through a complicated chemical refining process that uses genetically engineered enzymes and caustic acids. The resulting highly refined product, which contains a 70 percent or higher level of fructose, is actually chemically similar to high fructose corn syrup (HFCS) and like HFCS can cause mineral depletion, liver inflammation, hypertension and atherosclerosis, obesity, and insulin resistance (type 2 diabetes). Furthermore, the large quantities of toxic steroid derivatives known as saponins that are contained in agave syrups can disrupt red blood cells, cause diarrhea and vomiting, and contribute to miscarriage. Unfortunately, many health food stores have been fooled by this highly refined syrup, just as they have been by nonfermented soy products, and stock it liberally on their shelves. As food scientist Russ Bianchi recommends, consumers should avoid this toxic, unapproved, and mislabeled refined fructose agave syrup, as well as any products that contain it.[239]

Aspartame (also known as NutraSweet or Equal)

This widely used artificial sweetener is a neurotoxin (nerve poison) that has been linked to numerous disorders and diseases, including skin rashes, dizziness, visual impairment, severe muscle aching, numbness of the arms and legs, pancreatitis, gastrointestinal distress, nausea, menstrual disturbances, high blood pressure, retinal hemorrhage, seizures, depression, headaches, memory loss, Alzheimer's, Parkinson's disease, brain tumors, mood swings, panic disorders, insomnia, hyperactivity, and birth defects.[240] Aspartame is a genetically engineered chemical that is most often (~70 percent) used in the soft drink industry (e.g., Diet Coke, Diet Pepsi, Diet Snapple, and Sugar Free Kool-Aid), but it is also found in over 9,000 other foods and pharmaceuticals, including many low-fat products (e.g., jelly, yogurt, candy), chewing gum, and even children's vitamins and medicines. Furthermore, it is found in small packets on the tables of almost every restaurant in the United States packaged under the name NutraSweet or Equal as an "alternative" to white sugar.[241]

Despite the "damning evidence" from the original safety studies on aspartame conducted by the pharmaceutical giant G. D. Searle and Company, as well as formal objections by two of Searle's own scientists, the FDA tentatively approved the use of this sweetener in 1974. Later, in 1980, on the same day that Ronald Reagan took office, Searle—under the leadership of its new CEO Donald Rumsfeld, who had vowed that "no matter what, he would see to it that aspartame would be approved"—reapplied for full FDA approval. In 1985, when Searle was sold to Monsanto, the FDA granted full approval for aspartame. The acting head of the FDA at the time, Michael Friedman, M.D., was later given a high-level position at Monsanto.[242]

When aspartame is digested it breaks down into phenylalanine, aspartic acid, and methanol. Methanol, also known as wood alcohol, is a known poison and breaks down into formaldehyde in the body, while phenylalanine decomposes into diketopiperazine (DKP), a known carcinogen.[243] In fact, Dr. Morando Soffritti, a cancer researcher in Italy who oversees 180 scientists and researchers in thirty countries and has spent twenty-eight years conducting research on potential carcinogens, reported in February 2006 that an extensive seven-year study had revealed that this sweetener was associated with "unusually high rates of lymphomas, leukemias, and other cancers."[244] The widespread and serious effects of this synthetic sweetener are also clearly illustrated by the fact that, as of 1995, *over 75 percent* of the complaints reported to the Adverse Reaction Monitoring System (ARMS) of the FDA were due to aspartame ingestion. That same year, the United States Department of Health and Human Services published a report that listed ninety-two categories of symptoms attributed to aspartame, with the frequency of each reported complaint. Obviously, a sweetener that requires the use of chemical goggles, protective gloves, a chemical apron, and an air-purifying dust respirator by all those who produce and handle it (per NIOSH/MSHA regulations) should be avoided like the plague.[245]

Finally, recent research has revealed that diet drinks don't even do what they're primarily purported to do, which is to prevent weight gain. In a massive study of 600 people over an eight-year period conducted by the University of Texas Health Science Center at San Antonio, researchers found that individuals who consumed diet sodas gained more weight than those who consumed regular soft drinks.[246]* Although the researchers were perplexed over this outcome, it is likely that these statistics primarily reflect the normal weight gain that naturally occurs anytime the digestive, metabolic, and neurological systems are impaired and dysfunctioning, which, as previously described, have all been linked to the habitual ingestion of aspartame.

*In this study, approximately 33 percent of those drinking one to two cans per day of regular soda became overweight or obese, as compared with 54 percent of those drinking diet soda. For those who drank more than two cans per day, 47 percent of the regular soft drink consumers became overweight or obese, as compared with 57 percent of those drinking diet soda.

KICKING THE SOFT DRINK HABIT

Organic fruit juices with no extra sugar added that are diluted with San Pellegrino or other quality sparkling waters can be an excellent alternative to soda for those who are trying to kick the soft drink habit. Individuals should increase the dilution over time, until they can be satisfied with simply sparkling water and a lime or lemon slice, and they no longer crave the sugary drink fix.

Barley Malt Syrup

This syrup is made from sprouted grains and is an acceptable sweetener in small doses for those who don't have, or have significantly cleared, dysbiosis (overgrowth of intestinal pathological microorganisms—see chapter 7). Barley malt syrup has few nutrients, but its maltose content—a disaccharide containing two glucose molecules, is a less stressful sugar than fructose.[247] It has been a popular sweetener for thousands of years, especially in Asia.

Brown, "Raw," "Natural," Turbinado Sugar or Florida Crystals

These sweeteners are nothing more than coarse white sugar with small amounts of molasses added to them for coloring.[248]

Brown Rice Syrup

This thick and mildly sweet syrup is formed by culturing brown rice with enzymes. Because it contains 50 percent complex carbohydrates, it is a slow-digesting sweetener and therefore an excellent alternative to white sugar. Of course, in cases of significant dysbiosis, it should be avoided, as should all added sweeteners.

Concentrated Fruit Juice

This highly refined and concentrated sweetener contains 68 percent soluble sugar.[249] Unfortunately, it is used extensively by many health food companies and can be found in packaged cookies, cake and pastry mixes, jams and jellies, and other supposedly "alternative" treats. Concentrated fruit juice (e.g., grape, apple, or pear) can cause aberrant blood sugar fluctuations like those caused by refined white sugar, and they should be avoided.

Date Sugar

This sweetener, made from dehydrated dates, has a high tryptophan content that has a calming effect on hyperactive children.[250] Nevertheless, it is a highly concentrated sweetener and its use should be limited to rare desserts, and avoided altogether for those who have significant intestinal dysbiosis.

Dehydrated Cane Juice

This category includes the products Rapadura and Sucanat, which are sold primarily in health food stores.

Rapadura is a type of dehydrated cane sugar, similar to Sucanat, that claims to retain many minerals, unlike refined sugar. However, Dr. Nancy Appleton, a renowned expert in the field of nutrition, believes that this new sugar being sold at health food stores causes just as much harm in the body as table sugar.* Like regular sugar, Rapadura contains four grams of sugar per teaspoon, which Appleton asserts can cause an elevation in blood glucose and insulin, suppress the immune system, and disrupt the body's chemistry, similar to the effect of refined white sugar.[251]

Sucanat is dehydrated organic cane juice (its trade name is the acronym of *sugar cane natural*).[252] As is the case for Rapadura, its drying process does not strip away all the vitamins and minerals. However, also similar to Rapadura, it is a concentrated form of sugar and should be used in very limited amounts, if at all.

Fructose and High Fructose Corn Syrup

In 1976, the sugar industry discovered that it was cheaper to make sugar from corn than from beets or sugarcane and started producing dextrose, dextrine, corn syrup, fructose, and high fructose corn syrup (HFCS). Since then, the cheaper HFCS has replaced sucrose as a sweetener in most soft drinks, baked goods, and processed foods.[253] Fructose, as well as HFCS, is even more harmful than white sugar, or sucrose, especially in growing children.[254] Although all cells in the body can metabolize glucose, the liver must metabolize fructose. Individuals who ingest a lot of soft drinks, and therefore HFCS, should take note that the livers of rats on a high fructose diet have been found to be identical to the livers of alcoholics—plugged with fat and markedly cirrhotic. Furthermore, the corn and enzymes used to make HFCS are genetically modified, or GMO, foods—linked to cancer, developmental abnormalities, and immune system dysfunction.[255]

*Furthermore, Rapadura and Sucanat have not tested well energetically on patients in my clinical experience.

cirrhosis: Cirrhosis comes from a Greek word meaning "orange yellow" and refers to severe liver disease in which fibrosis (scarring) and nodular formation are common.

Fructose and HFCS have been linked to heart disease, elevated blood triglycerides and cholesterol, and excessive blood clotting and can cause the white blood cells of the immune system to become "sleepy" and unable to defend against foreign invaders.[256] Other disorders associated with HFCS ingestion are an increase in intestinal gas and bloating, diarrhea, elevated uric acid levels, and gout. Although advocates for fructose have espoused its use in a diabetic diet, it has also been shown to reduce insulin's affinity for its receptor site, which is the cardinal sign for type 2 diabetes.[257]

The addition of the inexpensive HFCS to not only cakes, cookies, and soft drinks but also thousands of other foods—from low-fat yogurt to chicken noodle soup—has been singled out by many health experts as one of the chief culprits for the rising trend of obesity. Researchers reported in a 2004 *American Journal of Clinical Nutrition* that HFCS causes more weight gain than sugar, through a process called "de novo lipogenesis," where large amounts of fructose cause fatty acids to be stored as fat in the tissues or released as triglycerides in the bloodstream. If weight gain isn't enough to convince consumers not to drink this poison, then perhaps statistics on excessive aging will tip the decision-making scale. Scientists have further found that rats fed fructose demonstrated significantly more aging markers such as cross-linking in the collagen of their skin.[258] Thus, if vanity has driven the consumption of HFCS drinks, then scientific proof of *weight gain* and *accelerated aging* with these products should certainly begin to take the wind out of the sails of this Madison Avenue–propagated fallacy.

CHILDHOOD OBESITY

A recent study conducted by Harvard pediatrician David Ludwig of 548 schoolchildren found that for each additional sweet drink (soft drink) consumed daily, the odds of obesity increased 60 percent. In fact, one out of every five calories in the U.S. diet is liquid, thus bestowing on soft drinks the designation of the nation's single biggest "food."[259] Based on these statistics and a study published in the *International Journal of Pediatric Obesity,* researchers predicted that by 2010, almost 50 percent of U.S. children would be obese, followed closely by an estimated 38 percent of European children.[260]

Honey

Raw honey (not heated over 117°F) is considered a health food and can be used in moderation by those who don't have, or have significantly cleared, dysbiosis. Unheated, unfiltered, unsmoked raw honey is loaded with amylase enzymes (which digest carbohydrates), vitamins (especially B and C), some minerals, and numerous antimicrobial and anti-inflammatory phytonutrients (plant nutrients). Most conventional grocery stores carry honey that has been heated, robbing it of enzymes and other nutrients. Buy only honey labeled "raw." Honey has been used in medicine since antiquity. It was the first known antiseptic and antibiotic in recorded history, and in ancient Egypt it was used daily as well as in battle. Honey has been shown to be excellent topically in healing wounds and superior to silver sulphadiazine (antibacterial ointment) in controlling infection in burn victims.[261]

► Three excellent sources of raw honey are Y. S. Organic Bee Farm (www.ysorganic.com), the Synergy Company's Healing Honey (www.thesynergycompany.com), and Honey Gardens Apitherapy (www.honeygardens.com).

Raw honey should not be given to infants under the age of twelve months, however, because they lack sufficient stomach acid to deactivate the naturally occurring bacterial spores.[262] Honey is also a high-glycemic-index food that is quickly absorbed and metabolized in the body. Therefore, it is best tolerated in combination with other foods such as whole-wheat breads and whole-grain cereals, so it can be more slowly absorbed and utilized for fuel. On the other hand, honey is a monosaccharide (single-sugar molecule), and it is much more digestible than disaccharides (two-sugar molecules) and polysaccharides (starches) for individuals who have difficulty digesting carbohydrates.

HONEY AND THE SPECIFIC CARBOHYDRATE DIET

Honey, as well as other monosaccharides such as those found in fruits and nonstarchy vegetables, is allowed in the specific carbohydrate diet (SCD), which was initially developed by Dr. Merrill Haas and later popularized by Elaine Gotschall in her book *Breaking the Vicious Cycle: Intestinal Health Through Diet.*[263] The gluten-free SCD diet has recently been shown to be effective in treating autistic children, especially when dairy products are also omitted. Dr. Natasha Campbell-McBride's GAPS (gut and psychology syndrome) diet, which is a combination of SCD guidelines with the probiotic supplementation popularized by the body ecology diet (BED) and the fermented foods and meat broths central in the Weston A. Price (WAP) diet, has been effective for a significant percentage of children as well as adults suffering from a wide spectrum of neuropsychological disorders including autism, ADD, ADHD, dyspraxia, dyslexia, depression, and schizophrenia.[264]

Maple Syrup

Maple syrup comes from the sap of maple trees, and like honey, when used in small amounts it is a healthy sweetener high in minerals and a variety of B vitamins for those who don't have, or have significantly cleared, dysbiosis. Avoid commercial, nonorganic maple syrups produced with formaldehyde or "maple-flavored" syrups containing as little as 3 percent maple syrup, with the remainder being primarily corn syrup. Syrup is graded according to its color and strength of flavor; therefore "light," "medium," or "dark amber" (all Grade A), or the richer Grade B, describes these characteristics and does not refer to the quality of the syrup.[265]

Maple syrup is also a high-glycemic-index food (very quickly absorbed and metabolized in the body). Therefore, it is best tolerated in combination with other foods such as whole-grain cereals and pancakes, so it can be more slowly absorbed and utilized for fuel.

Molasses

This is the "waste" product spun out of the centrifuge during the production of refined sugar. If it is extracted from sugarcane grown in organic well-fertilized soil—versus the typical depleted soil sprayed with massive amounts of chemical fertilizers and pesticides—it contains many minerals, especially iron, calcium, zinc, copper, and chromium. Again, like honey and maple syrup, blackstrap molasses is a familiar sweetener to health-conscious shoppers, and it can be healthfully ingested in moderation for those who don't have, or have significantly cleared, dysbiosis.

Refined Sugar (White or "Table" Sugar)

The deleterious effects of refined white sugar (whether produced from sugarcane, sugar beets, or corn) have been discussed in the beginning of this section. Although not as damaging as high fructose corn syrup or artificial sweeteners such as aspartame, it should still be avoided due to the degenerative effects it has on immune system functioning, the pancreas and liver, and the rest of the body.

Saccharin

This sugar substitute, 300 times sweeter than table sugar, was the first artificial sweetener. It was discovered by a research chemist at Johns Hopkins University in 1879. Used initially as a food preservative, saccharin wasn't used as a sweetener until 1901, when John F. Queeny founded a new company called Monsanto to produce and sell it in the United States. Just two years later, Monsanto began to ship its saccharin to another little-known company at that time in Georgia—Coca-Cola.[266] With the help of these two growing and future corporate giants, as well as the dearth of table sugar due to rationing during both world wars, saccharin became well entrenched in the U.S. diet.

In 1977, Canadian scientists found that saccharin caused cancer in laboratory rats and banned it immediately in all food and beverages. However, once again, corporate interests won out in the United States, and Congress passed moratoriums seven times over the next twenty-six years on the banning of saccharin until further research was conducted, but also mandating a cautionary warning label to be placed on the product. In 1991, because no definitive link was found between saccharin consumption and cancer *in humans,* the FDA conferred on it "probationary status," thereby allowing its continued sale; however, it is still classified as an "anticipated human carcinogen."[267] Saccharin has been shown to cause bladder cancer in male rats, probably since this artificial sweetener is so foreign to our bodies that it is not metabolized by our digestive system at all, but is quickly excreted through the urine. In fact, frequent urination in healthy individuals is not uncommon after the ingestion of even small amounts of saccharin. Additionally, saccharin-sweetened infant formula has been linked with irritability, hypertonia (abnormal muscle tension), insomnia, opisthotonus (rigidity and severe arching of the back), and strabismus (eye muscle focusing deviation).[268]

Stevia

This sweet powder is made from an herb found in Paraguay, *Stevia rebaudiana,* and is an excellent choice even for those who are sensitive to natural sweeteners.[277] In fact, studies have shown that stevia helps regulate pancreatic functioning in diabetics and hypoglycemics by helping to balance blood sugar levels.[278] Furthermore, this herb has antimicrobial properties and can even be used topically to fight acne, speed wound healing, and reduce scar tissue formation.[279] Unfortunately, many don't like stevia's bitter aftertaste. However, if stevia is used in small amounts for baking, this bitterness is greatly reduced.

The newer stevia-based sweeteners on the market—Truvia from Coca-Cola and PureVia from Pepsi Co.—have been deemed "generally recognized as safe" by the FDA. These sweeteners, however, are derived not from the whole plant but from two active ingredients synthesized from the plant. When active ingredients are extracted, the synergistic and balancing effect of the whole plant is often lost. Thus, until further testing is done, it would be prudent to use the whole stevia plant, which has been used as a natural sweetener for more than 1,500 years, rather than trust these new sugar substitutes from the two companies that brought us Coca-Cola and Pepsi.[280]

Sucralose (also known as Splenda)

This artificial sweetener, known chemically as 1,6-dichloro-1,6-dideosy-BETA-D-fructofuranosyl-4-chloro-4-deoxy-alpha-D-galactopyranoside, is a chlorinated white sugar known by the trade name Splenda. About 600 times sweeter than table sugar, sucralose was fully approved by the FDA in 1999. However, independent scientists have deemed the safety tests that were conducted by the primary producer of this sweetener, Johnson and Johnson Corporation, "inadequate and methodologically flawed."[269] Furthermore, in lab animals sucralose has caused shrinking of the thymus (up to 40 percent), liver and kidney enlargement, atrophy of the spleen, reduced growth, decreased red blood cell count, hyperplasia of the pelvis (abnormal growth), longer pregnancies, decreased fetal and placental body weights, and diarrhea. In fact, despite its approval, in the FDA's "Final Rule" report, sucralose was considered to be "weakly mutagenic" in mice.[270]

Sugar Alcohols

This class of sweeteners includes sorbitol (from glucose), mannitol (from glucose syrups), xylitol (from birch tree bark), erythritol (from corn), lactitol (from lactose), maltitol (from maltose), isomalt (from sucrose treated with enzymes), and hydrogenated starch hydrosylates or HSH (from corn, wheat, or potato starch). These sweeteners are called "sugar alcohols" because half of their chemical structure resembles a sugar and half resembles an alcohol. They are manufactured through hydrogenation, a process that is a known problem in the production of fats and oils; however, it is relatively unknown how these sugar alcohols are affected.[271] Although these noncaloric sweeteners are considered more or less indigestible, they can be broken down by some intestinal bacteria, resulting in diarrhea and cramps, especially if ingested in large amounts as in the case of chewing "sugar-free" gum or sucking on breath mints all day.[272] Additionally, in excessive consumption, sorbitol has been implicated in cataract formation and xylitol has caused tumors and other organ damage in animals.[273] Dr. Douglas Hunt, author of the book *No More Cravings,* claims that sugar alcohols can increase hunger and cause allergies.[274]

On the positive side, xylitol has been shown in some studies to increase the absorption of B vitamins and calcium, help mineralize tooth enamel, and prevent ear infections.[275] Due to its antibacterial effects, xylitol, as well as sorbitol, has been used in chewing gum, breath fresheners, mouth sprays, and toothpastes.[276] Thus, as compared to artificial sweeteners, sugar alcohols are a better alternative, especially in small amounts in dental products. However, like all synthetically produced products, sugar alcohols should be used with caution.

Miscellaneous

There are numerous artificial sweeteners that are still just a vision in the eye of a pharmaceutical corporation research chemist. However, there are many poised to enter the marketplace as this book is going to press. Some of these include Pfizer's alitame or Aclame (L-aspartic acid, D-alanine and 2,2,4,4-tetramethylthietanyl amine), Monsanto's neotame or "superaspartame" (N-[N-(3,3-dimethylbutyl)-L-a-aspartyl]-L-phenlalanine 1-methyl ester), and the attempted reentry by Abbott Laboratories of the sweetener cyclamate after it was banned for causing cancer in laboratory mice in 1969.[281]

For more information on these artificial sweeteners, order "Sugar-Free Blues" by Jim Earles, which was published in the *Wise Traditions* Winter 2003 journal. This fascinating exposé of the history and ill effects of artificial sweeteners should be read by every would-be dieter who purchases these dangerous chemicals in individual packets, soft drinks, and packaged goods in a misguided attempt to lose weight. No short-term weight loss is worth the havoc that these chemical sweeteners can wreak in the body.

▶ To order the *Wise Traditions* journal or a reprint of the "Sugar-Free Blues" article, call (202) 363-4394 or e-mail info@westonaprice.org.

Best Bets for Sweeteners

Natural sweeteners such as raw honey, maple syrup, stevia, and brown rice syrup that have been in use for centuries are superior when used in moderation for those who have reasonably cleared their dysbiosis (pathological intestinal bacteria and fungi). In contrast, refined white sugar, fructose, or high fructose corn syrup, which have been proven to cause numerous disorders and disease, are not wise choices. Finally, the artificial sweeteners such as aspartame, saccharin, and sucralose are no alternative at all, and are even more risky to ingest than refined white sugar.

CONCLUSION

Food and nutrition are hotly debated topics in holistic communities. Too often individuals blindly follow dietary regimens espoused by popular and charismatic nutritional gurus, rather than through their own personal experience discovering the diet that most favorably serves their health and well-being. However, there are also dietary commonalities that can be endorsed and incorporated into everyone's food choices. Following the wise traditions of our ancestors who enjoyed optimal mental and physical health just makes sense, especially when Dr. Weston Price's observations and dietary guidelines about these traditional cultures continue to be validated by modern research findings.

Throughout history, dietary changes have brought about many profound cures. However, this is rarely the case today. Individuals burdened by a history of excessive antibiotics and other prescription drugs, DNA-damaging vaccines, toxic chemicals in their home and environment, and a mouthful of mercury amalgam fillings can no longer cure or prevent future degenerative disease simply by eating well. These modern-day toxic insults are too overwhelming for the body, and without effective holistic intervention the system typically degenerates over time into the more depleted reaction modes—the exhausted tuberculinic and the destructive luetic miasms. It's important to note that this understanding is not new, but that even in the eighteenth and nineteenth centuries toxic and suppressive allopathic practices observed by Dr. Samuel Hahnemann,* the founder of homeopathy, caused him to echo this same belief:

> After it [the illness from a toxic insult] has once advanced and developed to a certain degree it can never be removed by the strength of any robust constitution, it can never be overcome by the most wholesome diet and order of life, nor will it die out of itself . . . [without the correct homeopathic remedy]."[282]

However, for those who are actively detoxifying and have endeavored to find and receive quality holistic care, an organic and nutrient-dense diet is essential. As was discussed in the introduction to this part, although diet *alone* can no longer heal the majority of individuals suffering from chronic dysfunction and disease, *without a clean diet individuals can never fully heal.*

*See chapter 14 for information on Dr. Samuel Hahnemann and constitutional homeopathy.

NOTES

1. R. Williams, *Biochemical Individuality (*New Canaan, Conn.: Keats Publishing, 1998), viii.
2. Ibid., 53–72.
3. J. DeCava, "Food Fights–Part 2," *Health and Healing Wisdom* 25, no. 4 (Winter 2001): 5.
4. R. Williams, *Biochemical Individuality* (New Canaan, Conn.: Keats Publishing, 1998), 22–23.
5. S. Fallon, "The Right Price: Interpreting the Work of Dr. Weston A. Price," *Wise Traditions* 6, no. 3 (Fall 2005): 18.
6. S. Fallon, *Nourishing Traditions* (San Diego: ProMotion Publishing, 1999), 15, 33–34.
7. Ibid., 35.
8. F. Lyman, "MSNBC Reopens Debate on Safety of Bovine Growth Hormone in Milk," www.organicconsumers.org/rbgh/msnbconrbgh.cfm.
9. S. Fallon, "A Campaign for Real Milk," www.realmilk.com.
10. W. Douglass, *The Milk Book* (Atlanta: Second Opinion Publishing, 1994), 67.
11. Ibid.
12. S. Fallon, *Nourishing Traditions* (San Diego: ProMotion Publishing, 1999), 34.
13. B. Jensen, *Goat Milk Magic: One of Life's Greatest Healing Foods* (Escondido, Calif.: Bernard Jenson, 1994), 17–23.
14. C. Kilham, *The Whole Food Bible* (Rochester, Vt.: Healing Arts Press, 1991), 55.
15. C. Masterjohn, "On the Trail of the Elusive X-Factor," February 13, 2008, www.westonaprice.org/abcs-of-nutrition/175-x-factor-is-vitamin-K2.html.
16. S. Fallon, *Nourishing Traditions* (San Diego: ProMotion Publishing, 1999), 16–17.
17. C. Masterjohn, "On the Trail of the Elusive X-Factor," February 13, 2008, www.westonaprice.org/abcs-of-nutrition/175-x-factor-is-vitamin-K2.html.
18. Ibid.
19. S. Fallon, *Nourishing Traditions* (San Diego: ProMotion Publishing, 1999), 16–17.
20. Ibid., 17.
21. E. Lipski, *Digestive Wellness* (Los Angeles: Keats Publishing, 1996), 54, 239–40.
22. Verner Wheelock, "Raw Milk and Cheese Production—A Critical Evaluation of Scientific Research" (September 1997), www.rawmilk.org/pdf/raw-milk-critical-evaluation.pdf
23. C. Kilham, *The Whole Food Bible* (Rochester, Vt.: Healing Arts Press, 1991), 58.
24. S. Fallon, *Nourishing Traditions* (San Diego: ProMotion Publishing, 1999), 31–32.
25. R. Cummins and B. Lilliston, *Genetically Engineered Food* (New York: Marlowe and Company, 2000), 107.
26. C. Kilham, *The Whole Food Bible* (Rochester, Vt.: Healing Arts Press, 1991), 56.
27. S. Fallon, *Nourishing Traditions* (San Diego: ProMotion Publishing, 1999), 81.
28. C. Kilham, *The Whole Food Bible* (Rochester, Vt.: Healing Arts Press, 1991), 61.
29. S. Fallon, *Nourishing Traditions* (San Diego: ProMotion Publishing, 1999), 4–15.
30. Ibid., 5.
31. Ibid., 6.
32. C. Kilham, *The Whole Food Bible* (Rochester, Vt.: Healing Arts Press, 1991), 62.
33. "Great Egg-spectations," *Natural Home,* March/April 2004, 34.
34. Paavo Airola, *Are You Confused?* (Phoenix: Health Plus Publishers, 1971), 61–62; M. Kennedy, "Green Corner," *Naturopathic Doctor News & Review,* May 2006, 17.
35. S. Fallon, *Nourishing Traditions* (San Diego: ProMotion Publishing, 1999), 11.
36. M. Gershon, *The Second Brain* (New York: Harper Perennial, 1998), 154.
37. Paavo Airola, *Are You Confused?* (Phoenix: Health Plus Publishers, 1971), 61–62; A. Vonderplanitz, *We Want to Live* (Santa Monica, Calif.: Carnelian Bay Castle Press, 1997), 146.
38. G. Meinig, *"New"trition* (Ojai, Calif.: Bion Publishing, 1987), 147.
39. C. Kilham, *The Whole Food Bible* (Rochester, Vt.: Healing Arts Press, 1991), 62–63.
40. G. Meinig, *"New"trition* (Ojai, Calif.: Bion Publishing, 1987), 148.
41. A. Vonderplanitz, *We Want to Live* (Santa Monica, Calif.: Carnelian Bay Castle Press, 1997), 146.
42. M. Schmidt, *Smart Fats* (Berkeley: Frog, Ltd., 1997), 48, 56.
43. J. Hattersly, "Eggs Are Great Food!" *Health and Healing Wisdom* 26, no. 2 (1996): 22.
44. U. Erasmus, *Fats and Oils* (Vancouver, Canada: Alive Books, 1986), 63, 228.
45. C. Kilham, *The Whole Food Bible* (Rochester, Vt.: Healing Arts Press, 1991), 87.
46. S. Fallon, *Nourishing Traditions* (San Diego: ProMotion Publishing, 1999), 258–59.

47. A. Jetter, "How Safe Is Your Food?" *Reader's Digest,* August 2003, 69.

48. Ibid.

49. C. Kilham, *The Whole Food Bible* (Rochester, Vt.: Healing Arts Press, 1991), 82.

50. P. Lecky, *Primal Nutrition* (Clarcona, Fla.: Primal Nutrition, 1997), 13.

51. M. Schmidt, *Smart Fats* (Berkeley: Frog, Ltd., 1997), 48–49, 54, 115–16.

52. C. Masterjohn, "The Cod Liver Oil Debate: Science Validates the Benefits of the Number One Superfood," *Wise Traditions* 10, no. 1 (Spring 2009): 19; S. Fallon, "A Response to Dr. Joe Mercola on Cod Liver Oil," *Wise Traditions* 10, no. 1 (Spring 2009): 42–43.

53. C. Masterjohn, "The Cod Liver Oil Debate: Science Validates the Benefits of the Number One Superfood," *Wise Traditions* 10, no. 1 (Spring 2009), 18–19, 20.

54. D. Wetzel, "Cod Liver Oil Manufacturing," *Wise Traditions* 6, no. 3 (Fall 2005).

55. Ibid.

56. S. Fallon, "December 2008 Update on Cod Liver Oil" (November 30, 2008), www.westonaprice.org/cod-liver-oil/171-2008-dec-clo-update1.html.

57. D. Wetzel, "Cod Liver Oil Manufacturing," *Wise Traditions* 6, no. 3 (Fall 2005).

58. L. Forristal, "Is Something Fishy Going On?" *Wise Traditions* 1, no. 3 (Fall 2000): 43–46.

59. D. Wetzel, "Update on Cod Liver Oil Manufacture," *Wise Traditions* 10, no. 1 (Spring 2009): 32.

60. Ibid.

61. L. Forristal, "Is Something Fishy Going On?" *Wise Traditions* 1, no. 3 (Fall 2000): 43–46.

62. A. Mosness, "Letters," *Wise Traditions* 1, no. 4 (Winter 2000): 5.

63. L. Miller, "Fish for Thought," *Marin Independent Journal,* May 22, 2002, C1, C4.

64. C. Kilham, *The Whole Food Bible* (Rochester, Vt.: Healing Arts Press, 1991), 87.

65. J. Carper, *The Food Pharmacy* (Toronto: Bantam Books, 1988), 269–72.

66. S. Fallon, *Nourishing Traditions* (San Diego: ProMotion Publishing, 1999), 32.

67. C. Kilham, *The Whole Food Bible* (Rochester, Vt.: Healing Arts Press, 1991), 41–42.

68. S. Fallon, *Nourishing Traditions* (San Diego: ProMotion Publishing, 1999), 47.

69. J. Trowbridge and M. Walker, *The Yeast Syndrome* (New York: Bantam Books, 1986), 131.

70. S. Fallon, *Nourishing Traditions* (San Diego: ProMotion Publishing, 1999), 52.

71. G. Meinig, *"New"trition* (Ojai, Calif.: Bion Publishing, 1987), 252.

72. J. Brostoff and S. Challacombe, *Food Allergy and Intolerance* (Philadelphia: Balliere Tindall, 1987), 423, 556, 562, 808.

73. S. Fallon, *Nourishing Traditions* (San Diego: ProMotion Publishing, 1999), 52.

74. Ibid., 584–85, 585–96.

75. Ibid., 89–91.

76. P. Airola, *How to Keep Slim, Healthy and Young with Juice Fasting* (Phoenix: Health Plus Publishers, 1971), 11, 15.

77. P. Kouchakoff, "The Influence of Food Cooking on the Blood Formula of Man," Proceedings from the First International Congress of Microbiology, Paris (1930): 782 (translated by the Lee Foundation for Nutritional Research, Milwaukee, Wis.).

78. Ibid., 780–84.

79. S. Fallon, *Nourishing Traditions* (San Diego: ProMotion Publishing, 1999), 175.

80. W. Fischer, *How to Fight Cancer and Win* (Baltimore: Agora Health Books, 2000), 130–36.

81. S. Fallon, *Nourishing Traditions* (San Diego: ProMotion Publishing, 1999), 366.

82. S. Fallon, "The Right Price: Interpreting the Work of Dr. Weston A. Price," *Wise Traditions* 6, no. 3 (Fall 2005): 20.

83. J. DeCava, "Food Fights," *Health and Healing Wisdom* 25, no. 3 (Fall 2001): 6.

84. S. Fallon, *Nourishing Traditions* (San Diego: ProMotion Publishing, 1999), 452.

85. Ibid., 452–53.

86. J. Thym, "Ancient Grains," *Marin Independent Journal,* October 30, 2002, C1.

87. S. Fallon, *Nourishing Traditions* (San Diego: ProMotion Publishing, 1999), 430.

88. J. DeCava, "Food Fights," *Health and Healing Wisdom* 25, no. 3 (Fall 2001): 6–7; Chek, "Vegetarianism Inside-Out," *Health and Healing Wisdom* 32, no. 3 (Fall 2008): 7.

89. C. Masterjohn, "Dioxins in Animal Foods: A Case for Vegetarianism?" *Wise Traditions* 6, no. 3 (Fall 2005): 43.

90. P. Pitchford, *Healing with Whole Foods* (Berkeley: North Atlantic Books, 1993), 95–96.

91. Ibid., 95.

92. S. Fallon, *Nourishing Traditions* (San Diego: ProMotion Publishing, 1999), 212.
93. Ibid., 30.
94. Swami Nikhilananda, *Vivekananda: A Biography,* www.ramakrishnavivekananda.info..
95. J. DeCava, "Food Fights–Part 2," *Health and Healing Wisdom* 25, no. 4 (Winter 2001): 6.
96. C. Kilham, *The Whole Food Bible* (Rochester, Vt.: Healing Arts Press, 1991), 71.
97. L. Gay, "Meat from Diseased Animals Approved for Consumers," Scripps Howard News Service, July 14, 2000, 1–2.
98. J. DeCava, "Food Fights–Part 2," *Health and Healing Wisdom* 25, no. 4 (Winter 2001): 6.
99. S. Fallon, *Nourishing Traditions* (San Diego: ProMotion Publishing, 1999), 31–32.
100. Ibid., 116.
101. S. Fallon and M. Enig, "Wise Choices, Healthy Bodies," *Wise Traditions* 1, no. 4 (Winter 2000): 39.
102. Ibid.
103. F. Pottenger, "Hydrophilic Colloidal Diet," *Health and Healing Wisdom* 21, no. 1 (Spring 1997): 17.
104. S. Fallon, *Nourishing Traditions* (San Diego: ProMotion Publishing, 1999), 116.
105. F. Pottenger, "Hydrophilic Colloidal Diet," *Health and Healing Wisdom* 21, no. 1 (Spring 1997): 17–18.
106. F. Pottenger, *Pottenger's Cats* (San Diego: PPNF, 1995), 9–13.
107. S. Fallon, *Nourishing Traditions* (San Diego: ProMotion Publishing, 1999), 231.
108. Ibid., 32, 330.
109. S. Fallon and M. Enig, "Vitamin B12: Vital Nutrient for Good Health," *Wise Traditions* 6, no. 1 (Spring 2005): 15.
110. S. Fallon, *Nourishing Traditions* (San Diego: ProMotion Publishing, 1999), 330.
111. S. Fallon, "The Right Price: Interpreting the Work of Dr. Weston Price, *Wise Traditions* 6, no. 3 (Fall 2005): 20.
112. S. Fallon, *Nourishing Traditions* (San Diego: ProMotion Publishing, 1999), 29.
113. Ibid., 512.
114. Ibid., 112.
115. Ibid., 113; I. Bell, *Clinical Ecology* (Bolinas, Calif.: Common Knowledge Press, 1982), 31.
116. M. Schmidt, *Smart Fats* (Berkeley: Frog, Ltd., 1997), 10, 45.
117. S. Fallon, *Nourishing Traditions* (San Diego: ProMotion Publishing, 1999), 114–15.
118. Ibid., 4, 336; U. Erasmus, *Fats and Oils* (Vancouver, Canada: Alive Books, 1986), 3–11.
119. S. Fallon, *Nourishing Traditions* (San Diego: ProMotion Publishing, 1999), 5.
120. Ibid.
121. Ibid., 4.
122. B. Fife, "Nature's Miracle Oil," *Health and Healing Wisdom* 26, no. 1 (Spring 2002): 8.
123. S. Fallon, *Nourishing Traditions* (San Diego: ProMotion Publishing, 1999), 8–9, 11.
124. M. Enig, *Know Your Fats: The Complete Primer for Understanding the Nutrition of Fats, Oils and Cholesterol* (Silver Spring, Md.: Bethesda Press, 2000), 213–14.
125. S. Fallon, *Nourishing Traditions* (San Diego: ProMotion Publishing, 1999), 159.
126. Ibid., 20.
127. Ibid., 19.
128. S. Fallon and M. Enig, "The Great Con-ola," *Wise Traditions* 3, no. 2 (Summer 2002): 19.
129. "Olive Oil's Secret," *Press Democrat,* September 13, 2005, D–1.
130. S. Fallon, *Nourishing Traditions* (San Diego: ProMotion Publishing, 1999), 20, 135, 454.
131. W. Fischer, *How to Fight Cancer and Win* (Baltimore: Agora Health Books, 2000), 130–36.
132. The Grain and Salt Society, *The Value of Real Celtic Sea Salt* (Asheville, N.C., n.d.)
133. P. Pitchford, *Healing with Whole Foods* (Berkeley: North Atlantic Books, 1993), 162–63; The Grain and Salt Society, *The Value of Real Celtic Sea Salt* (Asheville, N.C., n.d.).
134. S. Fallon, *Nourishing Traditions* (San Diego: ProMotion Publishing, 1999), 48–49.
135. "Himalayan Pink Salt," http://himalayanpinksalt.net.
136. Ibid.
137. R. Fogoros, "Salt Wars—Is Salt Restriction Necessary? A New Spin on an Old Problem," 2009, http://heartdisease.about.com/cs/hypertension/a/saltwars.htm.
138. Salt Institute, "Salt and Cardiovascular Health Outcomes," www.saltinstitute.org/issues-in-focus/Food-salt-health/Salt-and-cardiovascular-health.
139. Dr. Mercola, "Are You Eating Too Much Salt?" February 28, 2004, http://articles.mercola.com/sites/articles/archive/2004/02/28/sodium.aspx.
140. R. Fogoros, "Salt Wars—Is Salt Restriction Necessary? A New Spin on an Old Problem," 2009: http://heartdisease.about.com/cs/hypertension/a/saltwars.htm.

141. S. Fallon, *Nourishing Traditions* (San Diego: ProMotion Publishing, 1999), 540–41.
142. S. Schechter, *Fighting Radiation and Chemical Pollutants with Foods, Herbs, and Vitamins* (Boston: Vitality Ink, 1992), 72, 74.
143. S. Fallon, *Nourishing Traditions* (San Diego: ProMotion Publishing, 1999), 21, 62.
144. *Soy Alert!* (brochure on soy), Weston A. Price Foundation, Washington, D.C.
145. S. Fallon, *Nourishing Traditions* (San Diego: ProMotion Publishing, 1999), 201.
146. M. Murray, class notes at Bastyr University in Seattle, "Botanical Medicine," February 16, 1989.
147. R. Buist, *Food Chemical Sensitivity* (Garden City Park, N.Y.: Avery Publishing Group, 1986), 126, 165; S. Fallon, *Nourishing Traditions* (San Diego: ProMotion Publishing, 1999), 261.
148. T. Reid, "Caffeine," *National Geographic,* January 2005, 11.
149. R. Cummins and B. Lilliston, *Genetically Engineered Food* (New York: Marlowe and Company, 2000), 2.
150. Ibid., 21–22.
151. Ibid., 21.
152. Ibid., 30.
153. E. A. Belongia et al., "An Investigation of the Cause of the Eosinophilia-Myalgia Syndrome Associated with Tryptophan Use," *New England Journal of Medicine* 323, no. 6 (August 9, 1990): 357–65.
154. R. Cummins and B. Lilliston, *Genetically Engineered Food* (New York: Marlowe and Company, 2000), 30–31.
155. Ibid.; J. Smith, "All Thumbs Book Reviews," *Wise Traditions* 4, no. 3 (Fall 2003): 43.
156. R. Cummins and B. Lilliston, *Genetically Engineered Food* (New York: Marlowe and Company, 2000), 31–34.
157. Ibid., 34; J. Smith, "All Thumbs Book Reviews," *Wise Traditions* 4, no. 3 (Fall 2003): 43.
158. R. Cummins and B. Lilliston, *Genetically Engineered Food* (New York: Marlowe and Company, 2000), 34.
159. Ibid., 35; J. Smith, "All Thumbs Book Reviews," *Wise Traditions* 4, no. 3 (Fall 2003): 43.
160. C. Kilham, *The Whole Food Bible* (Rochester, Vt.: Healing Arts Press, 1991), 53.
161. Ibid.; R. Cummins and B. Lilliston, *Genetically Engineered Food* (New York: Marlowe and Company, 2000), 39.
162. S. Fallon, *Nourishing Traditions* (San Diego: ProMotion Publishing, 1999), 34.
163. C. Kilham, *The Whole Food Bible* (Rochester, Vt.: Healing Arts Press, 1991), 53; R. Cummins and B. Lilliston, *Genetically Engineered Food* (New York: Marlowe and Company, 2000), 41.
164. S. Talbott, "The Trouble with Genetic Engineering," *NetFuture.org* 31 (November 5, 1966): 6.
165. Ibid., 5.
166. C. Holdredge and S. Talbott, "Golden Genes and World Hunger: Let Them Eat Transgenic Rice?" *Wise Traditions* 2, no. 4 (Winter 2001): 21.
167. S. Talbott, "Is Genetic Engineering 'Natural?'" *NetFuture .org* 75 (1998): 2.
168. A. Gittleman, *How to Stay Young and Healthy in a Toxic World* (Los Angeles: Keats Publishing, 1999), 145.
169. J. Smith, "All Thumbs Book Reviews," *Wise Traditions* 4, no. 3 (Fall 2003): 43.
170. R. Weiss, "Biotech Seeds Pervasive," *Press Democrat,* February 24, 2004, A3.
171. Ibid.
172. S. Mills, *Turning Away from Technology* (San Francisco: Sierra Club Books, 1997), 79.
173. C. Wilson, ed., "Continuing Debate Over Labeling of Genetically Modified Foods," *Our Toxic Times* 13, no. 9 (September 2002): 23, 24.
174. R. Cummins and B. Lilliston, *Genetically Engineered Food* (New York: Marlowe and Company, 2000), xv, 65–67.
175. J. Smith, "All Thumbs Book Reviews," *Wise Traditions* 4, no. 3 (Fall 2003): 43.
176. J. Lanzendorfer, "The Food Biz," *Pacific Sun,* June 17–23, 2005, 11–14.
177. "The American Academy of Environmental Medicine Calls for Immediate Moratorium on Genetically Modified Food," press advisory, May 19, 2009, www.aaemonline .org/gmopressrelease.html.
178. S. Fallon and M. Enig, "Cold Pasteurization," *Wise Traditions* 3, no. 1 (Spring 2002): 9–10.
179. Ibid.; Organic Consumers Association, "Frequently Asked Questions about Food Irradiation," www.purefood.org/ irradfaq.cfm.
180. C. Kilham, *The Whole Food Bible* (Rochester, Vt.: Healing Arts Press, 1991), 38.
181. Ibid.; S. Fallon and M. Enig, "Cold Pasteurization," *Wise Traditions* 3, no. 1 (Spring 2002): 9–10.
182. T. Valentine, "Microwave Ovens . . . The Dangerous Price of Convenience," *Gerson Healing Newsletter* 11, no. 3 (n.d.): 2.
183. A. Wayne and L. Newell, "The Hidden Hazards of Microwave Cooking," 11–13, www.mercola.com/article/ microwave/hazards.htm.
184. "Food Prepared in the Microwave Oven Leads to Changes

in the Blood," www.xpressnet.com/bhealthy/microwave.htm.

185. L. Chaitow, *Amino Acids in Therapy* (Wellingborough, U.K.: Thornsons Publishers, 1985), 79, 88, 89.

186. J. Samuels, "MSG Dangers and Deceptions," *Health and Healing Wisdom* 22, no. 2 (Summer 1998): 3, 4, 5.

187. Ibid., 3, 4.

188. P. Lecky, *Primal Nutrition* (Clarcona, Fla.: Primal Nutrition, 1997), 6.

189. D. Schwarzbein and N. Deville, *The Schwarzbein Principle* (Deerfield Beach, Fla.: Health Communications, 1999), 278–79.

190. S. Fallon, *Nourishing Traditions* (San Diego: ProMotion Publishing, 1999), 10.

191. Ibid., 10–11.

192. M. Schmidt, *Smart Fats* (Berkeley: Frog, Ltd., 1997), 10, 45.

193. Ibid., 19–20; M. Enig, *Know Your Fats: The Complete Primer for Understanding the Nutrition of Fats, Oils and Cholesterol* (Silver Spring, Md.: Bethesda Press, 2000), 119–21.

194. S. Fallon, *Nourishing Traditions* (San Diego: ProMotion Publishing, 1999), 19; M. Enig, *Know Your Fats: The Complete Primer for Understanding the Nutrition of Fats, Oils and Cholesterol* (Silver Spring, Md.: Bethesda Press, 2000), 111.

195. Ibid., 196.

196. S. Fallon, *Nourishing Traditions* (San Diego: ProMotion Publishing, 1999), 19; M. Schmidt, *Smart Fats* (Berkeley: Frog, Ltd., 1997), 187–88.

197. S. Fallon, *Nourishing Traditions* (San Diego: ProMotion Publishing, 1999), 19.

198. Ibid., 11, 15.

199. L. Litin and F. Sacks, "Trans-fatty Acid Content of Common Foods," *New England Journal of Medicine* 329, no. 26 (December 23, 1993): 1969–70.

200. C. Wilson, ed., "Acrylamide Found in Food," *Our Toxic Times* 13, no. 11 (November 2002): 21.

201. R. Rabin, "Study Links Breast Cancer, Fries," *Press Democrat,* August 18, 2005, A3.

202. S. Fallon, *Nourishing Traditions* (San Diego: ProMotion Publishing, 1999), 14; P. Lecky, *Primal Nutrition* (Clarcona, Fla.: Primal Nutrition, 1997), 12.

203. W. Schmitt, *Get These Out of Your Family's Kitchen!* (brochure).

204. M. Schmidt, *Smart Fats* (Berkeley: Frog, Ltd., 1997), 88.

205. Ibid.

206. K. Severson and M. Warner, "Food Industry Targets Trans Fats," *Press Democrat,* February 13, 2005, A-1, A-12.

207. Ibid.

208. S. Fallon and M. Enig, "The Ploy of Soy: A Debate on Modern Soy Products," reprinted from *Nexus Magazine,* "Tragedy and Hype: The Third International Soy Symposium," April/May 2000, 3–4.

209. Ibid., 5, 9, 50.

210. "Russian Scientists Find that GE Soy Affects Rat Posterity," November 16, 2005, 3, www.beyondpesticides.org/news/daily.htm.

211. S. Fallon, "Phytoestrogens in Soy Depress Immune Function," *Wise Traditions* 3, no. 2 (Summer 2002): 50.

212. S. Fallon and M. Enig, "The Ploy of Soy: A Debate on Modern Soy Products," reprinted from *Nexus Magazine,* "Tragedy and Hype: The Third International Soy Symposium," April/May 2000, 9.

213. K. Daniel, "Soy Alert!" *Wise Traditions* 7, no. 1 (Winter 2005/Spring 2006): 63.

214. S. Carson, "The Shadow of Soy," *Pacific Sun,* May 15–May 21, 2002, 25.

215. A. Gittleman, *How to Stay Young and Healthy in a Toxic World* (Los Angeles: Keats Publishing, 1999), 22–23; J. Locke, "Sugar Menace," *Pacific Sun,* April 21–April 27, 2004, 16.

216. N. Kristoe, "Mike Huckabee Lost 110 Pounds. Ask Him How," *New York Times,* January 29, 2006, www.nytimes.com.

217. N. Appleton, *Lick the Sugar Habit* (Garden City Park, N.Y.: Avery Publishing Group, 1996), 17.

218. A. Gaeddert, "Herbal Treatments for Diabetes and Syndrome X," *Health Concerns* 12, no. 1 (2004): 200.

219. Jeffrey Norris, "Sugar Is a Poison, Says UCSF Obesity Expert," June 25, 2009, www.ucsf.edu/science-cafe.

220. N. Kristoe, "Mike Huckabee Lost 110 Pounds. Ask Him How," *New York Times* January 29, 2006, www.nytimes.com.

221. Centers for Disease Control and Prevention, "Fast Stats A to Z: Overweight Prevalence," www.cdc.gov/nchs/fastats/overwt.htm.

222. C. Kilham, *The Whole Food Bible* (Rochester, Vt.: Healing Arts Press, 1991), 108.

223. N. Appleton, *Lick the Sugar Habit* (Garden City Park, N.Y.: Avery Publishing Group, 1996), 16–17, 25.

224. S. Fallon, *Nourishing Traditions* (San Diego: ProMotion Publishing, 1999), 24

225. N. Appleton, *Lick the Sugar Habit* (Garden City Park, N.Y.: Avery Publishing Group, 1996), 23.

226. Ibid., 24, 25.

227. C. Dean, "Sweet Conspiracy," *Natural Health,* January/February 2001, 75.

228. Ibid., 76; R. Mestel, "Heat Is on Juice, Soft Drinks," *Press Democrat,* September 27, 2005, D-1.

229. C. Dean, "Sweet Conspiracy," *Natural Health,* January/February 2001, 59–109; J. Locke, "Sugar Menace," *Pacific Sun,* April 21–April 27, 2004, 15.

230. A. Gaeddert, "Herbal Treatments for Diabetes and Syndrome X," *Health Concerns* 12, no. 1 (2004): 199.

231. A. Gittleman, *How to Stay Young and Healthy in a Toxic World* (Los Angeles: Keats Publishing, 1999), 22–24.

232. J. Locke, "Sugar Menace," *Pacific Sun,* April 21–April 27, 2004, 17.

233. Ibid., 17, 18.

234. C. Kilham, *The Whole Food Bible* (Rochester, Vt.: Healing Arts Press, 1991), 105.

235. C. Dean, "Sweet Conspiracy," *Natural Health,* January/February 2001, 79.

236. J. Earles, "Sugar-Free Blues," *Wise Traditions* 4, no. 4 (Winter 2003): 25–26.

237. Ibid.

238. S. Morell and R. Nagel, "Worse than We Thought: The Lowdown on High Fructose Corn Syrup and Agave 'Nectar,'" *Wise Traditions* 10, no. 1 (Spring 2009): 49.

239. Ibid, 49–51.

240. S. Fallon, *Nourishing Traditions* (San Diego: ProMotion Publishing, 1999,) 51; R. Golan, *Optimal Wellness* (New York: Ballantine Books, 1995), 66; A. Gittleman, *How to Stay Young and Healthy in a Toxic World* (Los Angeles: Keats Publishing, 1999), 28–29; C. Dean, "Sweet Conspiracy," *Natural Health,* January/February 2001, 125; M. Warner, "The Lowdown on Sweet?" *New York Times,* February 12, 2006, www.nytimes.com.

241. R. Cummins and B. Lilliston, *Genetically Engineered Food* (New York: Marlowe and Company, 2000), 107.

242. J. Earles, "Sugar-Free Blues," *Wise Traditions* 4, no. 4 (Winter 2003): 21–22.

243. Ibid., 22.

244. M. Warner, "The Lowdown on Sweet?" *New York Times,* February 12, 2006, www.nytimes.com.

245. J. Earles, "Sugar-Free Blues," *Wise Traditions* 4, no. 4 (Winter 2003): 22, 23.

246. T. Mitchell, "Diet Soda? Fat Chance," *USA Weekend,* July 22–24, 2005, 10.

247. S. Fallon, *Nourishing Traditions* (San Diego: ProMotion Publishing, 1999), 537.

248. Ibid.; C. Kilham, *The Whole Food Bible* (Rochester, Vt.: Healing Arts Press, 1991), 107.

249. B. Skinner and D. Skinner, "How Sweet It Is!" Cypress Natural Medicine Newsletter, www.cypressnaturopathic.com.

250. S. Fallon, *Nourishing Traditions* (San Diego: ProMotion Publishing, 1999), 536–37.

251. N. Appleton, "From Our Readers: New Sugar, Old Problems," *Health and Healing Wisdom* 26, no. 2 (Summer 2002): 25.

252. S. Fallon, *Nourishing Traditions* (San Diego: ProMotion Publishing, 1999), 536.

253. N. Appleton, *Lick the Sugar Habit* (Garden City Park, N.Y.: Avery Publishing Group, 1996), 57.

254. S. Fallon, *Nourishing Traditions* (San Diego: ProMotion Publishing, 1999), 52, 537.

255. L. Forristal, "The Murky World of High Fructose Corn Syrup," *Wise Traditions* 2, no. 3 (Fall 2001), 61.

256. N. Appleton, *Lick the Sugar Habit* (Garden City Park, N.Y.: Avery Publishing Group, 1996), 57.

257. S. Morell and R. Nagel, "Worse Than We Thought: The Lowdown on High Fructose Corn Syrup and Agave 'Nectar,'" *Wise Traditions* 10, no. 1 (Spring 2009), 46.

258. M. Santora, "East Meets West, Adding Pounds and Peril," *New York Times,* January 12, 2006, www.nytimes.com=2006=01=22=nyregionspecial5=12diabetes.html.

259. A. Marchione, "AP Studies: Sodas a Cause of Obesity," *Press Democrat,* March 6, 2006, A3.

260. M. Burns, "Childhood Obesity to Bloat Manifold by 2010: Study," March 6, 2006, 1, www.earthtimes.org/articles/news/5628.html.

261. National Honey Board, "Honey as Healer," *Health and Healing Wisdom* 24, no. 3 (Fall/Winter 2000): 9.

262. S. Fallon, *Nourishing Traditions* (San Diego: ProMotion Publishing, 1999), 536.

263. J. Matthews, *Nourishing Hope for Autism* (San Francisco: Healthful Living Media, 2008), 99.

264. N. Campbell-McBride, "Gut and Psychology Syndrome," *Wise Traditions* 8, no. 4 (Winter 2007): 13–23.

265. C. Kilham, *The Whole Food Bible* (Rochester, Vt.: Healing Arts Press, 1991), 110.

266. J. Earles, "Sugar-Free Blues," *Wise Traditions* 4, no. 4 (Winter 2003): 23.

267. Ibid.

268. Ibid.

269. Ibid., 27.

270. Ibid.
271. Ibid., 30, 31.
272. A. Gittleman, *How to Stay Young and Healthy in a Toxic World* (Los Angeles: Keats Publishing, 1999), 29–30.
273. Ibid.; C. Kilham, *The Whole Food Bible* (Rochester, Vt.: Healing Arts Press, 1991), 106.
274. A. Gittleman, *How to Stay Young and Healthy in a Toxic World* (Los Angeles: Keats Publishing, 1999), 29.
275. J. Earles, "Sugar-Free Blues," *Wise Traditions* 4, no. 4 (Winter 2003): 31.
276. B. Skinner and D. Skinner, "How Sweet It Is!" *Cypress Natural Medicine Newsletter,* www.cypressnaturopathic.com.
277. S. Fallon, *Nourishing Traditions* (San Diego: ProMotion Publishing, 1999), 536.
278. C. Dean, "Sweet Conspiracy," *Natural Health,* January/February 2001, 125.
279. J. Earles, "Sugar-Free Blues," *Wise Traditions* 4, no. 4 (Winter 2003): 34.
280. Dr. Mercola, "FDA Approves Two New Stevia-based Sweeteners," January 10, 2009, www.mercola.com.
281. Ibid.
282. G. Vithoulkas, *The Science of Homeopathy* (New York: Grove Press, 1980), 123.

6

FOOD ALLERGIES: A HIDDEN EPIDEMIC

Food sensitivities and allergies have become such a major and universal problem that they have necessitated their own chapter in this book. Whether it's wheat, milk, corn, soy, eggs, or chocolate, avoiding one or more of these common offenders for months or even years is often an essential step in restoring optimal digestive and immune system functioning. Considering what we learned in chapter 5 about corn sweeteners, pasteurized milk, and (unfermented) soy products, it is not surprising that these common foods can cause allergic reactions and should be avoided by health-conscious individuals. Other foods, however, such as fertile eggs from free-range chickens or raw butter from grass-fed cows, are a shame to eliminate from anyone's diet. Fortunately, these products and other healthier forms of the past-adulterated foods can often be reintroduced into the diet after a reasonable period of abstinence when combined with effective holistic therapies.

The word *allergy* derives from the Greek words *allos,* meaning "other," and *ergon,* meaning "work," which suitably describe the immune system's function or "work" of protecting against foreign or "other" invaders.[1] In fact, the father of medicine himself, Hippocrates, observed that milk could cause gastric upset and urticaria (hives).[2] Despite this recognition of food allergies since antiquity, most individuals equate the term *allergy* only to the immune system's *acute* response to seasonal environmental allergies—immediate sneezing, weepy eyes, and a runny nose from pollen, grasses, house dust, mold, animal hair, and so forth. In actuality, allergies to food are more common than seasonal sensitivities; however, they are the most underdiagnosed. In fact, Arthur Coca, M.D., a pioneer in the allergy field who has been called the "dean of American immunologists," asserted even in the mid-1950s, before processed foods had gained the momentum they have today, that as many as 90 percent of Americans suffer from one or more food allergies.[3] And it has been further estimated that 80 percent of all these food allergy reactions are not the immediate or acute (IgE) type, but the delayed or "hidden" (IgG) type.[4] Understandably, these delayed food allergy reactions are difficult to correlate to the offending food, which might have been ingested hours or even days before. Thus, for the vast majority of individuals, food allergy symptoms are often misdiagnosed or entirely overlooked.

TYPES OF FOOD ALLERGY REACTIONS

Acute Reactions

The well-known immediate or acute reaction to foods, generally occurring within seconds or less than an hour's time, is referred to as a *type I* response in immunology. This occurs when an offending food, known as an *antigen,* binds to a defending *antibody,* specifically the immunoglobulin IgE type circulating in the blood. An acute food allergy reaction is apparent by precipitating typical histamine reactions such as hives, edema (lip or body swelling), redness, itching, gastrointestinal distress (e.g., pain, cramping, and diarrhea), asthma, and even anaphylaxis (severe shock, collapse, and sometimes even death). These first-line defense responses are most often induced by histamine-releasing foods such as peanuts, egg whites, fish, shellfish, chocolate, alcohol (especially red wine), and some fruits (e.g., strawberries and tomatoes).[5] Other immediate food allergy reactions can be precipitated by tyramine-containing foods* (chocolate, yeast, fermented cheeses, white wine), food additives (monosodium glutamate or MSG), coloring agents (tartrazine and erythrosine), preservatives (benzoates and sulfur dioxide), and synthetic antioxidants (sodium nitrite in pork).[6]

antibodies: *Antibodies* are specialized proteins that are produced by lymphocytes in order to neutralize an offending foreign protein or toxin referred to as an *antigen.* Antibodies are also referred to as *immunoglobulins,* abbreviated as *Ig,* which are divided into five classes: IgA, IgD, IgE, IgG, and IgM. IgE antibodies are involved in acute food allergy reactions, and IgG, IgM, and IgA antibodies participate in delayed food allergy reactions.†

Delayed Reactions

Less well known is the second type of food allergy known as the delayed or "hidden" allergy reaction. This type of allergy stimulates the response of other circulating antibodies—primarily IgG immunoglobulins, but also IgM and IgA immunoglobulins and "T cells" (lymphocytes that develop in the thymus gland)‡—that trigger symptoms over an hour or so after consumption of the offending food, as well as *up to two to three days later.*[7] Based on this lengthier timeline, delayed food allergy reactions are less frequently diagnosed than acute ones, because symptoms that typically arise much later are rarely attributed to the food eaten a day, or even several days, before. Additionally, this more common food allergy reaction can involve any organ system and cause myriad symptoms, not just the classic skin and respiratory responses associated with acute food allergy reactions.[8] For example, such diverse and seemingly non-digestive-related symptoms as panic attacks, bladder infections, or even an increased severity of monthly menstrual cramps are rarely correlated with food allergies in most people's minds—and even by the majority of physicians. Finally, the symptoms of delayed food allergy responses are in most cases much more subtle than with acute reactions. For example, classic delayed responses include mild fatigue and depression, intermittent joint pain, and periodic headaches. Unfortunately, when most patients present in the office of their allopathic practitioner with chronic symptoms such as these, an NSAID (non-steroidal anti-inflammatory drug) such as ibuprofen or aspirin or an SSRI (selective serotonin reuptake inhibitor) antidepressant such as Prozac, Zoloft, Paxil, or Luvox is typically prescribed, rather than an in-depth history-taking and a well-considered working diagnosis.

allergy/sensitivity: In classical immunological terminology, an *allergy* is defined as the immediate, IgE-mediated type of reaction, and the delayed responses are most typically referred to as food *sensitivities.* However, as more and more holistic practitioners have observed, delayed allergic reactions are actually much more insidious and debilitating than the more transient symptoms of IgE antibody-mediated responses—that is, a transient rash from strawberries, stomach cramps from sodium nitrite in pork, or a bout of sneezing from shellfish (unless of course it's a more rare but deadly anaphylactic shock reaction). Thus, this older "IgE-only" allergy definition has become somewhat obsolete. Therefore, in this chapter, the stronger appellation *allergy* will be used to characterize both acute and delayed food allergy responses. However, for the sake of avoiding redundancy and due to the fact that in general language the terms *allergy* and *sensitivity* are relative synonyms, these terms will be used rather interchangeably in various parts of the text.

working diagnosis: A *working* diagnosis is when a physician is not completely sure of the actual cause of the problem, but based on a patient's signs and symptoms, he or she postulates one or more diagnoses to be later confirmed or discarded depending on whether or not the proposed treatment shows them to be accurate. For example,

*Tyramine is produced from the breakdown of the amino acid tyrosine and causes noradrenaline release and a rise in blood pressure.

†IgD is found in low levels in serum; its role is uncertain. Research has indicated that this antibody may be involved in the pathogenesis of the measles virus. (M. I. Luster et. al., "Measles Virus-specific IgD Antibodies in Patients with Subacute Sclerosing Panencephalitis," *Proceedings of the National Academy of Sciences* 73, no. 4 [April 1976]: 1297–99.)

‡This delayed response can be mediated by the binding of IgG or IgM antibodies to antigens (type II), the binding of IgG antigens to antibodies to form immune complexes (type III), and the reaction of T cells, or T lymphocytes, to tissues sensitized by allergens (type IV).

a holistic practitioner may make two working diagnoses of a patient's depression, attributing it to the patient's load of mercury amalgam fillings and/or a suspected food allergy. Often both these working diagnoses will be confirmed if, for example, the patient's mood improves after she or he has avoided the allergenic food *as well as* had the fillings replaced with a less toxic alternative material.

CAUSES OF FOOD ALLERGIES

A food allergy is defined as an abnormal reaction to a generally harmless substance. One may wonder why circulating antibodies (IgE, IgG, IgM, and IgA) would react to "harmless" food substances, when the immune system is supposed to protect us only from harmful invaders such as bacteria, viruses, toxins, and other antigens. Unfortunately, in today's world, foods at conventional grocery stores are far from harmless.

Toxic Dairy Antigens

The two most common food allergens—milk products and wheat—are completely adulterated by modern processing methods. Homogenization and pasteurization not only denature milk proteins but also deplete the enzymes necessary for complete digestion. When these indigestible milk antigens are absorbed into the bloodstream, they are tagged as foreign by the immune system, in the same way as an invading bacterium or other toxin that the body must defend itself against.

THE MODERN COW

Modern farming practices have also wreaked significant damage when it comes to our relationship with dairy. For example, most commercial milk comes from the modern Holstein cow. Sadly, this animal has been bred to produce three times as much milk as the old-fashioned cow and usually is fed antibiotics and high levels of growth hormones.

One way to reduce dairy sensitivity is to buy milk from old-fashioned breeds of cows such as Jerseys, Guernseys, Red Devons, Brown Swiss, or older genetic lines of Holsteins. For more information, go to www.realmilk.com.

The Same Old Wheat—Over and Over

In former times, grains used to be partially germinated or sprouted by being left to stand in sheaves and stacks in open fields, which greatly increased their vitamin content and neutralized the phytotoxins that normally inhibit digestion.[9] Sadly, the faster and more efficient farming methods of the present day don't allow the time for this germination to occur, rendering modern wheat more difficult to digest. Additionally, as health-conscious consumers are aware, in most commercial grocery stores wheat is available only in a white flour state, and often "enriched" with B vitamins and iron, in a futile attempt to recover the nutrients lost through the refining process. Consumers should avoid these "enriched" grains like the plague, since the added vitamins and minerals are synthetically derived and often toxic, such as a metallic form of iron in "iron-fortified" foods.[10] Additionally, when the bran and germ that contain the vitamins and minerals are removed in the refining process, the body absorbs the refined carbohydrate too quickly and blood sugar rises too precipitously. Over time, this can lead to type 2 diabetes.

phytotoxins: *Phytotoxins* are naturally occurring toxins in plants, which many ancient cultures knew how to neutralize through sprouting, fermenting, soaking, dehydrating, and other methods.

THE "RISE" OF REFINED BREAD

Refined bread became popular in the early twentieth century, at the same time that many toxic metals (mercury amalgam fillings) and petrochemicals were introduced. In 1910, 70 percent of all bread eaten in the United States was baked at home, but by 1930 this percentage had dropped to 30 percent. After the Continental Baking Company introduced Wonder Bread in 1927, home bread baking became more and more rare in U.S. households.[11]

Furthermore, the majority of Americans tend to eat *only* wheat—from breakfast toast to sandwiches for lunch to rolls for dinner—in contrast to rotating into their diet other nutritious grains such as quinoa, amaranth, teff, and millet. In fact, of the more than 4,000 edible plant species (including vegetables and grains), only 150 are cultivated today, and just *three* of them provide 60 percent of the world's food. Additionally, out of the more than 200 varieties of wheat, only *three* account for *90 percent* of all the wheat grown in the world today.[12]

Thus, due to the overconsumption of the same species of wheat, as well as the refining process that strips away the nutrients embodied in the whole grain—not to mention the immunological havoc that comes with the genetic engineering of wheat—allergies to wheat and other gluten-containing grains have become more common today than dairy allergies.[13]

SEVERE DISORDERS HAVE MULTIPLE CAUSES

It's important to realize that in most cases, severe disorders are caused by many factors. For example, a child with autism often has a gluten allergy, vaccinosis after an MMR (measles, mumps, and rubella) vaccination (see chapter 15), and a narrow palate developmentally that is impinging on his pituitary and brain functioning (see chapter 16).

Refined Sugar's Toxic Influence

Another contributing cause to food allergies is the concomitant use of refined sugar. Dr. Nancy Appleton, whose expertise on the toxic effects of refined sugar was described in chapter 5, makes the point that it is *not* a coincidence that the foods that most people are allergic to—milk, wheat, corn, and chocolate—are the ones most commonly eaten with sugar.[14] Thus, eating ice cream, pudding, cookies, and cakes and drinking soft drinks in our younger formative and developmental years causes our immune systems to associate the indigestible toxic sugar with the dairy, wheat, and corn with which it was combined, and therefore we develop defensive allergic reactions over time to *both* substances. Dr. Appleton also believes that because eggs are also typically eaten at breakfast with sugary foods such as doughnuts, pastries, toast and jelly, orange juice, and other sweet fruit juices, the same immunological generalizing mechanism occurs with this common allergen.

Miasmic (Inherited) Allergenic Tendencies

There is also a significant familial (or miasmic) tendency to inherit a proclivity toward allergies. In fact, if both parents have allergies, their offspring have a 75 percent chance of developing allergies themselves, and most commonly to the identical foods. However, if only one parent has allergies, then the child's chance of developing the same sensitivity is reduced to 50 percent.[15]

Environmental Factors—Fetal and Infant Life

Food allergy tendencies can be developed during gestation (pregnancy) from exposure to undigested food proteins from the mother that pass through the placenta to the fetus.[16] Therefore, women who eat a clean and relatively allergenic-free diet during their pregnancy can greatly help reduce future allergic tendencies in their children. Furthermore, infants born vaginally begin life more often with healthy intestinal flora (good bacteria), which is essential for optimal immune system functioning and reducing the chance for future allergies. In fact, in one study of four- to six-day-old infants, 60 percent of those born vaginally had helpful *Bifidobacteria infantis* in their gastrointestinal tract versus only 9 percent of the babies born through cesarean.[17]

Additionally, short-term or, even worse, no breast-feeding at all has been highly correlated to the tendency to have food allergies. This omission in an infant's immunological development is often doubly compounded by the substitution of allergenic cow's milk, soy milk, or formulas containing toxic preservatives. At least four months of breast-feeding is the standard recommendation to help prevent allergies and other immunological weaknesses in infants and children, and six months is considered optimum. Another factor is smoking, which if done by one or both parents during pregnancy or during an individual's infancy or childhood greatly contributes to impaired immune responses and a tendency toward food and environmental allergies. Finally, taking excessive doses of antibiotics or breathing toxic household chemicals such as formaldehyde increases the chances that a child will suffer from allergies.[18] Thus, based on all these pervasive negative influences, it is easy to understand why an estimated 95 out of every 100 people in modern industrialized nations suffer from some type of adverse food reaction.[19]

A NOTE ON BREAST-FEEDING

Breast milk is still the optimal choice of nutrition for infants, despite the *very* distressing fact that it has become tainted with toxic chemicals, metals, and pathogenic microorganisms since the mid-twentieth century. The best a new mother can do is clean up her body as much as possible *at least* months—preferably years—before conception, and supplement with quality bifidobacteria. (More on probiotic supplementation with lactobacilli and bifidobacteria is provided in the next chapter. See "Treatment of Dysbiosis" on page 243.)

FOOD ALLERGY TESTING

Skin Prick and Blood Tests

You can save yourself considerable expense and time by skipping the classic skin prick or scratch test administered by many allergists. Its reliability is highly debated, because it is notorious for giving too many false positive (too many foods testing positive) as well as false negative (the allergenic food not testing positive) results.[20] Furthermore, indirect skin testing measures only the IgE-mediated immediate or acute food reactions; therefore, it is unsuitable for testing the majority of delayed food sensitivities.[21] This is also true for the radioallergosorbent test (RAST). The enzyme-linked serum assay (ELISA) and cytotoxic testing have both been criticized for giving too many false positives.[22] Furthermore, when told to avoid twenty to thirty foods based on the results of one of these tests, most individuals either will refuse to do it at all or will soon fail in their resolve, which can be both frustrating and self-defeating.

Additionally, the more subtle sensitivities that arise intermittently with excessive ingestion, such as sensitivities to some spices, fruits, or certain meats, which can show up on these blood tests, are often considerably reduced in occurrence and intensity when individuals avoid their primary allergenic food(s). This is also the case for environmental allergies. When individuals avoid their one or two primary allergenic foods, seasonal reactions to dust and pollen are greatly reduced, and sometimes completely eradicated. Although the enzyme-linked serum assay/advanced cell test (ELISA/ACT) was developed to measure delayed hypersensitivity reactions and give no false positives and less than 0.2 percent false negatives, clinical correlations with patients' actual reactions in these tests have not corresponded satisfactorily either.[23]

> **false positive/false negative:** In food allergy tests, a *false positive* is when a test yields a positive result but the patient is not allergic to the food. A *false negative* is when there is a negative test result but the patient is allergic to the food and has a genuine reaction to it—immediate or delayed—after eating it.

According to nutritionist Alan Gaby, M.D., there has been little consistency among the different labs that attempt to identify food allergies, and even in the same lab when attempting to duplicate their own results on the same blood samples.[24] Recently, however, the ALCAT (antigen leukocyte cellular antibody test) has proved more reliable. This blood test measures the allergenic response of leukocytes (white blood cells) to foods and delineates which of the foods cause inflammation. This test has been found in scientific studies as well as clinically to be significantly more comprehensive and accurate at pinpointing allergenic foods (with very low rates of false positive or false negative readings) than other allergy testing currently used in holistic medicine. When it comes to identifying food allergies, kinesiologists and other practitioners who utilize energetic testing methods, combined with the ALCAT and/or the elimination-challenge test described in the next section, have had the most successful and consistent results.

The Elimination-Challenge Test

Considered to be the gold standard in determining food allergies, the elimination-challenge test has a number of benefits. First, it is absolutely free, unlike some of the pricier blood tests described in the previous section, which can run in the hundreds of dollars. Second, with some simple instructions, it can be done in the comfort of the patient's own home. Finally, and most essential, most immunology texts and experienced clinicians agree that it is the most reliable testing method of food allergies.[25]

The directions for the elimination-challenge test are described in this section in two ways. First the instructions are briefly outlined to convey a generalized sense of the test. Then the directions are described in more depth to anticipate any questions for those who plan on using the elimination-challenge test themselves.

THE ELIMINATION-CHALLENGE TEST OUTLINE

Please feel free to photocopy this outline for personal use or for your patients.

1. *Eliminate:* Do not eat the suspected allergenic food—or foods if more than one is suspected—for 2 weeks (5 days for children). Be sure to eliminate the food (or foods) *completely* from your diet.
2. *Challenge:* Day 1—Eat a moderate amount of the suspected allergenic food (if more than one food has been eliminated, choose only one to test first) with each meal. (If you get an unpleasant reaction minutes to hours afterward, *stop* the challenge. This is a positive test.)

   Days 2, 3, and 4—On these three days again eliminate the suspected allergenic food from your diet. Continue to monitor yourself physically and emotionally for symptoms of a delayed allergy reaction. If you have any symptoms during these four days, it is a positive test strongly indicating that the food is an allergen.
3. *Repeat:* If there is more than one food you need to test, repeat this procedure (steps 1 and 2) for each new food, waiting approximately 1 week (or 3 days for children) after Day 4 of the last food challenged.
4. *Avoid:* If a food you challenged has tested positive, you should avoid it for an estimated two to six months before rechallenging it.

Deciding Which Foods to Challenge

This decision can be greatly aided by energetic testing—kinesiology, arm length testing, or electroacupuncture methods. However, if you do not have a holistic practitioner nearby who does quality energetic testing, it is important to be aware that the great majority of individuals are significantly allergic only to one, two, or at the most three major food categories. Thus, most people are allergic only to one or two of the "big five": wheat, milk products, corn, soy, and eggs. Furthermore, of these five, wheat and milk products are most commonly the two biggest culprits. Another good tip when deciding on what to eliminate first is to consider which foods you most crave and typically overconsume. (See the "Masking and Craving" box, page 217.) For example, if you crave lattes in the morning but wouldn't touch an espresso (that has no milk in it), and you love eating ice cream, cheese, and yogurt, there is a good possibility that you're allergic to dairy (milk) products. On the other hand, if your weakness is fresh bread, croissants, rolls, cookies, and cake, you could have a chronic wheat allergy. If you crave and eat a lot of foods from both these categories, it is wise to eliminate both at once, and then challenge them one at a time to identify whether they are both truly major allergens.

dairy/milk products: The terms *dairy* and *milk products* are used synonymously in this chapter. A dairy allergy includes milk products derived from a cow, goat, sheep, or buffalo (or, in some parts of the world, llamas, camels, mares, water buffalo, or reindeer!).

MULTIPLE ALLERGIES

There are individuals who cannot tolerate ten to twenty or even more foods, but these aren't all major food allergens, but primarily incompletely digested foods due to major intestinal dysbiosis and leaky gut (see chapter 7), heavy metals, toxic chemicals, and so forth. These individuals are often reacting in the tuberculinic (exhausted) and/or luetic (anxiety, insomnia, and so on) miasmic levels, and are also often extremely environmentally sensitive. Very sensitive and ill patients with a multitude of allergies can heal, but they need to be under the long-term care (one to two years or more) of an experienced holistic practitioner.

Slightly less common allergenic foods that you might also choose to eliminate include chocolate, citrus fruits, pork, beef, fish, shellfish, peanuts, nuts, yeast, and nightshade foods. Although sugar is often mistakenly thought of as a primary allergen, it actually acts more as a toxin in the body.* Thus, no one can afford *not* to eliminate, or at least greatly reduce, refined white sugar, and *entirely* eliminate high fructose corn syrup, artificial sweeteners, and other systemic poisons from their diet.

*Since sugar has no protein content, there is not a classic antibody/antigen immune response in the body because antibodies primarily couple with protein antigens.

NIGHTSHADE FOODS

Allergies to foods from the nightshade (Solanaceae) family (tomatoes, potatoes, peppers, eggplants, and tobacco) most typically cause chronic joint and muscle pain. Sweet potatoes (from the morning glory or Convolvulaceae family) and yams (from the wild yam or Dioscoreaceae family) do not generally need to be excluded because they are not in the Solanaceae group. In my experience, however, nightshades are usually a more minor and transient food allergy, which resolves as the digestive system is healed. The exception is if the patient's chief complaint is severe rheumatoid arthritis or other forms of significant muscle and joint disease. In these cases, nightshades may need to be avoided for years.

Dr. Garrett Smith's excellent article in the Spring 2010 *Wise Traditions* journal highlights this point.[26] In fact, this naturopathic physician has found that his patients can experience exceptional pain relief by avoiding nightshade foods.

All individuals who suffer from chronic pain should eliminate and then challenge the following nightshade foods commonly found in the Western diet:

- tomatoes
- potatoes
- eggplant
- peppers (bell peppers, chilis, paprika, and bottled hot sauces, but not peppercorns)
- goji berries
- ashwagandha
- Cape gooseberries
- ground cherries
- garden huckleberries

Eliminating the Chosen Food

The elimination-challenge method consists of avoiding the selected food(s) for two weeks if you are an adult, and five days for an infant or child (generally under twelve years old). Some individuals may need to eliminate the allergenic food for longer, for example, for a three-week period, if the withdrawal symptoms during the elimination period are still occurring even at the end of two weeks (or five days for children). If you suspect you may be allergic to two or three major foods, it will be necessary to eliminate *all* of these foods during this elimination phase too. Although this takes more willpower, your results will be clearer when you later challenge each of these foods to determine which one is a primary allergen.

During the elimination period, food cravings often arise as well as withdrawal symptoms—and sometimes severely so. If distressing withdrawal symptoms arise—such as achy flulike symptoms, including headaches and joint pain, or debilitating fatigue—taking large doses of buffered vitamin C* (or even Alka-Seltzer Gold) can quickly alkalinize a too-acidic system and help reduce the symptoms significantly. Other helpful therapies such as Epsom salt baths, frequent naps, taking an enema, or receiving a colonic may also be valuable in reducing uncomfortable withdrawal symptoms. Finally, remember that if you are ill, it is important to do the elimination-challenge protocol under the guidance of an experienced holistic practitioner.

Challenging the Suspected Food

Often the withdrawal symptoms—as well as the subsequent relief from avoiding the offending dairy, wheat, soy, or corn—are so dramatic and obvious during the two-week challenge test that many individuals choose to continue avoiding this food until they are well enough to try reintroducing it once again into their diet. However, if the withdrawal or relief during these two weeks was not noteworthy, then challenging the offending food at this point is often dramatically clear and extremely helpful in galvanizing your will to continue avoiding this disturbing food.

To challenge the suspected allergen after two weeks of avoidance (or five days in infants and young children), simply eat a moderate amount of the food for one day. For example, if you avoided wheat, you might have one piece of toast for breakfast, a sandwich at lunch, and a roll with dinner. Of course, if you immediately get a negative reaction, such as a runny nose, itchy throat, or diarrhea, that is in itself a positive test and no further

*Buffered vitamin C has a laxative effect and should therefore be taken to "bowel tolerance." For example, you could take 500 milligrams every 30 minutes until the symptoms are relieved, stopping as soon as your bowel movements begin to be soft or with the onset of diarrhea.

MASKING AND CRAVING

When we ingest daily our allergy food—such as wheat or dairy—we often actually feel better after eating it. This phenomenon is called "masking" and is why food allergies are often referred to as "hidden."[27] Closely related is the addiction and craving cycle. That is, when we crave our breakfast scone or creamy after-dinner dessert, we often feel better (for a while) after eating these addictive foods—in the same manner that an alcoholic or cigarette smoker feels better after the first sip of gin or puff on that Marlboro.

The addictive nature of allergenic foods is dramatically demonstrated in the population of individuals with the most severely damaged digestive systems—autistic children, who suffer from vaccinosis (see chapter 15). The large proteins in wheat (gluteo-morphines) and in dairy (caseo-morphines) are very difficult for these children to digest. When autistic children (and other children and adults) with damaged and leaky gut walls eat these allergenic foods, most of the gluteo-morphine and caseomorphine proteins are only partially broken down into peptide chains. The resulting partial protein chains are similar in structure to opiate-like drugs such as heroin and morphine, and they exert a morphinelike effect on the brain, with resulting neuropsychological symptoms and behaviors (e.g., hyperactivity, irrational anger, poor memory and attention span, and dyslexia).[28] Furthermore, these morphinelike chemicals from gluten and dairy set up a vicious cycle of craving for more of these addictive foods.

In her book *Nourishing Hope for Autism*, Julie Matthews describes the most effective diets to reduce the symptoms in this devastating disorder.[29] Autistic children, as well as those on the autism spectrum, need to remove from their diets the foods that inflame the already weakened and leaky gut. In addition to gluten and dairy foods, this includes other common allergens such as soy, corn, and eggs.

challenge is necessary to know that you have a wheat allergy. In this case, since the body has now become more sensitized to the allergenic food, it can respond more quickly to this "known toxin," as it does in acute or immediate food allergy reactions. This type of dramatic and immediate response is a nice confirmation of a suspected food allergy.

It can also be further diagnostic at this point to employ Dr. Coca's pulse test.[30] This procedure involves taking your pulse before the ingestion of the suspected food, and then again afterward. If your pulse either drops (decelerates) or increases (accelerates) ten beats or more per minute after eating the food, immunologists consider it a positive response indicating that the food is quite likely allergenic.[31]*

If you have avoided more than one food, pick the one you are most suspicious of and challenge it first. For example, if you avoided both wheat and dairy but you strongly suspect that dairy is your major food allergy, challenge it first. Then wait a week (or three days for infants and children) after the last day of the four-day challenge period (described in the next paragraph), and challenge the second suspected food.* During this next week you should avoid the first suspected food if it has tested positive, as well as the second suspected food that you are presently testing. Continue in this pattern until you have challenged all suspected allergenic foods.

If you don't get an immediate reaction, however—that is, a pulse change or symptomatic reaction—go ahead and eat the suspected food with all of your meals the first day, and then *avoid it again* for the next three days. During this four-day period consisting of eating the suspected food on the first day and then not eating it for three more days, it is important to carefully observe how you feel, and compare this experience to the two weeks of abstinence. For example, if you feel worse during the four-day challenge period (excluding the elimination period, when you may have suffered

*Dr. Coca's pulse test has been criticized as being too labile because everything from the weather to your dinner companions can affect the pulse rate. Therefore, it is considered unreliable by many allergists. However, at this point—after two full weeks of eliminating the suspected allergenic food—it can be valuable in confirming the suspected allergen.

*Note: You may need to wait longer than one week—for example, ten days to two weeks—if you're still experiencing symptoms from challenging the first suspected allergenic food.

from withdrawal symptoms) and old familiar symptoms return, you may accurately conclude that you are indeed allergic to the food you have chosen to test. For example, if you feel nothing on Monday while you are eating the suspected food allergen, but you wake up with diarrhea on Tuesday, have joint pain on Wednesday, or experience a migraine headache on Thursday, these signs and symptoms are all positive indicators that the suspected food is indeed a major allergen.

A further benefit to the elimination-challenge test, besides price, convenience, and reliability, is that you can *directly* experience which particular symptoms are associated with each suspected allergenic food. For example, dairy foods may make you feel tired and depressed, whereas wheat could give you abdominal pain and diarrhea. In this way you gain an understanding of the specific harm and particular symptoms each food triggers, and you become more sensitive to your body's signals when you ingest the offending food in the future.

Avoiding the Foods That Test Positive

If the challenge test is positive, you should completely avoid the food for at least two to six months, depending on your particular level of health. After this period, you can rechallenge the food again; however, it is most beneficial to challenge the healthiest form of the food, in its unadulterated form. For example, if you have tested positive to dairy, challenging raw butter, organic cultured cottage cheese, or small amounts of organic goat or sheep yogurt is wise, since a negative test to these healthy foods will allow you to begin to eat them once again, albeit in moderation. Or if you have a wheat allergy, a not-overused wheat moiety like kamut or spelt bread, or more digestible sprouted bread, may not elicit a positive test, and that food can then be eaten in amounts within reason, such as one small serving two or three times a week.

The important thing to remember is not to overeat one particular food, and furthermore, to practice rotation of all the foods that you do eat. The classic rotation diet protocol is to eat tolerated (nonallergenic) foods no closer together than every four days. Extremely sensitive patients may need to wait a week or more, but with less sensitive patients, foods can be spaced out at closer intervals—for example, every two to three days. The reason is to avoid resensitizing your system to new food groups or the same allergenic food again. Thus, patients are often instructed to remember the term "V & R"—that is, variety and rotation, which are both essential in healing food allergies.

In cases of long-term illness and other signs of compromised health, individuals may need to strictly avoid their allergenic food throughout their life. However, most people can eventually eat small amounts of their allergenic food intermittently, especially if they achieve more optimal functioning through detoxifying their toxic metals and chemicals, clearing their chronic foci, and taking their constitutional homeopathic remedy. It is important to note that as you go through the ups and downs of *unpeeling the onion* through various drainage and detoxifying measures, sensitivity to your primary food allergy also varies. For example, while you are treating a major tonsil focus, your primary dairy allergy may become quite strong again even if you have reasonably avoided milk products for years. During this tonsil focus clearing time, which can last for months or years, you may not even be able to eat any goat or sheep's milk products until the focus—and the related intestinal dysbiosis—is significantly cleared.

Limitations of the Elimination-Challenge Test

For all its merits, the elimination-challenge test does have a few limitations. First, if you don't assiduously abstain from *all* foods containing the suspected allergen, then the challenge test results may not be obvious or positive because of this incomplete avoidance. For example, many margarines are labeled "non-dairy" because they don't contain lactose, but they still typically contain casein—the protein in dairy foods that is even more allergenic than the lactose sugar. Thus, it's important that you consult the list of foods and ingredients in the "The Five Most Common Allergenic Foods" section (see page 221) to avoid unknowingly consuming your allergenic food during the two-week period of abstinence.

Another complicating factor is that toxins, such as a mouthful of amalgam fillings or years of "polypharmacy" (the prescription of multiple drugs), can often mask any positive responses gained from either avoiding or challenging the suspected allergy. This false negative response—that is, no discernible response at all—often occurs in ill individuals who don't feel well most of the time anyway. For example, if chronic constipation, bloating, and related fatigue are primarily caused by taking three or more prescription drugs and *only secondarily* influenced by a food allergy, then any symptoms elicited by the challenge test of the suspected allergenic food might not be readily apparent. Or, if chronic arthritic joint pain is secondary to mercury toxicity from amalgam fillings as well as toxic chemicals from painting houses for a living, then the effects of avoiding or challenging an allergic food will often be superseded by these two stronger toxic influences. In these cases of impaired homeostasis or *blocked regulation,* the disturbing food allergy symptoms are "drowned out" by the stronger wave of toxic influence operating in the body.

homeostasis/blocked regulation: *Homeostasis,* as previously defined, is the state of healthy functioning that occurs when normal functioning and control of the body is properly maintained, so the body can react to external stressors appropriately. Abnormal homeostasis, often referred to as *blocked regulation* in Europe, is when the system has been so disturbed and overloaded with toxins for such a significant period that the body can no longer respond appropriately to external challenges. Suffering from a cold for months, typical of the tuberculinic reaction mode, and chronic insomnia, classic in the luetic miasm, are examples of blocked regulation.

However, if a patient in this situation then goes to a holistic practitioner who uses energetic testing and finds that the patient is testing positive to the suspected allergenic food, the practitioner will often suggest retaking the elimination-challenge test. If this second attempt results in another negative response, it is often left to the patient to decide whether to continue avoiding—or reasonably avoiding—the suspected allergenic food. After the mercury amalgam fillings, toxic chemicals, prescription drugs, or other "obstacles to cure" are reduced, two scenarios are then possible: the challenge response may now be obviously positive, or, because of the decreased toxic load, the challenge response will be either still negative or somewhat equivocal, now that the patient's immune system is functioning more appropriately and therefore is responding less intensively to food allergens.

SYMPTOMS

Allergy Symptoms Change as We Age

It is a common misconception that we outgrow our allergies. In fact, just the opposite occurs in the majority of individuals. That is, with inadequate holistic care as well as typical allopathic drug suppression (e.g., antibiotics, vaccines, and antihistamines), our childhood symptoms often simply move deeper into our body tissues and start affecting more vital tissues as we age. Thus, the common childhood psoric and sycotic signs of allergies—colds, earaches, tonsillitis, and eczema—eventually move into more serious tuberculinic and luetic symptoms such as chronic fatigue, depression, anxiety, and arthritis. In fact, it has been estimated that over fifty medical conditions are associated with food allergies.[32]

The Same Food Can Cause Different Symptoms in Different People

Although there are some generally related symptoms associated with particular foods—for example, dairy allergies tend to cause chronic upper respiratory symptoms, whereas gluten is often the primary cause of serious intestinal distress such as ulcerative colitis and Crohn's disease—for the most part *any food can cause any symptom.* Therefore, two people can experience completely different symptoms from the same food. The particular organs and tissues that are affected can be influenced by numerous factors, including a person's inherited constitution (miasm) as well as environmental factors (e.g., nutrition, lifestyle, vaccines, or drugs).

Crohn's disease: *Crohn's,* or *regional enteritis* or *ileitis,* is a chronic inflammatory condition of the gastrointestinal tract, commonly involving the terminal ileum (the end of the small intestine just before the large intestine, the appendix area). Symptoms include chronic diarrhea, weight loss, and abdominal pain.

The reason for this great variability is best illustrated by the following scenario of how food allergies can manifest. When individuals eat too much of any one specific food, over time they can exhaust the enzymes needed to digest that particular food.[33] When subsequently undigested particles of this food enter the bloodstream and travel to the head, headaches, fatigue, dizziness, memory loss, depression, or anxiety can ensue. If these microparticles lodge in the joints, pain and swelling can occur. If they localize in the skin, there can be subsequent reactions of hives and other types of rashes, hair loss, dandruff, acne, and eczema. Thus, *any* organ or tissue can be adversely affected by the same food, because the location of the injured tissue depends primarily on the particular miasmic tendency—that is, the inherited and environmental weakness or disease predisposition that is unique to each individual. This great variability in disorders and illnesses that can result from food allergy is further illustrated in the following section.

Common Signs and Symptoms of Hidden Food Allergies

The symptoms of hidden food allergies listed in this section are grouped according to the area of the body or the body system they most affect. Doctors and health practitioners are encouraged to photocopy this list and use it in their offices to discuss their patients' possible allergy-related symptoms. This list was compiled from many sources, but most notably from Dr. Sherry Rogers's book *The E.I. Syndrome* and the *Textbook of Natural Medicine* by Dr. Pizzorno and Dr. Murray.

Skin. Rashes, urticaria (hives), acne, rosacea, eczema, psoriasis, edema (swelling), sweating, redness, paleness, hair loss, dandruff, chills, sweats.

Brain and Nervous System. Autism, minimal brain dysfunction (MBD), hyperactivity, learning disorders, attention deficit disorder (ADD), attention deficit/hyperactivity disorder (ADHD), multiple sclerosis (MS), schizophrenia, stuttering, mental confusion, poor concentration, memory loss, "brain fog," spaciness, lethargy, depression, undue fatigue and sleepiness, poor coordination, irritability, anger, mood swings, insomnia, sluggishness in the morning, restless leg syndrome, anxiety, nervousness, hallucinations, seizures, twitching, slurred speech, drug addiction, chronic alcoholism, pediatric autoimmune neuropsychiatric disorders associated with streptococcal infections (PANDAS).

Head. Headaches (e.g., tension, migraine, or sinus), dizziness, faintness, motion sickness, seasickness, unsteadiness.

Eyes. Dark circles under the eyes, swelling around the eyes, watery eyes, bloodshot eyes, itchy eyes, burning eyes, blurred vision, photophobia (sensitivity or intolerance to light), dilated pupils.

Ears. Tinnitus (ringing in the ears),* earaches and recurrent infections, blocked ears (fullness and pressure), fluid in the ears, deafness, itchy ears, motion sickness.

Sinuses. Sinus congestion and pain, recurrent sinusitis, sinus headaches.

Nose. Runny nose, stuffy and congested nose, frequent colds, itchy nose, postnasal drip, sneezing, hay fever, sores in nose, nosebleeds.

Mouth. Itchy palate, bleeding gums, coated tongue, bad breath, cracked lips, swollen lips, canker sores (aphthous ulcers).

Throat. Tonsillitis and frequent sore throats (chronic tonsil focus), swollen glands, chronic cough or tickle in the throat, chronic tonsil focal infections, dry cough, hoarseness, gagging.

Thyroid. Hypothyroidism (fatigue, cold hands and feet, weight gain, coarse and dry hair), hyperthyroidism, Hashimoto's thyroiditis.

Lungs. Chronic chest congestion, asthma, wheezing, dyspnea (difficulty breathing), bronchitis, pneumonia.

Heart. Chest pain, tachycardia (rapid heartbeat), bradycardia (slow heartbeat), palpitations (skipped and irregular heartbeats), hyper- and hypotension (high and low blood pressure).

Gastrointestinal System. Sleepiness after meals, thirsty after meals, diarrhea, constipation, stomachache, abdominal cramps and pain, peptic (stomach) and duodenal (small intestine) ulcers, irritable bowel syndrome (IBS), Crohn's disease, heartburn, gas (flatulence, belching), bloating after meals, chronic candidiasis, gallstones, hypoglycemia (low blood sugar), nausea, vomiting, hemorrhoids, rectal itching, rectal mucus, being overweight, being underweight, compulsive eating.

Adrenals. Adrenal exhaustion, chronic fatigue syndrome, depression, faintness upon standing, back pain.

Musculoskeletal System. Arthritic joint stiffness and pain, muscle stiffness and achiness, muscle spasms, leg cramps, restless legs, muscle twitching, muscle weakness.

Genitourinary System (female). PMS (premen-

---

*Tinnitus can be miraculously easy to treat if it is caused simply by food allergies. Otherwise, it can be more difficult and may require the treatment of dental foci (see chapter 11), stabilizing dental malocclusions (see chapter 16), or finding the correct constitutional homeopathic remedy (see chapter 14).

strual syndrome), menstrual cramps, menorrhagia (heavy flow), scanty flow, mittelschmerz (mid-cycle pain), irregular menses, vaginal itching, vaginal burning, vaginal discharge, urinary tract infections (cystitis), bed-wetting, incontinence, kidney failure, depressed or excessive sex drive, frigidity (difficulty with arousal or orgasm).

Genitourinary System (male). Prostate inflammation and infection, burning of the penis, frequent urination, difficult urination, dribbling, urinary tract infections (cystitis), bed-wetting, incontinence, kidney failure, depressed or excessive sex drive, frigidity (difficulty with arousal or orgasm), impotency.

THE FIVE MOST COMMON ALLERGENIC FOODS

In order to thoroughly avoid your allergenic food or foods during the two-week elimination period, it is essential to be aware of *all* the foods and ingredients in which the suspected allergen is contained. The following section describes the five most typical allergenic foods—wheat (gluten), dairy, corn, soy, and eggs—in depth. At the end of each explanation is a brief summary of the foods and ingredients to avoid, which can be copied and used as a reference while shopping.

Wheat and Gluten

When the endosperm (innermost part) of the wheat kernel is milled, it yields a flour comprised by 6 to 8 percent of the protein known as gluten. Gluten is made up of two smaller proteins, *glutenin* and *gliadin,* which occur in approximately equal amounts. Gluten is the gelatinous agent in baking that imparts elasticity and strength to bread. However, this Janus-like wheat protein has another face that has caused untold suffering. Gluten intolerance is so damaging that it has warranted its own disease classification. It was first termed *celiac disease* by a British physician, Samuel Gee, in 1888, but the condition was not correlated with wheat ingestion until 1950 by a Dutch doctor, W. K. Dicke.[34] Celiac disease, or gluten intolerance, may present initially in infancy or childhood (often between six months to six years), or it may not show up symptomatically until the adult years when a person's nutritional state and immune system are depleted.

Celiac Disease Symptoms and Diagnosis

The classic symptoms of celiac disease are gastrointestinal bloating, diarrhea, fatty stools, muscle weakness, and weight loss.[35] Gluten intolerance is also associated with a family history of alcoholism, arthritis, Down syndrome, schizophrenia, and dementia, and it has been correlated with a chronic B_6 deficiency.[36] As discussed earlier in this chapter, both gluten and dairy sensitivity have been linked to autism.[37] In one study, opioids derived from casein (caseo-morphines) and gluten (gluteo-morphines) were found to cross the blood-brain barrier in animals and mimic the "social indifference" symptoms seen in autistic children.[38]

Diagnosis of celiac disease is based on these classic signs and symptoms and confirmed by jejunal (second part of the small intestine) biopsy, where the normally healthy fingerlike villi projections will appear inflamed and flattened.[39] However, instead of subjecting an infant, child, or adult to this invasive endoscopic procedure requiring toxic anesthetics, where a tube is threaded down the throat and into the intestine, it is simpler and far less traumatic to first do the elimination-challenge test for gluten foods. If this test is dramatically positive, then the diagnosis of celiac disease can be confirmed without surgery.

BIOPSIES AND BLOOD TESTS

The biopsies used to diagnose celiac disease have the reputation of being rather hit-or-miss, because the area biopsied may not have the extensive damage that a neighboring intestinal section might. Additionally, blood tests to determine celiac disease have an estimated 40 percent false positive rate. Testing by the Enterolab company, however, has recently been more successful by utilizing stool samples to test for anti-gliadin antibodies.[40] (Learn more at www.enterolab.com.)

Additionally, more recent research has found that gluten sensitivity and celiac disease can be present even in the absence of gastrointestinal signs and symptoms. In fact, since 1996 scientific evidence has been mounting that gluten sensitivity can present itself in multiple organ and tissue systems, including as autoimmune disorders, myocarditis, osteoporosis, ADHD, and autism.[41]

Gluten-Containing Grains

In descending order of quantity, gluten-containing grains are wheat, spelt, triticale (a hybrid of wheat and rye), kamut, oats, rye, barley, teff, and corn.[42] However, teff has *very* little gluten in it. Since it has not been overeaten and is traditionally soaked and fermented before being made into delicious morning porridges or breads, it should be tested by each gluten-intolerant person on a case-by-case basis to determine if there is a reaction to this ancient Ethiopian grain. Corn also has a *very* small amount of gluten and should be tested via the elimination-challenge test to determine individual sensitivity to it.[43] Furthermore, recent research suggests that the gluten protein found in oats, called *avenin,* is dissimilar enough to wheat gluten that it may be tolerated by some individuals with celiac disease.[44]

Although buckwheat is *not* a grain but the seeds of an herb similar to rhubarb, and millet has no gluten in it at all, both contain a substance (called *proloamine*) that is similar to the protein gliadin found in wheat.[45] However, rarely do millet and buckwheat cause allergic reactions, even in those with acute celiac disease.[46] Finally, although there is no gluten connection, 10 to 15 percent of celiac patients also have a coexisting hypersensitivity to soy—but this is most likely non-fermented soy that no one can digest well.[47]

Teff, corn, and oats are among the foods that gluten-allergic individuals should first avoid, along with the other classic gluten-containing grains (wheat, barley, rye, kamut, triticale, and spelt). And individuals with serious celiac disease should test the gluten-related grains—buckwheat and millet—on a case-by-case basis. On the other hand, individuals with a less serious gluten allergy, after a period of abstinence and holistic support, may be able to tolerate small amounts of oats, teff, or corn on a rotational basis (every few days).

It should be noted that in an Italian study from 2004, published in the *Applied and Environmental Microbiology* journal, celiac patients did not react adversely to bread made from wheat, oat, millet, and buckwheat flours that had been naturally fermented for twenty-four hours. In comparison, this same group of seventeen celiac patients who had been gluten-free for at least two years had significant gut-permeability changes when they (bravely) ate nonfermented bread, made to rise with baker's yeast. The authors of this study, based on the premise that natural lactobacilli fermentation can hydrolyze or sever allergenic gliadin proteins and thus neutralize allergic reactions in celiac patients, were "cautiously enthusiastic" about the dramatic results.[48]

A Wheat or Gluten Allergy?

When determining a wheat allergy, it is essential to determine whether you are simply allergic to wheat or to *all* gluten-containing grains. Fortunately, there is not significant cross-reactivity in the grass family in which cereal grains like wheat are included. Thus, you may have a wheat allergy because of the overconsumption of this grain, but not a (more serious) allergy to *all* gluten-containing grains or celiac disease. In the case of a simple wheat allergy, you may still be able to eat oats or rye, but only sparingly and preferably in the highest quality possible. This may include soaked and fermented oat groats as a morning cereal or sprouted rye bread (found in the refrigerated section of the health food store). However, in the case of a gluten allergy, you must avoid all gluten-containing products assiduously.

OAT GROATS PREPARATION

Eating unrefined oats, or oat groats, is preferable to eating the refined oat flakes commonly used today to make oatmeal. To properly ferment them, oat groats can be soaked in water and a little whey (juice from yogurt) overnight and then cooked slowly the next day for breakfast. Grinding them up briefly in a blender in the morning is an alternate preparation method that can quicken the cooking process.

In the following sections, wheat and gluten allergies are separated to delineate between the two different types of sensitivities. If you don't have a practitioner nearby who can energetically test for this distinction, avoid all gluten products during the elimination period, and then first challenge with oats, rye, or barley. If you test positive to one of these three grains, you should avoid all gluten-containing grains. If you don't test positive, you are probably sensitive only to wheat products.

Wheat Avoidance

Specific Grains to Avoid: wheat, kamut, spelt, triticale.

KAMUT AND SPELT

Although many health food consumers are heralding these two ancient nonhybridized grains—kamut from Egypt and spelt lauded by St. Hildegard from Germany—as nonallergenic, in most holistic practitioners' experiences even they must often be avoided for a significant period of time. However, after one to three months, many patients can digest small to moderate amounts of these grains, especially if they are fresh and fermented before cooking.

What May Be Listed on the Label: bulgur, gluten, gliadin, flour (enriched, white or whole), durum flour, farina, graham flour, modified food starch, semolina, vegetable gum, vegetable protein (hydrolyzed), wheat bran, wheat germ, wheat (or vegetable) starch.

Typical Foods to Avoid: bread and rolls, bakery goods (e.g., cakes, cookies, muffins, pastries, and pies), (many) cereals, ice cream cones, couscous, crackers, croutons, dumplings, fried food batters (unless corn), (some) gravies and sauces, (some) hot dogs and sausages, pasta (macaroni, noodles, et cetera), pretzels, (some) soups, soy sauce, (many) alcoholic beverages (bourbon, gin, vodka, whiskey, and most beer and ales).*

▶ For a more complete list of hidden sources of gluten, see page 24 of the Summer 2006 *Wise Traditions* journal.

Wheat-Free Grains: amaranth, barley, buckwheat, corn, millet, oats, quinoa, rice, teff.

QUINOA PREPARATION

Quinoa contains more protein than any other grain. It should always be rinsed thoroughly prior to cooking to remove its natural coating of saponin, which appears frothy in the rinse water. Quinoa should be cooked similar to rice, at a ratio of 2:1 (water to quinoa), for approximately twenty minutes.[49]

---

*Tequila, rum, and wine are wheat-free. Beer is usually made from wheat or barley.

Substitute Foods: wheat-free crackers, breads, cereals, pasta, flours; corn (e.g., tortillas, popcorn); rice; (wheat-free) tamari; tapioca.

Avoidance of *All* Gluten-Containing Grains

Specific Grains to Avoid: wheat, barley, kamut, rye, oats, spelt, triticale, corn, and teff (perhaps buckwheat and millet as well).

What May Be Listed on the Label: barley malt, bulgur, gluten, gliadin, flour (enriched, white or whole), durum flour, farina, graham flour, modified food starch, semolina, vegetable gum, vegetable protein (hydrolyzed), wheat bran, wheat germ, wheat (or vegetable) starch.*

Typical Foods to Avoid: bread and rolls, bakery goods (e.g., cakes, cookies, muffins, pastries, and pies), (many) cereals, ice cream cones, couscous, crackers, croutons, dumplings, fried food batters, (some) gravies and sauces, (some) hot dogs and sausages, oatmeal, licorice, pasta (e.g., macaroni, noodles), pretzels, (some) soups, soy sauce, (many) alcoholic beverages (bourbon, gin, vodka, whiskey and most beer and ales).†‡

▶ Determining whether a product is gluten-free or not can be quite complicated because manufacturers often change formulas and labels do not always reflect *everything* used in the production of the product. If you are severely gluten-allergic, you should use an even more extensive list such as in the book *More from the Gluten-Free Gourmet* by Bette Hagman.

Gluten-Free Grains: amaranth, buckwheat, millet, quinoa, rice.

Substitute Foods: gluten-free crackers, breads, cereals, pasta, flours; rice; (wheat-free) tamari; tapioca.

*This is the exact same list as under "Wheat Avoidance," except barley malt has been included because it is a common additive.

†Tequila, rum, and wine are wheat-free. Any drink containing "barley malt" or "grain neutral spirits" has gluten in it.

‡This is the same list as under "Wheat Avoidance," except licorice and oatmeal have been added and all fried food batters need to be avoided since they are usually made up of wheat or corn. Furthermore, sometimes commercial ketchups, vinegars, candies, seasoned French fries, and even the glue on envelopes and stamps can have added gluten. (Cider, wine, and rice vinegars are completely gluten-free.)

Dairy

When individuals are not breast-fed and/or are exposed to (pasteurized) cow's milk during the first six months of life, they are much more likely to have a dairy sensitivity than someone who has had no exposure.[50] The two most classic dairy allergy signs are upper respiratory (colds, sore throats, swollen glands, and ear infections) and gastrointestinal (bloating, spasm, and constipation or diarrhea) symptoms.[51] However, like all primary food allergies, dairy sensitivity can cause myriad diverse symptoms, from asthma to eczema.

What's less well known is how often dairy allergies contribute to joint and muscle pain. A California chiropractor, Dr. Daniel Twogood, has found that the protein casein in milk does the same thing in joints and muscles that it does in cheese and ice cream—thicken and congest. Casein in dairy products therefore is often the major underlying factor in the onset of chronic arthritis, muscle pain and stiffness, and muscle tension headaches.[52] In the experience of many practitioners, eliminating dairy has been dramatic in alleviating or even completely curing patients' chronic headaches or muscle and joint pain. Furthermore, there is often an obvious viscerosomatic (organ to joint) relationship occurring between the dairy-disturbed stomach, pancreas, and small intestine and the mid to lower spine; the organs neurologically reflex into and cause pain in the spine. In these cases, chiropractic and osteopathic manipulative treatments provide only palliative and temporary relief. (See chapter 17 for more information.)

The Allergenic Casein Protein

There are actually more than twenty-five different proteins in cow's milk that can potentially cause allergic reactions.[53] However, the most common are the sugar/protein combinations of lactalbumin, lactoglobulin, and casein.[54] The majority of the protein in dairy products is casein—in fact, approximately 77 percent of the protein in cow's milk is made up of casein.[55] However, because of the strong focus on only lactose over the years, many products in commercial grocery stores are falsely labeled "non-dairy," even though they are loaded with the much more allergenic caseinate.

Lactose Intolerance Mitigated by Fermentation

Classically, allergists have claimed that the primary allergenic substance in milk is the lactose milk sugar due to a congenital lactase enzyme deficiency.[56] Lactase deficiency is common in non-Caucasian peoples, averaging from 85 to 90 percent in Asians, 80 percent in Arabs, from 60 to 80 percent in Jews, and 70 percent in blacks.[57] However, these statistics do not account for the traditional methods of fermenting milk that many cultures have practiced for centuries, including the Masai in Africa and Indians, who both consume cultured milk products as their principal food. Once again, it's the loss of traditional wisdom that has contributed to the plethora of dairy allergies seen today. In fact, consuming pasteurized and denatured milk products is relatively new. Before the industrial age and widespread refrigeration, fermented milk products such as yogurt, cheese, and curds and whey were consumed liberally. This culturing process breaks down the difficult-to-digest protein casein, as well as increasing (or restoring after pasteurization) the lactase enzyme that helps digest the milk sugar lactose.[58]

Many Allergic to Milk Products from All Animals

As with wheat and gluten allergies, there is a continuum of severity with milk allergies. That is, some people must avoid all cow dairy, but they can eat goat and sheep products, while others must completely abstain from all cow, goat, sheep, and even buffalo milk products for a specified period of time. However, since it has been demonstrated that there is a 70 percent occurrence of cross-reactivity between goat's and cow's milk, *all* dairy products are listed in the following "Typical Foods to Avoid" section.[59] Then, during the challenge period, goat, sheep, or buffalo milk products can be tested on an individual basis to determine if there is a sensitivity to one or more of these slightly less allergenic foods.

Whey Is Less Allergenic than Most Other Dairy Products

Although whey is listed below under "What May Be Listed on the Label" as a food to avoid, for most people a little whey (or juice from unsweetened yogurt) added to the soaking water for grains, vegetables, raw meats, or beverages rarely causes any allergic reactions. Milk consists of curd (the solid part) and whey (the liquid part). The curd is mostly composed of casein, the primary allergenic and aggravating factor found in milk. However, whey, the thin serum of milk after the curd has been removed, is much less reactive.

Cultured Milk Products and Food Rotation Are Helpful

After a healing period of elimination (from two to six months, generally), many individuals can enjoy raw butter or cultured (fermented) raw butter, as well as other cultured products such as cottage cheese, raw goat and sheep cheese, and yogurt and kefir, as long as these are eaten in moderation. The words *in moderation* should be strongly noted here. Many individuals eat yogurt in excess, primarily because it is such an emotionally consoling food, like pudding. However, yogurt is often a strong allergenic food in dairy-sensitive individuals, even more so than raw butter, cultured cottage cheese, and raw cheeses. Thus, individuals with a primary dairy allergy who can tolerate yogurt should eat it only in small amounts, and never daily. Varying as well as rotating these foods—for example, eating them once every two or four days—is a helpful habit to practice in order to avert the reactivation of allergenic defensive responses in the immune system. Thus, as described earlier, variety and rotation should always be kept in mind while grocery shopping and preparing meals at home.

▶ Cultures may be obtained from G.E.M. Cultures at (253) 588-2922 or www.gemcultures.com, and from www.culturesforhealth.com/Piima-Yogurt-Starter.html.

Dairy Avoidance

Specific Foods to Avoid: cow, goat, sheep, and buffalo milk products.

What May Be Listed on the Label: butter, milk or non-fat milk, cream, cheese, margarine, whey, casein, caseinate (calcium or potassium), lactalbumin, lactoglobulin.

Typical Foods to Avoid: butter, cheese, cottage cheese, milk (e.g., condensed, evaporated, dried, whole, skim, 2 percent), cream (e.g., whole, half-and-half), yogurt, ice cream, baked goods made with milk, (some) baking powders, (many) candies, chocolate,* cocoa, creamy salad dressings, soups and sauces, custards and puddings, doughnuts, junket,† kefir, (some) margarines, (some) "non-dairy" products, sherbet.

DAIRY-FREE COCOA

Ah!Laska, as well as some other health store brands, makes an unsweetened organic baker's cocoa with no milk that can be mixed with coconut milk, coconut oil, nuts, and honey or maple syrup to make various sugar-free and milk-free drinks and desserts.

Substitute Foods: almond milk, rice milk, milk-free baked goods (e.g., French bread, "kosher," and many health food store brands), carob treats (without milk), coconut milk, margarine (non-caseinated, non-hydrogenated, e.g. Spectrum's brand), sorbet, tofu.

MILK ALTERNATIVES

Almond, rice, oat, and other substitute "milks" are fair substitutes for dairy milk, but they have been packaged "aseptically" (subjected to high temperatures for a brief period) in order to preserve shelf life and therefore have been somewhat "deadened" and adulterated. (Of course, as described in chapter 5, soy milk is not recommended at all.) It's therefore better to make these milks at home fresh. For example, almond or hazelnut (filbert) milk can be made by pouring two cups of boiling water over one cup of organic almonds (or hazelnuts), letting the mixture cool, pulverizing it in a food processor (or blender), and straining. For more information, consult Meredith McCarty's book *Sweet and Natural,* pages 242–43.

*Bittersweet chocolate (usually) contains no milk; however, it always contains some form of sugar.

†Junket is sweetened milk, flavored and thickened into a curd with rennet. (Rennet or rennin is an extract of the membrane lining the stomach of an unweaned animal, especially the fourth stomach of a calf, which curdles milk and may be used in making cheeses and junket.)

Corn

Predisposition to Corn Allergies in Spanish and American Indian Cultures

Corn, also known as maize, originated in Central and South America and is thought to have grown wild in Mexico more than 9,000 years ago.[60] It is still a staple food in these regions. Therefore, patients of Mexican and Central and South American Indian descent are more susceptible to corn allergies and should include corn as one of the likely allergens for the elimination-challenge test.

Corn Allergies from High Fructose Corn Syrup

Because of the ubiquitous use of corn in processed foods, everyone from "modern" industrialized nations must also consider the possibility of having a mild to major corn allergy. As mentioned previously in the discussion of sugar, the use of fructose and high fructose corn syrup (HFCS) has exploded since 1976, when the sugar industry figured out that it was cheaper to make sugar from corn than from beets or cane.[61] Add to this the common use of corn oil, corn starch, and corn syrup, and it's very possible that many junk-food-addicted teens (and adults) are possibly just as hooked on the stimulatory effects of ingesting corn as they are on the sugar high from soft drinks or candy. Of course, these euphoric food-drug reactions are always transient, and the later withdrawal reactions of irritability and fatigue just continue to fuel the cyclic craving and the need for another "fix."

Corn Is Highly Hybridized and Genetically Engineered

Like wheat and other grains, corn is an extremely exploited plant. Most of the modern corn grown today is in the form of highly refined hybrid strains, developed for high yields and resistance to pests. Most of the corn grown today in Ohio, Illinois, Indiana, Iowa, Kansas, Missouri, and Nebraska is from the same few strains, and therefore causative in stimulating stronger allergic reactions than corn from a variety of strains.[62] Furthermore, much of the corn crop has been genetically modified, and as discussed previously, the toxic aspects of these new genetically engineered strains are quite serious.

Niacin Deficiency

Modern food processing methods have also ignored much of the important traditional wisdom in the preparation of corn. Although corn has notable quantities of the B-complex vitamins, the niacin (B_3) in corn is largely in a chemically bound form, which makes it unavailable for assimilation and absorption.[63] Traditional Native American and Central and South American recipes obviate this problem by soaking corn or corn flour in lime water to release vitamin B_3 and improve the amino acid quality of the proteins in the germ.[64] When this traditional wisdom is ignored, eating excessive amounts of corn products has the potential of creating a niacin deficiency, termed *pellagra*. This syndrome is mnemonically remembered by both holistic and allopathic medical students as being characterized by the four D's: dermatitis, diarrhea, depression, and dementia. These latter two symptoms are possibly why corn allergies have sometimes been associated with neurological symptoms such as irritability, restlessness, and oversensitivity, and in severe cases with delusions, disorientation, and hallucinations.[65] Therefore, it is important to keep in mind that those individuals testing positive to corn products during the elimination-challenge test may also require niacin supplementation.

► The niacin found in Thorne's Niasafe-600 is a non-flushing form that many individuals prefer. To order, contact Thorne Research at (800) 228-1966.

Corn Avoidance

Specific Foods to Avoid: corn.

What May Be Listed on the Label: corn (e.g., alcohol, flour, meal, oil, starch, sweetener, syrup), dextrin, dextrose, food starch, fructose, corn syrup, high fructose corn syrup, MSG, sorbitol, vegetable (broth, oil, starch).

Typical Foods to Avoid: corn, cornmeal, soft drinks, many commercial baked goods, baking powders, many mixes (cake, pancake, waffle), some breading, popcorn, many alcohols (most American beer and ales, gin, Canadian whiskey, corn whiskey, bourbon whiskey), candy, club soda, coffee creamers, some cold cereals, some creamy sauces, soups and salad dressings, distilled vinegar, fruit juices, grits, gum, hominy, infant formulas, instant coffee, jelly and preserves, ketchup, medications (aspirin, cough syrup, laxatives), (not pure) maple syrups, most table salt, many vitamins, adhesives (stamps, stickers).

Substitute Foods: arrowroot, kuzu, or tapioca (to replace cornstarch); baking soda or cream of tartar (as leavening agents); other flours (potato, quinoa, rice, spelt); wheat products and flour (if not sensitive to the small amount of gluten in corn); pure honey and maple syrup.

HIDDEN CORN PRODUCTS

In the mid-1990s, an estimated 1,500 prescription and over-the-counter drugs contained cornstarch. Although foods must be labeled, "trade secrets" legislation allows cornstarch, as well as lactose, to be labeled as "inert substances."[66] Many cardboard containers, such as milk cartons, are also powdered with cornstarch.

Soy

Toxic and Allergenic

As discussed in chapter 5, *nonfermented* soy is difficult to digest not because of its primary allergenic components but because it contains large quantities of enzyme inhibitors, strong phytoestrogens, goitrogens, and other "antinutrients." Thus, like sugar, nonfermented soy is a toxic food that should be avoided. However, *unlike* sugar, soy has a high protein content that also renders it a potential allergen. Sensitivity to soy's proteins is exemplified by individuals who can't even ingest properly fermented soy products like tamari or miso without adverse reactions. Similar to the adulteration of dairy and wheat, it's difficult to know how much a soy allergy has been influenced by past ingestion of nonfermented soy (as well as other improperly prepared legumes) cross-reacting with fermented soy products. Regardless, reactions to soy are prevalent enough that it must be included here in the top five group of primary food allergens. Fermented soy products such as miso, tamari, or tempeh should be the first ones eaten during the challenge period of the elimination-challenge test, to see if these appropriately prepared soy foods can be tolerated in moderation.

PEA FAMILY ALLERGENS

The pea family is an important source of food allergens and includes soybeans, peanuts, lentils, garbanzos, alfalfa, beans, guar, and licorice.[67]

Soy Avoidance

Specific Foods to Avoid: soy.

What May Be Listed on the Label: soy (e.g., flour, oil, protein, sauce), soya, lecithin, textured vegetable protein (TVP), vegetable starch.

Typical Foods to Avoid: bakery products with soy flour or oil, Bragg's Liquid Aminos, many canned soups, some coffee substitutes, lecithin, imitation meat products (hot dogs, burgers, sausage, lunch meats, vegetarian chili), miso, natto, phytoestrogen products, shortenings (e.g., Crisco, Wesson), many salad dressings, soy formula, soy milk, edamame, protein bars, protein powders, soy sauce, tamari, tempeh, teriyaki sauce, tofu, fish and other products packed in soy oil, Worcestershire sauce.

Substitute Foods: other milks (almond, coconut, cow, goat, oat, rice), other oils (coconut and olive), other protein powders (rice, et cetera), potatoes (as a thickening agent in place of tofu).

Eggs

Immediate and Delayed Allergic Reactions

In pediatric practices, eggs are among the foods that most frequently cause hypersensitivity reactions. The primary offender is the albumin in egg whites, which binds primarily to IgE antibodies that cause immediate reactions, and sometimes severe anaphylaxis.[68]* However, delayed allergy reactions are also seen, especially when commercially produced eggs are eaten in excess for long periods of time.[69] Egg allergies are the most common cause of infantile eczema, which has been linked to a greater predisposition to bronchial asthma later in children and adults (especially with allopathic suppressive drug intervention such as steroid creams).[70] Other typical manifestations of egg hypersensitivity are urticaria (hives), angioedema (swelling of the skin), headaches, excessive flatulence, vomiting, and diarrhea.[71]

Egg-Related Allergens

Since the albumin protein in other bird species is antigenically similar to that hen's eggs, allergy to the eggs of ducks, turkeys, and other fowl is common. Some children (or adults) may also be sensitive to chicken meat.[72]

*Unfortunately, it is impossible to separate the yolks from the whites so that every trace of albumen is removed.

Furthermore, since several vaccines—including measles, influenza, and yellow fever—are grown on chick embryos or eggs, extremely sensitive children may react allergenically to them.[73] For this and other reasons, including possible reactions to the toxic preservatives such as formaldehyde in vaccinations, resuscitation equipment should always be available when administering vaccines to infants and children.

Adulterated Commercial Eggs Most at Fault

As in the case of wheat, dairy, corn, and soy, the toxification of eggs—through the use of antibiotics, toxic feed, and the extra hormones stimulated from the daily torture of being imprisoned in a small cage—is currently one of the primary causes of subsequent allergic reactions. Therefore, for an individual who has tested positive to eggs in the elimination-challenge test and avoided them for a reasonable period of time (for, example, two to six months), the first challenge should be a cooked fertile egg from an organic free-range hen. (Cooking denatures the albumin protein, rendering it less allergenic, so a hard-boiled egg is the least allergenic of all.) Possible tolerance to eggs at this time is further enhanced if you have been undergoing holistic care, including digestive enzyme and probiotic (acidophilus and bifidus bacteria) supplementation. Of course, if you have a history of severe reactions to eggs, it is important to check with your holistic practitioner first before challenging this food.

Egg Avoidance

Specific Foods to Avoid: eggs (hen, duck, or turkey).

What May Be Listed on the Label: albumin (or ovoalbumin), egg whites or yolks (powdered or dried), livetin, lysozyme, ovomucin, ovomucoid, ovotransferrin, vitellin (ovovitellin).

Typical Foods to Avoid: eggs, omelets, quiches, custards, puddings, soufflés, many baked goods (bread, cakes, cookies, glazes, icings, meringue, muffins, pastries), some baking powders, some breaded foods, some candies, doughnuts, dumplings, egg noodles and some macaroni, French toast, hollandaise and other creamy sauces, some ice creams, marshmallows, mayonnaise, meat loaf, pancakes, salad dressings, tartar sauce, waffles.

EGG WHITE PROTEINS

The total protein content of egg white is approximately 10 percent and consists of about forty different proteins. The majority of protein content in egg whites (the yolk is not very allergenic) is ovoalbumin at 54 percent.[74] (*Ovo-* simply denotes "egg.")

Substitute Foods: mashed banana, extra flour, baking powder, ground flax, psyllium seed, or cornstarch (as binding substances); coconut oil or butter; Ener-G Foods Egg Replacer (contains potato flour).

HIDDEN EGG PRODUCTS

Surprisingly, some wines are "cleared" with egg white, and some pharmaceutical preparations such as nose drops and laxatives may contain egg.

THE VERY REAL BENEFITS OF IDENTIFYING AND AVOIDING A PRIMARY ALLERGEN

It's essential that every health-conscious individual is aware of the importance of identifying and avoiding for a period of time any possible food allergens. As the preceding text indicates, health issues arising from allergies can range from slightly annoying to severe and degenerative. However, whether the externally noticed symptoms are mild or major, it is important to realize that chronic allergies are never minor but an important indicator of systemic illness and of serious immune system dysfunction.[75] In fact, food allergies have even been linked to serious degenerative diseases such as multiple sclerosis (MS), amyotrophic lateral sclerosis (ALS) or Lou Gehrig's disease, and cancer.[76] Therefore, identifying a food allergy(s) and eliminating the offending food(s) from your diet can make the difference between a life lived fully and one marred by chronic symptoms and ill health. Furthermore, similar to the removal of mercury amalgam fillings, it is one of the best preventive measures to guard against the onset of future neurological and degenerative disease.

Other gains made from eliminating allergenic—and to the body's way of thinking *toxic*—foods include an often substantial decrease in chronic seasonal allergies and hay fever symptoms. Cross-reactivity, a well-researched area in immunology, occurs when an immune system antibody (IgE, IgG, IgM) mistakes a normally nonoffensive antigen as a threat and binds to it.* For example, in the case of a dairy allergy, IgG and IgM antibodies bind to cow's milk antigens, but quite often also to the similarly appearing goat's milk antigens. Thus, many dairy-allergic individuals cannot eat *any* milk products—cow, goat, sheep, or buffalo—due to this cross-reactivity. Less well understood is the often seen cross-reactivity between a peanut (a legume) and a walnut or a pecan in the completely different "tree nut" family. A few cross-reactions "seem to defy any explanation," such as the immune system error that confuses dust mites and kiwi fruit.[77]

These antibody blunders are the primary reason that many individuals react in a domino-type effect to more and more food and environmental antigens over time. However, by simply avoiding a daily dose of disturbing allergenic foods, people with hay fever and seasonal allergies invariably benefit greatly through this reduction of their total immunological load. Furthermore, as the immune system calms down and begins to function more effectively, the antibodies become more intelligent and discriminating. Therefore, cross-reactivity is reduced and more "advanced" patients are then able to eat their goat yogurt or spelt bread, even though they may still have a mild dairy or wheat allergy.

HOLISTIC CARE

After a period of avoidance that can range from one to two months or one to two years, most individuals can begin to eat small amounts of their allergenic foods on a rotation basis (every few days). This is especially the case in "cleaner" individuals, who have drained and detoxified their heavy metal load (mercury amalgam fillings and nickel- or palladium-laden crowns), use petrochemical-free personal care products and cleaning supplies, have treated their tonsil and dental focal infections and scar interference fields (described in part 4), and are on their constitutional homeopathic remedy (discussed in chapter 14). They may also be supplementing with digestive enzymes, an especially important "crutch" to facilitate the assimilation of needed nutrients while the digestive and immune systems are rebalancing and repairing. Additionally, they may employ herbal drainage (gemmotherapy or plant stem cell) remedies such as European Alder, Grey Alder, Fig, and Walnut, which are indispensable at draining gut toxins and regenerating gastrointestinal function. Finally, probiotics (acidophilus and bifidus bacteria) are essential at some point (after the gut pathogens have been reduced enough to allow implantation of good bugs) to help repopulate the intestine with protective and beneficial flora.

- **The digestive enzymes** Dipan-9 (pancreatin) and Bio-Gest or B.P.P. (pancreatin plus hydrochloric acid combinations) facilitate protein digestion to reduce allergy symptoms, as well as fat and carbohydrate digestion. To order, contact Thorne Research at (800) 228-1966. For those who have—or have had—ulcers, gastritis, gastroesophageal reflux disease (GERD), or simply undiagnosed chronic pain in the stomach or abdomen, Formula 601, also known as Gastric Comfort, is an excellent enzyme and herbal blend without HCL (hydrocholoric acid) protease (which can be irritating to an inflamed stomach or intestinal mucosal lining over time). To order, contact Enzymes, Inc., at (800) 637-7893.

When individuals ingest milk or wheat products every day, symptoms of allergic reactions often blur with their particular personality traits and may become an accepted and even unnoticed part of their everyday life.[78] Therefore, eliminating these consoling as well as stimulating allergenic foods can take as much courage and willpower as taking that first step toward self-understanding by walking into a psychotherapist's office or joining a psychospiritual path. It is therefore important to get the support needed to take this step—from family or a significant other, from a holistic practitioner,

*This is because the antibody recognizes only a small part of its antigen. This "chemical handshake" between the antibody (IgE, IgG) and the antigen molecule (e.g., milk, wheat) occurs on a particularly small site of the antigen called the *epitope*. The epitope binding and recognition site may look similar to that of another antigen, and the antibody can then mistake this small area of a normally nonreactive food like halibut for a shrimp. (L. Gamlin, *The Allergy Bible* [Pleasantville, NY: Reader's Digest, 2001], 15.)

and through self-study on this subject—to become *absolutely* convinced of the serious effects of hidden food allergies. Only through avoiding and treating these major insults to immune and digestive system functioning can individuals realize the physical and emotional equilibrium enjoyed by those who have essentially cleared their food sensitivities and enjoy the very gratifying rewards of optimal health.

NOTES

1. P. Austin et al., *Food Allergies Made Simple* (Sunfield, Mich.: Family Health Publications, 1985), 1.
2. J. Pizzorno and M. Murray, *Textbook of Natural Medicine,* 2nd ed., vol. 1 (New York: Churchill Livingstone, 2000), 454.
3. K. Daniel, "Soy Alert!" *Wise Traditions* 7, no. 1 (Winter 2005/Spring 2006): 63.
4. J. Nowicki, "Food Allergies—an Unrecognized Epidemic," *Priority One Newsletter* 6, no. 2 (July 10, 2006): 2.
5. T. Randolph and R. Moss, *Alternative Approach to Allergies* (New York: Harper and Row, 1990), 4, 35.
6. J. Brostoff and S. Challacombe, *Food Allergy and Intolerance* (London: Balliere Tindall, 1987), 428–29.
7. Ibid.
8. P. Austin et al., *Food Allergies Made Simple* (Sunfield, Mich.: Family Health Publications, 1985), 39–40.
9. I. Bell, *Clinical Ecology* (Bolinas, Calif.: Common Knowledge Press, 1982), 31–32.
10. Chris Gupta, "Enriched Food Deception," August 24, 2004, www.newmediaexplorer.org/chris/2004/08/24/enriched_food_deception.htm.
11. K. Czapp, "Against the Grain," *Wise Traditions* 7, no. 2 (Summer 2006): 21.
12. S. Fallon, *Nourishing Traditions* (San Diego: ProMotion Publishing, 1999), 57.
13. Ibid., 463.
14. J. Brostoff and S. Challacombe, *Food Allergy and Intolerance* (London: Balliere Tindall, 1987), 808.
15. N. Appleton, *Lick the Sugar Habit* (Garden City Park, N.Y.: Avery Publishing Group, 1996), 34.
16. P. Austin et al., *Food Allergies Made Simple* (Sunfield, Mich.: Family Health Publications, 1985), 3.
17. N. Trenev, *Probiotics: Nature's Internal Healers* (New York: Avery, 1998), 55.
18. L. Gamlin, *The Allergy Bible* (Pleasantville, N.Y.: Reader's Digest, 2001), 21, 241–43.
19. J. Nowicki, "Food Allergies—an Unrecognized Epidemic," *Priority One Newsletter* 6, no. 2 (July 10, 2006): 2.
20. L. Gamlin, *The Allergy Bible* (Pleasantville, N.Y.: Reader's Digest, 2001), 65, 91; J. Brostoff and S. Challacombe, *Food Allergy and Intolerance* (London: Balliere Tindall, 1987), 368.
21. A. Rowe, *Elimination Diets and the Patient's Allergies* (Philadelphia: Lea and Febiger, 1944), 13.
22. D. Thom, *Coping with Food Intolerances* (Portland, Ore.: JELD Publications, 1995), 41–43.
23. Ibid.
24. A. Gaby, "Letter to the Editor," *Alternative Medicine Review* 9, no. 3 (September 2004): 238.
25. J. Brostoff and S. Challacombe, *Food Allergy and Intolerance* (London: Balliere Tindall, 1987), 915; A. Rowe, *Elimination Diets and the Patient's Allergies* (Philadelphia: Lea and Febiger, 1944), 134.
26. G. Smith, "Nightshades: Problems from These Popular Foods Exposed to the Light of Day," *Wise Traditions* 11, no. 1 (Spring 2010): 48–54.
27. J. Brostoff and S. Challacombe, *Food Allergy and Intolerance* (London: Balliere Tindall, 1987), 808–9.
28. N. Campbell-McBride, "Gut and Psychology Syndrome," *Wise Traditions* 8, no. 4 (Winter 2007): 21.
29. J. Matthews, *Nourishing Hope for Autism* (San Francisco: Nourishing Hope, 2008), 95–98.
30. A. Rowe, *Elimination Diets and the Patient's Allergies* (Philadelphia: Lea and Febiger, 1944), 30.
31. J. Brostoff and S. Challacombe, *Food Allergy and Intolerance* (London: Balliere Tindall, 1987), 815.
32. J. Nowicki, "Food Allergies—an Unrecognized Epidemic," *Priority One Newsletter* 6, no. 2 (July 10, 2006): 2.
33. N. Appleton, *Heal Yourself with Natural Foods* (New York: Sterling Publishing Company, Inc., 1998), 33.
34. J. Brostoff and S. Challacombe, *Food Allergy and Intolerance* (London: Balliere Tindall, 1987), 521–22.
35. R. Berkow et al., eds., *The Merck Manual,* 15th ed. (Rahway, N.J.: Merck Sharp and Dohme Research Laboratories, 1987), 792–93.
36. S. Fallon, *Nourishing Traditions* (San Diego: ProMotion Publishing, 1999), 56.
37. P. M. Kidd, "Autism, an Extreme Challenge to Integrative Medicine. Part 1: The Knowledge Base," *Alternative Medicine Review* 7, no. 4 (August 2002): 305.
38. K. Reichelt and A. Knivsberg, "Can the Pathophysiology of Autism Be Explained by Discovering Urine Peptides?" in "DAN! (Defeat Autism Now!) Spring 2002 Confer-

ence Practitioner Training," B. Rimland, ed. (San Diego, Calif.: Autism Research Institute, 2002).

39. R. Berkow et al., eds., *The Merck Manual,* 15th ed. (Rahway, N.J.: Merck Sharp and Dohme Research Laboratories, 1987), 792–93.
40. K. Czapp, "Against the Grain," *Wise Traditions* 7, no. 2 (Summer 2006): 18.
41. A. Vojdani, T. O'Bryan, and G. H. Kellermann, "The Immunology of Gluten Sensitivity Beyond the Intestinal Tract," *European Journal of Inflammation* 6, no. 2 (2008): 1–4.
42. S. Rockwell and L. Bondi, *Dr. Sally's Blood Sugar Blues* (Seattle: self-published, n.d.), 24.
43. S. Fallon, *Nourishing Traditions* (San Diego: ProMotion Publishing, 1999), 56.
44. J. Pizzorno and M. Murray, *Textbook of Natural Medicine,* 2nd ed. (New York: Churchill Livingstone, 2000), 1159.
45. S. Rockwell and L. Bondi, *Dr. Sally's Blood Sugar Blues* (Seattle: self-published, n.d.), 24.
46. S. Fallon, *Nourishing Traditions* (San Diego: ProMotion Publishing, 1999), 459; L. Gamlin, *The Allergy Bible* (Pleasantville, N.Y.: Reader's Digest, 2001), 177.
47. J. Brostoff and S. Challacombe, *Food Allergy and Intolerance* (London: Balliere Tindall, 1987), 541.
48. R. DiCagno et al., "Sourdough Bread Made from Wheat and Nontoxic Flours and Started with Selected Lactobacilli Is Tolerated in Celiac Sprue Patients," *Applied and Environmental Microbiology* 70, no. 2 (2004): 1088–96.
49. S. Petusevsky, *The Whole Foods Cookbook* (Nottingham, UK: Clarkson Potter, 2002), 155.
50. D. Thom, *Coping with Food Intolerances* (Portland Ore.: JELD Publications, 1995), 5–6.
51. P. Austin et al., *Food Allergies Made Simple* (Sunfield, Mich.: Family Health Publications, 1985), 9.
52. D. Twogood, *No Milk* (Victorville, Calif.: Wilhelmina Books, 1991), 73–75, 248.
53. J. Brostoff and S. Challacombe, *Food Allergy and Intolerance* (London: Balliere Tindall, 1987), 347.
54. Ibid.
55. D. Twogood, *No Milk* (Victorville, Calif.: Wilhelmina Books, 1991), 73.
56. J. Brostoff and S. Challacombe, *Food Allergy and Intolerance* (London: Balliere Tindall, 1987), 591, 973.
57. F. Oski, *Don't Drink Your Milk* (Brushton, N.Y.: TEACH Services, 1983), 10.
58. S. Fallon, *Nourishing Traditions* (San Diego: ProMotion Publishing, 1999), 80, 81.
59. J. Brostoff and S. Challacombe, *Food Allergy and Intolerance* (London: Balliere Tindall, 1987), 592.
60. E. Roehl, *Whole Food Facts* (Rochester, Vt.: Healing Arts Press, 1988), 64–65.
61. N. Appleton, *Lick the Sugar Habit* (Garden City Park, N.Y.: Avery Publishing Group, 1996), 57.
62. C. Kilham, *The Whole Food Bible* (Rochester, Vt.: Healing Arts Press, 1991), 26.
63. E. Roehl, *Whole Food Facts* (Rochester, Vt.: Healing Arts Press, 1988), 64–65.
64. S. Fallon, *Nourishing Traditions* (San Diego: ProMotion Publishing, 1999), 454.
65. P. Austin et al., *Food Allergies Made Simple* (Sunfield, Mich.: Family Health Publications, 1985), 13.
66. N. Appleton, *Lick the Sugar Habit* (Garden City Park, N.Y.: Avery Publishing Group, 1996), 125.
67. P. Austin et al., *Food Allergies Made Simple* (Sunfield, Mich.: Family Health Publications, 1985), 17.
68. J. Brostoff and S. Challacombe, *Food Allergy and Intolerance* (London: Balliere Tindall, 1987), 368.
69. T. Randolph and R. Moss, *Alternative Approach to Allergies* (New York: Harper and Row, 1990), 29.
70. P. Austin et al., *Food Allergies Made Simple* (Sunfield, Mich.: Family Health Publications, 1985), 16; J. Brostoff and S. Challacombe, *Food Allergy and Intolerance* (London: Balliere Tindall, 1987), 368.
71. P. Austin et al., *Food Allergies Made Simple* (Sunfield, Mich.: Family Health Publications, 1985), 16; D. Thom, *Coping with Food Intolerances* (Portland, Ore.: JELD Publications, 1995), 113.
72. P. Austin et al., *Food Allergies Made Simple* (Sunfield, Mich.: Family Health Publications, 1985), 16.
73. L. Gamlin, *The Allergy Bible* (Pleasantville, N.Y.: Reader's Digest, 2001), 249.
74. J. Brostoff and S. Challacombe, *Food Allergy and Intolerance* (London: Balliere Tindall, 1987), 370.
75. R. Francis, *Never Be Sick Again* (Deerfield Beach, Fla.: Health Communications, Inc., 2002), 189.
76. Pat Lazarus, "Multiple Sclerosis and Amyotrophic Lateral Sclerosis: More Hope Than We Think?" *Let's Live,* April 1980, 70–77; J. Diamond et al., *An Alternative Medicine Definitive Guide to Cancer* (Tiburon, Calif.: Future Medicine Publishing, Inc., 1997), 144, 220.
77. L. Gamlin, *The Allergy Bible* (Pleasantville, N.Y.: Reader's Digest, 2001), 15.
78. G. Null, *The Egg Project* (New York: Four Walls Eight Windows, 1987), 80.

7

DYSBIOSIS

All disease begins in the gut.

HIPPOCRATES, FATHER OF MEDICINE (460–370 BCE)

If the probability of serious disease from eating sugar and allergenic foods doesn't "scare you straight," then this section on the pandemic putrefaction of everyone's gut from these foods (and drugs) just might. In the early part of the twentieth century, Professor Elie Metchnikoff (1845–1916), a Russian scientist at the Pasteur Institute in Paris, coined the term *dysbiosis,* which comes from the term *symbiosis,* meaning "living together in mutual harmony," and the prefix *dys,* meaning "not." *Dysbiosis* describes bowel toxicity arising from a deranged intestinal terrain due to the overgrowth of pathogenic microbes. Bowel toxicity is as old as poor dietary choices and overindulgence. However, with the twentieth century's exceptional abuse of antibiotics and refined sugar, *dysbiosis* has been embraced by holistic practitioners as a perfect term to characterize this resulting epidemic of pathogenic microbial overgrowth. Furthermore, as Dr. Metchnikoff believed and described in detail, gastrointestinal *endotoxins*—the toxins produced from pathogenic microbes—greatly contribute to chronic and serious disease and the resulting shortened life spans.[1*] In fact, the expression "Death begins in the colon" was apparently originated by Metchnikoff, who was echoing Hippocrates' assertion two centuries earlier that disease—and death—truly begin in the gut.[2] In 1908, Dr. Metchnikoff won the Nobel Prize for his work researching lactobacilli and demonstrating their role in preventing and reversing intestinal dysbiosis.[3]

gut: The term *gut* refers to the intestine or the bowel—both the small and large aspects.

"FRIENDLY" BACTERIAL FLORA

The digestive tract, from the mouth to the anus, has two major functions: (1) digestion and absorption of food nutrients and (2) protection and maintenance of normal immune system defenses (see figure 7.1). Within this tract literally *trillions* of bacteria reside—*millions* in the mouth, few to none in the stomach due to its highly acidic environment, *millions* in our small intestine, and *trillions* in our large intestine. These friendly bacteria are called intestinal *flora,* derived from the Latin word for "flower." This term was first adopted by the Swedish botanist Carolus Linnaeus in 1745 to characterize the plants (and flowers) of a specified region or time. Thus, *intestinal flora* is used to designate the plant life, or bacteria and other microbes, which reside in the region of the intestine. And this plant life is exceptionally numerous and diverse. For example, there are an astounding 400 to 500 different kinds of bacteria in our intestines, *each* of which has numerous types of different strains. However, out of these literally thousands of different bacterial species, two groups have been identified as "friendly" and essential to health—the lactobacilli bacteria that reside primarily in the small

*Near the end of the nineteenth century, renowned naturopath Louis Kuhne proposed that excessive or wrong food intake caused the fermentation and toxic overgrowth of intestinal bacteria, which over time resulted in disease. (J. Hawrelak and S. Myers, "The Causes of Intestinal Dysbiosis: A Review," *Alternative Medicine Review* 9, no. 2 [June 4, 2004]: 180–81.)

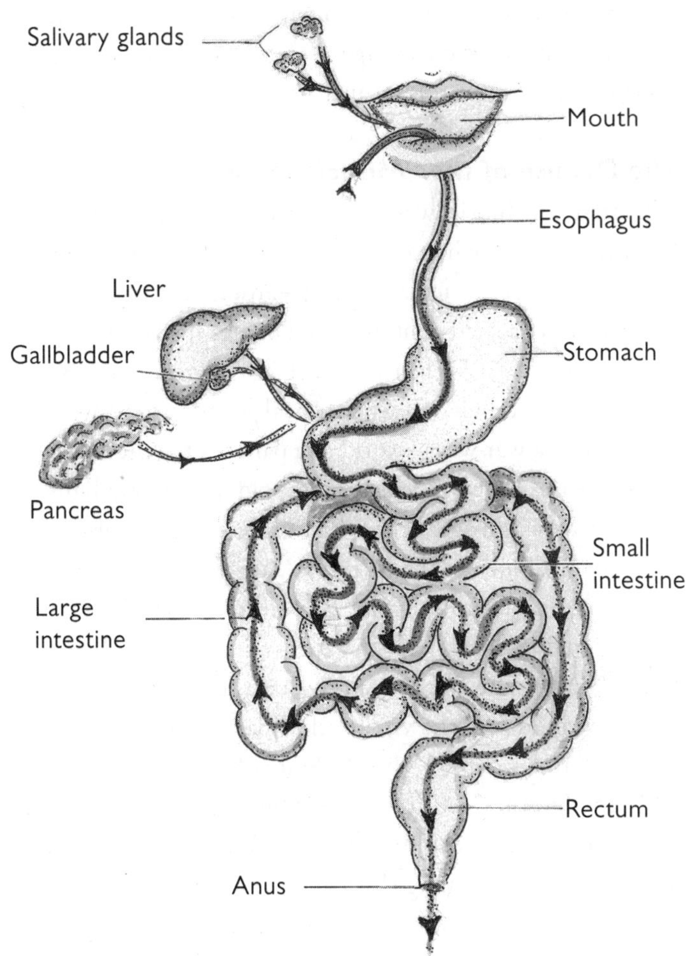

Figure 7.1. A schematic representation of the digestive system. Food travels in one long tube from the mouth to the anus, assisted by the four ancillary glands and organs—the salivary glands, the gallbladder, the liver, and the pancreas.

intestine, and the bifidobacteria bacteria found primarily in the large intestine.[4]

These "friendly" flora are indeed *very* good friends, and they perform a multitude of functions. Lactobacilli produce their own natural antibiotic substances (acidophilin, lactocidin, and acidolin) to fend off bacterial pathogens such as salmonella, shigella, staphylococcus, *E. coli,* clostridia, and *H. pylori.*[5] These friendly bacteria also secrete acids (acetic, formic, and lactic) that through "competitive exclusion" make the intestinal area unsuitable for the overgrowth of yeast, such as *C. albicans,* and other pathogenic microorganisms.[6] Lactobacilli and bifidobacteria also manufacture essential B vitamins (B_1, B_2, B_3, B_5, B_6, B_{12}), as well as the important fat-soluble vitamins A and K.[7] Furthermore, they are required in the synthesis of essential fatty acids as well as the valuable short-chain fatty acids, which provide 10 percent of the body's energy needs and have powerful antimicrobial properties.[8] These friendly flora additionally break down and rebuild hormones, protect us from xenobiotics such as mercury, pesticides, and radiation, and have antitumor and anticancer effects. Finally, lactobacilli and bifidobacteria are essential for normal digestive functioning by regulating peristalsis for regular bowel movements, digesting lactose in dairy products, and digesting protein into free and utilizable peptides and amino acids.[9]

> **peristalsis:** *Peristalsis* is the wormlike movement of the digestive tract that propels its contents along, resulting finally in defecation.

ANTIBIOTICS

Ecological Marauders

Antibiotics, like other drugs, have no innate wisdom directing them in the body. Therefore, as their name implies—*antibiotic* meaning "against life"—they indiscriminately kill harmful pathogenic bacteria *and* the friendly and essential lactobacillus and bifidobacterium species.* For example, the cephalosporin and erythromycin families of antibiotics are capable of eliminating 99 percent of lactobacillus species over the standard ten-day course of antibiotics.[10] Although these friendly bacteria have the potential to recolonize in the intestine afterward, this is often an uphill battle with the current widespread ingestion of sugar and other junk foods, the lack of fermented foods in the standard American diet, and the repeated rounds of antibiotic prescriptions for recurrent infections.

Antibiotics and Leaky Gut Syndrome

Not only is the population of friendly flora often devastated, but after several courses of antibiotics, only the

*Another reason antibiotics have such a devastating systemic effect on the body is that when they kill a bacterium it explodes into fragments of endotoxins. Dr. Hal Huggins clearly describes this process: "Endotoxins present a huge challenge to the immune system, for now, instead of facing one bacterium, it has to process and eliminate perhaps one hundred endotoxins." (Hal Huggins, "Root Canal Dangers," *Wise Tradtitions* 11, no. 2 [Summer 2010], 50.)

most hardy and resistant bacteria, parasites, viruses, and yeasts remain. These pathogenic microbes produce poisonous chemicals—such as amines, ammonia, hydrogen sulfide, indoles, phenols, and secondary bile acids—that cause extensive harm to the vital "brush border"* intestinal lining. After numerous courses of antibiotics as well as dietary abuse, this intestinal lining can become so irritated and inflamed that the normally protective tight junctions (*desmosomes*)—that is, the tiny intestinal wall holes that allow only properly digested fats, proteins, and starches to pass through—become quite damaged. As these deranged junctions grow larger and larger, they allow undigested food particles, as well as toxic chemicals, metals, and disease-causing bacteria and yeast, to move directly into the bloodstream. Then this formerly protective intestinal mucosa functions no longer as an adequate barrier but as a primary portal of entry for both foreign and *autogenous* (self-generated) toxins.[11] This intestinal hyperpermeability has been termed "leaky gut syndrome," and it is a prime factor in the causation of food allergies discussed in chapter 6. Leaky gut syndrome is also one of the key reasons allergic individuals don't respond well to treatment and must avoid their particular food allergy for an extensive period—that is, from three to five years or even more. (This time frame can be less with "radical" medical intervention from a knowledgeable holistic practitioner.)

autogenous: *Autogenous* means self-generated or originating within the body, including the amines, ammonia, hydrogen sulfide, indoles, phenols, and secondary bile acids that were just described.

The most serious cases of dysbiosis and resulting leaky gut syndrome are caused by overuse of antibiotics. How this medication, which was once championed as the "miracle drug," has deteriorated into what the world-famous homeopath George Vithoulkas has called "one of the greatest curses of our modern civilization" is a long odyssey indeed.[12] However, it boils down to twentieth- and twenty-first-century scientific materialism thinking: excessive blind faith in modern technology and the concomitant frenetic seeking for the quickest and easiest "magic bullet" to restore health.

*This important epithelial border, covered with microscopic villi, is where absorption of essential nutrients takes place in the small intestine. This essential mucosal barrier also protects the body from foreign antigens.

The Demise of the "Miracle Drug"

The first antibiotic was discovered by Sir Alexander Fleming in 1928, when he noticed a clear ring indicating no staphylococcus bacterial growth around a mold spore (penicillin) that had contaminated one of his laboratory culture plates.[13]* Within the next few decades, antibiotics came to be viewed as chemical wonders and were "grasped by a war-weary world as a panacea for the infectious diseases that had killed more soldiers and civilians in the two world wars than had bullets and bombs."[14] Due to antibiotics, the survival rate for pneumonia increased dramatically from 20 percent in 1937 to 85 percent in 1964. In 1962, the Australian immunologist Frank Macfarlane Burnet wrote that the late twentieth century would see "the virtual elimination of infectious disease"; and in 1967, United States Surgeon General William Stewart told a White House gathering that infectious disease would soon be completely eradicated from the planet. During this time the accolade "miracle drug" entered America's vocabulary, and the family doctor became a hero.[15]

Amid this wave of unbridled optimism few listened to any words of caution, even ironically from Alexander Fleming himself. In fact, in 1945 the honest and forthright British scientist actually stated his misgivings over this antibiotic in a *New York Times* article. Fleming accurately prophesized that the "misuse of penicillin could lead to the selection and propagation of mutant forms of bacteria resistant to the drug"—an occurrence he had *already witnessed* in his own laboratory.[16] But not even Fleming, nor anyone else at that time, could have predicted the devastating assault resistant bacteria would wage—and continues to wage—against humankind.

*Contrary to the popular myth surrounding Fleming, he himself was never able to reproduce these first results and as late as 1939 was inclined to write off penicillin as a useful antibiotic. It was actually Dr. Howard Florey and a colleague, Dr. Chain, who proved penicillin's effectiveness and were able to produce it in a utilizable form. (S. Shakman, *The Autohemotherapy Reference Manual* [Santa Monica, Calif.: Institute of Science, 1998], ch. 5, p. 4.)

Bacterial Resistance

When bacteria reproduce through a process called *conjugation,* they share their genetic material with each other, including pieces of DNA that are referred to as *plasmids.* These plasmids carry supplemental genetic information to ensure the survival of bacteria. Some of this information includes how to adapt when subjected to various temperatures, shade versus sunlight, and acidic or alkaline pH in soils; how to adhere to the cells lining the intestinal mucosa and not be displaced by the digested food passing by; and, finally, *how to survive and resist antibiotics.*[17] This ability to adapt and resist pernicious influences, which is conferred by and carried in the plasmids, is referred to as resistance factors or *R factors.* This ability is not particularly unusual, but simply a fact of life for all living things and part of normal evolution.[18] However, unlike human beings, who transfer this survival information from one generation to the next, bacteria can transfer this information from one to another as quickly as they reproduce, which in optimal growth conditions can occur in *less than one hour's time.*[19] In the face of this fantastic ability to adapt and survive, the efforts of the pharmaceutical giants, who have tried mightily to keep up with this bacterial resistance by introducing new antibiotics at a rate of *five to ten per decade,* are rather futile. In the reality of the world of microbes, bacteria's mutative ability to evolve in ever-harsher conditions against more and more lethal antibiotic drugs seems to know no bounds.[20] Dr. George Jacoby of Harvard Medical School summarizes this point quite succinctly: "Bugs are always figuring out ways to get around the antibiotics we throw at them. They adapt, they come roaring back."[21]

This astounding ability to resist antibiotic drugs has been most dramatically witnessed in hospitals, which have become the greatest bacterial breeding grounds of all. For example, as of 1997, hospitals reported that one of the most dangerous microbes, *Staphylococcus aureus,* which originally was 100 percent *sensitive* to penicillin in 1950, had become 95 percent *resistant* to penicillin (as well as methicillin, dicloxacillin, nafcillin, and oxacillin) and currently could be treated by only one antibiotic (vancomycin).[22] Many readers are familiar with the evolved variant of this bacterium dubbed MRSA, for methicillin-resistant *Staphylococcus aureus,* since it has become a major plague in hospitals. Patients with open wounds and weakened immune systems are particularly at risk for MRSA. Visitors and hospital staff are advised to follow stringent sanitary procedures when they are near patients with MRSA infections, including isolation protocols requiring donning gloves, gowns, and masks.

Similar to the staphylococcus example, although rheumatic fever was considered completely eradicated through penicillin and erythromycin by 1970, in 1985 a new mutant strain of the primary causative bacterium of this illness, *Streptococcus pyogenes,* was discovered to be responsible not only for the recurrence of rheumatic fever but for an eighty-fold increase between 1982 and 1985. Jim Henson, the famed puppeteer and inventor of the Muppets, was a well-known victim of this more virulent and mutant strain of streptococcus in 1990.[23]

Furthermore, pathogenic *enterococci* (*E. faecalis* and *E. faecium*) bacteria have presently become resistant to *all* known antibiotics, even to what some physicians refer to as "the last big guns"—that is, powerful antibiotics like vancomycin and quinolone.[24] Many who suffered from acne and the resulting intestinal dysbiosis from years of antibiotic use will recognize the medication tetracycline, which is yet another example of drug failure since bacteria have become resistant to this family of broad-spectrum antibiotics as well. In fact, staphylococci bacteria have evolved a kind of "pump mechanism" that pumps out tetracycline medications as fast as they enter in through the cell walls.[25]

Another example of nosocomial (hospital-induced) infections is the growing adaptability of *Clostridium difficile.* These bacteria, largely due to their resistance to the broad-spectrum antibiotic ciprofloxacin, cause one of the most common infections occurring in hospitals and long-term care institutions, prolonging hospital stays by an average of nearly three weeks.[26] The toxins from clostridium are so virulent that they literally peel off the lining of the colon, resulting in an explosive, debilitating, and often lethal form of diarrhea.[27]* In fact, illness initiated by *Staphylococcus, Streptococcus, Enterococcus,*

---

*The fact that diarrhea—mild to major—is reported in one out of every eight to ten patients who have taken antibiotics demonstrates the damage that is done internally to the intestinal mucosa and normal flora. (M. Lappé, *When Antibiotics Fail* [Berkeley, Calif.: North Atlantic Books, 1986], xv.)

TYPICAL ANTIBIOTICS AND ANTIBACTERIALS USED IN ALLOPATHIC MEDICINE

Cephalosporins, 1st generation: cefadroxil, cefazolin, cephalexin, cephalothin, cephapirin, cephradine

Cephalosporins, 2nd generation: cefaclor, cefamandole, cefmetazole, cefonicid, cefotetan, cefoxitin, cefprozil, cefuroxime, loracarbef

Cephalosporins, 3rd generation: cefdinir, cefixime, cefoperazone, cefotaxime, cefpodoxime, ceftazidime, ceftibuten, ceftizoxime, ceftriaxone

Cephalosporins, 4th generation: cefepime

Penicillins/Natural: penicillin G aqueous, penicillin G benzathine, penicillin G benzathine/procaine, penicillin V potassium

Penicillins/Aminopenicillins: amoxicillin, ampicillin, bacampicillin

Penicillins/Extended spectrum: carbenicillin, mezlocillin, piperacillin, ticarcillin

Penicillins/Penicilinase-resistant: cloxacillin, dicloxacillin, methicillin, nafcillin, oxacillin

Penicillins/Beta-lactamase inhibitor: amoxicillin/clavulanate potassium, ampicillin/sulbactam, piperacillin/tazobactam, ticarcillin/clavulanate potassium

Carbapenems: imipenem/cilistatin, meropenem

Monobactams: aztreonam

Aminoglycosides: amikacin, gentamicin, kanamycin, neomycin, netilmicin, paromomycin, streptomycin, tobramycin

Macrolides: azithromycin, clarithromycin, dirithromycin, erythromycin, troleandomycin

Quinolones: nalidixic acid, oxolinic acid

Fluoroquinolones: cinoxacin, ciprofloxacin, gatifloxacin, gemifloxacin, levofloxacin, lomefloxacin, moxifloxacin, norfloxacin, ofloxacin, pefloxacin, sparfloxacin, trovafloxacin

Tetracyclines: chlortetracycline, demeclocycline, doxycycline, methacycline, minocycline, oxytetracycline, tetracycline

Antituberculosis agents: capreomycin, cycloserine, ethambutol, ethionamide, isoniazid, para-aminosalicylic acid, pyrazinamide, rifabutin, rifampin, rifapentine

Sulfonamides: sulfadiazine, sulfamethizole, sulfamethoxazole, sulfisoxazole

Oxazolidinones: linezolid

Streptogramins: quinupristin/dalfopristin

Methenamines: methenamine

Nitrofurans: furazolidone, nitrofurantoin

Lincosamides: clindamycin, lincomycin

Folate antagonists: trimethoprim

Drug combinations: erythromycin ethylsuccinate/sulfisoxazole, trimethoprim/sulfamethoxazole

Other antibiotics: bacitracin, chloramphenicol, colistin, fosfomycin, metronidazole, novobiocin, polymyxin B, spectinomycin, vancomycin

Adapted from *The Antibiotic Paradox: How the Misuse of Antibiotics Destroys Their Curative Powers* by Dr. Stuart B. Levy.

Clostridium, and other pathogenic bacilli have become so prevalent that they have gained the notorious distinction of being the number one cause of nosocomial infections.[28]

Serious Illnesses on the Rise

In 1994, a *Time* magazine article reported that because bacteria have "outwitted antibiotics," both new and old infections are once again on the rise, including streptococcus A ("flesh-eating bacteria"), cholera (*Vibrio cholerae*), gonorrhea (*Neisseria gonorrhoeae*), leprosy (*Mycobacterium leprae*), Legionnaire's disease (*Legionella pneumophila*), tuberculosis (*Mycobacterium tuberculosis*), and even AIDS and cancer.[29] In fact, in a study of more than 10,000 Washington State women, a clear link was discovered between breast cancer and the amount of antibiotics these women had taken in their life. The researchers concluded from the data that women who had used the most antibiotics had *double* the chance of getting breast cancer, and furthermore, that this association was consistent for all forms of antibiotics and that the cancer risk was increased by the number of courses of antibiotics taken.[30]

EXAMPLE OF ANTIBIOTIC RAMIFICATIONS

One tragic example of the ramifications of antibiotic damage was illustrated by the suicide of Hannelore Kohl, wife of former German Chancellor Helmut Kohl, in 2001 after she had suffered since 1993 from a painful and untreatable allergy to sunlight triggered by a severe reaction to penicillin. This photo-allergy, which caused rashes and fever, forced her to remain indoors every day until dark and to take painkillers for the last fifteen months of her life, before her untimely death.[31]

This serious drug resistance and resulting pathogenic microbial overgrowth is not just a problem in modern, industrialized nations but also in poorer countries where self-medication from antibiotics sold on the black market or over the counter commonly occurs. As researcher Laurie Garrett states in her book *The Coming Plague:*

> This state of affairs [excess antibiotic use] guaranteed that a sizable percentage of the human population were walking petri dishes, providing ideal conditions for accelerated bacterial mutation, natural selection, and evolution. Whether one looked in Spain, South Africa, the United States, Romania, Pakistan, Brazil, or anywhere else, the basic principle held true: overuse or misuse of antibiotics, particularly in small children and hospitalized patients, prompted [the] emergence of resistant mutant organisms.[32]

The chronic dysfunction and serious illnesses resulting from excessive antibiotic use are greatly influenced by each individual's particular miasmic tendency, as discussed in chapter 1. For example, if an individual functions primarily at the psoric level, the toxins manufactured in the dysbiotic intestine and released through the leaky gut wall into the bloodstream often take up residence in this first reaction mode's vulnerable skin tissues. The results are chronic eczema, acne, rashes, hives, or any number of other skin complaints. However, in an individual predisposed to the tuberculinic diathesis, the toxins more typically travel to susceptible throat and lung tissues, resulting in intermittent or chronic upper respiratory symptoms such as sneezing, nasal congestion, and sinusitis, as well as bronchitis and pneumonia. The following list contains the various symptoms and illnesses that can result from dysbiosis and leaky gut syndrome.*

Associated Syndromes and Symptoms of Intestinal Dysbiosis and Leaky Gut Syndrome

Abdominal pain
Acne and cystic acne
Aging (e.g., loss of skin elasticity, thinning skin, puffiness)
Allergy, food and environmental (seasonal)
Anxiety
Apthous ulcers (canker sores)
Arthritis
Attention deficit disorder (ADD)
Autism
Autoimmune syndromes
B_{12} deficiency
Cancer (especially breast and colon)
Candidiasis
Cervical dysplasia
Cognitive and memory deficits
Constipation
Chronic fatigue syndrome
Chronic hepatitis
Chronic pelvic inflammatory disease (PID)
Chronic sinusitis
Chronic urinary tract infections (interstitial cystitis)
Colitis
Colon polyps
Crohn's disease
Depression
Diaper rash
Diarrhea
Dyslexia
Eczema
Emphysema
Excessive weight and obesity
Fevers of unknown origin
Fibromyalgia
Gas (flatulence)
Gingivitis and periodontal disease
Halitosis (bad breath)
Herpes
Human papilloma virus
Hyperactivity

*Compiled from lists authored by Dr. Mikhael Adams, Dr. Ralph Golan, Dr. Morton Walker, and Elizabeth Lipski, M.S., C.C.N.

Hypoglycemia
Infertility
Inflammatory bowel disease
Insomnia
Multiple food and chemical sensitivities
Osteoporosis
Otitis media (ear infections)
Poor exercise tolerance
Prostatitis
Psoriasis
Schizophrenia
Shortness of breath
Steatorrhea (fatty stool seen in malabsorption syndromes)
Ulcerative colitis
Ulcers
Vitiligo

"The Second Brain": Dysbiosis and Psychological Symptoms

As demonstrated by the inclusion of various mental and emotional disorders in the preceding list, brain and central nervous system disturbances such as anxiety, depression, and even schizophrenia are correlated with dysbiosis. These mental and emotional symptoms are caused not only by toxins passing through the gut wall and traveling to the brain, but also by the lack of assimilation of essential vitamins, minerals, *and* neurotransmitters in the altered intestinal terrain. This latter point is particularly well illustrated by the little-known but astounding fact that 95 percent of the body's serotonin—the neurotransmitter that plays an essential role in mood regulation—is synthesized in the intestine and stored under its mucosal lining.[33] Yes, this is the same intestinal wall that is damaged and rendered too permeable by antibiotic drugs, resulting in leaky gut syndrome. That the gastrointestinal tract synthesizes serotonin as well as *every other* neurotransmitter found in the brain, as well as the fact that the gut contains more nerves than any other part of the body and can even function independently from the central nervous system, prompted neurobiologist Michael Gershon to label this intestinal or *enteric* nervous system "the second brain."

serotonin: *Serotonin* is a hormonal neurotransmitter that works at the synaptic junctions, where one nerve communicates with another. In the thalamus, serotonin activates the formation of dopamine, which inhibits pain and produces a feeling of well-being, and even euphoria.

enteric nervous system: The term *enteric nervous system* (ENS) denotes all the nerves that regulate function in the small and large intestines. Astoundingly, the ENS can function on its own without any input from the central (brain and spinal cord) or the peripheral (sympathetic and parasympathetic) nervous systems.[34]

▶ *The Second Brain* is also the name of Dr. Gershon's excellent book, which is a highly recommended read.

Thus, in a great majority of cases, the widespread use of SSRI drugs such as Prozac, Zoloft, and Paxil that address the biochemical aspect of depression through a serotonin neurotransmitter deficiency theory are targeting the wrong "brain." In fact, the origin of serotonin deficiency in our pandemic dysbiotic world lies in the *gut*—not the brain. A recent report titled "The Emperor's New Drugs" clearly demonstrates that the pharmaceutical companies manufacturing these popular antidepressant drugs are on the wrong track.[35] In this comprehensive examination of thirty-eight well-controlled and peer-reviewed studies, the effectiveness of six antidepressant drugs—Prozac, Zoloft, Paxil, Serzone, Celexa, and Effexor—was analyzed. Astonishingly, *every one* of these popular antidepressant drugs was found to be "clinically negligible" in comparison to placebos (sugar pills with no medicinal value) in the treatment of depression and related mood disorders.[36] Moreover, taking SSRIs on a long-term basis, similar to antibiotics, although the latter have a much quicker action, contributes to the reduction of beneficial bacteria in the gut over time.[37] Thus, the long-term use of SSRIs can generate the need for more antidepressant drugs as the damaged intestine further fails to generate enough of the neurotransmitters essential for normal brain function and emotional equanimity.

It is important to point out that this brain-gut relationship is not new. As Dr. Thomas Cowen pointed out in a *Wise Traditions* journal article, Rudolf Steiner (1861–1925), the Austrian philosopher and founder of biodynamic agriculture, the anthroposophical spiritual movement, and Waldorf education, acknowledged this close relationship and even referred to the brain as just "smooshed up guts!"[38] The brain has the same receptors as the gut and works similarly to it both morpho-

SSRIs AND SEROTONIN SYNDROME

SSRI stands for "selective serotonin reuptake inhibitors." Today, an estimated 30 to 40 million Americans take SSRI drugs to treat depression, with U.S. sales in 2004 measured at $11.2 billion.[39] A more recent study published in the *Archives of General Psychiatry* reported that the use of antidepressant drugs actually doubled between 1996 and 2005, with the vast majority of these being SSRI medications such as Paxil and Prozac.[40] Adverse effects from these drugs have now spawned their own new disease category, known as serotonin syndrome, which is characterized by mental changes (confusion, agitation, fatigue and lethargy, suicidal or homicidal ideations), autonomic nervous system malfunction (sweating, shivering, diarrhea, hypertension, insomnia), and neuromuscular complaints (muscle jerks, tremors, clumsiness, extreme stiffness, seizures, coma).[41] After studying 1,000 patients, Ann Blake Tracy, Ph.D., found that the long-term effects of these SSRIs include impaired memory, impaired concentration, and mental disability, and—because a disruption of serotonin alters perception and creates a stronger hypersuggestible state than hypnotism—that Prozac patients, for example, are likelier to report false memories of abuse. Tracy points out that these mental abnormalities are understandable because elevated serotonin is the same type of chemical found in LSD, PCP, and other psychedelic drugs responsible for producing profound hallucinations. In fact, elevated levels of serotonin are found in schizophrenia, mood disorders, organic brain disease, Alzheimer's, anorexia, and autism.[42] Thus, once again, it is the natural balance of nutrients and neurotransmitters that creates mental and emotional harmony, not the mechanistic "more is better" attitude propagated by allopathic medical doctors who prescribe these drugs and the pharmaceutical companies that have popularized them.

logically and biochemically. More recently, Dr. Natasha Campbell-McBride has written about this relationship in her book *Gut and Psychology Syndrome,* where she describes the severe dysbiosis typically found in autistic children.

Excessive antibiotic use and the ensuing gut dysbiosis has a profound impact on brain functioning in children. The late Dr. Gérard Guéniot, a leading holistic French physician and expert on drainage, emphasized that the harm done to the normally protective intestinal mucosa by antibiotics has other repercussions besides leaky gut syndrome and the impaired synthesis of neurotransmitters. The intestinal lining is also richly endowed with lymphoid tissues, known in immunology as the mucosa-associated lymphoid tissues (MALT). These lymphatic tissues line the gastrointestinal tract—and are most significantly congregated in the Peyer's patches in the small intestine and the tonsils—and make up *70 percent* of a child's immune system. When this MALT, or intestinal mucosal barrier, is damaged from excessive courses of antibiotics as well as the ingestion of sugar and other junk food, the child's body has difficulty recognizing "self" (normal cells and tissues) from the "non-self" of the undigested food antigens, foreign microbes, and toxic metals and chemicals that are allowed to pass freely through the now-porous intestines. Guéniot asserts that this situation not only leads to a lack of immunological identity and a predisposition toward autoimmune disease (rheumatoid arthritis, Hashimoto's thyroiditis, diabetes, lupus, various anemias, and other chronic illnesses and syndromes) but also grossly truncates a child's sense of self and psychological development. This psychosocial truncation is especially significant when numerous courses of antibiotics are given before the child's immune system has reached its full maturity, which occurs around the age of seven.[43]*

Peyer's patches: *Peyer's patches* are masses of lymphoid tissue primarily located in the third part of the small intestine, the ileum. They monitor food antigens and determine which foods to accept and which to alert the lymphocytes to defend against. They are a source of B and T immune system cells that fight infection in the gut.

*This truncation of normal immunological development in pediatric populations also occurs with the injection of the toxic mercury preservative thimerosal and the foreign proteins contained in children's vaccines. See chapter 15 for more information on *vaccinosis*—that is, illnesses incurred from vaccinations.

Peyer's patches are located near another important lymphatic structure—the appendix.

ANTIBIOTICS AND ALLERGIES

Researchers at the Henry Ford Hospital in Detroit found that children who receive antibiotics within the first six months of their life were one and a half times more likely to develop allergies by age seven than children who didn't receive these drugs.[44]

Another leader in the field of drainage and dysbiosis, Mikhael Adams, N.D., of Toronto, has had remarkable success treating learning disabilities and attention deficit disorder in both children and adults through the diagnosis of dysfunction primarily in the *corpus callosum*, the brain structure that divides and coordinates information between the two cerebral hemispheres. Dr. Adams treats this brain dysfunction caused by dysbiosis primarily with drainage remedies, a sugar-free (anti-candida protocol) diet, nutritional supplementation, and auriculotherapy.

corpus callosum: The *corpus callosum* is approximately 10 centimeters (about 4 inches) long and is located between the two cerebral hemispheres. This large brain structure's role is to speedily transfer information between the two hemispheres to coordinate left and right brain activity. The corpus callosum can be damaged through head trauma, anoxia (lack of oxygen), vaccinations, dysbiosis, forcing a left-hander to be right-handed, toxic metals and chemicals, and emotional stress. This can result in various forms of cognitive disorders including dyslexia, inability to concentrate and retain information, attention deficit disorder (ADD), and memory loss. A common symptom of mild corpus callosum impairment is difficulty with map reading and following directions.

Thankfully, through the emerging field of psychoneuroimmunology, the twentieth-century-induced schism between neuroscience and psychology is finally being healed. Researchers are now discovering what William Philpott, Carlton Fredericks, Carl Pfeiffer, Abram Hoffer, and dozens of other nutritional pioneers have averred for decades—that the biochemical and physical causes of brain dysfunction and mild to major mental illness are *very* real, and fortunately very treatable.

Chronic Systemic Candidiasis

Fungi and yeast species, especially the widespread and opportunistic *Candida albicans,* have also emerged as major pathogens, primarily through the suppression of T-cell function by tetracycline and other overly prescribed broad-spectrum antibiotics.[45] Candida is normally present and harmless in small amounts in the mouth, esophagus, large intestine, and vagina. Under normal conditions, these saprophytic (surviving by consuming dead tissues) yeasts quietly reside in our intestines and dine on our waste material. However, these yeasts lose their commensal relationship with us whenever the intestinal ecosystem is deranged. Thus, when antibiotics are given and the beneficial bacteria that normally hold candida in check are killed off, these tiny, spherical-shaped yeasts are triggered into becoming invasive branching fungal forms that can invade and inflame the digestive tract, vagina, and adjacent tissues.[46] Pathogenic *Candida albicans* is extremely virulent, releasing exceptionally potent antigens and toxins that alter metabolic functioning, destroy cells, and damage tissues.[47] The resulting symptoms can range from vaginal infections and skin rashes to an invasion of the bloodstream (*candidemia*) and even death in individuals with severely compromised immune systems.[48]

commensal: *Commensal,* from the Latin roots meaning "together at the same table," describes a functional and noninjurious relationship between an organism and a microbe. *Symbiotic* is a synonym for *commensal.*

In abundance and overgrowth, candida colonies easily migrate through the bloodstream and tissues and can be absorbed anywhere in the body. However, there are five major systems that are primarily affected. These are the gastrointestinal system (gas, bloating, indigestion, and allergic symptoms); the genitourinary system (bladder irritability, recurring vaginal yeast infections, and menstrual disturbances); the neurological system (chronic fatigue, depression, irritability, memory loss, poor concentration, hyperactivity, and learning disorders); the immune system (creating or increasing preexisting allergy symptoms from both food and environmental antigens); and the endocrine system (autoimmune illnesses). In fact, research has shown that *Candida albicans* actually secretes humanlike hormones that can generate the release of anti-ovarian and anti-thymic antibodies.[49] The presence of these autoimmune anti-ovarian antibodies is one reason why a growing number of women with chronic candidiasis have menstrual irregularities and infertility, and the anti-thymic autoimmune antibodies help explain, at least in part, why immune system dysfunction has become so prevalent in the population.

Candida overgrowth can be challenging to treat because these yeasts induce a craving for sugar to feed on and grow. Yeasts feed on glucose and other carbohydrates and ferment them into alcohol, a phenomenon termed *auto-brewery syndrome* by a Japanese doctor in the 1970s.[50] This alcohol creates symptoms similar to those an alcoholic experiences (fatigue and lethargy, depression, and agitation and anxiety) when the liver converts alcohol into toxic acetaldehyde. As with alcohol, candida yeasts induce both a strong psychological as well as a physical craving for more sugar/alcohol to feed on, thus inducing a vicious cycle in which our microbes are actually more in control than we are.

Opportunistic Parasites

There is also substantial documentation that antibiotic overuse leads to the infestation and spread of intestinal parasites.[51] Like candida overgrowth, parasites can cause a diverse number of symptoms including abdominal cramping and gas, chronic fatigue, constipation, joint and muscle pain, nervousness, and insomnia.[52] The two most common parasites that primarily reside in the small intestine, *Giardia lambia* and *Entamoeba histolytica,* are the possible cause of up to 70 percent of the cases of chronic fatigue and immune dysfunction syndrome (CFIDS).[53]

Testing for these parasites can be quite challenging, however. In fact, because of the high inaccuracy of stool sampling and testing processes in many labs, parasitology research has not advanced as far as the studies of other microbes.[54] However, a few labs specialize in parasitology testing and can be trusted to obtain more consistent and accurate results. Whatever the results of the laboratory tests, *Candida albicans,* as well as parasitic overgrowth, is rarely the cause (unless you have just returned from a third-world country with an acute parasitic infection), but the result of the larger problem: the indiscriminate use of antibiotics and the consequential intestinal dysbiosis and leaky gut.

- Genova Diagnostics in North Carolina and Meridian Valley Lab in Washington State both specialize in testing for parasites. Physicians can contact Genova Diagnostics at (800) 522-4762 or www.genovadiagnostics.com; and Meridian Valley at (425) 271-8689 or http://meridianvalleylab.com.

Judicious Use of Antibiotics

Dr. George Vithoulkas, one of the most respected homeopathic physicians in the world, succinctly underscores the importance of intestinal flora: "The quality of our health depends almost entirely on the quality of the microorganisms that exist normally within our bodies."[55] Since the population of friendly intestinal microorganisms can be seriously reduced with even one course of antibiotics, Vithoulkas accordingly recommends that antibiotics should be given only in emergency situations when the life of the patient is threatened.[56]

However, due to the overuse as well as the misuse of antibiotics that has led to the great resistance of many bacterial species, these former life-saving drugs are no longer effective, even in many serious emergency situations. For example, the Centers for Disease Control (CDC) reported in 2001 that of the 235 million doses of antibiotics prescribed, an estimated 20 to 50 percent were *unnecessarily prescribed* for viral infections (colds, flus, and so forth).[57] It was additionally estimated in 2003 that $1.1 billion is spent per year on unnecessary adult upper respiratory infection antibiotic prescriptions.[58] This problem is further exacerbated by the commonplace practice of prescribing antibiotics for ear infections, of which 90 percent are viral.[59] In a revealing 1997 New Zealand study, no difference in treatment success rates was seen in 2,089 patients with otitis media who were treated with antibiotic drugs as opposed to those who were not treated with antibiotics.[60]

Despite an extensive advertising campaign waged by the CDC and FDA warning about the dangers of antibiotic overuse, antibiotic resistance is still a serious problem claiming more lives each year than the "modern plague" of AIDS.[61] Fortunately, a 2006 survey found that overall antibiotic prescribing has dropped 13 percent (based on comparing 2005–2006 prescriptions to those in 1997–1998), so the word is getting out, but the overprescribing of this medication is still excessive.[62] This is especially reprehensible since antibiotics cause damage to the gut flora and overall health of the body not only chronically but also acutely. In fact, antibiotics are the cause of nearly half of all emergency room visits; 80 percent of these antibiotic-caused "adverse events" were due to allergic reactions.[63]

The excessive use and abuse of these so-called miracle drugs has rendered them over time relatively impotent against emerging and reemerging resistant pathogenic bacteria. Therefore, knowledgeable individuals now realize that their best hope lies in prevention, by restoring the normal intestinal flora and good digestive system functioning. Furthermore, we need to limit the use of antibiotics only to rare acute and serious bacterial infections.

OTHER CONTRIBUTORS TO DYSBIOSIS

Sugar—A Close Second to Antibiotics

Chronic ingestion of sugar and other toxic and refined foods also greatly contributes to an unhealthy inverse relationship of intestinal bacteria—that is, the normal healthy ratio of friendly (lactobacilli) bacteria to unfriendly (*E. coli*) bacteria at 85 percent to 15 percent can actually become reversed, and the unfriendly bacteria outnumber the friendly ones.[64] Sugar is also a well-known promoter of *Candida albicans* fungal growth, not only intestinally but also vaginally.[65]

As described previously, it can be particularly difficult to eliminate sugar from the diet, because not only does an individual's mind and emotions crave the consolation and quick energy from this refined food, but the billions of pathogenic yeasts, bacteria, and parasites also need this daily fix to grow and replicate. These constant craving signals make it especially hard for overweight individuals to muster the willpower to lose weight or to maintain weight loss for long. Additionally, the dysbiotic structural degenerative changes of intestinal prolapse and megacolon that are typical in obese and ill individuals play a significant part in the difficulty and frustration many experience even on the most stringent diets. Thus, dysbiosis—and the antibiotics and sugar that have helped create it—are largely responsible for our country's epidemic weight problem: seven out of every ten adults in the United States are currently overweight, and approximately three out of every ten are obese.[66] Obesity not only has been correlated with an increased risk of heart disease, cancer, diabetes, and arthritis but also speeds aging by adding the equivalent of nine more years onto the body.[67]

> **intestinal prolapse:** *Intestinal prolapse* is when a part of the colon is displaced and sinks downward in an abnormal position. The horizontal-lying transverse colon is particularly prone to prolapse.
>
> **megacolon:** *Megacolon* refers to an abnormally large or distended colon and is often associated with chronic constipation or neurological deficit (dysfunction of the nerves that control colon function).

OBESITY AND ANTIBIOTICS

A 2005 article in *Medical Hypotheses* links the mass consumption of antibiotics since the mid-twentieth century with the explosion in obesity.[68] The growth-promoting effect of antibiotics was discovered in the 1940s and is one of the reasons that the use of penicillin-type drugs in farm animals has increased globally by 600 percent over the past thirty years. In the same period the use of tetracyclines has increased by 1500 percent. A fatter pig or cow yields more profit. In the same way, courses of antibiotics pack on pounds in human subjects.[69]

Other Drugs

Although antibiotics are by far the worst offenders, other drugs can also create a dysbiotic terrain. Sulfa drugs, oral contraceptives, painkillers (especially nonsteroidal anti-inflammatory drugs, or NSAIDs), corticosteroids, immunosuppressive drugs used in cancer therapy, antidiarrheal drugs, laxatives, and other medications can wreak havoc on the intestinal lining and contribute to dysbiosis and the related leaky gut syndrome.

Stress

Factors such as significant psychological and physical stress have been correlated to reduced lactobacilli and resulting intestinal dysbiosis. In one study, infant monkeys who were separated from their mothers demonstrated a decrease in healthful lactobacilli and an inverse increase in bacterial pathogens (shigella and campylobacter) in their feces. These negative alterations in the gut flora have also been observed in Soviet cosmonauts from the stress of space travel, in college students during and just after final exams, and in children who have a tendency toward recurrent colds and flus.[70]

The vast majority of studies on stress adversely affecting levels of gut flora have been conducted on subjects suffering from IBS (irritable bowel syndrome), a disorder highly correlated to an etiology of chronic mental and emotional stress.[71] Specifically, it has been found in several animal studies that chronic stress induces dysfunction of the intestinal barrier, resulting in the enhanced uptake of noxious substances (e.g., antigens, toxins, various pro-inflammatory molecules) and the concurrent reduction of healthy gut bacteria.[72]

More recent research from Yvette Tache of UCLA has revealed that when stress triggers cortisol-releasing factor (CRF) in our brains (a stress response), this has significantly adverse effects on digestion, including the reduction of small intestinal cleansing peristaltic waves, which favors pathogenic bacterial overgrowth. The stimulation of CRF, which increases adrenaline in the body, also increases the frequency of stool elimination, which exacerbates the symptoms of IBS.[73]

TREATMENT OF DYSBIOSIS

Clearing pathogenic microbes from a dysbiotic digestive tract and healing the "leaky gut" holes in the intestine is as challenging as detoxifying mercury from the body. This correlation is actually not accidental. As discussed in chapters 3 and 15, toxic mercury and pathogenic bacteria mutually potentiate each other in an unhealthy bodily terrain.* Mercury, pathogenic bacteria, and petroleum chemicals can be the most insidious, tenacious, and difficult-to-clear toxins in the body. Fungi, parasites, and even viruses typically arise secondary to these three primary bodily poisons. Acute infestations of parasites acquired from travel in foreign countries should be dealt with holistically with strong antiparasitic herbs, probiotics, homeopathy, and possibly (but rarely) medications. But in the case of chronic intestinal toxicity, the short-term gain experienced from antibiotic, antiparasitic, and antifungal drugs typically backfires, with clinical signs of dysbiosis returning later with a vengeance. Therefore, healing the gut requires a multipronged attack that includes the detoxification of heavy metals and petrochemicals, a clean diet, herbal drainage (gemmotherapy) remedies, a constitutional homeopathic remedy, and quality nutritional supplementation.

It should be noted that in the case of severe systemic candidiasis, the use of allopathic drugs such as nystatin have helped in the short term to greatly reduce symptoms. However, these popular antifungal medications have not proved to be ultimately healing to the gastrointestinal tract without significant concomitant changes in a patient's diet and supplementation with nutritional products. Furthermore, researchers have found that nystatin triggers mutation of the candida species, which can allow for the subsequent development of resistant forms, analogous to what has occurred in bacteria with the prescription of antibiotics. Additionally, nystatin does not penetrate the blood-brain barrier, so it is unable to reach and remove *Candida albicans* from one of the body's most damaged terrains—the central nervous system.[74]

Diet

For those who are only mildly to moderately dysbiotic—a diagnosis that can be obtained by observing digestive symptoms before and after eating, having lab tests done, and undergoing energetic testing*—following the dietary guidelines as described in chapter 5 and excluding primary food allergens as detailed in chapter 6 will be sufficient. However, for those who are more ill, a stricter diet is indicated. Dr. Mikhael Adams, who specializes in the treatment of dysbiosis, recommends Dr. John Trowbridge's four-phase yeast control regimen. This diet begins with the strictest phase-1 level that is limited primarily to meat, fish, chicken, eggs, and vegetables

*Inorganic metallic mercury in amalgam fillings mixes with the bacteria in the mouth, as well as in the gastrointestinal tract when the mercury is swallowed, to form methylmercury—a compound ten times more toxic than the original metallic mercury. (U. Heintze et al., "Methylation of Mercury from Dental Amalgam Mercuric Chloride by Oral Streptococci In Vitro," *Scandinavian Journal of Dental Research* 91 [1983]: 150–52.)

*When digestive organs continue to "therapy localize"—that is, test positive over and over again—it is another indication of probable dysbiosis and leaky gut. For more information on energetic testing (kinesiology, electroacupuncture, MRT or the reflex arm length method, et cetera), see appendix 3, "Energetic Testing Explained."

and excludes the sugar- and yeast-producing foods that candida thrive on such as wine, beer, fruit, mushrooms, bread, vinegar, aged cheese, and nuts.[75] In patients who are not as ill, Dr. Adams uses the guidelines from Dr. Trowbridge's less strict phase-4 protocol, with some exclusions.

However, the meat, fish, and poultry in every phase of these diets should exclude all commercial, nonorganic beef, chicken, pork, and other livestock, as well as farm-raised fish, due to the reckless use of antibiotics in animal feed as "growth promoters."[76] For example, the Center for Science in the Public Interest estimates that approximately *40 percent* of the antibiotics used in the United States are fed to animals.[77]

- Meridian Valley Lab and Genova Diagnostics are excellent labs that can assess dysbiosis, leaky gut, and other gastrointestinal disorders through stool, urine, and blood analysis. Physicians can contact Genova Diagnostics at (800) 522-4762 or www.genovadiagnostics.com, and Meridian Valley at (425) 271-8689 or http://meridianvalleylab.com.

- For more information on Dr. Trowbridge's yeast control regimen, read *The Yeast Syndrome* by John Trowbridge, M.D., and Morton Walker, D.P.M. For more information on Dr. Mikhael Adams's seminars, contact his office at (905) 878-9994 or Seroyal at (800) 263-5861.

Whatever your choice of a dysbiosis-clearing regime, the key points to remember are to always choose whole unprocessed foods, avoid sugar and even fruit in the case of serious dysfunction and disease, chew thoroughly, avoid your primary food allergen, practice V & R (i.e., choose a wide ***variety*** of foods when shopping and ***rotate*** potentially allergenic foods on a three- or four-days basis), and drink plenty of filtered water.

MORE ON THE IMPORTANCE OF CHEWING

Chewing food slowly allows enough saliva to be released in the mouth to thoroughly wet the food, as well as for amylase, the enzyme in saliva, to begin carbohydrate digestion. In Germany (the Mayr technique) as well as the United States ("Fletcherism"), the importance of chewing food slowly and thoroughly before swallowing has been understood and promoted for centuries. In fact, John Robbins, in *May All Be Fed,* noted that three men survived in a concentration camp during World War II by chewing their food very well, while their compatriots perished.[78]

- In 1989, Carlo Petrini founded the Slow Food organization in response to a fast-food chain opening in Rome's Piazza di Spagna.[79] This group now numbers more than 100,000 and has members in 153 countries. For information on how to join, go to www.slowfood.com.

Water

Filtered water is not an option—it's a necessity. According to the *New York Times,* at least one in five Americans, or 20 percent, drink tap water polluted with feces, radiation, or other pathogenic contaminants. Additionally, in most of the United States, the toxic chemicals fluoride and chlorine are added to drinking water. For example, according to the EPA, 75 percent of Americans drink chlorinated tap water. This chlorine, which was used as a toxic chemical weapon during World War I, sterilizes not only the water but also the intestinal tract, destroying many beneficial intestinal flora. Furthermore, fluoride, which was the principal active ingredient in rat poison for years before being added to our water after World War II, has been shown to increase the risk of hip fractures by 20 to 40 percent, as well as increasing the risk of heart disease and bone cancer in young men.[80] Thus, individuals who eat a scrupulously clean diet but still drink tap water are seriously sabotaging themselves and, depending on the quality of the local water, greatly impairing their progress in repopulating and repairing their digestive tracts.

- Reverse osmosis is considered the optimal water filtration by most health practitioners. Dennis Higgins, M.D., who has studied hydrology (the study of water) for over twenty years, recommends a fourteen-stage reverse osmosis unit he designed that scrupulously filters out toxic metals and chemicals, with a special filter inserted at the end of the process to slightly mineralize and alkalinize the water. This process renders water most akin to the optimum water that is found in clean mountain streams and lakes. For more information, contact Mary Cordaro at (818) 766-1787 or www.marycordaro.com, or the Radiant Life Company at (888) 593-9595 or www.radiantlifecatalog.com.

Nutritional Supplementation

Enzymatic Support

All individuals need to supplement their digestive enzyme production until their dysbiosis is considerably reduced. A dysbiotic and deranged intestinal ecology not only inhibits enzyme secretion from the small intestine but also impairs adequate enzyme and bile production from the stomach, pancreas, and liver. However, when a quality enzyme is ingested with meals, two benefits occur. First, the food is better assimilated and utilizable nutrients are more readily available to assist in energy production to strengthen these weakened digestive organs. Second, when these organs get somewhat of a "breather" in their effort to produce enough enzymes during and after every meal, they can expend more energy in detoxifying harmful microbes and toxins, repairing tissues and organs, and reregulating deranged metabolic pathways. Unlike medications that continually congest the liver and other organs over time, plant- and animal-derived enzymes have been observed clinically by holistic practitioners for decades to significantly strengthen digestive organs without any growing dependence on these supplements or toxic side effects. In fact, after six months to two years of supplementation (depending on the severity of the dysbiosis and food allergies), enzymes are no longer needed by advanced patients except for the rare celebratory occasions to assist with the overindulgence of food or drink. Thus, although the supplementation of enzymes can be seen as a "crutch" to bolster the action of weakened digestive organs, it is an essential component in the healing of dysbiosis as well as food sensitivities, and it is actually quite curative in the long run.

Enzymatic Support for Sensitive Stomachs

Before prescribing enzymes, practitioners need to ask whether the patient has (or ever had) ulcers, gastritis (stomach pain or inflammation), heartburn, acid reflux (GERD or gastroesophageal reflux disease), functional hiatal hernia syndrome, a history of long-term use of NSAIDs, or just simply intermittent but chronic abdominal pain (especially gnawing and burning pain).* If so, the supplementation of hydrochloric acid (HCL) or protease enzymes could possibly re-irritate the still raw mucosal tissue. The symptoms of this irritation may not occur for the first few days or even the first few weeks, and in fact, the patient may feel exceptionally better during this "honeymoon" stage of noticeably better digestion. However, in many cases, the protease or HCL will begin to erode dormant areas in the mucosa that are still raw and not entirely healed, and, after a few days or weeks, patients will complain of the reemergence of their old abdominal pain. Therefore, practitioners must be *extremely* cautious in the prescription of supplemental enzymes and HCL when patients have currently, or have had in the past, any type of ongoing abdominal pain.

In these ulcer or "subclinical" (no overt symptoms) ulcer cases, an enzyme product devoid of the two most irritating substances in most enzyme formulas—protease and HCL—is indicated. The product, Gastric Comfort (also known as Formula 601), has all the other needed enzymes (amylase, lipase, lactase, and so forth) as well as herbs such as papaya and plantain. It is an excellent formula that has held up clinically for over a decade. If a patient is presently in pain from ulcers or chronic gastritis, Formula SF734 is a time-tested naturopathic formula that can provide pain relief and also support the healing of the damaged gastrointestinal mucosal barrier.

- ▶ Gastric Comfort does an excellent job of digesting protein, even without HCL and protease, through the action of its herbal ingredients, as well as the help of all the other supporting enzymes included for the digestion of starch, sugar, fat, and fiber. It is available from Enzymes, Inc., at (800) 637-7893 or www.enzymesinc.com.
- ▶ Formula SF734 is available from Thorne Research; call (800) 228-1966 or go to www.thorne.com.

Another option for individuals with past or present ulcers or gastritis is a combination product of herbal bitters. Bitter herbs such as goldenseal, wormwood, fennel, gentian, dandelion, chamomile, prickly ash, and a host of others stimulate the secretion of digestive juices from the stomach, pancreas, and small intestine, as well as bile from the gallbladder for the emulsification of fats. Furthermore, many of these bitter herbs have significant antibiotic, antifungal, and antitumor actions.[81] Unfortunately, the bitter formulas prepackaged at most

*Many holistic practitioners have observed that the prescription of antibiotics and bismuth (e.g., Pepto-Bismol) for ulcers caused from *Helicobacter* (or *Campylobacter*) *pylori* bacteria has not been truly curative in the long run.

health food stores are more often designed to treat constipation, so they have too strong a laxative effect. (For instance, Swedish Bitters by Nature Works is very good for constipation but not as a digestive stimulant before meals.) Additionally, they are one-size-fits-all formulas, which may not be the right combination for many people. Thus, the best bitter formulas are custom-made by practitioners who utilize kinesiology and other energetic testing methods and who can test which specific herbs are right for each individual patient.

In preparing a treatment, practitioners should start with eight to ten bottles of herbal bitters from a good-quality company like Eclectic Institute, which carries the largest supply of organic herbals in the country. Then, from this "bitters kit," and a supply of one-ounce glass bottles, bitters formulas can be custom-made to gently stimulate function according to which digestive organs and herbs test positive using energetic testing. In my clinical experience, these custom bitter formulas usually contain five or so herbs, and the dosage is from three to seven drops in a half glass of warm water, from five to thirty minutes before (or even during) a meal.

For practitioners who don't want to custom make their bitters, Sweetish Bitters Elixir by Gaia tests well in appropriately stimulating hydrochloric acid (HCl) and digestive enzymes in the stomach, pancreas, and small intestine when taken just before (as well as sipped during) meals.

► You can reach Eclectic Institute at (800) 332-4372 or www.eclecticherb.com.

► Sweetish Bitters Elixir is available from www.gaia-herbs.com or by calling (800) 917-8269.

Pancreatic Enzymes for Digestion and Healing

If an individual has never had intermittent or chronic abdominal pain, or it occurred many decades before and there is reason to believe that the mucosa is now reasonably healed, pure pancreatin may be prescribed to support protein, as well as carbohydrate and fat, digestion. Pancreatin not only has strong proteolytic action to supplement protein digestion but also is important in repairing tissue by degrading and removing dead cells and microbes. In fact, pancreatic enzymes have been used in orthomolecular amounts (high dosages) in the treatment of many serious illnesses including multiple sclerosis, cancer, and autoimmune diseases.[82] Furthermore, they are excellent at reducing pain and inflammation from sports injuries, or even in the case of chronic degenerative or rheumatoid arthritis.

The product Dipan-9 from Thorne contains pancreatin in a 9X or 10X dilution, which closely resembles our human pancreatic digestive enzyme output, thus making it very assimilable and clinically effective. If gastric (stomach) HCL support is also needed, the combination broad-spectrum formulas Bio-Gest and B.P.P. from Thorne, which contain both HCL and pancreatin, are indicated. However, usually HCL supplementation is required for a shorter period of time—for example, only over a few months—whereas enzyme supplementation is often necessary for months, or even years in some cases, during a detoxification protocol. Furthermore, as patients eat a cleaner diet, receive their deepest constitutional homeopathic remedy, and detoxify their heavy metals and chemicals, enzyme supplementation is needed less and less, and is often only required while eating out at restaurants or after indulging in desserts during a celebratory occasion.

► Most commercial and even health food store brands sell pancreatin at a 2X to 3X potency, which means that it has been diluted, usually with lactose. Dipan-9 is made by Thorne Research; call (800) 228-1966 or go to www.thorne.com. Bio-Gest and B.P.P. are also available from Thorne Research. B.P.P. is Bio-Gest without ox bile.

Killing the Bugs: Antimicrobial Supplements

Dysbiosis can be so tenacious that it is often necessary to directly target the offending pathogenic bacteria, fungi, and parasites that have become entrenched in the gut. In fact, German physicians warn that in the case of chronic candidiasis, a yeast-free diet alone is not enough without the support of antifungal herbs and supplements. They argue that with just a clean diet the candida fungus is often simply driven into deeper tissues, where it is much more difficult to eradicate.[83]

Fortunately, there are herbal supplements that have strong antimicrobial properties but inhibit and kill *only* the pathogens, without significantly damaging healthy microbes the way that antibiotics and other drugs do. In the case of pathogenic bacterial overgrowth, which is characteristic of intestinal dysbiosis, the product Entrocap from Thorne is an excellent choice because it contains the proven broad-spectrum antimicrobials berberine and grapefruit seed extract. When the need to treat chronic parasitic overgrowth or acute parasitic infestation arises, Artecin from Thorne is a good choice because it contains *Artemisia annua,* an antiparasitic herb that also has a beneficial bitter and carminative (gas-relieving) action. In the case of major candidiasis, Formula SF722 contains undecylenic acid with significant anti-candida action, which, in conjunction with a clean diet, can provide exceptional relief and gastrointestinal healing. Finally, the gemmotherapy (plant stem cells) drainage remedies discussed in chapter 2, notably Fig (the major remedy for any gastrointestinal dysfunction), European Alder (detoxifies the entire gut and reduces food allergies), and Grey Alder (for severe food allergies and gut dysfunction), are exceptionally supportive in treating dysbiosis.

- Entrocap, Artecin, and Formula SF722 can be ordered from Thorne Research at (800) 228-1966 or www.thorne.com.

- Plant stem cell remedies, as well as educational seminars on their use, are available to healthcare practitioners from two companies in the United States: PSC Distribution at (631) 477-6696 or www.epsce.com and Gemmos LLC at (877) 417-6298 or www.gemmos-usa.com. Plant stem cell remedies should be prescribed by a knowledgeable practitioner, as they are contraindicated for some patients.

Probiotics

In contrast to the word *antibiotic,* meaning "against life," the term *probiotic* means "promoting life." Probiotics describes both the health-promoting good bacteria already existing in our gut and the supplements—primarily *Lactobacillus acidophilus* and *Bifidobacteria*—that are prescribed to replenish this population of healthy flora in a damaged and dysbiotic gut. Although lactofermented fruits, vegetables, and milk products have been a dietary cornerstone for centuries, few of us today have been raised on these healthful foods our ancestors enjoyed. For most of us, the supplementation of probiotics is crucial in replenishing this essential population of healthy bacteria in order to begin the process of truly healing and restoring optimal gut function.

Quality Products

Probiotics—primarily lactobacillus and bifidobacteria—are notoriously under-regulated in this country. Two research studies from Bastyr University, in fact, revealed that not only did the probiotic supplements in health food stores fall way short of having any viable bacteria as promised on their labels but that many products were actually *contaminated with significant amounts of pathogenic bacteria.*[84]

BioImmersion is one of the rare probiotic companies to scientifically prove the quality of their supplements. Each batch of their *Lactobacillus acidophilus* and *Bifidobacterium* is authenticated by the American Type Culture Collection (ATCC), which is a globally recognized bioresource center in Virginia and considered the gold standard. The specific ATCC probiotic strains are chosen by BioImmersion's scientists for their strength, compatibility, safety, and over forty years of proven ability to clinically perform most optimally in patients.* They have the ability to protect the integrity of the gastrointestinal tract's mucous membrane and to neutralize dietary toxins, carcinogens, and infectious microorganisms.

BioImmersion products test better than other probiotic products both energetically and clinically over time. Patients have reported that they have significantly less fatigue and more energy and stamina after taking these products and that their chronic gastrointestinal symptoms (e.g., constipation, diarrhea, bloating) were either greatly reduced or completely cleared.

BioImmersion's Original Synbiotic Formula is a powdered formula consisting of *Lactobacillus acidophilus, Bifidobacterium longum, Streptococcus thermophilus, Lactobacillus rhamnosus,* and *Lactobacillus plantarum.* It also contains *pre*biotics, that is, nondigestible dietary fiber such as inulin and other fructo-oligosaccharides that help stimulate the growth and activity of the five bacterial probiotic strains. The combination of prebiotics and probiotics results in a *synbiotic* formula, hence the name for this product. Inulin helps protect and improve

*For more information on these pedigreed strains of lactic acid bacteria, go to www.bioimmersion.com.

the survival of the probiotic bacterial organisms as they cross through the upper part of the GI tract. Butyric acid, an important energy source that facilitates healthy cell metabolism and reduces the risk of colon cancer, is produced in the gut from the fermentation of inulin by bifidobacteria. The large intestine also utilizes other short-chain fatty acids such as valerate, propionic acid, and acetic acid, but butyric is by far the most abundant and important of the four.

BUTYRIC ACID

Although most of the tissues in the body burn glucose as a fuel, the large intestine is relatively unique in that it is most dependent on butyric acid for energy.[85] This short-chain fatty acid is so vital to the health of the large intestine that it has been shown clinically to heal inflamed bowel tissues and to stop the growth of colon cancer cells in vitro. Butyric acid is normally produced in the colon by the fermentation of fiber by bifidobacteria and other beneficial bacteria. However, when fiber in the diet is deficient, or when bifidobacteria is depleted, not enough butyric acid is produced, so subsequently the colon cells don't have enough fuel to maintain normal functioning. In these cases, numerous intestinal conditions and illnesses can manifest, including constipation, diarrhea, diverticular disease, irritable bowel syndrome, ulcerative colitis, polyps, hemorrhoids, and colon cancer.[86] The best dietary source of butyric acid is found in butter. (For more information, see "Raw Butter Is a Health Food," page 158.)

One serving (½ tablespoon) of Original Synbiotic Formula provides 30 billion lactic acid bacteria and 5 grams of inulin. However, because these healthy flora are of such an optimal and pure grade, it may be better in some cases to start with reduced dosages (e.g., ¼ to ½ teaspoon) and build up over time. This allows for slower detoxification of the gut in sensitive and more heavily burdened toxic patients and therefore results in fewer healing reactions.

BioImmersion also specializes in providing antioxidant protection in their supplements in the form of pesticide- and herbicide-free fruits and berries. Their High ORAC Synbiotic Formula combines these antioxidants with the probiotic strains in the Original Synbiotic Formula. ORAC stands for "oxygen radical absorbing capacity," the scientific standard for measuring the anti–free radical potency of foods. Thus, a high ORAC score indicates a high total antioxidant capacity. BioImmersion's High ORAC supplement has exceptionally high antioxidant capability, derived from its constituents of wild blueberry extract, raspberry and raspberry seed extract, grape and grapeseed extract, wild bilberry extract, and cranberry, tart cherry, and prune extract, giving it 3,000 ORAC units per gram. The High ORAC formula has proven to be an excellent combination supplement of high-quality probiotic bacterial strains and potent antioxidant berry and fruit extracts. One capsule packs an impressive 25 billion *Lactobacillus acidophilus* and *Bifidobacterium longum* bacteria and 250 milligrams of berry and fruit extracts. The recommended dosage is 2 capsules per day.

BioImmersion has other potent supplements that have held up clinically over time and continue to test exceptionally well on patients. Wild Blueberry Extract is a powerful product that contains from twenty-five to thirty different anthocyanins and has potent antioxidant effects (most fruits contain only three or four types of anthocyanins). This extract comes from Nova Scotia, where the highest-quality blueberries in the world are known to grow. In addition to their significant anti-aging effects, blueberries are known for their ability to regenerate nerves and improve cognition. In one study, senile rats given Wild Blueberry Extract exhibited more physical agility and learned to run a maze within four months. This product is often prescribed to reduce the neuropsychological effects of severe gut dysbiosis.

Like High ORAC Synbiotic Formula, the Triple Berry Probiotic formula combines potent fruit and berry antioxidants and probiotics, but it is in a powder form that is particularly appropriate for children. Cranberry Pomegranate Synbiotic Formula is also a combination antioxidant/probiotic that is indicated for treating urinary tract infections as well as to support healthy cardiovascular and gastrointestinal health.

▶ For more information on any of the BioImmersion products, visit www.bioimmersion.com. Doctors and practitioners can order these products from BioImmersion, Inc., at (425) 451-3112 or through the website.

Contraindications

BioImmersion's probiotic products are generally very safe and are recommended even for the infants of women who breast-feed (because, unfortunately, there has been a decline in beneficial bacteria occurring simultaneously with the rise of pathogens and toxic metals and chemicals currently found in breast milk).[87]

It is essential to keep in mind, however, that probiotic supplementation may not be appropriate at first for those with major dysbiosis. That is, patients who have significant small intestine bacterial overgrowth, known as SIBO, will typically respond adversely to probiotic supplementation with symptoms such as gas, pain, and bloating.[88] In fact, an adverse reation to probiotics is a key sign of SIBO in patients suffering from GI dysfunction. An analogy to this reaction is that it would not be appropriate to sow seed in fields infested with weeds and toxins. In the same way, probiotics should be prescribed only when they can be well utilized. When prescribed prematurely, probiotics can actually increase an active or dormant autoimmune tendency in the intestine from years of sugar ingestion and past courses of antibiotics. Thus, *probiotic supplements may not* test positive for new patients initially, until the patients have detoxified reasonably enough—avoided their primary food allergens and avoided sugar—to begin effective and not-so-reactive colonization of their gut. The one exception to this rule is during acute crises. For example, when a patient is taking antibiotics, it can be quite appropriate to take probiotics concurrently during this crisis of "deflorestation" of the gut. However, the probiotic should be taken at another time during the day, because it can potentially reduce the killing action of the antibiotic when taken together with it.

CONCLUSION

It is important to conclude this chapter by reiterating to readers struggling with compromised health to try not to get discouraged, and to realize that almost everyone nowadays has significant gut dysbiosis and at least one, and often many, food cravings. Fortunately, the willpower to eat a clean and healthy diet does build in direct proportion to the amount of detoxification (emotional and physical) and effective holistic therapies a person receives. In fact, "advanced" patients (who have been treated for toxicity, have cleared their foci, and are on their deepest constitutional homeopathic remedy) report that their awareness of their nutritional needs becomes more and more apparent as their bodies heal. For example, food cravings in these dedicated patients can undergo a dramatic metamorphosis over time—away from the temporarily consoling and nutritionally empty ice cream and coffee and toward vine-ripened tomatoes, a perfectly ripe organic peach, or a nutrient-dense bone-broth soup.

As more sentient and perceptive beings, advanced patients also begin to experience on a personal level what the great homeopath George Vithoulkas succinctly stated, "What we place into our body affects *every* level of our being."[89] This increased sensitivity in cured individuals can be referred to as the yin/yang paradox of optimal health. That is, along with the experience of feeling stronger and more robust than ever before, there simultaneously exists an increased sensitivity to the more subtle states in our bodies, as well as other dimensions of consciousness. Thus, for an exceptionally healthy individual, accidentally eating a salad containing hydrogenated oil or politely indulging in (conventional) birthday cake may be noticed as mildly disturbing, but will not be debilitating.

This yin/yang law of having the capacity to be both highly sensitive and perceptive, and at the same time very strong and relatively invulnerable, has been known and taught since ancient times in the Far East as the sign of a highly developed human being. Furthermore, when individuals begin to notice that this principle is truly enriching their lives, the time, effort, money, willpower, and sheer determination it took to reach this higher level of functioning is most fully understood and appreciated.

NOTES

1. E. Lipski, *Digestive Wellness* (Los Angeles: Keats Publishing, 2000), 73.
2. B. Jensen, *Dr. Jensen's Guide to Diet and Detoxification* (Lincolnwood, Ill.: Keats Publishing, 2000), 1.
3. Ibid., 73–74.
4. E. Lipski, *Digestive Wellness* (Los Angeles: Keats Publishing, 2000), 59, 60–61.
5. R. Golan, *Optimal Wellness* (New York: Ballantine Books, 1995), 156.

6. E. Lipski, *Digestive Wellness* (Los Angeles: Keats Publishing, 2000), 62.
7. Ibid., 63.
8. N. Plummer, *Probiotics, Essential Fatty Acids and Antioxidants in Health and Disease,* a manual accompanying a workshop of the same title hosted by Seroyal Continuing Education in Portland, OR, February 26–27, 2000; S. Fallon, *Nourishing Traditions* (San Diego: ProMotion Publishing, 1999), 17; V. Branscum, "Intestinal Flora and Human Health," *Explore!* 7, no. 1 (1996): 48.
9. E. Lipski, *Digestive Wellness* (Los Angeles: Keats Publishing, 2000), 63.
10. N. Plummer, *Probiotics, Essential Fatty Acids and Antioxidants in Health and Disease,* a manual accompanying a workshop of the same title hosted by Seroyal Continuing Education in Portland, OR, February 26–27, 2000.
11. E. Lipski, *Digestive Wellness* (Los Angeles: Keats Publishing, 2000), 79, 95, 96–97.
12. G. Vithoulkas, *A New Model for Health and Disease* (Berkeley, Calif.: North Atlantic Books, 1991), 95.
13. M. Lappe, *When Antibiotics Fail* (Berkeley, Calif.: North Atlantic Books, 1986), 29–30.
14. Ibid., xi.
15. J. Robbins, *Reclaiming Our Health* (Tiburon, Calif.: H. J. Kramer, 1998), 328, 329.
16. S. Levy, *The Antibiotic Paradox* (New York: Plenum Press, 1992), 7.
17. Ibid., 10, 68, 78.
18. M. Lemonick, "The Killers All Around," *Time,* September 12, 1994, 66.
19. S. Levy, *The Antibiotic Paradox* (New York: Plenum Press, 1992), 10.
20. M. Lappé, *When Antibiotics Fail* (Berkeley, Calif.: North Atlantic Books, 1986), xiii.
21. M. Lemonick, "The Killers All Around," *Time,* September 12, 1994, 66.
22. N. Plummer, *Probiotics, Essential Fatty Acids and Antioxidants in Health and Disease,* a manual accompanying a workshop of the same title hosted by Seroyal Continuing Education in Portland, OR, February 26–27, 2000.
23. L. Garrett, *The Coming Plague* (New York: Penguin, 1994), 414, 416.
24. M. Adams, *Antibiotic Resistance, Biotherapeutic Drainage,* a manual accompanying a workshop of the same title, hosted by Seroyal Continuing Education in Toronto, 1998, 54; E. Dobb, "Growing Resistance," *Mother Jones,* November/December, 2000, 23.
25. M. Adams, *Antibiotic Resistance, Biotherapeutic Drainage,* a manual accompanying a workshop of the same title, hosted by Seroyal Continuing Education in Toronto, 1998, 54.
26. A. Schuld et al., "The True Story of Cipro," *Wise Traditions* 2, no. 4 (Winter 2001): 39.
27. M. Gershon, *The Second Brain* (New York: Harper Perennial, 1999), 149.
28. G. Vithoulkas, *A New Model for Health and Disease* (Berkeley, Calif.: North Atlantic Books, 1991), 7.
29. M. Lemonick, "The Killers All Around," *Time,* September 12, 1994, 62–69; E. Lipski, *Digestive Wellness* (Los Angeles: Keats Publishing, 2000), 76–77.
30. R. Stein, "Breast Cancer, Antibiotics Linked," *Press Democrat,* February 17, 2005, A6.
31. "Hannelore Kohl, 68, Ex-Chancellor's Wife; A Suicide After Illness," *New York Times,* July 16, 2001.
32. L. Garrett, *The Coming Plague* (New York: Penguin, 1994), 419.
33. M. Gershon, *The Second Brain* (New York: Harper Perennial, 1999), xii.
34. D. Noonan and G. Cowley, "Prozac vs. Placebos," *Newsweek,* July 15, 2002, 49.
35. I. Kirsch et al., "The Emperor's New Drugs: An Analysis of Antidepressant Medication Data Submitted to the US Food and Drug Administration," *American Psychological Association: Prevention and Treatment* 5, no. 23 (July 15, 2002): 1–11.
36. N. Campbell-McBride, "Gut and Psychology Syndrome," *Wise Traditions* 8, no. 4 (Winter 2007): 19.
37. E. Pringle, "Business Booming for SSRI Makers," Lawyers and Settlements.com, January 8, 2007, www.lawyersandsettlements.com/articles/00534/ssri-business.html.
38. T. Cowan, "Moods and the Immune System," *Wise Traditions* 9, no. 4 (Winter 2008): 32.
39. American Headache Society, "SSRIs, Triptans and Serotonin Syndrome: What Is the Risk of Serotonin Syndrome in Migraine?" 2007, www.achenet.org/education/patients/SSRIsTriptansandSerotoninSyndrome.asp.
40. D. Gutierrez, "Hooked on SSRIs: Antidepressant Use Doubles in U.S.," NaturalNews.com, June 17, 2010 www.naturalnews.com/029010_antidepressants_SSRI.html.
41. Ibid.
42. A. Tracy, "Prozac: Panacea or Pandora?" www.outlookcities.com/psych.
43. Transcript of Dr. Gerard Guéniot's seminar, "Drainage,"

prepared by Dr. Jonathan Miller, Toronto, November 19–22, 1998: 6–7.

44. S. Song, "Allergies: The Two-Dog Trick," *Time,* October 13, 2003, 93.

45. G. Vithoulkas, *A New Model for Health and Disease* (Berkeley, Calif.: North Atlantic Books, 1991), 7.

46. H. Buttram, "Overuse of Antibiotics and the Need for Alternatives," *Townsend Letter for Doctors,* November 1991, 868.

47. P. Yutsis, "Candida Albicans: A Fresh Look at the Existing Controversy," *Explore!* 7, no. 2 (1996): 18.

48. R. Golan, *Optimal Wellness* (New York: Ballantine Books, 1995), 208.

49. H. Buttram, "Overuse of Antibiotics and the Need for Alternatives," *Townsend Letter for Doctors,* November 1991, 869.

50. N. Campbell-McBride, "Gut and Psychology Syndrome," *Wise Traditions* 8, no. 4 (Winter 2007): 19.

51. E. Lipski, *Digestive Wellness* (Los Angeles: Keats Publishing, 2000), 71.

52. Ibid., 115.

53. H. Buttram, "Overuse of Antibiotics and the Need for Alternatives," *Townsend Letter for Doctors,* November 1991, 869.

54. E. Lipski, *Digestive Wellness* (Los Angeles: Keats Publishing, 2000), 115.

55. G. Vithoulkas, *A New Model for Health and Disease* (Berkeley, Calif.: North Atlantic Books, 1991), 9.

56. Ibid., 95.

57. D. MacKay, "Can CAM Therapies Help Reduce Antibiotic Resistance?" *Alternative Medicine Review* 8, no. 1 (2003): 28.

58. A. M. Fendrick, A. S. Monto, B. Nightengale, and M. Sarnes, "The Economic Burden of Non-influenza Related Viral Respiratory Tract Infection in the United States," *Archives of Internal Medicine* 163, no. 4 (2003): 487–94.

59. "Antibiotics Put 142,000 into Emergency Rooms Each Year," http://lloydwright.org/messages, February 25, 2010.

60. D. Page, *Your Jaws, Your Life* (Baltimore: SmilePage Publishing, 2003), 59.

61. Dr. Mercola, "Overuse of Antibiotics Spurs Vicious Cycle," www.mercola.com, June 10, 2010.

62. Centers for Disease Control and Prevention, "Get Smart: Know When Antibiotics Work," www.cdc.gov/getsmart/antibiotic-use/fast-facts.html.

63. "Antibiotics Put 142,000 Into Emergency Rooms Each Year," http://lloydwright.org/messages, February 25, 2010.

64. B. Goldberg, *Alternative Medicine* (Puyallup, Wash.: Future Medicine Publishing, Inc., 1994), 221.

65. J. Trowbridge and M. Walker, *The Yeast Syndrome* (New York: Bantam Books, 1986), 149.

66. R. Stein, "Study: Fat Speeds Aging," *Press Democrat,* June 14, 2005, A3.

67. American Heart Association, "Heart Disease and Stroke Statistics," 2005, www.AmericanHeart.org.

68. G. Ternak, "Antibiotics May Act as Growth/Obesity Promoters in Humans as an Inadvertent Result of Antibiotic Pollution?" *Medical Hypotheses* 64, no. 1 (2005): 14–16.

69. eMed Expert, "16 Interesting Facts About Antibiotics," www.emedexpert.com/tips/antibiotics-facts.shtml.

70. J. Hawrelak and S. Myers, "The Causes of Intestinal Dysbiosis: A Review," *Alternative Medicine Review* 9, no. 2 (1987).

71. H. Eutamene and L. Bueno, "Role of Probiotics in Correcting Abnormalities of Colonic Flora Induced by Stress," *Gut* 56 (2007): 1495–97.

72. J. Söderholm and M. Perdue, "Stress and the Gastrointestinal Tract II. Stress and Intestinal Barrier Function," *American Journal of Physiology, Gastrointestinal and Liver Physiology* 280, no. 1 (January 2001): G7–G13.

73. Mark Pimentel, *A New IBS Solution* (Sherman Oaks, Calif.: Health Point Press, 2006), 34–35.

74. P. Yutsis, "Candida Albicans: A Fresh Look at the Existing Controversy," *Explore!* 7, no. 2 (1996): 18.

75. J. Trowbridge and M. Walker *The Yeast Syndrome* (New York: Bantam Books, 1986), 191–227.

76. E. Dobb, "Growing Resistance," *Mother Jones,* November/December 2000, 23.

77. E. Lipski, *Digestive Wellness* (Los Angeles: Keats Publishing, Inc., 2000), 46.

78. J. Robbins, *May All Be Fed: Diet for a New World* (New York: Harper Perennial, 1993).

79. M. Holmes, "Slow Food: Inching towards Food Sovereignty?" www.foodfirst.org/node/1774.

80. D. Casper and T. Stone, *Modern Foods: The Sabotage of Earth's Food Supply* (San Diego: CenterPoint Press, 2002), 118–19, 121.

81. D. Hoffmann *The Holistic Herbal* (London: Harper Collins Publishers, 2001), 35.

82. B. Goldberg, *Alternative Medicine* (Puyallup, Wash.: Future Medicine Publishing, Inc., 1994), 221.

83. P. Yutsis, "Candida Albicans: A Fresh Look at the Existing Controversy," *Explore!* 7, no. 2 (1996): 18.

84. D. Ingels and A. Gaby, "Quality of Probiotic Supplements

Questioned," Bastyr Center for Natural Health, http://bastyrcenter.org/content/view/664.

85. E. Lipski, *Digestive Wellness* (Los Angeles: Keats Publishing, Inc., 2000), 54.
86. Ibid., 239–40.
87. N. Trenev, *Probiotics: Nature's Internal Healers* (New York: Avery, 1998), 59.
88. O. Zaidel and H. C. Lin, "Uninvited Guests: The Impact of Small Intestinal Bacterial Overgrowth on Nutritional Status," *Practical Gastroenterology* 27, no. 7 (2003): 27–34.
89. G. Vithoulkas, *A New Model for Health and Disease* (Berkeley, Calif.: North Atlantic Books, 1991), 4.

PART FOUR

BLOCKS TO HEALING: DOMINANT FOCI AND THEIR DISTURBED FIELDS

Because the concepts of foci and disturbed fields will be unfamiliar to many readers, a more in-depth introduction is included here to introduce some basic concepts before launching into the chapters that focus on the specific aspects of this widespread obstacle to healing.

Most modern-day conventional medical doctors have never heard of the terms *dominant focus* or *interference field,* or of the therapies that are used to treat them, such as *neural therapy* and *auriculotherapy.* In fact, even the majority of holistic doctors and other practitioners do not know how to accurately diagnose and treat chronic foci. However, much like the term *miasm* discussed in chapter 1, the word *focus* is not really obscure but rather forgotten. The definition of a focus in a recent edition of *Dorland's Medical Dictionary* demonstrates the prominent place this term once played in medical diagnosis: "[A focus is . . .] the starting point of a disease process."[1] Another descriptive definition comes from *Webster's Dictionary:* "a part of the body where a disease process, as an infection, tumor, etc., is localized or most active."[2]

A *dominant focus* is an area of chronic disturbance in the body that frequently goes undiagnosed because it causes no obvious localized symptoms. The most common dominant foci are teeth, tonsils, and scars. What makes foci so particularly insidious and difficult to detect is that although they are usually asymptomatic locally—meaning that an individual experiences no overt or obvious symptoms such as pain, swelling, numbness, and so forth—they can cause pain or dysfunction in other seemingly unrelated areas of the body. The areas that are secondarily disturbed by a focus are often quite distal from the focal site and are referred to as *disturbed fields.* For example, a woman may be prescribed a regimen of palliative anti-inflammatory drugs for her arthritic and painful joints (the disturbed fields), but the true cause of her chronic pain—a tonsil focus—usually goes undetected. Or a man may become desperate enough to submit to prostate surgery to alleviate difficult urination symptoms, when the primary cause of his prostate disturbed field is actually a failed root canal in one of his teeth. Thus, modern medicine often misses the mark by concentrating on relieving the symptoms emanating from a disturbed field, rather than treating the true cause of the problem, which is the dominant focus.

disturbed field/focal disease: *Disturbed fields* are also known as *burdened fields.* When a focus triggers a disturbed field, it is often referred to as a *focal disease.*[3]

In the United States, this silent "irritating thorn" that initiates a disturbance elsewhere in the body is primarily referred to as a *focus* or *focal infection,* while in Europe, the term more often used is *interference field.* However, there is a slight difference in the meaning of these two terms. The word *focus* describes a very specific and localized area such as a knee surgery scar or a single tooth that can be the primary focal or starting point of the problem, whereas *interference field* characterizes the obstruction to normal nerve conductivity and connective tissue integrity that these scars and chronic subclinical infections cause. This book will use the term *focus* (or *dominant focus*) as an umbrella term to describe all types of foci. However, when referring to a chronically infected focal region such as the teeth or tonsils, the more specific term *focal infection* will be used. Furthermore, when describing scar tissue (externally or internally) that is blocking normal nerve and connective tissue function and flow, the more descriptive term *interference field* will be employed.

subclinical: The term *subclinical* characterizes disturbances that cause no obvious symptoms such as unmistakable pain, swelling, numbness, tingling, itching, and so forth.

SCAR INTERFERENCE FIELDS

Scars on the external as well as the internal parts of the body are often completely asymptomatic. However, surgical scars from appendectomies, tonsillectomies, hysterectomies, and so forth are typically chronic interference fields. Irritating scars from surgeries to repair traumatized tissue such as torn ligaments in the knee, compound fractures (in which the broken ends of the fractured bone pierce through the skin), and stitches for deep cuts are also common interference fields. Nonsurgical scars that do not heal well can also become interference fields over time, such as cuts and tears (without stitches), severe bruises, major wounds (e.g., puncture or crushing), and even scars formed from past skin infections (e.g., cystic acne, boils, or abscesses), especially when they were highly charged emotionally, such as in the case of acne. The internal scarring to organs, bones, and tissues from surgery, trauma, or chronic infection can also act as a chronic interference field, although no visible scar shows on the skin. For example, blows to the head commonly cause interference fields, which are even more insidious than external scars because they are invisible in the scalp or buried under the hair.

Thus, whether scars are visible on the external skin or invisible in the deeper underlying tissues, they can act as interference fields that chronically, and often silently, disturb other seemingly unrelated areas of the body. In contrast to focal infections, scars are not areas of active and chronic infection, although they always have the potential to *generate* infection. Thus, a wide range of disturbance is possible in a scar interference field, whether this occurs in its symptomatic disturbed field or its *mother ganglia* (see page 300). These disturbances can range from mild neurological irritation to chronic inflammation with associated toxic by-products (e.g., histamine and lactic acid) to outright infection. For example, an inflamed intestinal disturbed field from an appendix scar can be a fertile environment for the growth of pathogenic microbes. In fact, an appendix scar focus can be just as culpable in contributing to chronic intestinal dysbiosis as excessive dietary sugar or antibiotic abuse.

FOCAL INFECTIONS

A dominant focus can also generate bacteria and other microbes that continuously spread, or metastasize, throughout the body, chiefly via blood and lymphatic channels, as well as along nerve fibers.[4] Focal infections are most typically found in teeth and tonsils; however, other sites include the sinuses, appendix, and genital organs—primarily the cervix (neck of the uterus) and prostate.[5] Over time, the chronic inflammation and infection generated in a focal infection degrades the surrounding tissue to create scar tissue. Although this hidden scar tissue does not show on the skin, its presence in the underlying deeper tissues is debilitating over time to the health of the body. Therefore tooth, tonsil, sinus, prostate, uterine, and other focal infections eventually also act as scar interference fields.

Dominant vs. Significant Foci

In German electroacupuncture testing methods, the term *dominant* describes foci that are major disturbances in the body. These disturbances most often include abscessed (but relatively pain-free) teeth, infected (but symptom-less) tonsils, and large or (unconsciously) emotionally upsetting scars from surgeries or serious injuries. The term *significant focus* refers to foci that are less of an issue or that have been mitigated through treatment. For example, a former dominant tonsil focus might be referred to as a *significant focus* after several treatments.

Example of an Appendix Focus

One example of a classic dominant focus is an appendix scar. Most people experience no pain or other symptoms from an appendix scar; however, these common scars are notorious among practitioners who treat foci for causing right hip and low back pain as the disturbed fields. Appendix scar interference fields also typically irritate the intestine and cause chronic irritable bowel–like symptoms such as gas, bloating, and alternating diarrhea and constipation. Furthermore, like other foci, appendix scars can cause disturbance in areas quite remote from their focal site (the appendix is in the lower right abdominal region). For example, the brain is a common appendix-scar-induced disturbed field, triggering symptoms such as chronic insomnia, headaches, or intermittent depression. (See the figure that follows.)

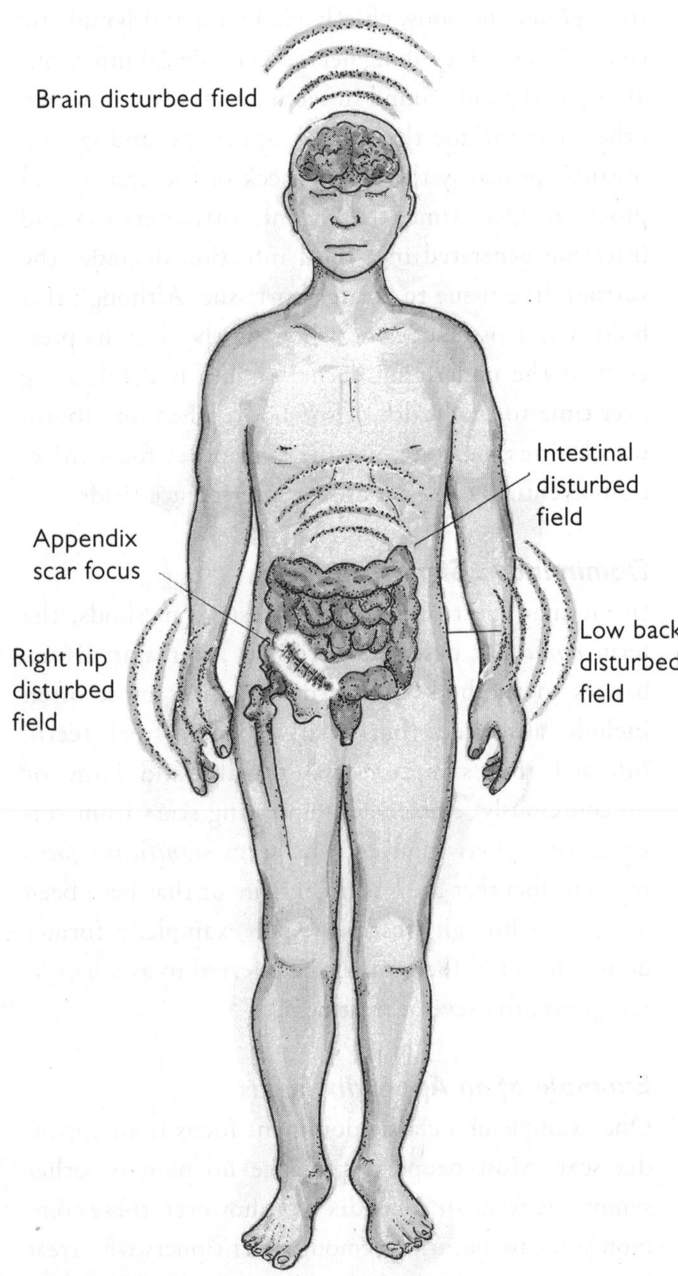

An appendix scar focus (or interference field) and some typical disturbed fields—the right hip and low back, the intestine, and the brain

CHALLENGES TO DIAGNOSIS

As noted earlier, what makes the diagnosis of foci so challenging is that they may be completely asymptomatic—or at least *very rarely* cause any pain or discomfort. Furthermore, because foci produce little to no inflammation, they remain under the radar of the immune system's surveillance. Thus, chronic foci form a gap in the crucial communications network of the body. If they are not recognized and directly addressed through effective treatment, foci continue to exist in the body permanently, all the while slowly and insidiously eroding our health and well-being.

As early as 1921, a brilliant researcher named Henry Cotton described the insidious nature of the chronic focal infection in a lecture series presented at Princeton University's medical school:

> The presence of pus, pain, and frequently swelling and the elevation of temperature differentiate acute infections from chronic infections. These symptoms leave no doubt in the mind of the patient or physician that infection is present in a given area. In the last few years, however, it has been found that there is another type of infection which has been designated as focal infection, or chronic infection, which frequently gives no evidence to the patient because of an absence of the symptoms, pain, pus, swelling and fever.[6]

Thus, while acute illnesses such as an ear infection can feel like a burning, painful fire, in contrast a chronic focal infection simply smolders—just beneath the patient's conscious awareness. A forest fire is readily seen and efforts are mobilized to put it out quickly; whereas smoldering embers, like silent chronic foci, are often overlooked and become much more dangerous over time because of the devastation wrought by their slow and relatively quiet destruction. Furthermore, chronically inflamed foci, like smoldering embers, have the possibility of erupting under stress into a fiery blaze at any point, which can engulf and overcome an entire forest—or an individual's life. This potential was addressed as early as the 1930s by Dr. Martin Fischer, who warned dentists about the clear morbidity (illness) and mortality (death) resulting from dental focal infections in his landmark book, *Death and Dentistry*.[7]

In his book, Fischer also discussed the characteristic of a generalized systemic sense of feeling unwell throughout the body that can mask the presence of a dominant focus. Although foci are classically recognized as causing *specific* disturbed fields—such as a failed root canal causing prostate dysfunction—they also adversely affect the health and vitality of the body as a whole. Thus, living with a chronic focal infection for many years can be debilitating because of the diminished level of efficient functioning in all of the body's systems—immune, circulatory, neurological, hormonal, and so forth. As Fischer commented,

> Patients with low-grade streptococcal infection [focal infections] are commonly of the ambulatory type. On certain days they are "bilious,"* feel themselves spent and are conscious of aches and pain; thus they drag along for weeks, months or years, never very ill, but never well either. They are often anemic, frequently adjudged neurasthenic,† many times, hypochondriacal. In this way, they may live out what looks like the allotted [life] span, though not infrequently, the more spectacular manifestations of a gastric hemorrhage, gall bladder disease or appendicitis are thrown as flare into the scene, or a "heart attack," or cerebral accident brings down the curtain.[8]

These generalized symptoms of feeling unwell rarely lead an inexperienced practitioner to an appropriate diagnosis because the majority of healthcare providers are completely unaware of the existence of focal infections. Additionally, blood and other laboratory tests are not exceptionally helpful because the body's immune system has usually adapted so greatly around a focal infection that these tests commonly come back negative. Although many practitioners honestly admit that they do not know what is wrong with the patient, others, less principled, may blame the patient and label the symptoms as being *psychosomatic*—that is, primarily emotionally based.

Finally, another confounding characteristic of foci is their *periodicity,* or their intermittent symptoms. For example, the symptoms in a disturbed field such as neck and shoulder pain originating from a dental focus may be relieved for weeks with a new dental appliance or splint, or an exceptionally clean diet, which often gives the patient false hope that the problem has been alleviated. However, as soon as this individual falls off the diet regimen or the appliance wears down, the familiar neck or shoulder pain soon returns. These intermittent symptoms are caused by what Fischer refers to as the "test tube permeability" of chronic focal infections:

> A chronic focus of infection which cannot heal for mechanical reasons, must be considered as a test tube with a permeable wall which affords not only abundant opportunity for the exit of bacteria and their products, but also for the conditions favoring the acquisition of various infective powers by the bacteria.[9]

This waxing and waning of various symptoms secondary to the intermittent migration of bacteria out of a focal area not only torments the recipient but also confounds practitioners. And when the typical examination and laboratory tests come back negative, they are once again tempted to dismiss the patient as a hypochondriac. Thus, the lack of an accurate diagnosis of the existence of focal infections prevents an appropriate treatment from being rendered.

❧

Because there has never been a complete history covering the "rise and fall" of the theory of focal infections that occurred in the United States and Europe in the late 1800s and early 1900s, chapter 8, "The History of Foci: A Major Historical Precedent," is purposely comprehensive in its description of this unique and exciting period in medical and dental history. Some readers may want to skim over this rather detailed chapter and move on to chapter 9, "Development of a Dominant Focus," which picks up where this introduction leaves off and describes how a focus develops in the body over time. Others, however, may find the history as well as the causes for the subsequent demise of the focal infection theory in the mid-twentieth century to be fascinating and enjoy the in-depth description of these forgotten figures in holistic medicine and dentistry.

**Biliousness* is a state characterized by nausea, abdominal discomfort, headache, and/or constipation.

†*Neurasthenia* is a form of nervous exhaustion, with symptoms such as insomnia, headache, back pain, feelings of constriction around the head, exhaustion after slight mental or physical exertion, increased sensitivity to noises, irregular heart actions, vertigo, dyspepsia, visual disturbances, and loss of memory. (J. Yasgur, *Homeopathic Dictionary* [Greenville, Pa.: Van Hoy Publishers, 1998], 29, 163.)

NOTES

1. J. Friel, ed., *Dorland's Illustrated Medical Dictionary,* 26th ed. (Philadelphia: W. B. Saunders Company, 1981), 631.
2. *Webster's New World College Dictionary,* 4th ed. (Cleveland: Macmillan, 1999), 548.
3. F. Kramer, "Focal Diagnosis in Dental Practice," *AABD Manual,* Spring 1989, 3.
4. P. Dosch, *Manual of Neural Therapy* (Heidelberg: Haug Publishers, 1984), 62; M. Fischer, *Death and Dentistry* (Springfield, Ill.: Charles C. Thomas, 1940), 14; F. Billings, *Focal Infection* (New York: D. Appleton and Company, 1916), 20–22; P. Störtebecker, *Neurology for Barefoot Doctors in All Countries* (Stockholm: Störtebecker Foundation for Research, 1988), 294–99.
5. M. Fischer, *Death and Dentistry* (Springfield, Ill.: Charles C. Thomas, 1940), preface.
6. H. Cotton, *The Defective Delinquent and Insane* (New York: Arno Press, 1980 [orig. pub. 1921]), 33–34.
7. M. Fischer, *Death and Dentistry* (Springfield, Ill.: Charles C. Thomas, 1940), 55.
8. Ibid., 17.
9. Ibid., 37.

8

THE HISTORY OF FOCI: A MAJOR HISTORICAL PRECEDENT

This chapter is divided into three main sections. The first introduces the key players in the rise of the focal infection theory in England and the United States. Next, we will explore the reasons for the downfall of this theory, before we conclude with a look at current European research on focal infection theory.

THE RISE OF FOCAL INFECTION THEORY IN ENGLAND AND THE UNITED STATES

The existence of dominant foci, and their subsequent diagnosis and treatment, emerged during a period from the late eighteenth to the early twentieth century. Both U.S. and European physicians and scientists contributed to the clinical and scientific research that resulted in the recognition of chronic foci—dental, tonsil, scar, and others—as a major field of study and a health disorder that was adversely affecting a significant percentage of their patients.

John Hunter: England's Father of Dentistry

Although German practitioners are primarily credited with the diagnosis and treatment of chronic foci, the recognition of dental focal infections was actually documented almost two centuries earlier. Sir John Hunter of England (1728–1793) first recorded the relationship between acute oral infections and systemic disease in his seminal textbook, *Natural History of the Human Teeth,* published in 1778.[1] Hunter, frequently referred to as the father of dentistry, noted that the pain and inflammation from problems with the eruption of teeth could cause dysfunction and disease elsewhere in the body. He found that by using a lancet to cut gum tissue that was impeding the eruption of wisdom teeth in adults or baby teeth in children, these teeth would then properly erupt.[2] Hunter observed clinically that not only would his patients' local dental pain and inflammation clear up (the focal infection), but simultaneously their *more distal* symptoms would also resolve (the disturbed fields), such as arthritis and bladder dysfunction.[3]

ANCIENT KNOWLEDGE

Although Sir John Hunter was the first to *document* an understanding of focal infections, examples from antiquity show awareness that dental focal infections can cause distal pain and dysfunction. For example, in 700 BCE physicians attributed the pain in the head, arms, and feet of an Assyrian king to his teeth and recommended extraction. Later, another Assyrian king, Ashurbanipal (669–626 BCE), was given this same advice by his physician for his bodily pains. In another region of ancient Assyria between 648 and 626 BCE, the court physician Arad-Nana recommended to King Aanapper that his teeth be extracted to cure the pains in his side and his feet.[4]

Benjamin Rush: America's Father of Medicine

Around this same period, Benjamin Rush (1745–1813), George Washington's physician and one of the signers of the Declaration of Independence, was also treating dental infections to heal remote symptoms in the body. In 1801, Rush cured a case of rheumatism in the hip (joint pain), dyspepsia (stomach indigestion), and epilepsy through extraction of the suspected causative teeth. In two of these cases, the teeth were obviously decayed. In the case of the tooth linked to the dyspepsia, however, he observed "no mark of decay appeared in it."[5] Rush, considered to be America's father of medicine, made the following conclusions about dental focal infections:

> I cannot help thinking that our success in the treatment of all chronic diseases would be very much promoted, by directing our inquiries into the state of the teeth in sick people, and by advising their extraction in every case in which they are decayed. It is not necessary that they should be attended with pain in order to produce disease, for splinters, tumors and other irritants . . . often bring on disease and death . . . and are unsuspected causes of them. This translation of sensation and motion into parts remote [disturbed fields] from the place where impressions are made [the focus], appears in many instances.[6]

Unfortunately, Rush's other insights were not as brilliant. As professor at the University of Pennsylvania's medical school for forty-four years (1769–1813), Rush taught radical allopathic procedures to approximately *three-fourths* of the educated and practicing physicians in the United States. These treatments included excessive bloodletting, the use of mercury lotion (calomel), strong emetics (bringing on vomiting), "violent purging of the bowels," and medicines made from lead. Although he was not present at the bedside of George Washington, the aggressive treatments futilely employed to save this first president—bloodletting (80 to 90 ounces), mercury-containing calomel, blisters, and emetics—were certainly popularized by Rush's teaching and his widespread influence in the development of allopathic medicine in the United States. In fact, after "various ineffectual struggles" to speak, General Washington was finally able to articulate "a desire that he might be allowed to die without interruption!"[7]

W. D. Miller: Father of the Focal Infection Theory

A century later, an American dentist and doctor, who has been referred to as "the greatest dental scientist of his day," recognized and published his research proving that the teeth are a major *focus of infection.*[8] Born in Ohio, Willoughby Dayton Miller (1853–1907) obtained his degree in dentistry at age twenty-six from the Dental School of the University of Pennsylvania. He later enrolled at a German medical school, from which he graduated at age thirty-four with an M.D. degree, after receiving one of the highest grades ever in the exhaustive final exam (in his non-native language of German).[9]

Miller has been credited with two major accomplishments in dentistry. First, based on his extensive clinical and laboratory research, he asserted that microorganisms (bacteria) cause dental cavities. Thus, his "chemico-parasitic" origin of dental caries was the first rational theory to explain the process of tooth decay, previously thought in antiquity as well as even as late as the 1600s to be caused by "fine worms" and even "earthworms." Miller's 1889 publication, *Die Mikro-organismen der Mundhole,* which was issued in the English translation the next year as *The Microorganisms of the Human Mouth,* revolutionized worldwide thinking about dental decay and advanced the cause of dental hygiene and prevention.[10*]

Second, Miller was the first to study in detail the microorganisms of the mouth and to describe an infected tooth as a *focus of infection.*[11] Adopting the rigorous and exacting research methods of Robert Koch, whose laboratory was in close proximity to his while he worked in Berlin,[†] Miller identified over twenty microbes in the human mouth and conducted exten-

*Miller's investigation into the decay-causing bacteria in the mouth was favorably commented on by Dr. G. V. Black in his 1884 book, *Formation of Poisons by Micro-organisms.* Black also noted, however, that Lieber and Rottenstein of Germany first suggested in 1868 that germs (microbes) caused cavities in teeth. (G. V. Black, *Formation of Poisons by Micro-organisms* [Philadelphia: P. Blakiston, Son and Co., 1884], 153–54.)

†Robert Koch (1843–1910), a German physician, began studying the anthrax bacillus in 1873. In 1882, he identified the tubercular bacillus. Koch is well known for his *Four Postulates,* outlining the scientific steps necessary to prove that a given organism is the cause of a given disease. (A. Castiglioni, *A History of Medicine* [New York: Jason Aronson, Inc., 1969], 808–9.)

sive research on their pathogenicity in the body. In one study that dramatically illustrated the toxicity of focal infections in the human mouth, Miller observed that 91 percent of 111 experimental mice died within forty days after being injected with one to two drops of saliva from one subject.[12] In his dynamic but relatively brief professional career,* Miller published more than 160 research papers. In 1891, his research published in the journal *The Dental Cosmos* established that infected teeth were major "foci of infection" that could cause disease in the body "adjacent to *or remote from the mouth*" (disturbed fields).[13] Miller accurately described the following three significant characteristics of dental foci:

1. *Microbes invade and infect both the external enamel and the underlying bone.* Miller accurately observed that microbes first cause "dissolution of the enamel as a result of acid produced by bacterial action" and that these "germs or their products, or both," pass into the dentin, to the pulp and periodontal ligament, and then into the bone: "Ostitis and osteomyelitis belong to the more common complications of decay of the teeth. Every severe inflammation of the pericementum [periodontal ligament] is naturally accompanied by more or less inflammation of the bone marrow [myelitis], or of the bone (osteitis), or of both together (osteomyelitis)."[14] As will be described later, *osteomyelitis*—that is, inflammation and ultimately necrosis or degeneration of the jawbone underlying a tooth—is characteristic of all chronic dental focal infections.
2. *Dental foci have multiple causes.* Miller recorded that dental focal infections can be caused by gum disease, general diseases such as syphilis, "traumatic injuries or impeded eruption of the wisdom-teeth," and "the incorporation of certain mineral poisons (mercury, phosphorus, lead, arsenic)."[15] These factors—and especially damage and decay from toxic mercury amalgam fillings, trauma, and the faulty eruption of the wisdom teeth—are still recognized today as the most common precipitating causes of dental foci.*
3. *Dental foci cause disturbed fields.* Miller recognized that dental focal infections often cause dysfunction in other parts of the body through blood or lymph channels "wherever a point of diminished resistance exists." Through extensive research, he found that microbes from a dental focus could migrate to the brain (encephalitis, meningitis), stomach and intestines (ulcers), lungs (pneumonia), sinuses (sinusitis), and tonsils (tonsillitis).[16] In 1891, Miller clearly described this "foci-disturbed field" progression: "During the past few years the conviction has grown continually stronger among physicians as well as dentists that the human mouth, as a gathering place and incubator of diverse pathogenic germs, performs a significant role in the production of various disorders of the body, and that, if many diseases whose origin is enveloped in mystery could be traced to their source, they would be found to have originated in the oral cavity."[17]

Because of Miller's exacting research methods and his great number of scientific studies investigating the cause of dental decay and disease, he has been lauded as "the pioneer who laid the foundation for modern dental research."[18] Furthermore, Miller's scientific investigation and extensive publications on dental focal infections laid the groundwork for other doctors, dentists, and researchers to build on during this scientific renaissance period at the turn of the twentieth century.

*W. D. Miller developed appendicitis and, "in spite of an operation," succumbed to peritonitis (inflammation of the membrane surrounding the abdominal cavity) at a Newark, Ohio, hospital on July 27, 1907, at the age of fifty-four. (M. Ring, "W. D. Miller: The Pioneer Who Laid the Foundation for Modern Dental Research," *New York State Dental Journal,* February 2002, 35.) Ironically, this brilliant man who understood so well both the pathogenicity of dental focal infections and their microbial metastatic tendency to move to remote parts of the body, such as the intestines, probably died either from an appendix disturbed field from the teeth or tonsils or from an appendix focus itself, stemming from a chronic but silent infection in this intestinal region.

*Although gum disease (e.g., gingivitis, periodontitis) is often blamed as the culprit, it is rarely the true underlying cause of dental foci. That is, gum disease is not initiated on its own but is a secondary symptom of mercury amalgam toxicity, the ingestion of sugar and other toxic foods, and the resulting chronic intestinal dysbiosis (pathogenic microbes) that continue to infect the inflamed oral mucosa.

G. V. Black: Father of Cavitation Surgery

As a prolific contemporary of Dr. Miller's, G. V. Black, D.D.S., M.D. (1836–1915)—known as the father of cavitation surgery—authored more than five hundred articles and several books. Published in 1908, his two-volume opus, *Work on Operative Dentistry,* was instrumental in standardizing operative procedures in dentistry.[19] In fact, years before the term *cavitation* was coined, Dr. Black had witnessed this phenomenon in the jawbone and called this new disease *chronic osteitis* (bone inflammation). He characterized this disease as a progressive "death of bone, cell by cell" that was able to "soften the bone, often hollowing out the cancellous portions of large areas of bony tissue" or alternatively producing a soft mass filled with dead bone material. Black was amazed that even the larger jawbone *osteomyelitic* (inflammation of the bone and bone marrow) cavitation areas full of necrotic (dead) debris could—unlike osteomyelitis in the body*—cause no visible redness, swelling, or increase of a patient's temperature.[20] Thus, even the most serious and pathological dental focal infections were often silent. Fortunately, Black found that when these bone cavitation lesions were "opened freely and every particle of softened bone removed until good sound bone forms . . . generally, the case makes a good recovery."[21] Thus, Black not only identified the serious pathological processes that are generated in infected teeth and bone but also pioneered the cavitation surgery methods that are still being emulated today in the removal of these dental focal infections.

> **cavitation:** *Cavitation* is the term used to describe both the holes in the jawbone that are generated from chronic infection and the type of surgery required for removal of the necrotic bone and tissue. (Cavitation surgery is covered in depth in "The Seven Most Effective Treatments for a Dental Focus" in chapter 11; see page 336.)

In 1936, Black's son Arthur D. Black, M.D., D.D.S., published a four-volume set, *G. V. Black's Work on Operative Dentistry,* that included his father's work as well as others', most notably a chapter on focal infection by Edward H. Hatton, M.D., in the fourth volume, titled *Pathology Treatment.*[22]

William Hunter and Oral Sepsis

Another renowned physician, Sir William Hunter (unrelated to John Hunter), was also investigating the dental focal infection during this period in England. In 1900, Hunter coined the term *oral sepsis* (infection), which more graphically described the danger of dental infections that often lead to systemic disease.[23] In an article published in the *British Medical Journal,* Hunter wrote that he had clinically observed that many illnesses, including endocarditis (heart disease), pleurisy (lung disease), cholecystitis (gallbladder inflammation), and anemia, were frequently caused by the hematogenous (via bloodstream) spread of bacteria from infected teeth.[24] The term *oral sepsis,* although descriptive of the serious toxicity of focal infections, did not hold up over time and was supplanted by Miller's term, *focal infection,* which is still used today.

Perhaps Hunter's most influential contribution to the focal infection field was a memorable speech at McGill University in 1910. In this rousing talk, Hunter soundly castigated his colleagues—dental and medical—for not recognizing the serious and widespread "ill-health associated with 'bad' mouths":

> Gold fillings, gold caps, gold bridges, gold crowns, fixed dentures, built in, on, and around diseased teeth, form a veritable mausoleum of gold over a mass of sepsis to which there is no parallel in the whole realm of medicine or surgery . . . There is no rank of society free from the fatal effects on health of this surgical malpractice.[25]

After the publication of this stirring speech in the *Lancet* journal the following year, dentists and physi-

*Osteomyelitis in the body causes fever, pain, and swelling, usually within hours or days after the onset of the infection. People most prone to osteomyelitic infections are young children and older adults, as well as postsurgical patients (especially those with artificial joint implants), individuals with cancer or postradiation therapy, and those with skin ulcers (especially in the foot). In fact, even conventional medicine allows that a sinus, gum, or tooth infection can spread to the skull and cause bone infection, although it doesn't recognize other typical disturbed fields from focal infections. Conventional treatment for osteomyelitis is antibiotics, especially those few that are still effective against *Staphylococcus aureus,* but if this fails, surgery can be required.

cians worldwide began to take more seriously the possibility that many syndromes and diseases were actually caused by the "intensely virulent" spread of infection from diseased jawbones silently residing in chronic dental focal infections.[26]

Frank Billings Furthers the Focal Infection Theory

At approximately the same time that Hunter recognized the gravity of oral sepsis in England, Frank Billings, M.D. (1854–1932), was researching dental and tonsil focal infections in Chicago.[27] In 1898, Dr. Billings was appointed head of the department of medicine at Rush Medical College, which was named for his predecessor, Benjamin Rush.* Billings and two other colleagues at the school, Ludvig Hektoen and Edward C. Rosenow, contributed so greatly to the understanding of foci and propagated this information so widely in scientific journals that many consider the period of collaboration among these three researchers to be the birth of focal infection theory.[28] In fact Billings, seemingly unaware of W. D. Miller's publications, was credited with coining the term *focal infection* in 1912.[29] Billings further cemented his place in this field of study by delivering a series of lectures on this subject to the Stanford Medical School in September 1915, which was published two years later and titled *Focal Infection: The Lane Medical Lectures.*[30]

Similar to Hunter and Miller, Billings found that the peripheral manifestations of disease (the disturbed fields) were not simply "vague systemic intoxications" but the "product of direct invasions" by microbes through the bloodstream from focal infections. Previous to the late 1800s, most scientists believed that microorganisms rarely circulated in the bloodstream—and if they did, the result was fatal.[31] Billings added to the growing understanding during this period that the blood was indeed *not* sterile and commonly carried streptococcus and other bacteria from dental and tonsil focal infections to remote parts of the body (disturbed fields).[32] Based on his exhaustive study and research in this field, Billings was the first scientist to definitively explain and fully characterize the nature of focal infections:

> [A focus of infection is] a circumscribed area of tissue infected with pathogenic microorganisms. Foci of infection may be primary or secondary. Primary foci are usually located in tissues communicating with a mucous or cutaneous surface [e.g., the teeth and tonsils]. Secondary foci [the disturbed fields] are the direct result of infection from other foci through contiguous tissues or at a distance through the bloodstream or lymph channels.[33]

Edward C. Rosenow's Scientific Confirmation of Focal Infections

Miller's laboratory finding that foci are infected with various forms of bacteria was confirmed by Billings's young protégé, Edward C. Rosenow, M.D. (1875–1966). Rosenow, who was influenced by Hektoen to study experimental bacteriology and by Billings to study internal medicine, joined the Rush Medical College faculty in 1904.[34] His laboratory research there was so well respected and renowned that later he was offered a post in bacteriology diagnosis at the prestigious Mayo Institute in Rochester, Minnesota, which he accepted in 1915.[35]

As a creative genius in research methodology and technique, Rosenow was instrumental in scientifically confirming the existence of focal infections. One of his most important contributions was the discovery that microorganisms thrive not in areas of high oxygen (aerobic) or in areas of no oxygen (anaerobic), but in areas with a "*partial tension* of oxygen."[36] For example, in rheumatic fever, the microenvironment of the heart valves has a particular partial oxygen concentration that favors bacterial growth and can result in damage to the mitral valves, which often manifests clinically as a heart murmur.[37] After becoming aware of this partial oxygen pressure state, Rosenow was able to culture live microorganisms from dental and tonsil tissue in patients suffering from chronic disease and prove that these microbes would reproduce the same disease in laboratory animals when injected or implanted in them.* This knowledge of a partial oxygen tension in foci was a key factor in the success of Rosenow's laboratory studies and his ability to

*Rush Medical College later merged with the University of Illinois Medical School.

*Surgically implanting a focal tooth under an animal's skin was the typical method of implantation.

reproduce the same type of environment experimentally. However, many researchers trying to replicate Rosenow's research have not understood the need to maintain these microorganisms in the same partial oxygen state in which they exist in patients' tissues. Therefore, they repudiated the existence of focal infections when their experimental studies using dead or otherwise altered microbes came back negative.

Pleomorphism: Bacteria Change Form and Pathogenicity

Rosenow further found that bacteria have *pleomorphic* qualities—that is, they change their shape, size, and pathogenicity according to the tissue in which they are residing. Like Billings and Miller, Rosenow observed that the bacteria that commonly reside in dental, tonsil, and other focal infections are often of low virulence; however, in the right conditions (e.g., stress, trauma, or toxicity), the number and pathogenicity of these bacteria can potentiate and they can migrate to other environments in the body that are favorable for bacterial growth. Rosenow was thus able to confirm Billings's clinical observations that microbes such as streptococcus from an "insignificant lesion" in dental or tonsillar tissue can actually *metastasize* in the bloodstream of laboratory animals and implant in an organ or tissue, causing serious dysfunction and disease in patients.[38] For example, Rosenow and Billings, confirming the previous work of Schottmüller, found that *Streptococcus viridans,* when isolated from patients with chronic heart disease (endocarditis), would *transmutate* into pneumococcus bacteria and cause acute (and more imminently life-threatening) pneumonia, as these strains of bacteria increased in virulence through successive inoculations (injections of bacteria) in laboratory animals. Rosenow proved this pleomorphic phenomenon of bacteria time and again through his research studies and with a multitude of diseases and syndromes including ulcers, arthritis, cholecystitis (gallbladder inflammation), appendicitis, pneumonia, bronchitis, and asthma.[39]

Streptococci's Role in Neurological Disease

Rosenow further proved that focal infections could cause symptoms in several diseases hitherto unsuspected as the result of a focus. For example, when he injected staphylococcus and streptococcus bacteria from the tonsillar and dental tissue of patients suffering from multiple sclerosis (MS) into animals, from 50 to 83 percent of these laboratory animals would reproduce signs and symptoms of this same neurological disease.[40] Dr. Patrick Störtebecker later corroborated Rosenow's findings through his research investigations. This Swedish scientist revealed that the transport of bacteria into the brain and spinal cord from dental foci such as failed root canals initiates the *disseminated sclerosis* (scars or plaques) seen in MS patients. Rosenow also replicated other viral diseases, including the flaccid paralysis of polio and the skin manifestations of herpes zoster, by injecting laboratory animals with streptococci obtained from the tonsils of patients suffering from these diseases—illnesses believed to be manifested solely through viral, not bacterial, origin.[41] He further developed a vaccine from streptococcus bacteria known as *thermal antibody,* which was significantly effective in curing, or at least greatly mitigating, the effects of polio as well as other focus-caused diseases.[42]*

DENTAL AMALGAM AND MULTIPLE SCLEROSIS

Through his clinical research, Störtebecker found that dental amalgam does not initiate MS but significantly potentiates the symptoms of the disease through the "double impact" of the corrosion of toxic amalgam fillings that releases mercury and the bacteria generated from dental focal infections. This highly toxic methylated mercury is transported—through the blood, lymphatic vessels, and nerves—directly into the brain just inches away.

Rosenow's Theory of Selective Affinity

Another monumental achievement from Rosenow was the discovery of the *selective affinity* or *elective localization* of all microorganisms, but most specifically, of the streptococcus bacteria.[43] This discovery, so significant that it has been labeled Rosenow's theory of selective affinity, is his finding that bacteria have a specific pathogenic affinity for certain tissues.[44] That is, when strep-

*Although this vaccine was used successfully for other streptococcus-related conditions, it is unfortunately not available today. However, the specific instructions for producing it were outlined by Rosenow in several published journal articles, so perhaps an enterprising holistic pharmacy will consider this undertaking at some point.

tococcus bacteria were taken from a patient's arthritic joint and injected into laboratory animals, these bacteria would also settle in the animals' joints, subsequently causing similar arthritic pain and deformities. Rosenow found that it didn't matter if the streptococci were isolated from the patients' arthritis-inducing teeth or tonsil foci or from the arthritic joints (disturbed fields) themselves—bacterial samples from any of these areas would initiate arthritis in 66 to 75 percent of the experimental animals.[45] He duplicated these same findings with appendicitis, ulcers, cholecystitis (gallbladder inflammation), rheumatic fever (heart disease and arthritis), erythema nodosum (skin disease), and myositis (muscle pain), as graphically illustrated in figure 8.1.[46]

Rosenow and Billings both believed that this selective affinity, characterized by one physician as similar to the "homing instinct of pigeons," is influenced by a patient's susceptibility, or *locus minoris resistentiae*.[47] That is, although the streptococcus bacteria in a tooth or tonsil focus may be of the subspecies that typically travels to the joints, if the patient has an inherited tuberculinic miasm, for example, in which he has a preexisting susceptibility toward arthritis, this tendency to cause joint disturbed fields is much more likely to occur and be more serious. However, in a luetic patient, these same arthritic-tending microbes could not only cause joint problems but also initiate a brain disturbed field, with resulting insomnia and anxiety characteristic of this reaction mode. Thus, these practitioners realized that the onset of disease was a *combination* of infection in the parts of the body where these focal microbes had an affinity and the predisposition of the host due to an inherited or acquired miasmic tendency.[48]

Dr. Russell Haden was among the many physicians who later corroborated Rosenow's theory of selective affinity. Through his research, he proved that streptococcus bacteria would replicate in animals the same eye infections, kidney disease, peptic ulcers, heart disease, and arthritis that his patients were suffering from.[49] Diseases of streptococcal origin, known as *rheumatic*

ELECTIVE LOCALIZATION OF STREPTOCOCCI

Source of Streptococci		Strains (220)	Animals Injected (833)	Percentage of Animals Showing Lesions in																
				Appendix	Stomach Hemor.	Duodenum Ulcer	Gall-bladder	Pancreas	Intestines	Joints	Endocardium	Pericardium	Myocardium	Muscles	Kidney	Lung	Skin	Tongue	Eye	Parotid
Appendicitis	When isolated	14	68	68	6	1	1	0	9	29	21	0	9	12	0	0	0	0	3	0
	Later	8	26	15	19	15	4	0	0	22	19	0	12	23	0	0	0	0	0	0
	After animal passage	7	22	45	45	30	40	0	20	36	20	0	20	25	10	0	0	0	0	0
Ulcer of stomach in man	When isolated	18	103	2	60	60	20	3	7	16	12	4	5	0	5	0	0	0	0	0
	Later	8	22	5	5	0	5	0	0	18	14	0	0	0	0	0	0	0	0	0
	After animal passage	7	39	0	23	33	30	15	15	21	5	0	3	3	8	15	0	0	0	0
Cholecystitis	When isolated	12	41	0	29	15	80	5	17	17	10	0	2	7	5	5	2	0	0	0
	Later	5	14	14	28	14	7	0	0	21	14	0	0	0	7	0	0	0	0	0
	After animal passage	4	16	0	31	13	56	19	13	25	19	0	13	0	13	6	0	0	0	0
Rheumatic fever	When isolated	24	71	8	23	18	3	3	13	66	46	27	44	27	39	4	6	0	10	0
	Later	8	14	0	14	21	0	0	0	21	21	0	28	0	21	0	0	0	0	0
	After animal passage	5	19	21	37	21	5	21	0	37	53	32	37	16	42	21	0	0	11	0
Erythema nodosum	When isolated	6	20	0	10	0	0	0	5	20	20	10	0	35	10	5	90	0	5	0
	Later	3	9	0	22	0	11	0	0	11	11	0	0	0	0	0	22	0	0	0
	After animal passage	6	14	0	21	0	50	0	7	50	14	7	14	50	7	43	43	0	0	0
Herpes zoster	When isolated	11	61	10	29	8	16	2	8	11	5	11	5	11	5	21	70	15	15	0
	Later	6	15	0	13	7	7	13	7	60	7	0	20	40	7	20	7	0	13	0
	After animal passage	4	7	0	28	10	0	0	0	43	0	14	0	28	0	43	28	14	0	0
Mumps	When isolated	9	19	15	21	5	21	42	10	42	15	0	37	3	5	15	15	0	0	73
	Later	5	8	12	0	0	0	12	12	24	24	0	12	12	0	12	12	0	0	24
Myositis	When isolated	3	40	2	4	10	2	7	7	20	10	0	35	75	2	0	7	0	8	0
Endocarditis	When isolated	8	44	0	7	0	5	0	15	15	84	4	20	0	20	20	2	0	0	0
Miscellaneous	When isolated	34	41	3	17	0	4	0	4	17	20	0	15	7	7	7	0	0	0	0
"Lab." strains	Before and after animal passage	5	100	2	18	5	2	2	2	45	49	0	15	12	10	17	2	0	6	0
Average percentage of animals injected with non-specific strains showing lesions in individual organs				5	20	9	11	6	8	27	14	2	10	12	9	11	2	1	3	0

NOTE. This table was used in a lantern slide to illustrate Lecture II. Since the lectures were delivered Rosenow has used the table in an article on Elective Localization of Streptococci, *Jour. A.M.A. LXVI, 1916, 1687.*

Figure 8.1. Rosenow's research proving the theory of selective affinity—that is, that streptococcus bacteria are attracted to specific tissues and will replicate the same disease in laboratory animals that had existed in human beings. (Reprinted from Frank Billings, Focal Infection: The Lane Medical Lectures *[1917], 36.)*

illnesses, are still recognized today, but Rosenow's important contribution—that they arise primarily from dental and tonsil focal infections—has sadly been forgotten. Only when more practitioners are educated on the subject of focal infections will the affected organs associated with these typically rheumatic disturbed fields—especially the heart, kidneys, joints, intestines, and brain—begin to be more thoroughly diagnosed and effectively treated. (Rheumatic illnesses are discussed in detail in chapter 12, see page 376.)

Weston A. Price: America's Father of Holistic Dentistry

Based on the clinical and experimental research of Billings and Rosenow in Chicago, whom he cited in his research articles, a dentist in Cleveland began making history in this field through exhaustively studying every aspect of the dental focus.[50] Weston A. Price (1870–1948), known as the father of holistic dentistry in the United States, spent over two decades in the early 1900s painstakingly researching dental focal infections and the disturbed fields that they cause in the body.[51] Price headed up a team of sixty leading scientists—including Dr. Frank Billings of Chicago, Dr. Milton Rosenau of Harvard, and Dr. Charles Mayo, who founded the Mayo Clinic—to study the cause of dental caries and focal infections at the first research institute of the National Dental Association in Cleveland.[52] In 1923, he published two definitive tomes covering his extensive research findings, titled *Dental Infections: Oral and Systemic* (volume 1) and *Dental Infections and the Degenerative Diseases* (volume 2).

► Price's *Dental Infections* books are out of print, but photocopied versions are available from the Price-Pottenger Nutrition Foundation at (800) 366-3748 or by e-mail at info@ppnf.org. This nonprofit foundation stocks all of Dr. Price's books as well as many others on holistic health, and it publishes an excellent quarterly journal titled *Health and Healing Wisdom*. Visit the website at www.ppnf.org.

X-Rays Are Not Always Reliable

Dr. Price's contributions to the dental focal infection field were enormous. He was one of the first practitioners to note that not only could typical dental foci such as infected root-canalled teeth visibly appear to be perfectly healthy, but even X-rays often failed to reveal the bone pathology surrounding them—a fact still misunderstood by many dentists today.[53] In fact, Price's first patient success story was with a female whose root-canal-filled tooth appeared perfectly normal and showed no evidence of infection on an X-ray. Nevertheless, suspecting that her severe arthritis was initiated by this tooth, Dr. Price received her permission to pull it. Indeed, Price's clinical intuition proved to be right on target, since this patient made a dramatic recovery after surgery. After suffering from crippling arthritis and being confined to a wheelchair for six years, the woman was able to walk again and even do fine needlework.[54]

Research Confirms Rosenow's Selective Affinity Theory

Furthermore, using the same methodology as Miller and Rosenow, Price observed that after embedding this woman's tooth under the skin of a rabbit, this animal developed the same kind of crippling arthritis as the patient, and died within ten days of the onset of infection.[55] Price duplicated these same results with other disorders, including eye diseases, heart disease, fatigue, gynecological dysfunction, and diarrhea and other intestinal dysfunction (see figure 8.2).[56] The conclusions of Price's seminal work—confirming Rosenow's theory of selective affinity—were summarized by the late Dr. George Meinig in his book *Root Canal Cover-Up:*

> One of the most important revelations of Dr. Price's research concerned how the bacteria in teeth act much like cancer cells that metastasize to other parts of the body. These bacteria in teeth similarly metastasize, and as they migrate throughout one's system they infect the heart, kidneys, joints, nervous system, brain, eyes—can endanger a pregnant woman, and in fact may infect any organ, gland, or body tissue.[57]

DR. PRICE'S ANIMAL EXPERIMENTATION

Unlike many modern research labs, Dr. Price took exceptional care of the approximately five hundred rabbits he required per year for his dental focus studies. They were well fed, "happily housed," and "privileged to die under chloroform." Price asserted that "for those who would criticize their use, I wish to state that many of these rabbits have in my judgment made a far greater individual contribution and service to the welfare of humanity than hosts of human beings." Actually, the most heartbreaking fact about this is that these animals may have died in vain, because the results from Price's important research studies on foci have been forgotten.

Modern Medicine Often Treats the Disturbed Fields, or Symptoms

Dr. Price recognized that modern medicine was "mistaking effect for cause."[58] That is, when doctors treat a patient's arthritis or heart disease without examining the strong possibility of a focal infection in the teeth or tonsils, they are often treating the effect—or the disturbed field—rather than the true cause. Thus, this holistic dental physician in the early twentieth century recognized what conventional doctors are still doing today—treating the symptoms of disease rather than diagnosing and treating the underlying cause of the disease.

Not All Root-Canalled Teeth Are Actively Pathogenic

Dr. Price also recognized the influence of miasms—that is, everyone has varying degrees of susceptibility to infection based on lifestyle and genetics, as discussed in chapter 1. He noted that a certain percentage of his patients didn't succumb to degenerative disease, despite having root canal fillings that could be classified as chronic foci. He concluded that the healthier immune systems of these (psoric) patients were able to engulf and control the bacteria generated from their focal teeth, thus preventing infection from being transferred to their more vital organs and tissues.[59] Demonstrating

SUMMARY OF ANIMAL REACTIONS AND PATIENTS' SYMPTOMS

Case Number	Patients' Chief Lesions	No. of Rabbits	Percentage with Major Lesions	Heart	Lungs	Liver	Gall-Bladder	Stomach	Intestines	Appendix	Kidneys	Urinary Bladder	Generative Organs	Joints	Muscles	ands	Spinal Cord	Brain	Eyes	Rheumatism Clinical	Chloroform
1124	Pelvic Inflammation and Discharge. Neur.	7	100	43	14	14			14		14		28	57	14	14				14	86
1087	Eyes. Nervous System	11	100	9	9	27	9		9	9	9			9	18		9		100		82
1094	Acute Rheumatism	12	42	33	8	33	8		33	8	33			25	16					16	75
1095	Heart. Rheumatism	2	100	100	100	50	50		50		100				50			50		100	0
306	Rheumatism	3	33	33									33		33					33	100
1098	Lassitude	6	67	67	33	33	17	17	33		50				50						50
381	Arthritis	2	50			50								50	50					50	50
1081	Neck and Shoulder Inv.	5	40	80		40			20	20	40		20		20	20	20	20		40	20
1085	Ovarian Pain	6	67T 100F	33		83	17		67	17	50	33	67T 100F								50
1050	Rheumatism. Heart. Uterine Pain and Discharge	13	55	23		31	8		8				8							8	85
1065	Lumbago. Myositis	3	100	67	33	100	33		67		67			33	33	33				100	33
581	Heart. Rheumatism	6	100	100	17	67	33	17	33	17	50			33	50					50	67
1049	Mild Rheumatism	4	0																		100
1057	Heart. Rheumatism. Emacia	6	83	50		33	33				17				17	17				33	67
1014	Neuritis. Myositis	10	20	30		80	50		60	20	30				10					20	30
1058	Heart	3	100	100	33	100		33	33		100			100	33					67	33
311	Heart. Rheumatism	2	100	100	50						50			50	50						50
1009	Heart. Arthritis	5	100	100		60			20		60				20				20	40	40
1048	Neuritis. Gall Stones	5	100		20	40	40	20	20	20	20				20	20	20	20	20	60	80
709	Arthritis	4	100	25		50	25		25		50			50	50	50		25	50	100	75
455	Rheumatism	9	78	22		11								22		11				78	100
1008	Eyes	13	62	38	8	54	31	23	69	15	54	8	15	23	31		8	8	62	8	23
1019	Diarrhea. Lameness in Shoulder and Arm	4	100			75	50	25	100			25			25	50				75	100
1005	Rheumatism	3	100																	100	100
987	Eyes. Rheumatism	12	83	58	25	42					33	33	25	33	25	17		8	58	50	58
955	Xerostomia. Rheumatism	12	83	33	42	33					33	8	8	17	8	83				8	67
1024	Rheumatism	10	60	30	30	30		20			40			20	30	10				50	60
433	Rheumatism	2	50	100	50	50		50			100			50	50	50				50	0
433	None	2	None																		100
938	None	4	None																		100
	None	1	None																		100

Figure 8.2. Dr. Price's research validating that bacteria from dental foci metastasize to specific organs and tissues in the body. The numbers under the organs indicate the percentage of rabbits that succumbed to disease in the given area. (Reprinted with permission from the Price-Pottenger Nutrition Foundation.)

the clinical discrimination characteristic of true holistic physicians, Price regarded each patient individually and *never* advocated the wholesale extraction of all root-canalled teeth. However, he did observe that under stress, a dormant root-canalled tooth could emerge as an active and disturbing focal infection. Dr. Price further noted that in his clinical experience the two most serious life stressors were pregnancy and lactation and influenza. He also noted other "overloads" to the body that could significantly increase both the pathogenicity of a dental focus as well as a person's immune susceptibility to these endogenous toxins. These stressors include trauma, chronic grief and worry, malnutrition, alcohol abuse, and exposure such as to severe cold.[60]

STRESS OF CHILDBIRTH AND NURSING

Of course, Price understood the importance of breastfeeding and encouraged it, but he also recognized the great stress a woman undergoes bearing a child and then nursing the baby for several years. This is especially true in modern societies, versus a culture like ancient China, for example, where women were given tonifying herbs and acupuncture to balance their bodies both before and after birth. Currently, the stress of pregnancy, birth, and caring for a new baby is still one of the most common precipitating events that can move a primarily psoric woman into a significantly weakened tuberculinic or luetic diathesis. However, with effective holistic care and lifestyle modifications—that is, the mother is financially stable and emotionally supported by her partner, family, and friends—the opposite is true, and it can be a time of great joy and fulfillment.

Major Dysfunction Can Arise from a Seemingly Minor Focus

Price also asserted that the tenet in conventional medicine that the "quantity and virulence of the organism (microbe) . . . determined in large part the danger to the host" could not always be applied to focal infections.[61] He elaborated on this subject in *Dental Infections: Oral and Systemic* (volume 1):

> When infected teeth produce disturbance in other parts of the body, it is not necessary that the quantity of infection be large . . . the evidence at hand strongly suggests that soluble poisons may pass from the infected teeth to the lymph or blood circulation, or both, and produce systemic disturbance *entirely out of proportion* to the quantity of poison involved. The evidence indicates that this toxic substance may under certain circumstances sensitize the body or special tissues so that very small quantities of the organisms, which produce that toxin, may produce very marked reactions and disturbances.[62]

The latter sentence seems to infer that focal infections can bestow an autoimmune-like reactive sensitivity in the bodies of susceptible patients. Indeed, holistic practitioners often witness that patients functioning in the more debilitated tuberculinic and luetic miasmic levels, who typically exhibit this hyper-reactive tendency to seemingly minor stresses, almost invariably have one or more major focal infections in their body. Frank Billings, who had also found host susceptibility to be of primary importance, echoed Price's beliefs by noting that the focal-generated microorganisms did not have to be particularly virulent to cause problems in the body. In fact, Rosenow, Billings, and Price all found that many of the microbes produced from focal infections, such as the *Streptococcus viridans* (mitis) strain, are normal harmless mouth flora (microbes) that become problematic only in a toxic oral environment.[63]* Therefore, the chronic effects of even mildly pathogenic bacteria over years—analogous perhaps to slow water torture—can be much more devastating to an individual's health than suffering through a strong yet short-lived acute illness. (Of course, this is true only if the individual *survives* a strong acute illness, such as pneumonia or influenza.) Through the slow, gradual, but steady release of these mildly toxic bacteria into the bloodstream and lymphatic channels and their slow but sure deposition into disturbed fields in the body, hidden tonsil and dental foci have greatly contributed to the growing list of chronic degenerative

*Price found that the majority of dental focal microbes were of the *Streptococcal fecalis* strain, a nonpathogenic bacteria that normally resides in the intestinal flora. This finding underscores the direct communication of the dysbiosis or pathogenic flora in the mouth and intestines, as well as how normal flora can develop into pathogenic forms in a toxic body terrain.

diseases. However, in the early 1900s, as they often are today, Price noted that the symptoms of these chronic degenerative diseases were frequently mistaken for "psychosomatic" or "normal aging" manifestations.[64]

> **autoimmune:** The term *autoimmune* refers to syndromes in which the body's immune system defenses react (mistakenly) to its own cells or tissues as if they were foreign invaders.

Price's Extraordinary Anthropological Nutritional Research

Price also recognized the pivotal role good nutrition plays in dental health. Based on the research of his extensive studies, he published many articles on the importance of proper calcium metabolism to prevent cavities and bone loss, predating another great dental expert on this subject, Melvin Page.[65] Price recognized that cavities in the teeth are just a first step along a continuum of degeneration, and that without proper treatment and dietary changes, they eventually lead to focal infections in the teeth and jawbone.[66]

In response to the need for nutritional prevention of tooth decay, Price toured the world studying firsthand the diet and health of fourteen isolated cultures living on their native foods. Invariably, he found that these natural and unrefined native diets consistently yielded excellent health and virtually no tooth decay or dental malformations.[67] For example, when Price examined the teeth of Indians living in remote parts of the Yukon Territory, he found only 4 out of 2,464 (0.016 percent) had cavities, in contrast to the Indians living closer to white settlements, who had dental decay ranging from 25 to 40 percent.[68] In 1938, Price published his findings in the book *Nutrition and Physical Degeneration,* which remains to this day one of the most definitive textbooks on anthropological nutritional research in the world. (For more information on Price's nutritional research, see chapters 5 and 16.)

Milton Rosenau and the Odontosomatic Relationship

As a member of Price's investigative team, Dr. Milton Rosenau also contributed greatly to the growing research literature on dental focal infections. Finding the same outcome as Miller, Billings, Rosenow, and Price, Rosenau published a journal article in 1939 on the results of his research with a focal infection in a patient's crowned tooth. He wrote that when he extracted streptococcus from an abscess in the root of a patient's crowned bicuspid tooth and intravenously injected this bacteria into laboratory animals, the animals would dramatically replicate symptoms of the same disease of mucous colitis (intestinal pain, diarrhea, or constipation, with excessive mucous secretion) that the patient had been suffering from.[69] This experiment not only reconfirmed Rosenow's theory of selective affinity but also demonstrated the additional influence of the acupuncture meridian relationship existing between the teeth and the organs in the body, referred to as the *odontosomatic relationship.*

In the 1950s, Reinhold Voll and Fritz Kramer of Germany were the first to observe that the Chinese five-element acupuncture system related not only to relationships in the body but also to the teeth. In their clinical research, the bicuspid teeth were found to be associated with the lung or the large intestine meridians. In Rosenau's case, this classic bicuspid-intestinal relationship was demonstrated through the colitis symptoms that both the patient and the laboratory animals experienced.[70] Rosenau observed identical findings when he transferred different strains of streptococcus bacteria from patients suffering from various diseases directly into the teeth of animals. Further corroborating the previous dental focus research of Rosenow and Price, he found that up to 75 percent of these laboratory animals would later develop the same disease that the patient was experiencing. These disorders included kidney disease (nephritis), bladder infections (cystitis), stomach ulcers, arthritis, and various central and peripheral nerve dystrophies.[71]

Martin Fischer's Landmark Text: Death and Dentistry

Another key player in focal infection research was Martin Fischer, a professor of physiology at the University of Cincinnati and a prolific medical writer.* Dr. Fischer warned dentists to consider the accumulating scientific evidence showing that not only were dental focal infections making patients sick, but these foci were greatly

---

*Holistic readers may be interested to know that Martin H. Fischer taught and inspired Henry G. Bieler at the University of Cincinnati. Dr. Bieler wrote the renowned book *Food Is Your Best Medicine* and was a well-regarded holistic practitioner in the mid-twentieth century to Hollywood movie stars as well as Pennsylvania coal miners.

implicated in the causation of chronic degenerative disease and patients' eventual death.[72] In 1940, Dr. Fischer succinctly presented the following fact in his book *Death and Dentistry*: "In addition to his slogan 'save the tooth,' the dentist has increasingly lost his patient."[73] Fischer further stated:

> Focal infection started in a tooth is obviously no trivial matter! From it are destined to flow into the periphery (other glands, organs, and tissues) [the disturbed fields] what amounts to unexpected and acute and chronic invalidism at the best; at the worst, death.[74]

Rhoads and Dick: The Harm Caused by Incomplete Tonsillectomies

Although much of the research at this time centered on the dental focus, focal infection research was not confined to the teeth. In 1928, an important new finding concerning the tonsil focus was reported in an article published in the *Journal of the American Medical Association*. Two Chicago physicians, Paul Rhoads and George Dick, discovered through their clinical analysis that even when tonsillectomies were performed by "specialists of established reputation," 73 percent of the time the surgery was incomplete. Through their laboratory experiments, they found that the remaining "stumps" and "tags" of tissue left over after these incomplete tonsillectomies often harbored *more* pathogenic streptococcus bacteria per gram than the original infected tonsils had contained before removal.[75] These astounding findings may have influenced the surgical movement during the pre- and postwar period to more thoroughly excise the tonsils during surgery. However, these more stringently performed tonsillectomies by less skilled (or less careful) surgeons often left visible scars, which generate another type of undermining foci—a tonsil interference field.

Even today, the allopathic surgical community seems to still be unaware of this important research conducted almost a century ago. Post-tonsillectomy patients can be just as prone to having a tonsil focus—from either the remaining infected tonsil stumps or tags left behind or the scars created from tonsil surgery—as those who have not undergone surgery.

OTHER TONSILLECTOMY COMPLICATIONS

Although many patients report that their chronic bouts of tonsillitis cleared after their tonsillectomy, other disorders often arise later—such as arthritis or heart disease—when the remaining tonsillar tissue continues to breed infection and these microbes migrate out to create disturbed fields. Furthermore, post-tonsillectomy scar interference fields—as well as internal scarring in nonsurgerized patients who have had many bouts of tonsillitis—commonly restrict blood flow to the brain and contribute to many neurological symptoms including insomnia, anxiety, depression, and memory loss.

During the early and mid-twentieth century, a great many other physicians and scientists contributed to both the clinical and empirical understanding of focal infection. However, their numbers and their research articles and publications are so great that they exceed the scope of this history. Perhaps this chapter will stimulate the publication of an all-inclusive text on this fascinating subject.

THE FALL OF THE FOCAL INFECTION THEORY

Although the experimental methods of all the focal infection researchers were exemplary and included large control groups of animals, warranting their publication in professional scientific journals, questions can still arise in many people's minds as to the veracity of focal infections. Namely, if these studies were respected enough to be published in scientific journals in the early 1900s, why is this body of research virtually unknown today?

DR. PRICE'S RESEARCH METHODOLOGY

Although double-blind studies were unknown at the time, Weston Price and others were extremely conscientious in their research methodology. For example, Dr. Price often transferred the same focal tooth into thirty different rabbits in succession. In one experiment, he even repeated the procedure in one hundred animals. In almost every case, the disease that the patient was suffering from was replicated in the animal. Furthermore, many *sham* items—healthy teeth (extracted for orthodontic purposes), sterile coins, glass, and so forth—were implanted in hundreds of animals as controls, to rule out the possibility that simply implanting a foreign object could cause the disturbance. In every case, these items caused no illness, nor did they shorten the life spans of any experimental animals.[76]

Over the years, many influences have led to the disregard—if not outright suppression—of this valuable research. Five of the most significant causes as to why this information was not propagated after the midpoint of the twentieth century are described here.

1. Research of Detractors Not Properly Conducted

As discussed previously, Rosenow's discovery that bacteria and other microbes could survive only in an environment with a small amount of oxygen allowed him and other researchers to trace the selective affinity—or attraction—of streptococci to certain tissues (disturbed fields). However, in subsequent studies, many researchers ignored this fact and therefore failed to reproduce the bacteria's affinity for certain tissues. Therefore, the research findings of Miller, Billings, Rosenow, Price, and others were often fallaciously declared invalid.[77]

2. Research Findings Fraudulently Manipulated

For almost a century, a single journal article has been quoted to discredit the numerous research papers supporting the validity of the focal infection theory. What is even more astonishing is that this paper's findings were based on clearly inaccurate data that was fraudulently manipulated.

Authored by W. L. Holman, this article was published in 1928 in the *Archives of Pathological and Laboratory Medicine.* It challenged the results of the focal infection theory through a "rearrangement of Rosenow's data." Based on frankly deceitful manipulation of his research statistics, Holman concluded that Rosenow's selective affinity (elective localization) theory of bacteria had not been proven.[78]

For example, Rosenow reported that 60 percent of 103 animals developed ulcerlike lesions in their stomach and duodenum after he had injected them with bacteria isolated from stomach ulcer patients. In a control group of 405 animals, he found that only 17 percent of those animals developed ulcerlike lesions when injected with bacterial strains from patients suffering from other diseases. Holman calculated (accurately) that 62 animals injected with bacteria from stomach ulcer patients (60 percent of 103) developed similar ulcers to these patients, as did 68 animals in the control group (17 percent of 405). However, Holman then falsely used the number 130 (62 + 68), to report that 48 percent (62 animals) developed ulcers and 52 percent (68 animals) did not, and he excluded the other 378 animals included in the study. Therefore, Holman erroneously concluded that "it is roughly a 50 percent chance" (48 percent and 52 percent) whether an animal succumbs to the same disease that the individual was suffering.[79]

Stuart Hale Shakman, an analyst and consultant in the health field for several government organizations, commented on this scientific debacle in his reference manual on the works of Dr. Rosenow:

> Holman's continuing legacy is exemplified in Paul B. Beeson's 1976 exclusive reference to a 1940 article by H. A. Reiman and W. P. Havens as concerns "decisive" rejection of Rosenow and "the focal infection fad"; Reiman and Havens, in turn, exclusively credited Holman with having refuted elective localization. Similarly, numerous works up to modern times, seemingly including virtually the whole of key supporting literature for modern endodontics [root canal specialty], are fundamentally reliant on Holman or works which themselves depend on Holman. For the most part, as a result of cumulative years of negative regard largely (directly or indirectly) traceable back to Holman, Rosenow's work has been generally maligned and consequently ignored.[80]

Even a later 1940 journal article in which Rosenow detailed the results of experiments conducted by himself and thirty-one other scientists involving more than 11,000 animals and confirming the validity of the focal infection theory did not stem the tide of this "negative regard."[81] Inconceivably, Holman's fraudulent article inflicted permanent damage to the focal infection theory, and it has been blindly utilized by generations of allopathic doctors and dentists ever since to continue to nullify the entire body of research conducted by the holistic pioneers in this field.

Dr. Weston Price's reputation also suffered from his own nemesis—an allopathic physician named Percy Howe. In an article composed of blatantly false data, Howe condemned Price's dental focal infection research and called him a fraud. The publication of this article threw doubt on Price's meticulous and scrupulous research and further contributed to the demise of the focal infection theory.[82]

3. Surgery Improperly Performed

When the clinical decision is made that a tooth must be surgically removed, simply pulling the tooth is not sufficient. *Cavitation surgery* is the term used to denote the appropriate and complete removal of *all* the infected tissue in and around a dental focal infection. This typically includes the removal of all infected soft tissue that may remain behind after a simple extraction, including the tooth's periodontal ligament as well as all infected necrotic (dead) jawbone areas that need to be carefully drilled out. Only when cavitation surgery is properly performed and supportive holistic care is rendered can a dental focus be completely resolved. Otherwise, the focal infection continues to exist in the jawbone and the illness in the disturbed field(s) remains unchanged.[83]

The same problem occurs with tonsillectomies. As described previously, the landmark study by Rhoads and Dick in 1928 found that the "stumps" and "tags" left after incomplete tonsillectomies often harbor even more pathogenic bacteria per gram of tissue than the intact tonsils had before surgery. And almost *three-quarters* of surgeons would fail to remove all of the infected tissue.[84] This large percentage of unsuccessful tonsillectomies was subsequently used as ammunition against the advocates of the focal infection theory. Thus, Dr. Martin Fischer's description in 1940 of the errors in tonsil and dental surgery is just as relevant today as it was then:

> Grossest error lies in the nonrecognition of obviously infected tonsils, teeth, and their surrounding tissues. Whereafter not merely incompetent but inadequate surgical attack makes for cropper.* The beneficent effects of proper diagnosis and effective surgery are so great that we teach our students that failure to stop progressive disease and thereafter to keep their patients symptomless is not to be written down as fault of the disease but of themselves. It is an unhappy fact that but few of throat or dental specialists are entitled to their designation. Their first shortcoming lies in an inability to see; their second, in operative fear—they do not go far enough because unversed in gross pathology. A tonsil shaved or the peritonsillar infected lymph channels and inflamed scar tissues not removed, a tooth extracted but its adjacent and similarly affected alveolar bone left standing, too frequently excite constitutional reactions compared with which the signs and symptoms that made the victim a patient were trifling [that is, the patient becomes worse after surgery].[85]

4. Saving the Tooth

Prevention through Nutrition

Over time, a growing number of dentists became more and more opposed to extracting suspected focal teeth, which was arguably rather excessive (by skilled and unskilled dentists) during this period. In fact, many holistic dentists, led by the work of Weston Price, began to advocate that more emphasis be placed on a healthy diet and good nutrition in order to prevent the decay and infections that often necessitated tooth extractions later on. As some dentists began to focus only on the preventive effects of a healthy diet on the teeth, the focal infection theory became less prominent.

*The term *cropper* refers to the action of cutting off only the tops of infected tissues, rather than thoroughly excising all of the focal area. The practice of surgically removing only a portion of the tonsils is not uncommon and is referred to in medical terms as a *tonsillotomy*. Peter Dosch has commented on this practice of cutting out only the tops of tonsil tissue: "In our experience, a tonsillotomy is never able to eliminate a tonsillar interference field but, on the contrary, is more likely to produce one." (P. Dosch, *Manual of Neural Therapy* [Heidelberg: Haug Publishers, 1984], 127.)

The Rising Popularity of Root Canals

Other dental groups espoused the use of root canals, despite the large amount of research evidence Dr. Price and others had amassed showing that many root-canalled teeth functioned as silent focal infections. This was especially true after the early 1940s, when the specialty of endodontics (dentists who perform root canals) had become a recognized branch of dentistry with its own professional association. This group exerted—and still does—a great deal of pressure among dentists and dental associations to choose root canal treatments over tooth extraction. In fact, based on journal articles by Holmans, Howe, and others repudiating the theory of the dental focal infection, a 1950s article in the *Journal of the American Dental Association* asserted the following: "The pulpless [dead] tooth is now no longer viewed with alarm and has been honored by the foundation of a specialty [the endodontic profession that specializes in root canals]."[86]

This false belief in the safety of all root canals was more recently evidenced by an article published in the 1994 fall/winter newsletter of the American Association of Endodontists (AAE): "Root Canal Therapy Safe and Effective." In their book, *The Roots of Disease,* Robert Kulacz, D.D.S., and Thomas Levy, M.D., reported that the authors of this AAE article dogmatically averred that root-canalled teeth do not serve as foci, and that their toxins do not spread to other parts of the body to create disturbed fields. However, in another confounding position statement, the AAE has also admitted that the formaldehyde-containing Sargenti paste that has been used in root canals *can* leak out of the tooth and "infiltrate the blood, lymph nodes, adrenal glands, spleen, liver, and brain."[87]* Kulacz and Levy point out the faulty logic of the AAE's two positions, since if chemicals from this formaldehyde paste can easily migrate throughout the body, then so too can bacteria and the chemical toxins that they produce.[88]

However, to the uninformed patient, a root canal—as unpleasant a picture as this conjures up in most people's minds—is still a more preferable choice than the loss of a tooth. Therefore, the majority of dental patients, especially those who were simply told they needed a root canal and not informed about the failure rates of this procedure or the focal infection theory, often opt for this alternative to the loss of a tooth. In fact, the number of root canal treatments performed in this country has grown exponentially since the middle of the last century; in 1999, an estimated 16 million of these controversial dental procedures were performed.[89] Even more alarming and seriously bordering on—if not squarely residing in—the arena of dental malpractice is the fact that many times root canals are recommended by dentists *prophylactically* on a noninfected tooth before a crown is placed. (Alternatives to conventional root canal treatments are discussed in chapter 11; see page 356.)

Antibiotic Use

The fact that antibiotics had been discovered and their use in both medicine and dentistry was increasing in the early and mid-twentieth century, simultaneous with the fall of the focal infection theory, was not simply coincidental. As discussed in chapter 7, this new "miracle drug" did indeed dramatically reduce the death rate from bacterial infectious diseases such as pneumonia, meningitis (inflammation of the membranes that cover the brain), and endocarditis (inflammation of the membranes lining the cavities of the heart).[90] It was therefore quite logical for doctors and dentists unaware of the drawbacks of this new drug to begin utilizing antibiotics in the treatment of *all* infections—including abscessed teeth and infected tonsils. The following quote illustrates the prevailing belief in the curative effects of this miracle drug in healing "oral foci" that had become extant by the mid-twentieth century:

> The discovery of antibiotic agents effective against a wide variety of organisms has lessened materially the general systemic danger of these oral foci . . . Today these oral lesions can be prevented or minimized by the use of the correct antibiotic . . . many systemic diseases which may arise from bacteria in the oral cavity can now be effectively and satisfactorily treated with antibiotics, lessening the systemic danger of oral infection.[91]

In acute dental and medical emergencies, the use of antibiotics can be appropriate. However, as the discoverer of penicillin, Sir Alexander Fleming, prophetically

*Sargenti paste has been denounced by the AAE and is now rarely used in root canals.

warned in 1945, the excessive use of antibiotics can eventually cause more harm than good.[92] Furthermore, the word *excessive* in many cases was indeed an understatement. Antibiotics in the twentieth century became the panacea for every ill, and even became the standard prophylactically *in case* of infection.[93] Therefore, doctors and dentists—then and now—excessively prescribed this drug *preventively* after tooth extractions and surgeries, liberally for bacterial infections, and often mistakenly for influenza and other virus-induced illnesses that don't even respond to antibiotic medications.

Taking a course of antibiotics is easy, painless, relatively cheap, and noninvasive—and an exceptionally more acceptable and attractive alternative to having a tooth pulled or getting a root canal. Therefore, patients often embraced this new wonder drug as enthusiastically as their allopathic physicians and dentists. Furthermore, patients' convictions over the effectiveness of antibiotics were often strengthened when there was an initial decrease or lasting change in their symptoms. And after witnessing the beneficial gain—albeit often short term—made from antibiotic therapy, dentists felt relieved from broaching the more difficult decision-making process of whether to extract a tooth. This decision was positively influenced by the fact that the use of antibiotics in the treatment of infections was (and still is) the "standard of care" in both the dental and medical professions. In fact, not prescribing antibiotics is still looked on askance by the dental boards, and dentists who don't prescribe them can even be subjected to severe disciplinary action.

The question that comes to mind, however—and was debated even at the beginning of their use—is whether antibiotics effectively kill the bacteria and neutralize the toxic excretions in a focal tooth or tonsil. In one particularly dramatic experiment that tested the possibility of *completely* sterilizing a dental focus, Dr. Weston Price washed with strong disinfectants, pumiced, and even placed in boiling water for an hour an infected tooth that had been removed from an experimental lab rabbit that had died of the patient's illness. Despite this rigorous process that was stronger than any antibiotic's effect, this tooth, when embedded in another rabbit, astoundingly caused this animal's death in twenty-two days.[94] In a subsequent study, focal teeth were subjected to the *ultimate* sterilization procedure of the high pressure and temperature of an autoclave (an instrument that sterilizes through steam under pressure). However, when these seemingly *completely* sterilized teeth were later embedded under the skin of rabbits, these animals began to lose weight and also died, within a thirty-five day period.[95]

Price's research additionally revealed that the enormously potent toxins that bacteria produce are more dangerous than the bacteria themselves.[96] In fact, he found that the injection of the excreted toxins of the bacteria into rabbits would cause the animals to get sick and die *sooner* than the implantation of the bacteria-containing tooth itself. Price theorized that the immune system had a greater "head start" to mount a defense when the bacteria were present, and when they were absent, it was less "primed" to fight their more potent excreted toxins.[97]

This same principle applies when antibiotics wipe out bacteria but fail to kill the bacterial poisons that remain behind in the tissues, which can set up the system for even more serious future immune dysfunction. Further evidence of the failure of antibiotics is that despite their liberal use, especially for childhood ear and tonsil infections, dental and tonsil focal infections are now epidemic and more common (based on the reports in the literature) than during the early part of the twentieth century. Although this fact is greatly influenced by the vastly increased modern-day ingestion of sugar and other degenerative foods, as well as the resistance of many bacteria species that has built up over the years, it suggests that antibiotics may not only be failing to treat but also *potentiating* the pathogenicity of chronic focal infections.

5. Turf Wars

Unfortunately, power struggles and turf wars occur just as often among health professionals as they do in politics. In fact, the titles of selected journal articles are listed in table 8.1 to illustrate the magnitude as well as the ferocity of the debate that occurred during this approximate fifty-year period of focal infection research (1886–1929). Internecine battles raged between dental groups who believed in extracting focal infection teeth versus those who believed in trying to save the teeth at all costs. There were also disputes between dentists and doctors—the latter felt that dentists were overstepping their scope of practice and should confine their treatments solely to the oral cavity. Dr. Weston Price, observing in his extensive research that over 95 percent of American adults had some form of dental focal infections, prophetically wrote in 1923:

> [U]ntil our dental colleges teach more of general medicine and clinical pathology, and the medical colleges teach more of dental pathology, both local and systemic [that is, both locally in the mouth and the effects of these dental microbes systemically in the body], humanity must wait and suffer.[98]

This tendency toward specialization versus general practice is still prevalent today. On one hand, one may reasonably argue that it is indeed imperative to have surgeons who are masters with a scalpel and skilled in advanced surgical techniques. On the other hand, this proclivity toward dividing up the patient pie into smaller and smaller sections so that everyone gets a piece of the healthcare dollar has resulted in so much specialization that the correct holistic diagnosis—and therefore the appropriate treatment—is often obscured by professional narrow-mindedness and self-interest. Dr. Peter Dosch, a German physician and renowned neural therapist, commented on this worldwide modern-day problem:

> Our specialized knowledge has become vast. There is no lack of facts. But there is a lack of synthesis of all this knowledge, a dearth of interconnected thinking that takes the natural laws of cybernetics [the science dealing with how the body functions as a synergistic unit] more effectively into account.[99]

TABLE 8.1. THE RISE AND FALL OF THE FOCAL INFECTION THEORY IN AMERICA, ILLUSTRATED BY SELECTED JOURNAL ARTICLES FROM 1886 TO 1929

The Rise	. . . and Fall
H. Judd, "The Retention of **Dead Teeth** in the Jaw (Oral Sepsis)," *Dental Items of Interest* 8 (1886): 403–4.	A. Gibson, "**A Plea for Moderation** in the Wholesale Extraction of Teeth," *Australian Dental Summary* 2 (1921–22): 210–11.
J. Crawford, "The Influence of the Wisdom Teeth in **Causing Diseases** of the Respiratory Tract," *Dental Items of Interest* 8 (1888): 490.	H. Schottmueller, "The **Doubtful** Interrelationship between Infected Teeth and General Disease," *American Dental Association Journal* 9 (1922): 668–71.
S. Spokes, "**Teeth and Appendicitis**," *British Journal of Dental Science* 43 (1906): 200–9 (selected).	C. Johnson, "Present **Rage** for Extracting Teeth," *Australia Dental Science Journal* 2 (1922): 38–40.
A. Underwood, "Two Cases of Serious **Constitutional Disturbance** of a Dental Origin," *British Journal of Dental Science* 53 (1910): 193–95. H. Upson, "Insanity Caused by Painless Dental Disease," *Dental Cosmos*, May 1910, 511–23 (abstract).	J. Tomlinson, "**Ruthless Extractions**," *Australia Dental Science Journal* 3 (1923): 269–71 (selected).
E. Rosenow, "Elective Localization of Bacteria in **Diseases of the Nervous System**," *Allied Journal* 11 (1916): 727–28 (abstract).	W. Meyer, "**Useless Extraction** of Teeth," *Australian Dental Science Journal* 5 (1925): 286–87. C. Johnson, "**Fads** and Their Effects (Re: Extraction of Pulpless Teeth)," *Australian Dental Science* 5 (1925): 368–71.
E. Schmitt, "Foci of Infection within the Oral Cavity and Their Relation to **Systemic Disease**," *American Dentist* 5 (1917): 1–3.	"The **Swing of the Pendulum** (Focal Infection)," *American Dental Association Journal* 15 (1928): 1791–94.
W. Price, "Dental Infection and Related Degenerative Diseases," *American Dental Association Journal* 11 (1924): 497–98 (selected). J. Buckley and W. Price, "Resolved, That **Practically All Infected Pulpless Teeth Should Be Removed**" (debate), 1303, 1468–1524, 28 illus., 16 tables, 1540–42.	"This Is Refreshing (The Inconsistent **Craze** for Removal of Teeth)," *American Dental Association Journal* 16 (1929): 917–19.

Bold emphasis in journal article titles added by author.

As figure 8.3 depicts, patients are often bewildered by all of the different diagnoses they receive from myopic practitioners. This increasing professional pressure and general movement toward specialization was also greatly instrumental in the decline of holistic dental practitioners who, like Weston Price, were able to correlate dental issues with the patient's overall health and functioning. Fortunately, this situation is beginning to reverse itself as the numbers of holistic dentists are growing as satisfied patients increasingly demand that natural medicine and biological dentistry be recognized forms of healing.

EUROPEAN RESEARCH

During the explosion of focal infection research in the United States in the early and mid-twentieth century, there was a simultaneous acceleration of investigation in this area in Europe, primarily in Germany. Most of this European research was centered on the treatment of foci through neural therapy. Neural therapy is traditionally (and most narrowly) defined as the injection of local anesthetic into a focus or scar interference field to restore normal functioning—or *healthy regulation*—in the focal area as well as its disturbed field. Due to the growing popularity of this *regulating* or rebalancing therapy, as well as the greater freedom holistic European practitioners have always enjoyed, significant advances and contributions to the focal infection theory have been made. In fact, just as U.S. interest was waning in the mid-twentieth century, European research in this holistic field was flourishing.

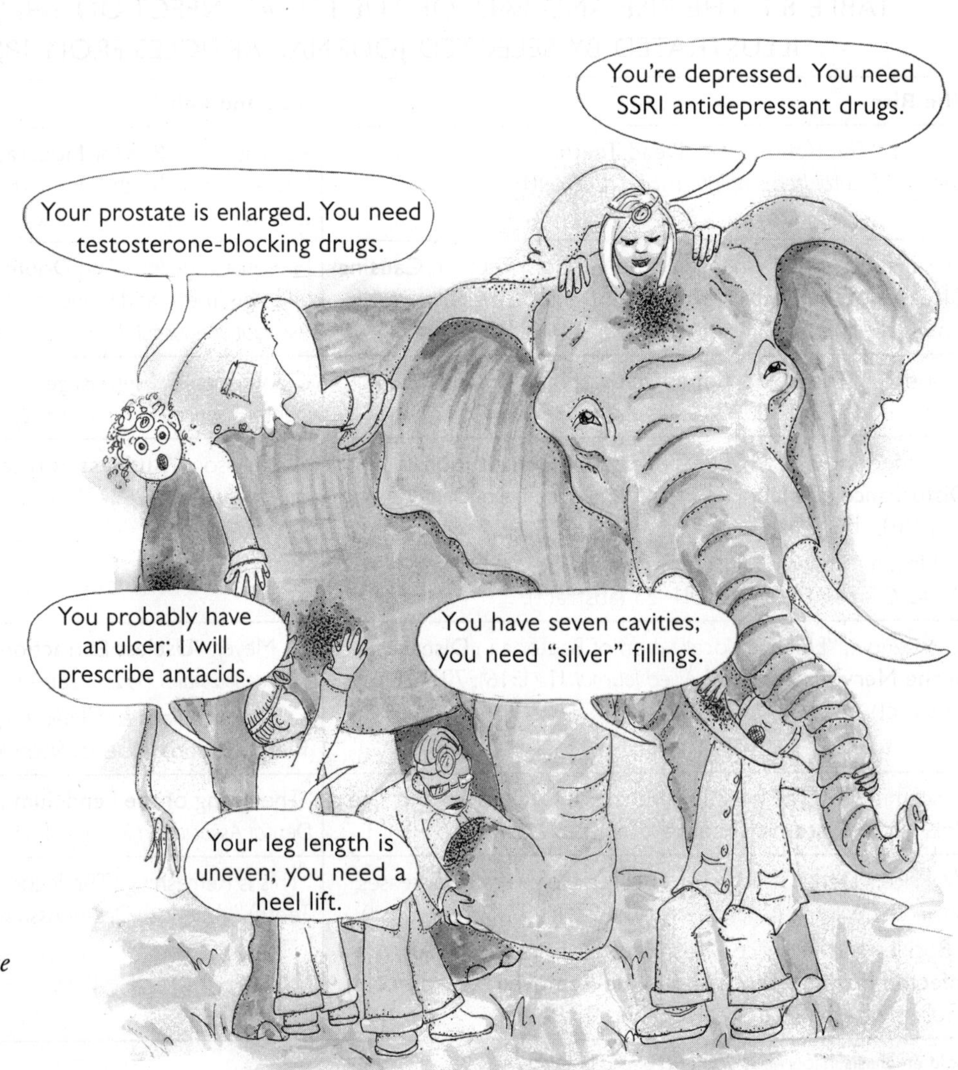
You're depressed. You need SSRI antidepressant drugs.
Your prostate is enlarged. You need testosterone-blocking drugs.
You probably have an ulcer; I will prescribe antacids.
You have seven cavities; you need "silver" fillings.
Your leg length is uneven; you need a heel lift.

Figure 8.3. Specialists diagnose a patient's fatigue symptoms.

The Huneke Phenomenon

The origins of neural therapy are primarily credited to the Huneke brothers in Germany. From 1925 to 1940, Drs. Ferdinand and Walter Huneke practiced what they termed *therapeutic anesthesia*—the injection of local anesthetics either intravenously or intramuscularly to treat all types of painful conditions and disorders.[100] In 1940, however, Ferdinand Huneke accidentally witnessed a new phenomenon on a female patient who had chronic right shoulder pain. The patient was suffering from frozen shoulder, or *adhesive capsulitis,* which greatly limits the shoulder's range of motion and causes chronic pain and stiffness. This woman's pain was of five years' duration, and it was so severe and intractable that the suspected causative sites—her tonsils and most of her teeth—had already been removed by German dentists and physicians who were knowledgeable about focal infections.

Ferdinand Huneke initially injected local anesthetic in and around the right shoulder area, but it was to no avail; the patient experienced no relief in pain and was discharged "uncured."[101] Fortunately for this patient, however, she returned a few weeks later because an old osteomyelitis* surgical scar on her left shin had suddenly become inflamed and painful.[102] Huneke, again utilizing his therapeutic anesthesia method, injected local anesthetic around the patient's leg scar to ease the pain. What was astonishing about this particular treatment was that not only was the scar pain alleviated locally but the patient's seemingly unrelated chronic and intractable right shoulder pain was also immediately relieved, within seconds after Huneke's injection. Furthermore, she was able to begin moving her arm more normally, without pain. Huneke recorded this unique event with the following revelation:

> This experience was so startling that I could have no doubt that I was looking at a fundamentally new piece of knowledge and that I was on the track of a hitherto unknown law in the field of focal processes.[103]

Huneke's serendipitous treatment was the first demonstration of a neural or scar interference field, where a scar on the leg was significantly inflaming nerves located far away in the opposite shoulder region.* This initial precedent-setting neural therapy treatment dramatically exhibited the following three phenomena:

1. Scar interference fields can cause distal symptoms (disturbed fields) through the *nervous system* (and the matrix connective tissue—discussed in chapter 9), because inflammatory pain from a bacterial focus such as the teeth or tonsils could not disappear so instantaneously.
2. An old scar can remain dormant and be triggered through some kind of stress to cause pain in a remote disturbed field years later (this patient's osteomyelitis surgical scar was thirty-five years old, yet her shoulder pain was only five years in duration).
3. A disturbed field, such as this patient's shoulder pain, can be alleviated through neural therapy.

The instantaneous relief of the patient's shoulder pain came to be known in neural therapy parlance as the Huneke phenomenon, the seconds phenomenon, or the lightning reaction.[104]

Other Contributions

Dr. Ferdinand Huneke, as well as his brother, Walter, continued to research the injection of local anesthetic into scars and other focal areas. Other German professors such as Dittmar, Kohlrausch, and Lampert significantly contributed to this new area of study, as did physicians practicing neural therapy during this period of intense clinical investigation, including Gross, Kibler, and Siegen.[105] Through their research and the subsequent formalization of the field of neural therapy, German physicians and researchers originated many of the expressions that are currently used today to describe the various effects of focal disturbances. For example, the term *interference field* (a synonym of the term *focus*

*Osteomyelitis is an infection of the bone usually caused by *Staphylococcus aureus.* Treatment with antibiotics is most typical, but sometimes surgery is necessary to remove the devitalized bone tissue.

*Ten years before, in 1930, Dr. Leriche of France had written about the disappearance of pain from a remote site in the body after the injection of local anesthetic into a scar. However, he did not widely propagate this information or draw any therapeutic conclusions from it; therefore, Peter Dosch attributed the primary discovery of interference fields and neural therapy to Dr. Huneke. (P. Dosch, *Manual of Neural Therapy* [Heidelberg: Haug Publishers, 1984], 74.)

most often used to describe noninfected scars) and the term *disturbed* or *burdened field* (the area secondarily disturbed by a focus) arose out of the necessity to clarify terms in the growing field of neural therapy.[106]

Other European physicians and scientists were also instrumental in researching and discovering the pathogenesis underlying the formation and perpetuation of a chronic focus, as well as formulating and testing neurological and connective tissue theories as to why neural therapy was successful. The work of the famous French surgeon R. Leriche; the Russian physiologists and neurologists Ivan Pavlov, A. D. Speransky, and A. W. Vishnevski; the British surgeon Sir Henry Head; the German scientists and physicians G. Spiess, Werner Scheidt, Peter Dosch, Jochen Gleditsch, and Hartmut Heine; and the Austrian professors and physicians Alfred Pischinger, Franz Hopfer, Felix Perger, and G. Kellner are just a few of the many past and present researchers who have significantly contributed to the scientific understanding of the effect of interference fields and focal infections on the body.[107]

Presently, holistic practitioners study and learn about foci chiefly from Europeans, typically the Germans, Swiss, and Austrians. This is because neural therapy, originated by the German Huneke brothers, has grown to be the most popular treatment modality for healing chronic foci in these Germanic-speaking countries.[108] In fact, the book *Manual of Neural Therapy According to Huneke,* written by German physician Peter Dosch, has been the only text extant for decades that has comprehensively described the diagnosis and treatment of foci. However, a Canadian physician, Robert Kidd, has recently written a reference book for physicians, called *Neural Therapy: Applied Neurophysiology and Other Topics,* that details the treatment of various foci and their related ganglia.*

Since the early 1990s, interest has been growing worldwide in this field of study. Dietrich Klinghardt, a German-born physician living in the United States, has been largely responsible for spreading the word about this important cornerstone of holistic medicine. Klinghardt, who has both a clinical and neurological mastery of the treatment of foci by neural therapy, has educated hundreds of practitioners in the understanding and application of this specialized school of healing.

*Ganglia are knotlike groups of nerve cell bodies located outside the central nervous system (the brain and spinal cord).

NOTES

1. J. Hunter, *The Natural History of the Human Teeth and a Practical Treatise on the Diseases of the Teeth* (Birmingham: The Classics of Medicine Library, 1980).
2. M. Fischer, *Death and Dentistry* (Springfield, Ill.: Charles C. Thomas, 1940), 200–201, 229.
3. J. Hunter, *The Natural History of the Human Teeth and a Practical Treatise on the Diseases of the Teeth* (Birmingham: The Classics of Medicine Library, 1980), 121–22, 126–28.
4. S. H. Shakman, *E. C. Rosenow and Associates: A Reference Manual* (Santa Monica, Calif.: Institute of Science, 1998), B2-1.
5. N. Goodman, *Benjamin Rush* (Philadelphia: University of Pennsylvania Press, 1934), 235–36.
6. Ibid., 236–37.
7. H. Coulter, *Divided Legacy: The Conflict between Homoeopathy and the American Medical Association* (Berkeley, Calif.: North Atlantic Books, 1999), 7, 17, 90; G. Null, *Germs, Biological Warfare, Vaccinations* (New York: Seven Stories Press, 2003).
8. M. Ring, *Dentistry: An Illustrated History* (New York: Harry N. Abrams, Inc., 1985), 285; W. Miller, "The Human Mouth as a Focus of Infection," *The Dental Cosmos* 33, no. 9 (September 1891): 689.
9. M. Ring, "W. D. Miller: The Pioneer Who Laid the Foundation for Modern Dental Research," *New York State Dental Journal,* February 2002, 35, 36.
10. Ibid., 35–37.
11. W. Miller, "The Human Mouth as a Focus of Infection," *The Dental Cosmos* 33, no. 9 (September 1891): 689.
12. Ibid., 789–805.
13. Ibid., 689–713.
14. Ibid., 690–91.
15. Ibid., 692.
16. Ibid., 691, 694–99.
17. E. Hatton, "Focal Infection," in G. Black, *Operative Dentistry* (Woodstock, Ill.: Medico-Dental Publishing Company, 1948), 417.
18. M. Ring, "W. D. Miller: The Pioneer Who Laid the

Foundation for Modern Dental Research," *New York State Dental Journal,* February 2002, 34.

19. A. Black, *G. V. Black's Work on Operative Dentistry,* vol. 1 (Chicago: Medico-Dental Publishing Company, 1936), 4.
20. J. Bouquot, *In Review of NICO (Neuralgia-Inducing Cavitational Osteonecrosis), G. V. Black's Forgotten Disease,* 3rd ed. (Morgantown, W.Va.: The Maxillofacial Center, 1995), 1.
21. M. Ring, *Dentistry: An Illustrated History* (New York: Harry N. Abrams, Inc., 1985), 276; J. Bouquot, *In Review of NICO (Neuralgia-Inducing Cavitational Osteonecrosis), G. V. Black's Forgotten Disease,* 3rd ed. (Morgantown, W.Va.: The Maxillofacial Center, 1995), 1.
22. E. Hatton, "Focal Infection," in G. Black, *Operative Dentistry* (Woodstock, Ill.: Medico-Dental Publishing Company, 1948).
23. W. Hunter, "An Address on the Role of Sepsis and of Antisepsis in Medicine," *Lancet,* January 14, 1911, 79.
24. R. Haden, *Dental Infection and Systemic Disease* (Philadelphia: Lea and Febiger, 1936), 14–15.
25. W. Hunter, "An Address on the Role of Sepsis and of Antisepsis in Medicine," *Lancet,* January 14, 1911, 81, 82.
26. Ibid., 83.
27. F. Billings, "Chronic Focal Infections and Their Etiologic Relations to Arthritis and Nephritis," *The Archives of Internal Medicine* 9 (January 30, 1912): 484–98.
28. M. Fischer, *Death and Dentistry* (Springfield, Ill.: Charles C. Thomas, 1940), 12, 198.
29. Ibid., 13–14, 26; P. Dosch, *Manual of Neural Therapy* (Heidelberg: Haug Publishers, 1984), 26.
30. F. Billings, *Focal Infection* (New York: D. Appleton and Company, 1916), 1–166.
31. M. Fischer, *Death and Dentistry* (Springfield, Ill.: Charles C. Thomas, 1940), 13, 14.
32. F. Billings, *Focal Infection* (New York: D. Appleton and Company, 1916), 20–22.
33. E. Hatton, "Focal Infection," in G. Black, *Operative Dentistry* (Woodstock, Ill.: Medico-Dental Publishing Company, 1948), 414.
34. M. Fischer, *Death and Dentistry* (Springfield, Ill.: Charles C. Thomas, 1940), 15–16.
35. R. Ziemer, coordinator, Mayo Historical Unit, personal correspondence to author, January 6, 2003.
36. M. Fischer, *Death and Dentistry* (Springfield, Ill.: Charles C. Thomas, 1940), 27.
37. R. Kulacz and T. Levy, *The Roots of Disease* (Bloomington, Ind.: Xlibris Corporation, 2002), 37.
38. M. Fischer, *Death and Dentistry* (Springfield, Ill.: Charles C. Thomas, 1940), 23.
39. Ibid., 26–33.
40. Ibid., 37.
41. P. Störtebecker, *Mercury Poisoning from Dental Amalgam—A Hazard to the Human Brain* (Orlando, Fla.: Bio-Probe, 1985), 33–34, 36–37, 118–21.
42. B. Rappaport, "Acute Poliomyelitis Treated with Thermal Antibody," *Lancet* 68 (1948): 395.
43. E. Rosenow, "Elective Localization of Bacteria in Diseases of the Nervous System," *Journal of the American Medical Association,* August, 26, 1916, 662–66.
44. R. Haden, "Elective Localization of Streptococci," *Orthodontia and Oral Surgery, International Journal* 12 (1926): 711.
45. F. Billings, *Focal Infection* (New York: D. Appleton and Company, 1916), 33–47.
46. Ibid.
47. E. Rosenow, "Elective Localization of Bacteria in Diseases of the Nervous System," *Journal of the American Medical Association,* August, 26, 1916, 665–66.
48. S. H. Shakman, *E. C. Rosenow and Associates: A Reference Manual* (Santa Monica, Calif.: Institute of Science, 1998), 1–2.
49. R. Haden, "Elective Localization of Streptococci," *Orthodontia and Oral Surgery, International Journal* 12 (1926): 711–13.
50. W. Price, "The Prevention of Systemic Diseases Arising from Mouth Infections and the Purpose and Plan of the Research Institute of the National Dental Association," *Cleveland Medical Journal* 14 (October 1915): 1, 2, 11.
51. G. Meinig, *Root Canal Cover-Up* (Ojai, Calif.: Bion Publishing, 1994), 8.
52. W. Price, "The Prevention of Systemic Diseases Arising from Mouth Infections and the Purpose and Plan of the Research Institute of the National Dental Association," *Cleveland Medical Journal* 14 (October 1915): 6–10.
53. W. Price, *Dental Infections: Oral and Systemic,* vol. 1 (Cleveland: The Penton Press Company, 1923), 47, 54; J. Bouquot, *In Review of NICO (Neuralgia-Inducing Cavitational Osteonecrosis, G. V. Black's Forgotten Disease,* 3rd ed. (Morgantown, W.Va.: The Maxillofacial Center, 1995), 3.
54. G. Meinig, *Root Canal Cover-Up* (Ojai, Calif.: Bion Publishing, 1994), 3.
55. Ibid.
56. W. Price, *Dental Infections: Oral and Systemic,* vol. 1 (Cleveland: The Penton Press Company, 1923), 287–90.

57. G. Meinig, *Root Canal Cover-Up* (Ojai, Calif.: Bion Publishing, 1994), 1.
58. W. Price, *Dental Infections: Oral and Systemic,* vol. 1 (Cleveland: The Penton Press Company, 1923), 19.
59. G. Meinig, *Root Canal Cover-Up* (Ojai, Calif.: Bion Publishing, 1994), 54.
60. W. Price, *Dental Infections: Oral and Systemic,* vol. 1, (Cleveland: The Penton Press Company, 1923), 268–74, 275–84.
61. Ibid., 19.
62. Ibid., 228.
63. F. Billings, *Focal Infection* (New York: D. Appleton and Company, 1916), 26–32.
64. W. Price, *Dental Infections: Oral and Systemic,* vol. 1 (Cleveland: The Penton Press Company, 1923), 622.
65. S. Fallon, *Nourishing Traditions* (Washington, D.C.: New Trends Publishing, 1999), 24.
66. W. Price, *Dental Infections: Oral and Systemic,* vol. 1 (Cleveland: The Penton Press Company, 1923), 358–63, 416–20.
67. G. Meinig, *Root Canal Cover-Up* (Ojai, Calif.: Bion Publishing, 1994), 8.
68. M. Ring, *Dentistry: An Illustrated History* (New York: Harry N. Abrams, Inc., 1985), 21.
69. G. Meinig, *Root Canal Cover-Up* (Ojai, Calif.: Bion Publishing, 1994), 139–40.
70. R. Voll, *Interrelationships of Odontons and Tonsils to Organs, Fields of Disturbance, and Tissue Systems* (Uelzen, Germany: Medizinisch Literarische Verlagsgesellschaft MBH, 1978), 27, 111.
71. Ibid., 139–40.
72. G. Meinig, *Root Canal Cover-Up* (Ojai, Calif.: Bion Publishing, 1994), 163.
73. M. Fischer, *Death and Dentistry* (Springfield, Ill.: Charles C. Thomas, 1940), 55.
74. G. Meinig, *Root Canal Cover-Up* (Ojai, Calif.: Bion Publishing, 1994), 150.
75. P. Rhoads and G. Dick, "Efficacy of Tonsillectomy for the Removal of Focal Infection," *Journal of the American Medical Association* 91, no. 16 (October 20, 1928): 1153–54.
76. G. Meinig, *Root Canal Cover-Up* (Ojai, Calif.: Bion Publishing, 1994), 157–61.
77. H. Robinson, "Systemic Relation of Dental Health and Disease," *Journal of the American Dental Association* 40 (June 1950): 656–58; M. Fischer, *Death and Dentistry* (Springfield, Ill.: Charles C. Thomas, 1940), 27; R. Haden, "Elective Localization of Streptococci," *Orthodontia and Oral Surgery, International Journal* 12 (1926): 711.
78. S. Shakman, *E. C. Rosenow and Associates: A Reference Manual* (Santa Monica, Calif.: Institute of Science, 1998), 2–3.
79. Ibid.
80. Ibid.
81. Ibid.
82. G. Meinig, "Do Root Canals Cause Serious Illness?" *Townsend Letter for Doctors and Patients,* May 1997, 101.
83. M. Fischer, *Death and Dentistry* (Springfield, Ill.: Charles C. Thomas, 1940), 135.
84. F. Billings, *Focal Infection* (New York: D. Appleton and Company, 1916), 52.
85. M. Fischer, *Death and Dentistry* (Springfield, Ill.: Charles C. Thomas, 1940), 52.
86. H. Robinson, "Systemic Relation of Dental Health and Disease," *Journal of the American Dental Association* 40 (June 1950): 657.
87. R. Kulacz and T. Levy, *The Roots of Disease* (Bloomington, Ind.: Xlibris Corporation, 2002), 46.
88. Ibid.
89. Ibid.
90. J. Robbins, *Reclaiming Our Heart* (Tiburon, Calif.: H. J. Kramer, 1998), 328; W. Price, *Dental Infections: Oral and Systemic,* vol. 1 (Cleveland: The Penton Press Company, 1923), 148.
91. H. Robinson, "Systemic Relation of Dental Health and Disease," *Journal of the American Dental Association* 40 (June 1950): 658.
92. S. Levy, *The Antibiotic Paradox* (New York: Plenum Press, 1992), 7.
93. H. Robinson, "Systemic Relation of Dental Health and Disease," *Journal of the American Dental Association* 40 (June 1950): 658.
94. G. Meinig, *Root Canal Cover-Up* (Ojai, Calif.: Bion Publishing, 1994), 148.
95. Ibid., 161.
96. R. Kulacz and T. Levy, *The Roots of Disease* (Bloomington, Ind.: Xlibris Corporation, 2002), 45.
97. Ibid.
98. W. Price, *Dental Infections: Oral and Systemic,* vol. 1 (Cleveland: The Penton Press Company, 1923), 23, 28.
99. P. Dosch, *Manual of Neural Therapy* (Heidelberg: Haug Publishers, 1984), 32–33.
100. Ibid., 75.
101. Ibid.

102. Ibid., 76.

103. Ibid.

104. D. Klinghardt, "Neural Therapy," *Journal of Neurological and Orthopaedic Medicine and Surgery* 14 (1993): 111.

105. K. Kretzschmar, "Neural Therapy," *Medical Times* 84, no. 5 (May 1956): 517.

106. P. Dosch, *Manual of Neural Therapy* (Heidelberg: Haug Publishers, 1984), 28–29.

107. Ibid., 25–30.

108. P. Dosch, *Manual of Neural Therapy* (Heidelberg: Haug Publishers, 1984), 11.

9

DEVELOPMENT OF A DOMINANT FOCUS

Foci can manifest anywhere in the body and can be generated by various disturbances to the system. In fact, a dominant focus can be caused by virtually any insult to the body—structural, chemical, or emotional—in which the disturbance is greater than the system can defend against or later repair. Furthermore, a focus can arise in any part of the body—from the head to the toes—if that area has been ill or traumatized. This is especially true for scar interference fields that can manifest literally anywhere in the body that has been injured. In contrast, focal infections are most commonly located in tissues communicating with a mucosal surface where bacteria have been allowed to enter, such as the teeth, tonsils, sinuses, and genital organs.[1]

THE FORMATION OF FOCI

Foci develop over a period of time. For example, if a child falls and cuts himself, that cut (with or without stitches) is not by definition an immediate interference field. It is an *acute*—or recent—injury that will or will not sufficiently heal over time. If appropriate treatment is rendered just after a trauma, then a focus may never form. The same principle applies to a focal infection. Infected tonsils can resolve completely without any *sequelae* (aftereffects). However, when they don't, the lingering low-grade inflammation, infection, or tissue scarring remains as fertile ground for future reinfection—and the eventual formation of a chronic focal infection.

sequelae: The term *sequelae* refers to any remaining disease or dysfunction after an illness. Thus, if an area heals "with no sequelae," it has resolved completely with no remaining symptoms (e.g., pain, numbness, or tension) or signs (e.g., infection, inflammation, tissue contraction, or scarring).

Example of a Scar Interference Field

Let's take, for example, the case of a child who falls off his bike and cuts his arm. If this child receives appropriate treatment—a homeopathic remedy, nutritional supplements, structural realignment (adjustments and massage), emotional support, or stitches (if they are needed) afterward—then full healing of this injury may occur. However, if the child receives no treatment or inappropriate treatment, and the injury was significant enough, then the resulting scar from the cut has the potential to develop into an interference field. The time period in which injuries, inflammations, or infections have the potential to move from the acute infected or traumatized stage into a chronic focus status is estimated at three weeks to three months, depending on the degree of injury and the level of the individual's immune system defense.

Example of a Tonsil Focus

When a child receives a course of antibiotics for acute tonsillitis, the tonsil area has the potential to coalesce into a chronic focus over the next few weeks or months. This is especially likely if the tonsils and the neighboring cervical lymphatic tissues are already littered with killed bacterial carcasses and their toxins that remain from frequent past infections accompanied by numerous courses of antibiotics. Furthermore, re-irritation or reinfection is bound to occur when the true cause of the tonsil infection—physical or emotional—is not addressed.

COMMON CAUSES OF A TONSIL FOCUS

In children, tonsillitis is most often triggered by the lymphatic response of the tonsillar tissue to an undiagnosed food allergy. Other causes include bacterial invasion from a nearby dental focus, toxic mercury from amalgam fillings, and chronically suppressing—or "swallowing"—major emotional issues.

After several bouts of tonsillitis and accompanying doses of antibiotics, the tonsils no longer, or very rarely, have the capacity to manifest the appropriate immune system defenses to become actively infected. Thus, teens and adults often begin to assume that they have "grown out of it" and that their tonsils are now fine. However, this is rarely the case. In actuality, the tonsillitis of the child has simply transformed into the chronic tonsil focus of the teen or adult. And, similar to food allergies that often cause dramatic symptoms in children but more subtle signs in adults, the problem is still there but the symptoms have changed. For example, instead of frequent colds and sore throats, the adult may suffer from intermittent but chronic low back pain, fatigue, memory loss, or depression. Thus, the psoric- and sycotic-like tonsillitis symptoms triggered by bacterial invasion of the more superficial tonsil mucosal surfaces in the child have actually moved deeper into the system and begun to manifest more serious tuberculinic- and luetic-like signs in the joints, brain, and nervous system of the adult.

THE PSYCHOLOGICAL COMPONENT OF A CHRONIC FOCUS

Often, traumatic emotions unconsciously associated with a chronic focus are the most significant factors underlying its initial development as well as perpetuating its continued existence. This development is known as the *psychogalvanic reflex.*

The Psychogalvanic Reflex

The psychogalvanic reflex refers to the increased *galvanism*—or electrical current of the autonomic sympathetic nerves—that can be measured on the skin overlying a scar or other focus.[2] Clinically, the scar's increased galvanic current, as compared to the normally innervated surrounding skin, causes a muscle to weaken in kinesiology testing when the doctor touches or *therapy-localizes* it. For example, using the previous scar interference field example, the child's arm scar could show up decades later in a holistic doctor's office as a chronic focus. Kinesiology testing might reveal that it was the persistent subconscious feeling of deficiency after being teased for falling off a bicycle, for instance, that was the primary reason for this interference field's formation and longevity.

> **therapy localization:** *Therapy localization* is a kinesiological term that describes when a practitioner firmly touches an area of skin, such as a suspected scar interference field, and simultaneously challenges a strong muscle. If this previously strong muscle weakens with the therapy localization (TL) challenge, the result is referred to as a positive TL, indicating that the scar is testing as a problem. Scars, however, typically need to be *ischemically* therapy-localized—that is, they need to be touched with a significant amount of pressure to summate enough nerve action potential to cause a change in muscle strength. This scenario is especially true with "older and colder" scars that have neurologically dissociated from the rest of the body to such a degree that the normal pressure from a therapy localization is not sufficient to elicit an appropriate positive response.[3]

Episiotomy Scar Example

Another typical focus, an *episiotomy* scar, can hold the cellular memory of excruciatingly painful labor contractions, fear of death (the mother's as well as the child's), shame for not having an easier birth or just "not doing it right," and myriad other negative emotions. Unless appropriately treated, this subclinical (relatively silent and symptom-free) episiotomy scar can adversely affect the surrounding nerves and tissues and interfere with the woman's bladder and bowel functioning, as well as the full expression of her sexuality and ability to orgasm. This clinical observation was definitively confirmed by a study published in the *Journal of the American Medical Association,* which concluded that episiotomies not only have *no* benefits but can actually *increase* the risk of tissue tears during delivery. These tissue tears have been shown to cause more pain, more stitches, and a longer recovery after childbirth. As an allopathic tradition since the 1930s, episiotomies are conducted in an estimated one-third of all vaginal births despite mounting evidence in the past two decades of their harm. This practice can also increase the risk of later sexual dysfunction in women.[4] And because scar interference fields also affect remote areas of the body, this emotionally charged scar might significantly contribute to the common symptom of postpartum depression, which has been traditionally associated only with hormonal imbalance.

episiotomy: An *episiotomy,* a surgical incision into the perineum (the skin between the vaginal opening and the anus), is commonly given during childbirth to avoid excessive stretching and tearing of the perineum and vagina just before the baby is delivered. From a surgeon's point of view, this incision is easier to repair than a tear. From the experience of many holistic practitioners and midwives, a perineal tear is a less disturbing interference field than an episiotomy. Beginning in the 1980s, this latter point of view has been borne out by an increasing number of published research studies that have been calling this procedure into question.

Psychogalvanic Autonomic Nerve Pathway

Every negative thought or emotion—fear, sorrow, or anger—is mediated and conducted by the *autonomic* nervous system through its primary emotional centers in the brain (the hypothalamus and limbic system). Scar interference fields have a direct influence on these nerves because sympathetic autonomic nerves densely innervate the skin. In fact, approximately 90 percent of all autonomic nerve substance has been estimated to reside in the skin.[5] Thus, scars can not only continuously irritate the sympathetic autonomic nerves that densely invest all layers of the skin but also continually irritate the emotional limbic system in the brain that these sympathetic fibers also innervate. Over time, this irritation becomes an insidious negative feedback cycle, through the conduction of habitual negative thoughts and feelings originating in this disturbed limbic area in the brain through these same sympathetic nerve pathways into the charged scar interference field. In the absence of effective holistic intervention, these disturbing neurological scar-brain-scar psychogalvanic cycles can perpetuate themselves indefinitely (see figure 9.1).

autonomic nervous system: The autonomic nervous system consists of sympathetic nerves that have a primary stimulating function in the body ("fight or flight") and parasympathetic nerves that restore and conserve body energy ("rest and repose"). There is also a third division, the enteric nervous system, which regulates digestive function.

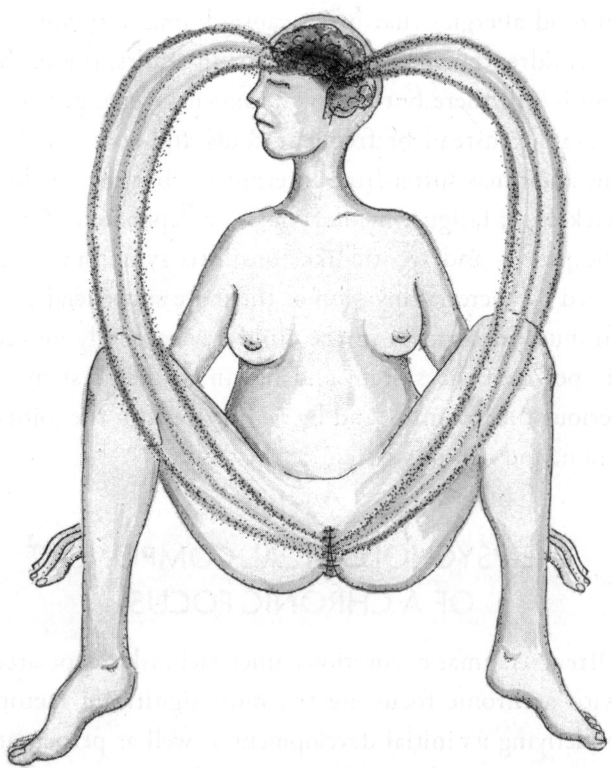

Figure 9.1. The chronic negative feedback cycle between an episiotomy scar interference field and the emotional limbic center in the brain

Scar Interference Fields Are Chronically Enervating

After a few years, or even a few decades, this episiotomy scar in our example—or even more subconsciously a circumcision scar given to a male in infancy—can be likened to an island of chronic neurological stress that emits disturbing signals throughout the body, but just under the threshold of awareness of the conscious mind. The effects of this low-level but chronically enervating emotionally charged scar interference field are similar to the effects unconscious anxiety has on the body. Thus, similar to mild but chronic anxiety, scar interference fields may be in the background or foreground of the autonomic nerves' radar throughout the day, but they are always present at some level. Although most individuals live a lifetime consciously unaware of their interference fields, this ignorance results in anything but bliss. These generators of subtle but chronic stress, analogous to slow water torture, continually sabotage any hope for a relaxed mind and body, and further block spiritually minded individuals from sustaining higher states of consciousness.

DORMANT VERSUS ACTIVE FOCI

The case of Dr. Ferdinand Huneke's patient (see chapter 8) shows that while scars can be dormant and therefore not significantly disturbing to the body, they always have the potential to be triggered by some kind of stress into an active interference field state. For example, his patient's right-shoulder disturbed field did not begin to cause pain until *five years* before she first consulted him. Yet the actual cause of her pain, which was her left-leg surgical scar, occurred *thirty-five* years before. What exactly triggered this dormant leg scar to emerge as an active interference field is unknown, which is often the case. When questioned, patients are usually completely unaware of what could have activated a dormant scar, because they were never aware of the scar as an interference field in the first place. Furthermore, the factors that can potentially activate old, dormant foci may be as seemingly innocuous as a minor argument, teeth cleaning, getting a new filling, or a bout of the flu.

ACUTE CONDITIONS OR CHRONICALLY WEAK AREAS?

Some holistic practitioners have ventured that perhaps there is no such thing as acute disease (except in the case of acute trauma, which may also be argued to be *psychically* triggered from unresolved karma), but only the activation of chronically weak areas such as focal areas and their disturbed fields, through the triggering factors of toxins, microbes, and other stressors.

The Trigger Factor

A. D. Speransky, the renowned Russian neurologist, used the term *trigger factor* or *second insult* in the early twentieth century to describe the stimulus that often activates the "tissue memory" in a focus even decades after the initial trauma.[6] Taking a careful history initially, as well as during subsequent treatments, is essential for practitioners to be able to ascertain if there were any significant changes in the patient's condition that may signal the emergence of a dormant focus. If there are no obvious signs or symptoms that implicate the arising of an active focus, then suspected scars, teeth, tonsils, sinuses, and so forth should be left alone for the time being. In holistic circles where practitioners use energetic testing methods (e.g., kinesiology, electroacupuncture, and reflex arm length), this decision-making process is made infinitely easier through specific positive indicators.

Treating the "Forest" before the "Trees"

The classic case of new patients presenting with both multiple amalgam fillings and root canals is a useful illustration of this clinical decision-making process. The majority of the time, energetic testing directs the practitioner to first clear the systemic toxicity from the amalgam fillings, before ascertaining if any of the root-canalled teeth are possible active focal infections. This process can be likened to first clearing the "forest"—that is, mercury poisoning of the entire body—before dealing with the individual "trees"—that is, one or more potential root canal dental foci. Typically, after the amalgam fillings are removed (or even from just a couple of quadrants), one or more of the failed root-canalled teeth (or other dental foci) emerge and begin to test positive, in the patient's "cleaner" body and clearer energetic field.

Conditions for Removal of Dormant Foci

If root-canalled teeth, as well as all other suspected foci, do not test positive or seem to be causing any signs or symptoms after a thorough history and exam, they should not be disturbed from their dormant and inactive state. The one exception is when a patient is suffering from a major illness or has just tested positive for a serious disease such as cancer. In this case, time is precious and the expeditious removal of *all* suspected toxic foci should be thoroughly considered and evaluated. It is further essential that holistic physicians and dentists work together in these cases and in close communication with the patient. Ultimately, the decision of whether to sacrifice a tooth is always exclusively the choice of only one person—the well-informed patient.

THE PATHOGENESIS OF A FOCAL INFECTION

Note: Radical Medicine *is written for holistic patients as well as for practitioners. The next two major sections, however, offer an in-depth and technical explanation of the pathogenesis of foci and their disturbed fields as well as scar interference fields. Therefore, readers who are not health professionals may choose to simply skim over or skip these sections entirely and begin reading again at the "Focal Chains, Frozen Regulation, and Toxic Ganglia" section (page 298).*

The pathogenesis of a focal infection—that is, how dental, tonsil, sinus, genital, and other foci are caused and develop over time—is relatively straightforward. Dominant foci that chronically harbor microbes are initiated through inflammations or infections that never completely resolve because of inadequate, ineffectual, or inappropriate treatment. Although it is possible that a focus may form after a single severe infection—for example, a major ear infection—more commonly foci arise over time. For example, a tonsil focus may form after a child suffers three or four bouts of tonsillitis over several years. These infections can occur through lowered immune system resistance from the chronic ingestion of sugar and other devitalized foods, overeating an allergenic food(s), multiple courses of suppressive and nontherapeutic pharmaceuticals such as antibiotics or steroids, exposure to toxic metals and chemicals, or trauma (psychological or structural), as well as the individual's hereditary "Achilles' heel"—that is, the person's primary miasmic predisposition. Dental focal infections, in particular, often arise from a toxic diet, which over time results in cavities in the teeth. When these cavities are drilled and filled by nonholistic or technically unskilled dentists, the trauma and toxicity (mercury amalgam; nickel, palladium, or aluminum-containing crowns) from these procedures can initiate inflammation and infection in the root of a tooth that can either immediately or eventually coalesce into a dominant focus.

How Focal Infections Cause Disturbed Fields

How these focal infections initiate a secondary site of disturbance elsewhere in the body was uncovered through the clinical and laboratory research of Miller, Hunter, Billings, Rosenow, Price, and others, first discussed in chapter 8.

Blood and Lymph Circulation

These researchers found that bacteria and other microbes from infected tonsils or the root of a tooth are readily absorbed into the bloodstream and lymphatic channels and may then circulate throughout the body. Streptococcal bacteria in particular have been shown to have a strong pathogenic affinity to specific tissues, especially the heart, kidneys, brain, intestines, and joints.[7] When bacteria reach a tissue in which they recognize an environment for them to survive and even thrive, they migrate out from the blood and lymphatic vessels and invade this tissue. Frank Billings first characterized this seeming magnetic attraction of potential disturbed fields to bacteria disseminated from focal infections during his 1917 Stanford Medical School lecture series:

> It appears that the cells of the tissues for which a given strain shows elective affinity take the bacteria out of the circulation as if by a magnet-adsorption.[8]

These newly created disturbed fields can be obviously symptomatic, such as in the case of a recently inflamed and painful rheumatic joint, or insidiously quiet, as with chronic endocarditis (heart disease). In fact, Fischer prophetically asserted as far back as the late 1930s that this bacterial affinity to the heart was the *primary causative factor* underlying what still remains today as our number one silent killer—chronic heart disease:

> Here are described the pathological backgrounds for that slowly progressive "chronic" heart disease that kills so many of the human species after forty—and "idiopathically" [of unknown origin].[9]

Axonal Transport Along Nerves

Another manner of specific microbial transport is through traveling along nerve fibers. This discovery, termed *axonal transport,* was made simultaneously in both Paris and the United States in 1923. Axonal transport describes the fact that nerves do not simply act as electrical cords in our bodies conducting impulses to and fro; they also have the capacity to transport chemicals along their axons (nerve shafts).[10] This transporting capability is a double-edged sword, however, because *both* nutritional as well as toxic chemicals may be transported along a nerve. In fact, bacteria, heavy metals, and other toxic microbes are commonly axonally transported along nerves from a focus into its neighboring *ganglia*—clusters of autonomic nerve cells that act as "little brains" to regulate functions throughout the body.[11]

ANATOMY OF A NERVE

A nerve is made up of three distinct portions: (1) the cell body, made up of the nucleus and the cytoplasm that contains organelles such as lysosomes, mitochondria, and Golgi complexes; (2) the dendrites, highly branched and thick extensions of the cytoplasm of the cell body, which conduct a nerve impulse to the cell body; and (3) the axon, a single long, thin process that conducts nerve impulses away from the cell body.

Why Disturbed Fields Form

Why does Mother Nature—or the innate wisdom of the body—create these secondarily disturbed fields? In other words, is there a positive life-enhancing aspect to this process? The transport along the axons of nerves from a focus to its "mother" ganglion could be one way the body adapts and reduces infection or toxicity, through sharing the toxic overload with other tissues. (See "Sharing the Stress with Mother Ganglia" on page 300.) Rosenow mirrored this observation in 1913, when he wrote that streptococcal invasions into the heart and other tissue did "not transgress . . . a certain maximum."[12] That is, the number of microbes that metastasize to various disturbed fields is somehow directed by the body to remain at a reasonably low level. Billings underscored this finding by noticing that the bacteria in foci and their disturbed fields were typically of very low virulence.[13] Thus, by sending out the overload of bacteria to its various disturbed fields, foci reduce the number of microbes in each area, which often has the added benefit of diminishing their pathogenicity as well. This diluting or "sharing the stress" effect allows the body to survive another day, without succumbing to the serious morbidity and even mortality that a major infection can cause.

THE PATHOGENESIS OF A SCAR INTERFERENCE FIELD

The migration of microbes from a focus through blood and lymph channels and along nerve fibers to a disturbed field is a relatively simple concept to grasp. However, how a scar interference field specifically disturbs the body, especially one that is triggered twenty or thirty years after its formation, is not as easy to comprehend. In fact, even knowledgeable holistic practitioners and researchers do not have all the answers to this rather astounding phenomenon. However, two primary theories have emerged from the decades of debate among European neural therapists on this subject—the *autonomic nervous system theory* and the connective tissue or *matrix system theory.*

The Autonomic Nervous System Theory

The autonomic nervous system is primarily made up of two divisions—a sympathetic generally excitatory part and a parasympathetic generally sedating part.* The dual innervation of these yang and yin aspects of the autonomic system governs digestion, respiration, urination, circulation, metabolism, body temperature, musculoskeletal function, hormonal balance, emotional responses, and other complex functions in the body.[14] Contrary to what is still taught in medical schools, the autonomic system does not consist simply of motor fibers that "automatically" stimulate target tissues; it is actually composed of a greater number of sensory nerves.[15] This dense network of autonomic sensory nerves constantly monitors the body's internal and external environment to maintain normal homeostasis (healthy functioning). When needed, this network can make necessary adjustments within milliseconds through feedback circuits to the hypothalamus in the brain. In fact, the conduction of information about literally everything—movements, actions, thoughts, and emotions—is transmitted along the billions of nerve fibers in our bodies at a mind-boggling speed of over 250 miles an hour, "a speed which makes the traverses of the body very nearly instantaneous."[16] The influence of the autonomic nerves is so vast that European researchers call it the *neurovegetative system,* referring to the supremacy of these nerves in all of our unconscious and involuntary (vegetative) functions such as blood circulation, lymphatic flow, and hormonal regulation. This system is so ubiquitous that it is considered by many neurologists to function as "a single entity, a great syncytium,"† in which every nerve cell is constantly aware of what is occurring in every other nerve cell.[17] Dr. Peter Dosch, the German neural therapist and author, expounds on this subject further:

> When we refer to the neurovegetative system, we mean by this not so much an anatomical entity as a functional concept which comprises the whole of the neurohumoral [the nerves and all the fluids in the body including the blood, lymph, and bile] regulating system working under the control of conditioned reflexes, i.e., that which comprises not only central but also peripheral regulation . . . The whole of the endocrine system is integrated into these autonomic interrelationships. The entire neurohumoral functional structure is so intimately interlinked that a disturbance in any part of it immediately causes the whole of the functional unit to become altered and react. Thus, it is never an organ that becomes ill, but always the whole human being! Every irritation, every stimulus strikes the whole, and the whole organism responds.[18]

NERVES: SENSORY AND MOTOR

Sensory nerves (afferent) send messages from the body to the brain and spinal cord (central nervous system), while motor nerves (efferent) send messages from the central nervous system to the body. The autonomic nervous system is not simply a peripheral efferent system (motor nerves outside of the brain and spinal cord) concerned primarily with the automatic regulation of the viscera (organs), as is taught in (holistic and allopathic) medical schools. New research on cadavers and in neurology studies has found that "at least 80 percent of the vagal fibers (the primary nerve of the parasympathetic system) are afferent (sensory)."[19] Furthermore, autonomic nerves not only control visceral and homeostatic functions (e.g., temperature, pH, sweating, vasomotor changes) but are the primary regulators of pain, joint and muscle function, and the emotions.[20]

As previously described, scars have extremely high sympathetic nerve activity as measured in neurology laboratories by electrical skin resistance meters, or dermometers.[21] If a scar's effect is strong enough, it can cause a chronic and "sustained sympathicotonia" (sympathetic nerve hyperactivity and dysregulation) that constantly affects every part of an individual's life, and greatly contributes to the onset of future disease and dysfunction.[22] Irvin Korr, who has researched the autonomic nervous system perhaps more than any other scientist, reported that this chronic sympathicotonia profoundly disrupts

*A third aspect—the enteric nervous system—has become recognized in recent years as a separate division of the autonomic nervous system. The vast enteric system regulates function in the digestive system—the esophagus, stomach, and small and large intestines. However, for simplicity's sake, the two classic divisions of the autonomic system—the sympathetic and the parasympathetic—are briefly defined here. Furthermore, currently only the sympathetic nerves that densely innervate the skin have been demonstrated in neurological research to conduct aberrant messages from scars.

†The term *syncytium* is used in this instance to characterize a group of nerve cells that are so closely allied that they function together as if they were a single unit.

the *ergotropic* system, that is the "housecleaning" and body maintenance functioning, of the autonomic nervous system.[23] Thus, the chaotic and "noisy" sympathetic nerve activity in a scar focus adversely affects the ergotropic moment-to-moment adjustments that the autonomic nerves must make in the visceral (organs), circulatory (blood and lymph), and metabolic systems to maintain normal function.[24]

> **dermometer:** Dermometers are instruments that measure the electrical current of the skin. Because the sympathetic nerves control this conductivity through sweat gland activity and vasodilation or vasoconstriction (increased or decreased blood flow), measurement of this skin current is also a direct measurement of sympathetic activity. Therefore, neurology laboratories often use dermometers to measure the activity of the autonomic nervous system, especially over skin areas that are known to reflex to vital organs, such as the heart. In fact, the high sympathetic nerve activity measured in the areas of skin that reflex to specific organs is the scientific rationale for utilizing the technique of therapy localization in kinesiology. For more information on kinesiology, see appendix 3, "Energetic Testing Explained."

Based on the previous description, it is obvious how a scar interference field can be systemically (affecting the whole body) disturbing through the autonomic nervous system. But how does a scar cause a disturbed field in a specific location in the body? Why some of these secondary disturbed fields form is obvious, while for others—especially the more remote ones—the reason is less readily apparent. Dosch has made the following observations about the varied locations a scar interference field can chronically disturb:

> After tonsils and teeth, scars figure as the next most common interference fields. Any scar, no matter how insignificant, even if it dates back to earliest childhood, whether healed by first or second intention,* can in later life become the cause of a therapy-resistant and potentially fatal angina pectoris [heart attack], severe rheumatoid arthritis, [spinal] disk lesions, hearing loss, glaucoma, sciatica, asthma, or other serious disorders of almost any kind. Thus, a scar said to be "nonirritating" can clearly act as a substantial neural irritant. But why one scar but not another should in such a case turn into an interference field still remains a mystery.[25]

The following three examples illustrate how a scar interference field may cause a disturbed field elsewhere in the body through autonomic nerve pathways.

Cutaneosomatic Reflex Pathways—An Ephapse "Electrical Short-Circuit" Example

Let's return to the previous example of the boy who fell off his bike and cut his arm. If this boy began experiencing left-sided tension headaches a short time later (or even years later), then his left arm scar should be considered as a possible causative factor. When the skin is cut in a traumatic injury, so are the densely packed sympathetic nerve fibers and blood vessels. The tearing of the blood vessels restricts the supply of blood and oxygen to the wound—a major limiting factor to healing. However, the sympathetic nerve disruption has even more long-term and serious consequences. When the sympathetic nerves are cut, they do not always heal well, creating a type of electrical short circuit between the severed nerve fibers. This has been referred to as an *ephapse,* as opposed to a *synapse*—the normal gap between two nerve fibers in which an impulse is transmitted from one neuron to the other.[26] In an ephapse, either signals are not transmitted across the neuronal gap properly or they hook up in an aberrant fashion to nerve fibers to which they should not be connected. Either way, an ephapse, described by Florida neurologist Hooshang Hooshmand in his book, *Chronic Pain: Sympathetic Dystrophy Prevention and Management,* as "focal nerve damage," creates what Hooshmand refers to as an "island of turbulence" in the scar area.[27] And with the concomitant torn blood vessels that limit the nutrient and oxygen supply to the area, this focal scar has no chance of fully healing without significant holistic intervention.

This chronic sympathetic nerve disturbance additionally causes skin temperature changes, a function also

*Healing by "first intention" or by "primary union" is when the edges of the tissue around the wound heal in close apposition (close together), there is no infection present, and a minimum of scar tissue is formed. Healing by "second intention" or by "secondary union" occurs in larger wounds or wounds complicated by infection, in which the healing process is more delayed and greater scarring results.

regulated by the autonomic nervous system. Although both increased and decreased skin temperatures have been measured over scar interference fields, the most common pathological phenomenon that has been observed is colder scar tissue area due to the eventual loss of normal sympathetic nerve innervation.[28] These well-entrenched "older and colder" noninflammatory scars are often the most insidious, and greatly contribute to autonomic nervous system chaos and loss of homeostasis.

SKIN TEMPERATURE CHANGES

Sympathetic nerves maintain relatively constant temperatures in the body through the regulation of blood vessel diameters. When blood vessels constrict, their heat is preserved, and when they dilate, heat is lost. Normally the sympathetic nervous system maintains a consistent symmetry of temperature on the surface of the skin, with only slight—from 0.5 to 0.9°C—variations. A scar interference field, however, can exhibit a 1 to 2°C difference in comparison to the surrounding skin. This small but neurologically significant variation can be detected only by thermography. When a practitioner senses a skin temperature difference over a scar, she is probably relying more on her psychic sense developed from years of clinical experience, because the human tactile ability to detect skin temperature differences occurs only in the 5 to 6°C range.[29]

When the chronic aberrated nerve signals from ephapse formations in these scar interference fields reach a certain threshold level of stress, a secondary site of distress—a disturbed field—will form. This is probably another example of the "sharing of stress" mechanism described earlier, where the neurological "noise" from a scar is greatly reduced by spreading out the nerve irritation to two sites.

In the example of cutaneosomatic pathways shown in figure 9.2, the left cervical (neck) area is the disturbed field of the left arm scar. The scar-induced aberrant sensory sympathetic signals travel into the upper thoracic sympathetic ganglia and spine. These sensory fibers irritate sympathetic motor nerves that emerge from upper back spinal ganglia and travel into the upper thoracic and cervical muscles. These disturbing sympathetic motor signals cause blood vessel vasoconstriction that triggers chronic muscle contraction, which can often result symptomatically in intermittent tension headaches and muscle spasm. This example of a scar interference field causing tension headaches is referred to as a *cutaneosomatic,* or "skin-muscle," reflex. Medications may relieve the headache, and chiropractic or osteopathic spinal manipulation may temporarily decrease the muscle tension. However, without appropriate diagnosis and treatment of the scar interference field, a complete cure is impossible.

Cutaneovisceral Reflex Pathways—Another Ephapse "Electrical Short-Circuit" Example

Scar interference fields can also disturb organs, or *viscera.*[30] This typical occurrence was described previously with the example of an episiotomy scar after childbirth. It is common for this interference field to chronically disturb the bladder, causing frequent urination and incontinence. It may also adversely affect the uterus by contributing to menstrual cramps (dysmenorrhea) or

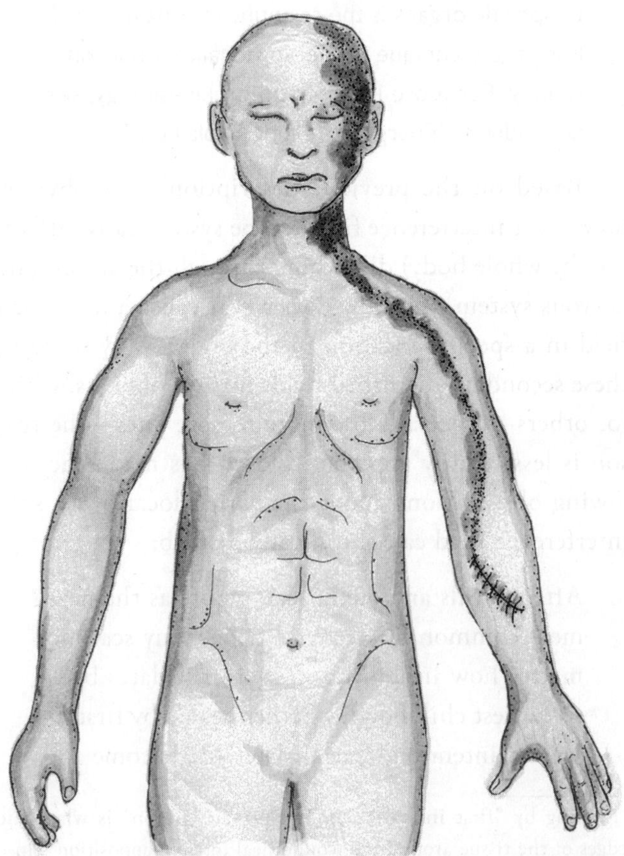

Figure 9.2. Left tension headaches initiated by a left arm scar interference field through a cutaneosomatic nerve reflex

excessive menstrual blood flow (menorrhagia), or the descending colon and rectum with resulting irritable bowel symptoms. Hernia scars are also culpable in creating disturbance in this genitourinal and lower intestinal area.

The previous sympathetic nerve ephapse example shows how the formation of disturbed fields can cause chronic neurological and vascular irritation in related areas. In this case, the disturbed fields can affect the parasympathetic nerves, which normally increase blood flow as well as stimulate erection in both sexes (penis and clitoral). Therefore, this interference field can adversely affect a woman's ability to orgasm after childbirth, and especially after several difficult births. In the same way, a circumcision scar can subtly but chronically contribute to a man's sexual dysfunction. When an episiotomy, hysterectomy, circumcision, hernia, or other scar interference field is chronically irritating an organ such as the bladder, uterus, penis, clitoris, or colon, this is referred to as a *cutaneovisceral,* or "skin-organ" reflex (see figure 9.3).

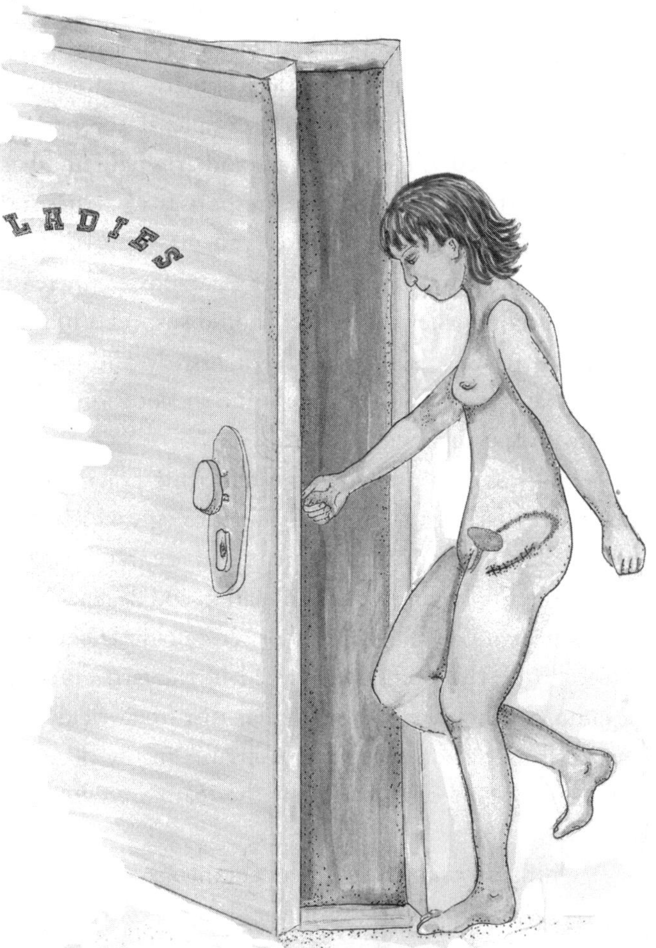

Figure 9.3. Chronic bladder dysfunction generated by an episiotomy scar through a cutaneovisceral nerve reflex

Viscerosomatic Reflex Pathways via "Thermatomes"—A Liver-Shoulder or "Viscerosomatic" Reflex Example

Scar interference fields are caused not only by scars on the external skin but also by internal scarring. In 1828, Dr. Thomas Brown of Scotland and Dr. Thomas Pridgin Teale of England almost simultaneously first described *viscerocutaneous* (organ affecting skin)—more broadly known as *viscerosomatic* (an organ affecting the skin, muscles, joints, ligaments, and so forth)—reflexes. In Europe, these reflexes are called "Head's zones";* in the United States, they are simply called "areas of referred pain." An example of a classic viscerosomatic reflex is the left shoulder, arm, and central chest pain that often signals cardiovascular stress and an impending heart attack.

Internal scar adhesions can result from surgery or from chronic inflammation and infection. For example, when someone with liver degeneration from abuse of alcohol, refined sugar, and/or drugs (street or prescription) begins to experience right shoulder and arm pain that is not amenable to structural treatment, it could be the result of a *viscerosomatic* manifestation. The chronically inflamed nerves from the damaged liver (*viscero-* or organ) reflexively disturb the joints in the thoracic spinal nerves (upper and mid-back). Because these thoracic nerves also innervate the shoulder, pain is eventually referred to this joint (*-somatic*). Thus, when the internal scarring from chronic degeneration of the liver becomes significant enough, it begins to act as an interference field and causes dysfunction in a remote disturbed field area—in this case the spinal vertebral joints, triggering pain in the right shoulder and arm. Therefore, not just the external skin but any organ or tissue that is chronically congested and inflamed may reach what may be referred to as a "neurological tipping point" and disturb secondary sites. If this organ or tissue is also infected, it can also function as a focal infection and transfer pathogenic microbes to its disturbed fields.

*Named after Sir Henry Head; see page 548.

A chiropractor or osteopath knowledgeable and experienced in the field of dominant foci first begins to suspect the possibility of a viscerosomatic relationship from the patient's history. For example, if the patient has experienced years of shoulder and arm pain and has had consistently inappropriate responses to structural therapies such as manipulation and massage—that is, no relief, only short-term relief, or a paradoxical increase of symptoms—the practitioner should suspect a hidden focus. In these cases, an in-depth history and quality energetic testing can help determine the location of the likely underlying focus.

Holistic chiropractic and osteopathic practitioners are particularly knowledgeable in neurology, which supports their making an appropriate and accurate diagnosis. For example, chronic inflammation and degeneration of tissue can create ephapse short circuits in the nerves innervating the liver, as described in the two previous examples. However, the particular disturbed field that arises from the damaged nerve circuits in the degenerated liver tissue can also follow the *thermatomal* reflex pathways.

Unlike *dermatomes,* or the cutaneous pathways of the general sensory nerves on the skin, *thermatomes* are *thermal* pathways, reflecting the cutaneous distribution of blood vessels.[31] As described previously, sympathetic nerves run with every blood vessel and regulate body temperature by vasoconstricting or vasodilating. Any thermal sympathetic nerve pathology, such as in the case of a chronic focus, can be measured by *thermography,* an imaging instrument that evaluates skin temperature differences as subtle as 1 to 2°C apart.[32]*

Because the sympathetic nerves that innervate the liver also innervate the skin over the liver, thermatomal pathways can also reflect deeper organ dysfunction. The liver (and related gallbladder) receives sympathetic nerve innervation from the upper and middle thoracic spinal cord—the second through the seventh thoracic segments, or T2 through T7. When a toxic liver chronically irritates and inflames the T2 through T7 sympathetic nerves, these nerves can irritate other areas innervated by these same thoracic nerve fibers, such as the right shoulder and arm tissues (the liver is situated primarily on the right side in the body). In fact, the right shoulder area is such a classic disturbed field from chronic liver dysfunction that it is included as a referred-pain liver reflex area in all neurology texts.[33] This viscerosomatic reflex example of a liver focus affecting the right shoulder and arm through sympathetic nerve pathways is depicted in the thermatome map pictured in figure 9.4.

SHOULDER DYSFUNCTION

Try to take your right shoulder through a normal range of motion (e.g., try to touch your opposite shoulder blade). Compare it to your left shoulder's range of motion. Often the right side is more restricted due to chronic liver dysfunction, which is ubiquitous in our modern culture of fast food and toxic drugs, chemicals, and metals. However, dental foci also commonly cause ipsilateral (same-side) dysfunction in the body. Therefore, right shoulder pain or dysfunction—or left—can also be secondary to a dental focal infection on the same side.

- Dr. Hooshang Hooshmand's book, *Chronic Pain: Sympathetic Dystrophy Prevention and Management,* is highly recommended reading for all practitioners.

The Matrix System Theory

The second hypothesis as to how a scar interference field affects the body is the *matrix system* theory. The matrix is the semi-liquid part of the connective tissue in our bodies.

Connective Tissue Defined

There are four main categories of tissue in our bodies: epithelial (skin), muscle, nerve, and connective tissue. *Connective tissue* is a broad term that encompasses many cells and tissues that provide structural, nutritive, and immune support to the body. Bone, cartilage, ligaments, tendons, and fascia all provide stability and shape, and

*In most cases, increased sympathetic nerve irritation causes chronic vasoconstriction and thus colder skin areas overlying a focal organ or scar interference field. However, a more pathological scar can become warmer than the surrounding skin over time due to the eventual paralysis of the thermoregulating ability of the sympathetic nerves in the region (Cannon's phenomenon). However, the skin immediately surrounding the warmer scar will still be colder than the normal skin temperature in the rest of the body. (H. Hooshmand, *Chronic Pain* [Boca Raton, Fla.: CRC Press, 1993], 16.)

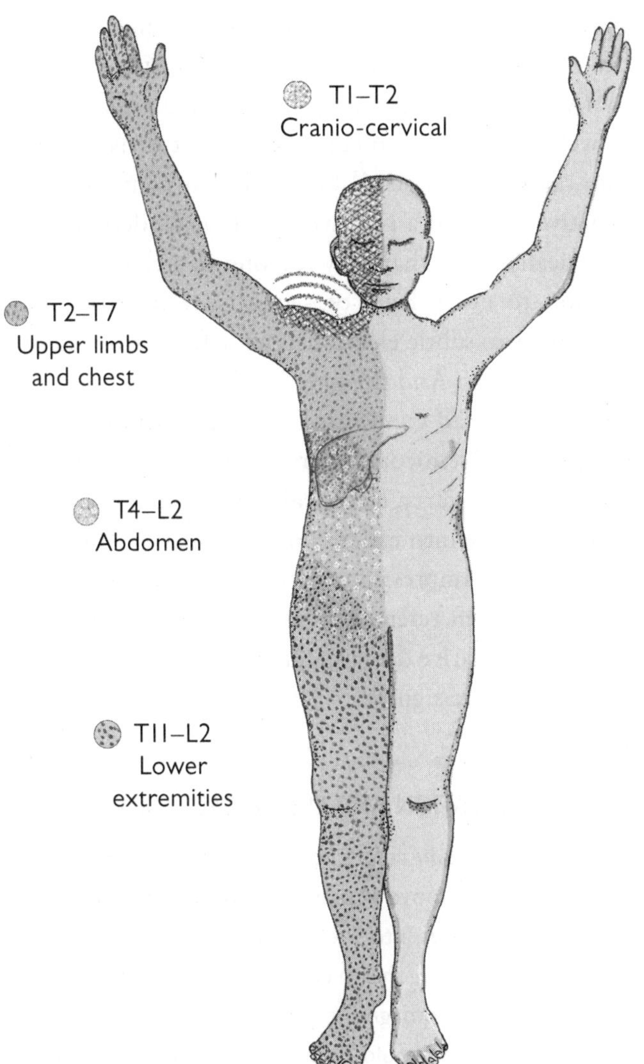

Figure 9.4. An example of a liver-shoulder viscerosomatic reflex through sympathetic nerve pathways, or thermatomes. (This adaptation is reproduced by permission of Routledge/Taylor and Francis Group, LLC, from Dr. Hooshmand's book Chronic Pain: Sympathetic Dystrophy Prevention and Management, *1993.) See plate 5 for a color rendition.*

they serve to protect our internal organs. Nutrients are transmitted through the blood supply and stored in adipose (fat) tissue, which also provides thermal insulation. This vast connective tissue system also includes immune defensive cells such as neutrophils, lymphocytes, eosinophils, and mast cells, as well as macrophages that phagocytize (eat up) invading bacteria. All of these various types of connective tissues are derived from the same embryonic mesenchyme tissue (a subdivision of the middle layer or mesoderm) and are more ubiquitous than any other tissue in the body. In his book *Job's Body,* Deane Juhan emphasizes the "connectedness" of this vast system:

> It [connective tissue] binds specific cells into tissues, tissues into organs, organs into systems, cements muscles to bones, ties bones into joints, wraps every nerve and every vessel, laces all internal structures firmly into place, and envelops the body as a whole. In all of these linings, wrappings, cables, and moorings it is a continuous substance, and every single part of the body is connected to every other part by virtue of its network; every part of us is in its embrace.[34]

Although connective tissue is continuous throughout the body, it varies greatly in consistency from place to place, as described by Juhan in his book:

> It [connective tissue] can be quite diffuse and watery, or it can form a tough flexible meshwork. In the tendons and ligaments, its tensile strength is superior to steel wire; in the cornea of the eye, it is as transparent as glass; it accounts for the toughness of leather, the tenacity of glue, the viscosity of gelatin. Invest it to various degrees with hyaline, a nylon-like substance exuded by chondroblasts, and it becomes the various grades of cartilage; invest it with mineral salts, and it becomes bone.[35]

Matrix Tissue Defined

The diffuse aspect of connective tissue is referred to as the *matrix tissue.* Also called *loose fascia, ground substance,* or *basic tissue,* matrix tissue is ubiquitous throughout the body and surrounds every single cell—all 75 trillion of them.[36] In fact, this tissue, which can change its consistency from watery (sol) to viscous (gel) as conditions dictate, has been compared to "an internal ocean" because it "bathes every nook and cranny in our body."[37]

All Extracellular Exchanges Take Place within the Matrix

The spongelike matrix has other functions besides filling space in the body and providing shape and protection to organs and tissues. In fact, far from being simply a "mute filling material," matrix tissue functions as the all-important liquid medium in which *every* extracellular function takes place.[38] This viscous tissue has a consistency and appearance much like raw egg whites. It is in this semi-fluid medium that *all* exchanges occur between cells and their external environment.[39] Furthermore, the state of the matrix itself—that is, the temperature, the relative liquidity (sol- or gel-like), the chemical makeup, and the presence of foreign toxins—has a crucial impact on the efficiency of all extracellular metabolic exchanges that take place in the body. For example, whether nutrients can cross from the capillaries to the cells, or how well cells expel their waste products, is highly dependent on the state—whether clear and healthy or congested with toxins—of the surrounding matrix. This functionality of the matrix tissue also affects the passage of essential hormones, antibodies, immune system cells, and various gases.[40]

MASSAGE'S EFFECTS ON THE MATRIX

Deep-tissue massage methods such as Rolfing cause the matrix to change from a gel to sol state, which allows toxic substances—as well as stored memories—to be released from this tissue. Dr. James Oschman has described how toxins trapped in the connective tissue meshwork—such as ether from someone who has been anesthetized and insecticides from farm workers and others who have been sprayed—can often be detected by massage therapists. The process of traumatic memories being released through the gel-sol warming and manual manipulation of the matrix has been referred to as a "somatic recall" or even a "flashback" experience, which massage therapists have witnessed countless times in their clinical practice.[41]

The Matrix Electrically Transmits Information from Head to Toe

The matrix not only provides shape and transports nutrients and wastes in the body but also generates electrical currents that carry information to every part of the body. This property, termed *piezoelectricity* from the Greek root *piezo-,* meaning "to press or squeeze," describes the spontaneous electrical current that is generated from any type of pressure or movement in the body.[42] This piezoelectrical nature stems primarily from protein-sugar complexes, called *proteoglycans,* as well as from the collagen fibers that densely innervate the matrix tissue.[43] Proteoglycans contain both a negative pole and a positive pole that renders them so electrically labile that they respond in a chain-reaction fashion to every level of stimuli—from gross body movement to subtle electromagnetic fields from electrical power lines. And the long white collagen fibers that densely invest all connective tissue are themselves considered to be "semiconductors of energy," meaning that they not only carry electrical currents but transform this electricity into energy and information.[44] Because of the highly impressionable nature of the matrix tissue, it has been referred to as "a delicately tuned and extremely sensitive detector, amplifier, and processor of electromagnetic signals."[45]

OSCILLATION AND ELECTRICAL LABILITY

The term *oscillation* refers to the coherent vibrations or frequencies that move rapidly throughout the matrix tissue and radiate out into the environment. These laserlike oscillations occur in the microwave and visible light portions of the electromagnetic spectrum.[46]

A form of what could be referred to as "noncoherent or pathological oscillation" has been observed in ill patients during various methods of energetic testing, including Auriculomedicine, arm length testing (AR), and the Matrix Reflex Testing (MRT) techniques. Dr. Paul Nogier of France, as well as Dr. Mikhael Adams of Canada, have hypothesized in Auriculomedicine that oscillation is mediated primarily through the corpus callosum (the structure that separates and organizes information transfer between the two hemispheres of the brain). However, the newest research reveals that this noncoherent oscillation emanates fundamentally from the matrix tissue—specifically from the highly electrically labile collagen fibers and proteoglycan (protein-sugar) molecules that are in electrical chaos because of a disturbing factor.

In my MRT technique, oscillation has been demonstrated by the body's inability to compensate for stress through one of Chinese acupuncture's six channel adaptation patterns. Thus, the body may oscillate between a Greater Yang and a Sunrise Yang adaptation pattern, for example, instead of stabilizing in one or the other. This pathological oscillation represents a significant disturbance—such as a dominant focus, mercury amalgam toxicity, or a major food allergy—for which the body is attempting to compensate.[47]

Scar Interference Fields Transmit Aberrant Signals through the Matrix

Considering how responsive this semi-fluid tissue is to stimuli, it is not difficult to understand how scars engender electromagnetic chaos in this energetically sensitive tissue. For example, a long-term scar interference field continuously propagates aggravating rhythmic patterns of contraction in this gel matrix, which subtly but chronically can disturb every aspect of our being. This chronic disturbance may not be perceptible to most individuals consciously, but it can sabotage our ability to deeply relax, as well as slowly but surely contribute to the onset of future disease simply by monopolizing the immune system's attention over time. The debilitating effect of this "slow torture" of a scar interference field conveyed through the matrix tissue to every cell in the body is illustrated in the following quote from a review of the book *Matrix and Matrix Regulation* by Austrian researcher Dr. Alfred Pischinger:

> The mesh [matrix tissue] is the first structure to react to any change of environment, and that reaction affects everything else that goes on in the matrix. It has a remarkable ability to develop rhythmic patterns of contraction that promote the best possible adaptation to adverse conditions. Those patterns can spread throughout the entire matrix, and they can be self-perpetuating. The effect of a pinprick can be traced as it spreads—it takes about four hours to go from head to toe. A very small but constant irritation, such as a badly healed scar, can set the stage for chronic disease.[48]

Recently, Mae-Wan Ho and other researchers have proposed that the liquid-crystal-like continuum of the collagen fibers of the matrix tissue is directly responsible for the direct current (DC) electromagnetic field that surrounds the entire body of all animals—a phenomenon Robert Becker detected in his book *Cross Currents*.[49] Thus, the weak electromagnetic signals constantly emitting from a scar interference field not only affect the body through the aberrant incoherent waves triggered in this liquid-crystal-like continuum, but also constantly disturb the body's energy or electromagnetic field. Furthermore, this DC electromagnetic field mediated by the liquid crystal conduction of the matrix tissue constitutes a "body consciousness" that is even faster than nervous system conduction—a half second faster, in fact, than sensory nerve signals can reach the brain. Thus, Ho has concluded that the "instantaneous coordination of body functions is mediated, not by the nervous system, but by the body consciousness inhering in the liquid crystalline continuum [of the matrix tissue] of the body."[50]

Focal Infections Can Transmit Microbes through the Matrix

Besides suffering the electrical chaos that disrupts normal conductivity and communication, the matrix connective tissue can "become saturated with toxins, much like an old sponge that has not been wrung out between uses."[51] Although the firmer fascial aspects of connective tissue can assist in preventing the spread of infection by walling them off in specific compartments in the body, when the load becomes overwhelming, microbes can metastasize throughout the body.[52] Although there is always some systemic microbial migration from chronic focal infections such as a tonsil or the abscessed root and bone of a tooth, with enough stress—such as a toxic diet, emotional upheavals, or the placement of amalgam fillings or nickel crowns—the fascial boundaries begin to break down and can no longer compartmentalize the focal microbes adequately, so they are released en masse through the fibrous connective tissue walls and throughout the fluid matrix tissue. However, the dysfunction and illnesses that often ensue are rarely accurately diagnosed and are often labeled as an "acute flu," or simply "catching a bug." According to German physician Hans-Heinrich Reckeweg, "This deterioration reduces the matrix's ability to transmit information and leads to chronic illnesses."[53] Thus, when major stress triggers a substantial release of these pathogenic microbes from chronic focal infections, more serious conditions such as pneumonia or heart attacks can result.

Research Proves the Supremacy of the Matrix Tissue in the Body

In 1945, Austrian professor and physician Alfred Pischinger (1899–1982), along with O. Bergsmann, Hartmut Heine, Franz Hopfer, Felix Perger, A. Stacher, and other research colleagues, began conducting laboratory research into the role of matrix connective tissue.[54] They found that the lightning reaction, or seconds phenomenon, that can occur after a profoundly affecting neural therapy injection is conducted primarily through the bioelectrical matrix tissue—*not* the autonomic nerves.[55] In addition, the matrix connective tissue is phylogenetically older than the autonomic nerves and is the only system found in single-celled and multicellular beings that breathe oxygen such as protozoans, bacteria, and viruses. Using electron microscopic research, Pischinger's team of researchers discovered that nerves as well as blood vessels *do not actually even touch* the cells in organs and other tissues but communicate only through the matrix tissue.[56] The ubiquitous nature of the matrix system is further illustrated by the following quote:

> Every cell in the body is embedded in a thin layer of semi-liquid gel . . . It is the matrix that enables us to adapt to a changing environment. Cells are not adaptable; each one is a closed system, with fixed behaviors that are set by their genes. The matrix, on the other hand, is an *open dissipative system,* able to juggle many interacting influences so that they function together, defying the forces of chaos.[57]

Based on their research findings, Pischinger's team concluded that the matrix is the most primal and fundamental tissue in the body that readily reacts to these disturbing foci and interference fields. They concluded that the matrix acts as a "ubiquitous synapse" for the autonomic nerves and blood vessels to communicate to all the organs and tissues and that the matrix tissue is therefore "primarily affected in every type of disease process, and that it plays [the most] significant role in healing processes."[58] Mae-Wan Ho, James Oschman, and other current researchers have further underscored Pischinger's assertions, finding that the liquid crystalline matrix is faster than nerve conduction, is responsible for creating our DC electromagnetic field, stores both memory and toxins, and can be said to be primarily responsible for our sense of "body consciousness."

> **synapse:** A synapse is the junction or gap between two neurons. Nerve impulses are usually transmitted across the synapse through chemical neurotransmitters (e.g., norepinephrine, acetylcholine). In the previous quote, Pischinger is stating that all the nerves in the body actually communicate via the "ubiquitous synapse"—the systemic and unified communicating nature—of the matrix tissue.

MIASMS AND DISTURBED FIELD LOCATIONS

Clearly, the highly sensitive matrix tissue is profoundly affected by any adverse stimulus—and certainly by an irritating scar. Nevertheless, how this chronic interference field *chooses* a particular area, or disturbed field, to secondarily disturb is not always clear. The following hypothesis by Dr. Peter Dosch helps clarify this phenomenon. It applies to both scar interference fields and focal infections:

> In my view, at least *two factors* must combine for an illness [disturbed field] to result from an interference field: firstly, the escalation of diseased tissue to the stage of becoming an active interference field and, secondly, an organ or organ system that has been previously damaged by hereditary or acquired factors to make it more susceptible to the action of an interference field.[59]

Thus, Dosch observed that the vulnerable tissues that were the primary disturbed field targets of a scar were largely based on an individual's miasmic weakness, through hereditary or acquired influences. For example, a primary tuberculinic individual with rheumatic joint tendencies might manifest the classic chronic cervical (neck) tension headaches typically seen in this miasm from a hernia surgery scar interference field. Whereas a luetic, who has a tendency toward destruction of tissue, might develop a stomach ulcer from this same hernia scar, and a sycotic may manifest a tendency to loose stools and intermittent diarrhea.

Contralateral Disturbed Fields Explained through Matrix Tissue

All of the previous examples of autonomic nerve pathways were *ipsilateral*—that is, the focus formed a disturbed field on the *same side* of the body. This is understandable from a neurological perspective, since the peripheral nervous system is arranged so that the general and autonomic nerves that exit the spinal cord do not cross the midline but innervate organs and tissues on the same side of the body. (This is in contrast to the brain, which, in most cases, sends neurons to the opposite side of the body.*) This ipsilateral tendency is commonly seen in practice, especially with dental foci, and assists greatly in diagnosing the most culpable focus.

This ipsilateral rule does not *always* apply, however, because scar interference fields are notoriously unpredictable. Dr. Huneke's now-famous example (see chapter 8) of the female patient who experienced instant relief—the Huneke or seconds phenomenon or lightning reaction—from the injection of a distant scar dramatically demonstrates this unpredictability. Just how did a *left* leg scar cause *right* shoulder pain? No one really knows. One probable explanation was that the right shoulder area was previously injured, as Dosch theorized, perhaps when this patient was a child, and the subtle tissue memory of that trauma made the region a likely candidate to be reactivated years later.

Another possible influence is that structural tissues typically adapt contralaterally. This contralateral compensation is a biomechanical imperative to maintain a balanced posture and to stand without falling over, or to be able to walk without tilting to one side. For example, a left leg scar interference field causes both electrical chaos in the surrounding matrix tissue and contraction in the neighboring muscles. In order to counterbalance this one-sided contraction pattern, muscles in the patient's opposite shoulder region need to compensate and contract. Over time, the patient's right shoulder tissues became inflamed and adhesed, resulting in a chronic adhesive capsulitis (frozen shoulder) condition (see figure 9.5).

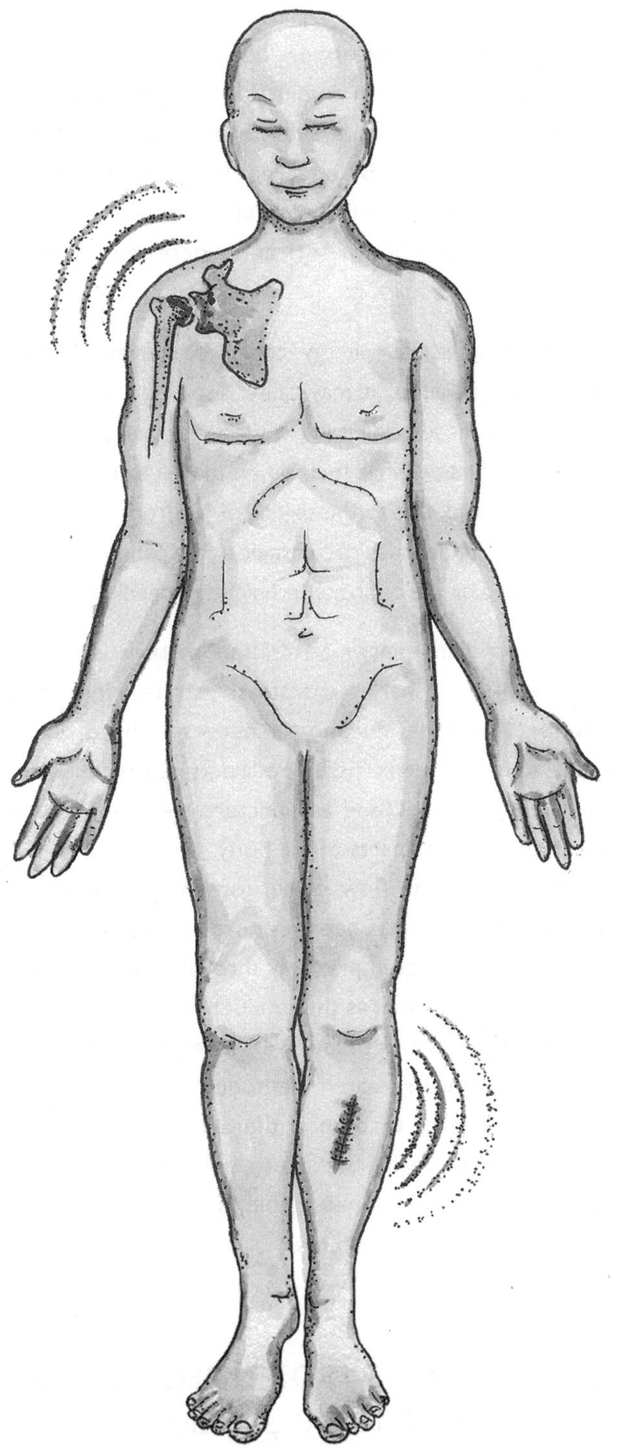

Figure 9.5. Another right-shoulder disturbed field, but this one is an example of a contralateral compensation to maintain a balanced posture due to aberrant matrix and muscular contraction patterns initiated by a chronic left-leg scar interference field.

*The notable exception to this rule is the cerebellum, which sends proprioceptive fibers to the ipsilateral aspects of the body.

CONTRALATERAL PATTERNS AND ACUPUNCTURE

Chinese medicine also recognizes contralateral patterns. For example, when excess or "perverse" energy invades an acupuncture meridian on one side of the body, a related meridian on the opposite side of the body can become deficient in energy.[60] By needling this opposite deficient meridian, acupuncturists help rebalance the disturbed equilibrium of the body. Ancient Chinese texts describe this treatment as follows:

> When the vicious energy comes to reside in the meridians as guest, it may cause disease on the right side while the left side is in excess; it may cause disease on the right side while the pain on the left side has not yet recovered, due to the shifting of Yin from Yang and vice versa; under such circumstances, the patient should be treated by the opposite technique of needling . . .[61]

This meridian energy adaptation pattern is another example of the "sharing the stress" strategy previously described—that is, autonomic nerves redirect excess nerve activity, matrix tissue redirects excess electrical contraction patterns, and acupuncture meridians redirect excess chi to other parts of the body.

Interestingly, the flow of chi (or energy) along acupuncture meridians has been proposed in recent research studies to be regulated primarily through both autonomic nerve pathways as well as the conductive liquid-crystal-like network of the matrix tissue.[62] However, these assertions based on modern research methodology do not impugn the importance or wisdom of the ancient Chinese masters, but rather verify that these energetic pathways in the body are real, are measurable, and can be explained through *many* various systems.

FOCAL CHAINS, FROZEN REGULATION, AND TOXIC GANGLIA

Focal Chains—Foci Generate Other Foci

Without appropriate treatment, foci generate other foci. When the disturbed field of a focus becomes chronically irritated and infected by bacteria over a period of time, it can become a primary focus itself and cause disturbance in a new, tertiary site. Billings noted that this focal chain tendency was a chief contributing factor underlying the chronic nature of infection in the body:

> Secondary foci [disturbed fields] may appear in various tissues as a part of the general or local disease which results from a primary focus. As we shall see, systemic and local diseases may occur through infection from a focal point by way of the bloodstream. This mode of infection is often embolic in character [i.e., microbes can travel through the blood similar to that of an *embolus,* or blood clot]. The tissues so infected may constitute new foci [i.e., the disturbed fields become focal infections], which in part explains the chronicity of many local and general infections."[63]

These focal chains can become so rooted in the body's terrain that they cannot be easily interrupted,

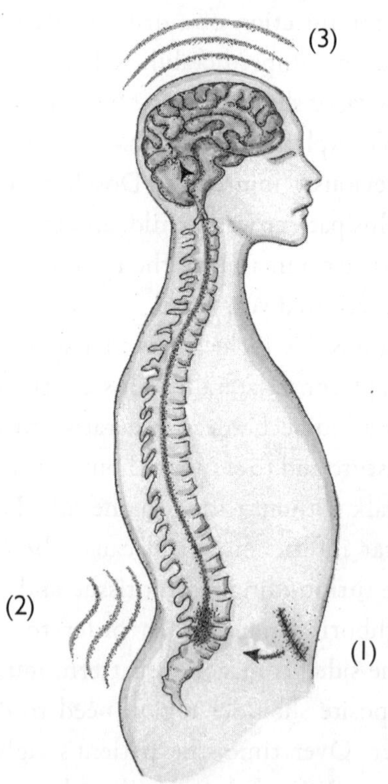

Figure 9.6. An example of a focal chain pattern: an appendix scar interference field (1) initially causes a lumbosacral joint disturbed field (2), which eventually coalesces into an active focus itself and which over time triggers disturbance in the brain (3), contributing to chronic depression.

even by holistic therapies, and *particularly* when practitioners are not knowledgeable in this field of study. William Kenneth Livingston commented on the phenomenon of chronic habit patterns becoming implanted in the body in his 1947 book, *Pain Mechanisms:* "[T]he longer the 'habit' . . . the harder the impulse needed to 'break the circle,' for the habit has become independent of the original cause."[64]

For example, an appendix scar interference field often causes a disturbed field in the lumbar vertebrae and sacroiliac joints, with resulting low back pain. Over time, these chronically irritated joints begin to act like a self-perpetuating focus themselves and—through the spinal cord nerve tracts, matrix tissue, and acupuncture meridian pathways—may then begin to affect the brain. This newly created brain disturbed field can cause symptoms of fatigue, depression, memory loss, or headaches (see figure 9.6). Unfortunately, when a patient presents for the treatment of chronic depression, rarely will a practitioner take into account the influence of an appendix scar interference field in the differential diagnosis.

A thorough and detailed history, referred to as an *anamnesis* (see the upcoming "Diagnosis of a Dominant Focus" on page 303), can help uncover this scar-joint-brain chronology. Those practitioners who combine the information obtained from the patient's history with their energetic testing results (e.g., kinesiology, reflex arm length, auricular medicine, and electroacupuncture) have the most success in unearthing and treating these focal chain patterns—especially the very long and complicated ones.

Frozen Regulation or Regulation Paralysis

Almost everyone has one focus, and most of us have more than one. Individuals who have had a lot of dental work, surgeries, major infections, or injuries can have multiple foci. Because foci generate other foci, it is not hard to envision how these focal chain patterns can multiply over a lifetime. In fact, it is common in our modern world for patients to have foci in the double digits.

The propagation of an increasing number of focal infections and interference fields can become so overwhelming to the system that it results in what the German neural therapists refer to as *frozen regulation,* or *regulation paralysis*. This condition occurs when the body becomes so inundated with aberrant signals that normal functioning, or homeostasis, is lost. In these typically tuberculinic- and luetic-functioning individuals, autonomic nerves are continuously receiving and sending abnormal signals, the chi energy of the acupuncture meridians is chronically imbalanced, and the liquid crystal conductivity of the matrix tissue is in chaos (with resulting incoherent oscillation patterns). Furthermore, in the case of focal infections, bacteria and other microbes are circulating through the blood and lymphatic channels, while continually saturating the matrix mesh with their toxic excretory products. (See figure 9.7.)

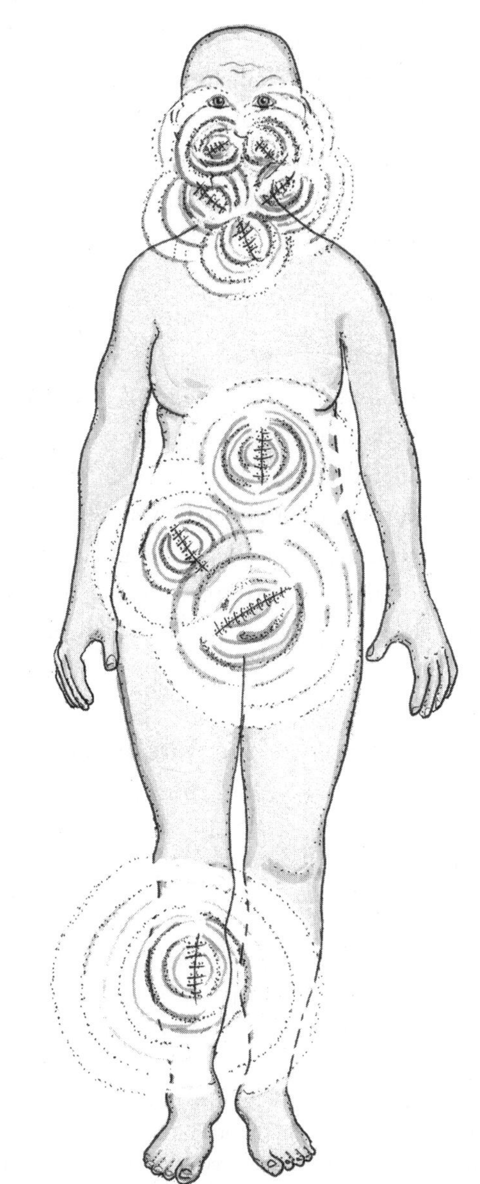

Figure 9.7. An example of frozen regulation or regulation paralysis from multiple foci and their disturbed fields

This systemic regulation paralysis, also affected by other factors such as steroids and toxic metals and chemicals, can become so pervasive that the system is constantly (dys-)functioning in survival mode. Even more problematic is that the very ill individuals with regulation paralysis, who need holistic care the most, can be the most challenging to appropriately diagnose and treat.

Every holistic practitioner who uses energetic testing methods has witnessed regulation paralysis, which forces practitioners to use various methods to clear this initial adaptation presentation before accurate testing is possible. In Neural Kinesiology (NK) or Autonomic Response Testing (ART), this frozen state is identified by an initial "blocked regulation" test, which signals that the autonomic nervous system is unable to respond to normal muscle testing challenges. In reflex arm length testing, also known as Matrix Reflex Testing (MRT), which is a direct measurement of the state of the matrix connective tissue, this frozen regulation can be indicated by an oscillating pattern.

In these difficult cases, precise diagnosis is required to assess the source of this initial "hyper-defensive" and aberrant pattern and to render appropriate treatment. Unfortunately, in this age of "endarkenment" where synthetic allopathic drugs and invasive surgeries are considered appropriate and even optimum, and herbs and homeopathics are eschewed as secondary and even "quackery," positive blocked regulation tests and incoherent oscillation patterns resulting from a multitude of foci in the body are the norm rather than the exception.

The Essential Role of the Autonomic Ganglia

The word *ganglion* is derived from the Greek word for "knot" or "knotlike mass."[65] In the body, a ganglion is a knotlike group of nerve cell bodies located outside the central nervous system (the brain and spinal cord).[66]* The majority of ganglia in the body's periphery are made up of either sympathetic, parasympathetic, or enteric (gut) autonomic nerves.†

Ganglia Act as "Little Brains"

Dr. Dietrich Klinghardt, a leading authority on the autonomic nervous system, has referred to these ganglia as "little brains," because they consist of masses of nerve cell bodies similar to the mass of the billions of nerve cell bodies that make up the brain.[67] Like the brain, these smaller brains, which are located throughout the body, help direct function in the peripheral organs and tissues. Autonomic ganglia relieve much of the workload of the brain by controlling and regulating automatic and unconscious functions in the body such as respiration, heart rate, digestion, urination, and defecation.

These ganglia are similar to thermostats that can increase or decrease autonomic *outflow* as needed, depending on the requirements of the individual.[68] For example, when you eat, the parasympathetic sensory neurons innervating the pancreas send messages up to the *vagus,* the chief parasympathetic ganglion that regulates digestion. This activates nerve impulses in the parasympathetic motor fibers that travel through the vagus to the pancreas, which stimulate the pancreas to produce digestive enzymes. At the same time, sympathetic nerve fiber impulses from the *celiac,* the primary sympathetic ganglion regulating digestion, are reduced to allow more blood flow in the abdominal area (see figure 9.8).

Sharing the Stress with Mother Ganglia

Besides regulating function in organs and tissues in the body, the autonomic ganglia play another major role—they seem to act as primary adaptive structures that *download* toxins from congested focal areas. As previously discussed, axonal transport—the movement of both healthy nutrients and pathogenic molecules such as microbes and toxins along nerve fibers—was first discovered in 1923.[69] Since then, the axonal transport of viruses such as herpes, polio, and rabies, as well as bacterial toxins from tetanus, has been extensively studied and well documented. In fact, the time delay individuals experience between feeling the classic prodromal neuralgic symptoms and the actual

*The term *ganglion* has also been used to refer to the basal ganglia, which are paired structures of the brain (the caudate nuclei, putamen, and globus pallidi) primarily involved in controlling voluntary body movement, muscle tone, and posture. They are located in the upper brain stem and posterior cerebral hemispheres.

†The posterior or dorsal root ganglia—sensory nerve cell bodies located posterior to the spinal cord—are composed of general sensory peripheral nerves. Ganglion cysts—benign cystic tumors that grow out of a joint, classically on the wrist or dorsum (top) of the foot—are not made up of nerves at all but of a thick, slippery fluid similar to the synovial fluid in the joints. When these cysts are large enough, they can press on local nerves and cause pain.

genital herpes outbreak is due in large part to the time required for the virus to be axonally transported from the sacral ganglia out to the skin.[70]

In 1975, studies conducted in both the United States and Sweden found that axonal transport of toxins could occur between the root of a tooth and its trigeminal ganglion, which is located at the base of the skull.[71] Later, in 1987, further studies proved that mercury from amalgam fillings can be directly transported from the teeth into the trigeminal ganglion, as well as from the tongue into another ganglion located in the skull—the hypoglossus.[72]

For over a decade, my colleagues (notably Dr. Dietrich Klinghardt) and I have tracked the axonal transport of various toxins from foci into ganglia—and witnessed the clinical success from treating both regions. Using energetic testing methods, specifically Neural Kinesiology (NK), Autonomic Response Testing (ART), and Matrix Reflex Testing (MRT) techniques, we have observed that the facial and cranial (head) ganglia can become congested with mercury axonally transported from amalgam fillings in the teeth, or with bacteria from dental or tonsil focal infections. In addition, we have seen that the by-products (e.g., lactic acid, substance P, histamine, kinins, and rogue oxygen) of chronic low-grade inflammation from scar interference fields are often transported to their primary regulating neighboring ganglia. For example, recently a patient presented with chronic prostatis, as well as symptoms of intermittent sexual dysfunction and mild urination difficulties. Examination found that two scars were contributing to the chronic congestion of his inferior hypogastric ganglion* that surrounds and regulates function in the prostate—one from a severely torn muscle injury in his right leg, and the other from the circumcision scars he received in the first week of life. After two auriculotherapy treatments to these scars and ganglia, as well as accompanying drainage and nutritional remedies, his prostate symptoms cleared.

Dr. Klinghardt coined the term *mother ganglia* to illustrate both the regulating and the coordinating function of ganglia, as well as the sacrificial role they play by receiving and accumulating the overload of toxins from a focus.[73] Thus, as with the formation of disturbed fields in the body, foci also "share the stress" with their mother ganglia, as a way to spread out and dilute the toxic load. Although this causes various levels of dysfunction in both the ganglia and the disturbed fields, the focal organ or tissue is saved from complete degeneration that could ultimately cause its demise. Thus, through this adaptive sharing of toxins, individuals fulfill their biological imperative and—albeit with impaired functioning—survive another day.

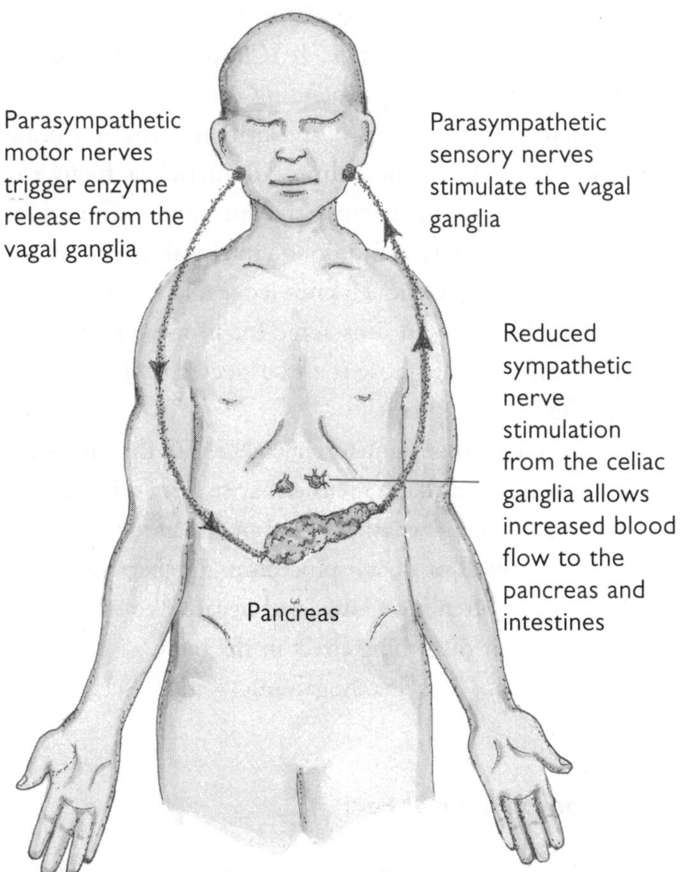
Parasympathetic motor nerves trigger enzyme release from the vagal ganglia
Parasympathetic sensory nerves stimulate the vagal ganglia
Reduced sympathetic nerve stimulation from the celiac ganglia allows increased blood flow to the pancreas and intestines
Pancreas

Figure 9.8. Autonomic ganglia—the parasympathetic vagus and the sympathetic celiac—regulate digestion by stimulating the production of pancreatic enzymes and blood flow.

TYPES OF DOMINANT FOCI

As described previously, typically foci are found primarily in the teeth, tonsils, and scars. This section

*The inferior hypogastric ganglion surrounds the prostate, rectum, and bladder. Its primary role is the regulation of bladder and prostate function. It often tests positive on patients who have sexual or bladder dysfunction.

provides a comprehensive list of the most typical foci found in clinical practice. It is important to keep in mind, however, that depending on each individual's particular state of health and primary reaction mode (psoric, sycotic, tuberculinic, or luetic), a focus can range from being completely dormant and nondisturbing to an active and dominant focal infection. An experienced practitioner knowledgeable in this field—preferably one who uses some form of energetic testing—can help diagnose these suspected foci and begin appropriate treatment.

It is also important to remember that this list is not all-inclusive and that a focus can arise from virtually *any* type of trauma—whether from an illness or injury, or from a surgical or dental procedure. Furthermore, long-lasting foci often have associated negative emotions that prolong their disturbing effect in the body, as previously described in "The Psychogalvanic Reflex" section (see page 283).

Common Dental Foci

Impacted teeth (e.g., wisdom teeth)
Root-canalled teeth
Dental implants
Devitalized teeth (e.g., from deep fillings, crowns, or trauma)
Abscessed teeth (often subclinical—i.e., without pain or obvious swelling)
Galvanic current (e.g., a gold crown on an amalgam filling)
Incomplete extractions (bone fragments or pieces of ligament remaining in the gum and alveolar bone)
Foreign bodies (e.g., a mercury "tattoo" in the gums)
Cysts, granulomas, or jaw osteitis (bone infection)

DENTAL IMPLANTS

Dr. Vera Stejskal, Ph.D., an expert in the allergic and autoimmune aspects of toxic metals as well as their role in the onset of premature aging, Alzheimer's, Parkinson's, and multiple sclerosis (MS), has found that from 25 to 50 percent of patients develop an autoimmune disease within eight years of receiving titanium implants.[74] Although the newer zirconium implants are being hailed in Europe as a better alternative, they too will always be registered by the nervous, matrix, and immune surveillance systems as a foreign body. Thus, any implant, no matter what material it is made up of, is by definition a focus (an "irritating thorn" and often the starting point of a disease process).

Tonsils and Other Ear, Nose, and Throat Foci

Chronic tonsillitis or past chronic tonsillitis
Past diphtheria or scarlet fever
Tonsillectomy and adenoidectomy scars
Chronic sinus infections or past chronic sinus infections
Sinus surgery scars
Chronic ear infections or past chronic ear infections
Ear tubes (myringotomies)
Mastoiditis or past mastoiditis (infection of the mastoid bone, just posterior to ear)
Mastoidectomy (removal of mastoid bone)

Body Foci

Umbilicus (belly button) scar from birth
Forceps delivery scars from birth
Scars from trauma (e.g., cuts, tears, wounds, severe bruises, or fractures)
Scars from surgery to repair traumatic injuries (e.g., knee surgery, episiotomies, compound or comminuted fractures,* wounds, or cuts)
Scars from other surgery (e.g., appendectomies, hysterectomies, hernias, cholecystectomies, circumcisions, cosmetic surgeries, spinal disk surgeries, heart bypass surgeries, cesarean sections, or abortions)
Scars from removal of skin growths (e.g., warts, moles, cysts, boils, or tags)
Scars from illness or infection (e.g., cystic acne or severe chicken pox)
Scars from vaccinations (especially from multiple puncture vaccines such as smallpox or BCG—tuberculosis)
Chronic unresolved inflammation or infections (e.g., a liver focus from chronic hepatitis or cirrhosis, a lung focus from chronic bronchitis or asthma, or a small intestine focus due to major dysbiosis, colitis [chronic intestinal inflammation in various locations

Compound refers to fractures in which the bone ends or fragments are sticking out of the skin. *Comminuted* refers to fractures in which the bone is splintered or crushed.

in the colon], pelvic inflammatory disease,* prostatitis, or interstitial cystitis [chronic bladder inflammation and irritation, considered an autoimmune syndrome])

Major past infections (e.g., a lung focus from past pneumonia, asthma, or chronic bronchitis)

Past or present IUD (intrauterine birth control device)

UMBILICUS SCARS

Sometimes, the umbilical cord is cut or clamped too close to the neonate, which can subtly pull too tightly on the umbilicus area and not allow complete healing. Through its attachment to the teres ligament that connects the umbilicus with the liver, this umbilicus scar interference field can chronically pull on the liver and the right side of the diaphragm that overlays the liver. This habitual tension can adversely and permanently affect liver metabolism and diminish full inspiration and expiration subtly over the years. Therefore, when an umbilical focus arises, the liver and right side of the diaphragm should also be therapy-localized. If these areas test positive, a massage of this ligament's course from the umbilicus to the liver is often necessary to clear this contraction. The umbilicus focus should also be treated through neural therapy or auriculotherapy, but usually this alone is not sufficient to release the chronic abnormal ligament constriction issue, without directly addressing it through massage or other deep tissue bodywork.

THE CULPABILITY OF ALLOPATHIC PRACTICES

As shown by the previous list, the hand of culpability in regard to the formation of foci points heavily toward modern-day allopathic medical and dental practices. Besides surgeries, root canals, dental implants, and other invasive procedures, the widespread use of antibiotics, antihistamines, steroids, and other drugs—while temporarily allaying the symptoms—only prolongs the illness in the long run by not diagnosing and treating the cause.

*Pelvic inflammatory disease (PID) usually refers to infection of the fallopian tubes but can also include infection of the cervix, uterus, or ovaries. It is most often transmitted by intercourse, and cultures typically reveal an underlying infection by gonorrhea or chlamydia organisms.

Thus, tonsillitis, sinusitis, rhinitis, appendicitis, and so forth are not diagnoses but descriptions of symptoms—that is, inflammation of the tonsils, sinuses, nose, and appendix. True diagnoses define the cause of the illness, such as a dairy allergy causing repeated tonsillitis, a dental focus inflaming the maxillary sinus just above it, or chronic intestinal dysbiosis from sugar ingestion and antibiotic abuse creating an inflamed appendix.

Furthermore, the common practice of repeated courses of these drugs to suppress the external signs of excretion and infection is not only detrimental to accurate diagnosis but actually *instrumental* in the creation and duration of these chronic foci, by driving the mutated pathogenic microbes and their toxins ever deeper into the more degenerated and scarred underlying tissues.

DIAGNOSIS OF A DOMINANT FOCUS

History Taking, or the "Anamnesis"

Many physicians were taught in college that taking a good history often far exceeds the physical exam and laboratory findings in achieving an accurate diagnosis. The Greek word *anamnesis,* meaning a "thorough and painstaking history," is often used to emphasize the important role taking an in-depth history has in holistic medicine.[75]

In searching for the patient's probable dominant foci, the practitioner pays close attention to the question of "when"—that is, the relationship of the onset of symptoms and the subsequent suspected illness, trauma, procedure, or surgery. For example, if a patient's migraine headaches began at age thirty-seven, the practitioner wants to know what changed in her life in the months—or even years—previous to this onset. Did she get a new crown or root canal, give birth to a child, or have a serious sinus infection? It is important to keep in mind that even a seemingly mild stress can activate an old focus. Dr. Ernesto Adler, a renowned European neural therapist, often found that simply traveling in a foreign country could trigger a dormant focus:

> The fortuitous "climatic provocation" in Spain often activates these "mute focal points" in our foreign patients, since the sun, the sea, and the wine draw them to the surface. The focal points "rejoice" much to the misery of their owners.[76]

Thus, illness after foreign travel is not always the result of intestinal parasites—the most typically suspected culprits when patients return home ill after vacationing in an exotic country—but also the possible activation of dormant foci.

Laboratory Testing

Unfortunately, blood, urine, and other laboratory tests cannot reliably predict the presence of chronic and adaptive focal infections, much less scar interference fields. Insidious chronic foci rarely initiate major immune system responses, so blood and urine testing are often negative. However, in one study of 200 patients with "clear-cut cases of [dental or tonsil] focal infection," some 63 percent showed a definite leukopenia (decreased white blood cell count) typical of chronic infection, as well as a definite albuminuria (increased albumin or protein in the urine), indicative of chronic liver and kidney dysfunction.[77] Therefore, when these blood cell count indicators are abnormal, a focal infection should be considered in the differential diagnosis.

The Value of Energetic Testing

Skillful energetic testing—when combined with a careful anamnesis, exam, X-rays (e.g., dental), and laboratory findings—is essential to accurately determine the dormant from the active foci and to determine which focus (if any) presently requires treatment. In most cases, foci, like dormant miasms in homeopathy, should not be treated until they reach a certain threshold level of disturbance in the body.* Before that, the system is either adequately compensating for the focus or unaware of any focal disturbance. And without adequate awareness, the body cannot initiate the necessary healing mechanisms—even when assisted by holistic therapies—to successfully resolve the focal disturbance.† Therefore, it is extremely valuable for holistic practitioners to use some form of energetic testing to help determine how, in what order, and when to treat the multiple potential foci.

Ascertaining and addressing the focus's related ganglia and specific disturbed fields can be almost impossible without some form of energetic testing that demonstrates cause and effect proficiently. Furthermore, while judging which came first—that is, differentiating between which tissue is actually the focus and which is the disturbed field—can be very important, it is sometimes quite challenging. For example, judging whether a third molar (wisdom) tooth is a focus or simply a disturbed field from a dysbiotic small intestine focus is an important clinical decision.* Pulling a tooth is a permanent measure that can't be reversed. Thus, in the face of critical decisions involving surgery, the practitioner's clinical judgment is greatly assisted by energetic testing methods informed by a thorough anamnesis and physical exam. (See appendix 3, "Energetic Testing Explained," for a list of the most widely used energetic testing methods.)

*I have never observed any lasting or profound effects from the injection of all the scars on a patient's body at once simply because they were there, as is the practice of some rather aggressive neural therapists. However, the more gentle treatment of massaging all the scars with various substances (essential oils, isopathic remedies, and shea butter) over a period of weeks can be valuable. For more information, see "Neural Therapy without Needles" in chapter 10, page 309.

†Of course, when necessary, there are energetic testing methods referred to as "cold-booting" to bring a focus up to the body's awareness. In the case of a serious disease such as cancer, the decision process of whether to extract a suspected focal tooth is often expedited due to the possible serious consequences of waiting.

*In chronic cases, both the tooth and the small intestine may ischemically therapy-localize—that is, test positive.

NOTES

1. E. Hatton, "Focal Infection," in G. Black, *Operative Dentistry* (Woodstock, Ill.: Medico-Dental Publishing Company, 1948), 420.
2. C. Richter, "Physiological Factors Involved in the Electrical Resistance of the Skin," *American Journal of Physiology* 88, no. 4 (February 15, 1929): 596.
3. D. Klinghardt and L. Williams, Neural Kinesiology Course, Germany (November 1994).
4. R. Stein, "Study Faults Episiotomy," *Press Democrat,* May 4, 2005, A5.
5. P. Dosch, *Manual of Neural Therapy* (Heidelberg: Haug Publishers, 1984), 439.
6. Ibid., 62, 432.
7. F. Billings, *Focal Infection* (New York: D. Appleton and Company, 1916), 20–22, 33–35.
8. Ibid., 44.
9. M. Fischer, *Death and Dentistry* (Springfield, Ill.: Charles C. Thomas, 1940), 25.
10. P. Störtebecker, *Mercury Poisoning from Dental Amalgam—*

A Hazard to the Human Brain (Orlando, Fla.: Bio-Probe, 1985), 46–47.

11. Ibid.; B. Arvidson, "Mercury Accumulates in Hypoglossal Ganglion," *Experimental Neurology* 98 (1987): 198–203; P. Störtebecker, *Neurology for Barefoot Doctors in All Countries* (Stockholm: Störtebecker Foundation for Research, 1988), 294–97.
12. M. Fischer, *Death and Dentistry* (Springfield, Ill.: Charles C. Thomas, 1940), 25.
13. F. Billings, *Focal Infection* (New York: D. Appleton and Company, 1916), 44–45.
14. I. Korr, "Sustained Sympathicotonia as a Factor in Disease" in *The Neurobiologic Mechanisms in Manipulative Therapy* (New York: Plenum Publishing Corporation, 1978), 229–68.
15. S. Porges, "Orienting in a Defensive World: Mammalian Modifications of Our Evolutionary Heritage. A Polyvagal Theory," *Psychophysiology* 32 (1995): 304; P. Dosch, *Manual of Neural Therapy* (Heidelberg: Haug Publishers, 1984), 439.
16. D. Juhan, *Job's Body* (Barrytown, N.Y.: Barrytown, Ltd., 1998), 155.
17. P. Dosch, *Manual of Neural Therapy* (Heidelberg: Haug Publishers, 1984), 93.
18. Ibid., 93–95.
19. S. Porges, "Orienting in a Defensive World: Mammalian Modifications of Our Evolutionary Heritage. A Polyvagal Theory," *Psychophysiology* 32 (1995): 304.
20. I. Korr, "Sustained Sympathicotonia as a Factor in Disease" in *The Neurobiologic Mechanisms in Manipulative Therapy* (New York: Plenum Publishing Corporation, 1978), 229–68.
21. I. Korr et al., "Patterns of Electrical Skin Resistance in Man," *Acta Neurovegetativa* (Vienna: Springer Verlag, 1958), 78; D. Hubbard and G. Berkoff, "Myofascial Trigger Points Show Spontaneous Needle EMG Activity," *Spine* 18, no. 13: 1803–7; H. Hooshmand, *Chronic Pain* (Boca Raton, Fla.: CRC Press, 1993), 14–25.
22. I. Korr, "Sustained Sympathicotonia as a Factor in Disease" in *The Neurobiologic Mechanisms in Manipulative Therapy* (New York: Plenum Publishing Corporation, 1978), 229–68.
23. I. Korr, "The Spinal Cord as Organizer of Disease Processes: Hyperactivity of Sympathetic Innervation as a Common Factor in Disease," *Journal of the American Osteopathic Association* 79, no. 4 (December 1979): 232–36.
24. Ibid.
25. P. Dosch, *Manual of Neural Therapy* (Heidelberg: Haug Publishers, 1984), 142.
26. H. Hooshmand, *Chronic Pain* (Boca Raton, Fla.: CRC Press, 1993), 16.
27. Ibid.
28. Ibid., 16–17.
29. H. Hooshmand, *Chronic Pain* (Boca Raton, Fla.: CRC Press, 1993), 16.
30. H. Head, "On Disturbances of Sensation with Especial Reference to the Pain of Visceral Disease," *Brain* 16 (1893): 16–17.
31. Ibid.
32. Ibid.
33. G. Tortora and N. Anagnostakos, *Principles of Anatomy and Physiology* (New York: Harper and Row, 1987), 342, 343.
34. D. Juhan, *Job's Body* (Barrytown, N.Y.: Barrytown, Ltd., 1998), 62, 63.
35. Ibid., 63.
36. P. Rowan, *Some Body* (New York: Alfred A. Knopf, 1995), 6.
37. D. Juhan, *Job's Body* (Barrytown, N.Y.: Barrytown, Ltd., 1998), 64.
38. P. Dosch, *Manual of Neural Therapy* (Heidelberg: Haug Publishers, 1984), 64; D. Juhan, *Job's Body* (Barrytown, N.Y.: Barrytown, Ltd., 1998), 64.
39. Ibid.
40. Ibid.
41. J. Oschman and N. Oschman, "Healing 101 Workshops: Somatic Recall Part I: Soft Tissue Memory," www.healing101.org/somaticrecall1.html.
42. Ibid., 359; P. Dosch, *Manual of Neural Therapy* (Heidelberg: Haug Publishers, 1984), 64.
43. A. Pischinger, *Matrix and Matrix Regulation* (Brussels: Haug, 1991), 19.
44. D. Juhan, *Job's Body* (Barrytown, N.Y.: Barrytown, Ltd., 1998), 359.
45. Ibid.
46. J. Oschman and N. Oschman, "Healing 101 Workshops: Somatic Recall Part I: Soft Tissue Memory," www.healing101.org/somaticrecall1.html.
47. L. Williams, "Matrix Response Testing Method," www.radicalmedicine.com/MRT_technique.html.
48. P. Horn, "The Extracellular Matrix," *Townsend Letter for Doctors and Patients,* May 1997, 134.
49. M. Ho, "Quantum Coherence and Conscious Experience," www.i-sis.org.uk/braindde.php.

50. Ibid.
51. P. Gosch, *Vital Energy Medicine* (Provo, Utah: Chronicle Publishing Services, 2003), 16.
52. D. Juhan, *Job's Body* (Barrytown, N.Y.: Barrytown, Ltd., 1998), 83.
53. P. Gosch, *Vital Energy Medicine* (Provo, Utah: Chronicle Publishing Services, 2003), 16–17.
54. A. Pischinger, *Matrix and Matrix Regulation* (Brussels: Haug, 1991), 18.
55. P. Dosch, *Manual of Neural Therapy* (Heidelberg: Haug Publishers, 1984), 65.
56. H. Heine, "New Insights into the System of Basal-Regulation," manual from a lecture given during the 14th Austrian Neural Therapy Symposium, Baden (October 18, 1986), 161–62, 163.
57. J. Yasgur, *Homeopathic Dictionary* (Greenville, Pa.: Van Hoy Publishers, 1998), 146.
58. A. Pischinger, *Matrix and Matrix Regulation* (Brussels: Haug, 1991), 17.
59. P. Dosch, *Manual of Neural Therapy* (Heidelberg: Haug Publishers, 1984), 128.
60. R. Low, *The Secondary Vessels of Acupuncture* (Wellingborough, Northamptonshire, England: Thorsons Publishers Limited, 1983), 130.
61. Ibid.
62. D. Juhan, *Job's Body* (Barrytown, N.Y.: Barrytown, Ltd., 1998), 360; Z. Xiangtong, *Research on Acupuncture, Moxibustion, and Acupuncture Anesthesia* (Beijing: Science Press, 1986), 359; S. Shakman, *The Autohemotherapy Reference Manual* (Santa Monica, Calif.: Institute of Science, 1996), 8.
63. E. Hatton, "Focal Infection," in G. Black, *Operative Dentistry* (Woodstock, Ill.: Medico-Dental Publishing Company, 1948), 419.
64. K. Kretzschmar, "Neural Therapy, Parts II and IV," *Medical Times* 84, no. 6 (June 1956): 643.
65. J. Friel, ed., *Dorland's Illustrated Medical Dictionary,* 26th ed. (Philadelphia: W. B. Saunders Company, 1981), 537.
66. Ibid.
67. D. Klinghardt, lecture notes from Neural Therapy Advanced Course, Albuquerque, N.Mex., (May 1993).
68. D. Klinghardt and L. Williams, *Neural Therapy without Needles* (Seattle: AANT, 1994), 7.
69. P. Störtebecker, *Mercury Poisoning from Dental Amalgam—A Hazard to the Human Brain* (Orlando, Fla.: Bio-Probe, 1985), 46–47.
70. G. Tortora and N. Anagnostakos, *Principles of Anatomy and Physiology,* 5th ed. (New York: Harper and Row, 1987), 266.
71. Ibid., 47–48.
72. B. Arvidson, "Mercury Accumulates in Hypoglossal Ganglion," *Experimental Neurology* 98 (1987): 198–203; Nilner et al., "Effect of Dental Amalgam Restorations on the Mercury Content of Nerve Tissues," *Acta Odontologica Scandinavica* 43 (1985): 303–7.
73. D. Klinghardt, lecture notes from Neural Therapy Advanced Course, Albuquerque, N.Mex. (May 1993).
74. D. Klinghardt, "Biological Dentistry: What Is It? Why Do We Need It?" International Academy of Biological Dentistry and Medicine Conference (March 31–April 2, 2006).
75. J. Friel, ed., *Dorland's Illustrated Medical Dictionary,* 26th ed. (Philadelphia: W. B. Saunders Company, 1981), 80.
76. E. Adler, *Neural Focal Dentistry* (Houston: Multi-Discipline Research Foundation, 1984), 94.
77. A. Crance, "A Review of Blood and Urine Examinations in 200 Cases of Chronic Focal Infection of Oral Origin," *Dental Digest* 27 (1922): 625–26.

10

CLEARING FOCI: NEURAL THERAPY AND AURICULOTHERAPY

There are two primary treatments for a dominant focus: *Neural Therapy* from Germany and *Auriculotherapy* from France. Drainage (gemmotherapy or "plant stem cell") remedies are often also required to help encourage the efficient clearance of the newly "unearthed" toxins associated with each focus (see chapter 2). And the use of a single constitutional homeopathic remedy (according to the Sankaran system) that effectively treats every aspect—physical, emotional, and mental—of an individual has a profoundly healing effect on all chronic foci in the body (see chapter 14).

If repeated sessions of auriculotherapy and/or neural therapy, along with supportive drainage and homeopathy, fail to clear the focus, then surgery should be considered. In the case of devitalized or abscessed teeth, correctly performed cavitation surgery to remove the tooth and dead jawbone tissue has been proven effective. Tonsillectomies have not been as successful, but this could be due in part to the lack of knowledgeable and artful surgeons performing this procedure, as well as the fact that most physicians do not address the chronic intestinal dysbiosis and related food allergies that feed into and perpetuate the tonsil focus. Thus, because tonsil foci are more a sign of systemic dysfunction, systemic treatments such as constitutional homeopathy and drainage are better options, with specific neural therapy and auriculotherapy. In the case of scar interference fields, surgical or laser excision of large scars (keloids) is rarely indicated and rarely successful clinically, although this procedure may be appropriate for cases of serious cosmetic surgery.

Chapters 11 to 13 cover the specific treatment protocols for each of the major focal areas. For now, we will discuss the rationale for using either neural therapy or auriculotherapy.

NEURAL THERAPY

As mentioned in chapter 8, neural therapy originated in the early twentieth century through the clinical work of Ferdinand Huneke. In a neural therapy treatment, local anesthetic is injected in and around a focus and its related ganglia to temporarily block the abnormal neuronal signals emitting from the pathologically disturbed tissue. Hypotheses on why neural therapy is effective chiefly center on the theory of encouraging a more functional cell membrane and autonomic nervous system.

The Scientific Rationale

During the one to three hours of respite that the anesthesia provides, the cells in the focal area begin to function more effectively primarily due to the improved polarity of the cell membranes. Analogous to a moat around a castle, the function of the membrane that surrounds a cell is to allow helpful nutrients in and keep toxic invaders out. However, this gate-keeping mechanism can only function properly when the cell membrane is operating within a certain range of normal electrical conductivity.

This conductivity is measured to be approximately –70 to –90 millivolts. The local anesthetic used in neural therapy temporarily *hyperpolarizes* the cells in a focal area; these diseased cells are often barely functioning, usually at –15 millivolts or even lower.[1] With the hyperpolarizing effect the local anesthetic provides, the cells in the focal area come closer to their normal and healthier membrane electrical potential. Additionally, this rest period temporarily interrupts chronic pathological neural reflexes.

When the anesthetic effect has worn off after a few hours, much of the therapeutic effect gained from neural therapy continues to last.[2] The cell membrane's electrical polarity in the focal region has moved closer to normal, which allows more nutrients to enter the cell and more toxic wastes to be expelled. Additionally, the interruption of abnormal nerve reflexes can often remain relatively permanent, which results in overall healthier cellular functioning through a more balanced autonomic nervous system.[3]

▶ For more information on neural therapy, refer to Dr. Peter Dosch's *Manual of Neural Therapy according to Huneke* (Haug Publishers). Additionally, Robert F. Kidd, M.D., has recently published an excellent book on the subject, *Neural Therapy: Applied Neurophysiology and Other Topics.*

A Major Drawback: Carcinogenic Anesthetics

Despite the positive-sounding nature of neural therapy treatments, a major drawback to this therapy is the carcinogenicity of local anesthetics.

As discussed in chapter 3, by 1994 researchers discovered that the local anesthetic lidocaine was "clearly carcinogenic" because it breaks down into aniline—a cancer-causing coal tar substance—in the body.[4] However, this toxic aniline breakdown is not confined to lidocaine. *All* popular local anesthetics including procaine (Novocain)—also widely used in neural therapy—can break down into this carcinogenic substance.[5] The extremely toxic nature of aniline has been well known since the 1700s, when it was first noticed that chimney sweeps were succumbing to cancer after chronic exposure to chimney soot.[6] Anilines are also a cause of cardiac arrest (heart attack), asthma, dementia, and neuromuscular diseases.[7]* Thus, toxic aniline buildup from numerous neural therapy injections could be significantly harmful, especially in weaker patients with reduced liver clearance.

Unfortunately, although a new aniline-free anesthetic was approved by the FDA in April 2000, Septocaine (articaine) contains a toxic preservative as well as epinephrine—a drug that can cause adverse heart and neurological symptoms. Therefore, this new anesthetic is not an ideal substitute in neural therapy.

My colleagues and I have corroborated the laboratory research on the toxic effects of aniline buildup in clinical practice by using energetic testing methods. Over the years, both lidocaine and procaine have consistently tested negative—that is, as stressful and toxic—when challenged. They have also triggered stress responses in "cleaner" patients, who would often immediately respond to the toxicity of these local anesthetics.

Due to these findings, many holistic practitioners began to use only homeopathic and herbal remedies in neural therapy injections, which seemed—despite the lack of anesthetic effect—to be reasonably effective. Sometimes a small amount of epinephrine-free, preservative-free bupivacaine (Marcaine) is included in these herbal or homeopathic injections for a beneficial anesthetic effect. Bupivacaine is the least toxic type of local anesthetic because it leaves 80 percent less aniline residue in the body than other local anesthetics.[8] These herbal or homeopathic remedies, when combined with a small amount of bupivacaine, seem to be the most satisfactory method, until a petroleum-free, natural anesthetic is produced.

Although certain plants have anesthetic properties, such a large amount of the plant is needed to produce even a small amount of local anesthetic that it has not been economically feasible so far for anyone to manufacture a (preservative-free) naturally derived local anesthetic.

---

*It makes one wonder if there is a neuro*lytic* (nerve destruction) aspect to these local anesthetics, similar to the destructive effect of nerve blocks purposefully done with neurolytic agents such as phenol and ethyl alcohol in cases of chronic severe pain. That is, perhaps some of the relief patients receive from neural therapy by the nerve-blocking effect is due to the *destruction* of some of the nerve tissue, rather than the anesthetizing effect on nerve tissue. (For more information on nerve blocks with neurolytic agents see John Bonica, *The Management of Pain* [Philadelphia: Lea & Febiger, 1990], 1,980.)

- Preservative-free, epinephrine-free bupivacaine is available to medical and licensed naturopathic doctors from the holistic pharmacy Apothecure at (800) 969-6601. Sensitive (and holistically oriented) patients can request that their dentists use this less-toxic form of local anesthetic during their dental procedures.

Neural Therapy without Needles

This problem of carcinogenic local anesthetics can be easily surmounted through noninjectible forms of neural therapy, referred to as "neural therapy without needles." Dr. Peter Dosch, one of the German masters of neural therapy, has quoted the founding Huneke brothers, who discovered that many types of effective treatment could be classified under the neural therapy "umbrella":

> The brothers Huneke have made it clear to us that the healing action of physiotherapy, balneotherapy [baths], and of other peripherally acting therapies such as acupuncture, Ponndorf's vaccinations,* massage and all dermal stimulation and tonal therapy, including Kneipp's, shortwave, ultrasonic and X-ray therapy, and even the effects of chirotherapy, are all ultimately based on a single common principle. They all make use of the reflex pathways of the neurovegetative system by setting up a therapeutic stimulus in the nervous system whose response to this stimulus then releases the healing reaction. Seen in this light, all these therapies can also be considered "neural therapy" in the wider sense.[9]

KNEIPP'S WATER CURE

Father Sebastian Kneipp (1824–1897), one of the fathers of naturopathy, was famous in the nineteenth century for healing thousands of sick people with his Nature Cure. Kneipp originated and popularized many natural methods of healing, but he was most well known for his cold water cure. In fact, the long pools that still exist in many European parks, where visitors can walk knee-high in cold water, exemplify his widespread popularity. Even today these baths are popular, and many Europeans still use hydrotherapy treatments to stimulate health and vitality. (For more information on Father Kneipp and other pioneers in naturopathic medicine, read *Nature Doctors* by Friedhelm Kirchfeld and Wade Boyle.)

This type of injection-free (and pain-free) neural therapy is most typically accomplished through massage, either with an herbal cream or isopathic (homeopathic) drops, sometimes accompanied by soft laser therapy. Neural therapy without needles can be additionally quite effective in mitigating older scar interference fields and focal infections and helping to clear much of the negative effects from these chronic disturbances.

- Dr. Klinghardt and I have taught "Neural Therapy without Needles" courses for two decades. For more information, go to www.klinghardtacademy.com or www.radicalmedicine.com.

Massage with Creams or Oils

Because an oil or cream can be massaged into a scar at home, it is often a preferred treatment for scars located in more personal areas such as the genital region. Thus, scars from episiotomies or perineal tears after giving birth, hysterectomies, hemorrhoid or rectal fissure surgeries, hernia operations, and circumcisions are often effectively treated in this more private manner. A further benefit is that home treatments give patients a chance to observe and address some of the negative thoughts and feelings often associated with their particular scar—that is, to *reacquaint* and *make peace* with this area that was previously damaged and has been somewhat separated from their energy field. Some practitioners even test for the specific emotions connected to each scar by having patients think about these issues while they massage the scar. This practice can allow individuals to inquire into their underlying negative thoughts and feelings related to the focus, and therefore gain more self-understanding. Often this heightened awareness and consciousness can trigger a release of the chronic emotional contraction patterns (e.g., anger, fear, or sorrow) subtly but chronically associated with the scar interference field. The typical treatment schedule for massage is once a day for a month, but in some cases two weeks can suffice.

*Ponndorf's vaccination is an immune-stimulating therapy similar to the smallpox vaccination procedure where small cuts are made in the skin with a lancet. Often, isopathic remedies and other natural homeopathics or herbals are rubbed into this scarified area to stimulate immune system functioning.

After such treatment, the scar interference field often tests approximately 50 to 80 percent improved, and it can then be completely cleared with one or more auriculotherapy treatments.

The most clinically effective herbal cream is shea butter, which is the fat derived from the seed of the *Butyrospermum parkii* tree from Africa. Shea butter has been traditionally used to reduce inflammation and shrink swollen mucosal membranes.[10] Clinically, it can promote nerve tissue healing and reduce the number of damaged ephapses (neural contact points) in the scar area.

▶ Shea butter is available at most health food stores, but not all shea butters are equal. In my experience, the shea butter from a small northern California company, Organic Essence, has tested as far superior to any other brand. Organic Essence has figured out how to purify—but not refine—its shea butter, thus maintaining nutrients such as nonsaponifiable fatty acids (stearic and loeic acid) that moisturize and support the skin's elasticity. Therefore, unlike other shea butters, it spreads easily and actually smells good, without the need to add essential oils to mask the normally unpleasant scent. To order Pure Organic Shea Butter from Organic Essence, go to www.orgess.com, or check to see if your local health food store carries it.

Essential oils are also quite effective when massaged into scar interference fields. Although some enjoy dropping the oils directly onto a scar, it is safest to dilute them with almond oil, olive oil, or shea butter to avoid irritating more sensitive tissues. Many essential oils such as oregano, cinnamon, thyme, tea tree, and clove are highly microcidal and can reduce infection in dental, tonsil, and other focal infections.[11] However, it is essential to use *clean* essential oils from companies that do not extract their oils with an excess of heat or benzene, toluene, and other solvents. Additionally, because essential oils affect both the physical and etheric body—that is, the subtle emotional and mental planes that surround the physical body—they can sometimes stimulate strong healing reactions. Therefore, they should be used with caution and most optimally under the guidance of a well-trained practitioner. Essential oils can also antidote homeopathics—especially when used over a thirty-day period—and should therefore not be used on patients who are on an acute or constitutional remedy. Or, alternatively, those individuals should be instructed to redose their homeopathic remedy more often to reduce the antidoting effect these oils may have on their remedy.

▶ Good-quality essential oils, such as those from the Aura Cacia company, can be found at most health food stores. BioResource carries quality ORMED essential oils, such as Lavender, Niaouli, and Ravensare, which often test well in the treatment of both scar interference fields and chronic focal infections. Contact BioResource at (800) 203-3775 or visit the website at http://bioresourceinc.com. Finally, unlike many multilevel companies whose products often don't hold up over time, the essential oils from Young Living and MiEssence have continued to test well. To find them, go to www.youngliving.com or www.anniesorganics.mionegroup.com

The Use of Isopathic Microbial Remedies

In contrast to classic homeopathic remedies that are *similar* to a patient's symptoms, isopathic remedies are homeopathically prepared substances that are *identical* to and often causative of a patient's symptoms. Thus, isopathy is based on the principle of not *similarity* but *sameness,* and often it is even based on "the substance being identical to the etiological agent."[12] For example, homeopathic pollens can be used to treat allergies, the compound Arsenicum metallicum for arsenic poisoning, homeopathic streptococcus bacteria (also known as a *nosode*) for chronic strep throat and tonsillitis, or a potentized drug (also known as *tautopathy*) to treat the toxic side effects of the drug.[13] Isopathic-type remedies have been used for centuries and were notably first advocated by the holistic physician Paracelsus (1493–1541).[14]

Not all isopathic remedies are derived from pathogenic substances. Some are made from normal body fluids. For example, practitioners use blood (known as *auto-hemotherapy*) to treat anemia and immune dysfunction or urine to treat chronic bladder infections. Isopathic remedies made from benign bacteria and fungi that normally reside in the body can reduce the virulence of their pathogenic relatives and trigger immune system responses that combat infection. These remedies are especially efficacious in the treatment of chronic dental and tonsil focal infections, and even the mild inflammation (usually invisible) surrounding a chronic scar interference field. Although these remedies may be ingested, they are always rubbed into the skin in the treatment of scar interference fields (sometimes in addition to oral treatment).

In 1939, the German physician Karl Stauffer described the actions of isopathic remedies made homeopathically from microbes:

> Isopathy . . . directly addresses microbial pathogens or their toxins that cause damage to the body and cause illnesses. Isopathic-homeopathic remedies are homeopathically diluted and potentized. It is important to emphasize that these medications do not contain the actual active forms of the microbes, but stimulate the body to initiate a response to address pathogens and their toxins present in the body that have been acquired through infection or heredity.[15]

The German company SanPharma follows traditional European guidelines in the formulation of its isopathic remedies. The bacterial remedies are made of metabolic products that stimulate a gentler, nonspecific immune response. Isopathic remedies that use whole cell or cell wall products often contain bacterial antigens that can provoke a specific immune response with the potential to trigger an allergenic excess reaction or anergy (no immune response).[16] Many of my colleagues and I have found through both energetic testing and patients' clinical results that these microbial isopathic remedies are superior to other formulations in the treatment of chronic foci. For example, the SanPharma isopathic fungal remedy Notatum 4X (*Penicillium notatum*), known in holistic circles as a "natural antibiotic," can significantly reduce strep and staph bacterial infections without any of the side effects that antibiotics create. This remedy activates the natural killer cells that are the primary immune system cells that fight infection in the body.[17] Notatum 3X tablets can be prescribed to augment the treatment of chronic tonsil and dental focal infections, and the 4X drops can be rubbed into scar interference fields to reduce the low-grade but chronic inflammation in the area.*

*In sensitive or weak patients, only the Notatum 4X drops should be used on *chronic* focal infections because the tablets can sometimes be too aggravating. However, in the case of *acute* infections, the tablets are more often appropriate and rarely cause healing reactions.

Furthermore, this remedy is especially effective in treating any associated infection in the underlying tissues of interference fields, such as in the case of chronic dysbiosis secondary to an appendix scar, intestinal colic secondary to a cholecystectomy (gallbladder removal) scar, or chronic vaginal candidiasis secondary to a hysterectomy or episiotomy scar.

Another microbial isopathic remedy, *Aspergillus niger,* is commonly used in alternating doses with *Penicillium notatum* to stimulate soft-tissue and bone healing of a dental focus or after cavitation surgery. *Aspergillus niger* can also be effective in the treatment of arthritic pain, due to this remedy's immune-modulating effect that can reduce inflammation in the muscles and joints.[18] In Kombination 4X drops, Aspergillus 4X drops are combined with *Mucor racemosus,* a remedy that is used in augmenting normal blood flow and circulation. This product, in tandem with Notatum 4X, often tests positive after dental surgery, since the Aspergillus assists in bone and soft-tissue healing and the Mucor aids blood flow and reduces the effects of bruising.

Other commonly used microbial isopathics include Mucor 4X drops (used alone when the Aspergillus does not test positive) to reduce bleeding and bruising after dental cavitation surgery and Roqueforti/Candida 3X rectal suppositories to help treat vaginal yeast, prostatitis, or intestinal dysbiosis associated with appendix and genital focal infections.

However, practitioners should be aware that suppositories, and sometimes even the tablets and capsules, occasionally have strong healing effects, even with SanPharma's gentler production methods.[19] Therefore, the milder drop form of these medications is often more suitable for weaker patients, especially at the beginning of treatment when the goal is to simply reduce inflammation and reintegrate the estranged focus with the body. When capsules or suppositories are indicated, they often need to be prescribed in conjunction with an effective drainage protocol, using the more potent gemmotherapy remedies described in chapter 2. Finally, it should be noted that the most important step that practitioners can make to reduce the possibility of potentially strong healing effects is to receive thorough training in the use of these remedies before prescribing them.*

*For information on seminars as well as ordering SanPharma products, contact BioResource. (See resource box on page 310.)

NEURAL THERAPY WITHOUT NEEDLES MASSAGE PROTOCOL

This neural therapy massage protocol can mitigate 70 to 100 percent of the (often silent) nerve and tissue irritation generated from a scar, and it can be performed in the privacy of your own home. Any remaining disturbance not cleared by this peripheral nerve treatment can be treated with auriculotherapy (see page 314).

Since all the scars on the body resonate together in one sheet of skin, it is important to remember to include *all* scars in your treatment—from your first scar, the belly button or umbilicus, to the smallest arthroscopic surgical scar to acne and stretch mark scars and even ear-piercing scars.

Although this protocol is relatively mild and rarely causes any healing reactions, chronically ill patients should check with their holistic practitioner before attempting this home treatment. Scar formation is an intrinsic and necessary response to healing cuts and injuries and *should not be interrupted.* This massage protocol is only for old, *chronic* scars—not for recent injuries.

Step 1: Massage Notatum 4X (anti-inflammatory), Aspergillus 4X (soft-tissue healing), or Kombination 4X (soft-tissue healing and blood circulation) drops into *all* your scars.

Step 2: Rub Pure Organic Shea Butter into each scar.

Do this two-step treatment for three to four weeks, once or twice a day. It is best done after a shower or bath, since warm, soft skin absorbs drops more readily, and/or before bed.

Note: For tonsillectomy scars, place two drops of Notatum 4X, Aspergillus 4X, or Kombination 4X in the back of your throat where the tonsillectomy scars lie (try to keep the tip of the dropper sterile—i.e., don't touch it to the gums or teeth), then rub the shea butter into either side of your upper external throat area, just below the jaw line where the tonsils and lymph nodes usually swell. For dental extraction scars just place the drops on those sites.

Placing an X on a copy of the following diagram at each scar location and hanging a chart like this in your bathroom can be an excellent way to jog your memory and ensure that you don't forget any minor or hidden scars.

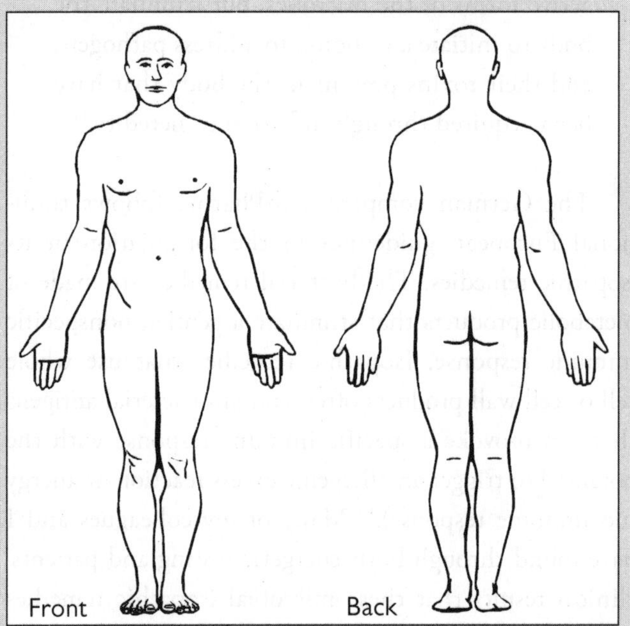

Laser Therapy

The effect of all of these remedies—isopathic microbial remedies, essential oils, and shea butter—can be intensified by *driving them* into scars and other focal areas through infrared light, or laser therapy. Low-level therapeutic lasers, as opposed to stronger *cutting* lasers used in surgical procedures, have proven to be both safe and efficacious in many forms of therapy, but especially in acupuncture, in dentistry, and in the treatment of pain.[20]*

Dr. Dietrich Klinghardt has proposed that the photons emitted from laser light hyperpolarize the depolarized "sick cell membranes" in the focal area and therefore change their electrical charge, which then allows for "easier in-flow and out-flow of the cell."[21] Thus, laser light can have a neural therapeutic effect similar to the injection of local anesthetic, but without the residual toxic aniline burden to the liver and kidneys. Furthermore, essential oils, microbial isopathics, herbs, and shea butter can all be driven deeper into the scar or focal area by the laser light, so that this *photophoretic* effect can enhance these remedies' absorption through the skin and into the deeper tissues.[22] For example, Notatum 4X drops can be rubbed into an appendix scar area and then

*Cell damage is possible with extended use of a 500-milliwatt (or higher) laser. Even soft therapeutic lasers should never be shone directly into the eye, because the lens will focus it on the retina, thus strengthening its intensity, which could possibly cause retinal damage. (D. Bartram, *Low Level Laser Therapy in General Dental Practice* [Australia: Biophoton Research Group Publication, 1993], 7.)

treated photophoretically by shining the laser light over this scar area. Beneficial clinical responses may include decreased inflammation and discomfort in the underlying dysbiotic intestinal region, as well as relief in the more distal associated disturbed fields.

laser: *Laser* is an acronym for "**l**ight **a**mplification by **s**timulated **e**mission of **r**adiation." The "radiation" aspect of this acronym refers simply to the expression of energy transmission by light, and not to harmful ionizing radiation.

electrophoresis: Electrophoresis is "the movement of charged particles suspended in a liquid under the influence of an applied electric field."[23] In electrophoresis, medications are rubbed on the skin and then a TENS or similar electrical instrument drives this medicine into the body through an electrode placed over the area. *Photophoresis* is the term coined by Klinghardt and Williams in 1993 to describe the effect of driving in remedies via the photon effect of laser light.

Laser therapy is especially efficacious in all phases of the treatment of dental foci. It can be used to prevent a future focus after a filling or crown is placed, by substantially reducing the inflammation caused by extensive drilling in the maxillary (upper jaw) or mandibular (lower jaw) nerves. It also has a significant therapeutic effect in the healing of the tooth and surrounding tissues. In fact, the laser's outstanding effectiveness in healing damaged nerves, gums, skin lesions, and other traumatized tissues has not only been observed by many practitioners clinically but well documented in scientific literature.[24]

Based on the magnitude of the positive clinical response, as well as the weight of the scientific research, many holistic dentists currently use a therapeutic laser after *any* stressful dental procedure. Thus, simply directing laser light to the root of a tooth or gum area after any type of drilling speeds healing in the inflamed tissues and can often arrest any damage incurred during this dental procedure that could potentially lead to a future devitalized tooth.[25] Furthermore, laser therapy is invaluable after dental cavitation surgery over the extraction site itself, as well as over any associated neighboring toxic ganglia.[26]

TYPES OF LASERS

Many types of therapeutic lasers are currently on the market. Not recommended are the types that have a pulsing light. I have observed clinically that these pulsing lasers cause stressful oscillation responses in patients (corpus callosum and pineal gland dysfunction and matrix tissue distress). For over a decade, the one laser that has worked well for my colleagues and me is the "Canadian laser," which has an 830-nanometer, 100-milliwatt output. One model has three milliwatt output choices—100, 200, and 400. The former 100-milliwatt laser can be loaned out to patients after they have had dental cavitation surgery (e.g., to be used six to ten times a day for approximately 60 seconds over the cheek of the surgery site for three to five days, to reduce pain and speed healing of the nerves, jawbone, and gum tissue). The stronger laser is ideal for clinical use in the office for a multitude of purposes—healing over new scars (e.g., 100 mw for 60 seconds or 200 mw for 30 seconds) and old scars (e.g., 200 mw for 30 seconds or 400 mw for 5 to 10 seconds), treatment of borderline focal teeth (e.g., 200 mw for 30 seconds or 400 mw for 5 to 10 seconds) and tonsil foci (e.g., 200 mw for 30 seconds or 400 mw for 5 to 10 seconds, to each side), a tooth with a new filling or crown that has been disturbing for months (e.g., 200 mw for 30 seconds), and auriculotherapy stimulation without needles (e.g., 100 mw for 5 seconds). Of course, milliwatt and times depend greatly on the acuteness or chronicity of the scar or focal infection, as well as on the sensitivity of the patient. (For more information on the Canadian laser, contact Rick MacKay at 250-474-3514 or e-mail him at jarek.mfg@shaw.ca.)

AURICULOTHERAPY

The term *auriculotherapy* is a combination of the Greek word *therapeuein,* which means "cure," and the Latin word *auricula,* which means "small ear."[27] Dr. Paul Nogier (1906–1996) of Lyons, France, coined the term in 1956 after exhaustively researching the diagnosis and treatment of ear reflex points in his patients. Nogier's odyssey had begun five years earlier in 1951, when he had observed the presence of a small scar in several of his patients that was located in the exact same area in the upper portion of the ear. His patients told him that they

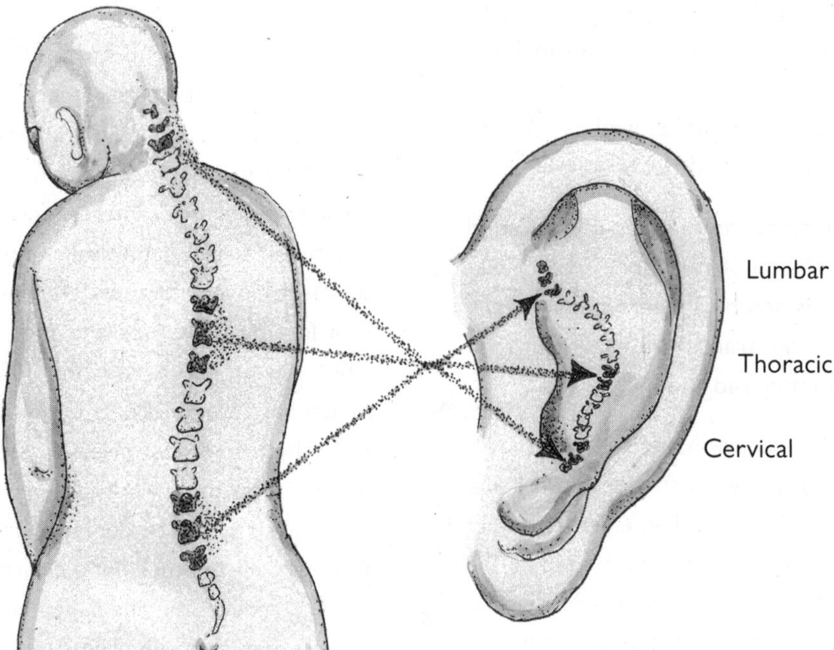

Figure 10.1. Beginning with the lumbar vertebrae, Nogier painstakingly linked areas of the spine with their corresponding points on the ear.

had been successfully treated for their sciatica (low back and leg pain) through the cauterization (slight burning) of this region of the ear.[28] This treatment was done by a lay practitioner in the area named Mrs. Barrin, who had been taught by her father, who had learned it from a man visiting from Manchuria.[29] When Nogier began to employ this same method on his patients with low back and leg sciatic pain, he had similar success.

> **sciatica:** *Sciatica* is the medical term for pain that follows the course of the sciatic nerve, radiating from the buttocks and down the leg.

One day, Nogier realized that this part of the ear might be related to the fifth lumbar vertebra—the spinal region that when misaligned, or when its intervertebral disc is prolapsed, puts pressure on the sciatic nerve and most often causes sciatica.* He began to research this possibility. After much clinical research with patients suffering from back pain in various areas of the spine, Nogier was able to correlate spinal areas with specific points on the ear (see figure 10.1). As this rudimentary map of the vertebral column projected on the ear developed, Nogier had the brilliant epiphany that these ear reflex points corresponded exactly to an inverted or upside down fetus (see figure 10.2).[30]

Working for decades with much perseverance and no doubt a psychic "sixth sense" aided by his extensive knowledge and understanding of the body, Nogier recorded every body point he found that consistently reflexed to a point on the ear. In 1956, he reported on the findings of his auriculotherapy research and treatments at a Premieres Journees d'Acupuncture congress in Marseilles, France.[31] Although small blood-lettings of ear points to treat impotency were recorded as far back as the fifth century BCE by Hippocrates (after he had studied in ancient Egypt for four years), Nogier was the first to originate and develop a complete ear acupuncture chart and a comprehensive system of treatment.[32] In fact, prior to 1956, only a few points on the ear were utilized by acupuncturists specializing in traditional Chinese medicine.[33] Later, after Nogier's articles had reached mainland China and had been studied by doctors of traditional medicine, the Chinese developed their own ear acupuncture charts.[34] However, the Chinese ear

*Dr. Nogier's previous study of acupuncture and manual medicine aided his intuition about auriculotherapy. Furthermore, Nogier's father had previously told him about an ear, nose, and throat doctor who had originated his own reflex microsystem called *centrotherapy,* which found that the turbinate bones in the nose corresponded to different parts of the body.

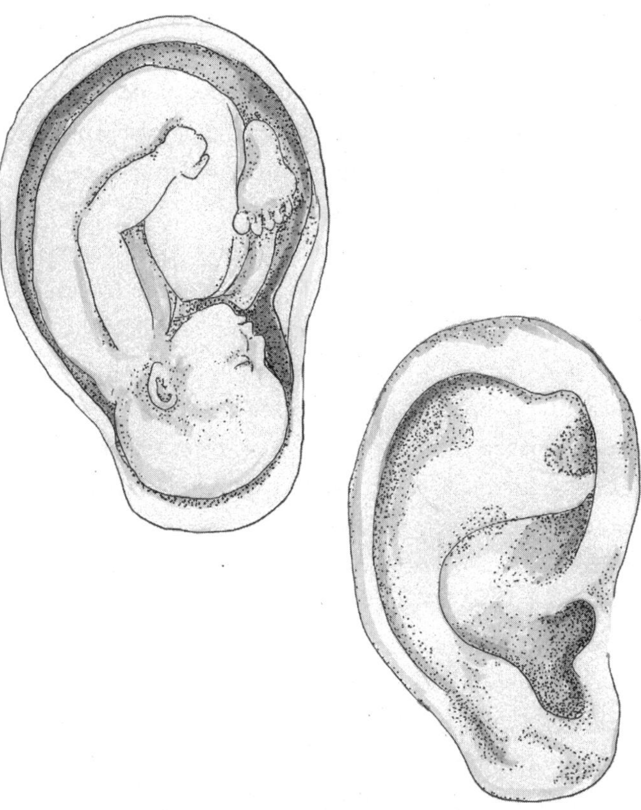

Figure 10.2. Dr. Nogier's startling epiphany that the shape of the ear and its related points resemble an inverted (upside-down) fetus

acupuncture charts are based on *functional* reflex disturbances, which differ greatly from Nogier's charts that are based on direct *anatomical* reflex points clinically correlated from specific areas of the body to the ear.[35]

Auriculotherapy has an advantage over neural therapy in that it can affect both the actual disturbed focus in the body's periphery as well as the memory of that focus, or *engram,* existing in the central nervous system (brain and spinal cord). Engrams are an important concept in the understanding of the etiology as well as the chronicity of foci.

While neural therapy treatments have more of a direct impact on the local nerves and tissues surrounding a focal region, or the peripheral nervous system, auriculotherapy has a more direct influence on the central nervous system, or the memory in the brain (engram) of a particular focus. In the following sections, two theories are postulated as to why auriculotherapy has such a direct and dramatic effect on the healing of foci through its connections to the central nervous system.

The Ear–Brain Connection

The ear is primarily innervated by the trigeminal (fifth), facial (seventh), glossopharyngeal (ninth), and vagus (tenth) cranial nerves and the superior cervical plexus (nerves in the upper neck), whose nerve fibers connect directly to the reticular formation in the brain stem.[36] The reticular formation is the oldest and most primitive nervous system in the body, and it has a powerful and widespread influence. For example, a single reticular neuron can descend from the thalamus and hypothalamus in the brain and travel through the brain stem and then down through the entire length of the spinal cord.[37] The unique feature of the reticular formation is that, when stimulated, it is affected *en masse,* and therefore it has the potent effect of arousing the entire cortex to instant wakefulness.[38]* This ability to alert and focus the brain's complete attention is proposed to be the chief means of how the reticular formation can instantly inform the cortex when a needle is placed in the ear. Thus, the auriculotherapist is "waking up" the brain to the dysfunction in the body through the stimulation of an ear point.

The particular dysfunctional area in the body, often a focus, is communicated to the ear through reflexes from the spinothalamic tract, which also synapses with the brain stem's reticular formation.[39] Running together in a tract from the spinal cord to the thalamus in the brain, the spinothalamic nerves convey sensory impulses of pain, temperature, pressure, and light touch.[40] Working in conjunction with the trigeminal nerves from the ear and the spinothalamic nerves from the body, this three-way brain-stem junction of the reticular formation confers profound consciousness and awareness in the body. It has been called the "junction zone of general and cephalic [head] somatesthesia."[41] *Somatesthesia* is the perception or consciousness of having a body. A focus negatively alters this body consciousness, which further strengthens the self-perpetuating aspect of the focal engram in the cortex. Auriculotherapy is effective

---

*This function of attentiveness is primarily regulated through the *locus cerueleus* region of the reticular formation in the brain stem. The locus cerueleus is also the region that has been identified as the primary area from which panic attacks emanate. Panic attacks, which can be thought of as "excessive attentiveness" to emotional fears, respond well to both auriculotherapy treatments and constitutional homeopathy.

ENGRAMS: "SECOND SCARS" IN THE BRAIN

With a long-standing focus, the body is constantly—albeit subconsciously—aware of its existence not only in the local focal region itself, but also in the central nervous system (CNS)—that is, the brain and spinal cord. The barrage of aberrant sensory *noise* generated from a chronic hernia scar—for example, in the peripheral nervous system (PNS)—informs the CNS of its continuous existence via the autonomic nervous system and the matrix tissue. After months and years of this constant sensory barrage, the focus actually creates a "second scar" in the brain. Referred to in neurology as an *engram,* it is "the lasting and permanent mark or trace left by a stimulus in nerve tissue."[42]*

Engrams are memory patterns that are learned over time. They allow us to master a skill such as riding a bike or playing the piano so thoroughly that we can eventually perform these functions almost unconsciously.[43] On the other hand, they also allow negative emotions to become embedded in our memory. These negative feelings can range from chronic deep-seated fears and hypervigilance linked to a psychologically traumatic childhood to an acute engram formation such as "I'm not safe" after being assaulted.

*Although engrams can be located anywhere in the body, the sensory area of the cerebral cortex in the brain appears to be "crucial to their organization." (D. Juhan, *Job's Body* [Barrytown, N.Y.: Barrytown, Ltd., 1998], 267.) Therefore, the cerebral cortex—where higher mental functions and reasoning, perception, and behavioral reactions emanate—is primarily where CNS engrams are established and perpetuated. These cortical engrams also chronically disrupt normal functioning in the corpus callosum, the approximately five-inch structure that separates the cortical hemispheres and regulates right and left brain activity. Incoherent or pathological oscillation patterns caused by the dysregulation of the corpus callosum have been clinically correlated through energetic testing to chronic foci and their well-entrenched cortical memory patterns, or engrams.

An engram associated with a chronic focus can be as difficult to clear as a psychologically induced trauma. This is especially the case because most individuals have never even heard of foci, so they are rarely diagnosed. Thus, little sympathy or further care is directed toward a root-canalled tooth or a scar once it has (seemingly) healed. Additionally, long-standing foci are always associated (directly or indirectly) with some form of suppressed and painful psychological memories, which only strengthen their grip on our subconscious and the chronicity of the resulting associated engram.

In his book *Job's Body,* Deane Juhan compares engrams to templates that produce different stitching patterns in a sewing machine.[44] Thus, every major focus is associated with a particular cortical "stitch pattern" in the brain. Over time, these focus-to-brain and brain-to-focus long-standing aberrant nerve and matrix tissue pathways coalesce into a chronic and vicious reflex cycle that only strengthens the pathogenicity and longevity of the focus. In fact, these engrams can become so *hardwired* in our central nervous system that even if a scar focus were magically entirely removed, many believe that the brain would eventually *restitch* another scar in the same location, dutifully following the same pattern.*

*Engrams also explain why "quick-fix" psychological techniques are only that—temporary and not lasting. (See chapter 18 for more information.)

because it communicates directly with *all* three of these areas: the somatesthetic junction of body consciousness in the brain stem, the engram or memory of the focus in the cortex, and the scar or focal infection itself in the body (see figure 10.3).

The Ear–Body Connection and Resonance with the Brain's Homunculi

A second essential factor in the efficaciousness of auriculotherapy in the clearing of chronic focal cortical engrams is that the cortex in the brain, like the ear, has a *somatotopic* relationship with the entire body. *Somata* is the Greek prefix for "body," and *topic* refers to "arrangement" or "place."[45] As previously described, and as the inverse fetus depicts (figure 10.2), every part of the body is represented and arranged on the ear in a configuration identical to the different anatomical parts of the body. In fact, when the ear is developing embryologically, it does so "in a mirror image fashion to the development of their associated brain structures at the same time."[46] Thus, as two leading auriculotherapists, Dr. Bryan Frank and Dr. Nader

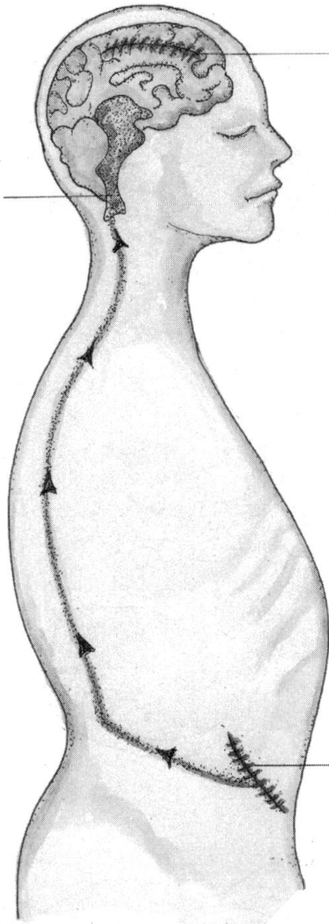

Figure 10.3. The three-way somatesthesia junction in the brain stem that allows auriculotherapists to treat chronic foci in the body, as well as to release their memory, or engram, in the brain

Soliman, describe this process, "the external ear develops as a 'mini copy' in exact conformity with the associated brain structures."[47] Both these parallel-developing structures—the embryonic ear and the embryonic brain—have a somatotopic, or body map, arrangement that "bear a striking resemblance" to each other.[48]

In the brain's cortex, this microrepresentation or map of the body is referred to as a *homunculus,* from the Latin word meaning "little man."[49] This homunculus represents both the position of the various tissues in the body and the degree of nerve innervation in the respective body parts—that is, how many nerves are committed to regulating each part of the body. According to Ralph Alan Dale, who developed the field of micro-acupuncture, homunculi, or microsystems, are "holographic reiterations of the body's qi."[50] For example, in humans the "little man" in the cortex has a *huge* face and hands because these strategic areas require the densest (and therefore most precise) nerve innervation (see figure 10.4). Other brain homunculi, or microsystems of nerve innervation in the body, are located in the thalamus (pain recognition and response) and the cerebellum (regulation of posture).[51]

Through his years of painstaking research, Nogier discovered and mapped out the ear's homunculus and discovered that it was strikingly similar to the homunculus in the brain. In his book *The Man in the Ear,* he described his years of painstaking auriculotherapy clinical research: "Little by little, I discovered that the various projections depend, not only on their anatomy, but also on their physiology. The auricular image of the thumb, for example, is clearly hypertrophied [enlarged]: one may remember how important its function is."[52]

Nogier had discovered that just like the cortex, the ear's homunculus mirrored both the *location* of the body's organs and tissues and their *importance* in the degree of nerve innervation. Furthermore, similar to the homunculi in the brain, the ear's homunculus is a major area for the densely innervated and strategic functioning of the thumb, as well as the other fingers and the rest of the hand (see figure 10.5). Because of these similar and parallel homunculi, it is possible that there is a direct morphogenetic resonance between the body map or "little man" in the ear and the body map or "little man" in the cortex of the brain. In fact, the ability of auriculotherapy to clear chronically disturbing scar interference fields and focal infections has been clinically proving this assertion in auriculotherapy offices all over the world for more than a century.

The ears—these "handles" sticking out on either side of our heads—have been clinically observed to be the most powerful of all the various microsystems in the body. In the body, or peripheral nervous system, there are other body maps that can be treated with pressure or needles, such as the well-known reflexology points in the feet and hands. Although treatment of these areas can be quite powerful, decades of clinical experience has revealed that the treatment of the points in the homunculus of the ear through Nogier's auriculotherapy methods is the *most* potent and lasting because of its direct communication with the inaccessible homunculi in the central nervous system (the brain and spinal cord).

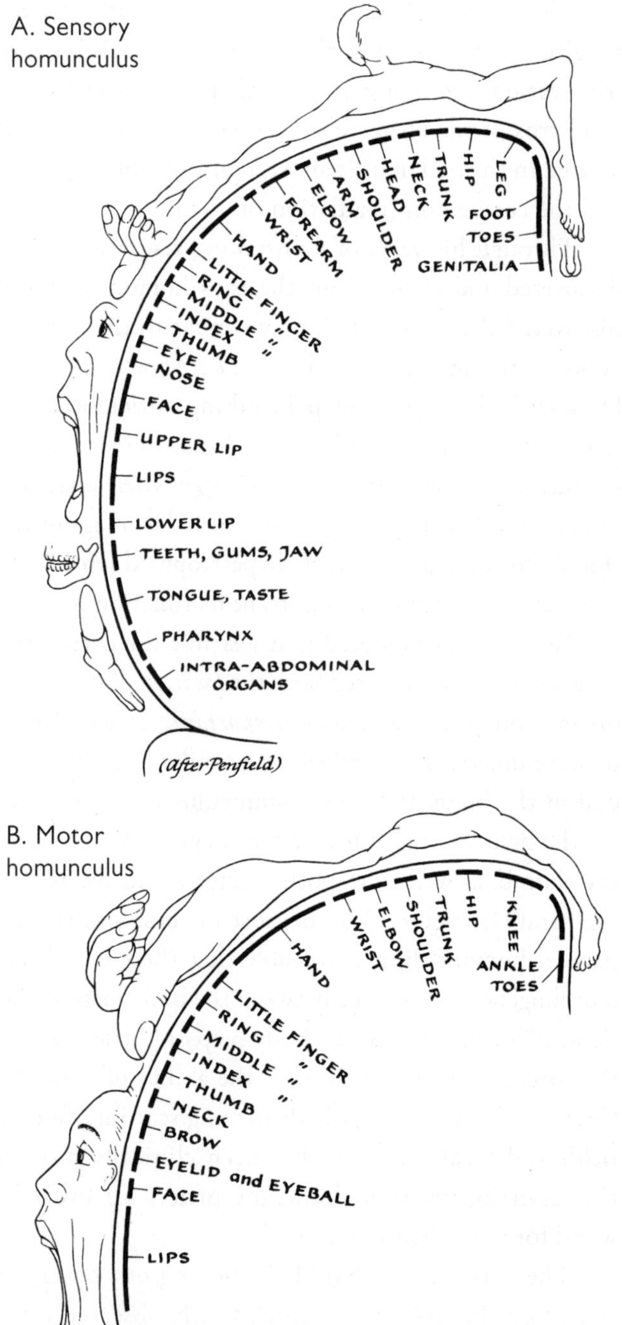

A. Sensory homunculus

LEG
HIP
TRUNK
NECK
HEAD
SHOULDER
ARM
ELBOW
FOREARM
WRIST
HAND
LITTLE FINGER
RING "
MIDDLE "
INDEX
THUMB
EYE
NOSE
FACE
UPPER LIP
LIPS
LOWER LIP
TEETH, GUMS, JAW
TONGUE, TASTE
PHARYNX
INTRA-ABDOMINAL ORGANS
FOOT
TOES
GENITALIA
(After Penfield)

B. Motor homunculus

KNEE
HIP
TRUNK
SHOULDER
ELBOW
WRIST
HAND
LITTLE FINGER
RING
MIDDLE "
INDEX "
THUMB
NECK
BROW
EYELID and EYEBALL
FACE
LIPS
JAW
TONGUE
SWALLOWING
ANKLE
TOES
(After Penfield)

Figure 10.4. The sensory and motor homunculi (body maps) in the cortex of the brain that represent how many nerves are committed to regulating each part of the body.

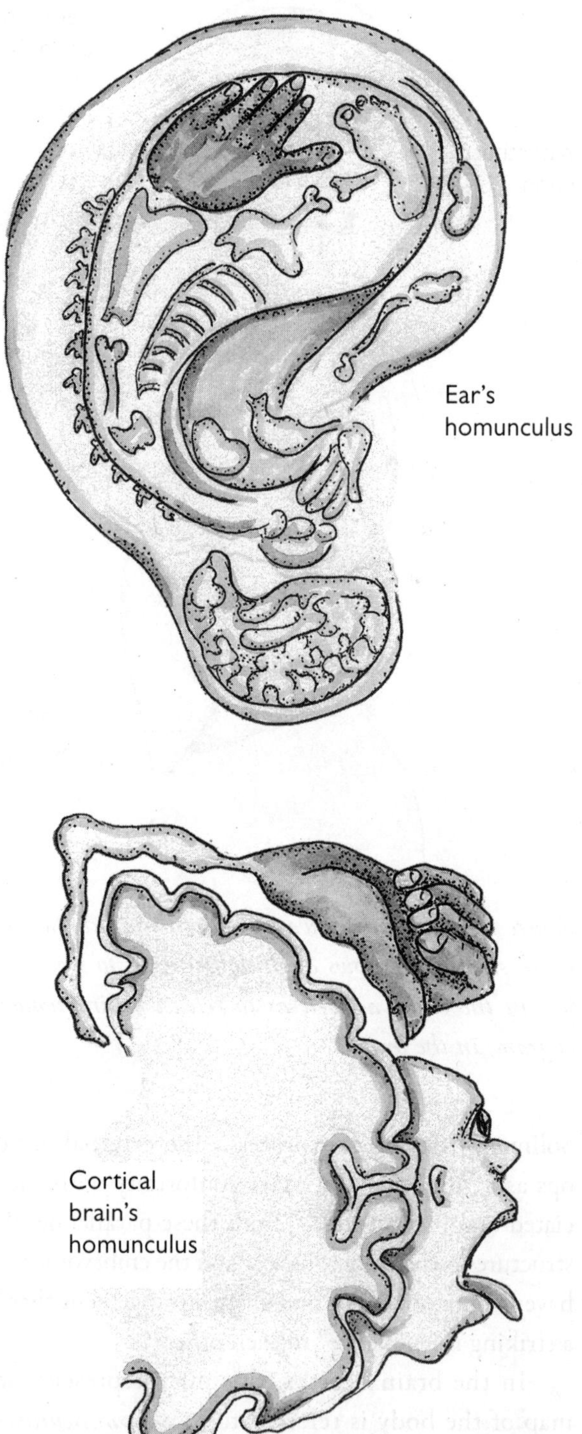

Ear's homunculus

Cortical brain's homunculus

Figure 10.5. The ear's homunculus has a large region directed to the hand, which mirrors the somatotopic organization of the brain's homunculus. (The motor homunculus is reprinted here with permission from the McGraw-Hill Companies from the book Principles of Neural Science, *by Eric R. Kandel, James H. Schwartz, and Thomas M. Jessell, published by Appleton and Lange, 1991, page 372.)*

WHEN TO USE NEURAL THERAPY AND WHEN TO USE AURICULOTHERAPY

Both neural therapy and auriculotherapy have their place in the treatment of chronic foci. Neural therapy is a direct method of healing because it specifically treats a scar or focus locally. Auriculotherapy is an indirect method because it treats a point on the ear distally that is anatomically representative of a focal area in the body.

The Benefits of Neural Therapy

Direct techniques such as neural therapy are effective in hooking up a patient's awareness to a focal area that has been neurologically and energetically somewhat separate and removed from the body's consciousness. This is especially the case when a focus is so old and degenerated that it has devolved into what has been referred to as an island of chronic unconscious distress, which (dys-) functions almost independently from *any* peripheral nervous system (PNS) or central nervous system (CNS) regulation. A woman's complete unawareness of the stress emanating from her fifteen-year-old hysterectomy scar and a man's unconscious irritation from his fifty-year-old hernia scar are examples of when individuals are completely unaware of any problem with the scar itself (in the PNS) or the disturbing memory pattern, or engram, of the scar interference field in their brain (in the CNS).

In these cases, it is often necessary to commence treatment with neural therapy—not with the goal of completely clearing the interference field but to allow the body to become more aware of the presence of this disturbing scar and to mitigate the chaos that it has caused locally in the PNS. Massage with shea butter, isopathic drops, and/or essential oils can be very effective in these cases to help "hook up" the disjointed and noncommunicating nerves (ephapses) and connective tissues (matrix) in the scar region. This initial "neural therapy without needles" has been found to be clinically effective in clearing from 70 to 85 percent of the disturbing effects of a scar interference field. This therapy is also effective in mitigating focal infections. For example, dropping Notatum 4X drops on a suspected dental focus can often mitigate from 60 to 75 percent of this disturbance (if surgery is not required).*

*The use of a 100-, 200-, or 400-milliwatt therapeutic laser to photophoretically "drive in" these isopathic drops can sometimes *completely* clear a dental focus (generally in one to four sessions), if the tooth is not already too devitalized. For more information, see the "Laser Therapy" box on page 312.

Auriculotherapy is then often indicated to clear the remaining impact of these foci—the engram, or memory pattern of the trauma of these foci in the brain, or CNS.

The Benefits of Auriculotherapy

There is a precedent in holistic health circles for the use of indirect techniques. For example, two of the most powerful therapeutic modalities in natural medicine—homeopathy and craniopathy—are indirect methods of healing. Indirect techniques are deeply potent in the same way that Jungian art therapy is powerful—that is, to release the subtle and chronic contraction and holding patterns "stuck" in our unconscious.

In fact, the protocol of treating initially with neural therapy and later with auriculotherapy can be compared to the classic practice in psychology of beginning therapy with counseling, and then later moving on to more potent techniques. Counseling and conventional cognitive forms of psychotherapy, similar to neural therapy, can connect individuals to their chronically held negative thoughts and feelings. However, after a certain level of understanding arises, many individuals seek out more potent methods to help further resolve remaining unconscious beliefs and sensations. At this point, indirect psychological techniques such as Jungian art therapy or breathwork* can be exceptionally effective in increasing their awareness and subsequent release of long-standing mental and emotional defensive contraction patterns. Analogous to auriculotherapy, indirect psychological techniques can more fully clear the traumatic and painful chronically held engrams in the central nervous system that perpetuate unconscious patterns of negative behavior and separate the individual from his or her true or essential self.†

Thus, because indirect techniques touch more of the unconscious origins of the formation of a particular

*Breathwork encompasses rebirthing as well as other types of methods used in the Ridhwan School, which uses breathing to "unearth" and inquire into deeply buried thoughts and emotions and to help release chronically held egoic contraction patterns over time. See chapter 18 for more information on breathwork.

†In his Clinical Kinesiology seminars, Gary Klepper, D.C., teaches that until a strong indicator *remains* strong when a patient thinks of a past trauma, there are still unresolved issues in his or her consciousness that need to be addressed. Therefore, any weakening is a positive response, indicating the need for more work—psychological or physical—on this particular issue. Scott Walker, D.C., also uses muscle testing in his Neuro Emotional Technique, or NET method. For more information, contact Dr. Walker at (800) 888-4638.

focus, they can more effectively release the most deeply held "cortical-stitch pattern," or engram, in the brain, unlike direct methods that effect change more locally. However, this is not to suggest that it is most advantageous to patients to simply skip neural therapy and be treated initially with auriculotherapy. Although there are instances where this approach might be appropriate, in most cases treating the PNS (body) disturbance first with neural therapy, and then later clearing the CNS (brain) engram with auriculotherapy, is the most efficacious process in the treatment of chronic foci. Similar to the "spiritual bypassing" practice described in chapter 18 where individuals try to engage in spiritual paths before having enough self-understanding and emotional maturity, "jumping" to auriculotherapy before neural therapy can be frustrating and ultimately unsuccessful.

THOROUGH TRAINING IS ESSENTIAL

Finally, a word of caution must be included for those who want to utilize auriculotherapy and neural therapy in their practice. Both of these systems can be quite powerful—and therefore also potentially harmful in the hands of an inexperienced practitioner, especially on a weak and compromised patient.

Neural Therapy Injections

Doctors

The art and skill required to diagnose and treat foci, their disturbed fields, and their neighboring ganglia through neural therapy injections necessitates comprehensive training and clinical expertise. So that they can gain the skills and clinical experience required to use neural therapy injections appropriately and successfully, doctors are encouraged to take several seminars, as well as to observe other physicians who use neural therapy in their clinics.

- Dr. Dietrich Klinghardt, a master in this field and a leading authority on the autonomic nervous system, teaches excellent courses on this subject in which participants not only learn neural therapy techniques but also come away with a greater understanding of anatomy, neurology, and biochemistry. Doctors interested in learning more can visit Dr. Klinghardt's website at www.klinghardtacademy.com. Dr. Robert Kidd also teaches neural therapy methods; contact him through www.neuraltherapybook.com.

Dentists

After placing a filling, inlay, onlay, or crown and at the end of cavitation surgery, dentists can help their patients greatly by injecting healing homeopathic or herbal remedies into the underlying tissues. Because the area is already anesthetized, often no additional local anesthetic is needed, just appropriate remedies to further healing after the trauma of drilling or surgery. Again, neural therapy seminars as well as holistic dental association conferences on this subject are recommended for dentists to learn this helpful form of dental neural therapy.

Neural Therapy without Needles

Although it may appear to be simple, the decision of which patients have the strength to initially treat their scars at home through massage and which require other systemic therapies first—such as avoiding their food allergy, removing amalgam fillings, or determining their homeopathic constitutional remedy—requires considerable clinical expertise. Furthermore, differentiating between the primary focus and its disturbed field, as well as identifying neighboring congested ganglia that need to be treated, necessitates significant study and hands-on experience. Finally, the skill necessary in using theraputic lasers—which milliwatt to use, for how long, when, and exactly where to place the probe—must also be learned before practitioners can use this modality confidently and correctly. Practitioners who wish to use neural therapy without needles in their practice should contact my office for a schedule of upcoming courses on this subject.

Auriculotherapy

Auriculotherapy is relatively complex and requires a considerable amount of study and clinical experience. For example, Paul Nogier discovered not just one set of points on the ear but four, which he termed *phases*.[53]* These four phases are "transitory holographic projections of the entire body, organs and tissues, onto the ear" that come into prominence based on the type and

*Chinese ear acupuncturists do not recognize the four phases of the ear.

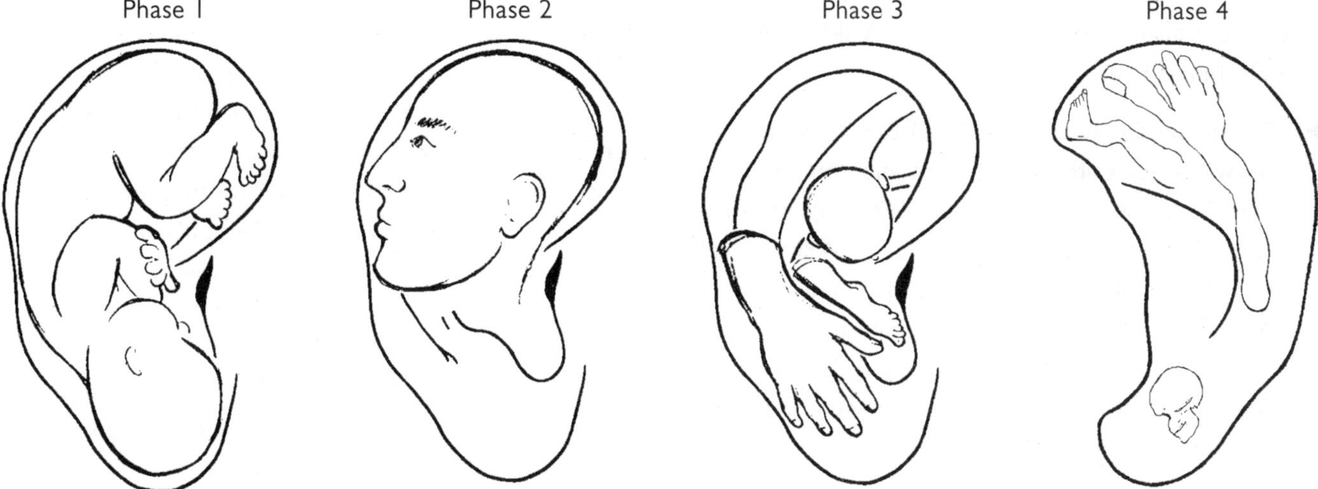

Figure 10.6. The four phases, or levels of dysfunction, in auriculotherapy. (Reprinted with permission from Bryan L. Frank, M.D., and Acupuncture Arts and Press, www.auriculartherapy.com.)

duration of the pathology of a particular focus, area of pain, or dysfunctioning tissue in the body through the integrative processing of the brain.[54] For example, when a phase 1 homunculus point tests positive with energetic testing, a nonpathological *functional* disturbance is occurring somewhere in the body. In contrast, a phase 3 point represents more *chronic* and *inflammatory* dysfunction, while a phase 2 point indicates frank *pathology* and *degenerative* conditions.* Thus, to diagnose and appropriately treat each of these phases, an auriculotherapist must thoroughly study and understand each of these phases and correctly identify the positive point(s) to treat the correct area of dysfunction in the body (see figure 10.6).[55] For example, a well-trained auriculotherapist knows that it is essential to treat a phase 3 point just after the treatment of a phase 2 point to avert a possible inflammatory healing crisis.[56]

Dr. Nogier also identified a fourth phase projected on the mastoid surface (back of the ear). However, treatment of this phase increases muscle tone and vasoconstriction (decrease of blood flow), so it is not as commonly used since most painful or dysfunctioning areas require the relaxing and vasodilating (increase of blood circulation) effects that occur with treatment of the first three phases on the external (outwardly facing) ear. Many modern auriculotherapists believe that phase 4 may actually represent the homunculi of each of the three phases of the ear as they are projected *through* the ear to the back side, possibly resulting in three mastoid phases, or six phases of the ear. Obviously, more clinical research needs to be conducted to more fully understand this fourth phase and the homunculi projected on the mastoid surface of the ear.

The practice of auriculotherapy is also complicated by Nogier's later discovery that these four auricular phases are further subdivided according to the three different embryonic tissue levels in the body—ectoderm, mesoderm, and endoderm.[57]* Therefore, an auriculotherapist must also determine which tissue aspect of a particular area is disturbed (e.g., the endodermal aspect of a tonsil focus), as well as its phase (e.g., the phase 3 inflammatory level of tonsil dysfunction), before he can determine the correct treatment point(s).

Auriculotherapy is an invaluable but complex system for the treatment of chronic foci. Practitioners who want to master auriculotherapy should be well trained in the art and science of this method to use it effectively in

*Dr. Nogier originally thought that pathology proceeded through a phase 1, then a phase 2, and last a phase 3 pattern. However, he later realized that the phase 2 homunculus projection on the ear was actually *more* pathological and degenerative than phase 3, so he changed the order. This is why the levels of dysfunction are currently counted in a nonordinal manner as "1, 3, and 2," with phase 1 being the least pathological and phase 2 the most pathological, while phase 3 is an intermediate inflammatory phase.

*Chinese ear acupuncturists do not recognize the different embryonic tissue types.

practice. In the United States, I recommend not only my courses but also courses taught by Dr. Mikhael Adams and Dr. Bryan Frank.

- To contact Dr. Adams, call (905) 878-9994 or go to www.integralhealth.ca. For information on Dr. Bryan Frank's courses, call (405) 623-7667 or go to www.auriculartherapy.com. To contact Dr. Williams, call (415) 460-1968 or go to www.radicalmedicine.com. Additionally, Dr. Frank and Dr. Soliman's new book on auriculotherapy, *Auricular Therapy: A Comprehensive Text,* is an excellent resource for both new and experienced auriculotherapists.

Techniques Not to Be Used Simultaneously

A further caveat that practitioners must be aware of is that neural therapy and auriculotherapy should never be done at the same time to treat the same focus.[58] That is, using an army analogy, it is confusing to issue simultaneous orders to both the privates in the army guarding the periphery (neural therapy) and the general who is normally in charge of commanding these soldiers (auriculotherapy). To do so could engender iatrogenic (doctor-induced) stress in the patient due to the neurological confusion resulting from the PNS-mediated stimulation from neural therapy concurrently with CNS-mediated auricular stimulation.

The one exception to this rule is in dentistry. As previously described, at the end of a dental drilling or surgical procedure when the area is already anesthetized, it is often appropriate to inject the site with homeopathic or herbal remedies. In these cases, it *does not* cause disturbance to inject these remedies locally and to treat the associated auricular points. The reason is that the neural therapy injection is experienced by the body as being part of the dental procedure, and not a separate (peripheral) therapy. Thus, after cavitation surgery, it is entirely appropriate for the holistic dentist to not only inject the site with homeopathic Arnica montana 200C or Notatum 4X but also to treat the related dental auricular point(s).

SPECIFIC TREATMENT PROTOCOLS FOR COMMON DOMINANT FOCI

Although it is beyond the scope of this book to describe and teach neural therapy and auriculotherapy in depth, a brief outline of the general treatment protocols for the most typical foci is included in chapters 11, 12, and 13. This outline will hopefully give potential patients a clearer "map" of what is entailed in healing dominant foci, as well as inform practitioners of the basic procedures. It should be noted that after reading the information addressing scars, individuals might become inspired to treat their scars at home through massage techniques. However, there should be a practitioner available as a backup before anyone attempts this form of neural therapy without needles, especially for those with moderate to major health problems, in case of strong healing reactions.

- For practitioners who would like to read further on the treatment of foci, the manuals *Neural Therapy without Needles* (Klinghardt/Williams) and *Neural Therapy for Naturopaths and Other Holistic Physicians* (Williams) are helpful. Although these two manuals focus only on neural therapy treatments, they are good resources for understanding the extent of dominant foci, their related ganglia, and their disturbed fields. To order these manuals, go to www.radicalmedicine.com.

This professional backup can also be helpful for those who experience the opposite effect—that is, *no* symptomatic change. A knowledgeable holistic practitioner can better ascertain whether the scar truly is active or, alternatively, whether it is quiescent and dormant—and therefore should be left alone. However, if the scar is an active interference field but does not respond appropriately to neural therapy, the practitioner should endeavor to discover what is blocking the therapeutic experience normally felt (to some degree) from this treatment. These "obstacles to cure"—typically toxic mercury amalgam fillings, major intestinal dysbiosis, the need for drainage remedies to clear congestion from chronic metabolic dysfunction, and so forth—often need to be addressed first. These cases are examples of the need to classically treat the "forest" (e.g., toxic metals, chemicals, or dysbiosis) before attempting to clear a specific "tree" (a focus).

However, there are always exceptions to this general rule. For example, a root-canalled tooth on the same meridian and same side as breast cancer should be considered a high priority and will often energetically test to be treated first. Even if it does not, the practitioner should always refer the patient to a holistic dentist for a second opinion when time is critical with a serious disease diagnosis. This unraveling of a patient's particular layers of pathology, often referred to as the "unpeeling of the onion," is best assessed by the detective-like prowess of a holistic practitioner who is skilled in energetic testing techniques and knowledgeable about foci, while working in conjunction with a similarly trained holistic dentist.

NOTES

1. P. Dosch, *Manual of Neural Therapy* (Heidelberg: Haug Publishers, 1984), 56–57, 195.
2. Ibid., 55.
3. D. Klinghardt, "Neural Therapy," *Journal of Neurological and Orthopaedic Medicine and Surgery* 14 (1993): 109.
4. T. Beardsley, "Take the Pain? Lidocaine Comes Under Suspicion as a Carcinogen," *Scientific American* 270, no. 5 (1994): 28–29.
5. A. Nickel, "Update on Heart Attacks and Cancer," unpublished paper, 2000, 1.
6. A. Nickel, "Aniline-Induced Toxicities from Local Anesthetics," self-published, 1996, 1.
7. A. Nickel, "Update on Heart Attacks and Cancer," unpublished paper, 2000, 1.
8. Ibid., 2.
9. P. Dosch, *Manual of Neural Therapy* (Heidelberg: Haug Publishers, 1984), 31.
10. Thorne Research, *Physician's Reference Guide* (Dover, Idaho: Thorne Research, Inc., 2002), 81.
11. P. Belaiche, *L'Aromatogramme,* vol. 1 of *Traite de Phytotherapie et D'Aromatherapie* (Paris: Maloine S. A. Editeur, 1979), 105–13.
12. J. Yasgur, *Homeopathic Dictionary* (Greenville, Pa.: Van Hoy Publishers, 1998), 127–28.
13. Ibid.
14. P. Gosch, "A Brief History of Bacterial and Fungal Isopathic-Homeopathic Remedies," *BioMed Report* 1, no. 2 (Winter 2002): 7.
15. Ibid.
16. R. Ullmann, "The Mode of Action of Bacterial Remedies," *BioMed Report* 2, no. 2 (Summer 2002): 15.
17. M. Sheehan, "Lab Study Proves That SanPharma Remedies Activate Natural Killer Cells," *BioMed Report* 5, no. 1 (2005): 1–3.
18. Ibid.
19. R. Ullmann and M. Sheehan, "The Benefits of Using SanPharma Isopathic Suppositories in Complementary Medicine," www.bioresourceinc.com/articles/benefits.php.
20. G. Lee et al., "The Application of Low-Power Laser Therapy and Its Rationale for Reviewing Pain Syndromes," *International Academy of Laser Dentistry* (Oct./Nov., 1992); X. Zhang, *Research on Acupuncture, Moxibustion, and Acupuncture Anesthesia* (Beijing: Science Press, 1986); D. Bartram, *Protocol for Combining Laser and Electrodermal Screening Techniques for Eliminating Interference fields from in and around the Jaw* (Hackney, South Australia: self-published, January 1992).
21. D. Klinghardt and L. Williams, *Neural Therapy without Needles* (Seattle: AANT, 1994), 91.
22. Ibid., 95–96.
23. J. Friel, ed., *Dorland's Illustrated Medical Dictionary,* 26th ed. (Philadelphia: W. B. Saunders Company, 1981), 427.
24. J. Kert and L. Rose, *Clinical Laser Therapy* (Copenhagen: Scandinavian Medical Laser Technology, 1989), 29–52; D. Bartram, *Low Level Laser Therapy in General Dental Practice* (Australia: Biophoton Research Group Publication, 1993), 15–47.
25. L. Williams, *Essentials of Cavitation Surgery* (Seattle: AANK, 1996), 24, 26.
26. D. Bartram, *Protocol for Combining Laser and Electrodermal Screening Techniques for Eliminating Interference Fields from in and around the Jaw* (Hackney, South Australia: self-published, January 1992); L. Williams, *Essentials of Cavitation Surgery* (Seattle: AANK, 1996), 21–40.
27. P. Nogier and R. Nogier, *The Man in the Ear* (Sainte-Ruffine, France: Maisonneuve, 1985), 41.
28. Ibid., 25.
29. B. Frank and N. Soliman, *Auricular Therapy: A Comprehensive Text* (Bloomington, Ind.: AuthorHouse, 2005), 6.
30. P. Nogier and R. Nogier, *The Man in the Ear* (Sainte-Ruffine, France: Maisonneuve, 1985), 28–29.
31. M. Adams, *Auriculotherapy Handbook* (Portland: self-published, 1984), 5.
32. P. Nogier and R. Nogier, *The Man in the Ear* (Sainte-Ruffine, France: Maisonneuve, 1985), 36–37, 41; P. Nogier, *Handbook to Auriculotherapy* (Sainte-Ruffine, France: Maisonneuve, 1981) 17; R. Bourdiol, *Elements of Auriculotherapy* (Sainte-Ruffine, France: Maisonneuve, 1982), 26–27.
33. M. Adams, *Auriculotherapy Handbook* (Portland: self-published, 1984), 5.

34. Ibid; P. Nogier and R. Nogier, *The Man in the Ear* (Sainte-Ruffine, France: Maisonneuve, 1985), 36–37.
35. M. Adams, *Auriculotherapy Handbook* (Portland: self-published, 1984), 5
36. J. Chusid, *Correlative Neuroanatomy and Functional Neurology,* 18th ed. (Los Altos, Calif.: Lange Medical Publications, 1982), 36; B. Frank and N. Soliman, *Auricular Therapy: A Comprehensive Text* (Bloomington, Ind.: AuthorHouse, 2005), 19–20.
37. E. Kandel et al., *Principles of Neural Science,* 3rd ed. (Norwalk, Conn.: Appleton and Lange, 1991), 692.
38. J. Chusid, *Correlative Neuroanatomy and Functional Neurology,* 18th ed. (Los Altos, Calif.: Lange Medical Publications, 1982), 36.
39. R. Bourdiol, *Elements of Auriculotherapy* (Sainte-Ruffine, France: Maisonneuve, 1982), 78.
40. G. Tortora and N. Anagnostakos, *Principles of Anatomy and Physiology,* 5th ed. (New York: Harper and Row, 1987), 346–47.
41. R. Bourdiol, *Elements of Auriculotherapy* (Sainte-Ruffine, France: Maisonneuve, 1982), 78.
42. J. Friel, ed., *Dorland's Illustrated Medical Dictionary,* 26th ed. (Philadelphia: W. B. Saunders Company, 1981), 444.
43. D. Juhan, *Job's Body* (Barrytown, N.Y.: Barrytown, Ltd., 1998), 268–69.
44. Ibid., 266.
45. M. Agnes, ed., *Webster's New World College Dictionary,* 4th ed. (New York: Macmillan, 1999), 1365, 1510.
46. B. Frank and N. Soliman, *Auricular Therapy: A Comprehensive Text* (Bloomington, Ind.: AuthorHouse, 2005), 22.
47. Ibid.
48. Ibid., 62.
49. J. Friel, ed., *Dorland's Illustrated Medical Dictionary,* 26th ed. (Philadelphia: W. B. Saunders Company, 1981), 616.
50. R. Dale, "The Principles, Systems, and Holograms of Micro-Acupuncture," *ICCAAAM '99 Conference Manual* (Las Vegas, August 12–16, 1999), 26–28.
51. E. Kandel et al., *Principles of Neural Science,* 3rd ed. (Norwalk, Conn.: Appleton and Lange, 1991), 371, 634.
52. P. Nogier and R. Nogier, *The Man in the Ear* (Sainte-Ruffine, France: Maisonneuve, 1985), 31.
53. S. Meeker, *Essential Auricular Reflexes* (Portland: Hollywood Clinic, 2002), 1–5.
54. B. Frank and N. Soliman, *Auricular Therapy: A Comprehensive Text* (Bloomington, Ind.: AuthorHouse, 2005), 45.
55. S. Meeker, *Essential Auricular Reflexes* (Portland: Hollywood Clinic, 2002), 1–5.
56. L. Williams, *Basic and Advanced AM/FM Manual,* part 2 (San Anselmo, Calif.: AANK, 1999), 53.
57. S. Meeker, *Essential Auricular Reflexes* (Portland: Hollywood Clinic, 2002), 1–5.
58. L. Williams, *Basic and Advanced AM/FM Manual,* part 2 (San Anselmo, Calif.: AANK, 1999), 54.

11

THE DENTAL FOCUS

In contrast to conventional medicine, dentistry has long recognized the term *focal infection*. In fact, the classic *Textbook of Pathology* by Dr. William Boyd thoroughly describes this term and the resulting disturbed fields that it causes in the chapter on dental pathology, as follows:

> The term *focal infection* as commonly used does not indicate merely a focus of infection but signifies the setting up of secondary infection at a distance from the original lesions [*disturbed field*]. With such a focus there are the following theoretical possibilities: (1) The bacteria may pass into the lymphatics and cause lymphadenitis [inflammation, pain, and swelling] of the regional lymph nodes. (2) They may enter the bloodstream, multiply there, and set up an acute or chronic septicemia.* (3) They may not multiply in the blood, but may settle in some distant part and multiply there. This is what is usually known as focal infection [again, for clarity this secondary site of infection is referred to as the *disturbed field*]. (4) They may remain localized, but their toxins may be absorbed and set up degenerative and fibrotic changes [scar interference fields] in distant organs.[1]

**Septicemia* is defined as a "*systemic* (whole body) disease associated with the presence and persistence of pathogenic microorganisms or their toxins in the blood." (J. Friel, ed., *Dorland's Illustrated Medical Dictionary,* 26th ed. [Philadelphia: W. B. Saunders Company, 1981], 1189.) An alternate term is *blood poisoning,* although this sounds rather alarming since most people think of acute blood poisoning with red streaks running up an arm or leg. However, chronic blood poisoning from focal infections is much more common, but so insidious that it is rarely accurately diagnosed.

To recap, the bacteria produced from a typical dental focal infection such as an impacted and infected wisdom tooth may travel to a joint and cause pain and stiffness, or to an organ like the heart and cause angina (chest pain) and intermittent palpitations. These bacteria may also pass into neighboring lymphatic tissues and initiate pain and swelling in the tonsils and surrounding cervical (neck) lymph nodes. All of these—the arthritic joint, the achy chest, and the sore throat—are typical *disturbed fields* that can result from this dental focus (figure 11.1).

DIAGNOSIS OF A DENTAL FOCUS

Signs and Symptoms

The following list includes significant history and symptoms indicating a possible dental focus.

1. The onset of the patient's present illness or health decline occurred *after* (days, weeks, months, or even years) a dental procedure (root canal, wisdom teeth extraction, implant, or a gold crown placed over an amalgam filling—that is, a "galvanic focus").
2. There was acute postextraction dry socket* or excessive pain, inflammation, or swelling.
3. Patient experiences chronic intermittent tooth or socket pain or sensitivity.
4. The patient has gingivitis (gum inflammation) with large pockets around the teeth or periodontitis (gum disease) with loose teeth.

**Dry socket* is the common expression used to describe the localized osteitis (bone infection) that can occur after an extraction. It occurs when the overlying blood clot is lost and the underlying bone becomes inflamed and infected. Symptoms are usually quite dramatic and include severe local as well as ear pain and a foul odor.

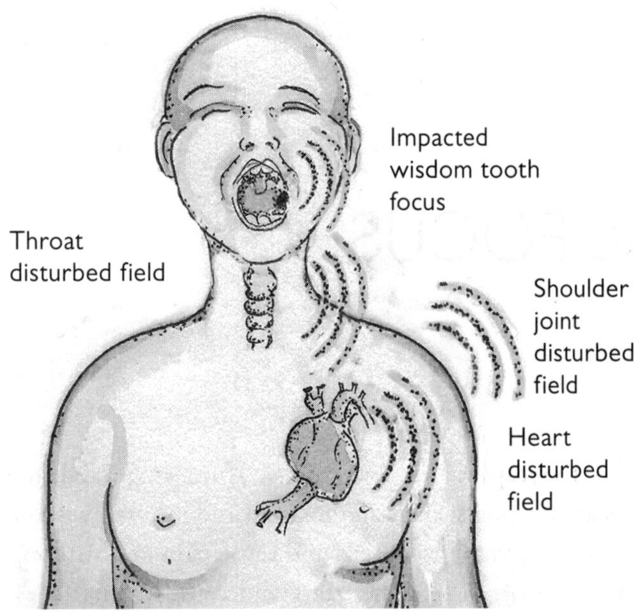

Figure 11.1. An impacted wisdom tooth focus and some typical disturbed fields—the shoulder joint, the heart, and the throat

5. There is an inability of a tooth to get numb before receiving a filling or crown, requiring large amounts of anesthetic.
6. There is previous shoddy dentistry and/or the use of military dentists.*
7. Trauma occurred to a tooth or the jaw area.
8. Chronic sinus infections occur above a suspected maxillary (upper jaw) dental focus.†
9. An ipsilateral (same side) chronically disturbed field, such as left shoulder pain and a suspected left upper first molar focus, is present.
10. Congenitally absent teeth sites are found.
11. Sometimes white blood cell counts are higher than normal.
12. X-rays are positive *or* negative for bone destruction (see next section).

*The military, especially during wartime with the need for expediency, has historically been notorious for providing very poor-quality dentistry.

†Of course, it is important to diagnostically differentiate whether the cause is a sinus focus or a dental focus. However, if both are chronically infected, each one then exists as an autonomous focus on its own. In patients with chronic sinus infections, it should also be determined if they have a primary (and secondary) food allergy. Strenuously avoiding one or more allergenic food groups can sometimes give chronically irritated and inflamed sinuses a chance to heal, if no dental focus is culpable.

13. Ultrasound diagnosis through the Cavitat device (see following section) or CAT scans or magnetic resonance imaging (MRI) was performed and indicated dead or dying areas in the jawbone.
14. Unhealthy-looking gums surround a tooth or cover an extraction site (e.g., inflammation, gums are boggy rather than firm, an abscess, bumps).
15. Pain or tenderness in the tooth or gum can be evoked by pressure, percussion, or vibration.*
16. (Unevoked) pressure occurs in the suspected area.†
17. Teeth are crowded, especially in the wisdom tooth areas, with little "retromolar space" behind them.
18. And very often, there are no symptoms at all. Again, it is important to reiterate that dental foci can be insidiously silent and may not engender any local symptoms. At times, the symptoms are so occasional and intermittent that an exact diagnosis of which tooth is disturbed and what is the exact problem is often difficult to make.

Diagnosis Through X-rays

From 30 to 50 percent of bone must be destroyed before signs become radiographically evident.[2] Therefore, X-rays can often appear perfectly normal and clear, even when there are frank symptoms and signs of a major dental focal infection. Furthermore, many radiographic appearances of bone destruction can be so subtle as to be virtually unidentifiable without extensive diagnostic experience.[3] However, many experienced holistic dentists have found that high-quality X-rays and multiple exposures at different angles can often reveal hidden bone infection that had gone previously undetected on poor-quality films or with only one exposure.[4]

*In 1995, Friedman elicited tenderness in the alveolar (dental) bone upon palpation in fifteen out of eighteen patients with dental foci. ("Maxillofacial Osteonecrosis, Signs & Symptoms," www.maxillofacialcenter.com/NICOclinical.html.) In a group of forty-eight patients with tender (to pressure) alveolar (jawbone) sites, all showed inflammatory or ischemic bone disease (focal infections) beneath the site. (McMahon et al., "Ischemic Osteonecrosis in Facial Pain Syndrome," *Journal of Craniomandibular Practice* 12 [1995]: 212.)

†Often patients complain of a pressure sensation in the area, which is consistent with the fact that internal bone pressures are much higher than normal in a dental focal infection site. ("Maxillofacial Osteonecrosis, Signs & Symptoms," www.maxillofacialcenter.com/NICOclinical.html.)

Positive X-ray Findings

Many holistic practitioners believe that if the X-ray findings are positive, cavitation surgery (tooth extraction and cleaning out the dead jawbone) should definitely be considered. Furthermore, if the patient is very ill or has recently been diagnosed with cancer or another grave illness, this surgery is *very seriously* considered to remove as much toxic material as soon as possible from the individual's compromised and failing system.

Negative X-ray Findings

However, if the X-rays are negative or ambiguous, dentists and practitioners should continue to be guided by one of the primary tenets of their holistic philosophy—*conservative care.* Thus, instead of diving into surgery or prescribing medications with side effects that can take up to two pages in a magazine *even* in fine print, they should utilize every appropriate holistic therapy available to strengthen the patient's immune system functioning to deal with the suspected dental focus. This approach can include any and all of the treatments described in this book, but *especially* the removal of all toxic metals in the mouth, a healthy diet, the avoidance of primary food allergens, and the prescription of the patient's constitutional homeopathic remedy. However, if these therapies fail and the decision is made to extract a suspected focal tooth, then the patient, practitioner, and dentist can be assured that despite their best careful and conservative efforts, dental cavitation surgery is indeed necessary and appropriate.

Of course, if the patient is seriously ill, time can be critical. In these cases, even when the X-ray findings are not clearly positive, as Dr. Hatton described in Dr. G. V. Black's landmark *Operative Dentistry* book from the 1930s, surgery may still be necessary:

> In cases of persons severely ill with heart disease, active diabetes, advanced anemia, leukemia, acute infectious processes, the acute stages of secondary focal infection, etc. [that is, the disturbed fields], it should be the rule to certainly eliminate all infection about the teeth, even though this may include the removal of a few treated teeth which appear to be negative, both in the X-ray and as a result of careful clinical examination.[5]

X-Rays Cannot Always Rule Out a Dental Focus

Thus, whether X-ray findings are positive or negative, they must always be considered as another tool to be weighed, along with the health of the patient, the physical exam findings, any pertinent lab tests, and the energetic testing results, in making a well-informed clinical decision. Because tooth and jawbone destruction is not always visible, X-rays are a good screening method for detecting more degenerative focal infections, but they cannot be used to *definitively* rule out the presence of a possible dental focus.

Diagnosis Through Ultrasound

The Cavitat instrument uses ultrasound technology to determine dead and dying areas in the jawbone. In February 2002, the FDA approved the Cavitat instrument for use in dental offices.[6] This instrument can identify areas of chronic ischemia (lack of blood supply) and low bone density characteristic of dental focal infections, which may not be visible on an X-ray.[7] In contrast to the false negative tendency of radiographs, the Cavitat instrument has been criticized for giving too many *false positive* readings. However, the use of a newer grading system—grade IV indicates dead bone, in contrast to grades I and II, which indicate that these might be healed nonsurgically simply by increasing blood flow—and improvements in the most recent model (Cavitat IV) have now purportedly reduced the level of false positives to approximately 2 percent.[8] Even with these reduced false positives, Cavitat research findings still reveal that dental jawbone osteonecrosis (dead bone) and chronic ischemia is truly epidemic. For example, in a recent study of more than 7,000 extraction sites, 94 percent were found to be positive for grade III and IV bone lesions.[9]

In light of this extremely high percentage, the question arises whether everyone should go out and have dental cavitation surgery performed on these sites. Many patients have done just that, with quite mixed results. These equivocal outcomes are due to many factors, but primarily because most of these individuals are not under the care of a holistic practitioner who is correlating the results of these imaging studies with the health of the patient, the history and physical exam findings, the X-ray findings (if any), and the energetic testing results before embarking on a permanent solution such as surgery. Furthermore, when it is clear that a socket needs to be treated or that teeth need to be removed, it is necessary that these surgeries be done in the correct order and by a skilled dentist or dental surgeon, with appropriate pre- and postoperative care. These decisions are best made through the coordinated efforts of an experienced holistic doctor and dentist, with the informed consent of a knowledgeable patient.

Other imaging instruments such as CAT scans or MRI have also been used with varying degrees of success to better determine the presence and level of infection in suspected dental foci.

The Ipsilateral Rule: Dental Foci Often Cause One-Sided Symptoms

One particularly helpful diagnostic clue is that in the vast majority of cases a dental focus causes *ipsilateral* symptoms—that is, symptoms on the *same side* of the body as the tooth is located. For example, if a patient presents with complaints of chronic right shoulder pain, right hip pain, and right-sided headaches, practitioners should immediately include a possible right-sided dental focus in their differential diagnosis (see figure 11.2). However, they must also keep in mind that these right-sided symptoms may be emanating not only from a right-sided tooth but also from a right-sided tonsil or sinus focus, a right-sided scar interference field,* or a chronically congested liver (which lies predominantly on the right side of the body).

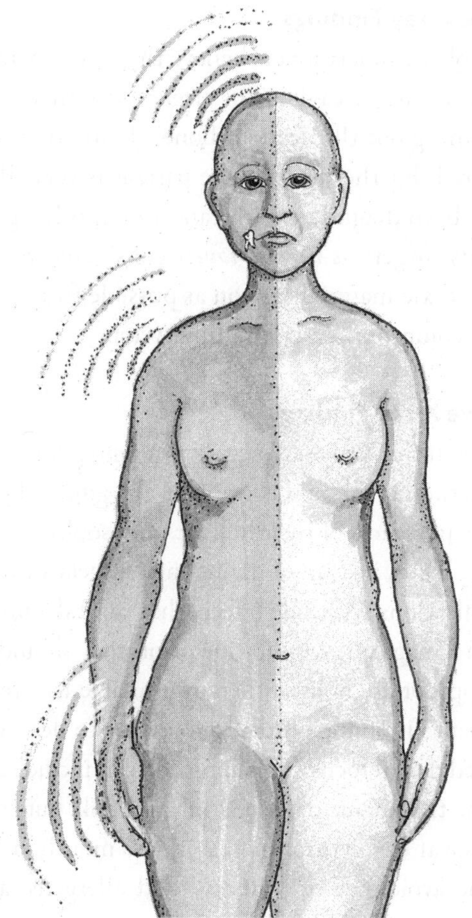

Figure 11.2. A typical example of a right-sided tooth causing right-sided disturbed fields

This ipsilateral rule is an important—and possibly life-saving—one to remember. For example, if a patient comes in with a diagnosis of left breast cancer, and she has an upper left second bicuspid tooth that has a gold crown placed over a root canal filled with mercury amalgam, then in biological dental circles this "corpse in a golden coffin" is a true holistic "code blue" (emergency), and the need for its expedient removal (with the consent of a well-informed patient) is quite clear (see figure 11.3).[10]

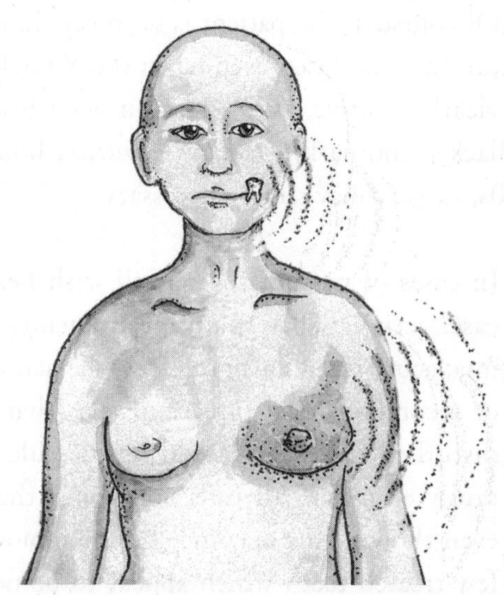

Figure 11.3. Another example of the ipsilateral rule: a left dental focus as a possible causative factor in left-side breast cancer

According to the research of Dr. Josef Issels, *thioether* (dimethyl sulfate) is the most dangerous toxin produced by root canals. This toxin is closely associated with the deadly combat gases used in World War I. Its gases have been proven to poison cellular respiration,

*However, scar interference fields can cause symptoms on the opposite side of the body too, as was described in the previous example with Dr. Huneke's famous patient whose surgical scar on the *left* leg caused a *right* frozen shoulder.

which forces the cell to produce energy through fermentation—thereby encouraging the growth of cancer.[11] Thus, in the face of serious degenerative diseases such as cancer, patients should be immediately referred to a qualified holistic dentist. In the majority of these cases, biological* dentists will recommend pulling the tooth and cleaning out the alveolar bone through cavitation surgery. However, if the suspected dental focus is on the right side of the mouth versus the left as in this example, the diagnosis and decision as to how to proceed is not quite as clear, and a secondary left-sided focus should be suspected.†

Homeopathic Remedies Also Treat "Sidedness"

It is also important to be aware that many constitutional homeopathic remedies treat this one-sided tendency of pain or dysfunction. For example, Belladonna and Lycopodium clavatum are treatments in cases of right-sided dysfunction, while Lachesis muta and Graphites naturalis treat more left-sided tendencies. Therefore, it is helpful clinically to determine (if possible) whether the patient's one-sided dysfunction or pain is due more to a focus or to a predisposing constitutional pattern that can be alleviated by homeopathy—*or* by both of these factors. If constitutional homeopathy is indicated, the patient should be referred to a well-trained and knowledgeable homeopath (see chapter 14).

Right- or Left-Sided Polarity and Emotional Patterns

Finally, a significant number of patients disclose that they experience vague right- or left-sided symptoms, such as muscle weakness, mild intermittent achiness, or simply just a heightened awareness of one side of their body. In modern neurological terms, this is a sign of sympathetic nerve dysfunction expressed by thermatomal patterns. Dr. Peter Dosch described this sidedness phenomenon in his *Manual of Neural Therapy:* "Some patients draw our attention to an autonomic asymmetry, which can be proved objectively from the blood picture (Bergsmann) by telling us that 'everything always happens to me on my right (or left) side.'"[12]

In more energetic terms, this laterality has been attributed to imbalanced or blocked life energy currents in the body, as described by the late Randolph Stone, D.C., D.O., in his field of expertise termed *polarity therapy*.[13] Additionally, in somatic-oriented psychological circles, right-sided polarity tendencies originate from a conflict with one's father, or with the powerful yang-like father forces. Problems on the left side spring from conflict with one's mother, or the more yin-nurturing mother forces.

These emotional and energetic lateralities often coexist with the ipsilaterally affecting focal infections or scar interference fields, making the diagnosis of pain or dysfunction on one side of the body even more challenging. Interestingly, individuals with major emotional issues with their mother, for example, also seem to attract numerous issues on their left side such as more dental cavities and abscesses, tonsil infections, and injuries that eventually coalesce into left-sided foci that further aggravate their chronic left-sided pain or dysfunction.

Impacted Wisdom Teeth Often Cause Bilateral Symptoms

When all four wisdom teeth are impacted or crowded, or at least one on each side of the mouth such as both of the mandibular (lower jaw) third molars, the patient will often present with bilateral (both sides affected) symptoms. These symptoms can include general leg weakness, intermittent abdominal pain (centralized pain, since both sides of the intestine are affected), or both right and left carpal tunnel wrist pain—with no (or very little) tendency toward laterality to one side or the other (see figure 11.4).

This is also the case whenever patients have dental focal infections on both sides of the mouth—whether they are the third molars or other teeth. Additionally, a focal infection arising in the midline teeth such as the front teeth can also cause midline or bilateral pain or dysfunction in the body, with very few lateralizing effects manifesting on one side or the other.

*The term *biological* is synonymous with *holistic*.

†In this example, although a right-sided dental focus and left breast cancer is not as clear-cut a causative relationship, simply the presence of dental galvanism (gold and mercury) mixed with the bacteria produced from a root-canalled tooth produces toxins that are disseminated everywhere in the body through blood and lymph channels. Thus, in any cancer patient, the systemic poison emanating from *any* major dental focus is a considerable load on an already compromised system, and the prompt removal of this dental focus should be seriously considered—no matter where it is located.

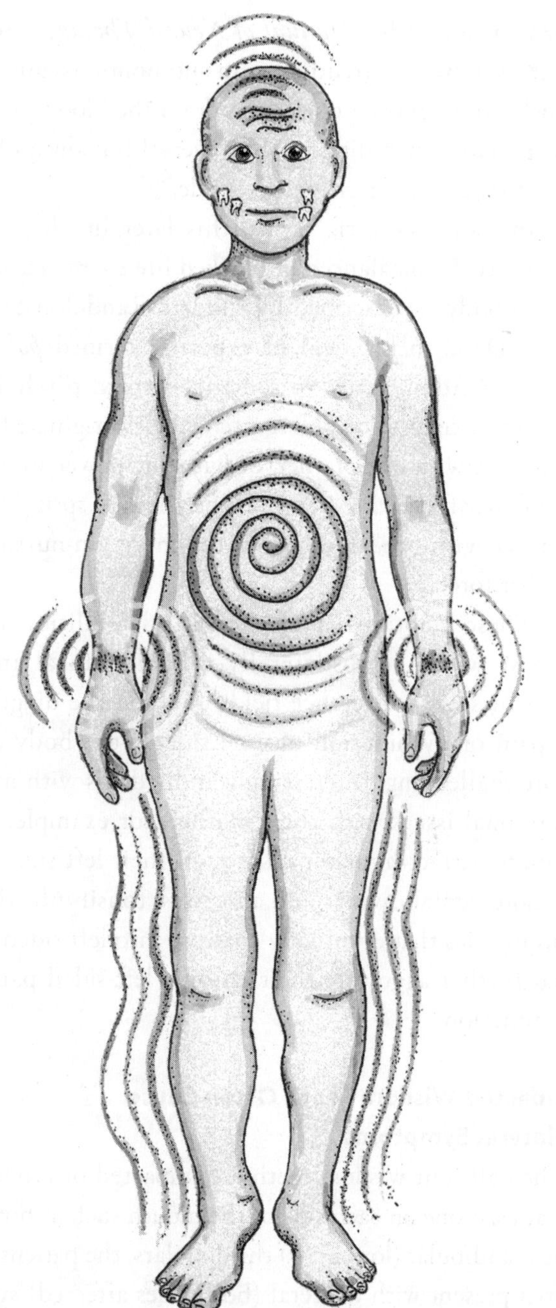

Figure 11.4. An example of bilateral symptoms (disturbed fields) from four impacted wisdom teeth foci

The Dental Relationship Chart

Another valuable diagnostic aid in assessing dental foci, as well as determining their disturbed fields in the body, was developed in the 1950s by Fritz Kramer, D.D.S., and Reinhold Voll, M.D.[14] As briefly described earlier, by using Voll's electroacupuncture instrument, Kramer found that based on Chinese medicine's five-element theory, each tooth correlated to an acupuncture meridian, as well as to that meridian's corresponding organs and tissues.[15] This discovery was termed the five-element odontosomatic relationship (*odonto* refers to the teeth and *soma* to the body).*

Holistic practitioners and dentists have used the dental-body relationship chart for decades as a helpful guide in diagnosing both the dental focus as well as its disturbed field in the body. The use of this chart helps identify not only general ipsilateral disturbed fields but also the specific ipsilateral tissues and organs that are particularly disturbed by the dental focus. For instance, using the previous example of a breast cancer patient with a left upper second bicuspid dental focus (tooth #13), the chart in figure 11.5 shows that this tooth relates to the left breast. In this case, knowledge of this chart should alert the practitioner to the possibility of a causative tooth-breast relationship, even if he or she knows nothing about focal infection theory. At the very least, this patient should be referred to a knowledgeable holistic dentist to have this suspected tooth thoroughly evaluated.

▶ Dental relationship charts are available to order through the www.radicalmedicine.com website.

Of course, like all linear measurements of dynamic living organisms, this chart should be used *only* as a guide, because other neurological and energetic influences can affect these five-element odontosomatic patterns. For example, in the case of chronic dental focal infections, secondary adaptation patterns may occur. That is, after years of "sharing the stress" with a disturbed field, a tooth may further compensate by disturbing other teeth. In the five-element theory, these secondary adaptation pathways are called *ko* (the destructive pattern), *mother-son* (the promoting pattern), and *counteracting* (the adaptative pattern). In a clinical setting, I have observed the *counteracting* relationship, which Chinese medicine has acknowledged for millennia, to be the most typical dental focus adaptive pattern. For example, this counteracting cycle explains why so many third molar focal infections (from incomplete and incorrectly performed extractions) not only adversely affect the small intestine and heart but also

*Actually, the term *odonton* refers to the entire structure of the tooth—the tooth itself, the pulp inside, the periodontal ligament, the nerves leading to the tooth, and the jawbone.

Dental Relationship Chart

Joints	Right: shoulder/elbow/hand (ulnar), S.I. joint, foot, toes	Right: TMJ, anterior hip/knee, medial ankle		Right: Shoulder/elbow/hand (radial), foot, big toe		Right: Posterior knee, hip, lateral ankle	Right: Posterior knee, sacrococcygeal joint, posterior ankle		Left: Posterior knee, sacrococcygeal joint, posterior ankle		Left: Posterior knee, hip, lateral ankle	Left: Shoulder/elbow/hand (radial), foot, big toe		Left: TMJ, anterior hip/knee, medial ankle		Left: shoulder/elbow/hand (ulnar), S.I. joint, foot, toes
Mammary Glands		Right breast											Left breast			
Endocrine Glands	Anterior pituitary	Parathyroid	Thyroid	Thymus	Posterior pituitary	Intermediate lobe of pituitary	Pineal		Pineal		Intermediate lobe of pituitary	Posterior pituitary	Thymus	Thyroid	Parathyroid	Anterior pituitary
Organs	Right heart, right duodenum, terminal ileum	Pancreas, right side of stomach, esophagus		Right lung, right side of large intestine		Right side of liver, gall bladder, right side of biliary ducts	Right kidney, bladder, uterus, prostate, rectum, anus		Left kidney, bladder, uterus, prostate, rectum, anus		Left side of liver, left side of biliary ducts	Left lung, left side of large intestine		Spleen, left side of stomach, esophagus		Left heart, left side of duodenum, jejunum ileum
Teeth Pictured	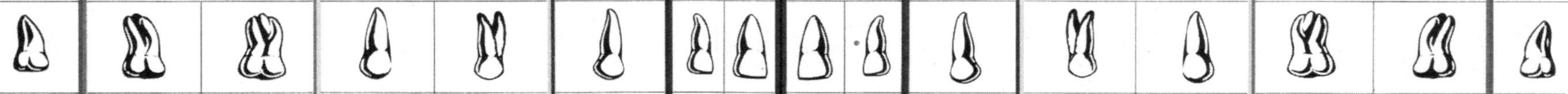 Retromolar															Retromolar
Names of Teeth	Right upper 3rd molar (wisdom)	Right upper 2nd molar	Right upper 1st molar	Right upper 2nd bicuspid (pre-molar)	Right upper 1st bicuspid (pre-molar)	Right upper canine (cuspid)	Right upper lateral incisor	Right upper central incisor	Left upper central incisor	Left upper lateral incisor	Left upper canine (cuspid)	Left upper 1st bicuspid (pre-molar)	Left upper 2nd bicuspid (pre-molar)	Left upper 1st molar	Left upper 2nd molar	Left upper 3rd molar (wisdom)
American Nomenclature	1	2	3	4	5	6	7	8	7	8	11	12	13	14	15	16
	32	31	30	29	28	27	26	25	26	25	22	21	20	19	18	17
Names of Teeth	Right lower 3rd molar (wisdom)	Right lower 2nd molar	Right lower 1st molar	Right lower 2nd bicuspid (pre-molar)	Right lower 1st bicuspid (pre-molar)	Right lower canine (cuspid)	Right lower lateral incisor	Right lower central incisor	Left lower central incisor	Left lower lateral incisor	Left lower canine (cuspid)	Left lower 1st bicuspid (pre-molar)	Left lower 2nd bicuspid (pre-molar)	Left lower 1st molar	Left lower 2nd molar	Left lower 3rd molar (wisdom)
Teeth Pictured	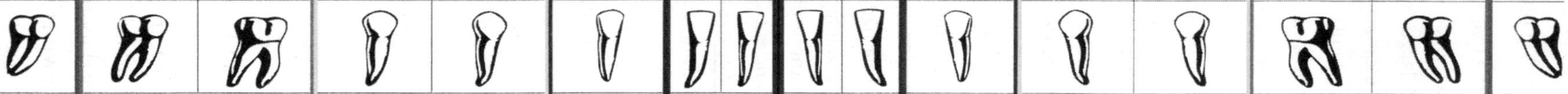 Retromolar															Retromolar
Organs	Right heart, terminal ileum, ileo-cecal	Pancreas, right side of stomach, esophagus		Right lung, right side of large intestine		Right side of liver, gall bladder, right side of biliary ducts	Right kidney, bladder, uterus, prostate, rectum, anus		Left kidney, bladder, uterus, prostate, rectum, anus		Left side of liver, left side of biliary ducts	Left lung, left side of large intestine		Spleen, left side of stomach, esophagus		Left heart, left side of jejunum, ileum
Endocrine Glands					Ovaries	Testicles	Adrenals		Adrenals		Ovaries	Testicles				
Mammary Glands				Right breast								Left breast				
Joints	Right: Shoulder/elbow/hand (ulnar), S.I. joint, foot, toes	Right: TMJ, anterior hip/knee, medial ankle		Right: Shoulder/elbow/hand (radial), foot, big toe		Right: Posterior knee, hip, lateral ankle	Right: Posterior knee, sacrococcygeal joint, posterior ankle		Left: Posterior knee, sacrococcygeal joint, posterior ankle		Left: Posterior knee, hip, lateral ankle	Left: Shoulder/elbow/hand (radial), foot, big toe		Left: TMJ, anterior hip/knee, medial ankle		Left: Shoulder/elbow/hand (ulnar), S.I. joint, foot, toes
	Fire	**Earth**		**Metal**		**Wood**	**Water**		**Water**		**Wood**	**Metal**		**Earth**		**Fire**

Figure 11.5. The dental relationship chart, based on the original chart developed by Dr. Fritz Kramer, with some changes by Klinghardt/Williams. (See plate 6 for a color rendition of this chart.)

REVISIONS TO THE DENTAL RELATIONSHIP CHART

There has been some controversy over the five-element dental relationship chart. As experienced practitioners may note in figure 11.5, the lung and large intestine meridians and the spleen (pancreas) and stomach meridians are *not* switched on the lower mandibular molars and bicuspid teeth, as was the case with Kramer's original chart. This change from the original chart is based on the clinical experience of my colleagues and myself, after years of correlating dental foci with disturbed fields in the body using kinesiological and reflex arm length testing. These findings were additionally confirmed by Dr. Van Benschoten, a California Oriental medical doctor. His research findings, published in the *American Journal of Acupuncture,*[16] documented what many kinesiologists have suspected—that the electric current induced into the body by electroacupuncture instruments can cause distorted readings in the patient. For example, Benschoten's research revealed that Voll had incorrectly switched the lung meridian to the ulnar aspect of the thumb from its classic location on the radial side, where it had been originally located by ancient Chinese acupuncturists. Benschoten discovered that this inaccuracy was due to electromagnetic distortion caused by the electrical current from Voll's Dermatron machine. In fact, all the electroacupuncture machines Benschoten measured in this study were found to cause distorted readings based on their high electrical currents. For example, the Voll instrument induces 900 millivolts, and Schimmel's Vegatest induces 1,500 millivolts into acupuncture test points, and thus into the patient's body. Considering that a nerve action potential has been measured to fire at 60 millivolts or less, it is understandable how these electroacupuncture instruments engender stress in the nervous system with resulting inaccurate readings. Additionally, the flow of natural energy currents along acupuncture meridians and throughout the matrix tissue is even subtler than in the nervous system, and therefore even more susceptible to electromagnetic stress induced by these electrical computer acupuncture instruments. Thus, based on years of energetic testing using autonomic nerve reflexes, acupuncture meridians, and matrix tissue reflexes (but not instruments utilizing electrical currents), I have found that patients most often test out based on the dental chart pictured in figure 11.5, which does not switch the mandibular meridian relationships.

over the years often start to impair prostate, bladder, and uterine function (see figure 11.6).

Is the Tooth the Focus or the Disturbed Field?

The dental relationship chart is also clinically invaluable in that it can help doctors and dentists determine where the culpable focus resides—in the tooth or the body. That is, pulling a tooth and having a root canal are both permanent measures that cannot be reversed. Therefore, it is essential that practitioners are cognizant of the possibilities of these dental relationships so that they can factor this information into the patient's history, exam, laboratory, and X-ray findings. By factoring in all the data, the practitioner can make a more informed decision and help ensure that a patient never needlessly loses a still vital tooth.

For example, if a patient has unknowingly eaten sugar as well as his major food allergen for years and thus depleted his pancreatic enzymes, his intermittent lower first molar pain (tooth #30) could be primarily due to a somato-odonton (pancreas-tooth) relationship (see the dental chart, figure 11.5). The pancreas may actually be the primary focus, and through this disturbance to the spleen meridian, the first molar eventually became a disturbed field. In many cases, this first molar has already been compromised and has a filling or crown on it. However, mild intermittent inflammation in this tooth should necessitate not an immediate root canal procedure as so many nonholistic dentists reflexively prescribe, but a careful diagnostic procedure to determine the underlying cause of this dental disturbance.

One positive aspect of this body-tooth causation is that individuals can be very motivated to avoid sugar as well as their food allergen to help save their tooth. These patients should also be prescribed the beneficial "crutch" of digestive enzyme supplementation for months or even years to restore pancreatic enzyme output, as well as save the tooth. Additionally, a patient's constitutional homeopathic remedy can be invaluable in restoring homeosta-

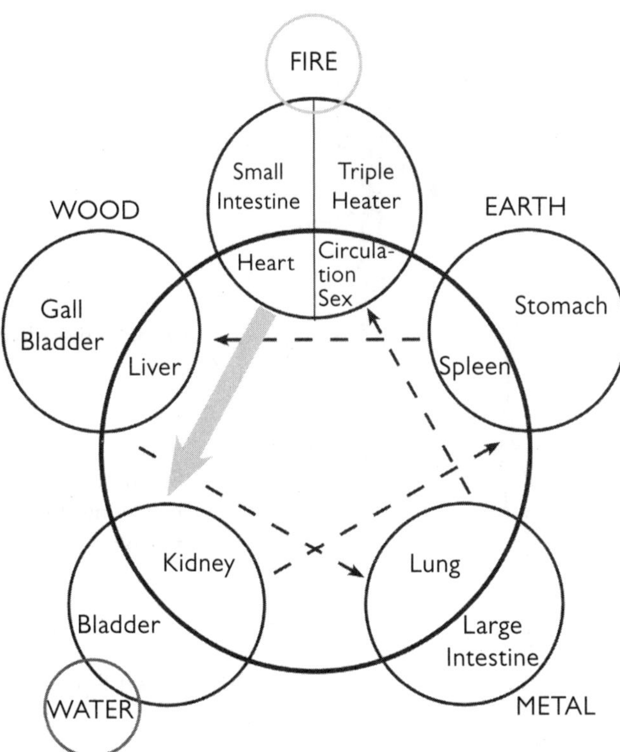

Figure 11.6. The counteracting cycle. Over time a third molar extraction-site focal infection may begin to trigger prostate, bladder, or uterine disturbance through the "counteracting" five-element adaptive pathway.

sis and more unimpeded and beneficial immune system functioning in the body, as well as to a borderline tooth. The inclusion of laser therapy, generally from three to seven sessions or so, can also heal the tooth, its roots, and the surrounding nerves and gums. Of course, if the filling or crown material is made up of a toxic metal, or if there is a suspected interference point (malocclusion*) on either of these restorations, a holistic dentist must promptly address these issues.

However, as discussed in chapter 9 regarding focal chains, over time this tooth disturbed field can become so inflamed and infected that it can begin to function as a primary focus itself. Over time, if this focal tooth becomes too devitalized, it will not respond to conservative care and may require extraction and cavitation surgery.

*Sometimes a tooth is chronically inflamed due to occlusal trauma, that is, a bad bite. In these cases, equilibrating, that is, drilling off the points of interference on a few teeth, can be appropriate when performed by a well-trained holistic dentist. However, when a patient has a major malocclusion, appliance or splint therapy is necessary. (For more information on the treatment of malocclusions see chapter 16.)

The Five Rheumatic Disturbed Fields

The word *rheumatism* might sound rather old-fashioned, but its effects are still predominant in many people's lives. Although *rheumatism* has developed over the years into a catchall term for all forms of joint and muscle diseases, it actually describes *all* the diseases and syndromes that are caused by streptococcus and staphylococcus bacterial infection, which are in no way limited to just the joints. Numerous researchers have observed through countless studies that not only do strep bacteria from a patient tend to migrate to the same tissues in lab animals in which the patient had shown dysfunction (the theory of *elective localization*) but also that these bacteria tend to migrate most often to the same five tissues.[17] These five areas are the heart (e.g., rheumatic fever, subacute bacterial endocarditis, mitral valve stenosis); the joints and muscles (e.g., rheumatoid arthritis, juvenile arthritis, fibromyalgia, myositis); the kidneys (acute and chronic glomerular nephritis); the stomach, duodenum (ulcers), and appendix (appendicitis); and the brain (e.g., chorea,* ADD, ADHD, Tourette's, PANDAS). Although the modern use of antibiotics has obscured the causal relationship between rheumatic diseases and dental and tonsil focal infections, these diseases still exist, although some of the names have changed.

Therefore, besides the previously described odontosomatic or tooth-body relationships, disturbed fields also form in the body according to these five primary areas where the microenvironment is most favorable for streptococcal bacterial growth. And often, both influences are at play. That is, a patient may suffer from a chronically painful arthritic left hip from a dental focus, rather than full-blown rheumatoid arthritis affecting all joints on both sides of the body. This left hip disturbed field example is caused by the migration of strep bacteria to a joint, as well as the odontosomatic relationship from, for example, a lower left second molar root canal focus (tooth #18) through the stomach and spleen meridians (see figure 11.7). Thus, in this example, two factors are at play: the normal metastasis of strep bacteria from a dental focus to joints in the body, and the energetic influence of the stomach and spleen meridians subtly directing these bacteria to coalesce more in the ipsilateral tooth-related

*Sydenham's chorea, also called rheumatic chorea or St. Vitus's dance, is a central nervous system (brain and spinal cord) disease caused by streptococcus infection, characterized by nonrepetitive, involuntary, and purposeless movements.

joint—in this case, the patient's left hip. Of course, with more allopathic dental treatment, other stressors in life, and the further degeneration of tissue, this patient may begin to experience systemic joint inflammation—that is, pain in all the joints on both sides of the body. At this point, the patient will be typically diagnosed with the autoimmune disease rheumatoid arthritis and be prescribed nonsteroidal anti-inflammatory drugs (NSAIDs) by an allopathic physician. However, when carefully questioned, even chronic rheumatoid arthritis patients can usually tell you which side is most painful or on which side the pain began, and this piece of history can be helpful in identifying the original culpable dental (or tonsil) focal infection.

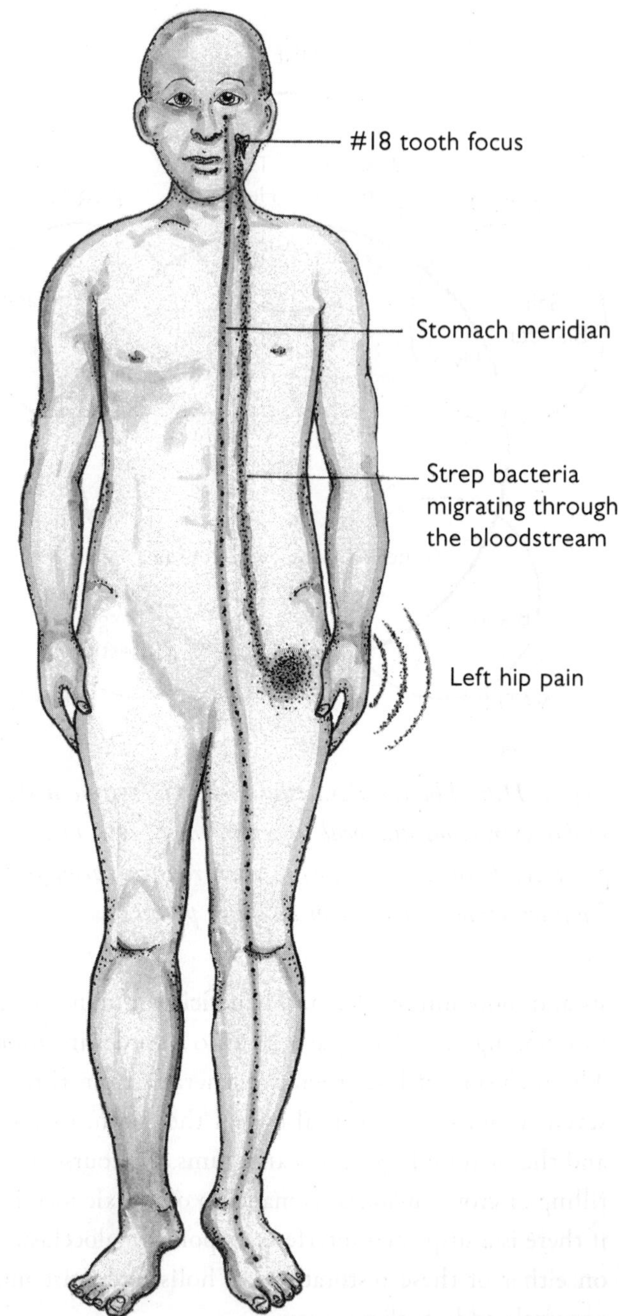

Figure 11.7. A left hip disturbed field caused by the general migration of streptococcus bacteria from tooth #18 (rheumatic relationship), as well as by the specific ipsilateral dental-joint pathway (odontosomatic relationship)

Determining Tooth Viability

Even with the help of the dental chart, energetic testing, and years of clinical experience, it often can be difficult for holistic practitioners to determine tooth viability. This section outlines some of the factors to keep in mind.

The Teeth's Sacrificial Role

Past indiscretions, such as in the previous example of the depleted pancreatic enzymes, are often the primary etiology (or cause) of dental foci. Children often have refined-sugar-laden diets, are given too many courses of antibiotics, and end up with rather intractable dysbiotic intestines and therefore impaired (mildly to greatly) pancreas and liver functioning as adults. Thus, besides the direct assault from refined sugar that causes cavities, the teeth also suffer reflexively through the various meridian (somato-odonton) relationships of these degenerated digestive (and other) organs. Dr. Hans Lechner, a renowned holistic dentist in Munich, has termed the role the teeth play in the body as *sacrificial*. That is, when the body has a choice, it will shunt the overload of toxic or neurological stress to less vital organs and tissues. Based on the work of renowned homeopath George Vithoulkas, figure 11.8 illustrates this innate hierarchy in the body's tissues, as defined by their essential value in preserving life and thus survival.[18] As can be seen by the preference pyramid, on a quantitative basis, with 32 teeth, 206 bones, and more than 600 muscles, the body can afford to lose function in some of these areas and still survive. Furthermore, our teeth are not only numerous but hard and tough tissues, just like bone tissue that is designed to defend and protect the softer tissues and organs in the body. Thus, on one hand, we *can afford* to lose a few of these very tough dental structures: witness the loss of teeth during pregnancy when women are calcium-deficient.

On the other hand, we *can't afford* to lose significant function in our solitary pancreas—or in our brain, liver, or heart.

THE LIVER-CANINE RELATIONSHIP

Although the liver is one of the most stressed organs in this toxic age, the liver meridian in the five-element theory is paired with the strongest teeth in the mouth—the canines or cuspids (teeth #6, #11, #22, and #27). From 1932 to 1942, Dr. Francis Pottenger scientifically validated this fact through his research on the effect of eating devitalized foods on subsequent generations of cats. He found that "in three to five years, all the incisors and most of the molars are missing" and that "the 'fangs' or canine teeth prove the most resistant to abscesses and loss."[19] Additionally, in my twenty-five years of practice, I have noticed that cuspid or canine focal infections are rare and often seen only in severely ill and degenerated patients. It seems to have been a wise choice of our innate intelligence to pair the much-beleaguered liver with the strongest teeth in our mouths.

Therefore, a major role that teeth play, along with the vertebrae and other bones, is one of adaptation. That is, besides protecting our softer organs and tissues structurally, these protective harder tissues will even *sacrifice* their vitality and health for the sake of the survival of the body's more life-sustaining organs. For patients who make the difficult and permanent decision to have cavitation surgery and lose a tooth, the preference pyramid can be very clarifying. When an individual understands the causes that underlie the loss of vitality—or death—of a tooth, and why sacrificing this now pathogenic dental focus can continue to benefit the health of a more vital organ or tissue, the decision to undergo cavitation surgery is made much easier. Furthermore, the peace of mind and resolve this knowledge can bestow only strengthen the immune system and thus support a better outcome from dental surgery.

Teeth Die Slowly

Teeth respond differently to trauma. Some teeth handle the stress and stay healthy for a lifetime; others lose their vitality over a few weeks or months, and some die years

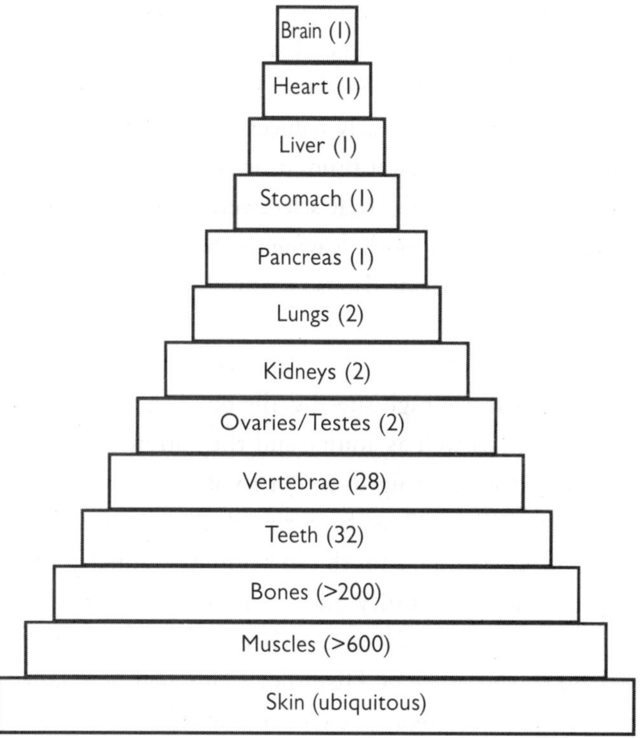

Figure 11.8. The preference pyramid: the body will sacrifice less vital tissues such as the teeth, bones, and muscles over more vital organs such as the brain, heart, liver, and pancreas. (This chart was inspired by the paradigm of healing detailed by George Vithoulkas in his book The Science of Homeopathy, *on pages 34–37.)*

after a trauma. Trauma is not confined to just accidents or blows. Trauma-induced death to a tooth can include orthodontic work (braces and retainers), an ill-fitting bridge or crown, and high-speed drilling.[20]

Conventional drills generate heat and cause microfractures in the tooth's enamel, allowing the ingress of bacteria into the dental tubules. Dr. Doug Cook, a leading U.S. holistic dentist, believes that high-speed drills also suck healthy tissue out of the tubules, which further aids bacteria in finding their way to the tooth's nerve, which can initiate a process of slow death in a filled or crowned tooth.[21] In the case of bigger restorations such as crowns and onlays, high-speed drills combined with plenty of water sprayed into the mouth are indeed necessary for drilling through enamel; otherwise, the tooth would suffer the stress of being open and vulnerable for hours with the use of a low-speed drill.[22] However, low-speed drills are indicated for use in smaller cavities, and especially in pediatric dentistry. Dr. Cook and other holistic dentists recommend using a slow-speed drill that is under 20,000 rpm, which eliminates the heat and vacuum effect and greatly reduces microfractures to the tooth.[23] An even newer innovation for smaller cavities is the use of laser drills that selectively vaporize only the decayed areas of a tooth, leaving the healthy tooth tissue intact. These laser drills also often obviate the need for toxic anesthetics.[24]

Unfortunately, the vast majority of conventional dentists still use high-speed drills on even tiny cavities in children as well as adults, and they often compound this vibratory beating to a tooth with a toxic mercury amalgam filling. Thus, from the placement of a child's first "silver" filling, a tooth can begin its gradual descent into the loss of vitality and eventual death. However, this process is usually so slow that the body adjusts and adapts to the problem. Disturbed fields are created, bacterial and metal toxins are hidden and stored away in the jawbone and neighboring ganglia, and little to no pain is experienced until a stressor in adulthood provokes the emergence of the underlying growing focus.

Dental Foci Can "Smolder" for Decades

Foci and potential foci can smolder quietly for years, as toxins are quietly released from the necrotic dying tooth, gum, and jawbone tissues.[25] Healthier individuals will quarantine these dentally produced toxins in the mouth—around the tooth, in the tonsils, and in the craniofacial ganglia.[26] Under significant stress, however, the body's defensive capacities become overtaxed, and microbes and their poisonous excretory products are released more quickly en masse into the systemic circulation, as well as into specific related organ and tissue disturbed fields. The holistic doctor and dentist at this point have the double diagnostic challenge of needing to assess both the state of the tooth and the state of the patient (psoric, sycotic, tuberculinic, or luetic). After weighing these two factors, practitioners, along with the patient, must decide how best to proceed. Sometimes it's important to spend time strengthening an individual's immune system through drainage, homeopathy, and nutrition before dental intervention, while at other times it is necessary to quickly intervene dentally.

TREATMENT OF A DENTAL FOCUS

This section of the chapter will cover the treatment of an *established* dental focus. However, it's important to emphasize that the *prevention* of a dental focus is always, of course, preferable.

Prevention

There are hundreds of ways to prevent a dental focus from forming—from good nutrition to good dental hygiene. However, one of the most overlooked measures is receiving care from both a knowledgeable holistic practitioner and a biological dentist—from early childhood and throughout your life. Through this conservative and nontoxic care, you can bypass the common iatrogenic foci induced by conventional dentists and allopathic physicians.

- To find a holistic dentist near you, contact one of the following organizations: DAMS at (651) 644-4572 or dams@usfamily.net; the HDA at www.holisticdental.org; IABDM at www.iabdm.org; or IAOMT at www.iaomt.org.
- To find a holistic practitioner knowledgeable about foci, contact Dr. Klinghardt through www.klinghardtacademy.com or Dr. Williams through www.radicalmedicine.com.

The Seven Most Effective Treatments for a Dental Focus

Neural therapy and auriculotherapy, as discussed in chapter 10, are the two most common and *specific* nonsurgical treatments for dental foci. However, nutritional supplementation, gemmotherapy, cell salts, and homeopathy can also be significantly therapeutic *generally,* and sometimes even curative. If these six treatments don't suffice, however, surgical intervention is often needed in the form of cavitation surgery. Using the pyramid model once again, these seven treatments, ranging from the most conservative and least invasive (nutritional and herbal supplementation) to the strongest and most invasive (cavitation surgery), are illustrated in figure 11.9.

1. Nutritional Supplementation

Although minerals, vitamins, and other nutritional supplements are usually not specific enough or quick enough alone to single-handedly heal a dental focus, they are excellent supportively. The supplement coenzyme Q10, which has been proven effective in fighting gum disease, can also be helpful in strengthening *all* of the tissues around a dental focus.[27] In fact, University of Washington researcher Dr. John Ely proposed that coenzyme Q10 might even obviate the need for cavitation surgery when taken at a megadose level (~400 milligrams per day).[28] Although I have not observed that level of success, a dosage of 60 to 120 milligrams per day of the antioxidant coenzyme Q10 can significantly increase blood circulation and oxygenate the gums, greatly supporting the healing of a borderline viable tooth. Be sure, however, to avoid cheap brands; only high-quality coenzyme Q10 from Japan is effective. Furthermore, the reduced form, ubiquinol, has been shown in scientific studies to be significantly more assimilable and bioavailable than the more commonly available ubiquinone, the oxidized form of coenzyme Q10. Ubiquinol is the antioxidant form of coenzyme Q10, which can neutralize free radicals; ubiquinone does not have this antioxidant effect.

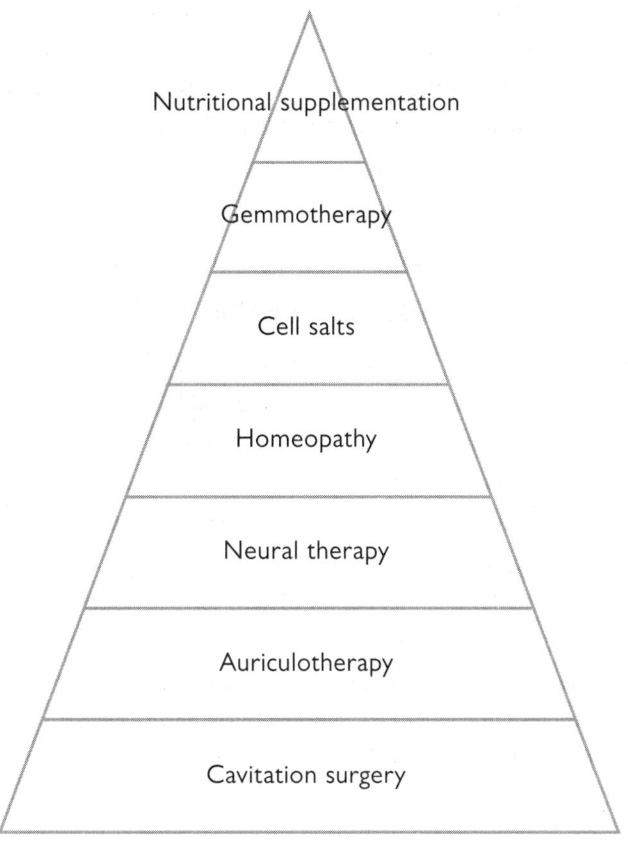

Figure 11.9. The seven most effective treatments for dental foci, ranging from the most general to the most specific and strongest intervention

▶ To order ubiquinol coenzyme Q10, practitioners should go to www.protocolforlife.com or call (877) 776-8610.

Other beneficial antioxidants are vitamin C, vitamin E, and alpha-lipoic acid. Calcium and magnesium supplementation may also reduce deterioration in the jawbones and teeth, when there is a tuberculinic miasmic tendency toward osteoporosis.

Probably the most superior mineral supplement for healing teeth, gums, and the jawbones, however, is the Quinton marine plasma product, which contains the full spectrum of minerals, trace elements, and organic micronutrients as they occur under natural oceanic conditions. This unique seawater harvested from pristine plankton blooms in an unpolluted water source not only helps remineralize but also speeds the healing of inflamed teeth and gums. Furthermore, since this marine plasma and the body's own plasma—the watery aspect of our blood in which the blood cells are suspended—are almost identical, the Quinton plasma is readily absorbed and assimilated in our bodies. Originally discovered by French physiologist Rene Quinton (1867–1925), this nutrient-rich cold-filtered and unheated seawater has been shown for over a century to support digestion and increase enzyme output; enhance immune system functioning; increase energy, stamina, and speed recovery in athletes; and improve mental focus and cognitive function.

▶ For more information on the Quinton marine plasma product, healthcare professionals should go to www.originalquinton.com, or call (888) 278-4686.

Finally, brushing teeth with organic sulfur can greatly reduce and even clear gingivitis and periodontitis, and it has even been seen clinically to heal a (nonsurgical) focal tooth.

▶ A good source of sulfur is Lignisul MSM Granular Crystals, available from www.msm-msm.com or by calling (800) 453-7516.

2. Gemmotherapy

As described in chapter 2, herbal remedies extracted from young plants, also known as gemmotherapy or plant stem cell remedies, are the most potent forms of botanical medicine known. One of these remedies, Silver Fir (*Abies pectinata*), can stimulate bone growth, help remineralize teeth and restore enamel, and reduce dental cavities. Silver Fir contains high amounts of the trace element silicon (found most often in a form called silica), which plays an essential role in bone formation by facilitating the absorption of calcium, as well as by reducing osteoclasts (bone-destroying cells) and increasing osteoblasts (bone-building cells). This gemmotherapy remedy is highly effective in reducing and preventing dental foci, as well as in the treatment of other bone and mineralization disorders such as osteoporosis and rickets. Other gemmotherapy remedies that support dental health and can therefore help prevent the formation of chronic focal infections include Oak (*Quercus pedonculata*), used in the treatment of bleeding gums and gingivitis (but contraindicated in cases of hypertension); White Willow (*Salix alba*), used as a mouthwash to reduce periodontal pockets (but contraindicated in children); and Boxwood (*Buxus sempervirens*), used topically to reduce inflammation and ease the pain from toothaches.

3. Cell Salts

Cell salts, or tissue salts, are homeopathic mineral remedies that are produced through trituration—that is, grinding, with lactose powder. Because these remedies are made at a very low potency (6X) and therefore still have micro amounts of minerals in them, they have both physical (biochemical) and energetic (homeopathic) effects in the body. In 1872, William Schuessler, a German homeopathic physician, developed the twelve cell salts because he believed that high amounts of minerals such as those prescribed in orthomolecular nutritional therapy were actually detrimental to the healthy functioning of cells.[29] He believed that the tiny micronutrients in cell salts could be more easily absorbed into sick cells, and furthermore, that these potentized micronutrients could catalyze the necessary biochemical reactions to reestablish healthy functioning in the cells. Schuessler found that his cell salts were even beneficial in cases of long-term and serious illnesses: "Long-standing, chronic diseases, which have been aggravated by overdosing, excessive use of such medicines as quinine, mercury, etc., can be cured by minute doses of cell-salts."[30]

In dentistry, cell salts are invaluable in helping to support the mineralization of the teeth, gums, and jawbone in childhood and after drilling, as well as to improve blood circulation. The following five cell salts are often prescribed to prevent the formation of a dental focus, as well as to heal a cavitation site after a dental focus has had to be extracted:

- *Calcarea fluorica 6X*—This mineral compound is found on the surface of bones (periosteum) and in the teeth enamel, the elastic fibers (ligaments and cartilage), and the cells of the skin. It is indicated for many dental abnormalities including the tendency toward decay and cavities, loose teeth, deficient or rough enamel, jawbone cavitations (holes in the bone), or exostoses (growths).[31] "Calc fluor" tablets are often prescribed to strengthen the teeth and stimulate delayed dentition in childhood, to assist healing the teeth and jawbone after dental drilling, to attempt to clear a borderline-surgical dental focus, and to help remineralize the jawbone and gums after cavitation surgery.

DENTAL FLUORIDE

Calcarea fluorica is the only safe source of dental fluoride, besides foods (e.g., brussels sprouts, cabbage, cauliflower, beets). Topical *stannous* fluoride used in conventional dental offices can actually be lethal if swallowed in large enough amounts, and sodium fluoride that is added to water supplies has been linked in numerous scientific studies to dental fluorosis (mottling of the teeth), bone pain, back stiffness, osteoporosis, bone fractures, immune deficiency, and cancer.[32] Additionally, sodium fluoride can accumulate in a child's developing brain and reduce IQ and contribute to many behavioral disorders.[33]

- *Calcarea phosphorica 6X*—"Calc phos," the most widespread mineral element in the body, is found in all tissues.[34] This tissue salt makes up 57 percent of bone and gives strength and solidity to the bones and teeth as well as the soft tissues. It is often prescribed in conjunction with Calc fluor to assist healing the teeth after dental drilling and to help heal the jawbone extraction site after cavitation surgery. Furthermore, it reduces tooth decay and is the chief remedy for all teething disorders in babies.[35] In older teenage patients, Calc phos can assist with the proper eruption of wisdom teeth (if there is a reasonable amount of room in the mouth for this to occur).

- *Ferrum phosphoricum 6X*—This cell salt is prescribed when patients exhibit signs of anemia (with or without positive blood tests) to activate the absorption of iron by the hemoglobin in the red blood cells.[36] If iron deficiency is demonstrable by blood tests, the combination of quality iron supplementation (e.g., Iron Picolinate or Ferrasorb from Thorne) and Ferrum phosphoricum 6X may be indicated. The iron directly supplements the deficiency, and the "Ferrum phos" enhances its absorption. Ferrum phos should also be considered before and after cavitation surgery if the patient has any signs of anemia, since good blood circulation is so important for healing of the bone.* Calc phos, helpful in cases of deficient blood coagulation and known as "the bone builder," is often prescribed in tandem with Ferrum phos before and after cavitation surgery. Additionally, Ferrum phos can be used after surgery or anytime there is excess bleeding or inflammation. This cell salt has also been used by mothers for over a century as a first-aid remedy for the initial stages of fever or inflammation—flu, toothaches, tonsillitis, sunstroke, bruises, injuries, and so forth.
- *Magnesium phosphoricum 6X*—This mineral salt is found in the blood, bones, teeth, nerves, and brain. It functions as an antispasmodic and is often prescribed for muscle spasms and menstrual cramps. In the same way, since much of pain is due to cramping and tension, "Mag phos" is indicated for pain reduction with teething, after dental drilling, or after cavitation surgery. It is also beneficial in hardening enamel and in cases of deficient bone and teeth mineralization in both the young and the old.
- *Silicea 6X*—Silica is found in connective tissue, bone, hair, nails, nerves, teeth, the pancreas, and the heart.[37] Silica cell salt, known as Silicea, breaks down scar tissue, both on the skin (scar interference fields) and internally (scar adhesions in a chronic focal infection). It also stimulates the elimination of pus in an abscess.[38] Thus, it can be an important remedy to treat abscesses in dental focal infections* or to help break down scar tissue after dental surgery.[39] Silicea can also stimulate the discharge of foreign materials and can therefore support the eruption of teeth in the case of delayed dentition (e.g., deciduous or baby teeth, wisdom teeth). However, because of this strong discharging quality, Silicea should never be prescribed to individuals with implants (hip, breast, dental, organ, etc.), with pins or screws, during pregnancy, or in the case of any "foreign body" that should not be encouraged to be pushed out from its location in the body.

Any of these five cell salts can be combined and taken together at the same time.† Cell salts should be taken at least fifteen minutes before or after eating and can be dissolved sublingually, under the tongue. Dosages vary but the following suggestions can be used as a general guideline:

Acute Dysfunction—2 tablets, every 10 minutes or every hour, for a few hours or a day, then reducing this dosage to three to six times a day, until symptoms abate.

Chronic Dysfunction—2 tablets, one or two times a

---

*Besides the classic signs of anemia—fatigue, weakness, and paleness—Dr. Gary Klepper found that a kinesiological method that tests for aerobic muscle fatigue could also be used to signal anemia, as measured by laboratory blood tests (serum iron and hematocrit levels). This test consists of testing a muscle repetitively at a rate of approximately once per second. Anemic subjects quickly tired within six repetitions or less, whereas nonanemic subjects were able to sustain their muscle contraction throughout the test. (G. Klepper, "The Relationship of Aerobic Muscle Fatigue Findings to Laboratory Measurements of Iron," *Applied Kinesiology Review* 3, 1 [1992], 33–39.)

*The homeopathic remedy Hepar sulphuris (30C or 200C) is also excellent for treating abscesses.

†There are some cell salts that should not be taken together since they counteract or inhibit the action of one another (e.g., Nat mur and Nat sulph), which is the reason that the combination cell salt formula Bioplasma rarely tests well energetically. However, the five cell salts described in this section can—and often should—be combined.

day, for two to three weeks to two to four months, or more.

Infants—1 tablet dissolved in warm water, sipped as needed.

Children (under 10)—1 or 2 tablets, one or two times a day.

Adults—2 tablets, from one to three times a day.

- Healthcare practitioners can order cell salts through Seroyal at (888) 737-6925 or at www.seroyal.com. Cell salts are also available at health food stores. Be sure they are in the 6X potency, because that is the level of resonance that consistently tests the best for holistic practitioners.
- Those who would like more information on cell salts in dentistry can order my handout *The Essential Role of Cell Salts in Holistic Dentistry* given at the March 2005 IABDM dental conference in Dallas, by calling my office at (415) 460-1968. *The Twelve Biochemical Salts of Dr. Schuessler,* available at www.seroyal.com, and *Dr. Schuessler's Biochemistry* by J. B. Chapman are also good resources. My two favorite books on this subject, however, are Dr. Skye Weintraub's *Natural Healing with Cell Salts* and *Homeopathic Cell Salt Remedies* by Lennon and Rolfe.

4. Homeopathy

Even the great pioneers of the focal infection theory and holistic dentistry—such as Miller, Price, Billings, and Rosenow—either were not aware of acute or constitutional homeopathy or did not comprehend the great potential for cure in this branch of holistic medicine. However, the practice of constitutional homeopathy (according to the Sankaran method; see chapter 14), even when the teeth are not directly addressed, is so curative that sometimes a borderline dental focus is healed simply through the enhanced immune system functioning that is facilitated with the correct remedy. In other cases, this correct homeopathic *simillimum* (most suitable remedy) can greatly assist in the diagnosis of a focal tooth. That is, after a few days, weeks, or months of processing this remedy, the body will begin to signal its deeper issues. In this "What's false arises" climate, a focal tooth (or scar, etc.) will begin to create symptoms in the body and test positive with energetic testing methods. At this time, a skilled practitioner can clearly determine if the tooth can be saved and simply requires a few sessions of neural therapy or auriculotherapy, or if surgery is indeed necessary. Thus, constitutional homeopathy can greatly assist physicians and practitioners in making that most difficult decision—whether a tooth is viable or whether it should be extracted.

simillimum: The simillimum is the *most* similar remedy, and therefore the most appropriate one, that best fits the totality of symptoms in a patient.

BACTERIAL VACCINES

Though the pioneers of focal infection theory seemed unaware of homeopathy, many of these early-twentieth-century physicians and scientists developed vaccines—dilutions of killed or deadened microbes—that are similar to nosodes in homeopathy without the succussion. In fact, E. C. Rosenow spent the last half of his life researching vaccine therapies, primarily at the Mayo Clinic. There he had phenomenal success in the treatment of multiple sclerosis, schizophrenia, and even the supposedly viral-induced disease of polio with his carefully prepared vaccines containing streptococcus bacteria.[40] Unfortunately, like his brilliant research on the focal infection theory, the art and science of making Rosenow's *thermal antibody* bacterial vaccines was forgotten in the fervor over the seemingly quick-fix antibiotic drugs in the mid and latter half of the twentieth century.[41] Fortunately, however, S. H. Shakman has compiled many of Rosenow's research studies in his book, *E. C. Rosenow and Associates: A Reference Manual.* Go to www.InstituteofScience.com to order this book. Perhaps someday a progressive holistic pharmacy will consider duplicating Rosenow's recipe for this successful vaccine and use it in a clinical trial to ascertain the results in a modern population of patients.

As described in chapter 14, constitutional homeopathy is the art and science of determining a specific single remedy for the treatment of the whole person—physically, emotionally, mentally, and spiritually. However, the profound sense of well-being that often results from the homeopathic remedy should not deter practitioners from continuing to be aware of a once-suspicious dental focus or a mouthful of amalgam fillings. In this modern age of toxic metals, chemicals, and allopathic medical and dental treatments, even the correct constitutional remedy is no guarantee against degenerative disease. Fortunately, with the deepest homeopathic simillimum, these degenerative silent foci areas will eventually "out" themselves so that energetic testing can reveal the need for their treatment at the appropriate time.

An *acute* homeopathic remedy—that is, a homeopathic remedy for a recent (in contrast to long-term and chronic) trauma or infection—can also be very effective in reducing, or even completely eradicating, the possibility of a future dental focus. Furthermore, although prescribing the correct constitutional remedy takes years of study, acute homeopathic remedies prescribed for *specific* purposes such as a dental trauma or infection are a little easier to evaluate and prescribe. An excellent reference in determining these remedies is the "Tooth Pain" section in Dr. Roger Morrison's *Desktop Companion to Physical Pathology.* The possibilities described here can then be further considered in other homeopathic materia medicas—Dr. Morrison's *Desktop Guide* is an excellent synopsis—and repertories, in conjunction with the knowledge gained at homeopathic seminars.*

The acute homeopathic remedy Arnica montana is well known for its extraordinary effectiveness in treating the pain and bruising that often accompanies dental drilling, extraction, or trauma. Arnica 30C (or 30K)† is therefore commonly prescribed from one to three times per day for three days (or more) after dental surgery or trauma. Arnica also greatly mitigates the "emotional injury" that may occur in sensitive patients after extensive drilling or surgery; therefore, giving this remedy is generally the best choice to mitigate all aspects of drilling. Hypericum perforatum 30C (or 30K), "the Arnica of the nerves," is also essential in case the drilling directly or nearly injures the nerves underlying the teeth in the maxillary and mandibular jawbones. In fact, when prescribed acutely (and quickly), Hypericum can even prevent the major side effect in the placement of deep fillings, crowns, or surgery—chronic numbness in the cheek and jaws. In these cases, Arnica and Hypericum can both be prescribed, given in alternating doses (e.g., Arnica in the morning and Hypericum in the evening, or more often), generally for three to five days. Finally, a couple drops of Rescue Remedy in a glass of pure water is an excellent remedy to give to patients chairside in the dental office after an emotionally stressful drilling or surgery.*

However, the dental physician should always ask first if the patient is on a constitutional homeopathic before prescribing Arnica, Hypericum, or Rescue Remedy. If the patient is indeed on a constitutional remedy—and is significantly better from it, indicating that it truly is his or her simillimum—then the patient should re-dose this constitutional remedy once or twice (or more as needed) after drilling, and not another homeopathic. The constitutional remedy will have the same or even better effects as an acutely prescribed homeopathic through stimulating the healing of tissue and emotionally rebalancing the individual. Remember that when a patient is happily on his or her constitutional remedy, Arnica, Hypericum, and even (although less likely) nonpotentized but diluted Rescue Remedy have the potential to antidote and interrupt the ameliorating effects of this remedy.

5. Neural Therapy

As discussed previously, isopathic drops can be used to prevent a dental focus from forming after extensive drilling or trauma, as well as after surgery to augment healing. Notatum 4X drops function well as an effective antibacterial in many cases. They can be dropped directly on a dental focus or an extraction site. Aspergillus 4X drops, commonly used in alternating doses with Notatum 4X, help stimulate soft-tissue and bone healing in a dental focus, or after cavitation surgery if it becomes necessary to pull the focal tooth and drill out the surrounding necrotic (dead) bone. Mucor 4X drops are additionally prescribed after dental surgery if there has been a lot of bleeding or bruising in the area. Kombination 4X drops,

*A homeopathic *materia medica* is a reference book that lists remedies and their therapeutic actions. A homeopathic *repertory* is also a reference book, with an index of symptoms and the remedies associated with these symptoms.

†K potencies, produced by UNDA in Belgium and distributed through Seroyal in Canada, are quite similar to C potencies. See chapter 14 for a description of the differences between C and K potencies.

*By definition, Bach flower remedies like Rescue Remedy are not strictly homeopathic. They are not succussed (potentized), nor were they developed through the use of homeopathic provings. Bach flower remedies are available at all health food stores.

a combination of Aspergillus and Mucor, are indicated when both these isopathic remedies would be beneficial (Aspergillus for soft-tissue healing and Mucor for increased blood circulation).

▶ To order isopathic remedies, practitioners can contact BioResource at (800) 203-3775 or visit the website at www.bioresourceinc.com.

Lasers can be used to "drive in" these remedies *photophoretically* in all phases of treatment. For example, laser therapy is very beneficial (with or without isopathy) after a filling or crown is placed to reduce inflammation and stimulate healing in the maxillary (upper jaw) or mandibular (lower jaw) nerve irritated by extensive drilling. Lasers are also invaluable over the extraction site after cavitation surgery, as well as over any associated toxic ganglia. The treatment of related positive craniofacial ganglia is best determined through energetic testing. However, for those who don't use energetic testing, a postcavitation surgery protocol of briefly treating all the common dental focus-related ganglia (e.g., 100 mw, for 10 seconds each, over each of the seven ganglia) can be quite beneficial. (See figure 11.10 for the seven most common ganglia requiring treatment after cavitation surgery.) The positive ganglia associated with a dental focus, like the tooth's disturbed fields, are always ipsilateral (same side) to the dental focus.*

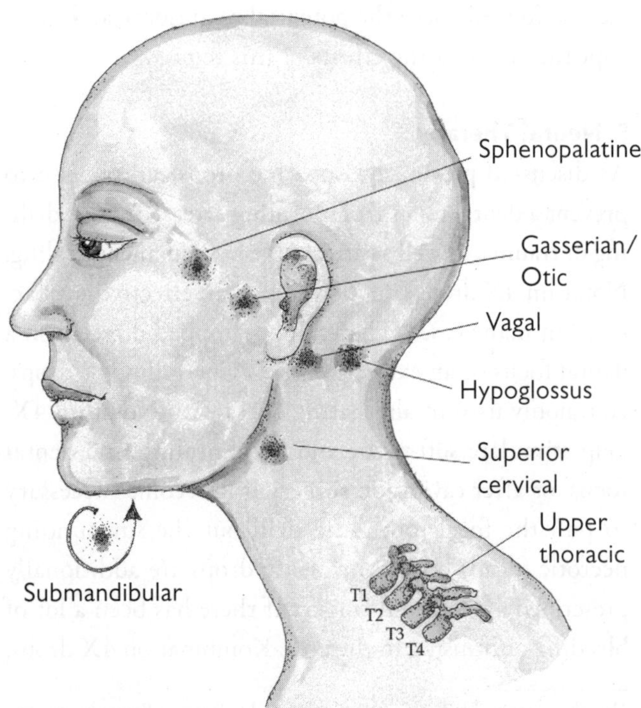

Figure 11.10. The seven most common ganglia requiring treatment after cavitation surgery

THE CANADIAN LASER

Because the Canadian laser's 100-milliwatt, 830-nanometer beam penetrates tissue up to approximately two inches, the postsurgery patient doesn't have to keep his mouth (uncomfortably) open for ten minutes but can just place the stylus on the cheek, pointing the beam into the extraction site area. Furthermore, according to Dr. Klinghardt, the beam "spreads out like an orange" once it penetrates the skin, so the patient doesn't have to worry about the angle of the laser's stylus needing to be perfectly pointing toward the site for it to be effective. With the Canadian laser with three milliwatt options, dentists can choose to use the stronger 200-milliwatt beam just after *extensive* drilling or surgery, or the 400-milliwatt beam over chronic focal sites. (For more on lasers, see page 313.)

An exceptionally popular and successful protocol has been to loan out the 100-milliwatt infrared laser for five days for patients to use at home while they are recuperating from their tooth extraction and cavitation surgery, or after a root canal treatment. During this five-day period, patients use the laser for one minute at a time, from six to ten (or more) times a day (more the first three days, and then less often the last two days).† This protocol not only greatly reduces the need for pain medication but also helps the gum and bone tissue heal more rapidly and effectively.

Neural therapy injections of homeopathic and isopathic remedies along with a small amount of local anesthetic in and around the tooth (or socket) can also be very effective in saving a (nonsurgical) tooth (or socket area).

*For example, when a lower right wisdom tooth (#32) is extracted and cavitated, the right vagal and sphenopalatine ganglia may need to be treated with laser therapy, whereas the left-sided ganglia will not test positive.

†Patients are always instructed never to shine the laser directly into their eyes. Additionally, I have never found any problem with multiple treatments—e.g., six to eight times a day after cavitation surgery—of the laser. The beam spreads out once it goes through the skin, so there is no danger of excess heating.

Functional Illness			Degenerative Conditions		
THE SIX PHASES					
Excretion	**Reaction**	**Deposition**	**Impregnation**	**Degeneration**	**Neoplastic**

THE FOUR MIASMS

Psoric	Sycotic	Tuberculinic	Luetic
skin issues (rashes, acne, eczema, psoriasis, and so on) overactive vital force—violent, brief eliminations (diarrhea, fever, sweating, vomiting, rashes, itching) good energy; quick to recover from illness active in evening, tired in morning mild joint pain allergy and hay fever symptoms parasites, hemorrhoids	deeper skin issues (warts, moles, lipomas, severe acne or eczema, and so on) intermittent fatigue and irritability chronic or intermittent joint pain intestinal dysbiosis/ digestive dysfunction more frequent colds, sore throats, sinusitis bladder, prostate, menstrual dysfunction	slow to recover from illness (frequent but inefficient fevers) susceptible to viruses recurrent colds, bronchitis, asthma, earaches, et cetera depression, anxiety, severe fatigue insomnia, exhausted in morning painful arthritis, scoliosis, osteoporosis	disturbed and imbalanced energy premature aging, memory loss anxiety, severe insomnia muscle cramps and achiness, especially at night and especially in the legs destruction of tissue—ulcers, acne rosacea, cancer, multiple sclerosis (MS), amyotrophic lateral sclerosis (ALS), Alzheimer's, Parkinson's, et cetera

Plate 1. The correlation between the four miasms and Reckeweg's six homotoxicology phases (see page 20 for text discussion)

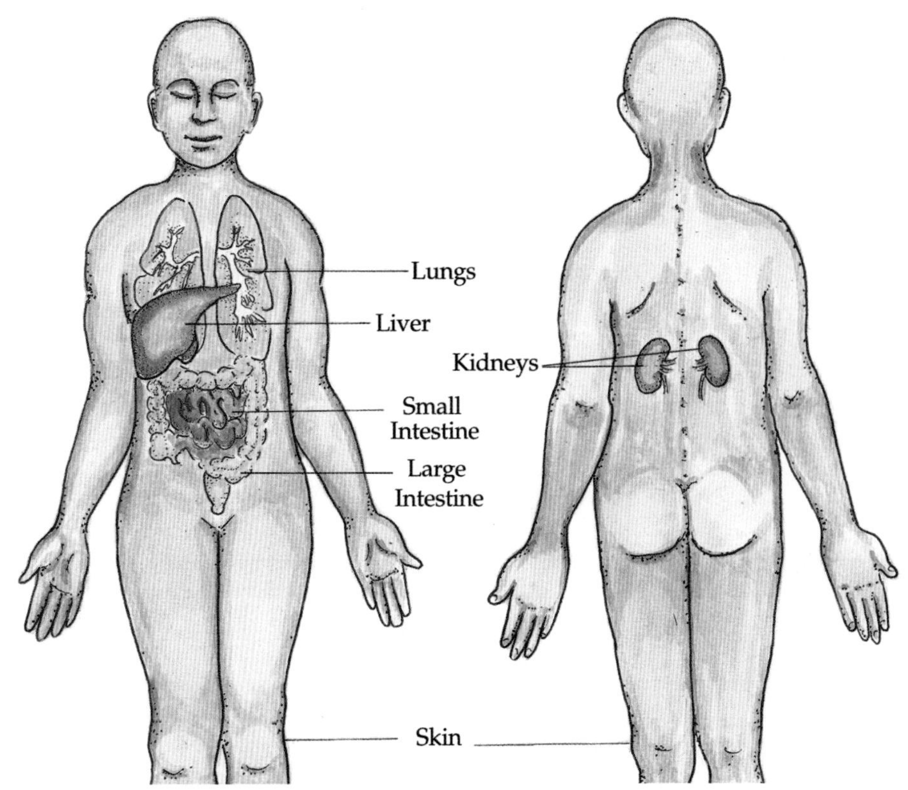

Plate 2. The primary emunctories (excretion organs and tissues) in the body (see text page 38)

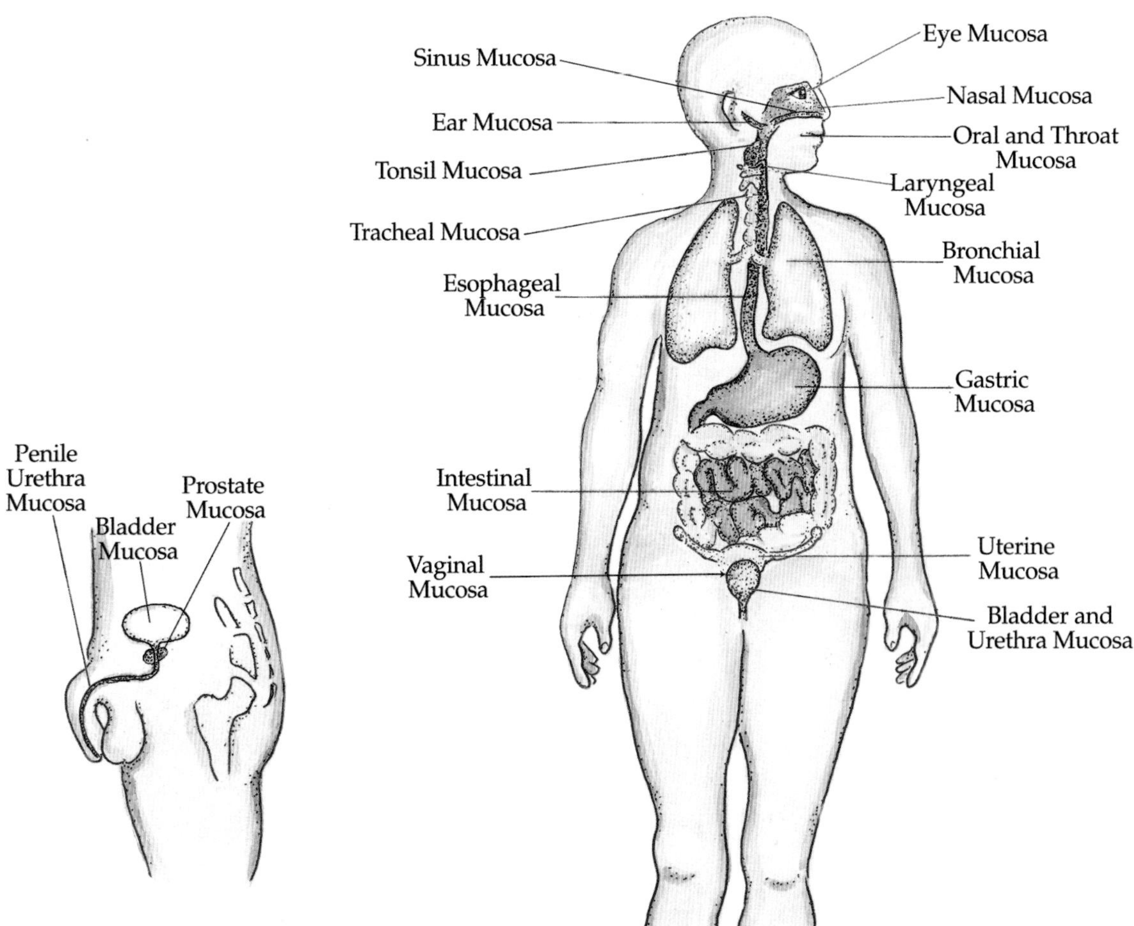

Plate 3. The secondary emunctories in the body (see text page 39)

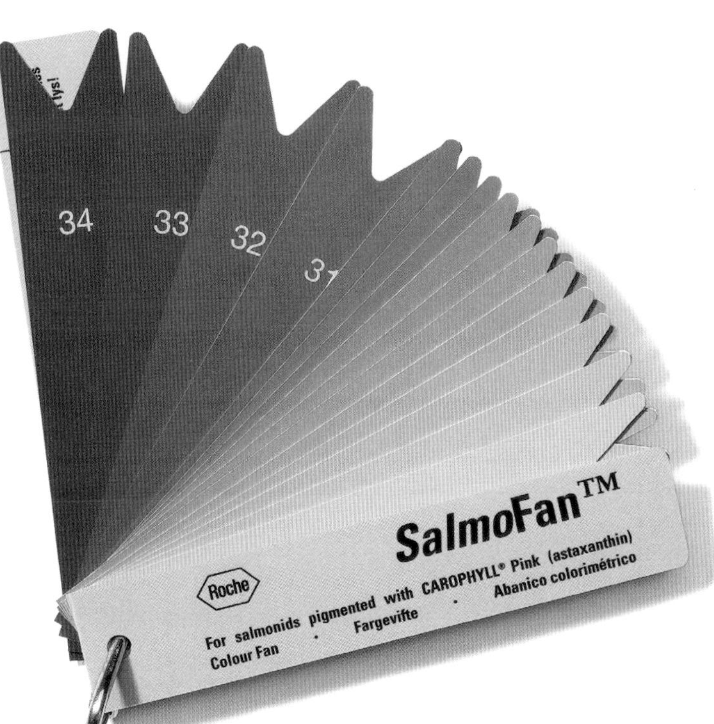

Plate 4. Farm-raised salmon is typically artificially colored with red food dyes (canthaxanthin or astaxanthin). See page 164 for the text discussion.

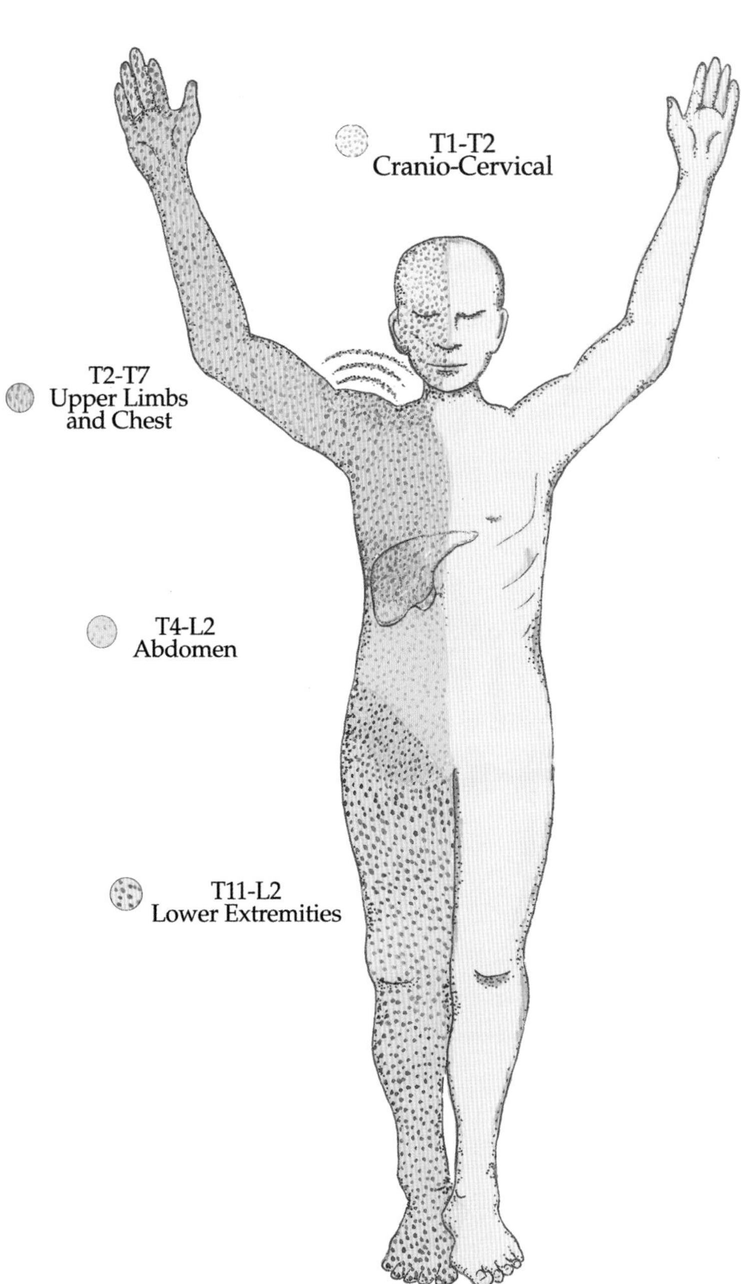

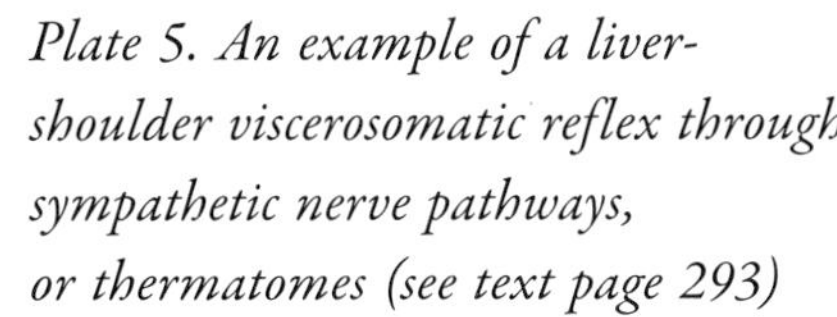

Plate 5. An example of a liver-shoulder viscerosomatic reflex through sympathetic nerve pathways, or thermatomes (see text page 293)

Dental Relationship Chart

Joints	Right: shoulder/elbow/hand (ulnar), S.1. joint, foot, toes	Right: TMJ, anterior hip/knee, medial ankle		Right: Shoulder/elbow/hand (radial), foot, big toe		Right: Posterior knee, hip, lateral ankle	Right: Posterior knee, sacrococcygeal joint, posterior ankle		Left: Posterior knee, sacrococcygeal joint, posterior ankle		Left: Posterior knee, hip, lateral ankle	Left: Shoulder/elbow/hand (radial), foot, big toe		Left: TMJ, anterior hip/knee, medial ankle		Left: shoulder/elbow/hand (ulnar), S.1. joint, foot, toes
Mammary Glands		Right breast											Left breast			
Endocrine Glands	Anterior pituitary	Parathyroid	Thyroid	Thymus	Posterior pituitary	Intermediate lobe of pituitary	Pineal		Pineal		Intermediate lobe of pituitary	Posterior pituitary	Thymus	Thyroid	Parathyroid	Anterior pituitary
Organs	Right heart, right duodenum, terminal ileum	Pancreas, right side of stomach, esophagus		Right lung, right side of large intestine		Right side of liver, gall bladder, right side of biliary ducts	Right kidney, bladder, uterus, prostate, rectum, anus		Left kidney, bladder, uterus, prostate, rectum, anus		Left side of liver, left side of biliary ducts	Left lung, left side of large intestine		Spleen, left side of stomach, esophagus		Left heart, left side of duodenum, jejunum ileum
Teeth Pictured	Retromolar															Retromolar
Names of Teeth	Right upper 3rd molar (wisdom)	Right upper 2nd molar	Right upper 1st molar	Right upper 2nd bicuspid (pre-molar)	Right upper 1st bicuspid (pre-molar)	Right upper canine (cuspid)	Right upper lateral incisor	Right upper central incisor	Left upper central incisor	Left upper lateral incisor	Left upper canine (cuspid)	Left upper 1st bicuspid (pre-molar)	Left upper 2nd bicuspid (pre-molar)	Left upper 1st molar	Left upper 2nd molar	Left upper 3rd molar (wisdom)
American Nomenclature	1	2	3	4	5	6	7	8	7	8	11	12	13	14	15	16
	32	31	30	29	28	27	26	25	26	25	22	21	20	19	18	17
Names of Teeth	Right lower 3rd molar (wisdom)	Right lower 2nd molar	Right lower 1st molar	Right lower 2nd bicuspid (pre-molar)	Right lower 1st bicuspid (pre-molar)	Right lower canine (cuspid)	Right lower lateral incisor	Right lower central incisor	Left lower central incisor	Left lower lateral incisor	Left lower canine (cuspid)	Left lower 1st bicuspid (pre-molar)	Left lower 2nd bicuspid (pre-molar)	Left lower 1st molar	Left lower 2nd molar	Left lower 3rd molar (wisdom)
Teeth Pictured	Retromolar															Retromolar
Organs	Right heart, terminal ileum, ileo-cecal	Pancreas, right side of stomach, esophagus		Right lung, right side of large intestine		Right side of liver, gall bladder, right side of biliary ducts	Right kidney, bladder, uterus, prostate, rectum, anus		Left kidney, bladder, uterus, prostate, rectum, anus		Left side of liver, left side of biliary ducts	Left lung, left side of large intestine		Spleen, left side of stomach, esophagus		Left heart, left side of jejunum, ileum
Endocrine Glands					Ovaries	Testicles	Adrenals		Adrenals		Ovaries	Testicles				
Mammary Glands				Right breast								Left breast				
Joints	Right: Shoulder/elbow/hand (ulnar), S.1. joint, foot, toes	Right: TMJ, anterior hip/knee, medial ankle		Right: Shoulder/elbow/hand (radial), foot, big toe		Right: Posterior knee, hip, lateral ankle	Right: Posterior knee, sacrococcygeal joint, posterior ankle		Left: Posterior knee, sacrococcygeal joint, posterior ankle		Left: Posterior knee, hip, lateral ankle	Left: Shoulder/elbow/hand (radial), foot, big toe		Left: TMJ, anterior hip/knee, medial ankle		Left: Shoulder/elbow/hand (ulnar), S.1. joint, foot, toes
	Fire	Earth		Metal		Wood	Water		Water		Wood	Metal		Earth		Fire

Plate 6. The dental relationship chart, based on the original chart developed by Dr. Fritz Kramer, with some changes by Klinghardt/Williams. *(See pages 330–32 for text discussion.)*

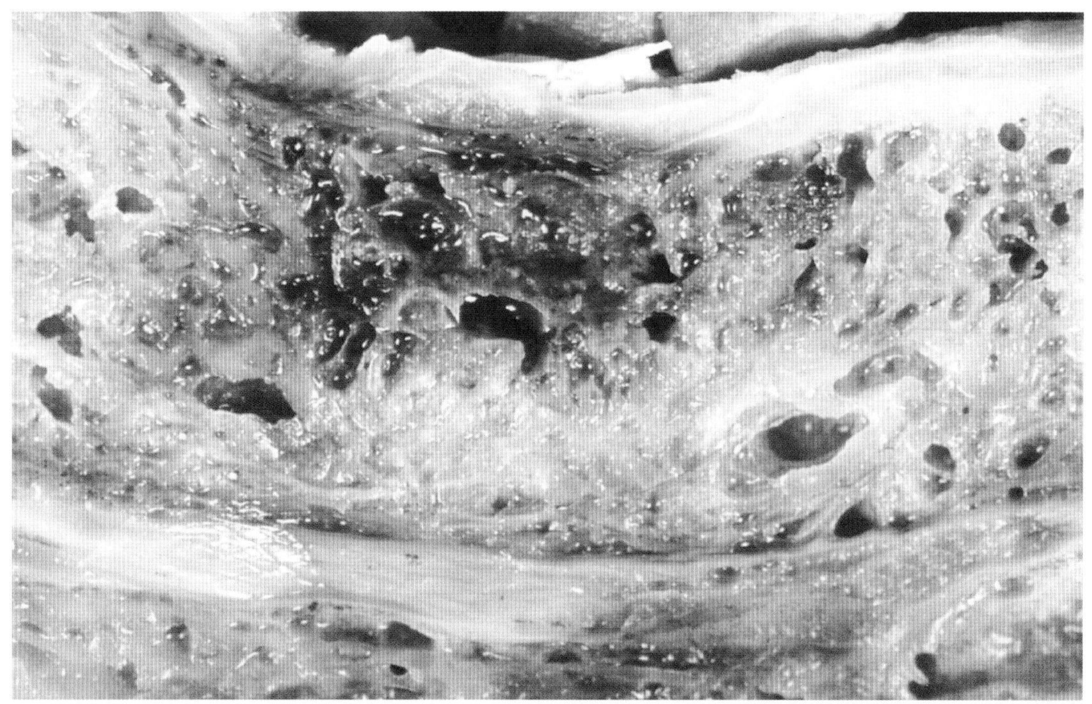

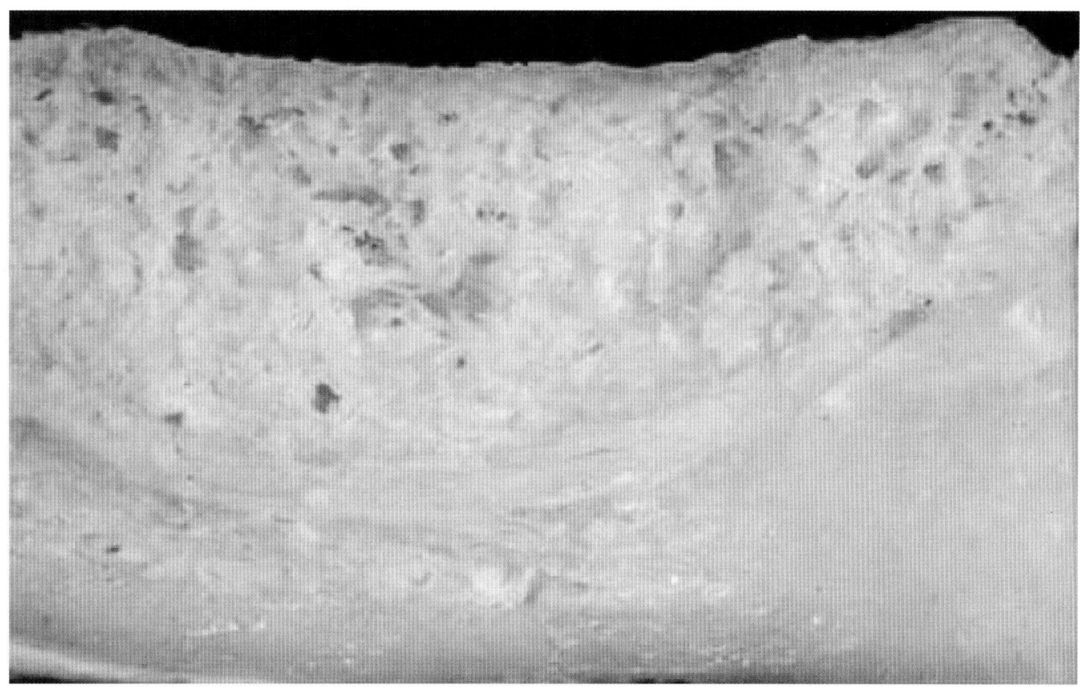

Plate 7. Cavitation (see text pages 344–47).
Top: A photograph of a jawbone cavitation site (focal infection) with a prominent osteonecrotic, or gangrenous area (in black), filled with dead bone.
Bottom: A photograph of a healthy jawbone.
(Photographs courtesy of Jerry Bouquot, D.D.S.)

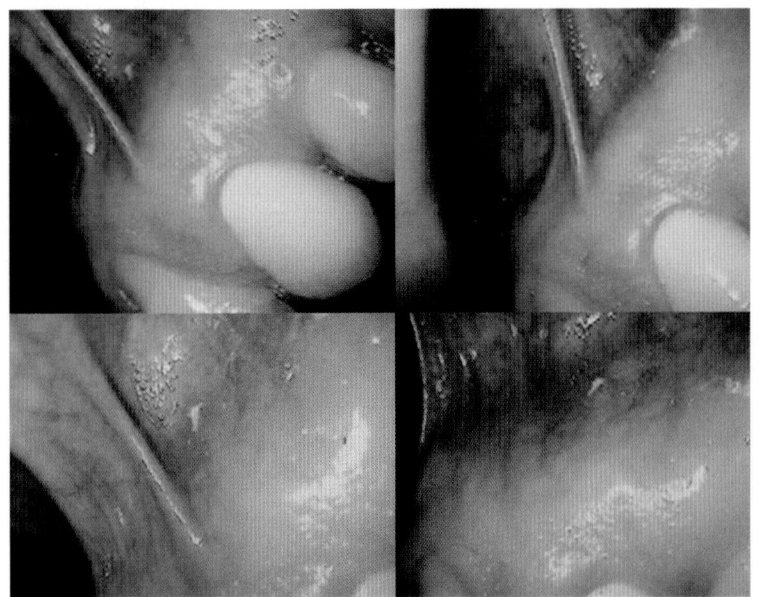

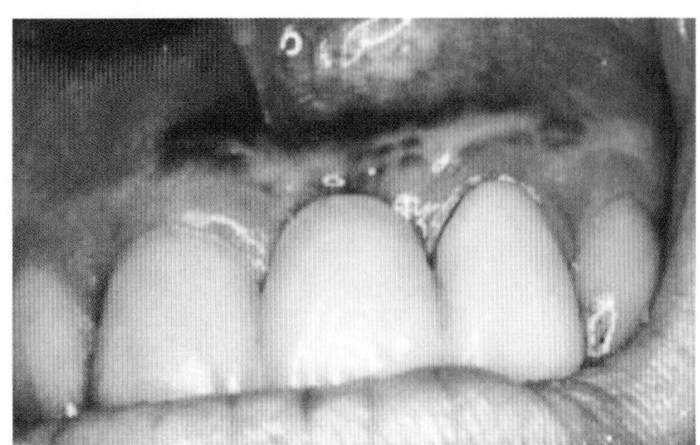

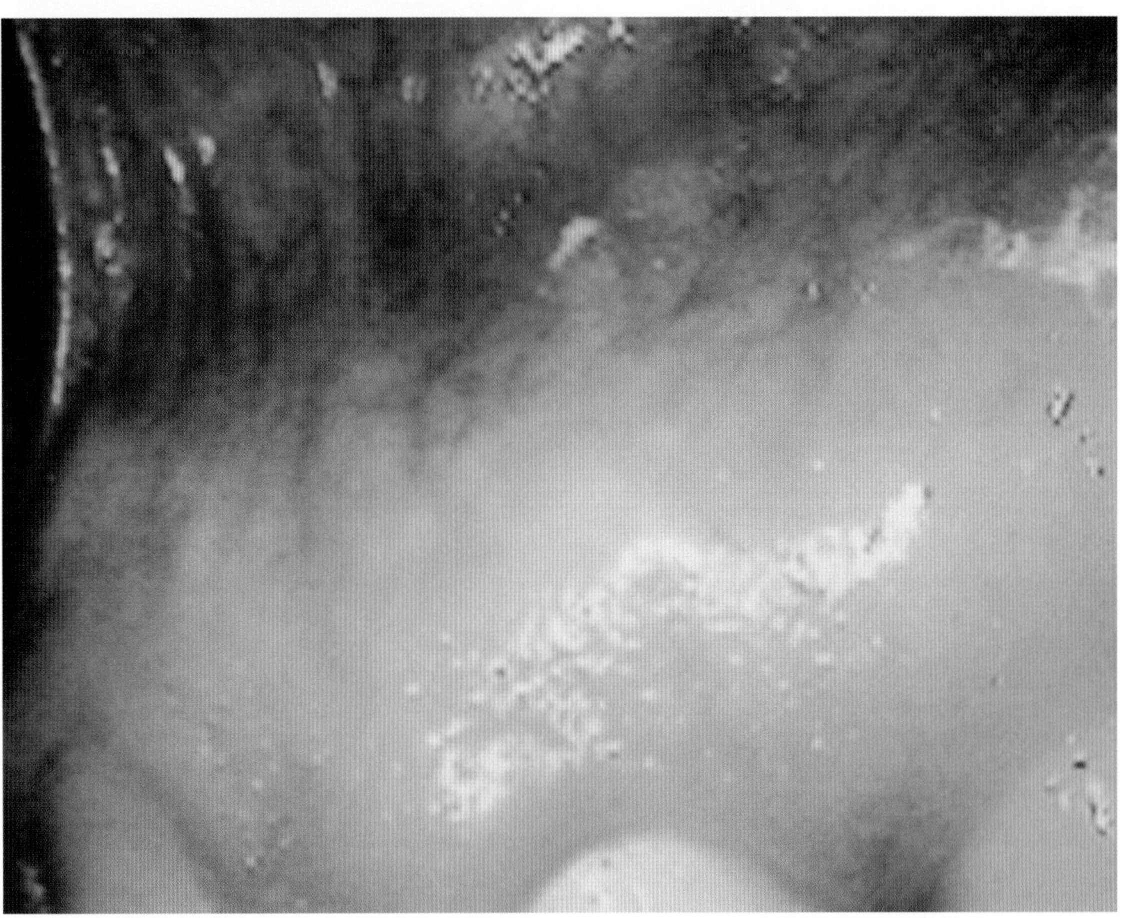

Plate 8. Examples of silver stain or "tattoo" in the gums (see text page 360). Photographs courtesy of Dr. William P. Glaros and Dr. Scott Loman.

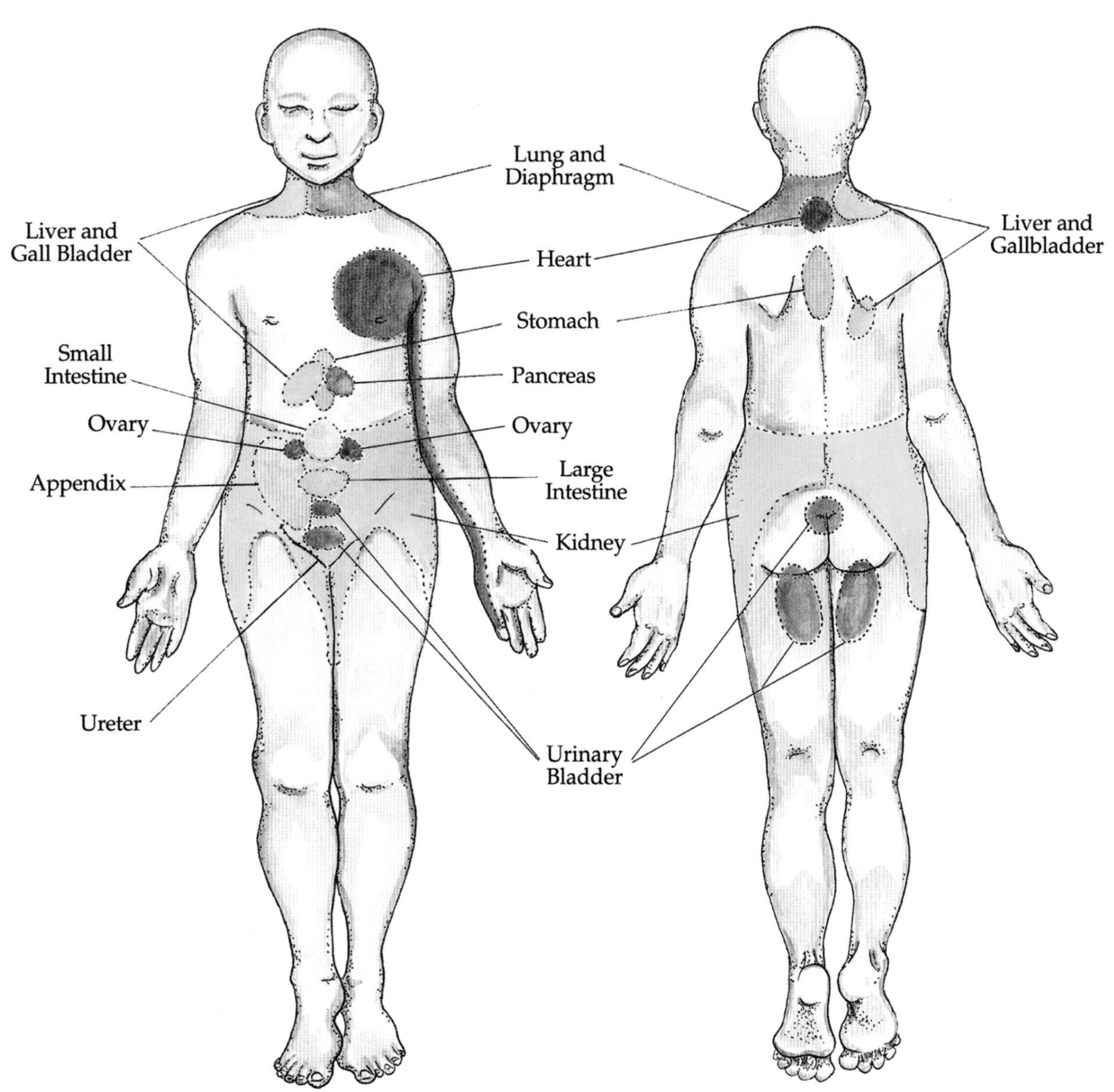

Plate 9. The areas of referred pain, also known as "Head zones," are generated from chronic visceral (organ) dysfunction and disease (see text pages 546–50).

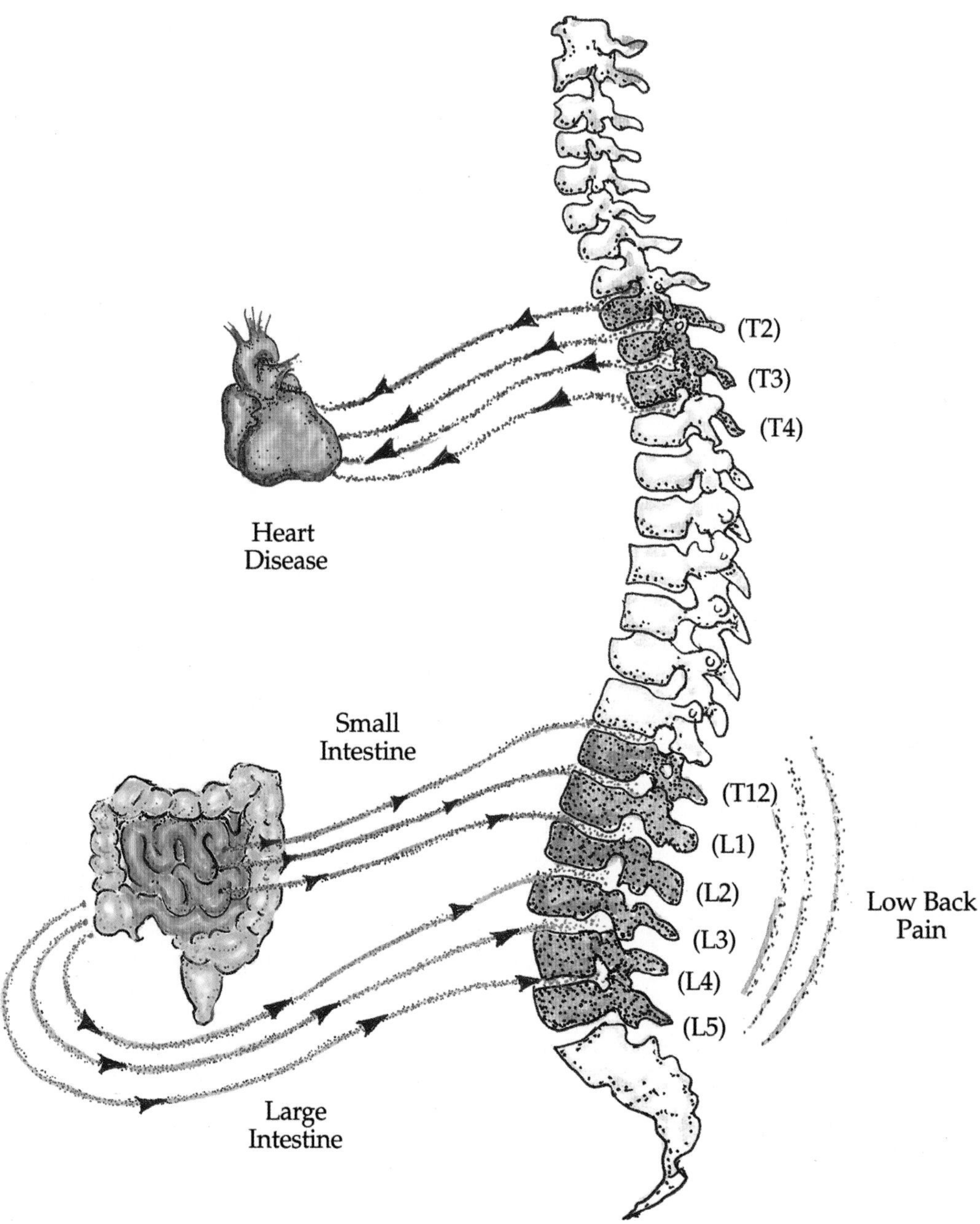

Plate 10. The somatovisceral reflex (spinal-organ referrals). Dentists who chronically strain their neck and upper back leaning over at work for years may eventually experience heart problems through inflamed autonomic somatovisceral (spinal-heart) nerve pathways. An individual who eats sugar and junk food may over time experience chronic low back pain through inflamed autonomic viscerosomatic (intestinal-spinal) nerve pathways. See text pages 553–55.

6. Auriculotherapy

As described in chapter 10, auriculotherapy is one of the most effective means for healing, or at least mitigating as much as possible, dental foci. Originating in France and often used in conjunction with a constitutional homeopathic remedy, this treatment is excellent preventively, as well as when attempting to save a dying tooth. There are numerous treatment modalities that can be applied to specific points, including visible red (CEPES) and infrared ("Canadian") laser light, electrical stimulation (Pointoselect DT), and needles.

Needle therapy ranges from small temporary acupuncture needles to the use of semipermanent (ASP) needles.[42] In his clinical practice, Dr. Nogier found that the transitory stimulation of temporary acupuncture needles was generally not sufficient with the more intractable and degenerative conditions in his patients. After some searching, he discovered that semipermanent needles—little harpoon-shaped cylindrical needles—that can remain in the ear from a few days to a week or more produced clinical results that were "ten times more significant than that realized with an ordinary needle."[43]

- ▶ The name of the ASP needle developed by Dr. Nogier is an acronym for Aiguilles Semi-Permanens. These needles can be ordered from Med Servi-Systems in Canada at (800) 267-6868.

However, just as Nogier replaced the more aggressive cauterization method with ASP needles, had he lived longer perhaps he may have found that even these strong semipermanent needles were not actually necessary after all. In my clinical experience, when patients have removed their toxic metals and (personal care and cleaning product) chemicals, are avoiding their primary food allergen and eating a cleaner diet, and are on their appropriate constitutional homeopathic remedy, ASP needles often begin to test as too strong energetically. In these cases, the less aggressive yet curative forms of auricular stimulation—temporary acupuncture needles, laser or electrical stimulation—are more clinically appropriate. In other words, on patients whose systemic toxicity (the "forest") has been addressed and reasonably cleared, specific auricular points relating to a particular focus (the "trees") do not need to be "hit over the head with a hammer" but can be more appropriately and even more effectively influenced through a gentler stimulus.

AURICULOTHERAPY TECHNOLOGY

The CEPES-Laser, originated by Dr. Wolfgang Ludwig of Germany, is a combination of visible red laser therapy and soft magnetic field therapy. It can be used as a gentle stimulation on auricular points. Although it has a very low milliwatt output (0.5), the visible red beam is combined with a 9 Hz frequency (between the 7.8 Hertz of Schumann waves and the 10 Hertz of the alpha rhythm of the blood circulation) and 64 trace elements. This yang (9 Hz) and yin (64 elements) influence on the laser beam yields a balancing and therapeutic resonance. To order, contact Med Servi-Systems in Canada at (800) 267-6868 or go to www.magnetotherapy.de.

The Pointoselect DT from Germany, unlike most electrical instruments, has a harmonic electrical signal and causes no detectable electromagnetic stress in the patient. Furthermore, it can be used for both diagnosis as well as treatment of auricular points. Unfortunately, it is only approved in Europe (CE) and does not have specific FDA approval at this time. To order the Pointoselect DT, contact Schwa-Medico in Germany at zentrale@schwa-medico.de or go to www.schwa-medico.de. Although most North American auriculotherapists use the Net II for electrical stimulation of ear points (available from Med-Servi Systems), this instrument has not energetically tested as well as the Pointoselect DT in my experience.

Another diagnostic instrument is the Pointer Plus point finder. It is excellent diagnostically to find the correct positive points and it is very inexpensive. However, it is not recommended for therapeutic use because it can cause subtle electromagnetic stress in patients (in the energetic testing experience of my colleagues and myself). However, new practitioners may want to begin with this inexpensive diagnostic instrument to help easily identify the positive auricular points, and then use one of the lasers—CEPES, Canadian, or the Pointoselect DT—to treat the point. Order the Pointer Plus from Lhasa OMS at (800) 722-8775, or go to www.lhasaoms.com.

- The MLI-2215 AcuGlide acupuncture needles are low in nickel and aren't sprayed with silicon and yet still insert easily. They can be ordered from Helio Medical Supplies, Inc. at (800) 672-2726 or www.heliomed.com.

Auriculotherapy is an excellent modality to use just after dental drilling, as well as after cavitation surgery. Therefore, holistic dentists and dental hygienists are especially encouraged to learn the art and science of this effective treatment of potential or active dental foci. In March 2004, I presented a brief lecture on how dentists can get started safely and effectively with auriculotherapy to the American Academy of Biological Dentistry (AABD), now known as the International Academy of Biological Dentistry and Medicine (IABDM), which can be ordered on DVD. After viewing and practicing with these introductory methods, dentists and hygienists who want to continue using auriculotherapy in their practice should pursue their training in auriculotherapy seminars.

- Dr. Williams's handout "The Benefits of Auriculotherapy in Dentistry" and DVD (about two hours long) can be ordered from the IABDM at www.iabdm.org. Recommended seminars in auriculotherapy include Dr. Mikhael Adams's (www.integralhealth.ca), Dr. Frank's (www.auriculartherapy.com), and Dr. Williams's (www.radicalmedicine.com).

7. Cavitation Surgery

The term *cavitation* has a dual meaning. In pathology terms, a *cavitation* is a cavity or hole within a bone. In surgical nomenclature, *cavitation surgery* is the term for the dental surgical procedure that is required to remove the dead and diseased bone from this cavity so that new healthy bone can fill it in as fully as possible.

Cavitation: Cavities within the Bone

In 1930, Dallas Burton Phemister coined the term *cavitation* to describe the "hollowed out" areas that can occur in various bones in the body.[44] Bone cavitations occur from both osteonecrosis and osteomyelitis. Osteonecrosis is degeneration of bone due to ischemia, or lack of blood supply. Besides the jawbone, it most commonly occurs in the hip joint (Legg-Calvé-Perthes syndrome), the knee joint (Osgood-Schlatter disease), and the spine (Scheuermann's disease). Osteomyelitis is an infection of the bone and bone marrow and is most often caused by *Staphylococcus aureus* bacteria. While osteomyelitis can occur in any bone, it most commonly occurs in the long bones (e.g., femur, tibia, and humerus), vertebrae, and pelvis—as well as the jawbone.[45]

However, as described in chapter 8, years before the term *cavitation* was coined, a dentist had already witnessed this phenomenon in the jawbone, which he called *chronic osteitis* (inflamed bone). In 1915, Dr. G. V. Black described this disease as a progressive "death of bone, cell by cell."[46] Black further witnessed that even the larger jawbone osteomyelitic cavitation areas full of necrotic debris could, unlike osteomyelitis in the body, cause no visible redness, swelling, or increase of a patient's temperature.[47] Besides identifying the chronic osteitis that is typical of serious yet silent dental focal infections, Black also pioneered the use of cavitation surgery to effectively clean out these bone lesions. He found that when these bone cavitation areas were "opened freely and every particle of softened bone removed . . . generally, the case makes a good recovery."[48]

Unfortunately—and quite analogous to the focal infection theory—pathological jawbone cavitations, coined as Black's disease by Dr. Jerry Bouquot, was forgotten by the dental profession for decades, becoming another statistic of the overzealous embrace of antibiotic medications in the mid-twentieth century. However, in the 1970s, it began to emerge again and has been reported under several different names, including Ratner or Roberts bone cavity, alveolar cavitational osteonecrosis, neuralgia-inducing cavitational osteonecrosis (NICO), and interference field (or focus).[49]

Osteonecrosis and osteomyelitis are similar in that they both cause bone (osteo-) degeneration and destruction, but in osteonecrosis this is due to ischemia (lack of blood supply) and in osteomyelitis this is due both to ischemia and infection. Thus, the term *interference field* more closely describes an osteonecrotic bone lesion, whereas the term *focal infection* more fully embraces an osteomyelitic bone lesion.

OSTEOMYELITIS IN THE BODY AND THE JAW DIFFER CONSIDERABLY

There is a distinction between an osteomyelitic infection in the jawbone versus one in the body. Because osteomyelitis in the body is often caused by *Staphylococcus aureus,* fever, swelling, pain, and demonstrable positive lab values (elevated white blood cells) usually occur within hours or days after the onset of the infection. Osteomyelitic infections in the body are conventionally treated through antibiotic therapy.[50] In contrast, an osteomyelitic infection in the jawbone is low-grade, silent, and subclinical, such that symptoms are often minimal or even nonexistent locally, and white blood cell (e.g., lymphocyte, neutrophil, or eosinophil) abnormalities are rarely seen in laboratory testing.

This identical type of infection responding in two different manners in two different parts of the body is an interesting phenomenon. Based on the principle of survival, one explanation is that infection can be better quarantined in the jaw, and the odonton (teeth and jawbone) can be sacrificed with no loss of life. Thus, in a somato-odonton (organ-tooth) relationship, perhaps the body wisely chooses the death of the tooth over the degeneration of the original organ focus. However, in the case of infection in the body, the osteomyelitic bone is closer to essential organs and tissues, and symptomatic adaptive measures that signal the need for help (e.g., pain, swelling, and redness) are necessary for survival. Furthermore, the more adequate blood supply in the body allows the passage of antibiotics to the bone infection, in contrast to the more ischemic areas in the jawbone, where antibiotics cannot readily reach and have little influence. Therefore, in chronic osteomyelitic jawbone cavitations, antibiotic therapies often fail.[51]

The primary cause of jawbone cavitations in extraction sites is the failure of the dentist or oral surgeon to remove all of the periodontal ligament when pulling a tooth. These remaining periodontal ligament pieces can later act as a barrier to the creation of new blood vessels and, therefore, to the regrowth of new bone.[52] Dr. Hal Huggins, likening the severity of this dental omission to the failure of removing the placenta (afterbirth) after delivering a baby, clearly explains this problem in his book *It's All in Your Head:*

> Bone cells will naturally grow to connect with other bone cells after tooth removal—providing they can communicate with each other. If the periodontal ligament is left in the socket, however, bone cells look out and see the ligament, so they do not attempt to "heal" by growing to find other bone cells.[53]

In addition to periodontal ligament fragments, particles of bone, root chips, and filling material left in the extraction site can also obstruct the regrowth of healthy bone tissue.[54] In these cases, Dr. Huggins and other researchers have found that approximately 2 to 3 millimeters of bone will superficially heal over the socket area; however, beneath the bone a hole, or cavitation, will remain (see figure 11.11). In these cases, giving antibiotics is rarely helpful because these antibacterial medications cannot fully reach the cavitation area due to the diminished blood supply.[55] In fact, during the extraction period itself, antibiotics may actually interfere with the healing process by converting osteoblasts (bone-building cells) to osteoclasts (cells that break down bone tissue), which further break down bone tissue and impede new bone formation.[56]*

Other contributors to cavitation formation include the introduction of bacteria into the extraction site, which is often caused by the lack of an adequate water filter on the dentist's water syringe,† and by clotting problems—either an increased tendency toward blood clots (thrombophilia) or a reduced ability to dissolve clots (hypofibrinolysis). In fact, the term for degeneration of bone tissue in these cavitation areas, *osteonecrosis,* is defined as the death of tissue due to poor blood supply.[57] Synonyms of osteonecrosis are *inflammatory liquefaction,* and, more familiarly, *gangrene.*[58] This

---

*The use of antibiotics during and after cavitation surgery is controversial. Dr. Christopher Hussar, a specialist in cavitation surgery, believes they are necessary to help immune-compromised patients "eradicate the residual bacterial infections." Dr. Jack Tips, a specialist on the candida syndrome, believes that antibiotics "encourage bacteria to mutate . . . [and that] the suppression of bacteria (and the immune system) with antibiotics may have opened the door to the more detrimental viral involvements." (S. Stockton, *Beyond Amalgam: The Hidden Hazard Posed by Jawbone Cavitations* [North Port, Fla.: Nature's Publishing, Ltd., 1998], 18, 19.) In my experience, antibiotics are almost always avoidable when the patient is prepared before and after surgery.

†ABC News *20/20* did a report on this subject, claiming that the water in most dental offices was dirtier than toilet water. (D. Ewing, *Let the Tooth Be Known* [Houston: Holistic Health Alternatives, 1998], 14.)

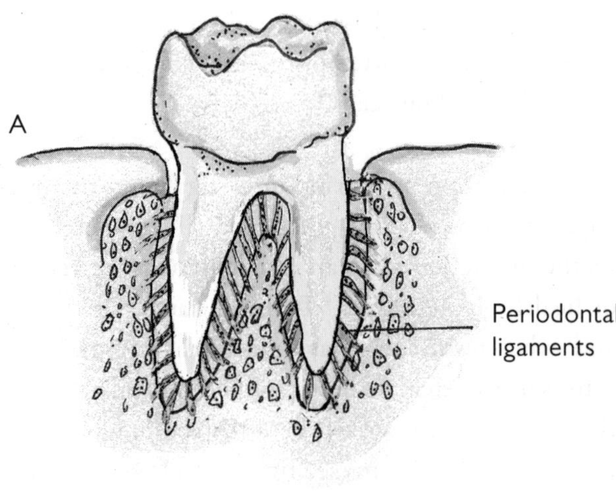

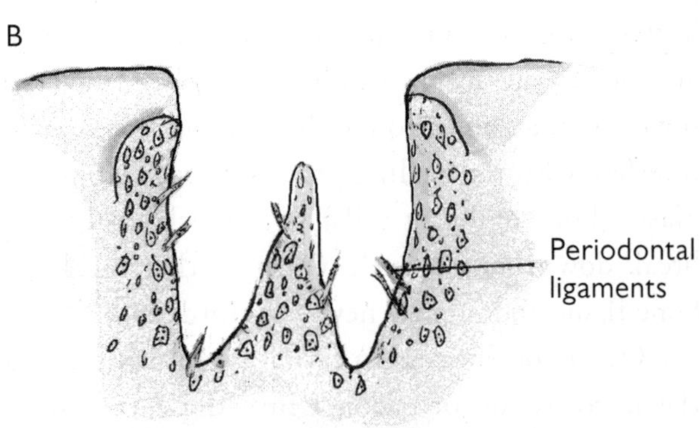

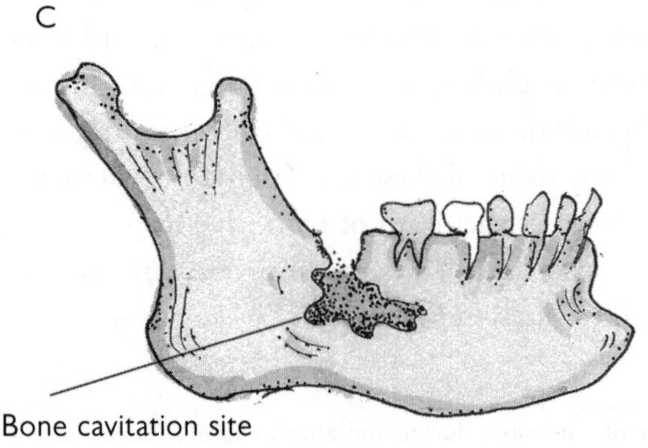

Figure 11.11. (A) Periodontal ligaments attach the teeth to the jawbone. (B) Nonholistic dentists may not drill out all the remaining pieces of ligament after pulling a tooth. (C) Cavitations, or holes in the jawbone, often form after these incomplete extractions.

latter term may seem too exaggerated since it primarily conjures up ghastly images of partial amputations on the battlefield. However, for those who have witnessed a dentist spooning out oily black mushy bone from an osteonecrotic cavitation site, the use of the term *gangrene* seems perfectly appropriate. (See figure 11.12.)

Other contributors to the formation of jawbone cavitations are abscessed teeth that infect the jawbone, failed root canals, and the use of mercury amalgam fillings. Mercury suppresses immune system functioning and suffocates intracellular respiratory mechanisms that can lead to cell death—organ cells, nerve cells, tissue cells, and bone cells.[59] The ingress of mercury into the body is primarily caused by the trauma of dental drilling to children's virgin teeth* and the subsequent spread of mercury through the microfractures made in the teeth.

Toxic mercury infiltrates the gums and jaws, as well as the rest of the body, through the bloodstream, lymphatic system, nerve fibers, and inhalation and swallowing. Chewing greatly enhances this spread of mercury, as well as the spread of bacteria from inflamed and infected teeth and gums. In fact, in one 1914 study, a researcher made cultures from the blood of twenty-five hospitalized senile patients with vascular disease and found a small streptococcus bacterium circulating in *three* of them. He then had these patients chew paraffin for thirty minutes and repeated his blood cultures. This time he observed the identical streptococcus in *twenty-one* of them, simply from that act of chewing.[60]

As discussed in chapter 3, inorganic mercury is *methylated* in the presence of bacteria to form possibly the most potent poison ever tested—organic mercury or methylmercury.[61] Within a short time after the implantation of mercury amalgam fillings, this toxic methylmercury is formed by mixing with the bacteria in the mouth. It then quickly invades vulnerable areas in the jawbone—compromised bone from dental drilling, abscessed teeth, and already existing cavitation areas. Unfortunately, this methylation process can occur even in a healthy mouth, because normal nonpathogenic bacteria in the mouth (and intestine) can also methylate mercury.[62] This newly formed organic mercury or methylmercury—substantially more toxic than inorganic or metallic mercury—necrotizes (destroys) bone cells at a much faster rate. Thus, the presence of mercury in the mouth and its ingress into the oral tissues is a primary generator of dental focal infections and jawbone cavitations.

*A "virgin" tooth is one that has never had any type of restoration—filling, inlay, onlay, crown, or root canal.

Cavitation Surgery Protocols

Pre-Cavitation Considerations. Before making the permanent decision to extract a tooth—whether a wisdom tooth or a front central incisor tooth—it is important to remove all of the factors that could be influencing the tooth's possible demise. In my experience, it is usually best to first remove an individual's amalgam fillings and other toxic metal restorations before undergoing cavitation surgery. Of course, there can be exceptions to this general rule, especially when a clear dental focus is apparent. However, even in these cases, if a suspected dental focus contains toxic metals such as a gold crown over a mercury amalgam filling, it is almost impossible even with skilled energetic testing to distinguish conclusively between a primary bacterial-induced dental focus and a galvanic-induced dental focus while these metals are still present in the tooth.* That is, this tooth may still have a chance to be saved by simply removing all of the toxic metals first.

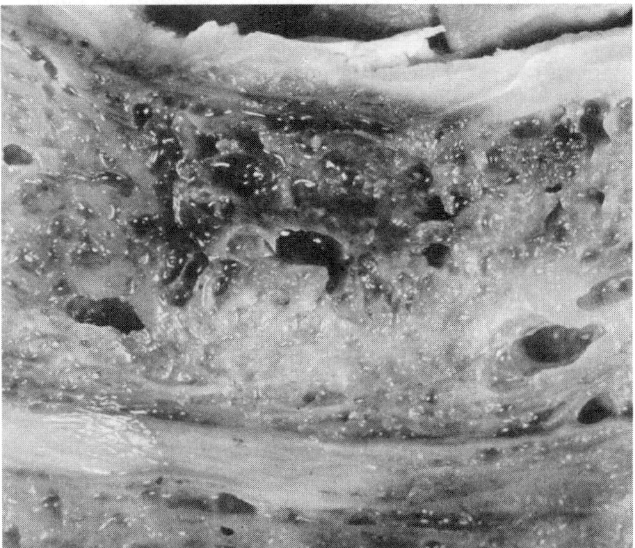

A. Gangrenous bone found in dental focal infections

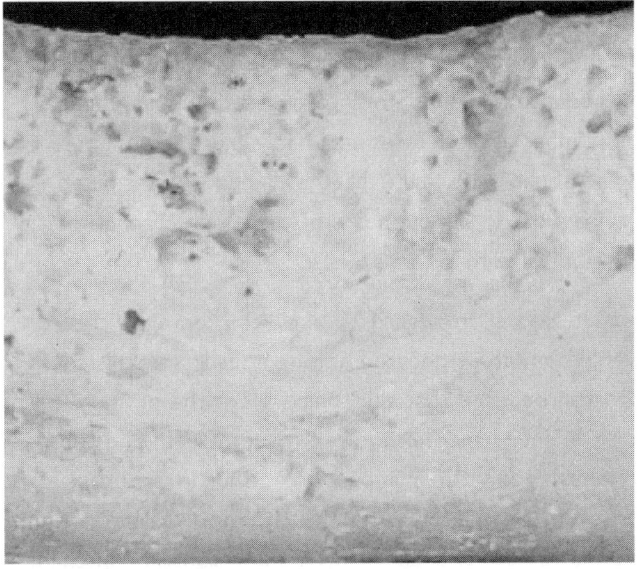

B. Healthy bone

Figure 11.12. (A) A photograph of a jawbone cavitation site (focal infection) with a prominent osteonecrotic, or gangrenous, area (in black), filled with dead bone, and (B) a photograph of a healthy jawbone. (Photos courtesy of Jerry Bouquot, D.D.S. See plate 7 for color renditions of these photos.)

In these instances, a temporary crown should be placed over the tooth for a few weeks or months to give the dentist and practitioner adequate time to determine if the tooth is viable. With this protocol, even if the tooth continues to show signs of a major dental focal infection and cavitation surgery is still indicated, the patient hasn't wasted money on a new crown and can rest assured that reasonable measures were made to attempt to save this tooth. On the other hand, if the tooth "settles down" symptomatically and no longer tests positive with energetic testing, and the X-rays show no visible signs of a cavitation, then at some point a permanent crown can be placed with more confidence.

Pre-Cavitation Support. Just as with amalgam filling removal, the individual must be strong enough to handle the stress of cavitation surgery. Therefore, since everyone has a unique history, each patient must be individually assessed for the appropriateness of the need for surgery in the first place, as well as the optimum time for it to be scheduled. In a significant number of cases, gemmotherapy remedies, constitutional homeopathy, nutritional support, Chinese medicines to tonify chi, and other holistic treatments are indicated weeks or months before scheduling surgery.

*However, if an X-ray is positive and reveals a large bone cavitation underlying the tooth, the patient may want to save the time and money spent on removing these metals and have the tooth extracted and the area cavitated, thus removing the toxic metals and the pathogenic bacteria in one stroke.

WISDOM TEETH

Wisdom teeth, or third molars, generally erupt between the ages of sixteen and twenty-one. Cavitations in the jawbone are most common around the wisdom teeth, and these teeth are the ones most commonly extracted. This tendency toward cavitations and extractions is due in part to the inaccessibility of the wisdom teeth; with the tight quarters at the back of the mouth, they're difficult to clean, and dentists have trouble maneuvering their fingers and instruments around them. This problem is amplified when the wisdom teeth are crowded or impacted—two extremely common conditions.

Fear of Injuring the Nerves

The delicate dental nerves (the trigeminal or fifth cranial nerves) that run below the teeth lie closer to the roots of the wisdom teeth than with any other teeth. Most dentists—although they have been taught virtually nothing in dental school about cavitation surgery—are well informed about the negative surgical side effects of injuring these nerves with conventional extraction methods. The most common side effect—chronic numbness of the cheek—can potentially last a lifetime.* Because this fact is often drilled into them in dental school (pun intended) and cavitation surgery is not, nonholistic dentists and oral surgeons often try to extract wisdom teeth as quickly and efficiently as possible and rarely risk nerve injury by removing any remaining pieces of periodontal ligament, necrotic (dead) bone, or other unwanted tissue.

Wisdom Teeth Are Often Infected

A large percentage of the wisdom teeth that are extracted are also impacted—that is, so embedded in the jawbone that their eruption is impossible. By definition, most impacted teeth are infected, which adds to the complexity of their extraction. In fact, in one study of impacted teeth in 600 patients, virtually *all* were found to be infected after the patients had reached a "certain level of maturity" (by the time they were teenagers).[63] One may wonder, then: are the impacted wisdom teeth creating inflammation and infection, or are they impacted and not properly erupting because they are already infected? Dr. Henry Cotton, an early-twentieth-century focal infection specialist in the treatment of the mentally ill, believed the latter.

> We have repeatedly shown that all impacted molars are infected—indeed it is probable that they are impacted because they are infected. The theory of pressure fails to explain the relation of impacted molars to arthritis, which has been found in so many cases. The only satisfactory explanation for the occurrence of impacted and unerupted molars and their influence on systemic disease is the one advanced by us that these teeth are infected early in their development and that by reason of this infection they fail to mature properly and continue to contaminate the system with micro-organisms . . . The question may well be asked, "How do these unerupted and impacted molars become infected?" Often, they are below the gum and embedded in the bone and have no connection with the oral cavity. From the fact that a number of these cases have badly infected tonsils it is reasonable to assume that the infection is transmitted from the tonsils by means of the lymph channels or blood stream to these teeth.[64]

Therefore, in regard to the "chicken-egg" controversy commonly debated among holistic specialists, Dr. Cotton believed that the tonsils were the primary culprit, infecting the neighboring wisdom teeth and subsequently causing their impaction and failure to erupt, or to erupt completely. And the common occurrence of numerous bouts of sore throats and tonsillitis in childhood helps explain why one dental researcher has found that "not a single patient (out of thousands) who had all four wisdom teeth removed was ever found to be cavitation-free and in fact, most had four cavitations, and nearly all the rest had three."[65]

*As previously discussed, homeopathic Hypericum perforatum 30C or 200C given quickly and intermittently after surgery for a few days or weeks can often mitigate and even cure numbness secondary to nerve injury.

The Effects of Poor Nutrition and Lack of Breastfeeding

The primary cause of crowded and impacted wisdom teeth is the nutritional habits of modern industrialized nations. Refined sugar and devitalized foods as well as the practice of replacing breastfeeding with bottle-feeding have greatly truncated the growth and development of our jawbones. The resulting lack of adequate jaw space leads to the common anomalies encountered in the third molar region—impacted teeth, abscessed teeth, and various malpositions, or teeth that grow in horizontally and even upside down (see figure 11.13). The crowding of our thirty-two teeth in our insufficiently sized jaws is a primary contributor to malocclusions, or bad bites, and temporomandibular joint dysfunction (TMD).

In the 1930s, Dr. Weston Price proved this point when he and his wife spent every summer for a decade visiting a total of fourteen different native cultures that did not have access to the foods of modern civilization. They found that in every case, not only was the rate of tooth decay extremely low—*less than 5 percent* in the cultures that were still eating only whole foods as compared with *greater than 90 percent* in modern cultures eating refined foods—but also that these people's traditional diets consisting of a variety of natural foods yielded straight teeth and broad facial structures that easily accommodated the four third molars or "wisdom" teeth.[66]

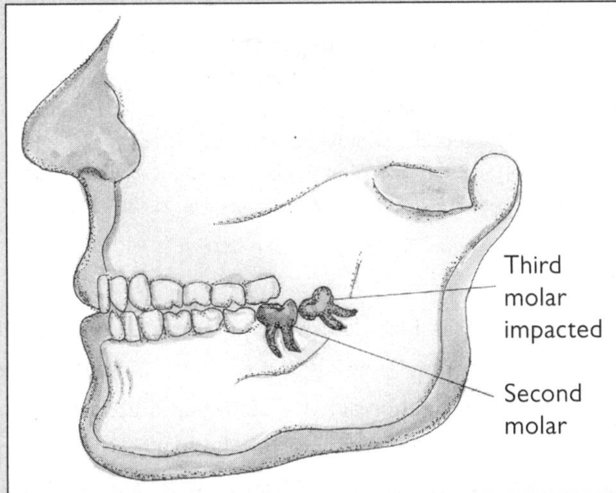

Figure 11.13. An example of a malpositioned third molar (wisdom tooth) due to the lack of jawbone growth and development

Before the third molars are extracted, the expansion of the jaws through orthopedic dental appliances should be considered if it is at all possible to make room for these four teeth to properly erupt. However, if the patient is older or if the third molars are already testing as focal infections, extraction and cavitation surgery are essential. Most holistic dentists suggest that the optimum time to remove these teeth is before the age of twenty, after they have come through the bone and are visible on X-ray but before they have cut through the gums.[67]

Wisdom Teeth Foci Linked to Neuropsychological Disorders

For more than fifty years Ernesto Adler, a holistic medical and dental physician, specialized in the study of the health effects of the wisdom teeth. As one of the most highly regarded experts in the field, this Spanish physician described the wisdom teeth as "terrorists" in our bodies and recommended early extraction.[68] Dr. Adler found a particularly high clinical correlation between the removal of wisdom teeth foci and subsequent relief from neurological disease. Using both neural therapy and cavitation surgery as treatments, he recorded many cured cases of epilepsy, stuttering, tremors, nervous tics, and multiple sclerosis, as well as manic depression and other neuropsychological disorders.[69] Both Adler and Jochen Gleditsch, a renowned German neural therapist, attribute the direct effect these third molars seem to have on brain and central nervous system functioning to the crowding of the *retromolar space* or *trigone* region just behind the wisdom teeth.[70] One diagnostic clue to this wisdom tooth crowding is the inability to place the tip of a little finger comfortably in this retromolar space. Although, as previously described, brain dysfunction is common with all streptococcus bacteria-related dental and tonsil focal infections, because of their direct central nervous system relationship, the wisdom teeth have a double impact—infectious and neurological—on the brain, and therefore tend to cause more serious cognitive disturbances.

The Worst Global Disease

Other classic disturbed fields arising from bacterial dental focal infections of the third molar teeth include arthritis, various forms of heart dysfunction and disease, and gastric and duodenal ulcers.[71*] In fact, as the dental relationship chart (figure 11.5 on page 331) depicts, the wisdom teeth have a direct acupuncture meridian reflex relationship with the heart and small intestine. Holistic practitioners and dentists experienced in the treatment of foci frequently see these two organ relationships and are especially aware of the serious impact wisdom teeth (or jawbone cavitations in the extraction site area) can have on cardiovascular function. Based on these relationships and resulting serious disease, Christopher Hussar, a holistic osteopath and dentist and a leading teacher in the techniques of cavitation surgery, asserted at a 1993 conference that incorrectly performed third molar extractions were actually the "worst global disease."[72]

Diagnosis of Wisdom Tooth Foci

As the previous information on wisdom teeth strongly suggests, alveolar or jawbone cavitations are not at all rare. Although estimates range greatly depending on the type of imaging used, the number of these chronic bone infections is indeed pandemic. After measuring more than 7,000 sites using the newest technology of the Cavitat instrument, one study found a whopping 94 percent of old extraction sites positive for bone cavitation lesions.[73†] Although not all of these areas were found to be the level III and IV lesions that often mandate surgery, this ninetieth-percentile finding is still staggering.

Many holistic dentists and practitioners rely on radiology, although they are aware that from 30 to 50 percent of bone must be destroyed before changes become radiographically evident. The most sensitive X-ray imaging technique is the simple periapical radiograph (an X-ray beam is focused around the root tip of the tooth). However, Dr. Jerry Bouquot, an expert on bone cavitations, has noted that the appropriate interpretation of these X-rays requires "considerable diagnostic experience . . . because changes are quite subtle and may mimic a number of other entities, including variations of normal anatomy."[74]

A thorough history (anamnesis), physical exam, clinical knowledge and experience, and quality energetic testing can greatly augment the diagnostic process when making a decision based on the more false-positive-tending Cavitat findings or the more false-negative-tending X-ray results.

Furthermore, the diagnosis of impacted wisdom teeth or malpositioned erupted wisdom teeth can often be distinguished from single dental foci through the presence of bilateral (both sides) symptoms rather than ipsilateral (same side) symptoms typically seen with single dental foci. These bilateral symptoms can include headaches on both sides of the head, hip pain in both joints, rashes not limited to one side of the body, or muscle aches and weakness in both arms or in both legs.

*In Appalachia, where more than 33 percent of elderly people have lost all their teeth, coronary heart disease is greater than anywhere else in the United States. (D. Page, *Your Jaws, Your Life* [Baltimore: SmilePage Publishers, 2003], title page.)

†In one new study of men, the biggest predictor for having a stroke was found to be not blood pressure, weight, stress, or activity level but having fewer than twenty-five teeth left in

(*continued*)
the mouth. These findings most probably indicate that when more than seven out of the original thirty-two teeth are (incorrectly) extracted, the amount of bacteria and toxicity generated from the remaining bone cavitations reaches a critical level and has a major impact on the survival of the individual. (S. Sinberg, *Pacific Sun*, January 15–21, 2003, 8.)

SUPPORT FROM CHINESE MEDICINE

Kidney (adrenal) chi (or qi) is bolstered by taking herbs according to the Chinese five-element body clock or according to the Law of Midday-Midnight. Taking kidney-supporting herbs during the kidney/bladder time of day, between 3 p.m. and 7 p.m., when these meridians are functioning at their peak energy, enhances the overall effect and uptake of these Chinese herbs (or gemmotherapy remedies such as Black Currant, Juniper, or White Birch Buds). Gently stimulating a hand or foot point related to the kidney can further aid the uptake and absorption of the herb into the organ. For a modified Su Jok hand chart developed by Dr. Yoshiaki Omura, who authored this selective drug uptake technique system, contact MIC at (201) 420-8988 or go to www.micint.com, or simply use a hand or foot chart available at your local health food store or in a Su Jok book. One of the gentlest kidney tonifying herbs that helps support both the yin and yang aspects of this organ is Jing; it is available from Dragon Herbs at (888) 558-6642.

It is also imperative to determine if a patient is taking any drugs that might contraindicate oral surgery. A recent article in the *Journal of Oral and Maxillofacial Surgery* reported that for patients taking oral (Fosamax or Actonel) or intravenous (Zometa or Aredia) bisphosphonate drugs, in a significant number of cases the jawbone did not heal properly after oral surgery.[75] Although this reported "osteonecrosis—or bone death—of the jaw" was most severe in cancer patients who had received the intravenous medications, about 10 percent of the sixty-three patients studied were taking Fosamax or Actonel—two extremely popular drugs that purportedly help prevent osteoporosis. Because bisphosphonates remain in bone indefinitely, the oral surgeon Salvatore Ruggiero (who coauthored the study) speculated that their long-term use could "upset the delicate balance between cells that put calcium in bone and cells that take calcium away."[76] Thus, in prospective patients for dental oral cavitation surgery it should be determined if they have *ever* taken these drugs, and if so, whether it is worth the risk to perform oral surgery on them.

OSTEOPOROSIS AND "DISEASE MONGERING"

In his book *Overdosed America,* John Abramson, M.D., asserts that "age-related osteoporosis is not a disease at all, but the quintessential example of successful 'disease mongering.'" He recommends that instead of taking drugs such as Fosamax and Actonel, women should engage in "constructive, evidence-based, inexpensive, do-it-yourself ways" to maintain bone health and prevent fractures, including regular exercise, a healthy diet, calcium and vitamin D supplements, and reducing the risk of falling. Additionally, Dr. Abramson reveals that taking Fosamax translates into reducing hip fracture by only a "tiny" margin (81 women with osteoporosis would have to take Fosamax for 4.2 years at a cost of more than $300,000 to prevent *one* hip fracture). The other drug, Actonel, didn't fare much better according to a study published in the *New England Journal of Medicine* in 2001, which disclosed that women with severe osteoporosis derived only a small benefit from taking this drug. Finally, a study in the Netherlands helps put into perspective the much touted bone mineral density (BMD) tests widely used to identify osteoporosis. This study found that the BMD score was only one of six factors identified for the risk of hip fractures. Other factors include the individual's level of frailty, muscle weakness, the side effects of other drugs, declining vision, and cigarette smoking. Dr. Abramson commented that "routine BMD testing may not be the best way to help women prevent hip fractures, but it is an excellent way to sell more drugs."[77]

As described previously, the cell salt Ferrum phosphoricum 6X should be prescribed with any positive signs of anemia—through physical exam, blood tests, or energetic testing—before (at least two weeks) and after cavitation surgery to augment healthy blood circulation, which is essential in the healing of surrounding jawbone and soft tissues. Calcarea phosphoricum 6X is helpful in cases of deficient blood coagulation. Known as "the bone builder," it is often prescribed in tandem with Ferrum phos before and after cavitation surgery. Additionally, Ferrum phos can be used acutely after surgery or anytime there is excess bleeding or inflammation. Because essential fatty acids (EFAs) are natural blood thinners, patients may want to stop their supplements of fish oil, borage oil, and evening primrose oil containing EPA, DHA, and GLA before surgery (at least for a week or two).

Cavitation Surgery Scheduling Considerations. Most patients opt to have one side extracted at a time (upper and lower third molars on the right or on the left), which requires less healing time than having all four teeth extracted at once. It also allows patients to chew on at least one side during the healing period. The time between these two extractions should be *at least* one month to allow full healing of the first two extraction sites.

Some patients opt to "get it over with" and remove all four third molars at once under general anesthesia. However, general anesthesia is more difficult for the liver to detoxify and requires more recuperative time than local anesthesia. Therefore, this quick removal option of all four third molars at once can be shortsighted, because the risk of one or more of these sites not fully healing and later fulminating into a chronic focus is greater.

One older tradition from Europe that some holistic dentists follow is not to perform surgery while the moon is waxing—that is, when it is full or almost full. It is said that surgeries are less successful during these "building" lunar cycles, and that they should be performed during the waning or "receding" lunar periods, when it is more appropriate to extract teeth.*

Cavitation Surgery Techniques. As already discussed, to avoid the future development of cavitations, the dentist or oral surgeon must remove all of the periodontal ligament and at least 1 millimeter of bone from the socket after tooth extraction. This cutting or "perturbing" of the bone not only removes the layers of bone that are infected with bacteria but also stimulates osteoblast cells (bone-producing cells) to lay down new healthy bone in the area.[78]

However, when dealing with healed-over sockets from previous incomplete extractions, cavitation surgery is more complex. Often, there are small tunnels or "worm holes"—up to 6 centimeters long in some cases—that are difficult to see and even more difficult to clean out.[79] Successful cavitation surgery of these older bone lesions requires great technical skill as well as sound judgment and good clinical instincts gained from extensive surgical experience.

For these deeper bone cavitations, it is helpful to use some form of energetic testing to determine when all of the necrotic (dead) bone and other matter has been adequately debrided.† Thus, a referral to a holistic dentist or oral surgeon who is knowledgeable about dental focal infections and has been well trained in cavitation surgery techniques as well as energetic testing is most optimal.

Finding a Well-Trained Dentist or Oral Surgeon. At this time, conventional dentists and even oral surgeons receive no education on the focal infection theory or cavitation surgery techniques in their dental schools or graduate training programs. Therefore, holistic dentists and oral surgeons must take specific postgraduate courses in these subjects in order to perform surgery accurately and effectively. If there is no one in your area, contact the dental associations listed below for a referral to a holistic dentist or oral surgeon skilled in the diagnosis of dental foci and treatment through cavitation surgery. Although you may have to travel some distance to visit a holistic dentist, it will probably be less expensive in the long run.

▶ To locate a holistic dentist or oral surgeon who specializes in cavitation surgery, contact one of the following organizations: DAMS at (651) 644-4572 or dams@usfamily.net; HDA at www.holisticdental.org; IABDM at www.iabdm.org; or IAOMT at www.iaomt.org.

The importance of choosing an experienced dentist or dental surgeon well versed in diagnosing and treating cavitations can be exemplified by Wilt Chamberlain's rapid demise after dental surgery. After having various dental foci—teeth damaged during his basketball career—removed, this sixty-three-year-old basketball legend lost approximately fifty pounds in one month and then died of an apparent heart attack.[80] His sister commented on his condition after his dental surgery: "He said it was the worst pain. I never heard him complain about pain ever," she said during a news conference. "He said he felt worse than he ever did . . . He looked worse than I have ever seen him."[81]

Although it's impossible to say exactly what caused this basketball legend's demise, the evidence strongly implicates that dental surgery probably liberated the bacteria from Chamberlain's chronic dental focal infections into his systemic circulation, and the bacteria then migrated to one of the five major rheumatic fields, in his case the heart, and overwhelmed this already weakened organ. (He was hospitalized in 1992 for an irregular heartbeat and possibly suffered a previous heart attack as early as 1964.) Dr. Henry Cotton explains in the following quote why these dental foci, which can be easily triggered and cause morbidity and even mortality relatively quickly, have been referred to as "silent time bombs":

> These chronic infections [dental and tonsil foci] are of a very low grade of virulence and show a very slow rate of progress. It usually takes years before the symptoms develop as the result of these infections and during this time the virulence of such infection is very slight,

*Another European custom is to place the extracted tooth in a solution of copper sulfate for a few days, which is said to allow healing to occur more effectively in the extraction site.

†The reflex arm length, or MRT, technique and auricular medicine are the most sensitive in determining when the cavitation surgery is complete. They are also the easiest to perform in the dental chair. Electroacupuncture instruments are also helpful, but they emit an electromagnetic stress that can cause distortions and false readings.

> or, indeed, may be negative. However, after having gained sufficient headway, any change in the individual—whether caused by mental or physical factors—may cause a latent infection to become virulent and bring about the death of the patient in a very short time.[82]

Postsurgery Procedures and Treatments. It is just as important to follow postsurgery procedures as it is to adequately prepare for surgery. The box on pages 354–55 compiles the postoperative instructions that holistic dentists often give to their patients. It is imperative that patients take *at least* three days off from work, and optimally five days off, to truly rest and relax. Even the vibration of extensive car and plane travel or the physical activity of long walks soon after surgery causes the blood pressure to rise and may renew bleeding in the wound and delay healing.

Additionally, the use of a therapeutic laser (830 nanometers and 100 milliwatts) is so effective in healing the inflamed nerves and soft (gums) and hard (bone) tissues that it has become a sine qua non in my postsurgical protocol. Patients generally use this laser by placing the probe next to the cheek over the surgery site for one minute at a time, anywhere from six to ten times a day for the first three days, and then tapering off to three or four times a day for the last two days. This laser often obviates the need for any pain medication, or can reduce the amount needed considerably. Through the protocol of loaning out this laser for five days after dental surgery, patients are saved the stress of making frequent trips to the doctor's office during this period when they should be resting and recuperating.

Also, as described previously, Notatum 4X, Aspergillus 4X drops, or Kombination 4X drops are often needed postsurgically to augment healing in the site. These isopathic drops can be dropped directly on the surgical site, often at a protocol of 2 or 3 drops three times a day for five days, and then one or two times a day for one week thereafter. (See "Neural Therapy," beginning on page 341, for more information about laser treatments and isopathic remedies.)

Acute homeopathic remedies are also essential for complete healing. As described previously, Arnica montana 30C is most commonly prescribed at a dose of 2 pellets, three times a day, for five days, and then once a day for one week thereafter. If the surgery was very extensive, then the higher potency of Arnica montana 200C should be used for the first two or three days, and then the patient can switch to the lower 30C potency. If the surgery was very deep and there is a chance that the maxillary (upper jaw) or mandibular (lower jaw) nerve was damaged, Hypericum perforatum 30C should also be taken, but at different times of the day than when the Arnica is taken, at a dose of 2 pellets, two or three times a day, for five days, and then once a day for a week thereafter. Again, if the nerve injury is suspected to be considerable, Hypericum perforatum 200C and even 1M should be used for the first two or three days.

There is one exception to the use of Arnica and Hypericum, however. When patients are already on their constitutional remedy, they should dose *this* remedy and not Arnica or Hypericum after surgery. However, the patient and the homeopathic practitioner must be very sure that this constitutional remedy is truly correct and is effecting *significant* changes in the individual's physical, mental, and emotional symptoms for the patient to utilize this remedy postsurgically. (These common homeopathic remedies are available at any health food store. See page 340 for more information.)

Additionally, one or more vials of Quinton marine plasma taken daily after surgery will further ensure the healing and appropriate mineralization of the gums, jawbone, and neighboring teeth. Patients should hold the contents of each vial in their mouth for approximately a minute to aid oral assimilation, and then swallow. Finally, 1 teaspoon to 1 tablespoon of organic sulfur taken one to three times a day can be very healing to the gums, nerves, and jawbone.

Following surgery, many dentists have the tooth and bone tissue samples analyzed through Dr. Jerry Bouquot's laboratory at the University of Texas Health Science Center at Houston. In one study of thirty-eight patients referred by me to Dr. Russ Borneman for cavitation surgery, 100 percent showed positive histological (tissue-related) signs of ischemic osteonecrosis (bone death) and osteomyelitis (bone infection).[83] In a larger clinical study of 175 operations conducted by Dr. Hans Lechner, a holistic dentist in Munich, laboratory analysis showed only one patient who had no positive bone findings (infection or destruction) postsurgically.[84] These histological findings are a good confirmation for the patient, as well as the dentist and doctor, that cavitation surgery was indeed necessary.

GENERAL POSTOPERATIVE INSTRUCTIONS AFTER DENTAL CAVITATION SURGERY*

Prepare in Advance

Food. A clear broth is best to drink when you first arrive home from surgery. After that, fresh or frozen soups, stews, and broths that can be well pureed before being served are nutritious and filling and don't require much chewing. Organic meat (lamb, beef), poultry (chicken, turkey), or fish broths along with vegetables (e.g., carrots, squash, turnips, onions, kale) supply the protein, vitamin, and mineral requirements needed for healing after surgery.

Also, stock up on oatmeal (pureed), rice, and millet (to make rice or millet cream cereal)† or buy prepackaged cream of rice or wheat. (Though if the incision site does not seem to be closing together well, you might want to avoid even these pureed grains until it adheres together appropriately.) Other easy-to-eat foods include applesauce, yogurt (if you are not allergic to it), soft tofu, and squash and potatoes (pureed). Additionally, make sure you have lots of pure water on hand.

Castor Oil Packs. At some point after surgery, the disturbed field—that is, the kidney, pancreas, stomach, liver, intestine, or other chronically disturbed organ or tissue—may begin to display healing signs through symptoms of pain or discomfort. By applying a castor oil pack to the area in the body that hurts, you can reduce "downstream" any dysfunction or toxicity in this chronically disturbed field that can reflex back "upstream" to the healing socket. In this way, the postsurgical socket can continue healing without interruption, and the disturbed field in the body can receive a regenerating and healing treatment.

For information on how to apply a castor oil pack, look under Therapies in the Edgar Cayce Health Database at www.edgarcayce.org. You will need a piece of soft cotton or flannel, a bottle of castor oil, and a heating pad or hot water bottle. In general, the directions are to pour castor oil onto the body part as well as the cloth, cover the body part with the cloth, then place the heating pad (or hot water bottle) over the cloth, with plastic wrap in between so the heating pad cover does not get stained. Turn the heating pad on low and relax for one to one and a half hours.

Things to Expect

Swelling. This is normal. It should reach its maximum in twenty-four to forty-eight hours, and then diminish by the fourth or fifth postoperative day.

Discomfort. The most discomfort that you will experience will be during the time when sensation returns to your mouth. However, homeopathic and the isopathic drops, infrared laser, and any needed pain medication should greatly reduce any discomfort.

Hemorrhage. Bleeding or "oozing" is expected the first twelve to twenty-four hours.

Indentation. There will be an indentation where your tooth was removed or where the extraction site was cavitated. It will have a spongy feeling for the first two or three days, and then it will gradually fill in with new tissue.

Things to Do

Bleeding. Bite gently on the sponges placed in your mouth for at least one hour after surgery. If bleeding is more than slight, follow these directions: With gauze remove all excess blood clots. Place gauze over the bleeding area only. Hold this pack in place firmly for twenty minutes, so that no blood escapes. Repeat this procedure if necessary. You can also use a moistened tea bag between gauze strips as an astringent. (Taking Ferrum phosphoricum 6X and Calcarea phosphoricum 6X cell salts at least 2 weeks before and after surgery can greatly reduce bleeding problems.)

Swelling. The amount of swelling is usually in proportion to the surgery involved, but it typically reduces in three to four days. The use of cold packs over the side of the face that was operated on can minimize swell-

*These instructions are a compilation of information provided by Dr. Gerry Becker, Dr. Russ Borneman, Dr. Robert Jarvis, and myself. The infrared Canadian laser is available from Rick McKay at (250) 474-3514 or jarek.mfg@shaw.ca. The homeopathic and cell salt remedies are available from health food stores or from Seroyal at (888) 737-6925 or www.seroyal.com. The isopathic remedies are available from BioResource at (800) 203-3775.

†Grind rice or millet in a grinder and then cook like oatmeal at a 2:½ ratio (water:grain). Grind to an absolute powder so no grains become stuck in the incision site.

ing. Cold packs should be applied for 15 minutes and then removed and left off for 15 minutes. Continue this procedure for a few hours. Prolonged use of ice is not useful. The infrared laser greatly minimizes swelling.

Pain. If you experience excessive pain, bleeding, or swelling, call your holistic dentist and practitioner.

Diet. After waiting one hour or so, you should be able to take fluids by mouth. A liquid or soft diet may be necessary for the first two days, such as soups, mashed potatoes, vegetable broths, and smoothies. Do not eat anything with small seeds or grains or other parts that could become stuck in your wound. Adequate pure water intake is essential.

Mouth Rinse. Do not rinse your mouth on the day of surgery. After the first day, rinsing your mouth with warm salt water (1 teaspoon of salt in an 8-ounce glass of water) following meals is helpful to speed healing by maintaining a clean wound. Do not brush your teeth for at least 24 hours, and after that period do so very gently, still avoiding the surgical area.

Rest. For optimum healing, completely rest the remainder of the day after surgery, using the infrared laser and taking the homeopathic (Arnica montana 30C or your constitutional remedy), isopathic (e.g., Notatum 4X), and cell salt remedies (Ferrum phos 6X and Calc phos 6X) as prescribed. Then continue resting and recuperating with very little activity over the next four days at least.

Sores at the Corner of the Mouth. This is common after surgery; apply a petroleum-free ointment to speed healing.

Things Not to Do

Avoid Heat. Do not apply heat to your face; this will increase swelling.

Avoid Spitting. This can create a negative pressure in your mouth and possibly dissolve the blood clot, leading to additional bleeding.

Do Not Drink from a Straw. This can dislodge the blood clot.

Avoid Strenuous Physical Activity. Physical activity causes the blood pressure to rise and may lead to a renewal of the bleeding.

Problems

Numbness. For a few days or weeks after surgery, you may have slight numbness of the cheek or lower lip, especially if a lower and/or impacted tooth was removed. This is usually a temporary condition. However, if the numbness is not subsiding or is significant, contact your dentist or practitioner, who will often prescribe Hypericum perforatum 30C (or 200C), at a dosage of 2 pellets, three times a day, for several days or so. (If your dentist had to come too close to the nerve, he or she may have already prescribed this treatment along with Arnica.)

Dry Socket. If a slight earache or sore throat develops initially, then goes away, but *then returns*—often with severe pain in the ear and socket, accompanied by a foul smell—your blood clot may be lost and you may have a condition referred to as "dry socket." This is a serious postoperative problem; call your dentist immediately. (In the vast majority of cases, dry socket can be avoided by closely adhering to all post-cavitation procedures, taking the prescribed remedies, and using the infrared laser.)

Sensitivity. Your surrounding teeth may be sensitive to cold for a while, but this sensation should subside over time.

Stitches. Not all of the self-dissolving stitches always dissolve in a timely manner. If you find yourself feeling somewhat irritable or tense on the sixth or seventh day after surgery, this could be due to the contraction the stitches are causing in the surgery site. Contact your dentist or surgeon, if this seems to be the case, to diagnose whether your stitches should be removed. (This most typically occurs in patients who have used the laser, which significantly speeds up the healing of the gums and bone.)

► Dentists and oral surgeons can order biopsy kits from Dr. Jerry Bouquot at (713) 500-4420 or jerry.bouquot@uth.tmc.edu.

It is important for the patient to return for a follow-up examination within one to two weeks after cavitation surgery. Cardinal signs that the cavitation surgery was a success and that healing is occurring in a timely and appropriate manner are that the patient is feeling much better and is experiencing little to no pain. Energetic testing signs include a negative therapy localization (gently made) over the extraction site and its disturbed field(s) and related ganglia, and the previously weak muscles associated with this dental focus and its disturbed field(s) now testing strong.

If the extraction site does not heal properly, it can become reinfected and dry socket can occur. The cause of a dry socket can be explained as follows. Just as with an injury on the skin, a blood clot is formed when a tooth is extracted. Unlike the skin, however, the mouth is full of saliva, so a clot never fully hardens into a dry scab. Dry socket, or "septic socket," happens when bacteria invade the area between the blood clot and the bone, and the blood clot is lost, thereby leaving the socket empty or "dry."[85] When this occurs, the exposed bone cannot heal because it can't form a new clot. Dry socket is usually signaled through pain, often severe—either in the extraction site or in the ipsilateral (same side) ear. Additionally, there is typically a foul odor, and sometimes swelling around the site or in the neighboring lymph glands. The standard treatment of antibiotics and eugenol from the oil of cloves for pain does little to help a new clot to form, and many believe the clove oil actually impairs healing in the area.[86] In these unfortunate cases, the holistic dentist or surgeon often needs to drill out the exposed infected bone and re-suture the site. If this procedure does not stimulate the formation of a new blood clot and subsequent healing, then cavitation surgery should be repeated. Thus, dry socket is a serious postoperative consequence. However, it can usually be prevented through adequate pre- and postsurgical therapies and protocols, and by using *only* dentists and surgeons well trained in cavitation surgery procedures.

Another traditional custom that should be mentioned is not to remove the stitches the following week on the same day of the week the surgery was performed. That is, if the cavitation surgery was performed on a Monday, the patient should have the stitches removed, not the next Monday, but on a Tuesday or Wednesday. It is generally believed that the immune system works on a seven-day cycle, and that the healing of the cavitation site will be interrupted if there is disturbance one week later. Dr. Hal Huggins, who has popularized this seven-day cycle concept, also cautions patients not to undergo any major therapies—more surgery or even more mercury amalgam removal—seven, fourteen, or twenty-one days after the first procedure has been completed.[87]

Finally, many dentists and oral surgeons currently use stitches that easily dissolve in the mouth. However, sometimes these stitches do not adequately dissolve as they should, and they need to be removed by the dentist or practitioner because they can constrict the tissue too much after a few days and thus impede healing. As previously described, this is especially the case with the use of the Canadian laser, when healing is so speeded up that stitches need to be removed sooner than usual.

THE ROOT CANAL CONTROVERSY

A root canal treatment that does not plant a focus does not exist!

SCHONDORF

A tooth-root-filling (root canal) is, according to Professor Kellner (1983) always a "scar with disturbed wound-healing," because it contains exogenous material . . . [similar to] shrapnel pieces after war injuries.

F. PERGER

Ninety-eight percent of our adult cancer patients have from two to ten devitalized teeth [both root-canalled and untreated].

JOSEF M. ISSELS, M.D.

The anti-root-canal sentiment espoused by these three European researchers is shared by many holistic U.S. practitioners and dentists based on their clinical experience. The focal-infection-inducing effect and the potential toxicity of root canals has also been well researched in many scientific studies.[88] In fact, most of the research on dental focal infections conducted by Billings, Rosenow, Rosenau, and Price previously described in chapter 8 was made on root-canal-filled teeth. In particular, Dr. Weston Price concentrated his studies on the effects of root canals and found that "practically zero" of these teeth were *not* infected with bacteria.[89] However, being the holistic dental physician that he was, he did not advocate the immediate extraction of all "pulpless teeth," as root canals were often referred to in the early 1900s. Here is his response to a colleague who accused him of that position in a spirited debate at a 1925 American Dental Association meeting in Louisville:

> . . . I must qualify the question as to the extraction of that [root canal] tooth by saying that a great deal depends on the danger of the overloads, the age of the patient and various contributing factors . . . a person at 55 years of age cannot be given the same treatment that would be given to a person 25 years of age. But all pulpless teeth, root filled or not, harbor so much danger of becoming infected that they should be extracted, though the time as to when they should be extracted will depend on several contributing factors. If the patient belongs to a family in which there is a low defense for streptococcal infection, it had better be soon . . . If the patient is in another group with a very high defense and not much in danger of overloads, and if it is a tooth that is greatly needed by that patient, I would advise you to do what I do: retain some of those root filled teeth, because I believe they are of more value to the patient in the mouth than out.[90]

Even today, the debate rages on whether root canals should be performed at all, and whether all existing root-canalled teeth should be extracted. Although root canal procedures and materials have improved since Price's era (although the typical filling material, gutta-percha, remains the same), they continue to be, along with incorrectly extracted wisdom teeth sites, the most culpable dental foci in existence and are implicated in a wide variety of diseases.[91] Due to the preponderance of clinical and scientific evidence that the root canal procedure is "fatally flawed," many holistic dentists and practitioners are soundly against them and do not recommend them to their patients.[92]

However, extraction of infected and devitalized teeth brings up other problems. Bridges destroy half of the two healthy neighboring teeth's structure, which can hasten the future demise of either or both of them.[93] Although a removable partial is the healthiest solution, many people object to the plastic appliance and/or the metal clasps, as well as to the "granny" image of false teeth.[94] Furthermore, the use of dental implants, even with the use of the "fairly biocompatible" titanium or newer zirconium, can continually leach some degree of metal into the body at a low and continuous rate. Additionally, implants often test as a focus just through their irritating effect as a foreign body in the jaw and the electromagnetic fields generated from the metal. They have also been implicated in the causation of several autoimmune syndromes.[95] Finally, if an individual opts to do nothing, over a number of years the neighboring and opposing teeth may (but not always) move into the space left from the extraction, leading to possible decay, gum problems, and malocclusions.[96]

Obviously, there are no good solutions to the loss of a tooth. Therefore, some patients opt for a root canal from a more holistically oriented dentist or endodontist (a specialist in root canals) who utilizes the best possible materials and the most up-to-date procedures. Once again, the quintessential holistic dental physician, Dr. Weston Price, always weighed the state of the tooth against the health of the patient, and he found that not all root canals create problems in the body:

> It is not proven that it is absolutely necessary that teeth be perfectly sterilized or that they be perfectly root-filled in order that an individual may not develop systemic involvement, since under favorable conditions the patient may provide an adequate defense or quarantine against these materials.[97]

That is, if an individual is healthy—in a dormant or rarely active psoric reaction mode—a root canal can be a viable option. In fact, in a recent study conducted by a leading amalgam and dental researcher, Dr. Boyd Haley, 25 percent of even conventional root-canalled teeth showed no obvious toxicity.[98] Of course, *obvious* is the key word here, since silent dental foci can cause considerable stress in the system before frank infection is apparent. However, when quality energetic testing methods render no apparent positive findings along with the history, laboratory, and general physical exam, then root-canalled teeth should be left alone in this dormant and quiescent state. However, if there are any adverse changes in an individual's health at some point in the future, this tooth should be thoroughly reevaluated, and extraction and cavitation surgery should be considered.

What Is a Root Canal?

Simply speaking, a root canal is a procedure in which the dentist or endodontist drills a hole through the crown (top) of the tooth and removes the pulp from the pulp chamber and the root canals. This pulp is the soft tissue of the tooth, which contains nerves, arteries, veins, and lymph vessels (see figure 11.14). After all the pulp is removed, most dentists flush the chamber out with an antibacterial solution. Some dentists fill the (now empty) pulp chamber and root canals immediately, while others wait for a second appointment.[99] The most common material used to seal off the tooth is called gutta-percha.

> **root canal:** The term *root canal* has two meanings: It is the anatomical term for the canals or pathways in the teeth from which the nerves, lymph, and blood vessels enter from the outside, and it is also the term for the procedure used to treat an infected tooth, primarily done by endodontists.

Drawbacks of the Root Canal Procedure

The main problem with root canals is that it is virtually impossible to completely seal off and sterilize a pulpless tooth, which Dr. Weston Price decisively proved almost a century ago.[100] The reason complete sterilization is impossible is that the tooth contains literally miles of tiny tubules (figure 11.15).[101] Although these dentin tubules are tiny, they are wide enough for bacteria to fit three abreast—a "virtual mansion" for these anaerobic (non-oxygen-breathing) bacteria.[102] Because these tubules run perpendicular to the root canals, they cannot be cleaned out during the procedure. And antibiotics are useless because there is no longer any blood supply to the tooth, since the blood vessels are entirely removed during a root canal procedure.[103] These anaerobic bacteria can then multiply in a root-filled tooth and produce toxic chemicals that leak out laterally through a microfracture in the tooth or through the apex (the tip of the root) from an ineffective seal in one of the canals.[104]

In addition, there are also drawbacks to the various filling materials used in root canals.

Gutta-Percha. Currently the most common root canal filling material, gutta-percha is a sticky substance made from the rubber tree.[105] However, only a minor portion of the gutta-percha is actually made up of natural rubber. The rest is composed of zinc oxide, barium (15 percent to make it show up on an X-ray), and traces of heavy metals such as lead and cadmium (up to 0.6 percent).[106]* Although a cadmium-free gutta-percha has recently been produced, random control testings of the product have shown that cadmium had not been actually removed from some samples. In my clinical experience, (supposedly) cadmium-free gutta-percha has not consistently tested as "clean" and inert. Additionally, because gutta-percha contains a synthetic type of latex, dentists and physicians have considered it to be potentially dangerous if the patient has a latex allergy.[107]

Gutta-percha is also problematic because it shrinks. Through his extensive research of this material in the early 1900s, Dr. Weston Price found that it was a "physical impossibility to fill a pulp chamber with gutta percha."[108] No matter what solvent or other chemicals are mixed with it, when the warm, rubbery gutta-percha cools and sets for a few days, shrinkage occurs, which then allows bacteria to multiply and escape through the apex of the tooth.[109]

Silver Point. Another material used to fill root canals is called silver point. These silver cones inserted into the roots of the tooth were notorious for leaching silver into the bone and body, producing symptoms similar to mercury poisoning (see figure 11.16).[110] Fortunately, silver point root canals are no longer the standard in modern endodontics. However, if individuals are older, have received dentistry from an older dentist trained in this procedure, or are from a third-world country, they may still have one of these toxic "time bombs" in their mouths.

Sargenti Paste. Another root canal filling material, called Sargenti paste, contains formaldehyde and lead and has been denounced even by the conservative ADA.[111] Although the current formulas have presumably removed the lead, tens of millions of these root canal treatments using the old formulas are still in people's mouths. Therefore, for your present and

*Although Dr. Hal Huggins and other authors have asserted in the past that gutta-percha contains mercury, this is probably no longer correct (although it may have been true in the 1930s or 1940s). The orange pigmentation of this material is more likely from an iron compound.

future well-being, anyone who has older root canals and is suspicious about the materials used should make an appointment with a holistic dentist.

A final drawback to conventional root canals is that from as early as the 1960s and even up to today, many nonholistic dentists packed mercury amalgam above the gutta-percha-filled roots as a filling material in a root-canalled tooth. Adding further insult to injury, typically a crown—often gold—is placed over the entire tooth. This triple threat of heavy-metals-containing gutta-percha (cadmium), mercury amal-

THE ANATOMY OF A HEALTHY TOOTH

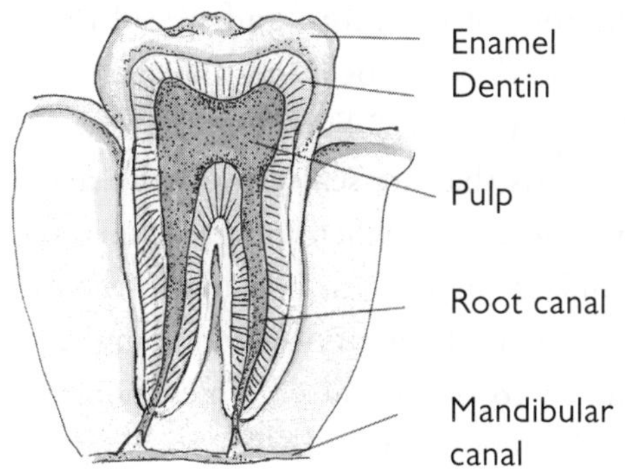

AN INFECTED TOOTH

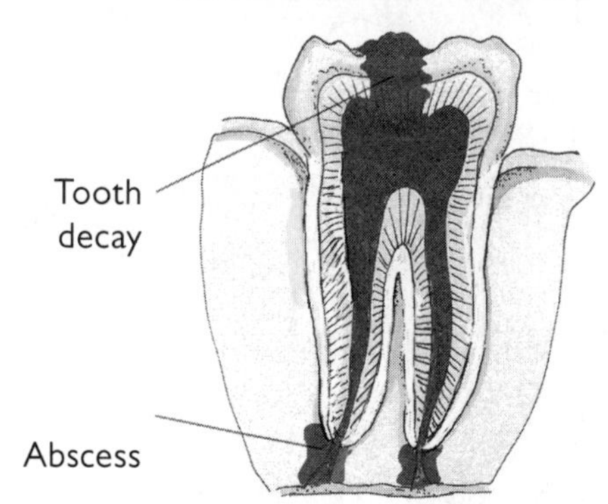

THE ROOT CANAL PROCEDURE

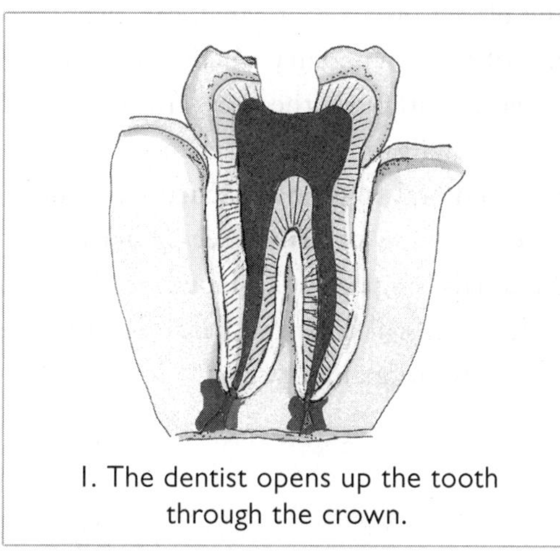

1. The dentist opens up the tooth through the crown.

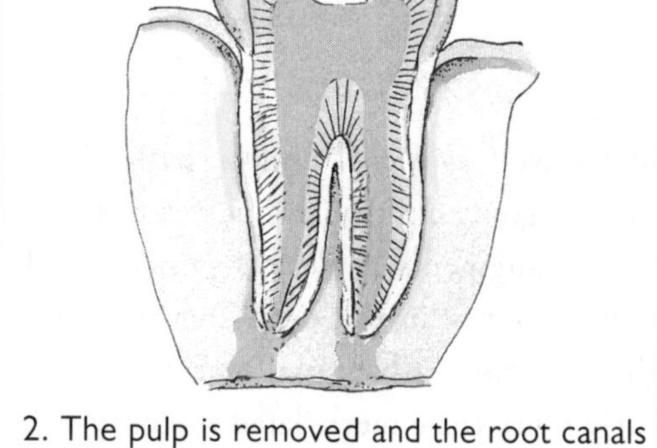

2. The pulp is removed and the root canals of the teeth are cleaned out and enlarged.

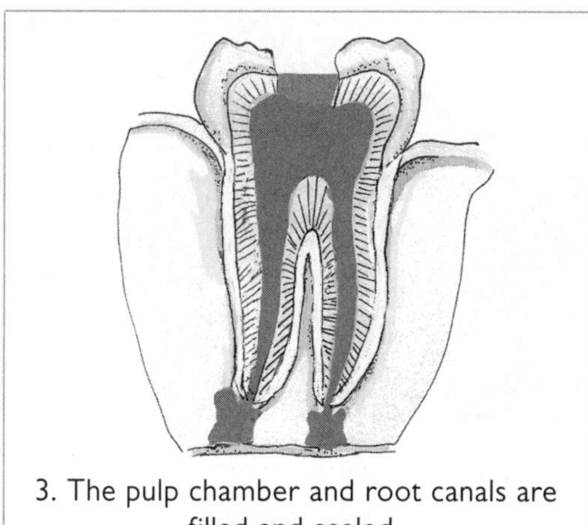

3. The pulp chamber and root canals are filled and sealed.

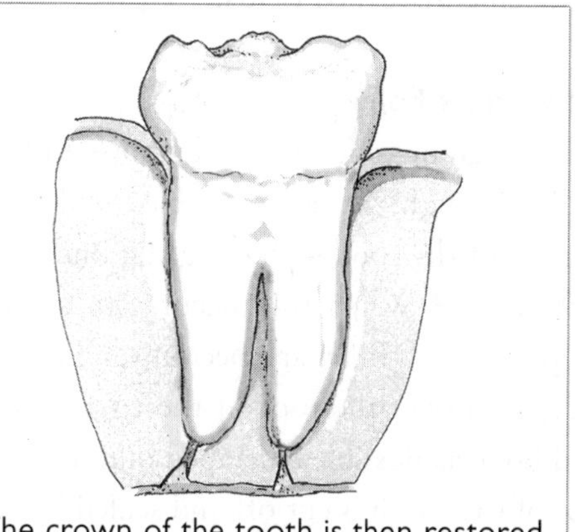

4. The crown of the tooth is then restored through a filling, inlay, onlay, or crown.

Figure 11.14. The anatomy of a healthy tooth and an infected tooth, and the root canal procedure

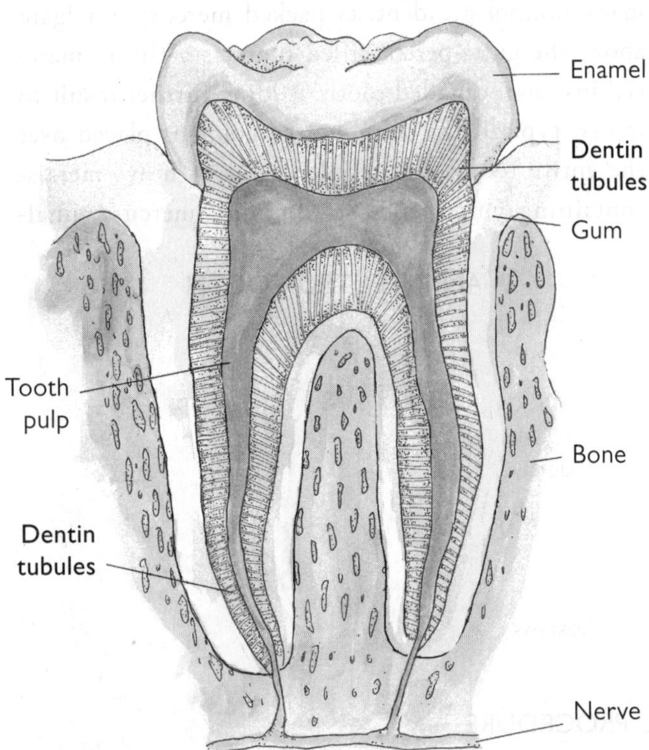

Figure 11.15. There are literally miles of dentin tubules in a tooth, and they are wide enough for anaerobic bacteria to live three abreast.

gam, and gold (as well as nickel and/or palladium) elicits instant and ongoing electrogalvanic stress in the mouth and greatly augments the pathogenicity and off-gassing of the mercury in the overlying amalgam filling through the action of bacterial methylation.[112] This significantly more toxic methylated mercury can metastasize to various parts of the body and establish seriously pathogenic disturbed fields.

When Root Canals Fail

A certain percentage of root canals obviously fail and abscess, usually through the egress of bacterial toxins through the apex of the tooth infecting the underlying alveolar (jaw) bone.[113] When this occurs, an apicoectomy is often performed. In an apicoectomy, an incision is made in the gum over the root of the tooth and as much infected bone as possible is scraped out. Then the tip of the root of the tooth is cut off and sealed.[114]

The problems with this procedure are twofold. First, the tooth and bone are still infected, because an apicoectomy cannot sterilize an infected tooth root and bone any more than a conventional root canal can. Second, the standard protocol has been to use amalgam to seal off the tip of the root. As unbelievable as this may seem, mercury—the second most toxic metal (next to plutonium) known—is directly implanted in the maxillary (upper jaw) or mandibular (lower jaw) alveolar bone! Unfortunately for the unsuspecting patient, pieces of this mercury often escape from this implant at the root of the tooth and spread through the jawbone, and they can be impossible to remove even if the tooth is extracted.[115] Furthermore, as was the case with root canals that are sealed over with amalgam, as previously described, when inorganic metallic mercury in an implant mixes with bacteria in the tooth, it forms organic methylmercury—a compound estimated to be from ten to one hundred times more toxic than the original metallic mercury.[116]

Through this electrogalvanic augmentation, the toxicity of an apicoectomy, or even simply an amalgam filling placed over a root canal, can rival that of an entire mouthful of mercury amalgam fillings. Fortunately, however, although the standard of choice has been the use of amalgam for decades, more and more endodontists and oral surgeons are currently using an alternative medical-grade cement. (See "Alternative Root Canal Materials" on page 362.) However, the apicoectomy procedure can still be just as hazardous to a patient's health as a conventional root canal.

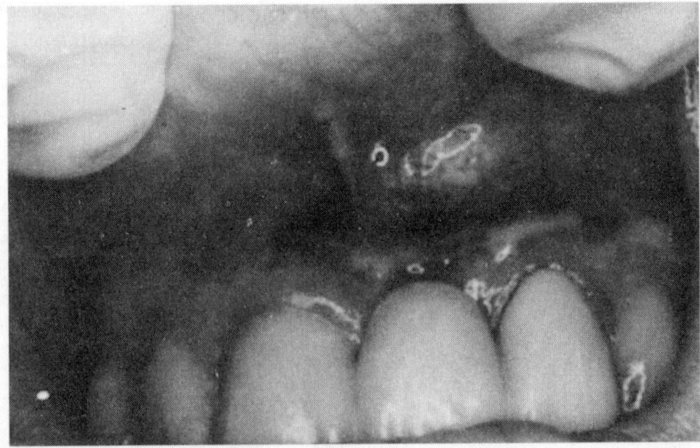

Figure 11.16. A visible silver stain or "tattoo" in the gums. Photograph provided courtesy of Dr. William P. Glaros of Houston, Texas. (See plate 8 for a color rendition of this photo.)

Preventing Root Canals

So, what do you do when your dentist tells you that you need a root canal? First of all, it is important to be aware that far too often conventional dentists prescribe root canal treatments for still viable teeth. Therefore, always get a second opinion from a holistic or biological dentist. (To locate a holistic or biological dentist, see the contact information on page 336.) In many cases a root canal is actually not needed, and a deep cavity can be effectively sealed with an inlay, an onlay, or, if necessary, a crown. Additionally, a holistic dentist who is trained in diagnosing malocclusions and treating temporomandibular dysfunction can also determine if the tooth is simply being structurally injured through a "traumatic bite" and prescribe a splint or oral appliance that can greatly reduce the trauma, and even save the tooth.

Another red flag that can signal you may be in the wrong dental office are dentists who "jump" from fillings to crowns. Individuals should be highly suspicious if their dentist suggests that a crown is needed for a virgin (never been treated) tooth, or a tooth that has only a filling. Holistic dentists take pains to remove as little tooth material as possible with the use of slightly larger fillings, inlays (laboratory-made restorations that fit inside the cavity), or onlays (laboratory-made restorations that cover the top of the tooth). Although restorations such as a larger filling, inlay, or onlay take more artistic skill and in most cases remunerate the dentist less than an expensive crown does, they remove much less vital tooth substance. For example, when a dentist places a crown on a tooth, from 40 to 75 percent of the tooth structure must be removed.[117] In light of this fact, it is understandable that 20 percent of crowned teeth (immediately or eventually) require root canals, because the tooth's nerve is vulnerable to permanent damage during the crowning procedure.[118]* Therefore, one of the best ways to prevent future root canals, besides good dental hygiene and a clean diet, is to consent to a crown only if you are absolutely sure it is necessary, and you have additionally consulted with a holistic dentist about this decision.

Furthermore, some conventional dentists actually suggest the need for "prophylactic" root canals. This abhorrent practice is often done before a crown is placed, so that this crown will not have to be removed at a future time when the patient may then be judged to need a root canal. Prophylactic root canals are obviously a form of gross malpractice, and patients should avoid dentists who recommend them like the plague.

Finally, knowledgeable holistic practitioners who use energetic testing can often determine if the decay was actually caused through a somato-odonton relationship—that is, an organ or tissue in the body. In these cases, where the original focus was an organ, and the tooth was, at least initially, simply the disturbed field, treating the original pancreas, stomach, lung, or large intestine may help arrest or at least slow the degeneration of the disturbed-field tooth. Other possible scenarios include teeth that have become chronically disturbed fields from a nearby tonsil focal infection. In these cases, the tonsil focus needs to be treated first—and this can be lengthy—before making a final decision about the viability of the tooth. Finally, Schuessler's cell salts, coenzyme Q10, an isopathic or homeopathic remedy, Quinton marine plasma vials, and organic sulfur can be very supportive and in many cases actually regenerative to bone and gum tissue.

Alternative Root Canal Materials

If the nerve in a tooth is positively beyond repair, and a root canal or extraction is required, the decision of how to proceed can be difficult. As discussed previously, none of the alternatives is perfect, and any eventual decision about this issue will always be a compromise. However, if an individual is in good health, the decision to have a root canal and to closely monitor this root canal—and its related disturbed fields and ganglia—over the following years is one viable choice.

If an individual chooses to have a root canal, there is one root canal filling material in use by holistic dentists that is considered to be a better choice than the conventional gutta-percha. Although no root filling can ensure complete sterility, U.S. dentists have recently begun using a mineral compound that has been in use in Europe for more than thirty years.[119] Primarily composed of calcium oxide and zinc oxide, the compound has the ability to gently expand into the root canals and even penetrate into the dental tubules, sealing off these areas from bacterial ingress better than gutta-percha.[120]

*The figure of 20 percent refers to the number of root canals needed within a year or so of the crown procedure and is probably a low estimate of the actual number of teeth that eventually die from the exposure of the nerve and the suffocation of the tooth's tissues.

Furthermore, this material has been shown in several studies to inhibit the growth of anaerobic bacteria.[121] Dentists can order this calcium-zinc compound, currently named EndoCal 10 (previously named Biocalex), from the Biodent company in Quebec, Canada.

- To order EndoCal 10, dentists can contact Biodent at (800) 363-2876 or go to their website at www.biodent.com.

One criticism of EndoCal 10 is that it doesn't expand into and reach the very apex, or tip, of the root. Alternatively, when it does reach the tip, it can sometimes fracture the filled root of the tooth.[122] To solve this problem, Dr. Richard Hansen and Dr. Scott Loman, two California holistic dentists, have pioneered the use of a material called mineral trioxide aggregate (MTA). Also known as medical-grade and modified Portland cement, this material was developed for use as the primary filling material in apicoectomies.* MTA cement is packed into the terminal 2 millimeters of the tooth's root, and then the rest of the roots and pulp chamber are filled with EndoCal 10. Research studies have shown that the bacterial regrowth after utilizing MTA is rare, and sometimes almost nonexistent.[123] This more effective seal of the roots can allow for the regrowth of the tooth's ligaments as well as that of the surrounding bone. Although the tooth is nonvital, Dr. Loman points out that it is still fulfilling a mechanical function in the body by "maintaining its viability as part of the masticatory apparatus."[124] That is, the patient's bite remains stable, unlike the malocclusions that can result from the extraction and nonreplacement of a tooth.

- To order MTA, dentists can contact Dentsply Tulsa Dental Specialties at (800) 662-1202 or go to www.tulsadental.com.

In the hands of a careful and technically skillful dentist or endodontist, these two new materials may render a devitalized tooth reasonably nontoxic and quiescent for some years in a healthy patient's body.† And the word *skillful* cannot be overemphasized. The more expert and precise the dentist or endodontist is in carefully filling the roots, the longer the root-canalled tooth will remain in a relatively dormant and nondisturbing state.

The intermittent use of the so-called natural antibiotic Notatum 4X, or the bone and tissue isopathic remedy Aspergillus 4X, can also help mitigate the negative effects of a root-canalled tooth. These drops can help reduce the pathogenicity of the bacteria being generated, as well as help heal and strengthen the tooth, gums, and surrounding bone. Additionally, cell salts—specifically Calcarea phosphoricum 6X and Magnesium phosphoricum 6X—and the Quinton marine plasma vials can both help mineralize and harden the teeth and bones and strengthen these structural tissues.

As will be discussed in chapter 14, constitutional homeopathy, according to Dr. Rajan Sankaran's new system of finding the most perfectly fitting remedy, heals and strengthens the body on every level—physically, emotionally, mentally, and spiritually. Therefore, individuals who are on their deepest constitutional remedy seem to "handle" the existence of one or two root canals in their mouth better than those who are not.

Before undergoing a root canal procedure, it is imperative that patients be well informed about their choices; this includes getting a second opinion with a holistic dentist to determine if the tooth is truly a nonvital (dead) tooth. Furthermore, a holistic dentist or practitioner who utilizes energetic testing may be able to determine if this tooth's disturbed fields or other toxic foci are actually the primary cause of the problem, and if treatment of these areas may be appropriate.

There are no easy solutions in the case of a nonvital tooth. Furthermore, the toxicity of the materials used in conventional root canals, combined with the lack of education and understanding about dental focal infections by the majority of endodontists, only adds to the difficulty in this decision making. If the patient is not seriously ill and does not want to lose a tooth, then the choice of a root canal treatment with the alternative mineral compound materials previously described can be a reasonable compromise if it is done as carefully and as skillfully as possible. This tooth should be monitored

*Nonrefined Portland cement has also been used in the building trades for years. MTA is a finely granulated modification of this cement.

†Nonendodontic dentists also perform root canals after special postgraduate training. This is especially true in the use of these alternative materials.

over the years, however, as well as the patient's state of health, and if any adverse changes arise, or the patient receives a serious diagnosis, then extraction and cavitation surgery should be seriously considered.

CONCLUSION

Ever since the original concept of focal infection led to an excess of extractions over 70 years ago, the theory has been in relative disrepute. And yet to ignore focal infection is to refuse to recognize an abundant literature, all of medical significance.

HUBERT NEWMAN, D.D.S., *JOURNAL OF DENTAL RESEARCH,* NOVEMBER 1992

Dental foci must be carefully diagnosed by knowledgeable, well-trained, and clinically experienced dentists and practitioners. When time is not a factor, all possibilities for saving the tooth should be exhausted, including constitutional homeopathy, isopathy, cell salts, nutrition, and auriculotherapy, as well as removing toxic metals and using orthopedic appliances to expand the dimensions of the jaw (e.g., to make room for wisdom teeth). If the tooth cannot be saved, the patient should be given a choice between a root canal or cavitation surgery, based on the knowledge of his or her present state of health and the clinical judgment of the holistic dentist and practitioner. In the case of a serious disease such as cancer, the tooth is often sacrificed in the hope of more quickly boosting the patient's immune system functioning by removing this chronic source of infection. In a 1930s journal article that extensively reviewed focal infection literature, Dr. Edward Hatton summarized the importance of careful clinical decision making on this subject:

> A conservative decision [whether to pull the tooth] is indicated where the patient is in good health and relatively immune to mouth and other infections. In cases of persons severely ill with heart disease, active diabetes, advanced anemias, leukemia, acute infectious processes, the acute stages of secondary focal infection, etc., it should be the rule to certainly eliminate all infection about the teeth, even though this may include the removal of a few treated teeth which appear to be negative, both in the radiograph and as a result of careful clinical examination.[125]

As with toxic metals, prevention is key. If dental schools simply trained dentists to remove all pieces of the tooth's periodontal ligament and at least 1 millimeter of bone after every extraction, bone cavitations would decrease precipitously. Furthermore, the history and theory underlying dental focal infections should be taught once again in both dental and medical schools, so that this important body of credible research is not lost to the profession and to humanity. Through this education, dentists and doctors could communicate with each other more fully about the profound impact dental foci can have on the body, as well as the reverse scenario—the impact dysfunction in the body can have on the teeth and gums. A final quote from a holistic dentist named Dr. A. Porter from Hornell, New York, once again from the first half of the twentieth century, when dental foci were well understood, describes the importance of a good working relationship between the holistic dentist and physician, especially before any surgical procedures:

> It is very evident that the dental consultant should be well-trained in oral diagnosis. He should be keenly aware of the danger of systemic disease through mouth infection, should know the oral cavity thoroughly in health and disease and should be able to take good roentgenograms and interpret them. Too often a physician refers his patient to a dentist who sticks a mouth mirror and an explorer into the patient's mouth and gives the patient a clean bill of health because there are no cavities, instead of exhausting all methods of diagnosis as he should . . . The physician should have a dental consultant in whom he has perfect confidence and from whom he demands full responsibility for the condition of the patient's oral cavity.
>
> The dentist in turn should make every effort to find and eliminate every possible focus of infection. In some hospitals every incoming patient has a thorough oral examination. This may not be necessary for every patient, but every patient that is to be operated on should have

every focus of infection removed, if possible, before they are placed on the operating table.

A patient's mouth should receive as careful preoperative attention as the heart and lungs. What good does it to keep the operative field sterile when the blood may bring in infection from a chronic alveolar abscess [dental focus] or a bad case of pyorrhea [gum disease] that has been overlooked?

In conclusion, let us hope that the near future will bring rapid advancement in the locating and control of focal infection and that our two professions may jointly carry on this good work.[126]

This hope is still alive in the hearts and minds of many holistic-thinking individuals.

NOTES

1. W. Boyd, *A Textbook of Pathology*, 8th ed. (Philadelphia: Lea and Febiger, 1970), 1439.
2. J. Bouquot, *In Review of NICO (Neuralgia-Inducing Cavitational Osteonecrosis), G. V. Black's Forgotten Disease*, 3rd ed. (Morgantown, W.Va.: The Maxillofacial Center, 1995), 3; D. Ewing, *Let the Tooth Be Known* (Houston: Holistic Health Alternatives, 1998), 48–49.
3. J. Bouquot and A. Roberts, "NICO (Neuralgia-Inducing Cavitational Osteonecrosis): Radiographic Appearance of the 'Invisible' Osteomyelitis," *Oral Surgery, Oral Medicine, Oral Pathology, Oral Radiology, and Endodontology* 74, November 1992, 202.
4. E. Hatton, "Focal Infection" in G. Black, *Operative Dentistry* (Woodstock, Ill.: Medico-Dental Publishing Company, 1948), 436.
5. Ibid.
6. L. Cashman, "Cavitat Approved by the FDA," *Dental Truth*, June 2002, 25.
7. J. Bouquot et al., "Computer-Based Thru-Transmission Sonography (CTS) Imaging of Ischemic Osteonecrosis of the Jaws—A Preliminary Investigation of 6 Cadaver Jaws and 15 Pain Patients," *Oral Surgery, Oral Medicine, Oral Pathology, Oral Radiology, and Endontology* 92 (April 2001).
8. J. Bouquot, "Through-Transmission Alveolar Sonography (TAU)—New Technology for the Evaluation of Low Bone Density and Ischemic Disease. Correlation with Histopathology of 339 Scanned Alveolar Sites," Presentation to the American Academy of Oral and Maxillofacial Pathology (April 2002); D. Ewing, *Let the Tooth Be Known* (Houston: Holistic Health Alternatives, 1998), 50.
9. Ibid., 48.
10. R. Voll, *Interrelations of Odontons and Tonsils to Organs, Fields of Disturbance, and Tissue Systems* (Uelzen, Germany: Medizinisch Literarische Verlagsgesellschaft MBH, 1978), 128–29, 131–32; J. Issels, *More Cures for Cancer*, translation from German (Bad Homburg, Germany: Helfer Publishing E. Schwabe, 1980), 14.
11. Ibid., 10.
12. P. Dosch, *Manual of Neural Therapy* (Heidelberg: Haug Publishers, 1984), 464.
13. R. Stone, *Polarity Therapy*, volume 1 (Sebastopol, Calif.: CRCS Publications, 1986), 42–49.
14. R. Voll, *Interrelationships of Odontons and Tonsils to Organs, Fields of Disturbance, and Tissue Systems* (Uelzen, Germany: Medizinisch Literarische Verlagsgesellschaft MBH, 1978), 111.
15. F. Kramer, "Bekannte und neue Erkenntnisse zum Thema Wechselbeziehungen zwischen bestimmten Zahn-Kieferstrecken und dem übrigen Organismus," *Deutxch Aeitschrift für Biological Zahnmedicin* 10, no. 3 (1994): 104–17.
16. M. M. Van Benschoten, "A Critical Investigation of Electrodiagnostic Instrumentation Using Omura's Bidigital O-ring Test," *American Journal of Acupuncture* 19, no. 3 (1991): 237–40.
17. R. Haden, "Elective Localization of Streptococci," *Orthodontia and Oral Surgery, International Journal* 12 (1926): 711.
18. G. Vithoulkas, *The Science of Homeopathy* (New York: Grove Press, Inc., 1980), 36–37.
19. F. Pottenger, *Pottenger's Cats: A Study in Nutrition* (San Diego: Price Pottenger Nutrition Foundation, 1995), 22.
20. D. Ewing, *Let the Tooth Be Known*, 2nd ed. (Houston: Holistic Health Alternatives, 2002), 31, 90.
21. Ibid., 90–91.
22. Personal communication with Dr. Scott Loman, February 19, 2003.
23. D. Ewing, *Let the Tooth Be Known*, 2nd ed. (Houston: Holistic Health Alternatives, 2002), 90.
24. R. Hansen, "Everything You Wanted to Know about Root Canals (and How to Avoid Them)," *Alternative Medicine*, November 1999, 32.
25. J. Bouquot, *In Review of NICO (Neuralgia-Inducing Cavitational Osteonecrosis), G. V. Black's Forgotten Disease*, 3rd ed. (Morgantown, W.Va.: The Maxillofacial Center, 1995), 2.

26. W. Price, *Dental Infections: Oral and Systemic* (Cleveland: The Penton Press Company, 1923), 20.

27. S. Sinatra, *The Coenzyme Q10 Phenomenon* (Los Angeles: Lowell House, 1998), 87–90.

28. J. Ely, "Micromercurialism and Coenzyme Q10," *Well Mind Association's Annual Scientific Symposium*, Seattle (1996): 1–2.

29. *The Twelve Biochemical Salts of Dr. Schuessler* (Toronto: Seroyal, n.d.), 1.

30. G. Carey, *The Biochemic System of Medicine* (New Delhi: B. Jain Publishers, 1989), 26.

31. Ibid., 35.

32. Whole Food Farmacy Wellness Center, www.wholefoodfarmacy.com/fluoride1.asp.

33. The Fluoride Debate: A Response to the American Dental Association's Booklet *Fluoridation Facts,* www.fluoridedebate.com.

34. *The Twelve Biochemical Salts of Dr. Schuessler* (Toronto: Seroyal, n.d.), 4.

35. G. Carey, *The Biochemic System of Medicine* (New Delhi: B. Jain Publishers, 1989), 40, 43.

36. Ibid., 53.

37. Ibid., 116.

38. *The Twelve Biochemical Salts of Dr. Schuessler* (Toronto: Seroyal, n.d.), 14.

39. Ibid.

40. S. H. Shakman, *E. C. Rosenow and Associates* (Santa Monica, Calif.: Institute of Science, 1998), A5C–A5E.

41. S. H. Shakman, *The Autohemotherapy Reference Manual* (Santa Monica, Calif.: Institute of Science, 1998), ch. 5, p. 3.

42. R. Sankaran, *The Sensation in Homeopathy* (Mumbai, India: Homeopathic Medical Publishers, 2005), 24.

43. P. Nogier, *Handbook to Auriculotherapy* (Sainte-Ruffine, France: Maisonneuve, 1981), 149.

44. J. Bouquot, *In Review of NICO (Neuralgia-Inducing Cavitational Osteonecrosis), G. V. Black's Forgotten Disease,* 3rd ed. (Morgantown, W.Va.: The Maxillofacial Center, 1995), 1.

45. R. Berkow et al., eds., *The Merck Manual,* 15th ed. (Rahway, N.J.: Merck Sharp and Dohme Research Laboratories, 1987), 1245, 2108, 2109.

46. J. Bouquot, *In Review of NICO (Neuralgia-Inducing Cavitational Osteonecrosis), G. V. Black's Forgotten Disease,* 3rd ed. (Morgantown, W.Va.: The Maxillofacial Center, 1995), 1.

47. Ibid.

48. M. Ring, *Dentistry: An Illustrated History* (New York: Harry N. Abrams, Inc., 1985), 276; J. Bouquot, *In Review of NICO (Neuralgia-Inducing Cavitational Osteonecrosis), G. V. Black's Forgotten Disease,* 3rd ed. (Morgantown, W.Va.: The Maxillofacial Center, 1995), 1.

49. Ibid.

50. R. Berkow et al., eds., *The Merck Manual,* 15th ed. (Rahway, N.J.: Merck Sharp and Dohme Research Laboratories, 1987), 1245, 1246.

51. J. Bouquot, *In Review of NICO (Neuralgia-Inducing Cavitational Osteonecrosis), G. V. Black's Forgotten Disease,* 3rd ed. (Morgantown, W.Va.: The Maxillofacial Center, 1995), 5; S. Stockton, *Beyond Amalgam: The Hidden Hazard Posed by Jawbone Cavitations* (North Port, Fla.: Nature's Publishing, Ltd., 1998), 18, 19.

52. Ibid., 16.

53. H. Huggins, *It's All in Your Head* (Garden City Park, N.Y.: Avery Publishing Group, Inc., 1993), 46.

54. R. Haden, *Dental Infection and Systemic Disease* (Philadelphia: Lea and Febiger, 1936), 25.

55. S. Stockton, *Beyond Amalgam: The Hidden Hazard Posed by Jawbone Cavitations* (North Port, Fla.: Nature's Publishing, Ltd., 1998), 18, 19.

56. G. Meinig, *Root Canal Cover-Up* (Ojai, Calif.: Bion Publishing, 1994), 194.

57. D. Ewing, *Let the Tooth Be Known,* 2nd ed. (Houston: Holistic Health Alternatives, 2002), 47, 51.

58. J. Issels, *More Cures for Cancer,* translation from German (Bad Homburg, Germany: Helfer Publishing E. Schwabe, 1980), 9.

59. D. Eggleston, "Amalgams and the Immune System Effect of Dental Amalgam and Nickel Alloys on T-Lymphocytes," *The Journal of Prosthetic Dentistry* 51, no. 5 (May 1984).

60. M. Fischer, *Death and Dentistry* (Springfield, Ill.: Charles C. Thomas, 1940), 38.

61. U. Heintze et al., "Methylation of Mercury from Dental Amalgam and Mercuric Chloride by Oral Streptococci In Vitro," *Scandinavian Journal of Dental Research* 91 (1983): 150–52.

62. I. Rowland et al., "The Methylation of Mercuric Chloride by Human Intestinal Bacteria," *Experientia (Basel)* 31 (1975): 1064–65.

63. O. Meyer, "The Eliminating Function of the Tonsils in Dental Infections," *Dental Digest,* December 1944, 557.

64. H. Cotton, *The Defective, Delinquent and Insane* (New York: Arno Press, 1980), 46.

65. R. Kulacz and T. Levy, *The Roots of Disease* (Bloomington, Ind.: Xlibris Corporation, 2002), 110.

66. S. Stockton, *Beyond Amalgam: The Hidden Hazard Posed by Jawbone Cavitations* (North Port, Fla.: Nature's Publishing, Ltd., 1998), 26.
67. F. Jerome, *Tooth Truth* (San Diego: ProMotion Publishing, 1995), 288.
68. E. Adler, "Wisdom Tooth—Unlucky Tooth" (monograph, Rambla Barnes 6, E-17310, Lloret de Mar, Gerona, Spain, n.d.), 1.
69. E. Adler, *Neural Focal Dentistry,* 2nd ed., trans. Javier Escobar (Houston: Multi-Discipline Research Foundation, 1984).
70. E. Adler, "Wisdom Tooth—Unlucky Tooth" (monograph, Rambla Barnes 6, E-17310, Lloret de Mar, Gerona, Spain, n.d.), 3.
71. J. Harrison, *The Periodontal Solution: Healthy Gums Naturally* (Delray Beach, Fla.: Corinthian Health Press, 2001), 13–18.
72. R. Shane and L. Williams, *A Manual of Dominant Focus Therapeutics* (Seattle: self-published, 1993), 10.
73. D. Ewing, *Let the Tooth Be Known,* 2nd ed. (Houston: Holistic Health Alternatives, 2002), 48.
74. J. Bouquot, *In Review of NICO (Neuralgia-Inducing Cavitational Osteonecrosis), G. V. Black's Forgotten Disease,* 3rd ed. (Morgantown, W.Va.: The Maxillofacial Center, 1995), 3, 5.
75. R. Rubin, "Drug Linked to Death of Jawbone," www.usatoday.com/news/health/2005-03-13-jawbone-deaths_x.htm.
76. Ibid.
77. J. Abramson, *Overdosed America* (New York: HarperCollins, 2004), 213–20.
78. S. Stockton, *Beyond Amalgam: The Hidden Hazard Posed by Jawbone Cavitations* (North Port, Fla.: Nature's Publishing, Ltd., 1998), 19.
79. Ibid.
80. Associated Press, "Chamberlain Had an Irregular Heartbeat," October 13, 1999, http://msn.espn.go.com/nba/news/1999/1012/110895.html.
81. Ibid.
82. H. Cotton, *The Defective Delinquent and Insane* (New York: Arno Press, 1980), 35.
83. R. Borneman and L. Williams, "Histological Signs of Dental Ischemic Necrosis and Osteomyelitis Correlated with Clinical and Kinesiological Testing Indicators" (unpublished research findings from the Head and Neck Diagnostics of America Laboratory, Seattle, 1995–96).
84. J. Lechner, "Biological Dental Seminar," transcript from a seminar in Bellevue, Wash., August 4–5, 1995, 3.
85. F. Jerome, *Tooth Truth* (San Diego: ProMotion Publishing, 1995), 282.
86. Ibid.
87. L. Williams, *Essentials of Cavitation Surgery* (Seattle: self-published, 1996), 9.
88. S. Gobel and J. Binck, "Degenerative Changes in Primary Trigeminal Axons and in Neurons in Nucleus Caudalis Following Tooth Pulp Extirpations in the Cat," *Brain Research* 132 (1977): 347–54; J. Issels, *More Cures for Cancer,* translation from German (Bad Homburg, Germany: Helfer Publishing E. Schwabe, 1980), 4–14; G. Meinig, *Root Canal Cover-Up* (Ojai, Calif.: Bion Publishing, 1994), 57–61; R. Kulacz and T. Levy, *The Roots of Disease* (Bloomington, Ind.: Xlibris Corporation, 2002), 223–33.
89. W. Price, *Dental Infections: Oral and Systemic* (Cleveland: Penton Press Company, 1923), 199–211.
90. A. Nichols, "The Virulence and Classification of Streptococci Isolated from Apical Infections," *The Journal of the American Dental Association* 13 (1926): 1227.
91. G. Meinig, *Root Canal Cover-Up* (Ojai, Calif.: Bion Publishing, 1994), 57–61; R. Kulacz and T. Levy, *The Roots of Disease* (Bloomington, Ind.: Xlibris Corporation, 2002), 42–51.
92. Ibid., 152.
93. F. Jerome, *Tooth Truth* (San Diego: ProMotion Publishing, 1995), 242–43.
94. D. Ewing, *Let the Tooth Be Known,* 2nd ed. (Houston: Holistic Health Alternatives, 2002), 85.
95. R. Kulacz and T. Levy, *The Roots of Disease* (Bloomington, Ind.: Xlibris Corporation, 2002), 118–23.
96. F. Jerome, *Tooth Truth* (San Diego: ProMotion Publishing, 1995), 245.
97. W. Price, *Dental Infections: Oral and Systemic* (Cleveland: Penton Press Company, 1923), 209.
98. V. Zeines, *Healthy Mouth, Healthy Body* (New York: Kensington Books, 2000), 150–51.
99. Ibid., 145, 146.
100. G. Meinig, *Root Canal Cover-Up* (Ojai, Calif.: Bion Publishing, 1994), 148.
101. D. Ewing, *Let the Tooth be Known,* 2nd ed. (Houston: Holistic Health Alternatives, 2002), 38.
102. F. Jerome, *Tooth Truth* (San Diego: ProMotion Publishing, 1995), 262.
103. D. Ewing, *Let the Tooth Be Known,* 2nd ed. (Houston: Holistic Health Alternatives, 2002), 38.

104. Ibid.
105. V. Zeines, *Healthy Mouth, Healthy Body* (New York: Kensington Books, 2000), 146.
106. F. Jerome, *Tooth Truth* (San Diego: ProMotion Publishing, 1995), 257.
107. R. Goldberg et al., "The Properties of Endocal 10 and Its Potential Impact on the Structural Integrity of the Root," *Journal of Endodontics* 30, no. 3 (March 2004): 159.
108. W. Price, *Dental Infections: Oral and Systemic* (Cleveland: Penton Press Company, 1923), 203.
109. D. Ewing, *Let the Tooth Be Known,* 2nd ed. (Houston: Holistic Health Alternatives, 2002), 39.
110. R. Marshall, *Toxic Teeth* (Austin, Tex.: Premier Research Labs, 1996), 4.
111. F. Jerome, *Tooth Truth* (San Diego: ProMotion Publishing, 1995), 257–58.
112. C. Eccles and Z. Annua, eds., *The Toxicity of Methyl Mercury* (Baltimore: Johns Hopkins University Press, 1987), 117.
113. Ibid., 41.
114. R. Kulacz and T. Levy, *The Roots of Disease* (Bloomington, Ind.: Xlibris Corporation, 2002), 64–65.
115. F. Jerome, *Tooth Truth* (San Diego: ProMotion Publishing, 1995), 270.
116. U. Heintze et al., "Methylation of Mercury from Dental Amalgam Mercuric Chloride by Oral Streptococci in Vitro," *Scandinavian Journal of Dental Research* 91 (1983): 150–52; C. Eccles and Z. Annua, eds., *The Toxicity of Methyl Mercury* (Baltimore: Johns Hopkins University Press, 1987), 117; H. Casdorph and M. Walker, *Toxic Metal Syndrome* (Garden City Park, N.Y.: Avery Publishing Group, 1995), 151.
117. F. Jerome, *Tooth Truth* (San Diego: ProMotion Publishing, 1995), 235.
118. Ibid., 271.
119. R. Marshall, *Toxic Teeth* (Austin, Tex.: Premier Research Labs, 1996), 5; R. Goldberg et al., "The Properties of Endocal 10 and Its Potential Impact on the Structural Integrity of the Root," *Journal of Endodontics* 30, no. 3 (March 2004): 159.
120. M. Ziff, "Root Canals—Friend or Foe?" *BioProbe Newsletter* 10, no. 6 (November 1994): 7.
121. M. Georgopoulou et al., "In Vitro Evaluation of the Effectiveness of Calcium Hydroxide and Paramonochlorophenol on Aerobic Bacteria from the Root Canal," *Endodontics & Dental Traumatology* 6, no. 9 (December 1993): 249–53; G. Cavalleri et al., "Comparison of Calcium Hydroxide and Calcium Oxide for Intracanal Medication," *Giornale Italiano di Endodonzia* 3, no. 4 (1990): 8–13.
122. R. Goldberg et al., "The Properties of Endocal 10 and Its Potential Impact on the Structural Integrity of the Root," *Journal of Endodontics* 30, no. 3 (March 2004), 159–62.
123. C. Bates et al., "Longitudinal Sealing Ability of Mineral Trioxide Aggregrate as a Root-End Filling Material," *Journal of Endodontics* 22, no. 11 (November 1996): 575, 577, 578; M. Torabinejad et al., "Histologic Assessment of Mineral Trioxide Aggregate as a Root-End Filling in Monkeys," *Journal of Endodontics* 23, no. 4 (April 1997): 225–28.
124. Personal communication with Dr. Scott Loman, February 24, 2003.
125. E. Hatton, "Focal Infection," in G. Black, *Operative Dentistry* (Woodstock, Ill.: Medico-Dental Publishing Company, 1948), 436.
126. A. Porter and S. Sweet, "Oral Focal Infection," *The American Dental Surgeon,* January 1930, 34–36.

12

THE TONSIL FOCUS

Whether the tonsil focus or the dental focus is more debilitating to the body is difficult to say. Nevertheless, no matter which one holds that dubious honor, there is no question that these two foci are the most pathological focal infections in the body.

W. D. Miller, Edward C. Rosenow, Frank Billings, Martin Fischer, and many other turn-of-the-twentieth-century focal infection researchers studied the effects of tonsil foci just as rigorously as those of dental foci. As discussed in chapter 8, Rosenow proved that the streptococcus bacteria that most commonly reside in the tonsillar region migrate through *elective localization* or *selective affinity* to various susceptible areas, or disturbed fields, in the body.[1] These disturbed fields can be located anywhere from the eyes to the toes, but the five typical target tissues, or "rheumatic disturbed fields," that provide the most hospitable environment for the chronic invasion of strep bacteria are the joints, the heart, the kidneys, the gut (stomach and small intestine), and the brain.[2]

THE ANATOMY AND PHYSIOLOGY OF THE TONSILS

Tonsils are large lymph nodes embedded in the mucosal membrane of the throat. The five tonsillar tissues include:

1. The paired **palatine** tonsils located in the back of the throat, most typically called "the tonsils." These may or may not be visible in the mouth.
2. The **pharyngeal** tonsil located in the nasopharynx area in the roof of the mouth, which cannot be seen without special instrumentation. Commonly called "the adenoids," this lymphatic tissue is approximately 10 millimeters in length (less than half an inch).
3. The **lingual** tonsil located at the base of the tongue, and bordering the palatine tonsil, which can be inspected only when the tongue is stuck far out of the mouth.
4. The **laryngeal** tonsil located near the vocal cords in the larynx (windpipe), which is not readily visible without special instrumentation.
5. The bilateral **tubal** tonsils located just posterior to (behind) the Eustachian tube opening in the nasopharynx, which is also not readily visible without special instrumentation.

These five lymphatic tissues are arranged in a ringlike formation in the throat (at the junction of the oral cavity and the pharynx) that is known as Waldeyer's ring (see figure 12.1).[3]

Tonsillar Ring Protects Body from Inhaled or Ingested Toxins

This strategically situated ring of protective lymphatic tissue guards against the invasion of foreign substances into the body. In fact, no food, breath, or microbe can enter the body without passing through the domain of the tonsillar ring.[4] Thus, whether toxins are inhaled or ingested, the job of the tonsils is to localize them and produce *phagocytes*—white blood cells that literally *phagocytize,* or eat, toxins—that can engulf and destroy these invaders. During these normal lymphatic defensive measures, the tonsils increase in size or swell. However, if the microbes or toxins are particularly virulent, the tonsils may become inflamed and the swelling, pain, and redness associated with a sore throat or tonsillitis ensue.

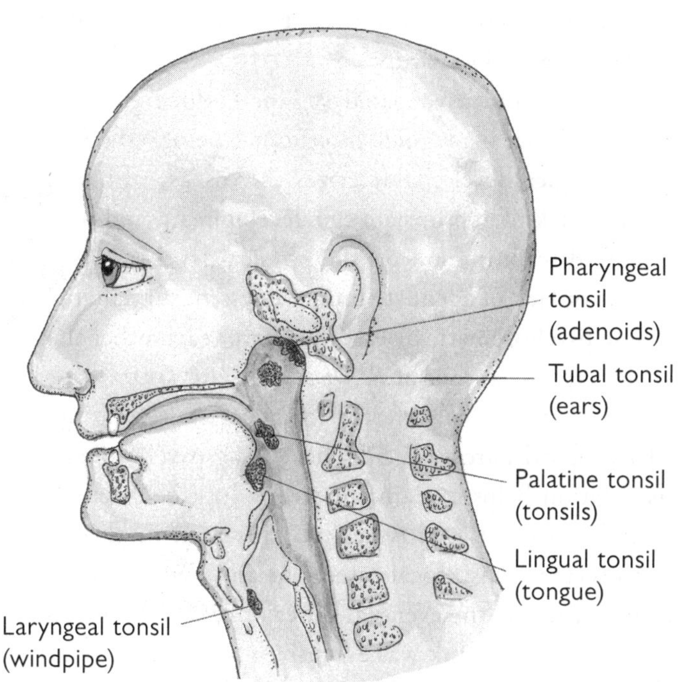

Figure 12.1. There are five tonsils arranged in a ringlike formation (Waldeyer's ring) in the throat that protect the body against pathogenic microbes and other toxins.

Tonsils Filter Toxins from the Teeth and Nose

The tonsils also act as an intermediary station of elimination between the head and the body. For example, when German researcher Henke injected small amounts of fine sterilized soot into the nasal mucosa of research subjects, he found that the soot would accumulate in the tonsils within a short period of time.[5] Later Henke, along with Permut and Roeder, proved that dental toxins are also quickly shunted to the tonsils. In a study conducted by the three researchers, when India ink was injected into the dental pulp (the center of the tooth) of test subjects, "punctate stipulation"—or little dots—of ink would appear on the tonsillar surface within twenty to thirty minutes.[6] Thus, the tonsils are responsible for filtering (if they can) the toxins and microbes from the nasal and oral mucosae.

Direct Communication Between Tonsils and Gut

The digestive system is one long tube from the mouth to the anus. The tonsils—or the remaining lymphatic tissue in the throat after tonsillectomies—are an integral part of that system. They stand like two pillars of defense and detoxification on either side of the mouth. Therefore, anything that is disturbing to the gut is disturbing to the tonsils. The communication between the tonsils and the digestive system is so closely linked that in immunology they have been termed the "gut-associated lymphoid tissue," or GALT. This system of lymphoid tissues consists of the tonsils and adenoids, the Peyer's patches (lymphatic aggregations in the ileum, the third part of the small intestine), and the appendix. However, the tonsils are more affected by ingested toxic foods and substances than the more distal lymphatic tissues in the gut, because they are the "site of first encounter (priming) of immune cells with antigens (toxic foods and substances) entering via mucosal surfaces."[7] Therefore, the tonsils filter not only toxins from the nose and mouth but also those ingested and digested by the gut.

THE FORMATION OF A TONSIL FOCUS

Tonsil foci usually develop in childhood from chronic infections. Occasional sore throats, colds, earaches, and fevers can be quite normal in children and, when not suppressed, allow the immune system to exercise and enhance its defensive capabilities. However, the more continuous—and in some cases constant—infections that tend to plague children nowadays are *not* normal and indicate that something is wrong with that child's immune functioning.

Three Major Allopathic Mistakes in the Treatment of Tonsillitis

1. Failure to Fully Diagnose

The mistakes modern allopathy makes in the treatment of tonsillitis are threefold. First, conventional doctors fail to adequately diagnose the true cause of the infection. Tonsillitis, strep throat, and other diagnostic labels only describe the outcome—not what caused the infection in the first place. Although the passage of germs in school-age children will occasionally overwhelm even the strongest immune system, chronic infections signal a deeper problem.

Dairy allergy. One of the most common causes of chronic tonsillitis is an undiagnosed food allergy. And of all the classic allergenic foods, the most typical culprit contributing to chronic upper respiratory infections is dairy. That is, although other food allergies can also chronically irritate and inflame the tonsils, milk, cheese, and other dairy products are by far the most culpable.* And when combined with sugar (ice cream, milk chocolate, milkshakes, etc.), as well as the ingestion of other junk foods (soda pop, fried foods, etc.) that have also been proven to reduce immune system functioning, the eventual formation of a tonsil focus in susceptible constitutions is almost ensured.

Suppressed emotions. Another major cause of chronic tonsillitis is emotional disturbance, such as the "lump in the throat" feeling that arises with sorrow and directly affects the tonsils. In fact, one German physician has asserted that she has never seen a tonsil focus in individuals who did not experience the effects of major parental discord as children.[8] Most notably, the chronic "stuffing of feelings" that occurs when individuals are not able to fully and authentically express their emotions can greatly block this throat chakra region. This unresolved emotional discord is often a major stimulus in the manifestation of more bouts of tonsillitis, and a chronic cyclical pattern of ill emotional and physical health.

These psychosomatic manifestations are no longer simply a New Age notion but have been incontrovertibly proven through psychoneuroimmunology research. Beginning as early as the 1950s and primarily stimulated by Dr. Hans Selye's work, studies have revealed that chronic emotional stress weakens immune system functioning, specifically through a decline in natural killer (NK) cells and monocytes (key defender cells). In the case of the tonsils, the classic pattern of the conscientious and sensitive child constantly repressing feelings of anger and sadness not only fuels the cycle of chronic tonsillitis and the eventual formation of a tonsil focus but also can contribute to the future onset of cancer, arthritis, asthma, chronic depression, and anxiety.[9]

Chronic tonsillitis and emotional repression are especially damaging during a child's formative years, when the immune system and the psyche are learning to discriminate "self" from "non-self." In fact, the syndrome PANDAS, discussed later in this chapter, is an example of autoimmune illness that arises directly from streptococcus-infected tonsils and round after round of damaging antibiotic drugs.

Author and psychoanalyst Jane Goldberg, Ph.D., has noted that inadequate discrimination of self on the psychological level characterizes the disease of narcissism or lack of appropriate ego development, and inadequate discrimination on the physical level results in cancer or lack of adequate immune system surveillance. These psychosomatic diseases so mirror each other that Goldberg, the author of *Psychotherapeutic Treatment of Cancer Patients,* has referred to cancer as "a condition of biological narcissism."[10] This strong psychosomatic association helps explain the strong link between the significant emotional issues typically seen in patients with serious tonsil focal infections and (without effective treatment) the eventual onset of cancer. This tonsil focus–cancer link was extensively researched by the German physician Josef Issels and will be covered later in this chapter.

Mercury amalgam fillings. As described earlier, tonsils receive and filter toxins from the teeth and oral cavity. Therefore, when chewing releases mercury from amalgam fillings, this toxic metal passes through the tonsils and remains there when the lymphatic organ is not fully functioning. This accumulation of mercury and other heavy metals in weakened tonsils is another major contributor to the formation of a tonsil focus. Furthermore, as with a dental focus, when the tonsil region becomes a chronic focus, the resident bacteria there continually complex with the metallic or inorganic mercury emitting from neighboring amalgam fillings. When this occurs, the mercury is "methylated" by the bacteria, which renders this newly converted organic mercury *ten to one hundred times* more toxic than the original metallic mercury in the amalgam filling.[11]

Susceptibility or miasmic tendency. Another cause of chronic tonsillitis is simply an individual's inherited weakness, or miasm, as discussed in chapter 1. That is, some people respond to stress—whether it's dairy, sugar, or emotional pain—with headaches, others with joint pain, and others with chronic upper respiratory infections. Those individuals who respond primarily in the sycotic reaction mode are most prone to frequent tonsillitis, otitis (ear infections), and sinusitis. However, after years of physical or emotional stress, numerous bouts of tonsillitis, and the excessive use of suppressive anti-

*One telltale keynote of a dairy allergy is chronically needing to clear the throat, especially after meals containing milk products. See chapter 6 for more information on food allergies.

biotics, individuals with a chronic tonsil focus begin to manifest more serious symptoms.

"Diseases of childhood, grown old." After many years of the infection/drug/immune response cycle, the tonsils become more and more degenerated and the individual begins to function primarily in the exhausted tuberculinic reaction mode. In these cases, fewer bouts of acute tonsillitis occur. This lack of reaction is often mistaken for "growing out of it" as children mature into their teens and twenties. However, these individuals often trade chronic tonsillitis for chronic fatigue, or other symptoms characteristic of a hidden tonsil focus in adults, as described by Dr. Martin Fischer in the mid-twentieth century:

> For it is said that the diseases of man's maturer years are naught but the "diseases of his childhood, grown old." What was acute sore throat in his teens is a pus-exuding or scarred tonsil later . . . All his diseases in fact are become but the manifestations in the upper decades of life of what in adolescence were "growing pains," stomach aches, vomiting spells, fever attacks, anemias, headaches, constipations, faintings and fits [seizures].[12]

2. The Nonjudicious Prescribing of Antibiotics

The excessive use of antibiotics is the second mistake allopathic medicine makes.* Approximately two-thirds of all infants in the United States receive antibiotics within the first two hundred days of their life.[13]

Mistakenly prescribed for viral infections. The widespread pediatric practice of prescribing anti*bacterials* to treat *viral* infections including the common cold, many sore throats, and the flu is particularly indefensible.† In fact, the Centers for Disease Control have reported that of the 235 million doses of antibiotics consumed in 2001, an estimated 20 to 50 percent of these doses were unnecessarily prescribed for viral infections.[14]

Antibiotic resistance. When a patient's sore throat is of bacterial origin, the overuse of antibiotics is still indefensible except in dire emergencies. The epidemic use of these antibacterial drugs has encouraged the emergence of dangerously mutated antibiotic-resistant strains that do not respond to any antimicrobial drugs.[15] In the case of chronic tonsillitis, the continual use of antibiotics almost ensures the formation of a tonsil focus by leaving the more virulent strains of bacterial carcasses and their toxins behind in the connective tissue.

Fortunately, medical students and residents are now taught that children with upper respiratory symptoms should not be treated with antibiotics unless drainage persists for ten to fourteen days. Unfortunately, there is a "striking dichotomy" between what is taught and what is practiced in the doctor's office. A recent survey of family practitioners and pediatricians revealed that doctors are often pressured to prescribe antibiotics by parents (often through the need of a working parent to more quickly return to work), by legal liability concerns in case the child does develop a more serious infection, and through drug promotion by pharmaceutical companies.[16]

Linked to autoimmune diseases. Bacteria and other infectious agents, as well as the previously described emotional repression in childhood, have also been implicated in inducing autoimmune disease.[17] That is, when bacterial proteins or *antigens* chronically invade the tonsils, the tonsillar tissue can become so altered that it is no longer recognizable as "self" to the body's immune system. Consequently, when the body's defensive antibodies mount an attack against these foreign bacterial invaders, they are not able to recognize "self" (the tonsil tissue) from "non-self" (the bacteria and bacterial toxins). Therefore, these immune system antibodies mistakenly attack *both* these tissues as if they were foreign invaders. This complication can occur *even after* the original inciting microbes have been killed.[18] Through this autoimmune miscommunication, the "smoldering" tonsil focus becomes even more firmly entrenched in the system, and it slowly but surely loses its capacity to repel foreign toxins from its tissues. Unfortunately, many researchers now believe that the chronic use of antibiotics for tonsillitis actually strengthens this autoimmune response.[19]

---

*In the early 1990s, penicillin caused an estimated 1.5 deaths per 100,000 doses. (K. Conroy et al., *Natural Approach to Ophthalmology and Otolaryngology* [Seattle: Healing Mountain Publishing, 2004], 378.)

†However, these prescriptions can sometimes alleviate symptoms, possibly validating Rosenow's theory that even so-called viral diseases such as polio have a bacterial origin.

3. Inappropriate and Ineffective Tonsillectomies

The third mistake modern medicine makes is the overuse of tonsillectomies. Although the common practice of prophylactically removing the tonsils as if they were simply vestigial tissues without function has been widely denounced, tonsillectomies are still the second most common surgery of childhood, with 600,000 being performed each year.[20] There are a number of reasons why these traditional tonsillectomies "miss the mark."

vestigial: The term *vestigial* refers to the remnant or trace of a structure that had been functional in a previous state of human development but currently serves little to no use in the body.

Inadequate diagnosis. First, surgery does nothing to shed any light on or treat the cause of chronic tonsillitis. Therefore, the damage that food allergies, suppressed emotions, mercury, and other toxic stressors cause is then simply shunted postsurgically to deeper immune system defensive organs—primarily the thymus and spleen.

Incomplete surgeries. Second, tonsillectomies are often performed incorrectly. As described earlier, the incomplete removal of these chronically infected lymphoid tissues can be more dangerous to the body than leaving them intact. In the landmark 1928 study by researchers Paul S. Rhoads and George F. Dick, the "stumps" and "tags" left behind from the surgeon's knife (or spatula) were found to harbor even *more pathogenic bacteria* per gram of tissue than the original tonsils contained before surgery.[21] To quote these researchers directly:

> It is shown by this work that tonsillectomy as usually done even by specialists fails to accomplish this end in 73 percent (!) of cases because of incomplete removal of infected tonsillar tissue . . . in many instances the condition resulting from incomplete tonsillectomy is worse than that existing before operation . . . Patients who with systemic diseases attributable to foci of infection failed to improve after their original tonsillectomy, improved strikingly after removal of the pieces of tonsillar tissues remaining from the first operation.[22]

TONSILLOTOMIES

A *tonsillotomy*—the excision of only the top part of hypertrophic tonsils—is an example of truly misguided surgery. The tonsils can function only when their surface mucosa with its superficial crypts can excrete toxins. Therefore, cutting off this excretory ability through a tonsillotomy is counterproductive. Dr. Peter Dosch stated, "A tonsillotomy is never able to eliminate a tonsillar interference field but, on the contrary, is more likely to produce one."[23]

In 1912, Dr. Frank Billings, another legendary researcher in the focal infection field, made the following remarks about ordinary tonsillectomies:

> Ordinary tonsillectomy leaves an abundance of lymphoid tissue which may be sealed over by the operative scar and leaves a *worse* condition than that for which the operation was made . . . in that foci of infection are frequently walled in.[24]

In his *Manual of Neural Therapy,* the German expert in the treatment of foci, Dr. Peter Dosch, reports that the more modern research statistics (mid-1980s) reveal little improvement:

> Extensive statistics compiled by university clinics have . . . shown that cures are achieved in only about 50 percent of all cases of those undergoing tonsillar surgery and relapses occur in exactly the same proportion amongst tonsillectomized cases as amongst the untreated. In light of this, Hoff described the results of surgical focus eradication as "shatteringly poor."[25]

Remaining scars become interference fields. Even when all of the infected tissue is effectively excised, the remaining surgical scars characteristically give rise to a chronic tonsil interference field with resulting disturbed fields in the body. Dr. Dosch saw so many cases of this condition that he would never discharge any chronically ill patient who had had a tonsillectomy before his or her tonsillectomy scars were tested—"even if the patient's previous history does not point in that direction."[26]

Natural Medicine: The Key to Preventing Tonsil Foci

Most holistic practitioners will say that infants and children are the easiest to treat. In the majority of cases, this pediatric population responds quickly to natural medicine. In fact, an array of holistic therapies have been proven to be safe and highly effective in the treatment of typical pediatric illnesses such as colds, sore throats, and ear infections.[27] These treatments include homeopathy (acute and constitutional), drainage remedies, herbal medicine (Western, Chinese, Indian, Brazilian, etc.), essential oils, spinal adjusting, craniosacral manipulation, hydrotherapy, and nutritional supplementation.

When a physician is aware of the clinical evidence as well as research studies that prove the effectiveness of natural and nontoxic therapies, treating upper respiratory infections and other common ailments in infants and young children initially with suppressive drugs is rather analogous to killing a flea with a sledgehammer, and borders on malpractice. Therefore, one key measure that could be taught to allopathic practitioners to help prevent future tonsil foci from ever developing is adopting the protocol to *first* utilize natural nontoxic therapies (through a referral to a naturopathic, chiropractic, acupuncturist, or other holistic practitioner if the allopathic pediatrician is not well versed in natural medicine) and to *reserve* the use of powerful antibiotics and other drugs only for when these initial measures fail or in the case of major emergencies. This clinical principle and practice was officially adopted at the 1992 American Association of Naturopathic Physicians annual convention:

> The use of antibiotics should be reserved for those patients who are unresponsive to naturopathic modalities and are not making significant improvement in a timely manner (i.e., no response after one week of naturopathic therapy).[28]

DIAGNOSIS OF A TONSIL FOCUS

Besides the all-important history, the first step in diagnosing a tonsil focus is to inspect the palatine tonsils in the back of the patient's throat for signs of infection such as redness, swelling, or scarring (from surgery or many past bouts of tonsillitis). However, even when tonsils visually appear to be pink and healthy, physicians should still test for the presence of a silent focus by following up this visual examination with energetic testing, assessing the presence of painful pressure points, or studying mucosal samples.

Inspection of the Palatine Tonsils

The palatine tonsils are bilateral almond-shaped masses located on either side of the back of the throat, between the palatoglossal arch and the palatopharyngeal arch. They may or may not be visible behind the palatine arches in the throat (see figure 12.2). The palatine tonsils are located at the level of the second cervical and the upper part of the third cervical vertebrae. Practitioners should note that simply laying the tongue depressor on the tongue and asking the patient to say "ahh" is often adequate to view the palatine tonsils. In fact, when force is applied to the tongue depressor, this pressure often initiates a spasmodic reflex in which the tongue tries to crowd against the roof of the mouth and thus blocks the view of the throat.[29]

If they are visible, healthy tonsils should be pale pink in color with an irregular surface area formed by *crypts*—invaginated blind cavities that extend throughout

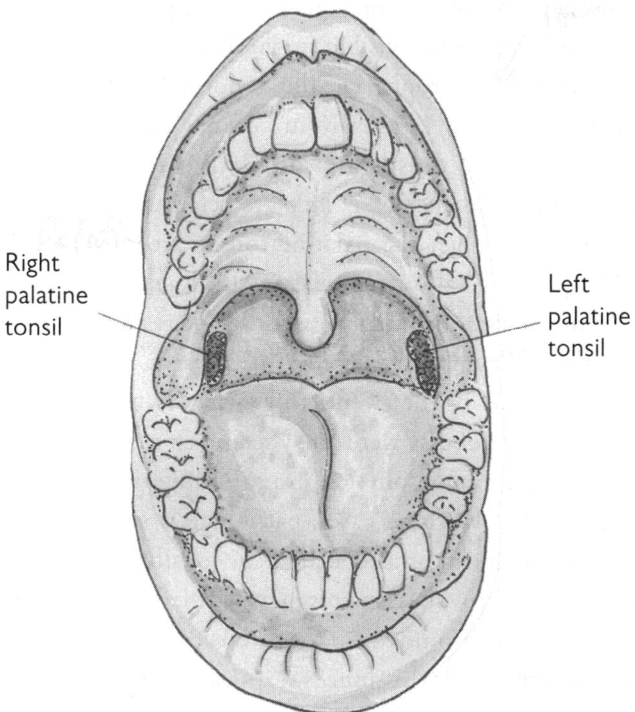

Figure 12.2. The palatine tonsils may or may not be visible.

the tissue. These tonsillar crypts, ranging from ten to fifteen in number, can fill with light-colored plugs that may then be secreted and swallowed, which is a normal lymphatic filtering process that occurs in healthy tonsils.

The shape of the palatine tonsil varies according to age, constitution (miasmic level), and tissue changes from past or present inflammation or infection. For the first five or six years of life, these lymphoid tissues increase in size and can often be readily seen upon inspection. At puberty the tonsils (and the thymus gland) begin to go through physiological involution, and thus diminish.[30]

Atrophied Tonsils

In many cases, the palatine tonsils can greatly decrease in size, or atrophy. Inspection is not helpful in these cases because the practitioner is unable to see whether the tonsils are normal and healthy or atrophied and degenerated. Many researchers including Frank Billings, Edward C. Rosenow, and Josef Issels have considered small atrophied tonsils to be the most dangerous type of tonsil focus and the most instrumental in the causation of serious diseases such as cancer.[31]

Hypertrophied Tonsils

The palatine tonsils may also be enlarged, or *hypertrophied,* and quite visible in the back of the throat. Tonsillar hypertrophy can be a normal response to acute infection, especially in infants and children. Sometimes the tonsils are so enlarged that they are touching, in which case they are referred to as *kissing tonsils.* When the palatine tonsils are chronically enlarged, especially after puberty, this is usually indicative of the establishment of a tonsil focus and the loss of effective lymphatic defense in the area. In fact, in the early part of the twentieth century, hypertrophied tonsils after puberty were rarely seen.[32] In contrast, they are now a common physical exam finding in teens and even adults. In these cases, pathological streptococci have invaded and proliferated in the tonsillar crypts. In acute tonsillitis, these crypts may be filled with pus. In the case of a chronic tonsil focus, however, these crypts are scarred and the mucosa appears wrinkled and contracted. When the tonsillar crypts can no longer excrete, streptococcus bacteria are deprived of their air supply and decompose into even more pathogenic toxic products. Furthermore, invading toxins are no longer able to be harmlessly secreted but are passed directly into the bloodstream.[33] Although many researchers believed that the smaller atrophied tonsils were the most degenerative and serious, Dr. W. D. Miller, as well as several of his Berlin colleagues, found the larger hypertrophied tonsils to be the most damaging, and "dangerous accumulators of pathogenic germs."[34] Hypertrophied tonsils have also been linked to hearing and speech dysfunction, sleep apnea (interrupted and/or shallow breathing during sleep), allergies, and dental malocclusions (bad bites).[35*]

Other Signs of Infection

In acute infections, as well as with chronic tonsil foci, the palatoglossal arch directly in front of the paired palatine tonsils can have a bluish tinge, and the uvula (the small fleshy process hanging down from the middle of the throat just above the back portion of the tongue) may be thickened and have gelatinous areas.[36†] The tongue may or may not be coated.[‡]

Inspection Cannot Rule Out a Tonsil Focus

However, even when none of these signs is apparent and the tonsils appear perfectly healthy, there may still be a silent focus or interference field. Dosch cautions that "even the most experienced eyes cannot tell by inspection alone whether the tonsils might be acting as a pathogenic focus or not."[37]

---

*Dr. Garretson has said that it is impossible to sing softly and finely with the tonsils enlarged. (J. Garretson, *A System of Oral Surgery* [New York: J. B. Lippincott Co., 1898], 563–64.) Thus, practitioners can also get clues from listening to the patient's voice; any rough or gravelly intonations can indicate a chronic tonsil focus.

†I have also often noted another sign in patients with a chronic tonsil focus—a small red or brown pigmented spot located on the alar portion of their nose, usually ipsilateral to the most hypertrophied tonsil. (The *alar,* or wing part of the nose, is that area that your finger touches when you occlude one nostril.)

‡Tongue diagnosis is an essential aspect of Chinese Medicine and requires much study to master. However, practitioners who have not studied the field of dominant foci and utilize this form of diagnosis should be aware that a coated tongue not only indicates chronic intestinal dysbiosis but also a possible tonsil focus that can be a major obstacle to cure in healing this dysbiosis—despite the patient's dutiful ingestion of a clean nontoxic diet.

Painful Pressure Points

Dr. Ernesto Adler, a renowned Spanish neural therapist, found that patients who had a chronic tonsil focus also had painful pressure points in the trapezius muscle of their upper back and shoulder area. He further correlated painful cervical (neck) pressure points to a wisdom tooth focus (see figure 12.3). Points lateral to the second cervical vertebra are related to upper wisdom tooth foci, while painful points next to the third cervical vertebrae are associated with lower wisdom tooth foci. However, the ipsilateral rule still applies whether the focus is in a tooth or a tonsil. That is, if a right lower impacted wisdom tooth is a chronic focus, then the pressure point just lateral to the right third cervical vertebra should also be tender. Alternatively, if the left tonsil is more degenerated than the right, then the left-sided trapezius points will be more chronically tender and painful.

Of course, sore neck and shoulders and painful trigger points in the upper back have become pandemic in recent times from various reasons—sedentary lifestyles, hunching over a computer for hours at a time, and chronic psychological tension. Therefore, the case for a tonsil focus cannot be based simply on pain elicited from these pressure points during a single examination. However, over time if one or more of these points continues to test positive and is exquisitely tender on deep palpation, the presence of a chronic dental or tonsil focus should be considered.

Mucosal Samples

A sample of the palatine tonsil mucosa can be sucked out with an instrument called the Roeder tonsil sucker.[38] This procedure can also be done at home by swiping a sample of the mucus overlying the tonsil with the end of a clean or gloved finger (whether you've had a tonsillectomy or not). Simply smelling this sample and monitoring it over time can help diagnose whether you have a chronic tonsil focal infection. If there is no real odor or even just a mildly stale smell, this is less diagnostic of a tonsil focal infection, although a tonsil interference field from tonsillectomy scars can still be present. However, a strong "carcasslike" smell indicative of chronic bacterial invasion and degeneration of tissue is strongly diagnostic of a chronic focal infection.[39] Surprisingly, this rotten smell elicited by a finger swab of the tonsils does not necessarily translate into chronic bad breath. Therefore, similar to a coated or

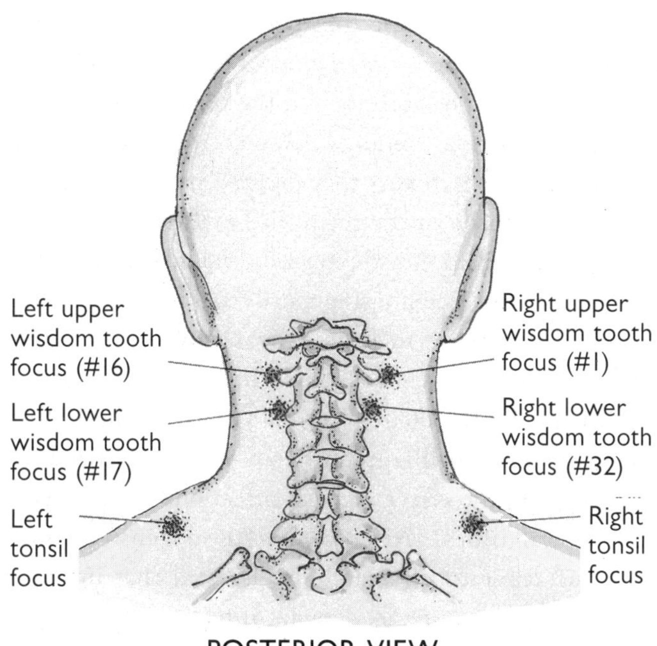

Figure 12.3. Adler's trigger points associated with chronic tonsil or wisdom teeth (third molar) foci

uncoated tongue, the absence of halitosis does not rule out the possibility of a tonsil focus.

Energetic Testing

Energetic testing is another method of physical examination relied on heavily by holistic physicians to determine the presence or absence of a tonsil focus, as well as to ascertain whether that focus is active or dormant. In fact, energetic testing in the form of kinesiology, reflex arm length testing, Matrix Reflex Testing, Auriculomedicine, or electroacupuncture (Voll, Vega, etc.) is essential to corroborate a suspected active tonsil focus, as well as to indicate how it should best be treated. Positive tests through a "therapy localization" of the tonsil area or through a filter such as a homeopathic vial, a sample of tonsil tissue, or a hand mudra are ways the patient's "inner physician" can signal that an area of focal stress needs to be treated. (See appendix 3, "Energetic Testing Explained," for more information.)

Is the Dental or the Tonsil Focus Most Culpable?

Energetic testing can help determine if the tonsil is the primary focus or if it is secondary—that is, the disturbed field of a dental focus. Based on research confirming that toxins from the teeth very quickly and directly migrate to the tonsillar tissue, many holistic physicians and dentists advocate the treatment of all dental foci before dealing with the tonsils.[40] However, this pathway is not simply a one-way street, because the bacteria and the toxins they excrete may also migrate from the tonsils to the teeth. For example, cavitation surgery of a third molar extraction site is less successful when there is a neighboring tonsil focal infection, especially if that tonsil focus was the original cause of the formation of the dental focus. This latter observation was made by Dr. Henry Cotton as early as the 1920s. Cotton was a brilliant physician who specialized in researching the effect of focal infections in the onset of mental illness. After conducting extensive clinical and laboratory research, he asserted that in most cases the wisdom teeth were not infected because they were impacted but were impacted because they were infected, and that this "infection is transmitted from the tonsils."[41]

Through clinical research (energetic testing, observing the effects of auriculotherapy and neural therapy treatments, taking a careful follow-up history each visit, etc.), my colleagues and I have found that the hypotheses of both Cotton and Henke are valid. That is, sometimes the originating focus is the *tonsils,* and at other times it is the *teeth*. Effective and sophisticated energetic testing methods are often required to make this relatively complex diagnostic differentiation in order to arrive at a more informed decision regarding appropriate treatment. When serious and permanent decisions must be made, such as the extraction of a tooth versus a tonsillectomy, the gathering of as much knowledge as possible is crucial to the final decision-making process.

Identifying the Disturbed Fields

Energetic testing can also assist with determining which areas of the body—that is, the disturbed fields—have been affected by the tonsil focus. This understanding of the primary cause of painful arthritic joints or chronic fatigue can be both relieving and inspiring. In the case of kinesiological methods, the direct experience of feeling the difference between a weak muscle before treatment compared with an incredibly strong muscle after treatment is empowering to the patient's subconscious mind and greatly adds to his or her capacity to heal.

Laboratory Testing

As with most foci, blood tests are not useful in determining the presence of a chronic tonsil focus because longstanding and insidious foci have lost the capability to initiate major immune system responses. Thus, standard blood and urine tests often come back negative. However, in one study of two hundred patients with "clear-cut cases of [dental or tonsil] focal infection," 63 percent showed a definite leukopenia (decreased white blood cell count) typical of chronic infection, as well as albuminuria (increased albumin or protein in the urine) indicative of chronic liver and kidney dysfunction.[42] Therefore, a complete blood count (CBC) may be worthwhile to test for an abnormal white blood cell count, and a urinalysis may elicit positive changes in the albumin count. On the other hand, negative blood tests can never rule out a focus. Dr. Martin Fischer's frustration with these chronic streptococcal focal infections in the mid-twentieth century are just as valid today for clinicians seeking positive laboratory confirmation:

> The streptococcal infections of greatest importance today present a far different front. Instead of acute, their disease manifestations occupy years, are practically afebrile [no temperature], without marked increase in leucocyte count [i.e., white blood cell count normal], and with only the vaguest of localizing signs and symptoms.[43]

Furthermore, the presence of strep bacteria from a throat culture has been deemed "neither reliable nor valid" in the diagnosis of chronic tonsillitis in numerous studies.[44] The "rapid strep test," which is not dependable even for use with acute infections, is not appropriate for determining the presence of bacteria in chronic tonsil focal infections either.

SYMPTOMS OF A TONSIL FOCUS—THE FIVE RHEUMATIC DISTURBED FIELDS

To most modern readers, the word *rheumatism* sounds rather passé. For many it may conjure up the image of a grandmother bundled up against the cold in her rocking chair, wringing her painful arthritic hands. However, rheumatic diseases are still very much alive and present in our modern world, and their effects continue to have both a subtle and not-so-subtle impact in most of our lives.

Rheumatism is a general term that refers to various disorders in the body marked by inflammation, degeneration, and derangement of the connective tissues. Rheumatism confined to the joints is known by its more common name *arthritis*. The related term *rheumatic fever* is the name for the "acute inflammatory complication of Group A streptococcal infections, characterized mainly by arthritis, chorea [brain disturbance], or carditis [heart inflammation] . . . with residual heart disease as a possible sequel of the carditis."[45] In focal infection terminology, the term *rheumatic* is used to characterize all the areas in the body—that is, the disturbed fields—where streptococcus bacteria typically metastasize. As previously discussed, Billings, Rosenow, Price, and other early-twentieth-century researchers found that the rheumatic disturbed fields emanating from chronic dental and tonsil focal infections centered primarily in five major areas: the joints, the heart, the kidneys, the gut (stomach and intestine), and the brain.[46]

Although antibiotics have been credited with a decline in cases of rheumatic fever, a significant decrease had begun even *before* the introduction of penicillin as a result of improved nutrition, hygiene, and standards of living.[47] Furthermore, the liberal dosing of antibiotics without first appropriately assessing the culpable microbe has rendered the diagnosis of streptococcus-induced acute rheumatic fever and its complications relatively obsolete.* However, over the decades as resistant bacterial strains have emerged, streptococcal infections have increased in virulence and rheumatic fever epidemics have reemerged with a vengeance in more recent times. Laurie Garrett elaborates on this phenomenon in her book *The Coming Plague:*

> In 1985 rheumatic fever broke out among white middle-class residents of the Salt Lake City region of Utah. In just three years' time the incidence of the disease skyrocketed eightyfold (between 1982 and 1985), and nearly a quarter of the patients suffered recurrences of the disease despite aggressive antibiotic therapy.[48]

This Pulitzer Prize–winning scientific writer further noted that "such ailments as rheumatic fever, strep pneumonia, and general respiratory infections with streptococcus in young children had never disappeared—or even significantly diminished—in the poor countries of the world."[49] Many knowledgeable holistic practitioners would argue that these streptococcal inflammatory syndromes have never significantly diminished in developed nations either but currently have other disease appellations such as fibromyalgia, Tourette's syndrome, and PANDAS. These more contemporary-sounding syndromes also result from chronic bacterial focal infections that are fueled by the toxic effects of sugar and other toxic foods, amalgam fillings, petroleum chemicals, and inherited and acquired miasmic susceptibility in the weakened progeny.

Countless research studies have proven that streptococcal bacteria have a marked affinity, or *tropism,* for specific tissues in the body, thus again proving Rosenow's theory of selective affinity or elective localization. The particular form of the streptococci microbes can vary, but Billings and Rosenow, as well as Price in separate studies, all found that they generally tend to be of the *Streptococcus viridans* or *Streptococcus hemolyticus* (pyogenes) species, or a hybrid of the two.* Billings described the research conducted by his protégé Rosenow in detail:

*Group A, beta-hemolytic streptococci bacteria are the most common pathogen in the causation of tonsillitis. Less common bacterial microbes that can infect the tonsils include *Staphylococcus aureus, Streptococcus pneumonia, Hemophilus influenza,* and *Escherichia coli,* as well as viruses. (K. Conroy et al., *Natural Approach to Ophthalmology and Otolaryngology* [Seattle: Healing Mountain Publishing, 2004], 378.)

*Through his extensive research, Rosenow found convincing evidence for the modification of microorganisms through their environment, or *pleomorphism.* He confirmed the earlier belief postulated by William B. Wherry that in a favorable environment, a streptococcus could biologically change into a pneumococcus or other type of bacterium. Rosenow further asserted that strep bacteria were the underlying causative microorganism for so-called viral diseases—polio, multiple sclerosis, and other central and peripheral nervous system disorders, and that in the right medium these bacteria could transform into viruses. This finding indicated a possible pleomorphic metamorphosis *between species* (viruses and bacteria)—a subject still hotly debated today. (M. Fischer, *Death and Dentistry* [Springfield, Ill.: Charles C. Thomas, 1940], 20, 36–38; S. Shakman, *E. C. Rosenow and Associates: A Reference Manual* [Santa Monica, Calif.: Institute of Science, 1998), C1–1, C2–4.)

> The dominant organism found in abscesses and sealed crypts of the faucial tonsil are *Streptococcus viridans* and *Streptococcus hemolyticus* (pyogenes). The *S. viridans* is usually a surface growth, while the *S. hemolyticus* is frequently found in pure culture in the deeper infected tissues. In acute rheumatism the bacteria obtained from joint exudates and rheumatic nodes have been studied by Dr. E. C. Rosenow, fellow of the Memorial Institute for Infectious Diseases, cooperating with us. He has found that organisms from rheumatism appear to occupy a position between *S. viridans* and *S. hemolyticus*. They are more virulent than the former and less virulent than the latter.[50]

As was previously described, this streptococcus bacteria disseminates out into tissues and organs from focal infections primarily by blood, lymph, and nerve (axonal) transport. The five major disturbed fields that the streptococcus bacterium most prefers—the brain, heart, joints, kidney, and gut—provide the most hospitable environment for this microbe's continued survival. In fact, the chill that often triggers the onset of an acute rheumatic illness (e.g., a cold or influenza) is one indicator of the change in the body's internal temperature that has the effect of altering tissue pH. This temperature change and pH alteration favors the growth of streptococcus bacteria in relatively avascular ("partial oxygen") environments that have the potential of becoming chronically disturbed fields. In fact, any change in environment (exposure, hard work, injury, amalgam filling, sugar bingeing, and so forth) can "alter the nutrient medium" and facilitate easier ingress of microorganisms from a focus to a disturbed field—or simply increase the pathogenicity of the microbes that are already comfortably settled into their tissue of choice.[51]

Where a microbe specifically chooses to settle in the body is also influenced by the individual's miasmic tendency, or reaction mode. For example, a rheumatic manifestation in an individual reacting primarily in the tuberculinic miasm is painful rheumatoid arthritis, whereas someone in the luetic reaction mode may succumb to chronic heart disease. However, simultaneous microbial metastasis to multiple areas is not uncommon, especially in the case of these five rheumatic disturbed fields. Dr. Cotton explained why heart disease and rheumatoid arthritis often occur together:

> There may be also repeated attacks [of rheumatic fever] from which the patient recovers, then finally a more severe attack occurs, from which the patient may not recover. As the heart lining is similar to that of the joints it is often attacked by these organisms. This explains the popular expression that "the rheumatism had gone to the heart."[52]

The Arthritic Joint Disturbed Field

The metastasis of streptococcus bacteria into the joints and muscles has probably been the most widely researched outcome of dental and tonsil foci.[53] In fact, the streptococcus-induced acute rheumatic fever that is characterized by red, hot, and swollen joints most often begins with tonsillitis.[54] As was previously discussed, the recognition and subsequent diagnosis of rheumatic fever is now less frequent because antibiotics often quickly reduce the early symptoms of acute ear, nose, and throat infections in school-age children (~ ages 4 to 18). Allopathic physicians herald this symptomatic reduction in *acute illness* as a modern-day scientific success; however, in light of the astounding proliferation of *chronic rheumatic illnesses,* the ultimate usefulness of antibiotics is hard to warrant. For example, in 1940 the seventh edition of the *Merck Manual* described only *four* arthritic manifestations—rheumatoid arthritis, osteoarthritis, gout, and gonorrheal arthritis.[55] In less than two generations, however, the fifteenth edition of this manual in 1987 described more than *one hundred*. Although the Merck editors boast that "increasingly effective drugs have been introduced" to combat these illnesses, this explosion of arthritic diseases and the concomitant proliferation of immunosuppressive drugs (e.g., corticosteroids) and new anti-inflammatories with "serious adverse effects"* such as Vioxx and Celebrex† hardly illustrates a success story for anyone—with the exception of the pharmaceutical drug companies.[56]

*These adverse effects encompass gastrointestinal, cardiovascular, and other complications that lead to hospitalization or death.

†More information on Vioxx, Celebrex, and other drugs with serious adverse effects can be found in appendix 4, "How Scientific is Allopathic Medicine?"

Every component of our musculoskeletal system is susceptible to streptococcal (as well as staphylococcal and gonococcal) infection. Microbes may travel to the muscles, causing myositis, fibromyalgia, tendonitis, or muscle strain; to the ligaments, contributing to acute and chronic sprains; and to the joint itself, with resulting rheumatoid arthritis, osteoarthritis (degenerative joint disease), adhesive capsulitis (i.e., frozen shoulder), synovitis, and bursitis. Through the extensive research of Rosenow, Price, Haden, and others, chronic and insidiously silent tonsil and dental focal infections were found to be the root cause of most—if not all—of these arthritic disorders.[57] Although no recent research has been conducted to determine how many individuals suffering from the "newer" rheumatism-related syndromes—fibromyalgia, Sjögren's, Raynaud's, systemic lupus erythematosus (SLE), and Lyme disease—have focal infections, in my clinical experience it has been in the ninetieth percentile.

The Cardiac Disturbed Field

Most focal infection research in regard to heart disease has been centered on dental foci as well as periodontal (gum) disease.[58] However, microorganisms from the tonsil region just as commonly migrate through the bloodstream to the heart muscle (myocarditis), the valves (endocarditis), or the pericardium (pericarditis).* And, as previously mentioned, acute rheumatic fever, in which the most common sequella (lingering sign or symptom) is carditis (heart inflammation), most commonly begins with tonsillitis.[59]

As is the case for arthritis, it is well documented that a bout of rheumatic fever can precipitate chronic heart disease.[60] However, since the heart area often causes no local pain or other symptoms, it can be even more insidious than joint disease and remain undiagnosed for years, or even a lifetime. This is especially true in children, in whom the cardiac symptoms "may be so mild that they escape notice" but later manifest as a valvular scar.[61] This classic "rheumatic heart disease without a history of rheumatic fever" affects primarily the mitral valve, and secondarily the aortic valve. In fact, the common diagnosis of mitral or aortic valve prolapse, regurgitation, or stenosis (from an incompetent bulging, thickened, and/or stenosed or narrowed opening disrupting normal blood flow) manifesting clinically in a (readily apparent or subtle) pericardial rubbing sound ("friction rubs") or valvular murmur or click most often develops from undiagnosed rheumatic fever that is typically considered at the time to be simply a bad cold or "the flu that's going around." Mitral valve disease can be so mild that it goes virtually unnoticed, or it may cause chronic palpitations, dyspnea (difficult breathing), chest pain (angina), and fatigue.[62] Tonsil and dental foci are not only instrumental in triggering rheumatic fever but are often the root cause of it and continue to sustain this chronic and insidious form of heart disease. The intermittent but continual translocation of bacteria from these undiagnosed oral focal infections can slowly degenerate the heart valve, cardiac muscle, and pericardial tissue and can be the underlying basis—along with mercury amalgam fillings—of "essential" hypertension (high blood pressure), myocardial infarctions (heart attacks), and cerebrovascular accidents (strokes).[63] Cor pulmonale—thickening of the right ventricle of the heart with resulting heart failure—has been specifically correlated to hypertrophied tonsils and adenoids, and successful treatment of this syndrome has been documented through tonsillectomy surgery in a pediatric population (children under age eight).[64]

> **essential hypertension:** *Essential hypertension* refers to cases of high blood pressure that are deemed *idiopathic*—i.e., they have no obvious diagnosable causation.

One negative aspect of any form of heart disease or extra heart sounds (friction rubs, valvular murmurs or clicks) is that this diagnosis can follow patients throughout their life and compel dentists to prescribe antibiotics for all their dental procedures—even for twice-a-year cleanings. Although the fear of potential bacteremia (bacteria circulating in the blood) is founded on accurate focal-infection premises as well as in some cases

*In the early twentieth century, a general correlation was found between a hard tissue focal infection (i.e., a tooth) and resulting endocarditis (heart valve infection); and a soft tissue focus (i.e., the tonsils) and resulting myocarditis (heart muscle infection), muscular rheumatism, ulcer, or appendicitis. This would be a valuable research study to conduct among current holistic practitioners who treat foci, to ascertain if these hard tissue/soft tissue relationships still hold true.

on active heart disease such as chronic infective endocarditis,* this dogmatic allopathic mandate ensures a life of chronic intestinal dysbiosis for millions, with all the attending immune system deficiencies that excessive antibiotics engender.

Recently, after five decades of endorsing prophylactic antibiotics, the American Heart Association (AHA) finally concluded that there's no evidence that they work:

> "We've concluded that if giving prophylactic antibiotics prior to a dental procedure works at all—and there's no evidence that it does work—we should reserve that preventive treatment only for those people who would have the worst outcomes if they get infective endocarditis," noted Chair of the new guidelines writing group Walter R. Wilson, M.D., from Mayo Clinic in Rochester, Minnesota, in a statement issued by the AHA. "This changes the whole philosophy of how we have constructed these recommendations for the last 50 years."[65]

The new AHA guidelines still include recommendations for prophylactic antibiotics in the case of more vulnerable populations—those with artificial heart valves, a previous history of infective endocarditis, or serious congenital heart defects.

Even before this change in policy, however, after some years of submitting to this practice, many holistically oriented patients chose to refuse these antibiotic prescriptions and substitute natural antibacterial herbs (e.g., Thorne's Entrocap) or homeopathic or isopathic remedies (e.g., SanPharma's Notatum 4X drops) during dental procedures.

▶ Order Notatum 4X from BioResource at (800) 203-3775, and Entrocap from Thorne at (800) 228-1966.

The Kidney Disturbed Field

The streptococcus microbe also has a special affinity for the kidneys, rendering the rheumatic renal disturbed field as prevalent as the heart and joint fields.[66] German ear, nose, and throat (ENT) specialist Dr. Gruner explains the relationship between ENT infections and these paired blood-cleansing organs:

> A special dependence exists between the kidneys and the area of the ear, nose, and throat, because damaging substances can penetrate the body via the skin and mucous membranes in the ear-nose-throat area of the body that the kidneys must eliminate.[67]

Additionally, in five-element acupuncture theory, the ears have been linked with the kidney meridian and the water element for millennia.[68]

Acute kidney infections—nephritis, glomerulonephritis, and pyelonephritis—occurring most commonly in children older than age three and in young adults, typically arise after the classic streptococcal infections of tonsillitis and otitis (ear infection).[69] That is, in focal infection terminology, these kidney infections manifest either as acute disturbed fields from throat and ear infections *or* from the acute exacerbation of chronic tonsil and ear focal infections. Renal (kidney) disturbed fields may also arise from gonococcus-infected genital foci such as the prostate and fallopian tubes.

As with heart disease, the relationship between the tonsil focus and the resulting kidney infection often goes undiagnosed because there is a latent period of one to six weeks (average of two weeks) between the upper respiratory streptococcal or genital gonococcal infection and the nephritis. Even more insidiously, about 50 percent of patients with kidney infections are symptom-free (or the mild bladder and back symptoms go unnoticed or unreported).[70]

In the early twentieth century, researchers Le Count and Jackson found that in animals, although the kidneys' "acute lesions heal," their place was taken "by scars, subcapsular retractions, retention (tubular) cysts, and other evidences of 'chronic interstitial nephritis.'"[71] That is, beyond the apparent (or nonapparent) acute signs and symptoms—oliguria (frequent urination), fever, and cystitis or urethritis (pain on urination)—the chronic manifestations of a renal disturbed field are rarely recognized. For example, chronic low back pain (mild to moderate) and fatigue, two of the most characteristic

*Infective endocarditis is an infection of the lining of the heart (endocardium) and usually also of the heart valves and often the heart muscle. When diagnosed, treatment consists of intravenous/oral antibiotics for two to six weeks, and possibly heart surgery.

symptoms, classically referred to in Chinese medicine as "deficient kidney chi," may never be correlated to bouts of childhood tonsillitis. In contrast to the acute kidney and bladder infections that can plague teenagers and young adults, the chronic—yet often mild and intermittent—symptoms from kidney disturbed fields linger for years in adults. The pervasive ENT infections that implant chronic foci in the body are possibly the explanation as to why "by the time the average person reaches age seventy-two, his or her kidneys are operating at only 25 percent of their capacity."[72] Focal infections also often underlie and even fuel interstitial cystitis, a relatively common autoimmune condition in women characterized by chronic bladder inflammation and irritation.

The Digestive Disturbed Field

The primary areas of disturbance in the digestive system are the stomach and small intestine. Dr. Cotton commented on the formation of these disturbed fields:

> The stomach and duodenum [first section of the small intestine] are very frequently the seat of secondary foci [disturbed fields]. The infection is conveyed to the stomach, either by means of constant swallowing of infected material from the mouth—teeth and tonsils—or through the lymph or blood circulation, more probably the former.[73]

One of the major rheumatic manifestations of these disturbed fields are gastric (stomach) and peptic (duodenal) ulcers.[74]* Gastric and peptic ulcers are often refractory to treatment, especially when the primary contributing focal infection is not diagnosed and addressed. Even the reported success of the relatively recent treatment of campylobacter-induced ulcers with bismuth (e.g., Pepto-Bismol) and antibiotics has been found by many practitioners to be lacking and to have a high rate of recidivism (recurrence of the ulcer).[75]

Appendicitis arising from infection in the ileum and ascending colon can be secondary to a tonsil or dental focal infection or to a genitourinary focus (prostate, fallopian tubes, etc.); however, it can also present independently as a primary focus itself due to major intestinal dysbiosis.

The large intestine and gallbladder are also frequently disturbed rheumatic fields emanating from tonsil focal infections.[76] The warm, wet, and enclosed sac of the gallbladder is an especially inviting environment for streptococcus microbes, as well as migrating of intestinal parasites. A major contributing factor to the microbial infestation of the large intestine is biomechanical. That is, as Dr. Cotton observed, we are still paying the price for "getting up on our hind legs."[77] This upright posture forces the bowel contents to "run uphill" in many parts of the colon and to constantly work against the effects of gravity. Furthermore, this bipedal position can seriously interfere with the circulation of blood and over time exhaust the organs, rendering them more prone to infection. This more posturally vulnerable large intestine in humans renders them more susceptible to diseases such as ulcerative colitis, Crohn's disease, and irritable bowel syndrome, which are often initiated and maintained by a focal infection and fueled by an undiagnosed food allergy.*

Stomachaches and appendicitis are often symptoms of focal infections, or disturbed fields from a focal infection, that are actively forming in childhood. These areas of infection and inflamed mucosa (the inner lining of the intestine, gallbladder, stomach, etc.) often manifest later in the adult as chronic ulcers, gastritis, cholecystitis (gallbladder inflammation), "heartburn," esophageal reflux, and colitis.

The Brain Disturbed Field

Mental conditions caused by tonsil and dental focal infections are relatively unique from the other four rheumatic syndromes in two primary ways. First, only in rare cases do the microorganisms themselves actually invade the tissues of the brain. However, the pathogenic

---

*The *duodenum* is the first part of the small intestine. The *jejunum* is the second or middle division, and the *ileum* is the third or last section. Peptic ulcers most commonly occur in the first few centimeters of the duodenum, but they also occur along the lesser curvature of the stomach that leads into the duodenum. Although ulcers are not currently identified as one of the five classic sequellae of rheumatic fever in present-day medical texts, abdominal pain is listed under "other manifestations." (R. Berkow et al., eds., *The Merck Manual,* 15th ed. [Rahway, N.J.: Merck Sharp and Dohme Research Laboratories, 1987], 2092.)

*A wheat or gluten allergic tendency is a little more common in the colon than a dairy allergy. See chapter 6 for more information.

streptococcal excretion products originating in the tonsils and teeth are easily transported through blood and lymphatic vessels, as well as along nerve pathways (axonal transport), to the central nervous system (CNS)—that is, the brain and spinal cord.[78] Billings, Rosenow, Upton, Cotton, and others identified this migration in numerous research studies in the early twentieth century and also recorded the resulting disorders—encephalitis (inflammation of the brain), meningitis (inflammation of the membranes that surround the brain), epilepsy, brain abscesses, insomnia, and various other "nervous and mental conditions."[79] Dr. Patrick Störtebecker of Sweden later confirmed these earlier studies through compelling evidence that the combination of mercury from amalgam fillings and bacteria from dental and tonsil focal infections is readily transported from the mouth to the brain and is instrumental in the causation of neurological disorders such as epilepsy, multiple sclerosis (MS), myasthenia gravis, and Parkinson's disease.[80]

A second phenomenon relatively unique to the CNS disturbed field is that when the brain is affected, rarely are the joints. That is, unlike the common specificity for some streptococcal strains that attack both the joints and the heart or the joints and the kidneys or gut, in many cases brain and other CNS disorders stand alone.[81]*

Chorea, PANDAS, and Tourette's—All the Same Disorder?

Chorea, a disorder characterized by involuntary movements, has been documented for over a century to be a common manifestation after streptococcal illness and can occur in up to 10 percent of rheumatic fever attacks.† This 10 percent estimate, however, is probably too low, because "choreic movements may merge imperceptibly into purposeful or semi-purposeful acts that serve to 'cover up' the involuntary motion."[82] And similar to the other insidious rheumatic manifestations, chorealike movements may not begin until much later—sometimes up to six months—after tonsillitis or other acute streptococcus infections.[83] Therefore, this and other CNS neurological disorders are rarely correlated to the original strep infection by the patient's general practitioner.

Chorea and other post-streptococcal-infection CNS manifestations have recently acquired a more modern appellation, PANDAS, which is the acronym for pediatric autoimmune neuropsychiatric disorders associated with streptococcal infections. PANDAS describes a wider spectrum of neurological and psychological disorders that can arise in children after a bout of strep throat.[84] The two hallmark manifestations of PANDAS—tics or chorea-like movements and obsessive-compulsive disorders (OCD)—are also seen in Tourette's syndrome.

OCD-like motor tics can include spitting, licking, touching, smelling, finger and foot tapping, piano-playing movements, kissing, jumping, kicking, hopping, turning, shoulder shrugging, eye blinking, wrinkling of the forehead, nose twitching, pursing of the lips, and other facial grimaces. Vocal tics include swearing, counting (usually inaudibly), coughs, grunts, and clearing the throat—which is also a classic indication of a likely chronic tonsil focus. Obsessive-compulsive concerns overlay the majority of these tics, especially in the area of symmetry—that is, needing to have things "even."[85] For example, an OCD child (or adult) may feel compelled to count out four taps with the right foot, and then four taps with the left.

Other OCD manifestations include constant hand washing and worries about dirt and germs; chronic worrying about any subject but especially religious and sexual issues, as well as safety (for oneself or for others) concerns; ritual arranging of things (stuffed animals, clothes, setting the table, etc.); and repeated "checking" compulsions (stove turned off? doors locked? etc.). Commonly associated symptoms include sloppy handwriting, slight slurring of the speech, separation anxiety (e.g., going to school), hyperactivity, and attention deficit disorder.[86] Of course, many of these signs can simply indicate a normal phase of childhood. However, when symptoms arise frequently and continue for long periods (even if they do wax and wane), children should be examined by a knowledgeable physician (a neurologist

*The observation that it is rare to have two diseases of sufficient strength afflict a patient, first made by Hippocrates, Hahnemann, and other giants in holistic medicine, was probably more true prior to the 1900s. (W. O'Reilly, *Organon of the Medical Art* [Palo Alto, Calif.: Birdcage Press, 1996], 81). With the current suppressive practice of *polypharmacy* (taking many prescription drugs, some prescribed to counteract the side effects of others), toxic diets, and weaker genetic inheritance, mental disorders and arthritic syndromes are more often seen in tandem.

†Chorea is also known as Sydenham's chorea or St. Vitus's dance. St. Vitus was a shrine that was frequented during the Middle Ages by religious zealots who danced in a wild and frenzied manner.

or holistic doctor aware of focal infections and familiar with PANDAS and Tourette's syndrome).*

Autoimmune Dysfunction in the Basal Ganglia

The letter "A" in the PANDAS acronym aptly describes the real "molecular mimicry"—or autoimmune tendency—of the strep bacterium, which is the primary underlying microbe that sustains a chronic tonsil focus.[87] Recently, neural imaging evidence has indicated that the basal ganglia are the areas of the brain most affected.[88†] These two "pistachio-nut-size areas deep within the brain" receive input from the cerebral cortex and thus have an effect in modifying behavior‡ and also act as an overall inhibitory "brake" on movement. Therefore, lesions (any pathological process or disturbance in function) in the basal ganglia nuclei have been linked with various movement disorders, including chorea, PANDAS, and Parkinson's.[89]

Allopathic Treatment for PANDAS

The current recommended treatments for PANDAS are typically allopathic—primarily antibiotics and even possibly *prophylactic* antibiotics (long-term use). In many cases, however, these medications do more long-term harm than good by further ensuring an autoimmune response in a chronic tonsil focal infection and its related streptococcus-infected CNS disturbed fields, as well as chronic intestinal dysbiosis. Other novel therapies undergoing clinical trials, including plasmapheresis (a "blood-cleaning" procedure) and intravenous immunoglobulin, are presently restricted to the treatment of very ill patients since the former treatment carries the risk of serious side effects and the latter can cause headaches, nausea, or vomiting.[90]

I have never seen a child diagnosed with Tourette's syndrome who *did not* have an accompanying tonsil focus, and usually a history of a previous significant streptococcal infection.* Therefore, Tourette's syndrome and PANDAS are very possibly simply new names for the present-day escalating rheumatic brain disturbances that often occur from increasingly resistant and virulent strep infections. This CNS-damaging tonsil focal infection can be implanted initially from an acute bout of tonsillitis, or it can be an exacerbation of a chronic tonsil focus from many past bouts of tonsillitis and accompanying rounds of antibiotics. Therefore, the current plethora of Tourette's diagnoses, along with the closely associated hyperactivity and attention deficit disorders, may very well reflect the devastating effects of the modern-day mode of excessively prescribing antibiotics and other allopathic drugs (as well as mercury-preserved vaccines—see chapter 15). In my experience, nontoxic natural treatments for tonsil foci and their associated CNS disorders are greatly superior to allopathic intervention.

Subclinical PANDAS?

Finally, it is interesting to ponder the subclinical (subtle) PANDAS effects that individuals may have been unaware of for years. In general, baby boomers who suffered from numerous childhood upper respiratory infections, whether or not the infections were diagnosed as strep throat at the time, received countless courses of antibiotics. And for the most part, this generation could certainly have been characterized as idealistic, daring, hedonistic—and also perhaps a little obsessive? In fact, many might recognize some of the aforementioned symptoms—counting for symmetry, constantly clearing the throat,† obsessive thinking, and compulsive tapping—as subtle but chronic behaviors they have intermittently engaged in for years. For those readers who can identify with one or more of these rheumatic CNS symptoms, the diagnosis and treatment of a possible chronic tonsil (or other) focal infection may be in order.

*Specifically, symptoms often come on abruptly after an infection (throat, ears, etc.) or exposure (cold, wet, etc.) and then slowly disappear over a few months' time, but can continue for years. This description of a typical PANDAS manifestation correlates with the episodic and periodic symptoms pathognomic of focal infections.

†Similar to the valves of the heart, the tissue in the basal ganglia has a molecular makeup that closely resembles the tissue in strep bacteria. When antibodies are mistakenly formed against these tissues, they attack the heart valves, resulting in mitral valve disease. When they attack, or "cross react," with the basal ganglia in the brain, the resulting symptoms are tics similar to Tourette's syndrome, as well as psychological symptoms such as obsessive-compulsive disorder. (R. Lahita, *Women and Autoimmune Disease* [New York: HarperCollins Publishers Inc., 2004], 90.)

‡Basal ganglia dysfunction has also been implicated in schizophrenia.

*Doctors should note that often a streptococcus-induced "mild cold, sore throat or flu" previous to the onset of the child's behavior disorder may not be remembered or reported during the history.

†Yes, it's also an allergy symptom, but if you have had allergies for years—especially dairy—it's likely you also have a tonsil focus.

Dr. Cotton, who had enormous success curing all types of mental illnesses as the medical director at the New Jersey State Psychiatric Hospital, discussed the physical nature of emotional disorders in his 1921 Princeton University lecture series:

> For years we have been content to consider mental disorders in two large groups, designated as "organic" [actual pathological changes found in the brain tissue] and "functional" [no pathology found in the brain] . . . This led to the erroneous viewpoint that certain mental diseases could occur independently of any changes in the brain . . . It should be said that the primary lesion which determines the abnormal mental state is most frequently not to be found in the brain itself. The brain cells are constantly influenced by abnormal conditions in other parts of the body through the circulation. Thus, frequently there is a direct action on the cerebral elements by the morbid agents carried directly through the circulation . . . We have seen many recoveries among the acute psychoses occur in a day or two after the removal of the chronic foci of infection . . . we have to recognize the physical nature of the disturbance . . .
>
> Psychoses arise from a combination of many factors, some of which may be absent, but the most constant one is an intracerebral, biochemical, cellular disturbance arising from circulating toxins, originating in chronic focal infections situated anywhere throughout the body.[91]

Thus, in a time when heredity was considered of "paramount importance in the causation of mental disease," Cotton was an outspoken and courageous pioneer in the field of psychiatry. In fact, even researchers currently working in the newly emerging mind-body field of psychoneuroimmunology have still not caught up to what Cotton observed countless times at the New Jersey State Hospital in the early 1900s: that chronic focal infections have a major, and sometimes *singular,* influence on the onset of all types of mental disease.[92]

Patients who have directly experienced relief from their depression, anxiety, panic attacks, tics, obsessive-compulsive ideations, and other psychological disorders through the clearing of their tonsil, dental, or other focal infection know the emotionally liberating experience effective holistic medicine can provide. In fact, just the psychological benefit derived from simply understanding that psychological disorders are not always *solely* caused by emotional tendencies resulting from a classic dysfunctional family background is profoundly empowering. And concurrent or future in-depth psychological work and spiritual understanding is immeasurably benefited when these psychophysical obstacles to cure are removed from a patient's body and consciousness.

The Tonsil Interference Field—Another Contributor to Brain Dysfunction

The brain is adversely affected not only by bacterial toxins but also by nerve dysfunction from a tonsil interference field. The scars in a tonsil interference field remaining after a tonsillectomy, or the scars generated from chronic streptococcal infection (i.e., the focus is both infected and scarred), are a constant disturbing "noise" to the sensitive nerve fibers flowing through this region.[93] The primary route of disturbance is cervicocranial—from the neck to the head—through sympathetic nerve dysfunction via the tonsil's neighboring ganglion.

As discussed previously, autonomic ganglia perform two major functions in the body: (1) they control autonomic—sympathetic and parasympathetic nerve—function, and (2) they act as "storage depots" to hold excess toxins. The palatine tonsils in the back of the throat lie 1 inch away from one of the most important ganglia in the body—the superior cervical. This upper neck ganglion is composed solely of sympathetic motor nerve fibers that control blood circulation in the entire head—the scalp, face, and the brain.[94] Tonsillar scars retract and compress the tissues in the nearby superior cervical ganglion, chronically disturbing sympathetic nerve flow. When these sympathetic motor nerves are irritated, they vasoconstrict and decrease the blood flow to all the organs and tissues they innervate. Thus, a tonsil scar interference field chronically deprives the brain of adequate blood flow, oxygen, glucose, and other nutrients. The resulting cerebral ischemia, hypoxia, and hypoglycemia can contribute to numerous neuropsychological disorders, including memory loss and "brain fog," depression and fatigue, and chronic anxiety. Furthermore, since the sympathetic nerves that innervate the pineal gland derive solely from the superior cervical ganglion, chronic insomnia also commonly results from a tonsil interference field. Other clinically observed cranial signs of a chronic tonsil focus include headaches, dizziness, and even balding from chronic scalp ischemia.[95]

The two most effective treatments for a tonsil scar interference field are auriculotherapy and constitutional homeopathy, which are described in the following section.

THE SEVEN MOST EFFECTIVE TREATMENTS FOR A TONSIL FOCUS

Similar to the dental treatment pyramid previously illustrated, the seven most effective treatments for a tonsil focus—both focal infections and scar interference fields—are depicted in figure 12.4. It should again be noted that although Rosenow, Billings, Cotton, and numerous other early researchers were truly giants in the field of focal infection diagnosis and treatment, not one of them was aware of the miraculous effects of the correctly prescribed constitutional homeopathic remedy. In fact, although dietary and other general holistic advice was given to patients, only two specific treatments were primarily employed to treat tonsil focal infections in the early and mid-twentieth century—surgery and streptococcal vaccines.* More information on these vaccines is included in the following nosodes section (the fifth suggested therapy), because vaccines and nosodes are closely related. Tonsillectomies are the last option, after all other avenues have been exhausted, and therefore are listed seventh in this list.

*Dr. Cotton was so impressed with the "powerful adjunct" of vaccines that he predicted that they would one day possibly "wholly replace" surgery. Unfortunately, these vaccines are not simple to make and no one at the time of publication is preparing them according to his and Dr. Rosenow's exacting standards. (For more information on these vaccine "recipes," see www.InstituteofScience.com/rosenow.html.)

1. Diet

To reiterate the central thesis of chapter 5, although a clean and conscious diet cannot cure a chronic tonsil focus, *without a reasonably clean and conscious diet a tonsil focus cannot heal.* In other words, without "plugging the dike" against chronic irritants—allergenic foods, refined sugar, and rancid hydrogenated oils—the tonsillar tissue will inflame daily and thus be unavailable for healing and repair.

The Gut and the Tonsils Work Synchronously

As previously described, the digestive system can be thought of as one long tube, from the mouth to the anus. The tonsils are the two lymphatic pillars that lie on either side of the entrance to this digestive system, and they act as the first defense against all toxic ingested substances. As part of the GALT (gut-associated lymphoid tissue), the tonsils and adenoids—or the remaining lymphatic tissue in the throat after tonsillectomies and adenoidectomies—work *so synchronously* with the

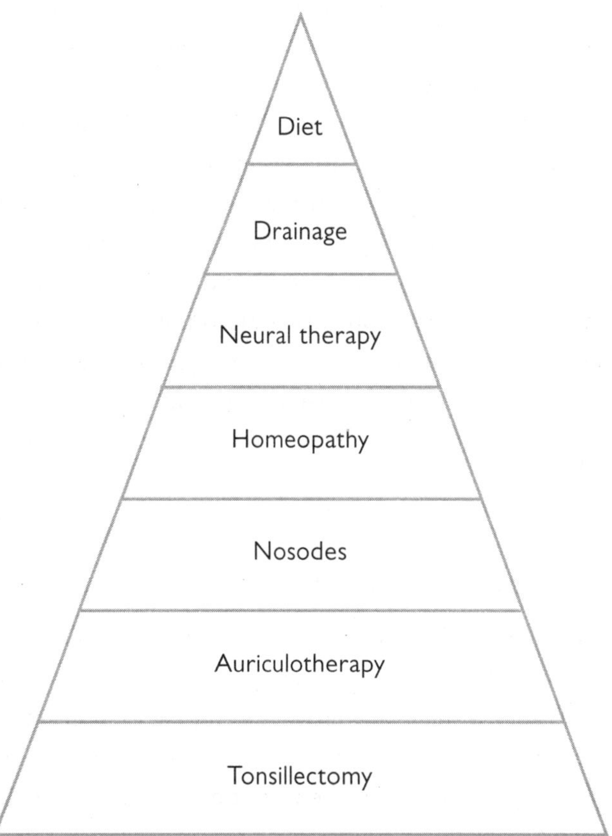

Figure 12.4. The seven most effective treatments for a chronic tonsil focus, ranging from the most general to the most specific and strongest intervention

Peyer's patches (in the third part of the small intestine) and appendix that they are functionally considered to be the same tissue. Therefore, any foods or substances that augment intestinal dysbiosis also augment the continued pathogenicity of a chronic tonsil focus. The opposite is also true—that is, any foods or substances that irritate and inflame the tonsils also irritate and inflame the lymphatic mucosa of the intestine.

Must Heal the Gut to Heal the Tonsils

Thus, in order to clear a chronic tonsil focus, individuals must also clear their chronic intestinal dysbiosis. In the case of major tonsil focal infection, an individual may need to adhere to a clean diet for many years. It is especially important to avoid a primary food allergen, since this has a direct adverse effect on the immune functioning of the GALT system. Almost everyone with a major tonsil focus has a dairy allergy, and many have secondary sensitivities to wheat, corn, soy (even properly fermented), and other foods. Although rigid adherence is not always necessary—that is, the use of organic raw butter, cultured cottage cheese, some raw goat and sheep cheeses, and occasional desserts and alcohol during celebratory occasions may not badly sabotage an individual's progress—the general axiom that "the cleaner one's diet, the faster one's healing" tends to hold true. In most instances, through trial-and-error testing, knowledgeable holistic patients become quite aware of what foods serve and do not serve their general well-being. Foods that are questionable can be energetically tested by a holistic practitioner and then double-checked by the patient through the elimination-challenge test at home. (See chapter 6 for more information on the elimination-challenge test.)

MILK FOR ULCERS—TREATMENT DEBUNKED

The past use of milk for treating ulcers has currently been debunked.[96] Furthermore, this practice is unwarranted for treating a rheumatic ulcer caused by a focal infection because it only exacerbates the dairy allergy that most probably contributed to the formation of the tonsil focus in the first place.

DEALING WITH CRAVINGS

It's important to note that being too rigid with a diet is never a good idea, especially since the opportunistic candida fungus that greatly proliferates in the presence of toxic microbes or mercury can *dramatically* magnify a person's sugar cravings. Do the best you can, and when cravings become too intense, indulge in low-glycemic-index treats that are easier on the pancreas—fresh fruit with nuts (soaked and dehydrated according to Sally Fallon's instructions); homemade muffins with raisins, apples, bananas, and nuts; French toast with cinnamon and honey or maple syrup; and so forth.

Additionally, patients with a chronic tonsil focus need to supplement their often-depleted digestive functioning with a quality enzyme supplement. For those individuals with a major rheumatic gut disturbed field, their chronically irritated stomach and small intestine mucosas require the gentle supplementation of a hydrochloric-acid-free and protease-free enzyme, such as Gastric Comfort (601) from Enzymes, Inc. Those with no significant history of ulcers, gastritis, or stomach or intestinal pain may choose to supplement with Dipan 9 from Thorne.

▶ Gastric Comfort, aka 601, is available from Enzymes, Inc., at (800) 637-7893. Dipan 9 is available from Thorne at (800) 228-1966.

2. *Drainage*

Gemmotherapy (plant stem cell) drainage remedies are essential components in the treatment of tonsil foci. Often basic drainage for the liver with Juniper (*Juniperus communis*) or Rosemary (*Rosmarinus officinalis*); the kidneys with Juniper or White Birch (*Betula pubescens*); and the pancreas, stomach, and small intestine with Fig (*Ficus carica*) or European Alder (*Alnus glutinosa*) is sufficient. However, specific drainage for the tonsils is also often needed.

White Willow (*Salix alba*), which is both anti-inflammatory and analgesic (pain relieving), makes an excellent gargle for painful throats. Another remedy indicated for tonsillitis is Black Poplar (*Populus nigra*), especially in cases with mercury amalgam fillings (past or present). The excellent Silver Fir (*Abies pectinata*) remedy is used most often in pediatric patients to treat tonsillitis, especially for children who suffer from chronic infections. It additionally helps remineralize bones and teeth, reducing dental cavities, strengthening the enamel, and therefore preventing future potential dental focal infections.

Specific drainage for rheumatic disturbed fields such as the joints with Mountain Pine (*Pinus montana*), the heart with Hawthorne (*Crataegus oxyacantha*), and the brain with Olive (*Olea europaea*) or Linden Tree (*Tilia tomentosa*) may also be indicated.

▶ Gemmotherapy remedies are available from PSC Distribution at (631) 477-6696 or www.epsce.com and from Gemmos LLC at (877) 417-6298 or www.gemmos-usa.com.

Natural drainage through the normal emunctories in the head—that is, through the various orifices—can also be enhanced. When toxins are released from the brain and face while the patient is receiving appropriate treatment, itching and redness may occur in the eyes, ears, nose, and throat. This is usually a positive sign, indicating that the prescribed drainage remedies, constitutional homeopathy, auriculotherapy, and other holistic treatments are working and releasing toxic metals or microbes.* To facilitate this transport, use an eyewash with eyebright (*Euphrasia officinalis*) herbal drops diluted with water in an eyecup, ear drops (e.g., mullein and garlic in olive oil), nasal and sinus washes (neti pots), and Karach's oil treatment for throat and tonsil detoxification (all available from health food stores).† Colonics or home enemas may also be indicated during this period.

*Often opportunistic candida fungus that proliferates as a defensive response to the presence of the more pathogenic and dangerous mercury or bacteria is discharged, with resulting symptoms of redness, irritation (physically and emotionally), itching, fatigue, and food cravings.

†Karach's oil treatment includes the gargling and swishing around the mouth of organic, unrefined sesame seed oil to absorb toxic chemicals and metals from the oral and throat mucosa. (See chapter 3 for more detailed information on this method.) Additionally, at the turn of the twentieth century, ground-up flaxseed gargles and ground-up grapefruit seed gargles in the form of warm teas were recommended. (J. Garretson, *A System of Oral Surgery* [New York: J. B. Lippincott Co., 1898], 559.)

EAR DRAINAGE/BRAIN FUNCTION CONNECTION IN ANIMALS

Holistic veterinarian Don Hamilton has noticed this phenomenon in animals. In his book *Homeopathic Care for Cats and Dogs,* he observes:

> There is an observed connection between the ears and the brain. Suppressed ear disease can lead to brain problems—and curative treatment of brain disease may be followed by an ear discharge. Suppressive treatment of the discharge may reawaken the brain illness.[97]

Finally, drinking adequate amounts of pure water (according to thirst) can further augment natural physiological drainage during this period. And since the tonsillar tissue in a focal infection is always (subtly or not-so-subtly) chronically inflamed, adequate pure water intake can reduce this heat, as well as dilute and help expel surface microbes. However, water should not be drunk in excess at meals to prevent diluting the stomach and intestinal juices and impairing efficient digestion.

▶ Effective reverse-osmosis water purifiers can be ordered from Radiant Life at (888) 593-8333, or go to www.radiantlifecatalog.com, and from Mary Cordaro at www.marycordaro.com.

3. Neural Therapy

The treatment of the tonsil focus through various neural therapy methods has been successfully utilized for almost a century. In children as well as adults with acute inflammation of this chronic focus, isopathic remedies can be very effective. For example, the SanPharma isopathic fungal remedy Notatum 4X, known in holistic circles as a "natural antibiotic," can significantly reduce strep and staph bacterial infections without any of the side effects that antibiotics create. Notatum 4X drops or the stronger 3X tablets are often indicated for acute tonsillitis or when a chronic tonsil focus acutely flares up.

As described for neural therapy treatment of a dental focus (page 341), a soft therapeutic laser can be employed to augment the effects of these remedies by driving them in photophoretically. The beam should be positioned just under the chin on either side of the upper neck (just anterior to the sternocleidomastoid muscle) and directed toward the tip of the opposite ear, commonly for one- to two-minute intervals on each side (depending on the patient's sensitivity), when using an 830-nanometer, 100-milliwatt laser.* If the practitioner has a laser with three different milliwatt options—100, 200, and 400—the stronger 200-milliwatt, and sometimes 400-milliwatt, beam, often energetically tests positive, since a tonsil focus is one of the toughest and most tenacious to treat in the body. In this case, the laser is used for a shorter period over each tonsil point, for example, for approximately thirty seconds with the 200-milliwatt beam, and for five seconds or less when utilizing the 400-milliwatt option. These treatments often need to be done intermittently, whenever the tonsils are testing positive, typically for months or even years, until this most challenging and chronic focus is cleared.

Essential oils such as lavender, peppermint, and frankincense can also be rubbed into the skin overlying the tonsil focus and driven in photophoretically with the laser. Niaouli oil from BioResource is especially good in the treatment of this chronic focus, as well as for acute respiratory infections. Patients can stock this oil at home so that it is always available for treating their tonsil focus as it flares up intermittently during the healing process, often accompanied by acute sore throats, colds, and bronchitis.†

▶ Niaouli oil is available from BioResource at (800) 203-3775.

Doctors and dentists who would like to use neural therapy injection techniques to treat the tonsil focus should contact Dr. Dietrich Klinghardt's office to learn these methods at his neural therapy seminars.

▶ For a schedule of Dr. Klinghardt's upcoming seminars, go to www.klinghardtacademy.com.

*The place where the stylus of the laser is positioned to treat each tonsil is the same point used to treat each side of the superior cervical ganglion, illustrated in figure 11.10. (See page 342.)

†These oils have the potential, however, to antidote the patient's constitutional remedy. Therefore, the patient may need to be instructed to intermittently re-dose (a gentle, liquid, daily, or "booster" dose) his or her remedy after utilizing these essential oils.

4. Acute and Constitutional Homeopathy

Along with auriculotherapy, homeopathy is the most effective healing modality for a chronic tonsil focus. Acute homeopathic remedies can be invaluable during a bout of acute tonsillitis, and a constitutional homeopathic remedy can be indispensable in the treatment of a chronic tonsil focus. Sometimes more than one constitutional homeopathic remedy is needed over the course of months and even years, as is typical in a complex, multilayered case. (See chapter 14 for more information on constitutional homeopathy, particularly the Sankaran system.) Furthermore, when treating a patient with a major tonsil focal infection, dosage requirements are often amplified, so the patient may need, besides the *initial* dose (e.g., 200C or 1M), a *booster* dose (e.g., 6C or 12C) weekly (or more often). Treatments that include additional booster doses help actively address the bacterial infection that usually becomes triggered during the "unpeeling" process of healing.

One of the most valuable aspects of constitutional homeopathy is its clarifying ability. That is, if a patient truly has an incurable tonsil focal infection, the correctly prescribed *simillimum*—or the deepest-acting remedy in a multilayered case—will allow that fact to be revealed during energetic testing. In other words, if constitutional homeopathy (in conjunction with the aforementioned therapies) cannot cure the patient, then often nothing can, and the body will recognize this fact.

If the tonsil tissues are truly degenerated, then they will continue to display as a focus in energetic testing and surgery may be indicated. The homeopathic simillimum helps the body function more effectively, and in this "clearer and cleaner" system, "what's false arises." However, because tonsillectomies are very hard on older teens and adults, surgery should be considered only in very serious cases when all other options have been exhausted.

5. Nosodes

The use of nosodes—homeopathic remedies made from diseased tissues, microbes, or toxins—can be another essential component of this multifaceted treatment protocol of a tonsil focus. In acute tonsillitis or in children where the vital force is still strong, nosodes can be very effective. However, in weakened adult patients who have been dealing with chronic tonsil focal infections for decades, nosode remedies are often too strong. For example, a homeopathic streptococcus nosode (e.g., 30C or 200C) is often given as an *intercurrent* remedy—that is, given for a brief period such as for one to three weeks—to allow the patient's body (the immune system surveillance) to become more conscious of the presence of unwanted strep bacteria residing in the tonsil tissues.* However, even a short-term or gentle dosage (e.g., 30C diluted in water, once a week for three weeks) can be too strong for PANDAS patients and activate a full-fledged immune system attack on this bacterial invader, which only fuels the chronic autoimmune dysfunction.

intercurrent: An intercurrent remedy is one that is given to "provide movement in a stalled case." Thus, an intercurrent nosode remedy can be prescribed for a few days or weeks to a patient who is already on a constitutional remedy, but whose tonsil focal infection is not showing signs of appropriate progress in healing.[98]

Therefore, when the need for a nosode does test positive while treating a tonsil focus in a weakened tuberculinic or luetic patient, many of my colleagues and I choose to make a subtler "energetic equivalent" of this remedy on a duplicating instrument or a radionics machine. These more subtle nosodes, when prescribed at a gentle dosage regimen, are less aggressive and therefore often more effective at treating chronic tonsil foci.

It is important to look at the previous success of a close cousin of nosodes—vaccine remedies developed in the early twentieth century.† These vaccine remedies, unlike the ones made today, were prepared freshly with natural products using no preservatives, such as the toxic mercury-containing thimerosal. Dr. Rosenow had particular success with his streptococcal thermal antibody vaccine, which was strikingly effective (82 percent) in the treatment of a wide variety of illnesses such as polio, multiple sclerosis, schizophrenia, coronary heart disease, cancer, and migraine headaches.[99] Unfortunately, the research on these seemingly incredibly effective bacterial vaccines declined to a virtual halt by the mid-twentieth century because of the precipitous decline of interest in focal infections. But in light of Rosenow's astounding results, a replication of Rosenow's vaccine and a research study measuring its effectiveness on individuals with chronic tonsil foci is particularly warranted. Unfortunately, at this time, no holistic pharmacy has yet attempted to reproduce it.* Hopefully, as the dominance of allopathic and pharmaceutical medicine in this country lessens and the holistic movement gains greater momentum, this will be accomplished, perhaps by our holistic colleagues in Mexico, Europe, and other parts of the world who enjoy more medical freedom than Americans.

6. Auriculotherapy

As with a dental focus, auriculotherapy is an essential component of the treatment protocol for a chronic tonsil focus. Auriculotherapy treatment of foci has already been described in the dental focus treatment section (see page 343). However, in the case of the tonsil focus treatment, the practitioner must keep in mind that many more aspects of this tissue may need to be addressed. That is, *all* three embryonic tissue layers may need to be treated: the endodermal layer that makes up most of the tonsillar tissue, the ectodermal layer for the superficial mucosal scarring from infection or surgery or the neighboring superior cervical ganglia, and the mesodermal layer for deeper tissue scarring or from damaged and degenerated blood vessels. Because tonsillectomy scars can block internal acupuncture pathways, these specific meridian points should all be treated. Dr. Frank Bahr of Germany, a colleague of Dr. Nogier and a great contributor to auriculotherapy, has mapped these points on the ear. Treatment of these points can increase meridian and blood flow to the points and the organs they represent.

Additionally, because the psychological aspect of a tonsil focus is often primary, the resulting chronically disturbed and imbalanced mental and emotional energy may need to be addressed through treatment

*In addition to the streptococcus nosode, a diphtheria or pertussis nosode—made from the disease products themselves or from the vaccine that is suspected to have been a primary cause of an individual's tonsil focus—should also be considered.

†Vaccines and nosodes are both made from diseased tissues, microbes, or toxins, but vaccines are simply diluted while nosode remedies are diluted and succussed, or potentized. See chapter 15 for more information.

*This information was made available to me by S. H. Shakman, who can be contacted through the www.instituteofscience.com website.

of auriculotherapy "master points" such as Point Zero, Shen Men, or the Master Cerebral Point.

▶ For information on seminars on auriculotherapy, contact Dr. Mikhael Adams at (905) 878-9994 or www.integralhealth.ca; Dr. Williams at www.radicalmedicine.com or (415) 460-1968; or Dr. Bryan Frank at www.auriculartherapy.com. Dr. Frank also has an excellent auricular chart, atlas, and book, titled *Auricular Therapy.* Bahr's auricular charts can be ordered from Dr. Williams.

7. Tonsillectomies

When all of the aforementioned conservative treatments still fail, even after many years of therapy, surgery may be indicated. Many physicians believe that surgery is necessary when the tonsillar tissue is so degenerated that it is simply no longer recognized by the body as "self," and in this chronic autoimmune state can no longer heal and regenerate. However, the decision about whether a chronic tonsil focus requires surgery is difficult. For one thing, in an older teen or adult, a tonsillectomy is a much more serious surgery than in a young child, so recovery can be long. Additionally, although many research studies have shown that tonsillectomies and adenoidectomies in young children often cure obstructive sleep apnea (insomnia due to breathing dysfunction), hearing and speech difficulties, and dental malocclusions (bad bites) and greatly improve school performance, no such studies on the effects of these surgeries have been conducted on an adult population.[100]* Furthermore, as early as the late 1800s, Dr. James Garretson, author of the seminal text *A System of Oral Surgery,* stated that at least with tonsillar *hypertrophy,* since it is more of an expression of systemic disease, "very little true benefit" has been derived from surgery, and it should be treated from a constitutional standpoint.[101]† Therefore, perhaps surgery should be seriously considered only in ill individuals with *atrophied* tonsils, which Dr. Josef Issels found to be the most pathogenic and dangerous.

Although it may seem strange to include tonsil surgery in a holistic book, throughout focal infection history tonsillectomies have been a primary treatment method. This surgery was not only the treatment of choice by American pioneers such as Billings, Rosenow, and Miller but also advocated by many European physicians.

German physician Josef Issels chiseled a place for himself in holistic medical history through uncovering the correlation between tonsil focal infections and cancer. In his 1954 book *More Cures for Cancer,* Dr. Issels explained how he discovered this tonsil focus–cancer relationship serendipitously. In his early years in practice in Germany, Issels had performed a tonsillectomy on a so-called incurable cancer patient suffering from severe rheumatic joint pain. The relationship between a tonsil focal infection and its rheumatic joint disturbed field was well understood at that time, so this was not an unusual surgical step. However, what occurred next astounded even this knowledgeable holistic physician. Not only was this patient's rheumatic joint pain relieved after surgery, but his tachycardia (excessively rapid heartbeat) and tumor size also began to diminish.[102] After observing this initial unexpected improvement and the eventual full recovery of this patient, Issels began to employ tonsillectomies more often. After many years of clinical experience, he found that not only cancer but also many other diverse illnesses responded to a carefully performed tonsillectomy. Issels documented the successful treatment of "intractable" tachycardia and hypertension, arthritis and chronic pain, and leukemia and other types of cancer.[103] He succinctly asserts the close link between tonsil and dental foci and cancer in the following quote: "We have never observed a malignancy, even in the young, in individuals not possessed of obviously bad teeth and tonsils."[104]

Thus, just as with dental focal infections, when a patient is diagnosed with a serious disease such as cancer, time is of the essence. If there is any question about the degenerative nature of a patient's tonsillar tissue, a tonsillectomy should be seriously considered. Based on this past research and experience, it is curious why surgeons in the medical profession haven't reinvestigated cavitation surgeries and tonsillectomies in the treatment of cancer, especially in light of the devastating side effects of chemotherapy and radiation. Hopefully, the renewed interest in focal infections will stimulate new research.

---

*Furthermore, no research studies have been made to compare the benefits of surgery with holistic measures in children or adults.

†In those days, cold saltwater bathing, a healthy diet, exercise, and lifestyle changes were generally prescribed, if the physician did not specialize in homeopathy.

For those who elect to have a tonsillectomy, the ENT surgeon should be aware of focal infections and willing to remove the tonsils even when the patient has not had a recent history of tonsillitis. Furthermore, he or she should be a skillful technician, and cognizant of the need to excise all the tonsillar tissue and not leave behind any "tonsillar tags or stumps," which were identified as early as 1928 in a *Journal of the American Medical Association* article of harboring *more* pathogenic streptococcus bacteria per gram than the original infected tonsils had contained before their removal.[105*] Furthermore, postsurgery protocols should be carefully prescribed, including the need for Arnica Montana 30C or 200C (or re-dosing one's constitutional homeopathic remedy), Notatum 4X drops or 3X tablets, and laser therapy or auriculotherapy to mitigate the scar formation.

The diagnosis of a chronic tonsil focus presents more of a challenge than a dental focus, and the decision to perform surgery even in a severely ill patient can be difficult to make. In adults tonsillectomies are serious surgeries with major risks and sometimes have painful and long recuperation periods. Furthermore, although holistic dentists have become more plentiful, holistic ENTs (those physicians specializing in ear, nose, and throat disorders) are almost nil. Therefore, a second opinion from someone who knows both the surgical procedure and focal infection theory is rare. Until medical schools review the focal infection literature and begin to teach this information in their curriculum, patients will need to rely on knowledgeable holistic practitioners for their diagnosis and conservative treatment. In the vast majority of cases, studiously avoiding food allergens, being on the correct constitutional homeopathic remedy, auriculotherapy treatments, *and* removing any neighboring dental foci are sufficient to heal a tonsil focal infection or to mitigate a tonsillectomy scar interference field.

*However, this surgeon must also take great care to avoid nicking the neighboring carotid artery.

NOTES

1. R. Haden, "Elective Localization of Streptococci," *Orthodontia and Oral Surgery, International Journal* 12 (1926): 711; F. Billings, *Focal Infection* (New York: D. Appleton and Company, 1916), 33–47; E. Rosenow, "Elective Localization of Streptococci," *Journal of the American Medical Association* 65 (1915): 1687–91.
2. E. Rosenow, "The Causation of Gastric and Duodenal Ulcer by Streptococci," *Journal of Infectious Disease* 19 (1916): 333–84; E. Rosenow, "Elective Localization of Bacteria in Diseases of the Nervous System," *Journal of the American Medical Association* 67 (1916): 662–65; E. Rosenow and W. Ashby, "Focal Infection and Elective Localization in the Etiology of Myositis," *Archives of Internal Medicine* 28 (1921): 274–311; E. Rosenow, "Nephritis and Urinary Calculi Following the Experimental Production of Chronic Foci of Infection. Preliminary Report," *Journal of the American Medical Association* 78 (1922): 266–67; E. Rosenow, "Microscopic Demonstration of Bacteria in the Lesions of Epidemic Lethargic Encephalitis," *Journal of Infectious Disease* 32 (1923): 144–52.
3. P. Williams et al., eds., *Gray's Anatomy* (New York: Churchill Livingstone, 1995), 1729.
4. D. Klinghardt, "The Tonsils and Their Role in Health and Chronic Illness" (paper presented at the American Academy of Biological Dentistry, Carmel, California, March 1999).
5. O. Meyer, "The Eliminating Function of the Tonsils in Dental Infections," *Dental Digest,* December 1944, 557.
6. J. Issels, *More Cures for Cancer,* translation from German, (Bad Homburg, Germany: Helfer Publishing Schwabe, 1980), 16.
7. I. Roitt et al., *Immunology,* 5th ed. (London: Mosby, 1998), 33.
8. Seminar notes from "Das Tonsillen Störfeld," Medicine Week, Baden-Baden, Germany, 1993.
9. L. Temoshok and H. Dreher, *The Type C Connection* (New York: Random House, 1992), 81–82, 204–7, 209–10.
10. J. Goldberg, *Deceits of the Mind* (New Brunswick, N.J.: Transaction Publishers, 1991), 163.
11. U. Heintze et al., "Methylation of Mercury from Dental Amalgam and Mercuric Chloride by Oral Streptococci in Vitro," *Scandinavian Journal of Dental Research* 91 (1983): 150–52.
12. M. Fischer, *Death and Dentistry* (Springfield, Ill.: Charles C. Thomas, 1940), 42.

13. D. MacKay, "Can CAM Therapies Help Reduce Antibiotic Resistance?" *Alternative Medicine Review* 8, no. 1 (February 2003): 29.
14. Ibid., 28.
15. Ibid.
16. Ibid., 29.
17. A. Vojdani, "The Role of Periodontal Disease and Other Infections in the Pathogenesis of Atherosclerosis and Systemic Diseases," *Townsend Letters for Doctors and Patients,* December 2000, 53.
18. S. Shakman, *E. C. Rosenow and Associates: A Reference Manual* (Santa Monica, Calif: Institute of Science, 1998), B2–24.
19. L. Verbist, "Antiobiotherapie de l'Angine de la Pharyngite: Necessaire, Utile, Superflue ou Nocive?" *Tijdschrift voor Geneeskunde* 48, no. 18 (1992): 1305–10.
20. American Academy of Otolaryngology, "Top Five 'Myths' of Tonsillectomy," www.entusa.com/pdf_downloads/TOP 5 MYTHS OF TONSILLECTOMY.pdf.
21. F. Billings, *Focal Infection* (New York: D. Appleton and Company, 1916), 52.
22. M. Fischer, *Death and Dentistry* (Springfield, Ill.: Charles C. Thomas, 1940), 52–53.
23. P. Dosch, *Manual of Neural Therapy* (Heidelberg: Haug Publishers, 1984), 127.
24. S. Shakman, *E. C. Rosenow and Associates: A Reference Manual* (Santa Monica, Calif.: Institute of Science, 1998), B2–5.
25. P. Dosch, *Manual of Neural Therapy* (Heidelberg: Haug Publishers, 1984), 127.
26. Ibid.
27. J. Pizzorno and M. Murray, *Textbook of Natural Medicine,* 2nd ed., vols. 1 and 2 (New York: Churchill Livingstone, 2000).
28. K. Conroy et al., *Natural Approach to Ophthalmology and Otolaryngology* (Seattle: Healing Mountain Publishing, 2004), 379.
29. J. Garretson, *A System of Oral Surgery* (New York: J. B. Lippincott Co., 1898), 559.
30. P. Williams et al., *Gray's Anatomy* (New York: Churchill Livingstone, 1995), 1728.
31. J. Issels, *More Cures for Cancer,* translation from German (Bad Homburg, Germany: Helfer Publishing E. Schwabe, 1980), 17–19; E. Rosenow, "Elective Localization of Bacteria in Diseases of the Nervous System," *Journal of the American Medical Association* 67 (August 26, 1916): 666.
32. J. Garretson, *A System of Oral Surgery* (New York: J. B. Lippincott Co., 1898), 563.
33. J. Issels, *More Cures for Cancer,* translation from German (Bad Homburg, Germany: Helfer Publishing E. Schwabe, 1980), 16.
34. W. Miller, "The Human Mouth as a Focus of Infection," *The Dental Cosmos* 33, no. 9 (September 1891): 697.
35. J. Garretson, *A System of Oral Surgery* (New York: J. B. Lippincott Co., 1898), 563–64; C. Oulis et al., "The Effect of Hypertrophic Adenoids and Tonsils on the Development of Posterior Crossbite and Oral Habits," *The Journal of Clinical Pediatric Dentistry* 18, no. 3 (1994): 197–201.
36. J. Issels, *More Cures for Cancer,* translation from German (Bad Homburg, Germany: Helfer Publishing E. Schwabe, 1980), 17.
37. P. Dosch, *Manual of Neural Therapy* (Heidelberg: Haug Publishers, 1984), 127.
38. O. Meyer, "The Eliminating Function of the Tonsils in Dental Infections," *Dental Digest,* December 1944, 557.
39. J. Issels, *More Cures for Cancer,* translation from German (Bad Homburg, Germany: Helfer Publishing Schwabe, 1980), 19.
40. O. Meyer, "The Eliminating Function of the Tonsils in Dental Infections," *Dental Digest,* December 1944, 557; J. Issels, *More Cures for Cancer,* translation from German (Bad Homburg, Germany: Helfer Publishing Schwabe, 1980), 16–17.
41. H. Cotton, *The Defective Delinquent and Insane* (New York: Arno Press, 1980 [orig. pub. 1921]), 46.
42. A. Crance, "A Review of Blood and Urine Examinations in 200 Cases of Chronic Focal Infection of Oral Origin," *Dental Digest* 27 (1922): 625–26.
43. M. Fischer, *Death and Dentistry* (Springfield, Ill.: Charles C. Thomas, 1940), 17.
44. A. Robinson et al., "Throat Swabs in Chronic Tonsillitis: A Time-Honoured Practice Best Forgotten," *British Journal of Clinical Practice* 51, no. 3 (April/May 1997): 138–39; M. Kurien et al., "Throat Swab in the Chronic Tonsillitis: How Reliable and Valid Is It?" *Singapore Medical Journal* 41, no. 7 (July 2000): 324–26.
45. R. Berkow et al., eds., *The Merck Manual,* 15th ed. (Rahway, N.J.: Merck Sharp and Dohme Research Laboratories, 1987), 2090.
46. F. Billings, *Focal Infection* (New York: D. Appleton and Company, 1916), 33–47; E. Rosenow, "Elective Localization of Streptococci," *Journal of the American Medical Association* 65 (1915): 1687–91.

47. K. Conroy et al., *Natural Approach to Opthalmology and Otolaryngology* (Seattle: Healing Mountain Publishing, 2004), 378.
48. L. Garrett, *The Coming Plague* (New York: Penguin Books, 1994), 416.
49. Ibid.
50. S. Shakman, *E. C. Rosenow and Associates: A Reference Manual* (Santa Monica, Calif.: Institute of Science, 1998), B2–7, 8.
51. M. Fischer, *Death and Dentistry* (Springfield, Ill.: Charles C. Thomas, 1940), 27; F. Billings, *Focal Infection* (New York: D. Appleton and Company, 1916), 17.
52. H. Cotton, *The Defective Delinquent and Insane* (New York: Arno Press, 1980 [orig. pub. 1921]), 71.
53. M. Fischer, *Death and Dentistry* (Springfield, Ill: Charles C. Thomas, 1940), 39; F. Billings, "Chronic Focal Infection as a Causative Factor in Chronic Arthritis," *Journal of the American Medical Association* 61 (September 13, 1913): 819–26; R. Cecil and D. Angevine, "Clinical and Experimental Observations of Focal Infection, with an Analysis of 200 Cases of Rheumatoid Arthritis," *Annals of Internal Medicine,* November 1938, 577–84; F. Billings, "Chronic Focal Infections and Their Etiologic Relations to Arthritis and Nephritis," *The Archives of Internal Medicine* 9 (January 30, 1912): 484–85.
54. S. Shakman, *E. C. Rosenow and Associates: A Reference Manual* (Santa Monica, Calif: Institute of Science, 1998), B2–9.
55. R. Berkow et al., eds., *The Merck Manual,* 15th ed. (Rahway, N.J.: Merck Sharp and Dohme Research Laboratories, 1987), 2090.
56. Ibid.; J. Abramson, *Overdosed America* (New York: HarperCollins Publishers Inc., 2004), 33, 35.
57. M. Fischer, *Death and Dentistry* (Springfield, Ill.: Charles C. Thomas, 1940), 16–17, 23–46.
58. S. Shakman, *E. C. Rosenow and Associates: A Reference Manual* (Santa Monica, Calif.: Institute of Science, 1998), B2–27; J. Harrison, *The Periodontal Solution: Healthy Gums Naturally* (Delray Beach, Fla.: Corinthian Health Press, 2001), 15.
59. S. Shakman, *E. C. Rosenow and Associates: A Reference Manual* (Santa Monica, Calif.: Institute of Science, 1998), B2–9.
60. R. Berkow et al., eds., *The Merck Manual,* 15th ed. (Rahway, N.J.: Merck Sharp and Dohme Research Laboratories, 1987), 2090–92.
61. F. Billings, *Focal Infection* (New York: D. Appleton and Company, 1916), 52–53.
62. R. Berkow et al., eds., *The Merck Manual,* 15th ed. (Rahway, N.J.: Merck Sharp and Dohme Research Laboratories, 1987), 524, 2091.
63. M. Fischer, *Death and Dentistry* (Springfield, Ill.: Charles C. Thomas, 1940), 24–27, 171–87; M. Ziff and S. Ziff, *The Missing Link* (Orlando: BioProbe, Inc., 1991), 77–113.
64. A. Skevas et al., "Cor Pulmonale due to Upper Airway Obstruction by Hypertrophied Tonsils and Adenoids," *Annals of Otology, Rhinology and Laryngology* 57, no. 9 (September 1978): 804–7; O. Brown, "Cor Pulmonale Secondary to Tonsillar and Adenoidal Hypertrophy: Management Considerations," *International Journal of Pediatric Otorhinolaryngology* 16 (July 1988): 131–39.
65. Medscape Medical News, "AHA Updates Recommendations for Antibiotic Prophylaxis for Dental Procedures," April 24, 2007, www.medscape.com/viewarticle/555596.
66. F. Billings, "Chronic Focal Infections and Their Etiologic Relations to Arthritis and Nephritis," *Archives of Internal Medicine,* April 12, 1912, 484–98; M. Fischer, *Death and Dentistry* (Springfield, Ill.: Charles C. Thomas, 1940), 30–32.
67. P. Gosch, *Vital Energy Medicine* (Provo, Utah: Chronicle Publishing Services, 2003), 76.
68. D. Connelly, *Traditional Acupuncture: The Law of the Five Elements* (Columbia, Md.: Traditional Acupuncture Institute, 1991), 79–80.
69. R. Berkow et al., eds., *The Merck Manual,* 15th ed. (Rahway, N.J.: Merck Sharp and Dohme Research Laboratories, 1987), 1589–90.
70. Ibid., 1590.
71. M. Fischer, *Death and Dentistry* (Springfield, Ill.: Charles C. Thomas, 1940), 31.
72. P. Gosch, *Vital Energy Medicine* (Provo, Utah: Chronicle Publishing Services, 2003), 76.
73. H. Cotton, *The Defective Delinquent and Insane* (New York: Arno Press, 1980 [orig. pub. 1921]), 64.
74. S. Shakman, *E. C. Rosenow and Associates: A Reference Manual* (Santa Monica, Calif.: Institute of Science, 1998), B2–20.
75. D. Klinghardt and L. Williams, "Biochemistry Seminar" (IAK GmbH-Forum International, Freiburg, Germany, April 1996).
76. M. Fischer, *Death and Dentistry* (Springfield, Ill.: Charles C. Thomas, 1940), 28; H. Cotton, *The Defective*

Delinquent and Insane (New York: Arno Press, 1980 [orig. pub. 1921]), 67.

77. Ibid., 66.
78. H. Cotton, *The Defective Delinquent and Insane* (New York: Arno Press, 1980 [1921 reprint]), 72.
79. S. Shakman, *E. C. Rosenow and Associates: A Reference Manual* (Santa Monica, Calif.: Institute of Science, 1998), B2–27; H. Cotton, *The Defective Delinquent and Insane* (New York: Arno Press, 1980 [orig. pub. 1921]).
80. P. Störtebecker, *Dental Caries as a Cause of Nervous Disorders: Epilepsy-Schizophrenia-Multiple Sclerosis* (Stockholm: Störtebecker Foundation for Research, 1982; Orlando: Bioprobe, Inc., 1986).
81. H. Cotton, *The Defective Delinquent and Insane* (New York: Arno Press, 1980 [orig. pub. 1921]), 73.
82. R. Berkow et al., eds., *The Merck Manual,* 15th ed. (Rahway, N.J.: Merck Sharp and Dohme Research Laboratories, 1987), 1419, 2109.
83. Ibid., 2108–9.
84. S. Swedo et al., "Pediatric Autoimmune Neuropsychiatric Disorders Associated with Streptococcal Infections: Clinical Description of the First 50 Cases," *American Journal of Psychiatry* 2, no. 155 (February 1998): 264.
85. S. Swedo and H. Leonard, *Is It "Just a Phase"?* (New York: Golden Books, 1998), 222, 249.
86. Ibid., 249.
87. Ibid.
88. R. Lahita, *Women and Autoimmune Disease* (New York: HarperCollins Publishers Inc., 2004), 90.
89. K. P. Bhatia and C. D. Marsden, "The Behavioural and Motor Consequences of Focal Lesions of the Basal Ganglia in Man," *Brain* 117, no. 4 (1993): 859–76.
90. S. Swedo and H. Leonard, *Is It "Just a Phase"?* (New York: Golden Books, 1998), 253, 254.
91. H. Cotton, *The Defective Delinquent and Insane* (New York: Arno Press, 1980 [orig. pub. 1921]), 12, 13, 16, 17, 18, 32.
92. Ibid., 19.
93. D. Klinghardt, "The Neural Therapy Advanced Course" (lecture, Albuquerque, N.Mex. May, 1993).
94. P. Williams, ed., *Gray's Anatomy,* 38th ed. (New York: Churchill Livingstone, 1995), 1300–1302.
95. D. Klinghardt and L. Williams, "Neural Kinesiology: American Academy of Head, Neck, and Facial Pain: Tenth International Symposium" (handout distributed at the symposium in Washington, D.C., July 29, 1994), 5.
96. J. Brody, *Jane Brody's Nutrition Book* (New York: Bantam, 1987), 256, 263.
97. D. Hamilton, *Homeopathic Care for Cats and Dogs* (Berkeley, Calif.: North Atlantic Books, 1999), 119–20.
98. J. Yasgur, *Homeopathic Dictionary* (El Paso, Tex.: Van Hoy Publishers, 2006), 125.
99. E. Rosenow, "Studies of Specific Prevention and Treatment of Diverse Diseases: Shown Due to Specific Types of Nonhemolytic Streptococci," in S. Shakman, *E. C. Rosenow and Associates: A Reference Manual* (Santa Monica, Calif.: Institute of Science, 1998), A5–D; B. Rappaport, "Further Observations on Acute Poliomyelitis Treated with Thermal Antibody," in S. Shakman, *E. C. Rosenow and Associates: A Reference Manual* (Santa Monica, Calif.: Institute of Science, 1998), A5–E.
100. D. Page, *Your Jaws, Your Life* (Baltimore: SmilePage Publishing, 2003), 84–85.
101. J. Garretson, *A System of Oral Surgery* (New York: J. B. Lippincott Co., 1898), 564.
102. J. Issels, *More Cures for Cancer,* translation from German (Bad Homburg, Germany: Helfer Publishing E. Schwabe, 1980), 18–19.
103. D. Klinghardt, American Academy of Biological Dentistry presentation notes, March 1999, from a translation of Josef Issels's book, *Mehr Heilungen von Krebs* (Bad Homburg, Germany: Helfer Verlag E. Schwabe, 1980).
104. M. Fischer, *Death and Dentistry* (Springfield, Ill.: Charles C. Thomas, 1940), 45.
105. P. Rhoads and G. Dick, "Efficacy of Tonsillectomy for the Removal of Focal Infection," *Journal of the American Medical Association* 91, no. 16 (October 20, 1928): 1153–54.

13

OTHER DOMINANT FOCI

Although the teeth and tonsils are by far the most common foci in the body, microbial infections that linger long after the acute stages and eventually coalesce into chronic foci can also occur elsewhere. The cavities in close proximity to the mouth—the sinuses and the ears—are the most susceptible. Additionally, there is a direct connection from the head to the pelvis, which readily allows the spread of bacteria to the urogenital organs, as well as the migration of microbes in the reverse direction, from the genitals to the head.

THE SINUSES

Any one of the three accessory or paranasal (next to the nose) sinuses can become a chronic focus—the maxillary, the frontal, or the ethmoid. These foci most often arise after one or more bouts of acute sinusitis usually secondary to upper respiratory infection. Sinus focal infections can be relatively silent or quite active, causing intermittent but chronic symptoms of pressure, pain, inflammation, and/or infections.

Sinuses Usually Secondary to a Maxillary Dental Focus

It should be noted that in many cases the sinuses are not the primary focus but the disturbed field of an upper dental focus (maxillary jawbone). As far back as 1891, Dr. W. D. Miller observed this relationship, writing in one research study that "in the vast majority of cases [maxillary sinus focus infections were] the result of the action of the mouth bacteria."[1] Later, in 1940, Dr. Martin Fischer also commented on the causal versus secondary nature of the sinuses in his book *Death and Dentistry:*

> Experience, too, is the basis for our belief that surgical attack upon the chronic infections of the accessory sinuses is not likely to prove curative of peripheral disease. Again, systemic infection from this source is not impossible; but we hold it improbable as indicated by the continuing lot of failures to recover after the most drastic types of accessory sinus manipulation. Our explanation is that the mucous membranes of the sinuses are flat and as such dispose with great difficulty to the development of nests chronically harboring low grade types of infectious organisms . . . Where signs and symptoms of peripheral disease have persisted after radical operation on the sinuses, we have seen relief only as the teeth were properly diagnosed, removed, and the infected state of the after-remaining bone of the jaws suitably cared for. In other words, the jaws were the first points for constitutional infection; but it was also from them that the sinuses were involved either by extension or otherwise.[2]

The spread of an infection from a dental focus into the sinuses is easily understood when we compare the bone structure between the upper (maxillary) and lower (mandibular) jaws. The maxillary bone is cancellous—that is, it consists of more porous bone, which allows toxins from the teeth to be readily absorbed into the sinuses. In contrast, the mandibular bone is made up of harder and denser osseous bone, which can absorb toxins more deeply, so that they are embedded into the bone. This characteristic is why the mandibular bone is one of the primary areas in the body that stores mercury residues long term (along with the lung, gut, kidneys, spine, and liver).[3]

Because of the porosity of the maxillary jawbone, the diagnosis of a primary sinus focus should be considered suspect until all the upper teeth have been examined and ruled out as the causative focus. If the patient suffers sinus symptoms primarily on only one side, then the ipsilateral rule should be kept in mind. For example, if the right maxillary sinus is a suspected focus, then all the upper maxillary teeth on the right side should be thoroughly evaluated.

Food Allergies a Major Cause

Suspected sinus foci often clear up considerably when individuals avoid their major food allergen. As with the tonsils, chronic irritation and infection in the upper respiratory system can be greatly mitigated by a change of diet. Thus, low-grade tonsil and sinus focal infections can often be completely resolved by simply removing all dairy and sugar products.

Other Holistic Treatments

Auriculotherapy to the sinus points, the correct constitutional homeopathic remedy, and drainage are essential to the successful resolution of a chronic sinus focus. Saline sinus washes (neti pots) and isopathic drops (Notatum 4X) can also be helpful in reducing bacterial infestations and their toxic excretions in these warm, wet, and microbial-hospitable cavities. Additionally, snorting a drop or two of Quinton marine plasma up each nostril daily (and drinking the rest of the vial) is especially healing to the nasal and sinus mucosae. Holistic measures can greatly reduce the amount of antibiotic drugs prescribed, or completely eliminate the need for them altogether, allowing for a quicker restoration of a normal sinus and gut terrain.

THE EARS

Childhood ear infections (acute, chronic or serous otitis media, and external otitis) have become so common that they are considered to be a normal rite of passage. Numerous infections are never normal, however, and several bouts per year are one of the cardinal signs of an inherited tuberculinic miasmic tendency. And when the true cause of the infection is unknown and symptoms are simply suppressed with course after course of antibiotics, the foundation for a future focus is firmly implanted in the body.

Symptomatic or Quiet

Like other insidious foci, an ear focal infection can be relatively quiet and not cause any obvious symptoms locally, or it can indicate its presence by recurrent itching, pressure, pain, vertigo, tinnitus (buzzing, ringing, roaring, whistling, or hissing sounds), hearing loss, or Ménière's disease (vertigo, hearing loss, and tinnitus combined).

Often Secondary to a Chronic Tonsil Focus

As with the sinuses, it's important to diagnose whether the ear(s) is a primary focus or simply secondary to a tooth or tonsil focus. And since the bilateral tubal tonsils (located just behind the Eustachian tube opening in the nasopharynx) make up part of Waldeyer's ring along with the palatine, pharyngeal (adenoids), lingual, and laryngeal tonsils, all of these lymphatic aggregations can easily become infected together and over time coalesce into a chronic focal infection lymphatic ring in the throat with a direct channel into the ear.

Often Secondary to a Dental Focus

If only one ear is problematic, this is often indicative of a dental (or a tonsil focus) located on that same side.* According to British neurologist Sir Henry Head, the lower second bicuspid and the first, second, and third (wisdom teeth) molars are the most culpable teeth to cause reflexive disturbance into the ear and auditory canal.[4] This relationship has been confirmed clinically by the numerous unfortunate individuals who have experienced sharp ear pain referred from a toothache (e.g., teething) or from "dry socket" after an extraction.†

*Although often both sides of the tonsils are infected in the case of a chronic focus, one side is usually more pathogenic than the other. For example, the left tonsil may be hypertrophied, but the atrophied right one is actually more degenerative and through its influence on the neighboring tubal tonsil it is fueling a chronic right ear focus.

†Dry socket, or "septic socket," happens when bacteria invade the area between the blood clot and the bone, and the blood clot is lost, which leaves the socket empty or "dry." When this occurs, the exposed bone cannot heal because it can't form a new clot. Dry socket is usually signaled through pain, often severe—either in the extraction site or in the ipsilateral (same side) ear.

Avoiding Food Allergies and Other Holistic Treatments

As with sinus infections, the formation of both tonsil and ear foci are best prevented through the diagnosis and avoidance of a child's primary food allergen. Furthermore, the use of alternative medicines—constitutional homeopathy, herbs, drainage, isopathic remedies, and nutrition, as well as cranial and spinal manipulation and auriculotherapy—can greatly reduce inflammation and infection as well as help prevent future infections. These natural remedies and treatments given in a timely manner can significantly decrease or even completely eliminate the need for antibiotics and other allopathic medications. Adults can also greatly benefit from natural medicine, although the treatment will take quite a bit longer to clear a decades-old ear (or sinus, tonsil, or dental) focal infection.

Scars from Surgery or Infection Can Act as Chronic Interference Fields

Ears can also be major scar interference fields with or without significant infection. These scars can occur naturally from a healed burst eardrum (perforated tympanic membrane) or from *myringotomies*—surgical excision of the tympanic membrane and the placement of tubes in the ears. Often these tubes fall out or are later removed, but if full healing of the tympanic membrane doesn't occur, the surgical scars can remain as a chronic irritant. Auriculotherapy is often effective to treat these internal scar interference fields. Fortunately, myringotomies are gradually falling out of favor, as new studies have shown that while they reduce inflammation in the short term they do not appear to improve children's speech and learning development, as compared to control groups who did not receive this surgical procedure.[5]

If a patient has had a mastoidectomy (surgical excision of the bone just behind the ear) due to past mastoiditis (an ear infection extending into the mastoid bone), then auriculotherapy is essential, along with constitutional homeopathy and other therapies, for this probable combination scar interference field and chronic focal infection.

THE UROGENITAL ORGANS

The Transport of Toxins Between the Head and the Pelvis

Among the many accomplishments made by physician and scientist Patrick Störtebecker of Sweden was his research and writing on the specific physiological mechanisms whereby focal infections as well as amalgam fillings cause widespread harm in the body. In his book *Neurology for Barefoot Doctors in All Countries,* he explains how certain veins in the head (cranial) and along the spine (vertebral) allow the two-way transit of toxins, primarily heavy metals and microbes, between the head and the pelvic regions. Citing the 1940 studies by the American researcher Oscar Batson, Störtebecker related that when Batson injected contrast medium into the dorsal vein of the penis, he was able to trace its direct pathway throughout the entire vertebral (spinal) venous (vein) system and then into the skull and face. Störtebecker observed through his own research that not only did microbes migrate from the pelvis to the head but that they also traveled in a *retrograde* (against the normal blood flow in the veins) manner, in the opposite direction—from the head to the pelvis (see figure 13.1).* Dr. Störtebecker explained that this retrograde transport is greatly augmented by the fact that craniovertebral (head-spine) veins have "few if any valves" to prevent the backflow of blood:[6]

> This cranio-vertebral venous system possesses a very peculiar characteristic: The flow in the system is unimpeded, as there are no valves directing the circulation!
>
> This fact implies that a transport of blood, including all its constituents, even various toxins, can freely take place in every direction.[7]

*Blood is returned to the heart by the veins. This flow is normally one-way, from the body and the head into larger veins that empty into the right atrium of the heart. This deoxygenated dark red blood then leaves through the right ventricle and goes to the lungs, where it loses its carbon dioxide and takes on oxygen again. Then this bright red oxygenated blood returns to the left atrium of the heart and reenters the systemic circulation through the left ventricle. This one-way flow of venous blood is aided by valves, the velocity of the blood flow, skeletal muscle contractions, and breathing.

Although this valveless state safeguards life in certain instances—for example, the final sprint by a long-distance runner doesn't cause a stroke and sneezes can't "blow your head off"—it also allows toxins to easily flow from the head down to the pelvis. Toxic metals and microbes from the teeth and tonsils can easily migrate "south" to the urogenital organs (uterus, bladder, prostate, etc.) in the pelvic region through this retrograde venous transport, as well as "north" from the urogenital organs to the head. Additionally, this two-way cranio-vertebral venous system has been implicated in the metastasis of cancer. Again, Dr. Störtebecker expounds on this subject:

> Studies by Robert Anderson in Chicago (1951) gave further confirmation of possible routes for spread of METASTASES via the valve-less vertebral venous system.
>
> He observed the close relationship of this venous system with veins of other structures, such as the prostate, kidneys, adrenals, lungs, breast, and thyroid.[8]

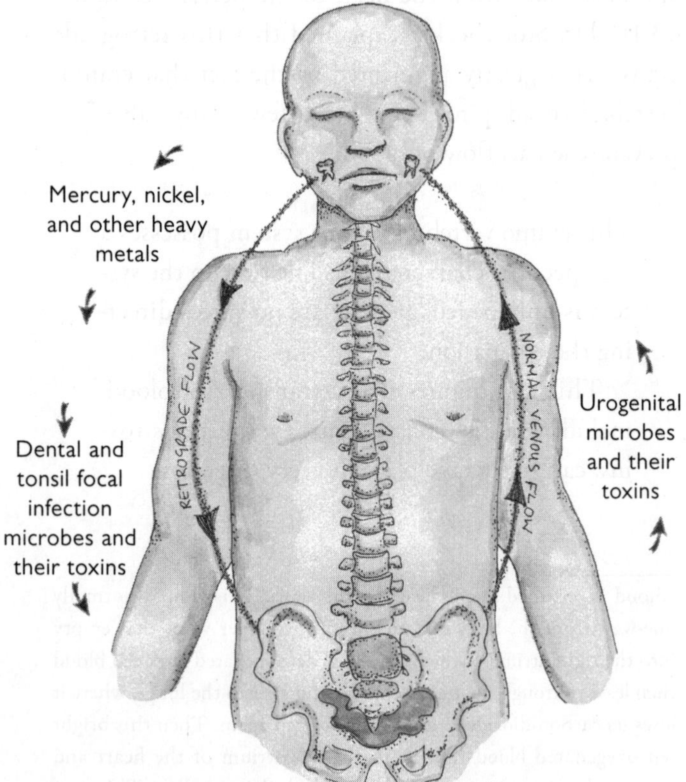

Figure 13.1. The two-way valveless communication of the cranio-vertebral (head-spine) venous blood flow

Toxins Transported through Nerve Pathways and Direct Sexual Contact

Störtebecker also researched another route for the migration of toxins in the body, called *axonal transport*—that is, the movement along nerve pathways. He cited studies wherein viruses, lead, and other toxins injected into the extremities (arms and legs) could be traced as they traveled up to the spinal cord and the brain along nerve axons in research animals, as well as in the opposite direction—from the head to the pelvis and legs.[9]*

Toxins can also be rapidly disseminated throughout the body by way of the blood and lymph channels. And microbes such as the *Neisseria gonorrhoeae* bacterium and the herpes simplex virus (HSV-2) can become implanted in the urogenital organs and associated ganglia through direct sexual contact with infected partners.

As with all focal infections, urogenital focal infections are initiated in three primary ways: (1) through blood (arterial) and lymphatic pathways, (2) via specific venous pathways through the cranio-vertebral valveless system, and (3) through axonal transport along nerve and spinal cord pathways. However, urogenital focal infections also commonly occur through direct transmission by sexual contact.

The Most Common Sites of the Urogenital Focus

Although any of the urogenital organs can become a chronic focus, the uterus and prostate are the most commonly involved areas. In women, the cervix (neck of the uterus) is the most typical site. According to Dr. Cotton, the ovaries and fallopian tubes are less common, and usually secondary to a primary uterine focal infection.[10] In men, the seminal vesicles and the prostate are most often involved. The bladder and the urethra can also be a focus in both sexes.

Symptoms Apparent or Silent

Like other foci, urogenital focal infections can be insidiously silent or cause intermittent symptoms. For women, these symptoms can be any number of menstrual difficulties—menorrhagia (excessive bleeding),

*These venous and nerve metastatic pathways are probably responsible for the common finding among holistic practitioners of mercury toxicity testing positive energetically in the urogenital organs.

dysmenorrhea (pain and cramping), or PMS (premenstrual irritability, anxiety, depression, breast cysts, etc.); intermittent genital pain or discharge; abnormal urinary symptoms (urgency, incontinence, frequent or painful urination); sexual dysfunction (frigidity or impotency); menopausal symptoms (insomnia, hot flashes, mood changes, etc.); gut dysfunction (constipation, diarrhea, irritable bowel, etc.); or low back or hip joint pain. For men, symptoms can include sexual dysfunction (premature ejaculation, impotency, etc.), urinary problems (dribbling, incontinence, retention, etc.), gut dysfunction (constipation, diarrhea, irritable bowel, etc.), and low back or hip joint pain.

However, as with many foci, symptoms are not always local; urogenital foci can trigger more remote disturbed fields such as distal joint pain (e.g., shoulder or neck pain), cardiovascular stress, or hormonal dysfunction in other endocrine organs (the adrenals, thyroid, pituitary, etc.). Furthermore, due to the aforementioned cranio-vertebral venous communication, disturbed fields in the head area are common, with resulting symptoms of insomnia, tension and migraine headaches, depression, anxiety, memory loss, and fatigue.

Treatment of the Urogenital Focus

Treatment of the urogenital focal infection can include all of the previously discussed methods (e.g., constitutional homeopathy, auriculotherapy), as well as a change of diet to reduce gut dysbiosis so that the migration of intestinal pathogenic microbes (bacteria, candida fungi, etc.) into the urogenital region is reduced. Additionally, when toxic metals test positive in these urogenital organs, herbal gemmotherapy remedies such as Black Poplar and Mountain Pine are an important component of the needed drainage protocol in the area. General drainage for the liver with Juniper (*Juniperus communis*) or Rosemary (*Rosmarinus officinalis*), the kidneys with Juniper or White Birch (*Betula pubescens*), and the gut with European Alder (*Alnus glutinosa*) or Fig (*Ficus carica*) may be indicated. Specific drainage alone, or in conjunction with general drainage, is also often needed. This can include drainage for the ureters, bladder, and urethra using Cowberry (*Vaccinium vitis-idaea*), Juniper, or White Birch, as well as drainage of the genital organs (e.g., Oak [*Quercus pedonculata*] for the prostate and Raspberry [*Rubus idaeus*] for the uterus).

Isopathic suppositories such as Notatum 3X and Aspergillus 3X are particularly powerful remedies for clearing toxins in the entire pelvic cavity. Dosage for these potent suppositories should be individualized, however, and varies considerably according to the patient's constitution. For example, a suppository inserted rectally before bed may be indicated on a once-a-week schedule or less for weaker patients who are functioning more in the tuberculinic or luetic miasmic levels. These suppositories have a much stronger antimicrobial action than a moving influence and therefore often congest the surrounding tissues and organs. Thus, it is essential that the patient is also on his or her constitutional remedy and/or a drainage remedy protocol to fully facilitate the clearance of microbes and other toxins in the region.

Since toxins are readily transported from the urogenital organs to the intestines, colonics or home enemas may also be indicated as part of the cleansing protocol.

Psychospiritual Work

Because the urogenital organs affect first-chakra issues of grounding, confidence, power, and potency (personal, social, financial, etc.), as well as second-chakra issues relating to emotional-sexual functioning, counseling and other forms of therapy are often needed in conjunction with holistic care. I have found that breathwork ("rebirthing") is particularly effective in clearing the unconscious painful memories associated with this sensitive area. Fear, sorrow, anger, or guilt engrams (stored memories) from past surgeries, abortions, miscarriages, rape, abuse, infections, divorce, or painful breakups between intimates readily arise as the breath is circulated throughout the whole body in the supportive environment provided by an experienced rebirther. In fact, these emotions are often evoked during treatment of the urogenital focal infection. It is important to remember that the release of these pent-up emotions after a perfectly placed auriculotherapy needle or a neural therapy treatment signals *progression* toward the freedom that real healing brings—and not *regression.* Often patients need to be reminded of this fact and encouraged to explore the fertile emotional ground of what Hameed Ali refers to as "the genital hole." Ali's psychospiritual school, named Ridhwan, or Diamond Heart, utilizes numerous approaches including breathwork and inquiry to further the release of an individual's egoic contraction pattern, often most strongly and unconsciously held in this genital area.

► For more information on rebirthing, go to the www.RebirthingBreathwork.com website. To locate a practitioner of holotropic breathwork (Dr. Stanislav Grof's form of breathwork), call (415) 383-8779, or go to www.holotropic.com. To contact the Ridhwan or Diamond Heart school, go to www.ridhwan.org.

Urogenital Scar Interference Fields

Pelvic-area scars from urogenital as well as from other surgeries are common interference fields. In fact, the numerous untreated abdominal and pelvic scars patients often present with dramatically illustrate the dearth of knowledge about foci among allopathic physicians. Whether it's an episiotomy scar that a midwife might have been able to circumvent or a large abdominal scar from a hysterectomy that might have been avoided with the use of natural medicine, these and other surgical scars graphically signal the need for more holistic instruction in our medical schools about the prevention of surgery and resulting interference fields through natural medicine, as well as the treatment of scars postsurgically and after a trauma.

SCAR INTERFERENCE FIELDS

Scars Can Be Symptomatic or Silent

As discussed previously, although the term *interference field* has been used to describe both external and internal scars, it is most often used to describe scars on the skin. Like deeper focal infections, scars are often silent, triggering symptoms in distal areas that have been referred to throughout this chapter as *disturbed fields*. However, there are certain clues that can indicate whether a scar is an active interference field or dormant (completely neutral and nondisturbing). If a scar has an abnormal coloration—that is, it is mildly pink, indicating chronic inflammation or whitish in areas, indicating ischemia (lack of blood flow)—or if it is lumpy in places, these signs can all indicate a probable scar interference field. A nondisturbing scar should be insensitive. When scars are continuously—or even just occasionally—painful, itchy, tender, numb, inflamed, or sensitive to weather changes, this is pathognomonic (extremely characteristic) of an active interference field. Furthermore, if you knead or roll a scar between your thumb and forefinger and it feels tender, painful, tingly, or numb—even in only one part—it is likely that this scar is a (mild to major) chronic interference field. Finally, it is important to remember that some asymptomatic scars are chronic interference fields, silently and insidiously causing disturbance in a distal site.[11]

Treatment through Auriculotherapy, Laser Photophoresis, or Massage

Treatment of skin scars was previously described in chapter 10; however, to reiterate briefly, auriculotherapy as well as neural therapy photophoresis—that is, when isopathic remedies are "driven in" by an infrared laser—are both very effective. However, for many other scars, patients can use "neural therapy without needles" methods at home by massaging the scar with isopathic remedies and/or shea butter or essential oils. This protocol is often prescribed daily from a two-week to one-month period. A further benefit to home massage is that adhesions—that is, the abnormal joining of connective tissue from a scar that has healed imperfectly—can be significantly reduced through thirty treatments of manual manipulation of this scar during a one-month period.

This massage protocol performed at home is particularly ideal for scars in the urogenital area. For example, a woman may need to treat her hysterectomy, episiotomy, or laparotomy scar, and a man may need to treat his hernia or circumcision scar. There is a positive side effect for individuals who treat these scars themselves. Often the shame, fear, anger, or sorrow that has subconsciously surrounded these chronic interference fields for years is released through patients "owning" this area once again, through literally taking it in their own hands and massaging it back "into the fold" of other healthy skin in the body.

Emotionally disturbing scars are not simply confined to the urogenital area. Gallbladder (cholecystectomy), appendix, triple bypass, thyroid, and many other types of surgical as well as traumatic scars from injuries can be highly charged. For example, I had one patient who didn't even want to touch her knee surgery scar, much less for a doctor to treat it. However, after being persuaded to massage Aspergillus 4X drops into the scar for a month, this patient's leg pain as well as her emotions about the scar were significantly reduced. Afterward, through a couple of auriculotherapy treatments and several sessions of rebirthing, the remaining symptoms associated with this emotionally charged scar interference field were fully cleared.

It's important to not forget the one scar we all share—the umbilicus scar from birth. This first scar interference field, along with food allergies, is one of the most common problems found in a holistic pediatric practice. However, adults can also benefit by treating the umbilical scar, especially if they had a difficult birth.

A NOTE ON BODY PIERCINGS

In my clinical research, scars that cross the central meridian, running from the perineum (between the genital organs and the anus) to the inner lower lip, are the most disturbing. Blocking the flow of chi energy along this *conception vessel* by scars—or piercings—seems to cause more stress in the body than when the flow from other noncentral acupuncture meridians is disrupted (although these other areas can also be significantly disturbed). When a ring in the umbilicus is removed, the treatment of the resulting piercing-hole scar is necessary in most cases, because the remaining disturbance from this interference field often lingers. Therefore, when teenage patients want to get body piercings, try to at least discourage umbilical and central lower-lip rings that disrupt the energy along this important central meridian.

Finally, it is important to remember that since ancient times, Chinese medical doctors have been aware of the energetic disturbance caused by scars crossing, and therefore blocking the flow of, acupuncture meridians. Another treatment option for this type of scar is to have a skilled acupuncturist "surround the dragon" by placing acupuncture needles in strategic points around the scar. In fact, home massage combined with acupuncture can be exceptionally effective in clearing the chronically disturbing effects of scar interference fields.

Preventing Scar Interference Fields

One caveat should be made regarding brand-new scars. Although the treatment of new scars is the best preventive medicine for obviating the future formation of an interference field, individuals should *never interrupt* the healing of a new scar because the closure of a wound by scar formation is a normal and necessary bodily function. Therefore, directly after surgery or a traumatic injury, nothing should be *rubbed* into a scar. However, isopathic drops such as Mucor 4X (helps restore normal blood circulation), Aspergillus 4X (aids soft tissue healing), Kombination 4X (a combination of Mucor and Aspergillus), or Notatum 4X (reduces inflammation and helps prevent infection) can be dropped directly on the scar to facilitate healing. Gentle application of aloe vera juice (gel or liquid) is also appropriate for a few days after surgery to take advantage of its anti-inflammatory constituents (primarily glycoproteins that break down bradykinin—a major mediator of pain and inflammation), as well as the wound-healing compounds of vitamin C, vitamin E, and zinc that are contained in this tropical plant.[12] Additionally, as after cavitation surgery, a 100-milliwatt, 830-nanometer laser beam applied just over (but not touching) the scar, approximately three times a day for two to three days, can be exceptionally healing in reducing keloid and interference field formation postsurgically.

- Isopathic drops are available from BioResource at (800) 203-3775.
- Aloe vera juice in liquid or gel form is available in most health food stores. Furthermore, you can simply break open a leaf from the plant and apply the fresh juice to the wound.
- The "Canadian laser" is available from Rick McKay at (250) 474-3514 or jarek.mfg@shaw.ca.

The use of Arnica montana 30C (heals inflammation and bruising), or simply re-dosing the correct constitutional homeopathic remedy, is also essential in the repair of tissue and should be done immediately after surgery or trauma at an accelerated dosage (e.g., three times a day for at least two to three days). The oral administration of vitamins such as vitamin A (essential in the replacement of epithelial tissue) and vitamin C (required for the manufacture of connective tissue and the formation of new blood vessels) is also an important adjunct to this scar treatment protocol. Finally, the herb gotu kola (*Centella asiatica*) has proven exceptionally efficacious in wound healing, and even in the reduction of keloids (hypertrophic large scars), when it is taken orally as a standardized extract (60–120 mg/day) or in tincture (alcohol solution) form (10–20 ml/day).[13]*

- Arnica is available from health food stores or can be ordered from Seroyal at (800) 263-5861.
- Although the Thorne product Venocap is designed to reduce varicose veins and hemorrhoids, it is also a helpful botanical support for wound healing. This gotu kola extract formula contains the flavonoid diosmin and the herbals witch hazel, horse chestnut, and butcher's broom, which all enhance the integrity and overall functioning of the surrounding blood vessels in the wound area. Order Venocap from Thorne at (800) 228-1966, or go to www.thorne.com.

Depending on the severity and size of the scar, after a few days or a few weeks, when the inflammation has been sizably reduced and the edges of the scar are closed together, you can begin gently rubbing shea butter and/or the oil from vitamin E capsules (opened with a sterilized needle) into the scar area to further assist healing and reduce the formation of adhesions (also called second-intention scar formation). Some people consider vitamin E to be too efficacious at wound healing and caution not to use it too soon after surgery, when the wound still needs "to breathe" and receive oxygen. Therefore, it is to be included later in the protocol, after the scar has healed sufficiently for a few days or weeks.

- Vitamin E (E-500) capsules are available from Thorne at (800) 228-1966, or go to www.thorne.com.
- Organic shea butter is available from www.orgess.com. It is also available at many health food stores, but not always in the organic form.

As with all foci, the knowledgeable holistic practitioner who uses energetic testing is the most valuable resource to determine which scars are major and active interference fields, in what order they should be treated, and how best to treat them.

*While the active ingredient in gotu kola, asiaticoside, has not proved toxic at high dosages when taken orally, the topical application has been reported to cause contact dermatitis, although infrequently. Therefore, gotu kola is only prescribed orally, not topically. (J. Pizzorno and M. Murray, *Textbook of Natural Medicine,* 2nd ed. [New York: Churchill Livingstone, 2000], 655.)

CONCLUSION

It is currently an appropriate time for the propagation of knowledge about some of the more esoteric aspects of holistic medicine, as more and more individuals are realizing the benefits of natural medicine. And dominant foci and their disturbed fields are still considered esoteric, even in holistic medical circles. In fact, few individuals or even doctors (allopathic or holistic) are aware of the existence of focal infections and scar interference fields. The dearth of knowledge in this crucial field of study is particularly difficult to reconcile when the successful cure of a multitude of illnesses through the treatment of these chronic "irritating thorns" was documented over a century ago in peer-reviewed scientific journals.

One of the generally accepted tenets underlying the scientific method is to always first review the literature before embarking on new research. Unfortunately, the allopathic medical community has completely ignored this tenet in regard to focal infection research in its drive toward funding more studies to discover a "cure" (read: another medication) for various syndromes and diseases. Particularly maddening is that many of these numerous diseases that allopaths are still battling derive from foci—such as breast cancer secondary to a dental focus or heart disease secondary to a chronic tonsil focal infection. This disregard of valuable scientific information is not only sloppy research methodology but borders on malpractice. As the British physician Sir William Osler (1849–1919) once stated:

> It can be said, regarding Medicine, that one who knows only current information about Medicine does not even know that.[14]

A vast number of common symptoms—joint pain, headaches, memory loss, fatigue, depression, insomnia, and so forth—are simply symptoms of the disturbed fields created by a chronic focus. Therefore, the recognition of dominant foci can save an individual significant time and money spent on both allopathic as well as many holistic forms of treatment. For example, for a woman suffering from postpartum depression, treatment of her episiotomy scar should be considered first before further burdening her liver with allopathic antidepressant medications. Or instead of investing hundreds of dollars as well as hours of time receiving joint manipulation from a (nonholistic) chiropractor or osteopath for chronic right hip pain, an individual should consider having her right-sided gold-crowned teeth evaluated by a holistic dentist. Or instead of seeing an acupuncturist once a week for years for chronic fatigue, an individual should be assessed for a possible tonsil focal infection, which is often the root cause of lifelong deficient kidney chi. Finally, instead of submitting to TURP (prostate) surgery,* a patient should be informed of the possibility of cavitation surgery for his upper incisor (front tooth) root-canalled tooth, which can affect the urogenital kidney meridian and its related organs (e.g., the prostate). These examples are just a few of the many possible benefits from accurately diagnosing and appropriately treating chronic dominant foci.

It is further hoped that the paradigm shift of viewing chronic enervating symptoms from a new perspective—that is, as simply arising from secondary disturbed fields—can convey a sense of relief and personal empowerment to many patients. In the case of individuals suffering from severe disease or faced with a serious diagnosis, the knowledge of a possible underlying causative focus is even more imperative. The diagnosis and treatment of chronic foci can often obviate the long-term use of prescription drugs, needless surgeries, and other debilitating allopathic procedures. In fact, an evaluation of the presence of dental, tonsil, and other foci should become the standard of care in all holistic clinics, especially for those who are scheduled for major surgery (heart, gallbladder, uterus, prostate, etc.), as well as those slated for chemotherapy or radiation treatments.

Finally, it is my expectation that while reading this part of the book many doctors, dentists, and practitioners have realized that the lack of awareness of the presence of dominant foci is a *big hole* in their diagnostic and treatment armamentarium. Especially in the case of those health practitioners who have become burned out and discouraged over the years, it is hoped that one or more of their former therapy-resistant patients have come to mind, and they are now anxious and excited to call them back into their office for a reevaluation of potential foci.

*TURP stands for "transurethral resection of the prostate," which is performed when there is bladder obstruction and the inability to urinate from benign prostate hypertrophy (BPH).

In conclusion, the turn of the twenty-first century is an opportune time to learn what Miller, Rosenow, Billings, Price, and other holistic pioneers tried so earnestly to teach us over a century ago. We now have the great opportunity to pick up the gauntlet and carry on where these courageous researchers left off in the scientific and clinical study of focal infections and scar interference fields. It is appropriate, therefore, to end this part with a quotation by one of these early holistic medical giants, Dr. Martin Fischer, from his book *Death and Dentistry:*

> If there is reason in nature for the need to every man of a life-long physician, it is written in these facts. All men sooner or later succumb to chronic focal infection; and most commonly, to one streptococcal in type. It is the principal cause of civilized man's break-up . . . The concept of the focal infection . . . marks the greatest advance and the greatest good that has come to a suffering world in this century.[15]

NOTES

1. W. Miller, "The Human Mouth as a Focus of Infection," *The Dental Cosmos* 33, no. 9 (September 1891): 699.
2. M. Fischer, *Death and Dentistry* (Springfield, Ill.: Charles C. Thomas, 1940), 49.
3. L. Hahn et al., "Dental 'Silver' Tooth Fillings: A Source of Mercury Exposure Revealed by Whole-Body Image Scan and Tissue Analysis," *The FASEB Journal* 3 (December 1989): 2641–46.
4. P. Dosch, *Manual of Neural Therapy* (Heidelberg: Haug Publishers, 1984), 108.
5. Associated Press, "Ear Tubes Do Not Improve Development, Study Says," *Marin Independent Journal,* April 19, 2001, A4.
6. P. Störtebecker, *Neurology for Barefoot Doctors in All Countries* (Stockholm: Störtebecker Foundation for Research, 1988), 271–86.
7. Ibid., 271.
8. Ibid., 275.
9. Ibid., 287–88.
10. H. Cotton, *The Defective Delinquent and Insane* (New York: Arno Press, 1980 [orig. pub. 1921]), 67–70.

11. P. Dosch, *Manual of Neural Therapy* (Heidelberg: Haug Publishers, 1984), 143.
12. J. Pizzorno and M. Murray, *Textbook of Natural Medicine* (New York: Churchill Livingstone, 1999), 582–83.
13. Ibid., 653–54.
14. J. McManus, *The Fundamental Ideas of Medicine* (Springfield, Ill.: Charles C. Thomas, 1963), 6.
15. M. Fischer, *Death and Dentistry* (Springfield, Ill.: Charles C. Thomas, 1940), preface, 45.

PART FIVE

THE MOST PROFOUND HOLISTIC TREATMENT AND ITS UGLY ALLOPATHIC TWIN

ꕤ

There have been two great revelations in my life.
The first was bebop, the second was homeopathy.

John Birks "Dizzy" Gillespie (1917–1993),
jazz trumpeter, bandleader,
singer, and composer

Constitutional homeopathy, which heals at all levels—physically, emotionally, mentally, and spiritually—is the single most powerful therapeutic modality in a holistic practice. In a perfect world—sans amalgam fillings, refined and devitalized foods, damaging vaccinations, and synthetic prescription drugs—homeopathy would be all we ever needed. Unfortunately, in our modern-day toxic environment, this is far from the case—hence the need for the other seventeen chapters in *Radical Medicine.*

Vaccinations, which can do irreparable harm physically, emotionally, mentally, and spiritually, are one of the most injurious practices utilized in allopathic medicine today. However, because vaccines originated soon after homeopathy and on the surface have some similarities to homeopathic remedies, they are included in this part.

Chapter 14 is devoted to the subject of constitutional homeopathy and chapter 15 to its ugly allopathic twin, vaccinations. Chapter 15 addresses the use of vaccines, describing their history and ingredients and offering natural alternatives and treatments, as well as resources to learn more about this controversial subject.

14

CONSTITUTIONAL HOMEOPATHY

Plus ça change, plus c'est la même chose.
"The more things change, the more they stay the same."

Samuel Hahnemann, the founder of homeopathy, recognized the damaging effects of toxic medications and foods over two hundred years ago. He particularly castigated his allopathic colleagues for using treatments that were in many cases more harmful to the patient than the original illness. Sadly, the practices criticized by this physician who lived in the eighteenth and nineteenth centuries are astoundingly similar to our current allopathic practices in the twenty-first century, in which adverse reactions to prescription drugs (ADRs) have been estimated to be between the fourth and sixth leading cause of death.[1]

allopathic: As described in previous chapters, the word *allopathic* literally means "other than, or against, disease." Hahnemann originated the term *allopathy* to describe the medicine practiced by the orthodox medical doctors of his time, in contrast to his own system of *homeopathy*. Allopathic physicians treat disease by using medicines antagonistic and suppressive to the disease symptoms, for example, through the use of *anti*histamines, *anti*biotics, or *anti*-inflammatories or through the removal (-ectomy) of diseased tissues through surgeries such as append*ectomies*, hyster*ectomies* and tonsill*ectomies*. In Hahnemann's day, opium, calomel, and bloodletting were three of the most common allopathic forms of medicine.

Hahnemann greatly cautioned his patients and holistic colleagues about calomel (a powder containing mercury), silver nitrate, opium, "bloodletting in torrents," leeches, and other common treatments used by medical practitioners in the late eighteenth and early nineteenth centuries.[2] In fact, he found that the chronic diseases "artificially induced" by these medical practices could so greatly weaken an individual's constitution that even the most perfectly chosen homeopathic remedy may "fail to cure."[3] In his book *Organon of the Medical Art,* which has stood the test of time for more than 200 years as the "homeopathic bible," Hahnemann wrote about the "diseases engendered by medical malpractice":

> Of all the chronic diseases, these botchings of the human condition brought forth by the allopathic calamitous art (at its worst in recent times) are the saddest and the most incurable. I regret to say that when they have been driven to some height, it seems to be impossible to invent or devise any curative means for them.[4]

Although Hahnemann's *Organon* has served as the foundation of homeopathic practice and principles since its publication in 1810, he could not have known that the above parenthetical phrase—"at its worst in recent times"—would be the one statement in his prophetic book that no longer holds true. That is, the present epidemic use of synthetic prescription drugs, excessive surgeries, heavy metals (amalgam fillings, nickel crowns, barium enemas, etc.), and toxic chemicals (anesthetics, chemotherapy, isopropyl alcohol, etc.) in modern allopathic medicine and dentistry has far eclipsed the intermittent use of caustic ointments, bloodletting, leeches, and other practices typical in the eighteenth and nineteenth centuries. In fact, bloodletting in moderation and the use of leeches can be valuable therapies and have come back into vogue, especially in European clinics and hospitals.

BLOODLETTING AND LEECHES

Both bloodletting and the use of leeches have merit and are still being used today. Bloodletting in *reasonable* amounts helps thin the blood and promotes detoxification, and it is used in both Europe and the United States for the treatment of hepatitis and hemochromatosis (excessive iron accumulation).[5] Leeches, another form of bloodletting, are prized for the heparin in their saliva that prevents blood from clotting. In the 1800s, leeches were a common treatment for "cerebral congestion," and when applied to a patient's temples they could relieve seizures. Leeches are presently used on puncture wounds to help dilate the blood vessels, allowing the wound to bleed for hours, which naturally disinfects the site and anesthetizes the area to decrease pain. Leeches are also used in modern plastic surgery, in reconstructive surgery (skin grafts), and on the inflamed nerve endings of amputated limbs. Recently, a French pharmaceutical firm received FDA approval to market leeches.[6]

Furthermore, in Hahnemann's day, because the "country people and the urban poor" were not privy to allopathic treatments, most still died of "natural diseases." In contrast, it is now rare to hear of anyone—rich or poor—dying peacefully in his sleep. And unfortunately, prescription drug use has become so prevalent that it is highly unusual for anyone over sixty-five not to be on at least one prescription drug. In fact, *polypharmacy*—that is, administering several drugs together—is currently the norm.

Through his recognition of the dangerous effects of allopathic medicine, as well as toxic foods and environments, Dr. Hahnemann coined the now famous phrase "obstacles to cure" or "obstacles to recovery."[7] In 1796, Hahnemann published an article on three different approaches to the treatment of disease in which he considered the removal of these obstacles a branch of healing in its own right, as well as the "most sublime."[8] The first approach was to remove the cause, that is, the obstacles to healing (e.g., replacing petroleum-laden cosmetics or removing amalgam fillings); the second was allopathy, or to suppress or palliate the symptoms (e.g., the use of medications such as antihistamines or steroids); and the third was homeopathy. Hahnemann utilized the first and third approaches to healing, and he denounced the second approach of using suppressive allopathic practices. Furthermore, at a time when advice on living a healthy lifestyle was relatively rare, this progressive physician advised his chronically ill patients to not only refrain from using toxic drugs and caustic ointments, but also to avoid excessive sugar and salt, alcoholic drinks, a sedentary lifestyle, and even quite prophetically (although petroleum chemicals were not in use at that time) many kinds of strongly scented colognes and sachets.[9]

Hahnemann's advice is as relevant today as it was then; only the names of the toxins have changed. That is, our current "obstacles to cure"—amalgam fillings and nickel-based crowns; toxic soaps, shampoos, and makeup; the excessive use of antibiotics; refined foods; the unwitting ingestion of food allergens; and chronic dental or tonsil focal infections and scar interference fields—must also be removed, or at least mitigated through treatment, to allow homeopathic remedies and other natural therapies to be able to fully act and effect a complete cure.

∞

Many books are available on constitutional homeopathy; therefore, this chapter will just briefly cover the history, definition, and scientific basis of this healing art, aiming for a clear overview rather than an in-depth analysis. In the recommended reading section at the end of the book, a number of excellent books on homeopathy for doctors and practitioners are listed, as well as books for interested readers who would simply like to understand more about this fascinating field of holistic medicine.

THE HISTORY OF HOMEOPATHY

One of the primary prerequisites for conducting solid scientific research is to initially do what is referred to as a "review of the literature." This review informs researchers about all the previous studies done on a particular subject so that they are knowledgeable about the important concepts and methods that have already been investigated and do not duplicate previous research that has already been well proved.

Samuel Hahnemann (1755–1843), a linguist who was conversant in at least eleven languages, probably conducted one of the most extensive reviews of the medical literature ever performed by a single individual. As early as the age of twelve, he was reading classical texts and tutoring other children in Greek and Latin.[10] Later, in college and medical school, Hahnemann supported himself by translating medical books in foreign languages and working as a medical librarian. By 1783, as a physician Hahnemann became convinced of the "danger and futility" of the allopathic healing methods of his day and "laid down the lancet and mercury," returning to his former profession and translating more foreign textbooks, including subjects on chemistry, toxicology, botany, alchemy, hydrotherapy, infant care and child rearing, nutrition and hygiene, philosophy, and psychology.[11]

In 1789, while translating the renowned Scottish physician William Cullen's text *A Treatise of the Materia Medica,* Hahnemann was struck by the similarity between the intermittent fever symptoms that occurred from poisoning by bark from the Peruvian cinchona tree, from which quinine was derived, and the intermittent fever symptoms of malaria that were treated by this quinine.[12] In a footnote in his translation of the text, Hahnemann noted that this similarity was probably not simply due to the bark's bitter and astringent properties as Cullen believed (since there were many more bitter and astringent plants and trees than cinchona), but possibly was indicative of the true curative powers contained in the cinchona bark itself.[13] Hahnemann's scientific mind and curiosity did not allow him to stop there, however. He endeavored to test his theory by conducting the first proving ever recorded, using himself as the subject. After taking "four drams of good bark twice a day," Hahnemann found his theory to be valid as he began to experience all the various symptoms of malaria—fever, chills, trembling, rapid heartbeat, weakness, and fatigue—in their typical "paroxysmal" or intermittent manner.[14] Through this self-testing with cinchona bark, Hahnemann tested concepts that would later become two of the most essential pillars on which the science and art of homeopathy stands: the law of similars and the law of proving. Based on Hahnemann's initial insight as well as his scientific testing of this bark from the cinchona tree, most historians consider 1789 to be the official year of the birth of homeopathy.[15] Hahnemann later proved cinchona bark formally with twenty-two provers, establishing it in the homeopathic materia medica as Cinchona officinalis or China.

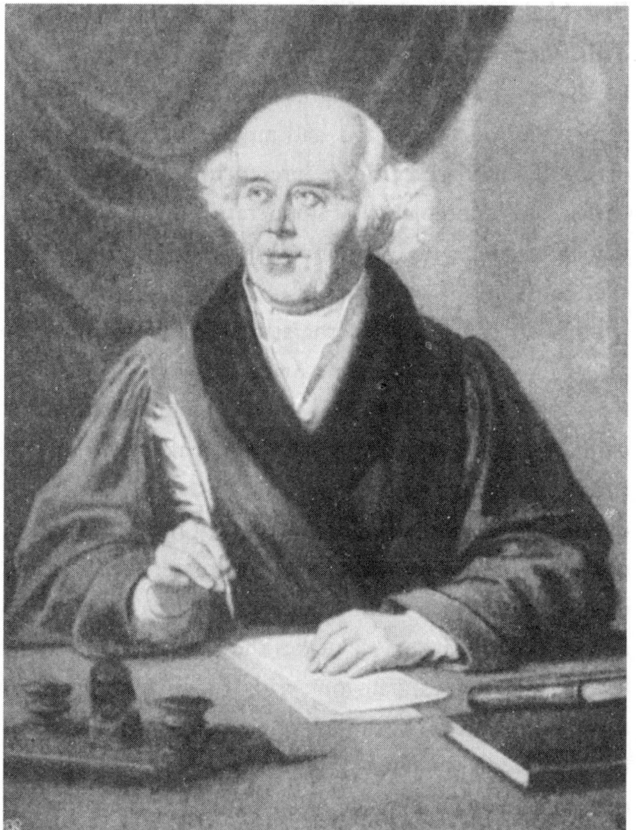

Figure 14.1. Samuel Hahnemann (1755–1843), the founder of homeopathy

Over the next twenty years, Hahnemann tested other medicinal substances on himself, as well as on his friends and relatives. Based on these "patient and meticulous" provings, he laid the foundation for his future *Materia Medica Pura,* published in 1821 in six volumes and containing sixty-six remedies.[16] Hahnemann published many other articles and books in his lifetime, the most notable being his complete text on homeopathy, the *Organon.* Although disputes have arisen over the interpretation of his teaching, the principles and methodologies outlined in the *Organon* have rarely been questioned and remain virtually intact to this day, which is a testament to Hahnemann as well as to the effectiveness of homeopathy.[17]

Pre-Hahnemannian Homeopathic Thinking

In the *Organon,* Hahnemann credited previous physicians who, he wrote, had had an "inkling" of the law of similars and therefore a "presentiment of homeopathy."[18] Most notable was Hippocrates (460–370 BCE), whose writings Hahnemann was able to read in the original Greek. This father of medicine wrote, "Disease is born of things, and by the attack of like things people are healed."[19] Later, the Swiss physician Paracelsus (1493–1541) also advocated the "like cures like" principle as well as a belief in "the minimal dose," and he further asserted that a poisonous substance that causes disease could also cure disease, if given in small enough dosages.[20]* Paracelsus succinctly characterized this law of minimum dose through the phrase *Dosis sola facit venenum,* "Only the dose makes the poison."[21] However, before Hahnemann, no one had recognized the magnitude of the law of similars or minimal dose, nor had they proceeded to systematize these laws—as well as the other homeopathic principles—in an organized manner and "carry it out" as a new field of healing science.[22] Thus, there has never been any question that Dr. Samuel Hahnemann is the true father and founder of the field of homeopathy.

Opposition to Hahnemann and Homeopathy

Unfortunately, Hahnemann's great revelations were not met kindly by everyone, especially jealous colleagues and pecuniary-minded pharmacists. The fact that he recommended small doses of medicine and was against multiple prescriptions made Hahnemann and his growing number of homeopathic colleagues a serious threat to the profits of the apothecaries (pharmacies). In fact, at one point he was arrested and charged with dispensing his own medicines—an act that was (and still is) illegal in Germany. Based on this and other harassment received from the medical establishment, Hahnemann was forced to leave Leipzig in 1820.[23]

The Worldwide Spread of Homeopathy Despite Opposition

Despite strong opposition from conventional medicine and pharmaceutical companies throughout his life, homeopathy was known and practiced in all the European countries (except Norway and Sweden), the United States, Mexico, Cuba, and Russia by the time of Hahnemann's death in 1843. And not long after that, homeopathy reached India and South America.[24] In fact, relatively soon after its introduction into the United States in 1825, homeopathy was offering severe competition to orthodox medicine, by as early as the 1840s.[25] This growing popularity and rapid spread of homeopathy, despite continuous opposition by orthodox medical practitioners, was primarily due to its phenomenal success rate in curing the sick—most dramatically demonstrated during epidemics. For example, Hahnemann himself successfully treated 180 men with only one death during the deadly typhus epidemic that attacked Napoleon's defeated troops in 1813. Furthermore, during a cholera epidemic in Cincinnati in 1849, only 3 percent of homeopathic patients died (35 out of 1,116), compared with the nearly 70 percent of patients who received conventional allopathic treatment.[26] Later, in 1854, the London Homeopathic Hospital had only a 16.4 percent death rate during a cholera epidemic, compared with a 53.2 percent mortality rate for patients treated in conventional hospitals.[27] Because of these and other dramatic successes that illustrated the distinct superiority of homeopathy, by the turn of the nineteenth century there were twenty-two homeopathic colleges in existence, twenty-nine homeopathic journals, and an estimated 15,000 practitioners in the United States.[28]

In the United States, despite even stronger opposition than Hahnemann and his followers had experienced in Europe, homeopathic physicians thrived. This was compounded by the fact that the rise in popularity of homeopathy coincided with a decline in the prestige

*Although Hahnemann credited many of his predecessors and "did not wish to incur the reproach of pretending to be the first and only discoverer of his method of healing," it is a mystery to this day why this learned man did not credit Paracelsus with the previous understanding and teaching of many of the main features of homeopathy. This omission is especially curious when one considers the fact that Paracelsus was one of the most famous and renowned physicians of the Middle Ages, and that he was born in the German-speaking part of Switzerland neighboring Hahnemann's German homeland. However, when he was queried about this issue in 1825, Hahnemann surprisingly replied that Paracelsus's teachings about homeopathy were unknown to him. (R. Haehl, *Samuel Hahnemann: His Life and Work,* vol. 1 [Fremont, Calif.: Jain Publishers, 1995], 81, 273–74, 425.)

of regular allopathic physicians and a "waning of public confidence in its procedures" in the mid- to late 1800s.[29] Harris Coulter, a medical historian, described this period in *Divided Legacy:*

> Dissatisfied patients switched back and forth until they found a physician in whom they had confidence, and, only too often, the homeopath was the ultimate victor. . . . Furthermore, the homeopaths were doing quite well without any bloodletting, and the doses of their medicines were extremely small—both of these aspects being very favorably regarded by the average patient.[30]

The allopathic physicians experienced the growing popularity of their homeopathic colleagues perhaps most painfully in their wallets, with the average doctor earning less than $1,000 per year in the last decades of the nineteenth century. In contrast homeopathic physicians, being much in demand, were said to earn from $3,000 to $7,000 a year. An in-depth analysis of the charges between homeopaths and allopaths revealed that there was no significant difference between the fees charged by these two groups, and that the relative prosperity of the homeopaths was due solely to their greater volume of business.[31]

AMA Formed to Eliminate Homeopathy

In response to this growing competition, the American Medical Association (AMA) was founded in the mid-1800s for two purposes: to improve the standards of medical education* and to combat homeopathy or "quackery in the profession."[32] This latter goal was not at all clandestine but clearly spelled out in its charter, which stated that the AMA was formed "to stamp out the scourge of homeopathy."[33] Dr. Nathan Smith Davis, the founder of the AMA and its leader for half a century, was a "bitter foe of homeopathy" and has been credited with being the single individual most responsible for the "extreme anti-homeopathic orientation of American medicine."* The first order of business for this new medical organization was an "ethical" ban on association and consultation by allopathic doctors with homeopathic physicians. Furthermore, the AMA required that all state medical societies purge themselves of homeopathic practitioners before they could be granted representation in their national organization. This edict was finally accomplished in the mid-1850s by every state medical society in the country, with the exception of that of Massachusetts.[34]

The success of this mandate was due in part to the weakness and vulnerability of the homeopaths themselves. Most homeopaths did not understand the practical wisdom of having a strong professional organization and "were too busy practicing medicine to countenance extensive involvement in medical politics." For example, out of the estimated 15,000 homeopaths practicing in the United States and Canada, only about 2,000 to 3,000 were members of their national organization. Furthermore, there was much internal strife among the homeopaths themselves, primarily over the subject of the appropriate level of potency. This internecine battle not only weakened the homeopathic profession but also confused the uninitiated public about this new and rather esoteric healing art. In 1947, the AMA fostered additional confusion and doubt about homeopathy during its national medical convention. Deciding that the public was not a "natural judge" of a qualified doctor, the AMA wrote a "Code of Ethics" that exhorted individuals to patronize *only* allopathic doctors, and this recommendation was extensively propagated in subsequent journals, magazines, and newspapers.[35]

Final Death Knell: The Flexner Report

Despite this fury of allopathic opposition and propaganda, however, homeopathic medicine continued to survive and even thrive until the publication of the infamous Flexner Report. In 1910, an educator named Abraham Flexner, accompanied by Nathan Colwell, who represented the AMA, made a comprehensive

*The majority of U.S. doctors in the nineteenth and early twentieth centuries had very little education. For example, as little as sixteen weeks of training, with some additional time as an apprentice in another doctor's office, was typical.

*Harris Coulter comments in his book that more on this historic period would be known today if it were not for the fact that the nineteenth-century files of the AMA, along with the personal papers of Dr. Davis (1817–1904), were destroyed in an unexplained fire shortly after Davis's death.

survey of medical schools in the United States and issued a report on their status. This report, which greatly favored the allopathic approach to medicine over the homeopathic, consistently gave a low rating to the existing homeopathic colleges. State medical examining boards accepted these findings and began to refuse acceptance of graduates of these (primarily homeopathic) schools—regardless of the candidate's knowledge or proficiency.[36]

The Flexner-Colwell Report became the final death knell for homeopathic colleges, as well as homeopathy itself, in the United States. In 1900, there were twenty-two homeopathic colleges in the United States, including Boston University and the University of Michigan; by 1923, however, only two schools were left.[37] Sadly, by 1950 there was not a single homeopathic college remaining in the Unites States. Furthermore, by this time the number of practicing homeopaths in the United States and Canada had declined from an estimated 15,000 to fewer than 100.[38] And the benefactors of this report, primarily Andrew Carnegie and John D. Rockefeller, continued to philanthropically pour money into the conventional medical schools and institutions in staggering amounts, thus ensuring the future existence and prosperity of allopathy in the United States.[39]*

Allopaths Co-opt Homeopathic Remedies and Principles

What's most striking about this blatant attack on homeopathy is that over the years the allopathic profession slowly began to include not only a large number of medicines that were first used in homeopathy but also some of its principles. Harris Coulter described this usurpation in his extensive documentary *Divided Legacy:*

> Throughout the nineteenth century the homeopaths employed a much greater number of different medicines in their prescribing than the orthodox physicians. This was one of the fundamental differences between the two schools, and its importance cannot be overestimated. The history of nineteenth-century therapeutics is essentially one of the progressive adoption by allopathic physicians of the numerous medicines originally introduced by homeopathy.[40]

Furthermore, as the allopaths witnessed the success of their homeopathic colleagues utilizing tiny doses of various medicaments, they slowly began to reduce their dosages, thus adopting in part the homeopathic law of minimal dose. (However, these smaller doses of allopathic drugs were still not minimal enough to obviate side effects, nor were they succussed.) Thus the AMA and its pharmaceutical accomplices successfully fulfilled their overt goal of eliminating homeopathic physicians in the United States, as well as their covert plan "to kill them with kindness" by co-opting much of homeopathic medicine into the (more profitable) allopathic school of medicine.[41]

The Worldwide Decline of Homeopathy's Influence and Its Recent Renaissance

This war on homeopathy and its practitioners greatly reduced the influence of this field of healing in Europe and the rest of the world, albeit not as completely as it was accomplished in the United States. With the rise in the holistic health movement in recent decades, however, homeopathy has slowly become more widespread and recently has enjoyed a massive renaissance movement through the propagation of new research emanating primarily from Europe and India. In England, visits to a homeopathic practitioner are increasing at a rate of 39 percent per year, and in a survey of 28,000 people in Britain, 80 percent reported that they used some form of alternative medicine.[42] Mahatma Gandhi was a great champion of homeopathy, and Mother Teresa introduced homeopathic care in many of the clinics in Calcutta. The first full-time homeopathic medical school in the United States since the 1920s, the American Medical College of Homeopathy, opened its doors in 2011. Homeopathy is also taught extensively in North American naturopathic colleges and universities, seven of which are fully accredited (and plans for an eighth are under way). There are also many schools and institutions in the United States and throughout

*It remains a mystery why John D. Rockefeller, who accepted *only* homeopathic treatment throughout his very long life (he died at age 97), permitted his millions to be used to undermine homeopathy in the United States.

the world that teach postgraduate courses to physicians, and many of these also accept lay practitioners.*

HOW HOMEOPATHY WORKS

Unlike vitamins, herbs, or prescription drugs, homeopathic remedies add nothing physical to the body. They do not supplement depleted nutritional stores like vitamins and minerals, nor do they contain therapeutic herbal components—alkaloids, glycosides, saponins, tannins, and so forth†—that are healing in botanical medicine.

Homeopathy simply acts on the patient's vital force, energetically removing the disturbing pattern. This *vital force* or *vital principle* that resides in every living being has been recognized for centuries in various cultures. It is known as *prana* in Hinduism and *chi* in Chinese medicine. Hahnemann believed that disease is not a physical phenomenon but arises from a disturbed vital force. In the *Organon,* he explained, "Human diseases rest on no material, on no acridity, that is to say, on no disease matter; rather they are solely spirit-like (dynamic) mistunings of the spirit-like enlivening power-force-energy (the life principle, the life force) of the human body."[43]

Hahnemann found that by pairing a patient's pattern of disturbances with a similar plant, animal, or mineral pattern, a correct homeopathic prescription could be ascertained. Healing is accomplished by using the nanotechnology of minute (often even nonphysical) amounts of these plant, animal, or mineral substances diluted in alcohol and water, and then shaken or *succussed.* In this way, the "hidden medicinal power" of the substance is revealed, and it can have a profoundly curative effect on the individual's "mistuned" vital force.[44] When the astute homeopath accurately finds the pattern of disease revealed in a patient's symptoms and characteristics and correctly matches this pattern with the pattern of the particular essence of a plant, animal, or mineral remedy, the life force of the organism is enlivened and can then initiate self-healing. Thus, homeopathy cures in the least invasive and yet most profound way possible, through communicating with that most subtle energetic force or spirit that maintains life in each individual.

> **succussion:** Succussion is the process in which the vial containing the remedy is hit a number of times against the palm of the hand or a book to liberate the energy and medicinal power within the substance.

In order to better understand how homeopathic remedies act in the body, it is essential to describe the four fundamental laws upon which homeopathy is based: the law of similars, the law of proving, the law of potentization and minimum dose, and the law of cure.

The Law of Similars: "Like Cures Like"

The law of similars is an ancient principle rediscovered and developed by Hahnemann that affirms that an individual's illness can be treated through the administration of medicine that is similar enough to the patient's symptoms to create a resonance and trigger healing. Although "traces" of this homeopathic *similia similibus curentur* ("let similars be cured by similars") or "like cures like" principle had been recorded for centuries, most notably by Hippocrates, Hahnemann credited a Danish army physician named Stahl with articulating it best in the early 1700s:

> The rule generally acted on in the medicinal art—to treat by opposite means (*contraria contrariis*)—is quite false and preposterous. On the contrary, one is persuaded that diseases yield to, and are cured by, means that engender a similar suffering (*similia similibus*)—burns by approaching the fire, frostbitten limbs by the application of snow and the coldest water, inflammation and contusions by distilled spirits.[45]

*It is important that practicing homeopaths study the basics of homeopathy before taking advanced courses, such as the recommended courses given by Dr. Rajan Sankaran and his Mumbai colleagues. For more information contact the North American Society of Homeopaths (www.homeopathy.org) or the National Center for Homeopathy (www.homeopathic.org).

†Herbal alkaloids such as reserpine treat mental illness, glycosides such as digitalis treat heart irregularities, saponins have emulsifying properties, and tannins can coagulate and detoxify heavy metals. (D. Kenner and Y. Requena, *Botanical Medicine: A European Professional Perspective* [Brookline, Mass.: Paradigm Publications, 2001], 2, 7.)

The law of similars, having the truth of a universal law, can also extend to other fields of healing.* Hahnemann cited the example of how grief can be greatly diminished or even extinguished upon hearing an account of another's greater loss. For example, grief at the death of a pet on September 10, 2001, might have been somewhat lessened by witnessing the holocaust-like scenes on television the next day in New York on September 11.

In the case of homeopathic remedies, the law of similars can best be illustrated through a few examples. When an individual is suffering from hay fever and has a profuse, watery discharge from his eyes and nose, he may be successfully treated with Allium cepa, a remedy made from red onions that stimulates these same symptoms in a healthy individual—as every cook can attest to when chopping onions before dinner.

An individual who suffers intermittently from hives—an allergic skin condition characterized by itching, burning, stinging, and the formation of swollen red patches on the skin—may benefit from the remedy Apis mellifica, made from the venom of a honeybee, which causes similar symptoms in an individual who has been stung.

This law of similars is not simply applicable to the healing of physical symptoms. For instance, in the latter example, Apis can be given as a long-term *constitutional* remedy to patients who manifest emotional symptoms of a beelike pattern. That is, Apis can be prescribed constitutionally to an individual who is obsessively busy, irritable when crossed, and jealous and has an excessively strong family orientation (as bees do with their hive). Thus, one rather dramatic but very clear way of understanding the law of similars is to realize that not only are ill individuals simply not themselves but that they are actually manifesting a pattern that is not human. As the renowned homeopathic physician Rajan Sankaran succinctly explained, a patient can be experiencing symptoms similar to the pattern of an animal (issues of competition, predator/prey, survival), a mineral (something is lacking or missing in his structure), or a plant (highly sensitive and affected by environment).[46]*

Healing occurs when the patient takes this stronger plant, mineral, or animal remedy that is similar to the weaker plant, mineral, or animal pattern of disturbance existing in him. This homeopathic remedy then resonates with the patient's similar pattern of disturbance, and because the energetic vibration of the homeopathic remedy is stronger, it annihilates the disturbance, analogous to when an opera singer hits the exact note (very loudly) to actually shatter a glass.[47] Hahnemann found that through potentization (diluting and succussing), his homeopathic remedies were gentle enough to not cause harm, yet at the same time powerful enough to overwhelm the existing pattern of disease in his patients. He described the potent action of these remedies in aphorism (section)† twenty-seven of his *Organon* text:

> The curative capacity of medicines therefore rests upon their symptoms being similar to the disease but with power that outweighs it. Each single case of disease is most surely, thoroughly, rapidly and permanently annihilated and lifted only by a medicine that can engender, in the human condition, a totality of symptoms that is the most complete and the most similar to the case of disease but that, at the same time, exceeds the disease in strength.[48]

When the correspondence between the symptom picture of the disease and the symptom picture of the given substance is most closely matched, the homeopathic remedy is referred to as the *simillimum*—that is, the most similar and most perfectly fitting medicine.[49] In order to identify the nature and effects of a particular plant, animal, or mineral remedy, Hahnemann originated specific types of experiments, called *drug provings.*

*Interestingly, the poet and writer Johann Goethe (1749–1832) was a supporter of both homeopathy and Hahnemann. After greatly criticizing the allopathic medicine of his day, Goethe wove the law of similars into the second act of his immortal drama *Faust:* "To like things like, whatever one may ail; There's certain help." (R. Haehl, *Samuel Hahnemann: His Life and Work,* vol. 1 [New Delhi: B. Jain Publishers, 2001], 170.)

*This will be discussed later in this chapter under the section titled "The New 'Sankaran System.'"

†Hahnemann called each section in which he made a specific point an *aphorism* in the *Organon.*

The Law of Proving: Single-Blind and Double-Blind Provings

Drug provings are performed by administering small doses of a particular homeopathic remedy to a healthy volunteer and then painstakingly recording all the symptoms that arise over the next few weeks or months. For example, using our two previous examples, the proving of Allium cepa (red onions) would create in a well individual all the symptoms of hay fever, and the administration of Apis mellifica (honeybee venom) would cause skin irritation and swelling, irritability, and the need to keep constantly busy. In this manner, by inducing an "artificial disease," the "natural disease" characterized by hay fever or irritability can be cured.[50]

Hahnemann laid out in detail the exact procedures necessary to conduct these proving experiments. As a strict and rigorous scientist, Hahnemann carried out these provings in a single-blind fashion—that is, the volunteers didn't know what remedy they were taking. He also used double-blind procedures—that is, the physician conducting the proving didn't know the identity of the remedy either. In fact, these provings in more recent years have fit the highest standards of scientific inquiry, by being conducted on a double-blind, placebo-controlled basis. (That is, some of the volunteers receive a sugar-pill placebo and others receive the actual remedy, but no one—the provers or the researcher conducting the proving—knows the identity of the remedy.)[51]

HAHNEMANN'S "PROVERS"

Hahnemann did not allow provers to drink wine, brandy, coffee, or tea, and he required that they give up any of these habits "long before the proving." Furthermore, provers had to avoid anything medicinal during the proving and eat a moderately bland diet, even avoiding "green vegetables and roots, all salads, and soup herbs" because "they always retain some disturbing medicinal power." Additionally, he required that a group of provers be both male and female, that they chart the symptoms that arise in detail, and that they be interviewed daily by the supervising homeopathic physician.[52]

A remedy must undergo one further test before being considered a valid medicine and allowed into the official homeopathic *pharmacopoeia*—it must show a proven ability to cure patients who have the same symptoms that have been observed during the drug provings. When a remedy has shown that it can cure a particular set of unique symptoms over time, it is included in homeopathic materia medicas—that is, encyclopedic books in which all the homeopathic remedies are listed and the particular symptoms that they can cure are described in detail.*

pharmacopoeia: The pharmacopoeia is the official "recipe book" that lists all proven homeopathic remedies and the exact method of their preparation, so that different laboratories and pharmacists can correctly duplicate them. In the United States the pharmacopoeia is the HPUS, or the Homeopathic Pharmacopoeia of the United States. In France it is the Codex, and in Germany it is the HAB This German HAB, based on Hahnemann's original prescriptions, is considered superior to all other pharmacopoeias. The HAB was used as a resource in preparing the U.S. pharmacopeia.

When homeopathy was in its infancy, the number of remedies in the materia medica was relatively small and easy to peruse. Over time, however, the number of proven homeopathic remedies rose into the hundreds, and therefore, an index called a *repertory* was developed. This book categorizes the numerous symptoms a patient may express according to the area—mind, head, throat, abdomen, extremities, skin, and so forth—where the symptom is experienced. An easy analogy to use to clarify the purpose of these books is to liken the materia medica to the white pages (listing the remedy and its action) and the repertory to the yellow pages (the various categories of symptoms are listed with the related remedies under each of these).[53] The first comprehensive and well-organized repertory was written by one of the great U.S. homeopaths, Dr. James Tyler Kent. Created in the early 1800s with more than 1,500 pages of information, *Kent's Repertory* still stands as "the bible" of all

*Although the ideal is to include only remedies that have been proven and also been shown to cure patients, this is not always the case. Some of the remedies listed in materia medicas have only been proven, while others have only been shown to cure one or more patients.

repertories, and it is usually bought first and referred to often by serious students of homeopathy.[54]

The remedies that are used in provings and listed in materia medicas and repertories are prepared according to exacting standards elucidated by Hahnemann in great detail in his book *Organon of the Medical Art.* The manner in which they are made through dilution and succussion is termed *potentization.*

The Law of Potentization and Minimum Dose

Potentizing, or the procedure of first diluting and then succussing (shaking) a remedy, was probably arrived at by Hahnemann through a combination of knowledge gained from translating and studying previous writings by such holistic medical luminaries as Hippocrates and Paracelsus, through practical considerations of reducing the side effects of potentially toxic substances, and finally through "sheer divine inspiration."[55]

Dilution and the Law of the Minimum Dose

Hahnemann discovered through clinical trial and error that if a patient needed a specific remedy, then he or she would be particularly sensitive to that remedy. Thus, he found that the amounts and doses sufficient to heal a sick patient were much lower than the amounts previously needed to stimulate a positive response during drug provings in healthy individuals who did not energetically resonate with the remedy. On the strength of these experiences, Hahnemann began to dilute a very small amount of the raw material of a remedy in water and alcohol solutions to find curative doses that did not produce unwanted side effects.[56] Later in the eighteenth century, this law of the minimum dose became an accepted pharmacology principle known as the Arndt-Schulz law, authored by Rudolph Arndt (1835–1900) and Hugo Schulz (1853–1932).[57] Also known as the theory of the reverse effect, this principle states that "weak stimuli excite physiologic activity, moderately strong ones favor it, strong ones retard it, very strong ones arrest it."[58]

This law of minimum dose is best exemplified through the use of extremely poisonous remedies such as arsenic or mercury. As a highly diluted homeopathic remedy, Arsenicum album can cure the toughest cases of acute gastroenteritis and vomiting as well as chronic anxiety.[59] However, in moderate to high dosages, this toxic metal is a deadly poison. An even more specific example of the benefits of homeopathy is with the remedy Mercurius vivus. When mercury is ingested, most commonly through the placement of mercury amalgam fillings, over time this poisonous metal can cause memory loss, night sweats, and tremors. However, as a homeopathic remedy, it has been proven in countless cases to heal these very same symptoms.[60] Another example of the benefits of the use of the minimum dose in homeopathy can be gleaned from the plant family with the remedy Conium maculatum. This ancient remedy made from poison hemlock was made famous by Plato's description of the death of the Greek philosopher Socrates. When taken internally, Conium maculatum causes an ascending paralysis, labored gait, trembling, and finally death through respiratory failure. However, when taken homeopathically, Conium maculatum is a primary remedy for the treatment of multiple sclerosis and other neurodegenerative disorders with the associated symptoms of trembling, paralysis, incoordination, and a difficult gait.[61] Thus, through the utilization of the law of the minimum dose as well as the law of similars, Hahnemann found that poisonous substances, which in larger amounts cause great harm, could be harnessed to cause great good in patients who are suffering from symptoms similar to the symptoms induced by these poisons.

Succussion

Another practical consideration led to the discovery of succussion—the other component in the process of potentization. At first, Hahnemann simply shook the vial in which he was preparing a remedy for homogenization purposes—that is, to mix the ingredients thoroughly.[62] Over time, however, he observed that "adding kinetic energy" to the remedy through this shaking greatly "liberated the energy contained within the substance" and made the homeopathic remedy more available to the vital force of the organism.[63] Hahnemann's succussion of remedies was more elaborate than simple shaking, however. He recommended that the homeopathic vial strike with an up-and-down motion against the palm of a hand or a leather-bound book (he used a bible).[64] Hahnemann expounded on the therapeutic benefits of this process of diluting and succussing, which he termed *dynamization** or *potentization,* in aphorism 269 of the *Organon:*

> For its own special purpose, the homeopathic medical art develops to a formerly unheard of degree the internal, spirit-like medicinal powers of crude substances. . . . This procedure [potentization] develops the latent *dynamic* powers of the substance which were previously unnoticeable, as if slumbering. . . . Therefore, this process is called *dynamization* or *potentization* (development of medicinal power).[65]

Preparing and Potentizing Homeopathic Remedies

As a fully qualified chemist, and being thoroughly acquainted with herbalism, botany, and metallurgy, as well as the field of alchemy that was popular at the time, Dr. Hahnemann had extensive knowledge on how to properly prepare plants, minerals, and other substances.[66] Furthermore, having an exacting and scientific nature, Hahnemann laid out in great precision and detail the method in which each remedy should be prepared and potentized in both his texts, *Organon of the Medical Art* and *Materia Medica Pura.*[67] In fact, his descriptions were so comprehensive and his standards so exacting that Germany's pharmacopeia, the HAB, was based entirely on Hahnemann's prescriptions. The German HAB is still considered the superior guide for making homeopathic remedies in the world, and it is utilized by many of the most respected homeopathic companies (e.g., UNDA in Belgium and Helios in England).

> **alchemy:** Alchemy was the form of chemistry and occultism popular in the Middle Ages and the Renaissance periods that concerned transmuting one substance of a lesser value (e.g., copper) into a more precious and valuable substance (e.g., gold). In medicine, alchemy referred to the transformation of natural substances such as plants into healing medicinals through specific therapeutic processes.

**Dynamis,* meaning "divine breath" in Greek, embodied the concept of life for the Greeks—that is, one of God breathing life into his creations. (V. McCabe, *Homeopathy, Healing and You* [New York: St. Martin's Griffin, 1997], 13.)

In brief, a homeopathic remedy begins with the raw material obtained from a plant, an animal, or a mineral.* Raw materials derived from soluble substances such as plants or animals—for example, the whole fresh plant of leopard's bane to make the remedy Arnica montana or the venom of the surukuku or bushmaster snake that makes up the Lachesis muta remedy—are extracted out in an alcohol and water solution for a period of days to weeks. The solution is strained, and after any remaining plant or animal material is discarded, the liquid portion, referred to as the *mother tincture,* is bottled and stored. This mother tincture is used as the starting point to make homeopathic remedies, and the strong alcohol percentage (~90%) of the solution preserves it almost indefinitely. If the substance is insoluble, such as in the case of carbonate of lime used to produce the remedy Calcarea carbonica, it is initially pulverized and triturated with lactose and then diluted in an alcohol and water solution.

The "C" Potencies

Hahnemann first potentized his remedies based on the *centesimal scale*—that is, based on a ratio of 1 to 100. These *C potencies* are made by dissolving one part of the mother tincture with ninety-nine parts of an alcohol and water solution. For example, when one part of a leopard's bane mother tincture is diluted in ninety-nine parts of an alcohol and water solution and succussed, this yields the remedy Arnica montana 1C. When one part of this 1C remedy is diluted in ninety-nine parts of another alcohol and water solution, it makes a 2C Arnica remedy. Repeating this procedure four more times produces Arnica 6C—a common homeopathic potency.† Succussion, or the number of times a

*For simplicity, only plant, animal, and mineral remedies are cited here as an example of the most typical homeopathic remedies. However, remedies can be made from other substances; for instance, *nosodes* are made from diseased material (Medorrhinum—gonorrhea, Tuberculinum—tuberculosis, Syphilinum—syphilis, etc.) and *imponderables* from electromagnetic energy (Sol—sunlight, Magnetis polus articus and Magnetis polus australias—the north and south pole of a magnet, etc.).

†To save on the expense of alcohol when making high-potency remedies, pharmacies often use double-distilled water in the intermediary steps but add alcohol in during the final step to preserve the remedy. This change does not adversely affect the remedy's quality. (G. Vithoulkas, *The Science of Homeopathy* [New York: Grove Press, Inc., 1980], 163.)

remedy is shaken, can range from twenty to one hundred times, and varies according to the laboratory making the remedy.

Less Is More: The Inverse Relationship of Substance to Power

Through the potentization process, Hahnemann made the startling discovery that the more dilute a remedy is—that is, the *less* the amount of physical substance actually remaining in the remedy after repeated dilutions and succussions—the *stronger* and more potent it becomes. This realization was consistent with the use of minute amounts in homeopathy, as discussed previously in the "Dilution and the Law of the Minimum Dose" section. For example, even in dilutions greater than a millionfold, atropine (an alkaloid of the belladonna nightshade plant) causes dilation of the pupil in humans and animal subjects. Furthermore, hydrochloric acid, when diluted a thousand-fold in water, has been found to easily dissolve fibrin and gluten. And this "solvent power" of hydrochloric acid does not increase but actually diminishes when the proportion of the acid is increased.[68]

However, Hahnemann's epiphany went even further. He found that this inverse relationship held true even when a homeopathic remedy was so highly diluted that it no longer contained *any* of the raw material of the original plant, animal, or mineral substance. The point at which this phenomenon occurs, referred to in mathematical nomenclature as *Avogadro's number,* corresponds to 12C in the centesimal scale potencies.* Thus, for example, the remedy Arnica montana 6C, which still has minute amounts of the original leopard's bane plant material in it, is not as strong-acting as Arnica 30C, which has no remaining material left in it at all. This inverse relationship—that is, that *decreasing* the quantity of raw material actually *increases* the power or potency of a remedy, even when no physical raw material remains in the remedy—is one of the primary principles in homeopathy. This law of potentization is illustrated in figure 14.2.

*In regard to other potencies that will be discussed here, Avogadro's number corresponds to 24X in the decimal scale (1:10) potencies and is estimated to be between LM2 and LM3 (Yasgur) or between LM3 and LM4 (Helios) in the LM scale (1:50,000) potencies.

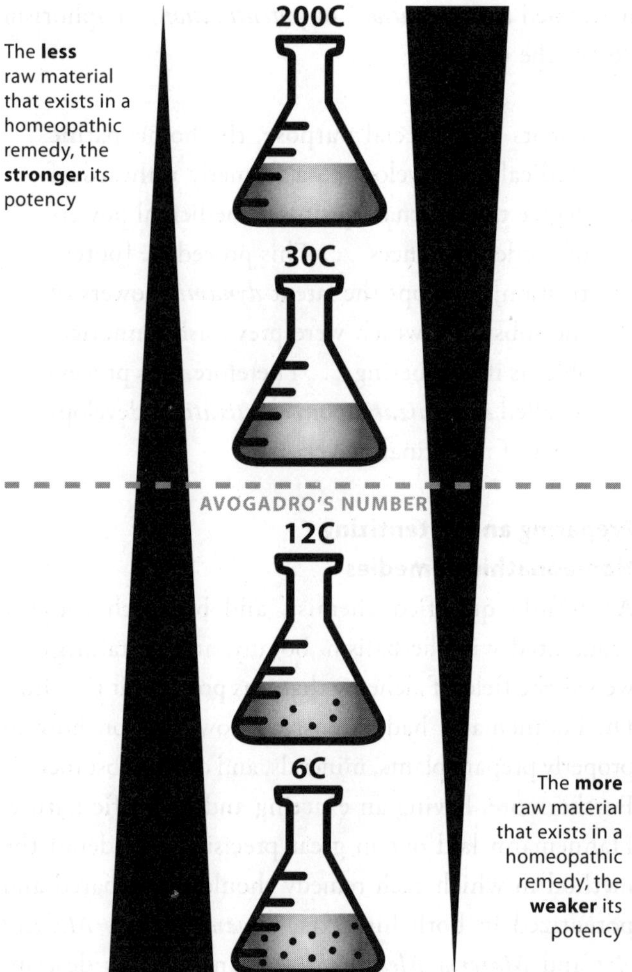
200C
The **less** raw material that exists in a homeopathic remedy, the **stronger** its potency
30C
AVOGADRO'S NUMBER
12C
6C
The **more** raw material that exists in a homeopathic remedy, the **weaker** its potency

Figure 14.2. The law of potentization: the amount of remaining raw material in a homeopathic remedy is inversely proportional to the strength and potency of that remedy.

Newtonian versus Quantum Physics

As a chemist and a contemporary of Amedeo Avogadro, Hahnemann was well aware of Avogadro's number.[69] However, it is an indication of his open mind as well as his advanced intuition of modern quantum physics that he continued to research the effect of the higher-potency remedies (whose dilution surpasses Avogadro's number, meaning they have no discernible remaining raw material in them). In fact, he found that in many cases these higher nonphysical potencies were more effective than the lower potencies and caused less adverse side effects, or healing reactions.*

*This is not to imply that the higher potencies are "better" than the lower potencies. The level of potency is prescribed according to the patient's symptoms and miasmic state (e.g., a strong versus a weakened constitution), as we'll discuss later in this chapter.

This belief, however, was completely at odds with the Newtonian theory of physics popular in Hahnemann's day. Sir Isaac Newton (1642–1727) viewed the world in a strictly materialistic manner, formulating principles "in which individual particles of matter followed certain laws of motion through space and time—[that is,] the universe as machine." Unfortunately, this more mechanistic and limited model continues to shape not only the science of physics but also all of modern medicine and biology.[70]

In contrast, through the advent of the new field of quantum physics that developed in the early twentieth century, the scientific explanation of non-mechanistic, subtle phenomena such as electromagnetic fields,* the property of "nonlocality" (e.g., that electrons as well as individuals can affect each other at a distance), and the particle/wave dualistic nature of subatomic molecules† has shaken the foundation of Newtonian physics, in which the laws of gravity are unchangeable when applied to large masses and distances—but fail at the atomic and subatomic levels. Thus, the twentieth-century field of quantum physics that sheds light on phenomena such as extrasensory perception (ESP), the collective unconscious, and, even to use spiritual terms, the transmission of Divine Consciousness, is entirely consistent with Hahnemann's eighteenth-century intuition of the intangible "spirit-like dynamis" inhabiting every living being, as well as his observations of the subtle effects of potentized homeopathic remedies.

Additionally, modern quantum physics research has demonstrated that once subatomic particles are in contact, they *always* remain in contact through all space and all time.[71] Through this model, it is easier to comprehend that even when the original raw material of the leopard's bane plant is no longer physically measurable in the higher-potency Arnica remedies, the water molecules "remember" the essence of this plant, can store this memory over time, and can "transmit" the energetic information of this plant to patients.[72] The subject of quantum physics is covered in more detail in "The Scientific Basis of Homeopathy" later in this chapter.

*All living things emit a weak radiation that creates an electromagnetic field surrounding them, as first elucidated by Michael Faraday and later validated by Albert Einstein and Rupert Sheldrake.

†Subatomic molecules are not solid objects behaving like little billiard balls; rather, they act sometimes as particles and sometimes as waves. (L. McTaggart, *The Field* [New York: HarperCollins Publishers, 2002], 10.)

Unfortunately, in the eighteenth and nineteenth centuries, the belief systems of a majority of physicians were firmly grounded in the materialistic principles of the newly emerging field of Newtonian physics, formulated a century before. Therefore, when Hahnemann began to use potencies that exceeded Avogadro's number, many of his followers could no longer follow.[73] This caused a major split in homeopathic circles that is still felt today.

"LM" Potencies: Gentle but Effective

Near the end of his life, Hahnemann developed one other homeopathic potency known as the *fifty-millesimal* or *LM* or *Q* potency. Hahnemann discovered this particular potency while searching for a dilution and succussion method that would cause the least amount of stress in a patient, known as an *aggravation* in homeopathy or a *healing crisis* in other holistic circles. The preparation of these potencies is complex and much different from the centesimal scale (1:100), but in brief, they are diluted at a ratio of one (plant, animal, or mineral substance) to 50,000 (alcohol and water) at each step during the potentizing process. Hahnemann found that through this much more dilute and therefore gentler ratio, he could succuss a greater number of repetitions—that is, 100 times instead of only 10 or 20 (as was often the case with the centesimal scale), and therefore bring about a "far greater development of power" of the remedy. He found that these "far more perfect dynamized medicinal preparations" could be given much more often and deliver a more profound impact on the patient, while causing no, or at least much more rare, healing aggravations than his C potencies.[74]

In the sixth and final edition of his *Organon,* Hahnemann recommended the use of these gentler but more powerful LM potencies over his C potency remedies. Unfortunately, when he died in 1843 this edition had not yet been published, and, purportedly due to Hahnemann's instructions not to publish it immediately, his wife never published it either.* Therefore, the new

*Some speculate that it was because Melanie Hahnemann was tired of being criticized by the allopathic community, and others believe she had more mercenary objectives and was waiting to publish this last edition at some later point to receive more money.

information about these important LM potencies was not known until nearly eighty years later (1921), when the sixth edition of the *Organon* was finally published.* Because of this delay in the propagation of Hahnemann's last ten years of research, most homeopaths learned to use only his original C potencies, as well as the *decimal* scale or "X" potencies† (i.e., 1:10 dilutions), which were developed in 1838 by a Philadelphia doctor named Samuel Dubs.[75‡] Even today LM potencies are still relatively uncommon, with the most typical potencies used in a homeopathic clinical practice being the decimal scale potencies: 6X, 12X and 30X; and the centesimal scale potencies: 6C, 12C, 30C, 200C, 1000C or 1M, 10M, 50M, and CM.§ However, over time, and especially during the past few years in which there has been an explosion of new investigation and research in the field of homeopathy, more and more homeopaths have come to appreciate the benefits of the powerful yet gently acting LM potencies, which are especially efficacious for the growing population of environmentally sensitive patients.

Liquid "C" Potencies

Another little-known aspect of *posology*—that is, the science of the dosages of homeopathic medicines—is that near the end of his life Hahnemann began to dilute his C potencies. Classically, homeopathic remedies were dispensed through little globules (tiny milk sugar pellets). However, just as with the LM potency, Hahnemann found that when the C potencies were diluted in water and alcohol, succussed, and then mixed in a glass of water from which a teaspoonful of this mixture was taken, the patient's vital force responded better and healing was much more effective. In 1837, he described this reaction in his Paris casebook:

> [O]ur vital principle cannot well bear that the same unchanged dose of medicine be given even twice in succession, much less more frequently to a patient. For by this the good effect of the former dose of medicine is either neutralized in part, or new symptoms proper to the medicine, symptoms which have not before been present in the disease, appear, impeding the cure. . . . But in taking one and the same medicine repeatedly (which is indispensable to secure the cure of a serious, chronic disease), if the dose is in every case varied and modified only a little in its degree of dynamization, then the vital force of the patient will calmly, and as it were willingly receive the same medicine even at brief intervals very many times in succession with the best results, every time increasing the well-being of the patient."[76*]

▶ Grateful appreciation is given to David Little and his encyclopedic mind on the subject of homeopathy for providing this information taken from Dr. Hahnemann's 1837 casebook. Little's new six-volume, 3,000-plus-page textbook, *Homoeopathic Compendium,* is recommended to all serious students of homeopathy (www.simillimum.com).

Hahnemann noted that this "slight change in the degree of dynamization" is favorably affected not only by the difference in the amount diluted with each dose (as the remedy bottle that contains the pellets, water, and alcohol reduces in volume), but also if it is "well shaken five or six times" each time before it is taken.[77]

C potencies that are diluted in water and alcohol and taken in liquid form are gentler to the system than when taken in globule form. Thus, just like LM potencies, practitioners often prescribe C potencies diluted in liquid for very weak and/or sensitive patients who cannot tolerate much aggravation (healing crisis symptoms) from taking the remedy. Also, these potencies can be dosed more frequently, which is often necessary in the case of ill patients suffering from chronic disease.

*At Melanie Hahnemann's death, the manuscript passed to the Böenninghausen family (Dr. C. Von Böenninghausen was a valued correspondent to Hahnemann and a famous homeopath in his own right). However, it was not until 1920 that the Böenninghausen family, financially ruined by World War I, agreed to sell the document to Dr. William Boericke of San Francisco, who had been trying to obtain it for more than twenty years. Subsequently, the German edition was published in 1921, and the English edition was published in 1922. (W. O'Reilly, ed., *Organon of the Medical Art* [Palo Alto, Calif.: Birdcage Books, 1996], 276.)

†Decimal potencies are labeled "D" potencies in Europe.

‡Constantine Hering, known as the father of American homeopathy, originally researched the decimal scale in 1833.

§"M" is the Roman numeral designation for 1,000. Thus, 1M is 1000C, 10M is 10,000C, and CM is 100,000C; these potencies are still considered part of the centesimal scale.

The "K" Potencies

Before leaving the rather complex subject of potency, the use of K potencies should be explained. In the 1820s, Hahnemann received a letter from a Russian physician, Dr. Korsakoff, who suggested the use of only one vial when preparing homeopathic remedies. He explained that allowing the solution left clinging to the walls of this vial to be considered one part, and then adding the required amount of alcohol and water and succussing in the usual manner for the next level of potency, would greatly save on the expense of vials.[78] Thus, with Korsakoff's method of preparation, the same vial was used throughout the process,* whereas with Hahnemann's method a vial was discarded after preparing each potency level (1C, 2C, 3C, etc.).[79] In the case of preparing a 200C potency through Hahnemann's method, 200 vials would need to be used and then discarded. Hahnemann gracefully received Korsakoff's suggestion and acknowledged his colleague's method by proposing that remedies made with a single vial be labeled *K* or *CK* (*centesimal Korsakovian*) potencies, whereas remedies made through the process of discarding each vial would be labeled *C* or *CH* (*centesimal Hahnemann*) potencies. However, based on the great expense—not to mention the ecological ramifications—of using hundreds and even thousands of vials when making higher-potency remedies, in actuality, most homeopathic pharmacies use the Korsakovian method when potencies are made above the 30C level.

Although the effect is very subtle, energetic testing sometimes reveals a discernible difference between, for example, a 30C remedy and a 30K remedy. According to Dr. Mikhael Adams, because the same flask is used, a 30K remedy better holds the information of all the lower potencies, whereas with a 30C remedy, the patient is receiving more of the specific 30C-level potency, with much less influence of the previous levels (29C, 28C, 27C, etc.). Therefore, a 30K potency might be prescribed when the lower and more physically acting potencies (6C, 12C, etc.) are needed to be included in the remedy, and a 30C potency is prescribed when that specific level of potency that accesses slightly more ("higher") psychological levels is required. However, in most cases, the difference between these two potencies is almost negligible.

The Law of Cure: "The Rapid, Gentle, and Permanent Restoration of Health"

Hahnemann devoted a large portion of his seminal text, *Organon of the Medical Art,* to detailing the principles of healing and cure. His most often quoted statements on this subject are from his first two aphorisms in the *Organon:* "the physician's highest and *only* calling is to make the sick healthy, to cure, as it is called," and "the highest ideal of cure is the rapid, gentle and permanent restoration of health."[80] This "rapid, gentle and permanent" cure continues to be every homeopath's goal, but the journey toward this ideal state is not always easy and rarely linear. Hahnemann recognized that even with the most perfectly fitting remedy, or simillimum, there could arise *aggravations*—the homeopathic synonym for "healing crises," when patients initially feel worse after taking a remedy through an increase in the quantity (amount of) or quality (intensity) of their symptoms.

Hering's Law

Dr. Constantine Hering (1800–1880), known as the father of American homeopathy, proposed a homeopathic principle in 1845, now known as Hering's law, to account for these aggravations and to more accurately measure true healing responses:[81]

> Cure proceeds from above downward [head to toe], from inside out [from the most important organs to the least important organs], and in the reverse order of the appearance of symptoms [e.g., a patient would first experience the musculoskeletal healing symptoms from a recent car accident before she would feel the detoxifying effects of living with asthma in her childhood].[82]

Through this law, Hering attempted to describe the appropriate "direction of cure" so that physicians could more accurately interpret whether their patients were truly getting well from the correctly chosen simillimum or if

*However, from time to time, it is desirable to set aside intermediate potencies for storage; therefore, when using Korsakoff's method, the actual number of vials can range from six to eight to make a 200K potency. (G. Vithoulkas, *The Science of Homeopathy* [New York: Grove Press, Inc., 1980], 162.)

they were *proving* an "imperfect" (not-similar-enough) remedy.[83] To this law, Dr. George Vithoulkas, a renowned modern homeopath from Greece, added this corollary in his book, *The Science of Homeopathy:* "Cure proceeds by amelioration on internal planes coupled with the appearance of a discharge or eruption of skin or mucous membranes."[84]

Thus, using the example of the preference pyramid based on Vithoulkas's teachings, it is clear that the best possible response to a remedy is for the system to heal the most vital and essential organs first (the brain, heart, liver, pancreas, etc.), while simultaneously discharging chronic toxic accumulations through the least important organs and tissues (the skin, muscles, teeth, vertebrae, etc.).* This level of hierarchy, or preference, in the body was illustrated in the pyramid figure in chapter 11 (see figure 11.8, page 335).

Moving in the Right Direction

Thus, if after taking a homeopathic remedy a patient reports that she has a rash over her abdomen (skin) and that she experienced a couple of bouts of diarrhea (intestinal mucous membrane), but her chronic depression and fatigue (brain, liver, heart) are greatly diminished, these symptoms would be most heartening to her homeopath and indicative that the prescribed remedy was most probably her simillimum. This direction of cure is also consistent with the principles of drainage outlined in chapter 2, wherein toxins are released through the primary emunctories of the intestine and skin. However, if a patient reports that after taking his new remedy, his eczema (skin) was improved but he was experiencing more severe insomnia (brain or liver) and anxiety (brain), then this would be a disturbing sign that the chosen remedy was acting somewhat suppressively and was therefore probably not the patient's correct simillimum.

Using Hahnemann's miasmic paradigm described in chapter 1,† it is clear that Hering's law charts the correct direction of healing through these four reaction modes. Thus, if a patient's luetic insomnia and anxiety or tuberculinic migraines and exhaustion were greatly reduced, with a concomitant increase in sycotic (nasal congestion and discharge) and psoric (skin rashes) discharges, then this patient is probably moving correctly in the direction of health from the more pathogenic to the least pathogenic miasmic levels. Dr. James Tyler Kent (1849–1916), known as the father of constitutional homeopathy,* perhaps restated this law of the direction of cure most succinctly: "The true homeopathic aggravation I say, is when the symptoms are worse, but the patient says, 'I feel better.'"[85]

Suppressive Allopathic Medicine Moves in the Wrong Direction

Hering's law of cure is important to understand because modern allopathic medicine is based on the opposite tenets of this law. That is, when steroid creams eliminate a skin rash, or anti-inflammatories reduce arthritic pain, these drugs are deemed "curative," and any subsequent depression, fatigue, or anxiety manifesting afterward in a patient is rarely considered at all, or it is considered to be completely unrelated.

A Modern Interpretation of Hering's Law

In recent years, primarily due to the current pandemic use of allopathic drugs (past or present in a patient's history), with their innumerable side effects that can greatly confuse and obscure the homeopathic healing picture, Hering's law has been criticized for not always being replicable.[86] However, Dr. Ahmed Currim, a modern-day homeopath in his third decade of practice, has proposed that according to logic, Hering's law should be read as follows:

Diseases get well:

1. from within outward and/or
2. above downward and/or
3. in the reverse appearance of symptoms.

*Hering's law is consistent with normal physiology. For example, after injury to the skin, new growth always takes place from in to out. In the same way, the internal organs also grow first from the internal aspects and then outward to the external aspects of the organ. (E. Marais, *The Soul of the White Ant* [New York: Productivity Press, 1986], 56.)

†However, the *tubercular* miasm originated from Antoine Nebel's clinical research.

*Dr. Kent introduced the concept of constitutional types and constitutional prescribing, in which both the physical and psychological characteristics of an individual are taken into account before a remedy is prescribed.

Thus, if any *one* of these three conditions is satisfied and the patient gets well, this can be judged as a positive indication of the correct direction of healing and a substantiation of Hering's law. For example, if the patient feels better emotionally and mentally (*from within outward*), but his knee pain improves before his neck pain (**not** *from above downward*), this result could still be a viable example of Hering's law of cure.[87]

Hering's Law Is a Good "Road Map"

In conclusion, as with any linear law applied to a complex system such as the human body and spirit, Hering's law, as well as the four-level miasmic paradigm discussed in chapter 1, should not be interpreted too narrowly but should be used only as a helpful guideline or "road map" to accurately interpret healing. The knowledgeable and experienced homeopath can use these principles to discern the difference between true healing responses, which may include some unpleasant aggravating symptoms, and symptoms that do not indicate healing. These can include uncharacteristic and unusual symptoms arising (*proving* the remedy), adverse responses (suppression of symptoms or moving in the wrong direction of cure), or no response at all (the chosen remedy is so dissimilar that it has no effect and the patient's disease progresses unchecked), which all indicate that the patient's case needs to be reevaluated and a new remedy chosen.

THE SCIENTIFIC BASIS OF HOMEOPATHY

Unfortunately, as many readers will notice, allopathic medicine's opposition to homeopathy (and just as notably chiropractic; see the box at right) has never really ceased, and still continues to this day. One of the most common methods used to discredit all forms of holistic medicine—then and now—has been to label them "unscientific." This charge is particularly ironic in the field of homeopathy in light of the fact that vaccinations, the allopathic modality that bears the closest resemblance to homeopathy, have *never* undergone a single scientific study—that is, placebo-controlled and double-blind,[88] whereas homeopathic remedies have undergone hundreds of scientific controlled trials and been proven significantly efficacious in many of them.[89] Fortunately, there have been a number of books published over the past several decades that have documented homeopathic research and thus refute the prevalent "unscientific" belief about this healing art and science. One outstanding example is the 2002 edition of *The Emerging Science of Homeopathy* by Paolo Bellavite, M.D., and Andrea Signorini, M.D., which is extensively referenced in the following two sections.

THE AMA AND CHIROPRACTIC

In 1976, the chiropractors in the state of Illinois filed suit against the AMA for restraint of trade based on more than *one million* documents that detailed the AMA's plans, actions, and strategies to eliminate the profession of chiropractic. The most infamous, known as the "Taylor memo," dated January 4, 1971, is quoted here:

> Since the AMA board of trustees' decision at its meeting on November 2–3, 1963, to establish a Committee on Quackery, your committee has considered its prime mission to be, first the containment of chiropractic and, ultimately, the elimination of chiropractic.

The Illinois chiropractors won their case, and in a similar suit, the AMA settled in 1981 with the New York attorney general's office out of court. The AMA further reworded its "Principles of Medical Ethics" in 1980 to allow medical doctors to refer a patient to a doctor of chiropractic without fear of discipline or sanctions.[90]

Challenges to Conducting Homeopathic Research

Financial Challenges

One of the primary practical challenges in the field of homeopathy for well over three centuries has been the lack of available research funds. Since the homeopathic colleges were entirely wiped out in the early 1900s and entrepreneurs such as Carnegie and Rockefeller channeled their funding solely into allopathic endeavors, there have been no centralized institutions with the financial wherewithal to sponsor research. Furthermore, from Hahnemann's time up to the present, non-holistically oriented pharmacies and pharmaceutical companies have been antagonistic to this relatively nonprofitable field of healing in which remedies cost only a few dollars and can last for years without the need for refills. Fortunately, since the 1960s, research in homeopathy has been greatly boosted through the support of homeopathic companies that have started financing university institutes (primarily European) or have set up their own research laboratories.[91]

Individualized Prescribing Challenges

Another major challenge specific to homeopathic research is that the remedies are prescribed on a highly individual basis. Thus, while scientists may conclude that a particular brand of antihistamine drug successfully suppresses hay fever symptoms in a significant number of subjects, a single homeopathic remedy may not test as effectively. That is, some of the research subjects may respond to the homeopathic red onion remedy, Allium cepa, whereas other hay fever–prone subjects may need Nux vomica (terrible sneezing and a fluent discharge), Pulsatilla nigricans (a thick, bland nasal discharge), or Arsenicum album (an acrid, watery discharge similar to that of Allium, but worse on the right side and often burning). Thus, because homeopathy treats the patient and not the disease, setting up an appropriate research design to accurately determine the effectiveness of remedies can be much more complex than testing out a new pharmaceutical drug.

For this reason, the most profound and dramatic successes of homeopathic prescribing have been seen during epidemics when large groups of people are afflicted with similar symptoms and a single remedy can be prescribed for the majority of those suffering from the same disease.[92] This was the case with the earlier examples of the typhus and cholera epidemics that were successfully treated in France, London, and Cincinnati. In one particularly well-conducted study (double-blind and placebo-controlled) in London from 1941 to 1942, homeopathy was found to be "statistically significant" for the treatment of burns from mustard gas.[93]

Homeopathic Research Studies

Homeopathy Significantly Reduces Muscle and Joint Pain

In order to address this need to individualize homeopathic remedies, a study conducted by the department of rheumatology at St. Bartholomew's Hospital in London on fibrositis (primary fibromyalgia) was the first to utilize a homeopathic history-taking method. The subjects selected to participate all had symptoms indicative of Rhus toxicodendron 6C, a classic remedy most often prescribed for this syndrome. After this trial was conducted using standard scientific testing protocols (double-blind, placebo-controlled, with a cross-over design method), results showed that the homeopathic remedy significantly reduced the subjects' muscular pain symptoms. In a similar trial studying rheumatoid arthritis symptoms in the Glasgow Homeopathic Hospital in Scotland, half the patients received their own prescribed remedy and half were treated with placebo. Again, the results measured by reduced pain, articular index (joint function), and stiffness showed a positive 82 percent improvement in the patients treated with their homeopathic remedy versus only 21 percent in the patients who received a placebo (sugar pill).[94]

> **fibrositis/fibromyalgia:** *Fibrositis* is the term used to describe acute inflammation and pain in the soft fibrous tissues—the muscles, tendons, and ligaments; *fibromyalgia* is the term for the more chronic condition, also accompanied by fatigue, sleep disorders, and flulike symptoms.

Homeopathy Effective in a Wide Range of Illnesses

Homeopathic research has not been confined only to the field of rheumatology. Homeopathic remedies are responsible for significant improvements in various syndromes such as migraine headaches, skin burns, diarrhea, influenza, and allergies. For example, in a Dutch study published by the *British Medical Journal* that rigorously reviewed 107 different homeopathic trials, 81 percent of these research studies yielded positive results as compared with taking a placebo. These 107 homeopathic studies covered a wide range of illnesses including the treatment of cardiovascular disease, respiratory infections, gastrointestinal diseases, hay fever, pain and/or trauma, and psychological syndromes.[95]

Homeopathy in Dentistry

Homeopathic remedies have also proved efficacious in the dental field. In a double-blind study conducted on patients with acute dental neuralgia (nerve pain) after tooth extraction, 76 percent experienced pain relief from either Arnica montana or Hypericum perforatum (St. John's wort), as compared with only 40 percent of the subjects who were on the placebo.[96]

Homeopathy Shown to Be Effective in Animal Studies

Homeopathy has also been tested on animals in veterinary medicine. For example, the remedy Sepia succus 200C, classically used to alleviate menstrual and pregnancy symptoms, has been shown to significantly reduce the number of typical postpartum complications in dairy cows after giving birth. In an experimental study, mice that had been subject to damaging radiation (100–200 rad) were "spectacularly" protected from these sublethal X-ray doses by taking remedies with radioprotective effects such as Ruta graveolens and Panax ginseng before and after radiation exposure.[97]

These and other well-conducted animal studies refute the common charge that homeopathic remedies act only through a positive placebo effect based on a patient's mental and emotional susceptibility. "Although a certain amount of suggestion is also possible in animals, it seems somewhat unlikely that simple psychological support measures can heal an abscess in a cat, skin disorders in a horse or mastitis in a dairy cow, and that this should be observed not just once in a blue moon, but repeatedly."[98]

The Negative Placebo Effect

The original Latin term *placebo* literally means "I shall please." Thus, when patients respect and trust their physician and unconsciously want to please him or her, even a placebo (sugar pill) can be highly effective in reducing their symptoms. So effective, in fact, that in one study placebos were almost as effective in reducing pain as the strongest pain analgesic of all—morphine.[99]*

However, in many cases homeopathic as well as other holistic practitioners battle the opposite effect, what might be termed a *negative placebo effect,* which can negatively affect the outcome of even a correctly prescribed remedy or treatment. This skeptical and pessimistic attitude toward natural medicine primarily stems from the pervasive allopathically influenced media that touts the use of prescription drugs and is further compounded by the nearly complete dearth of reporting on the success of homeopathic remedies (as well as other holistic modalities) in the media. Thus, the majority of the public still views "alternative" practitioners in a highly dubious light.

> **negative placebo effect:** The term for negative changes because of placebo therapy is called *nocebo.* However, I am using *negative placebo effect* to describe the generalized negative attitude still existing in many patients' minds even today about the effectiveness of their holistic practitioner's treatment.

Indeed, every homeopath knows well the negative vibe emanating from a skeptical husband dragged into the office by his wife, or the amused "scientifically oriented" new patient who claims to have come in primarily as a lark. This attitude of "I don't think this is going to work but I'll give it a try" (especially in less progressive parts of the country) can be psychologically debilitating over time to holistic practitioners. Furthermore, even when the correctly prescribed remedy does work, these skeptical patients often find it too egoically challenging to acknowledge that their symptoms were reduced or cleared through the auspices of an "alternative" practitioner. They typically attribute their healing to other factors (e.g., a change of diet, attitude, or exercise). Thus, this negative placebo attitude impairs the doctor-patient relationship even when the homeopathic remedy is effective, because it commonly results in the patient not returning for needed follow-up visits. After months or years, even the most perfectly fitting simillimum needs to be re-dosed to continue to be effective.

This negative placebo effect can also be greatly magnified when a practitioner does not exemplify the classic upper-class successful white male image that Madison Avenue has so vigorously sold to the public. Thus, it can double if a holistic physician is not associated with a modern clinic or hospital, triple if the practitioner is also a woman, and quadruple if she belongs

*In other studies, placebos have performed "comparably to, and sometimes better than, antidepressants," leading Richard DeGrandpre, the editor of the Vancouver-based magazine *Adbusters,* to bluntly state "the psychiatric drug industry is a sham." Based on these findings, *Adbusters* has recently announced plans to sell Placebo, a sugar pill with "minimal side effects, and a cost of mere pennies a dose." (L. Marsa, "Sleep for Sale: Get Ready for the Next Big Pharma Ad Blitz," *Mother Jones,* January/February 2005, 20.)

to a racial or ethnic minority. Thankfully, these attitudes and prejudices are changing as the public becomes more enlightened about other cultures and religions, as well as the various specialties in holistic medicine.

► For more information on the placebo effect, see Dr. Peter Bennett's article, "Placebo and Healing," in the *Textbook of Natural Medicine,* vol. I, by J. Pizzorno and M. Murray.

Quantum Physics' Research Validates High-Potency Remedies

Another positive aspect of modern-day knowledge on homeopathy is that the twentieth-century field of quantum physics—researched by such pioneers as Erwin Schrödinger, Werner Heisenberg, and Niels Bohr—has now proven the feasibility as well as the effectiveness of ultra-high homeopathic potencies. Thus, homeopathic potencies past Avogadro's number (e.g., 24X and 12C) have now been well proven in various research studies to have real physical effects, even when there are no actual physical molecules of the original plant, animal, or mineral remaining in the remedy. For example, in a 1966 study it was found that high dilutions (60X and 20M) of Sulphur, a common homeopathic remedy, had a significant effect on the growth of onions, as well as notably increasing their calcium, magnesium, potassium, and sodium content. In another experimental study that utilized high dilutions (up to 400X) of Arsenicum album, another common homeopathic remedy, there was a four times greater reduction in the death rate in a strain of fruit flies.[100] Besides these and other botanical and zoological experiments, studies conducted on humans and human tissues have also yielded significant results. For example, in several studies the remedy Apis mellifica significantly inhibited allergy responses (basophil degranulation, increased IgE production, etc.), even in high and ultra-high potencies (from 15C up to MM potencies).[101]

Homeopathy Consistent with Modern Holistic Medical Thinking

It is interesting to note that the centuries-old field of homeopathy is completely compatible with many of the emerging new frontiers of energetic medicine, in which disease is regarded not simply as a functional or structural abnormality but as a disturbance in the entire network of electromagnetic communication among elements (molecules, nerves, organs, etc.). This network of "information signaling systems," which was researched by the German biophysicist Fritz-Albert Popp, is the oldest communication system in our bodies, first developed in our ancestors millennia ago, evolving from earlier primordial organisms.[102] Thus, perhaps one reason why subtle energy medicines like homeopathy can effect such profound cures is that they resonate in some way with these ancient signaling systems and modify the ancestral "hardwired" patterns that have been transmitted for generations. This resonance paradigm helps explain in part the astounding phenomenon that can occur when a well-matched homeopathic simillimum causes dramatic transformations in an individual's physical, mental, emotional, and even spiritual well-being. In these cases, it can seem as if patients are literally reborn—free of the draining effects of their negative ancestral inheritance, and possibly even released from the negative karmic patterns of previous lifetimes.

THE INTERNECINE BATTLES AMONG HOMEOPATHS

Low Potency vs. High Potency Prescribers

As discussed in the previous section, modern quantum physics' research has only recently (since the relatively recent 1960s) begun to validate the use of high-potency remedies—that is, exceeding 24X, 12C, or LM4. Thus, many early homeopathic practitioners who utilized these "unproven" higher potencies—from Hahnemann on down—were often ridiculed as "being on a par with some kind of esoteric sect."[103] This caused a major schism in homeopathic circles that eventually came to be known as the split between the *low potency* and *high potency* prescribers.[104] Unfortunately for homeopaths and their profession, this internal acrimony within their own ranks was just as divisive and damaging as the attacks they experienced from their allopathic colleagues.

Higher Potencies Prescribed for Mental and Emotional Symptoms

This discord reached its zenith in the United States through the influence of the great American homeopath James Tyler Kent (1849–1916). Like Hahnemann, Kent believed that potencies of 200C or higher were often necessary to bring about a complete cure.[105] Influenced

THE ROLE OF WATER

One of the primary explanations for the action of these high dilutions is that the aqueous or water-alcohol solution* in a homeopathic remedy both "remembers" and stores the molecular imprint of the original plant, animal, or mineral substance. This memory of water theory was first proposed and later developed through the extensive research of French scientist Jacques Benveniste.[106] Although some have strongly criticized Benveniste's conclusions,† numerous other scientists have duplicated both his research findings and his conclusions.[107] A simple example of this "water memory" is the fact that ice cubes remain stable for a period of time at room temperature, demonstrating that there "exists in water a property which enables it to 'remember' for a certain amount of time that it has been kept in the freezer."[108]

This memory capability of water is also well known to chemists, who have observed that when a given compound is dissolved in water, the compound "informs" the collection of water molecules near to it and organizes them in such a way that they take on a configuration that reflects the compound itself.[109]‡ These water molecule configurations, referred to as *water clusters* or *IE crystals*, create incredibly stable electrical fields that have been shown to demonstrate unique biological effects. In fact, in one Italian study in which the researchers conducted over 500 experiments, homeopathic dilutions both below and above Avogadro's number (from 1C to 30C) proved significantly different from placebo dilutions 92 percent of the time.[110]

In the preparation of homeopathic remedies, the molecular transfer of information from the solute (the original plant, animal, or mineral substance) to the solvent (the alcohol and water solution) is greatly enhanced by the succussion of the remedy at each level of dilution. This shaking or succussion action is believed to communicate an "excess" of information to the molecules in the water.[111]

This "meta-molecular" transfer of information from the original plant, animal, or mineral substance to the water solution has been proposed to be the same mechanism that occurs when the homeopathic remedy is ingested by the patient. Furthermore, water, which is the natural medium of all cells, has been proven to not only conduct frequencies in all biological processes—cell division, protein replication, bone growth, and so forth—but also to *amplify* the signals that it receives and sends throughout the body.[112] Thus, these subtle electromagnetic signals that maintain homeostasis in the body are profoundly affected by all frequencies, and most significantly by the subtle resonances contained in the rarefied electromagnetic fields (EMFs) of homeopathic remedies.[113] In Lynne McTaggart's book *The Field,* she describes the functions of our EMFs as "responsible for our mind's highest functions, the information source guiding the growth of our bodies . . . [and] the force, rather than germs or genes, that finally determines whether we are healthy or ill, the force which must be tapped in order to heal." Einstein once characterized this phenomena most succinctly by stating that "the field is the only reality."[114]

It has been postulated that the "coherent vibrations" in the water in homeopathic remedies resonate with the noncoherent and discordant frequencies in the watery medium in our bodies. That is, the disturbing plantlike, animal-like, or mineral-like signals causing ill health in our bodies recognize and resonate with the plantlike, animal-like, or mineral-like signals in the homeopathic remedy, and these two similar

*In a remedy, alcohol is added to the water to preserve the solution and to thwart mold growth. (Globules and tablets are moistened with this alcohol-water solution; thus, they also last for years.)

†An inspection was organized of Benveniste's laboratory by the publisher of his original scientific article, the journal *Nature*, which consisted of a magician, a journalist, and an expert in statistics. After witnessing a number of experiments for only a week, this "scientific" panel wrote a very negative report. Benveniste's studies have since been replicated in over twenty studies in independent labs in France and other countries. For the most comprehensive information on this modern-day "witch hunt" that tried to refute Benveniste's findings, read pages 60 through 73 in Lynne McTaggart's book *The Field*.

‡These findings demonstrate why it's vital to have an effective water filtration unit in your home, because toxic chemicals and metals also hold memory in water. Radiant Life (888) 593-8333 has an excellent reverse-osmosis water filtration system that was originated by Dennis Higgins, M.D., who has been researching water for more than two decades.

frequencies can then begin to cancel each other out. This has been proposed to occur through the slightly stronger resonance of the homeopathic remedy communicating with the similar but slightly weaker resonance of the disturbing signals in the body, facilitating the dissolution of this latter discordant and "nonhuman" pattern of dysfunction. Hahnemann correctly described this phenomenon centuries before in a more poetic manner when he referred to disease as a "morbid mistunement" and to homeopathic remedies as "tunement-altering energies . . . acting upon our spirit-like force."[115] In homeopathy, healing occurs when, after ingestion of the remedy, this discordant yoke of chronic energetic disturbance is gradually removed and dissipated, and the organism is able to move from general disorder to increasingly coherent functioning. When this increasing coherency and clarity is experienced at all levels, individuals are able to function more optimally and begin to more fully actualize their own unique human potential.

by the Swedish scientist Emmanuel Swedenborg, Kent placed primary importance on the mental and emotional symptoms in a patient's case, while he considered the general (temperature, right- or left-sidedness, burning, etc.) and physical symptoms secondary. In what later came to be referred to as Kentian homeopathy, disturbance of these "higher" mental-emotional planes required the use of higher potencies, ranging from 200C up to 10M.[116] This principle, originally proposed by Hahnemann and elaborated on by Kent, that higher potencies are more appropriate for patients suffering on the mental and emotional planes and that the lower potencies are more suitable for treating physical symptoms continues to this day to be a primary tenet in modern homeopathy.*

EMMANUEL SWEDENBORG AND THE SWEDENBORGIANS

Emmanuel Swedenborg (1688–1772) was a Swedish scientist and inventor. After a religious vision in 1734, he undertook a new profession as a "seer of divine wisdom." From that time until his death at age 84, he devoted himself to spiritual studies, teaching, and writing. Many of the great homeopaths were Swedenborgians, including Hering, Farrington, Holcombe, and most notably Kent. In fact, Kent decided to arrange his famous repertory based on the Swedenborgian principle of "from above downward." The writings of Swedenborg became one of the major foundations of the Theosophy religion a century later.[117]

*Since Hahnemann's sixth edition was not published until five years after Kent's death, Kent was not privy to Hahnemann's "far more perfect" LM potencies, which had the benefit of being powerful high-potency remedies but at the same time being the gentlest and mildest in action.

Schism Broader than Simply Choice of Potency

However, this schism among homeopathic prescribers was centered not simply on the controversy of the level of potencies—especially since the "Highs" readily used low potencies when they were appropriate and the "Lows" were known to use high potencies at various times—but on far broader issues.[118]

Pathology-Based Prescribing vs. Individualized Prescribing

In general, the Lows, wanting to be more accepted by their allopathic colleagues, more often chose remedies based on pathology rather than on the individual patient's particular symptoms, while the Highs followed Hahnemann's teachings assiduously. Thus, the Highs maintained that the highly diluted remedy contained a stronger medicinal power to treat the deepest cause of disease—the disturbance in one's spirit—which required individualized, not simply pathology-based, case taking (history taking).[119] The following quote by Kent describes this concept of health and healing:

> There is no disease that exists of which the cause is known to man by the eye or by the microscope. Causes are infinitely too fine to be observed by any instrument of precision. They are so immaterial that they correspond to and operate upon the interior nature of man, and they are ultimated in the body in [the] form of tissue changes that are recognized by the eye. Such tissue changes must be understood as the results of disease only or the physician will never perceive what disease cause is, what

> disease is, what potentization is, or what the nature of life is.[120]

Differing Viewpoints on the Theory of Potentization

Many of the Lows, however, denied the theory of potentization and called it a "fanciful creation of Hahnemann" and an unsound "form of medical spiritualism." Furthermore, by choosing homeopathic remedies based on pathology rather than on the individual patient, the Lows greatly reduced the hundreds of possible homeopathic remedy choices in a patient's particular case to an easier-to-manage twenty to thirty remedies.[121] Additionally, to further simplify prescribing, many physicians and pharmacies began to mix homeopathic medicines together to form combination remedies.

"Lows" Prescribed More Allopathically

Prescribing in this more allopathic manner greatly streamlined history taking and case analysis—and yielded exceptional economic benefits. Thus, instead of two or more hours spent taking a patient's case and then analyzing the symptoms to arrive at the most perfect simillimum, many of the Lows realized that through spending less time on each case, they could see substantially more patients and enjoy significantly increased financial success. The Lows were also able to satisfy a growing number of patients who, after witnessing the action of suppressive allopathic drugs, often demanded immediate results for palliation of their symptoms. Furthermore, many Lows who sincerely wanted to heal the sick had become discouraged at the sheer difficulty of finding the correct remedy in homeopathy, especially since many of the earlier texts in the nineteenth century were inferior to the later published texts.[122]

"Highs" Characterized "Lows" as "Half Homeopaths"

The tension between the pure Hahnemannians and the rest of the homeopathic profession came to a head in 1870 when the Highs excluded the Lows from membership in their institute.[123] The Highs charged these "half homeopaths" with adulterating Hahnemann's law of similars by choosing remedies similar to a patient's disease state and not to the patient's unique symptoms. Although this practice was entirely consistent with the growing belief in Pasteur's germ theory of disease, it was entirely inconsistent with Hahnemann's law of similars and his belief in treating the patient's "mistuned" vital force rather than any disease label. Additionally, the growing practice of mixing several remedies together was a further refutation of another of Hahnemann's laws—that of the use of a single remedy at a time.

Hahnemann argued that single medicines are the only ones that have been fully proven; furthermore, it is impossible to predict how two or more remedies will alter each other's actions and effects on the body. Hahnemann, never a man to mince words, wrote about this subject in 1808:

> This motley mixing system is nothing but a convenient make-shift for one who, having but a slender acquaintance with the properties of a single substance, flatters himself, though he cannot find any one simple suitable remedy to remove the complaint, that by combining a great many there may be one amongst them that by a happy chance shall hit the mark."[124]

"Lows" Ridiculed "Highs" as Cultish

The Lows counteracted these charges by criticizing the Highs for being too rigid and dogmatic and having no tolerance for any new ideas formulated since Hahnemann's time. Furthermore, many of the Highs' religious-like fervor and ties to an unorthodox religion (Kent, Hering, Farrington, and other leaders were Swedenborgians) made them an easy target for ridicule, so they were often branded as unscientific and cultish. As discussed earlier, these nineteenth- and early-twentieth-century internecine battles greatly weakened the homeopathic profession, leaving homeopaths vulnerable to competing allopaths and the AMA, and eventually led to their near-extinction in the United States by the mid-1950s.

The Present

Knowledgeable readers will note that many of these controversies in homeopathy have still not been resolved. For example, anyone who has ever gone to a health food store desperate for a cold or flu remedy is aware that combination, or *complex,* homeopathic remedies are presently made in great abundance. In fact, many holistic practitioners prescribe combination remedies or use more than one homeopathic remedy at a time. To further add to this controversy as well as to patients' confusion, many various remedies—from combination remedies to nosodes to autohemotherapy (e.g., remedies made from the patient's own potentized blood)—are all included under the broad umbrella of homeopathy. It is particularly divisive among practitioners and confusing to patients when strict modern-day classical homeopaths (previously referred to as Highs)* not only legitimately restrict their patients from taking other possibly interfering remedies but also do not recognize the need for any other treatments such as the removal of mercury amalgam fillings or the treatment of chronic foci.

The primary problem—then and now—is due to a lack of understanding on both sides. This issue will be addressed through the explanation of three concepts in the following sections: acute versus chronic homeopathic prescribing, the subject of antidoting a homeopathic remedy, and modern-day obstacles to cure.

HOMEOPATHIC PRESCRIBING

Homeopathic prescribing is divided into two categories—*acute* prescribing and *chronic* (or *constitutional*) prescribing. As previously mentioned, in medicine, *acute* refers to the recent onset of illness, which lasts for a shorter period and is less deep-seated than in the case of *chronic,* or long-lasting, disease. Acute illnesses, although usually lasting only for a few days or weeks, can be relatively severe in action, such as when one succumbs to the influenza "going around" or experiences painful gastroenteritis (diarrhea) after a trip to Mexico.

Acute Homeopathic Prescribing

In these and other emergency situations, homeopaths take briefer case histories and prescribe remedies based both on the outstanding pathology and the patient's unique symptoms. Hahnemann, being a practical-minded physician, realized that since individual case taking could be a laborious and time-consuming pursuit, it was often not appropriate in the face of severe, acute disease when time was a crucial factor.[125] Nor, for that matter, is individual case taking always necessary in cases when the noxious agent is extremely intense. For example, in World War II, everyone in Hiroshima and Nagasaki would have required Radium bromatum (homeopathic radiation) after the nuclear explosions, and then later each would have needed an individualized constitutional remedy to address their own personal responses to the bombing—shock, fear, depression, anxiety, exhaustion, and so forth.

This method of prescribing was common in the eighteenth and nineteenth centuries in cases of widespread acute disease or contagions—that is, during epidemics. Hahnemann himself was the first to successfully prescribe Atropa belladonna as both a preventive and a curative remedy for scarlet fever in 1801.[126] This type of prescribing is termed *genus* or *genus epidemicus* prescribing.[127] Thus, when a large group is afflicted with the same acute and powerful disease, the combined symptoms can be sufficient to find the *epidemic simillimum,* which is often more appropriate than taking (valuable) time repertorizing each individual's case. Later, in 1835, Hahnemann recommended the use of camphor (Laurus camphor) as both preventive and curative for the violently acute disease of Asiatic cholera. Camphor so greatly reduced deaths that its price skyrocketed in France. It was later included in allopathic medical handbooks for its "almost magical effect" in the treatment of cholera.[128] Hahnemann recognized that many of these epidemic diseases were actually manifestations of acute miasms, particularly psora, and that individuals succumbing to these diseases that had their own particular nature and were of the same origin could often be treated with the same remedy. However, he also always took into mind each of his patient's individual reactions to these epidemic illnesses when there was time to take the case history. In fact, he noticed over time that Atropa belladonna, and later Aconitum napellus, were both no longer suitable for later cases of scarlet fever in which the nature of the symptoms had changed.[129]

Therefore, when time is vital during acute illnesses, most modern-day homeopaths condone the use of a self-prescribed single or combination remedy bought at the health food store when their patients are suffering and are unable to reach them. However, if the patient is able

*Note, however, that whether a modern-day homeopath prescribes a low-potency 6C or a high-potency 1M has nothing to do with his or her homeopathic philosophy. The terms *High* and *Low* had a specific connotation only in the nineteenth and early twentieth centuries.

to make contact, the homeopathic practitioner will usually do one of two things. First, if the patient is on a constitutional remedy already, the homeopath will often suggest that she re-dose her remedy. In many cases, this change is sufficient to animate the vital force and thus stimulate the patient's immune system to adequately fight off the acute infection. However, if this is not helpful after a few hours or a day, or if the noxious agent is extreme (e.g., radiation poisoning or a toxic chemical spill), or if the patient is not yet on her constitutional remedy, then the homeopath will take a brief case (over the phone or in the office) and prescribe an acute homeopathic remedy.

Chronic (or Constitutional) Homeopathic Prescribing

In the case of *chronic* disease that comes on gradually and dissipates a patient's energy and health slowly over time, however, neither combination homeopathic remedies nor single remedies that are self-prescribed or prescribed by a practitioner who has not studied homeopathy extensively have been proven to be efficacious. That is, they have rarely had any long-term curative effect. Chronic dysfunction and disease are best treated through *constitutional homeopathy*—that is, by a single homeopathic remedy prescribed for a patient's overall mental, emotional, and physical disturbances. In these cases, the most successful homeopaths adhere strictly to Hahnemannian principles, taking a lengthy history (case), analyzing the case in depth through referencing homeopathic materia medicas and repertories, and prescribing a single homeopathic remedy at the appropriate level of potency (-ies).*

One may wonder why more practitioners don't practice this curative field of healing. The primary reason is that constitutional homeopathy is absolutely the *most* complex and challenging field to learn in all of holistic medicine. Since at any one time there is only one correct remedy out of thousands—actually millions—it "imposes a very heavy responsibility upon the physician" to be skillful and knowledgeable enough to find each patient's simillimum in a timely fashion.[130] Homeopathic practitioners therefore must commit years to learning this challenging art and science, and since new remedies are being discovered every day, this learning never ends. Homeopathy can be so challenging, in fact, that even leading practitioners do not always find the patient's most appropriate remedy on the first try, but may require two, three, or even more homeopathic interviews to accurately determine the simillimum.[131] Thus, it is understandable why classically trained homeopaths become angry and can seem even dogmatically positioned when remedies are carelessly prescribed without an adequate case taking (homeopathic history), or without thorough analysis of a patient's case, by practitioners with no formal homeopathic training.

In conclusion, in acute illnesses or emergencies, or when an individual is not under the care of a qualified homeopath, low-potency single remedies (e.g., 6C or 30C) or combination remedies can be appropriate and sometimes remarkably healing—for example, the widespread use of Arnica montana after injuries or surgeries. However, constitutional homeopathy for long-term chronic dysfunction or illness should be left up to qualified practitioners who have devoted their lives to this challenging but curative field of medicine.

The New "Sankaran System"

A new and unique method of determining the correct remedy in the field of constitutional homeopathy has emerged over the past few years from Dr. Rajan Sankaran and his colleagues in Mumbai, India.* Sankaran, who graduated first in his class from the Bombay Homeopathic Medical College, has written over a dozen books on homeopathy and lectured internationally since 1986. Beginning in 1990, he began to teach that homeopathic remedies could be classified, and therefore more fully understood, according to their kingdom—that is, the plant, animal, or mineral

*Often nowadays, with so many antidoting factors (plane travel, toxic chemicals, coffee consumption, etc.), homeopaths prescribe "daily doses" (e.g., 6C or 12C) or "booster doses" (e.g., LM1 or higher) to guarantee that the resonance of the initial single constitutional dose (e.g., 200C or K or higher) is not disturbed.

*The Mumbai school is ever-expanding, but currently is made up of the following doctors: Rajan Sankaran, Jayesh Shah, Sujit Chatterjee, Divya Chhabra, Sunil Anand, Sudhir Baldota, Shachindra Joshi, and Bhawisha Joshi.

kingdom.[132] Furthermore—and quite similar to several current in-depth and effective psychological schools of healing (rebirthing, somato-emotional release, somatic experiencing, etc.)—Sankaran found that the "vital sensation"—that is, the deepest feeling sense of the patient, even beyond the mind and emotions—can most accurately identify the patient's central pattern of disturbance.

> **vital:** The word *vital,* in the context of the "vital sensation," refers to "the animating force, power, or principle present in all living things," rather than the common use of referring to things or people who are "full of life or energy"—that is, quite energetic and lively.[133]

By combining these two revelations, Sankaran found that a patient who needs a plant remedy lives with the vital sensation of a particular disturbance and feels vulnerable to it; that a patient who needs a mineral remedy has a chronic underlying sense of the need for structure and feels the incompleteness and lack of this structure; and that a patient who needs an animal remedy has issues surrounding survival and feeling like a victim (prey) or aggressor (predator). However, through the prescription of the correct homeopathic remedy, this overlying plant, mineral, or animal energy can be effectively released over time, freeing patients to become more fully human (and *not* plantlike, mineral-like, or animal-like), and thus capable of actualizing their own individual potential.

The "Other Song"

Sankaran describes this overlay of a nonhuman (plant, animal, or mineral) sensation or energy existing in patients as their "other song":

> If we pay attention to the energy in the case, we will realize that its pattern is similar to that of a plant/animal/mineral source in nature. Thus, it is completely out of place in the human being. The result is turmoil. This can be compared to two songs or melodies playing synchronously within us: one human and the other non-human. Most of the time the human melody plays louder and so is more audible; homeopathically speaking this can be translated as common emotions, aspirations, perceptions, struggles of all human beings. But time and again, from the background, the strains of a non-human melody surface. These represent what is "non-human specific" in man, the source of his inner turmoil.[134]

▶ Dr. Sankaran has most clearly described this amazingly curative phenomenon in his book *The Other Song: Discovering Your Parallel Self.*

The deepest inner conflict of individuals—that is, their disease—arises from the spirit of this nonhuman source that lives within them, which colors and clouds all of their human experiences. This is not to say that there is anything wrong with the plant, animal, or mineral "melody" it simply is not appropriate and creates disharmony in a human being. For example, a lion is a beautiful and majestic animal. However, the song of the lion is not harmonious in a human being and creates dissonance and stress in an individual's life when he behaves at times like this aggressive animal. Sankaran clarified his understanding of this underlying pattern or sensation:

> One melody is human and is in its proper place. The other melody, although also beautiful, is simply out of place inside the human being. Thus, these two voices sing together—what cacophony! This disharmony can be called "conflict" or "stress" in everyday parlance. . . . The non-human song has to be diluted till it ultimately fades and ceases and only the human melody is heard. This is the job of the remedy.[135]

The question that comes to many people's minds is, how did this "other song"—that is, other plant, animal, or mineral spirit—come to reside in us? Although ultimately this is a mystery, Sankaran suggests that this other energy pattern is "borrowed" during particularly stressful times in order to help us cope.[136] This strategy of survival may derive from inherited (miasmic) patterns, from what Carl Jung referred to as our archetypal unconscious, from past incarnations (past lives), or from all these influences. Whatever the derivation, this phenomenon has proven to be universal, as witnessed by the superlative clinical results gained when these plant/

animal/mineral "songs" are cleared through the prescription of the correct remedy by Sankaran-trained homeopaths worldwide.

Case Taking with a Nonhuman Focus and Six New Miasms

In order to identify which one of the thousands—actually millions—of possible plant, animal, or mineral remedies is needed for a particular patient, Sankaran pioneered a new way of case taking that involves a different way of listening and determining the appropriate remedy. In contrast to the classical method of listing all of the patient's symptoms and then rather mechanically categorizing them, Sankaran has found that the remedy can be found by listening to the more unconscious strains of the patient's pattern—demonstrated by words and gestures that are not distinct to humans. Through this specific nonhuman focus, a knowledgeable homeopath can ascertain which of the kingdoms the patient is speaking from, as well as from which of the subkingdoms the needed remedy should be chosen. For example, a patient describing a sensitivity and vulnerability that triggers the sensations of feeling tight, stiff, stuck, and caught with the desire to move is describing sensations from the Anacardiaceae, or poison ivy, family.[137]

To further help identify the correct remedy, Sankaran has researched and elaborated on six more miasmic levels, other than the four described in chapter 1, to differentiate among remedies that may seem similar but have different levels of energy, reactivity, and hope or desperation.* For instance, in the previous Anacardiaceae plant family example, if this patient additionally relates that when she feels tight, stiff, and stuck, she tries desperately to gain control over the situation, she is expressing aspects of the cancer miasm, indicating the need for the remedy Anacardium orientale.

*While these additional miasmic categories are extremely helpful to homeopathic practitioners, the four-miasm paradigm described in chapter 1 is an excellent model for use between patients and doctors. Through the four-miasm model, practitioners can determine the level of dysfunction and disease in their patients during the initial history taking, as well as note their progress back to healthy functioning through appropriate treatment.

"The Greatest Thing Since Hahnemann!"

Through correlating a patient's miasmic level with the appropriate kingdom (plant, animal, or mineral) and subkingdom (e.g., plant family), combined with a new, detailed, and specific case-taking interview method, this system enables homeopaths to find the correct simillimum much more consistently and accurately than ever before. Dr. Jeff Baker, who has practiced homeopathy for more than twenty-five years, describes in the journal *Homeopathic Links* the benefits of using the Sankaran system over the previous classical method that tended to be "woefully inadequate and inconsistent":[138]

> I now firmly believe that the fault or weakness [in the older classical method] lies in the fact that human phenomena are being given weight. Whereas in the new method, it is the non-human (not exclusive to the domain of humans), universal phenomena [that become] the basis for understanding and prescribing. Dr. Sankaran refers to these as "vital sensations."[139]

Many other experienced homeopaths have also confessed that compared with their past repertorization style in trying to find the correct remedy, Sankaran's system has truly revolutionized their practice. In fact, one student who has been a teacher of homeopathy himself for many years declared in one class that Sankaran's method is so effective that it is "the greatest thing since Hahnemann!"

It should be noted, however, that the Sankaran system requires in-depth study and years of clinical experience to master. Thus, all practitioners interested in learning this method should realize the commitment to thorough training that is required in mastering this complex but very curative and exceptionally satisfying field of study.

► Practitioners interested in Sankaran's courses given worldwide should visit his website at www.rajansankaran.com. For information on the school that teaches the Sankaran system in America, contact the California Center for Homeopathic Education at (760) 466-7581, or go to www.cchomeopathic.com.

Antidoting: When the Action of the Homeopathic Remedy Is Disturbed

Combination homeopathic remedies, as well as other factors, have the potential to *antidote* a constitutional remedy—that is, neutralize or counteract its effects. When a homeopathic remedy is antidoted, the healing effect it had in the patient's body diminishes and can eventually be entirely lost. Other major antidotes include strong scents (essential oils, perfume, fresh paint, coffee, etc.), disturbing electromagnetic influences (X-rays, CAT scans, MRIs, plane travel, etc.), and strong vibrations such as dental drilling.

> **antidote:** An antidote is a substance or other agent that has the potential to disrupt your homeopathic remedy.

A Controversial Subject

The issue of antidoting is another divisive factor existing between classical homeopaths and less-classical homeopaths as well as other holistic practitioners. On the one hand, it is true that other homeopathic remedies—single as well as combination formulas—can extinguish the action of the homeopathic resonance and should be avoided when patients are on a constitutional remedy. On the other hand, other holistic practitioners often become frustrated at the excessively long list of factors that some highly orthodox homeopaths insist that patients must avoid. These can include such seemingly benign treatments as herbal remedies, spinal adjustments, and even massage. In fact, these homeopathic restrictions can appear too rigid to patients as well as to other healthcare practitioners. However, homeopaths counter that the many other treatments "doctor-hopping" patients may receive make it exceedingly difficult to determine whether the constitutional remedy is working or has been antidoted, or if another treatment affected subsequent reports of improving or worsening health. This chronic conflict between classical homeopaths and other practitioners fosters ill feelings on both sides and is not unlike the hostilities between the Highs and Lows in the nineteenth century. However, if each camp understood more about the other, there would be considerably less animosity.

Antidoting Agents

There are two important factors to keep in mind on the subject of antidoting: the strength of the antidoting agent and the sensitivity of the patient. The strength of the antidoting agent is dependent on two primary factors—the power, intensity, or toxicity of the agent (e.g., toxic paint vs. "cleaner" VOC-free paint)* and the length of exposure (e.g., living in a newly painted house vs. simply walking through that house). Dr. Jeff Lester, a leading homeopathic physician and educator practicing in central California, has developed a list of possible antidotes and rated them according to their antidoting strength by the percentage of likelihood that a remedy will be antidoted from exposure to the agent (see table 14.1).[140†] For example, inhaling a strong essential oil such as camphor is a major antidoting factor and stands a 90 percent chance of neutralizing a homeopathic remedy. On the other hand, acupuncture treatments may or may not antidote a remedy and are listed as "30 percenters." The antidoting disturbance may occur within hours to weeks after exposure, depending on individual sensitivity. If you suspect you have antidoted your remedy, contact your homeopathic practitioner. It may be necessary to re-dose your constitutional remedy.

▶ To contact Dr. Jeff Lester, call his office in Watsonville, California, at (831) 724-1164, or go to www.lesterclinic.com.

The Sensitivity of the Patient

The capability of another medicine or disturbing agent to antidote a patient's homeopathic remedy is also based on another important factor—the patient's sensitivity. Hahnemann observed centuries before our present-day epidemic population of environmentally ill and highly sensitive patients that individuals had different responses to the same medicine. He wrote in his *Organon* that the response of sensitive or "fine-feeling" patients to homeopathy could respond "one thousand times greater than that of the most unreceptive ones."[141]

*VOC stands for "volatile organic compounds," which are normally found in paints and are toxic petrochemical distillates of solvents.

†Table 14.1 was adapted from Dr. Jeff Lester's patient handout; certain modifications were made based on my professional experience.

TABLE 14.1. ANTIDOTE RANKINGS

Possible Antidote	Neutralizing Strength
Strong essential oils (e.g., camphor, eucalyptus, etc.)*	90%
House paints, solvents, and pesticides (especially very toxic ones)	70%
Dental drilling	70%
Cigarette and marijuana smoking	60%
Coffee (the aroma)	60%
Antibiotics	60%
Other single homeopathic remedies (especially at the same potency level)†	60%
Combination homeopathic remedies	50%
Strong perfumes, colognes, aftershaves	50%
Commercial air travel	40%
Needles (vaccinations, acupuncture, auriculotherapy, neural therapy, etc.)	30%
Electric blankets	30%

*In homeopathic literature, camphor has historically been the most significant antidoting agent. Other essential oils—eucalyptus, peppermint, patchouli, sandalwood, lavender, etc.—can also potentially antidote. However, which oil has a particular antidoting effect on a remedy also depends on the sensitivity of the specific plant, animal, or mineral remedy to that oil (as well as the sensitivity of the patient).

†Schuessler cell salts (triturated at a 6X potency), isopathic remedies (diluted at 4X), flower remedies (diluted at approximately a 5X potency), and gemmotherapy remedies (diluted at 1X and 1C) are not succussed (potentized) and therefore are not classic homeopathic remedies. Thus, in my professional experience, they do not antidote constitutional homeopathic remedies.

Dr. Lester uses the term *filter* to describe this sensitivity tendency.[142] Highly sensitive patients have "thin" filters, while the more "unreceptive" patients who have greater immunity to external stimuli are referred to as having "thick" filters. This second aspect of antidoting must be considered when determining whether a patient should see his acupuncturist, have her house painted, or travel cross-country by plane. For example, a thin-filtered patient's homeopathic remedy might be antidoted by one acupuncture needle, by simply walking through a newly painted house, or by flying from San Francisco to Los Angeles, whereas a patient with a thick filter may receive multiple acupuncture needle sticks in several sessions, sleep in a newly painted bedroom, or fly to Europe without neutralizing the effect of his remedy.

A third key factor in whether a remedy will be antidoted is how perfectly fitting a patient's constitutional remedy is. A patient taking her simillimum will be less likely to antidote it, whereas another patient on a helpful remedy similar to but not exactly his simillimum will stand a greater chance of antidoting this remedy. Thus, knowledgeable homeopaths realize that when patients continue to easily antidote their remedy, it is probably not the most perfectly fitting remedy for them.

Guidelines to Antidoting and Prescribing for Sensitive Patients

The general consensus among most modern homeopaths is to ask patients to not do anything within the first month that could greatly upset their remedy. After that, when the homeopathic resonance is more imprinted in the vital force, the remedy is less easy to antidote.

Many homeopaths also give more sensitive patients "booster doses" of the remedy in a 6C or 12C potency, through an LM potency (e.g., LM1 or LM2), or in a C potency in solution (e.g., 30C) to continue the action in the body initiated by the one-time dose of the initial higher-potency remedy (e.g., 200C, 1M, or higher). Although many classical constitutional homeopaths abide rather strictly by the supposedly traditional rule of taking one dose and then waiting for months before re-dosing (depending on how the patient is doing at the follow-up appointment), more frequent dosing was advocated by Hahnemann himself in the case of chronic and serious disease. In his 1837 Paris casebook, Dr. Hahnemann described the benefits of both diluting C potencies and dosing patients more frequently—not only in acute disease (which is well known and accepted) but also in chronic disease (which is much less well known and understood):

> Experience has shown me, as it has no doubt also shown to most of my followers, that it is most useful in diseases of any magnitude (no excepting even the most acute, and still more so in the half-acute, in the tedious and most tedious) to give to the patient the powerful homoeopathic pellet or pellets only in solution, and this solution in divided doses. In this way we give the medicine, dissolved in seven to twenty tablespoonfuls of water without any addition, in acute and very acute diseases every six, four, or two hours; where the danger is urgent, even

> every hour or every half-hour, a tablespoonful at a time; with weak persons or children, only a small part of a tablespoonful (one or two teaspoonfuls or coffee spoonfuls) may be given as a dose.
>
> In chronic diseases I have found it best to give a dose (e.g., a spoonful) of a solution medicine at least every two days, more usually every day.

Sensitive and/or very weak and ill patients often need more frequent dosing of their remedy, most typically in low potency (e.g., LM1 or 2, 6C, 12C, or 30C) and in a liquid dosage. These booster doses are especially efficacious when patients feel that they have been significantly antidoted and begin to experience their old disturbing symptoms again. In these cases, they can re-dose their gentle low-potency liquid booster remedy in order to reinstate the healing resonance of their constitutional remedy. Of course, when there is any question about the effectiveness of the remedy, or the dosage guidelines, patients should always check with their homeopaths.

Intentional Antidoting

It is important to point out that antidoting can be used deliberately. For example, if a remedy is not the correct simillimum and is causing major proving symptoms, a patient can intentionally put camphor under the nose and inhale. This strong antidoting action, done once or twice, is usually sufficient to nullify the effects of the incorrect remedy. Of course, it is always best when patients can contact their homeopath and talk over this course of action to be sure they are correctly antidoting an incorrect remedy versus antidoting a simillimum that is simply causing a major aggravation or healing crisis.

In the latter case—that is, when a patient is experiencing significant and uncomfortable healing effects from her *correct* homeopathic remedy—it is often best to first try taking a lower potency of the remedy to help reduce these symptoms. For example, when a patient is feeling too strong an effect from a 1M potency, dosing with a 30C potency will typically greatly reduce and slow down these healing symptoms so that they are more tolerable.

൙

In conclusion, when other practitioners are knowledgeable about antidoting as well as whether a patient has a thin or thick filter, they can better judge whether their remedies or treatments will disturb or counteract the patient's homeopathic remedy. Or better yet, they can contact the patient's homeopath and discuss the value of their proposed treatment, or whether it would be wiser to put it off. Additionally, it is imperative that the classically trained homeopath is aware of the modern obstacles to cure, such as the need to replace toxic mercury amalgam fillings, and the valuable holistic treatments that specifically address these obstacles and can be administered in concert with the homeopathic remedy.

Obstacles to Cure

Factors that block the action of homeopathic remedies, referred to as obstacles to cure, were briefly discussed earlier. As previously described, Hahnemann was well aware of the interfering lifestyle aspects of a poor diet, alcohol, and a sedentary lifestyle, as well as allopathic "obstacles" such as mercury-containing ointments (calomel), extensive bloodletting, and the excessive use of painkilling opium.

However, it is a sad commentary that many modern-day homeopaths who claim to follow Hahnemann's methods often ignore our current obstacles to cure, especially in light of the fact that these modern obstacles are even more damaging to our vital force than the bloodletting and leeches of old. For example, many classically trained homeopaths do not recognize the well-propagated issue of toxic mercury amalgam fillings. It is the rare homeopath who is aware of the electromagnetic disturbance as well as the increased off-gassing of toxic metals elicited from dental galvanism—that is, a gold-nickel crown on or next to an amalgam filling. And few holistic practitioners, much less homeopaths who usually specialize in only this one modality of healing, have even heard of dominant foci, nor do they know how to recognize the symptoms that might necessitate their referring a patient with a major dental focus, for example, to a competent holistic dentist for treatment.

Lack of Homeopathic Education Regarding Obstacles

This tendency toward tunnel vision on the part of homeopaths arises primarily from two factors: First, homeopathic courses and training programs as a rule do not teach how to diagnose or treat artificially* induced diseases such as mercury amalgam poisoning, exposure to toxic chemicals, or chronic root canal or other focal infections. Dr. Heinz Pscheidl, a German homeopath with extensive experience in the diagnosis and treatment of amalgam poisoning, comments on this dearth of understanding in homeopathic education:

> During our homeopathic training most of us were/are not taught, how to diagnose the artificial diseases and how to handle them. Therefore, their immense spreading and influence is much underrated. This applies also to amalgam poisoning, especially to its chronic form. Artificial diseases cannot be cured by homeopathic means, the respective sources must be removed from the patient's body/environment.[143]

Needing to remove obvious toxins from the body should not be a new concept to homeopaths. Dr. Hahnemann recommended it three centuries before for another mercury-containing allopathic poison—calomel creams and powders.[144] Furthermore, because mercury and other metals and toxins possess "medication character"—that is, they create their own unique signature of disturbing symptoms in the body—Pscheidl asserts that "although the homeopathic remedy will often be able to eliminate those symptoms for which it fits according to similarity, the result will not be a cure (as in natural disease) but, at best, a 'scientific' passing palliation of poison takes place." For example, the homeopath may prescribe a remedy based more on the symptoms of mercury toxicity, rather on the deeper disturbance in the patient's unique vital force. In one case example, Pscheidl described how a past homeopathic remedy (Tuberculinum) he had prescribed for a patient's asthma symptoms had only palliated her symptoms and over time actually contributed to driving the toxins in deeper to her colon, where a tumor developed.* When this patient came back under his treatment, Dr. Pscheidl had the underlying cause of the patient's tumor removed—her mixed-metal alloy (gold, palladium, platinum, and silver) inlays and crowns.[145] Thus, although homeopathic remedies do not have the side effects of synthetic allopathic drugs, used unwisely, they can also be a form of suppression. Dr. Elizabeth Wright Hubbard, a renowned American homeopath, echoed this sentiment in the chapter "The Dangers of Homeopathic Prescribing" in her book *Homeopathy as Art and Science.* She wrote: "Never forget that to palliate a curable case is suppression."[146]

In contrast, when homeopaths recommend the removal of obvious obstacles to cure such as amalgam fillings, gold-nickel-palladium crowns, chronic exposure to toxic chemicals, and irremedial dental focal infections (requiring cavitation surgery), they can then prescribe a remedy based on a patient's deepest issues—that is, his or her individual miasmic response to these and other stressors—and not on the more superficial (albeit sometimes devastating) symptoms engendered by these toxic agents foreign to the body. However, in the case of less obvious foci—that is, the chronic "soft-tissue" infections seen in the tonsils, sinuses, and genitals—appropriate case management can be less clear. In many of these cases, a homeopathic remedy can greatly facilitate healing of these chronic foci (as it also can with curable dental foci), accompanied by other effective treatments including drainage through gemmotherapy and auriculotherapy.† In the case of scar interference fields, these foci almost always require one or more neural therapy or auriculotherapy treatments.

Excessive Faith in the Homeopathic Simillimum

The second reason why homeopaths often ignore toxic metals, chemicals, and foci is because many are taught

*In this case, *artificial* refers to amalgam or other toxins inducing disease, in contrast to Hahnemann's use of the term *artificial disease* to describe the effects of a homeopathic remedy in the body.

*The lung and large intestine are paired meridians in Chinese five-element theory and have been clinically correlated to the bicuspid teeth. (See figure 11.5, page 331.)

†In my professional experience, the 1X (diluted but not succussed) gemmotherapy drainage remedies have never antidoted my patients' constitutional homeopathic remedies. If several auriculotherapy needles are needed for a sensitive patient, that patient may require another dose of his or her booster remedy afterward.

PATIENT EDUCATION

It is critical that prospective patients become more knowledgeable about homeopathy and other forms of holistic medicine. As the growing army of knowledgeable holistic patients can attest, taking a synthetic medication to treat symptoms—despite the television ads filled with glowing models and handsome seniors enjoying idyllic days—ranks right up there with amalgam fillings as one of the most damaging effects of allopathy in both medical and dental practice. Hahnemann railed against this suppression of symptoms centuries ago, as illustrated by the following quote from his *Organon:*

> Whenever they can (in order to remain popular with patients) the adherents of the old school [allopathic doctors] employ means (palliatives) that, for a short time, immediately suppress and cloak the disease ailments through opposition (*contraria contrariis*)* but that leave the basis for these ailments (the disease itself) strengthened and aggravated.
>
> The adherents of the old school of medicine falsely deem the maladies located on the outer parts of the body as merely local and existing alone there by themselves, and they imagine them to have been cured if they have driven them away through external means, so that it is now necessary for the inner malady to break out at a more vital and critical place.[147]

Thus, when a psoric infant's eczema was treated with suppressive ointments, the infant often demonstrated her "inner malady" through other more serious means, most typically through the later onset of asthma characteristic of the more weakened tuberculinic reaction mode. Unfortunately, this understanding, although well known to homeopaths and a certain percentage of other holistic physicians and practitioners, is still foreign to the great majority of patients.

It is also essential to point out here that the suppressive effects of allopathic medicine are not always unwarranted. That is, they can sometimes be lifesaving—especially during emergencies. Currently, when many individuals are so weakened genetically and environmentally that their health is tenuous, they often react to any form of stress through the more pathological and serious illnesses characteristic of the tuberculinic and luetic reaction modes.

In the absence of emergencies, however—that is, in the case of chronic dysfunction and disease—individuals should strongly consider availing themselves of the best possible holistic medicine available. This care should always include constitutional homeopathy, which can most effectively free individuals from their current debilitating symptoms, as well as help prevent the future onset of degenerative disease.

**Contraria contrariis,* meaning "curing by opposites," is the philosophy of the allopathic doctor who utilizes treatments that are different or contrary to the disease, such as the use of an antihistamine in the case of hay fever. In contrast, homeopathy is based on the *similia similibus curentur,* or "like cures like" philosophy, in which hay fever would be cured by any number of potentized homeopathic remedies initiating reactions similar to the symptoms of the disease, and individualized according to the patient's particular symptoms (e.g., Allium cepa, Apis mellifica, Arsenicum album, etc.).

that the correct homeopathic simillimum is literally a panacea for every disturbance in the body. This relative arrogance can be understandable given that homeopathy is one of the top, if not *the* top, curative holistic treatments extant. However, there are too many present-day examples of long-term homeopathic patients, as well as leading homeopaths, who have succumbed to cancer, Parkinson's, Alzheimer's, and other toxin-induced diseases, despite being under extensive homeopathic care.[148] Furthermore, if Hahnemann himself recognized the need to remove toxic obstacles to cure back in the eighteenth and nineteenth centuries—before amalgam fillings, synthetic toxic chemicals, nuclear radiation, GMO and food irradiation, and so forth—then how can we expect to overcome our even stronger twenty-first-century toxins, especially with our more weakened genes? The fact is that, for the most part, we can't. As was discussed in the introduction to *Radical Medicine,* the great majority of us simply no longer enjoy the robust health that our grandparents and great-grandparents enjoyed (although we do enjoy greatly improved sanitation and less arduous physical labor). It is therefore crucial that homeopaths and other holistic physicians begin to work more closely together and respect each other's particular contributions toward their mutual aim: the healing of their patients.

Energetic Testing Augments the Treatment Protocol

Removing the "Obstacle" First

Toxic obstacles and blocks to healing can be better discerned with energetic testing—kinesiology, arm length testing, electroacupuncture, and so forth. That is, in conjunction with a thorough history, exam, and necessary laboratory work, energetic testing helps the practitioner determine which treatments are needed, as well as in what order they should be given. For example, often the chronic dental galvanism from a gold crown placed next to or over an amalgam filling can be so intoxicating and overwhelming to a patient's system that this major "obstacle to cure" must be dealt with first. After this obstacle is cleared, the determination of the correct homeopathic remedy is greatly facilitated, and the action of this remedy is much more effective in the less burdened body.

Giving the Remedy First

With energetic testing methods, the corollary is also true. That is, the correct homeopathic remedy can later bring up a major block that has been a chronic, yet perhaps more deeply buried, obstacle to healing. Thus, the correct homeopathic simillimum can *so* calm and stabilize the individual that "what's false then arises." For example, stores of mercury still residing deep in the kidneys may begin to test positive on a patient who had removed his amalgams and (presumably) detoxified heavy metals decades before. Or the damaging effects from vaccinations received when a patient was an infant or young child may display for the first time in treatment, even in a patient who has been treated holistically for years. Another example typically seen in practice is when scars (interference fields) that have been treated in the past test positive once again, but now reveal a subtle yet chronically debilitating emotion-related disturbance.

Therapeutic Guidance through Energetic Testing

Through effective energetic testing, modern holistic practitioners can witness a remarkable aspect of constitutional homeopathy unknown in Hahnemann's day (unless we include the highly developed psychic abilities, or *gnosis,* that many early holistic pioneers embodied),* since these modern forms of diagnostic testing were not developed until just after the mid-twentieth century.† As these layers of toxins and foci unlayer through the vast healing capacities of homeopathy, energetic testing can reveal whether it is best to do nothing and simply allow the constitutional remedy to continue to act, or whether other treatments (which don't interfere with the remedy) are appropriate. For example, auriculotherapy may be indicated to treat emerging foci, or the body may display the need to sacrifice an irremediable dental focus through cavitation surgery.

Case Management

When "unpeeling the onion"—that is, testing for the most appropriate treatment at each level of disturbance that arises in a patient—energetic testing can be invaluable. This is especially essential when the patient is very ill and weak. For example, it is important to determine in a new patient presenting with Crohn's disease whether it would be best to begin with a constitutional homeopathic remedy that could significantly alleviate the debilitating diarrhea or to first have the patient avoid and challenge her primary food allergen (gluten or dairy, etc.), or whether a primary factor in her illness is her right lower failed root-canalled bicuspid tooth that

***Gnosis,* from the Greek word meaning "knowledge" or "to know," is that special knowledge of spiritual and divine understanding that all individuals at times are privy to, but that is experienced by sages, saints, gurus, and other realized beings regularly.

†See appendix 3, "Energetic Testing Explained," for more information on this subject. The word *modern* was inserted into this sentence because another form of energetic testing, *dowsing* or *divining,* is as old as civilization itself. Evidence of dowsing for water with a forked branch has been found in Africa on wall murals that were carbon-dated to be at least 8,000 years old. Other ancient findings include etchings on Egyptian temple walls that reveal pharaohs holding dowsing devices in their hands and ceramic pendulums that have been found in this civilization's ancient tombs. Additionally, evidence of dowsing has been uncovered in China from 2,500 years ago and in Crete from around 400 BCE, and many passages in the Bible refer to the use of these dowsing devices in the Middle East. One of the founders of the American Society of Dowsers (ASD@dowsers.org), engineer Raymond C. Willey, defines this ancient art as "the exercise of a human faculty, which allows one to obtain information in a manner beyond the scope and power of the standard human physical senses of sight, sound, touch, etc." (L. Youngblood, "Dowsing: Ancient History," www.neholistic.com/articles/0008.htm.)

lies on the large intestine meridian, which should be further evaluated by a holistic dentist. Using an effective and sensitive energetic testing method and informed by a careful history, physical exam, and necessary laboratory tests or X-rays, the holistic practitioner can determine which one (or more) of these issues needs to be addressed first. When the practitioner provides these necessary treatments at the correct time and in the correct order, healing is greatly augmented and future treatment time periods are significantly reduced.

Sensitive energetic testing methods are also extremely helpful in later visits when a patient is on a constitutional remedy but comes in complaining of new symptoms. In many cases, classical homeopaths would interpret this change of symptoms as the need for a new homeopathic remedy—constitutional, acute, or intercurrent—which is often the case. However, sometimes the patient's previously prescribed homeopathic remedy is still acting and is the correct one, but it is now appropriately bringing up a focus or an area of chronic toxicity that needs to be addressed. Thus, in these "what's false arises" or "sunlight over the well"* cases, the remedy doesn't need to be changed but is actually functioning extraordinarily well in the body by strengthening the patient's vital force and spirit so substantially that she can then "face" her nemesis directly. This nemesis can be stores of toxic toluene and benzene in an artist, a wisdom-tooth-site focal infection from an incomplete extraction, an appendix scar that has recently begun to itch, or a deeply suppressed chronic emotional conflict. Whatever the arising issue, it is the highly curative aspects of constitutional homeopathy that allow these often deeply embedded toxic metals, chemicals, foci, or painful conflicts to emerge quite appropriately, in a body made significantly stronger and healthier by the remedy. Thus, the remedy's powerful healing action empowers an individual's immune system and vital force to both recognize as well as release deeply buried and adapted toxins—toxins that would in many cases be significantly instrumental in the person's eventual demise.

intercurrent: An intercurrent remedy is given to provide movement in a stalled case.[149] Usually, but not always, this homeopathic is a nosode remedy to treat a past intoxication that is currently emerging (e.g., a vaccine nosode such as pertussis, measles, or smallpox; a toxic chemical nosode such as toluene or propylene glycol; or Radium bromatum for past radiation exposure that is now arising). The need for nosodes often comes up concurrently with the unearthing and treatment of a chronic focal infection (dental, tonsil, sinus, genital, etc.), and they are usually prescribed for only a short period of time (e.g., days or weeks). After this treatment regimen, the patient resumes his or her constitutional remedy (unless it's early in the treatment regimen and the patient hasn't yet received one).

In these cases, the most appropriate treatment is through directly and efficiently addressing the arising issue. Treatment might be draining the chronic stores of toxic chemicals through gemmotherapy (already initiated by the draining effect of the homeopathic remedy), treating the appendix scar focus through neural therapy, or referring the patient to an experienced and skillful psychotherapist. Furthermore, since most of us have multiple layers of toxic accumulations and unresolved injuries, the patient may intermittently experience the onset of symptoms from many of these emerging issues while on the same remedy over a period of months and even years. A typical scenario of this process is shown in the line graph depicted in figure 14.3.

After these disturbances are cleared, the patient may sometimes need to re-dose or move to a higher level of potency of his or her homeopathic remedy, signifying the progress made energetically by clearing the focal or toxic issue appropriately. Therefore, when these aggravations or healing crises arise while the patient is on the correct constitutional remedy, the knowledgeable practitioner can assess through energetic testing what is arising and then explain to a worried or frustrated patient that the emerging toxin or focus is a sign of progression—not regression—through the homeopathic remedy's deeply healing and cleansing effects.

*This expression in spiritual traditions refers to sunlight, or divine consciousness, illuminating baser tendencies, and thus helping spiritual seekers to better observe and release chronic egoic personality patterns that hinder their reception of their soul, or true nature. In the present example, the correct homeopathic remedy (sunlight) brings up the chronic toxic accumulations in the body (e.g., mercury poisoning in our "well"), so that they can be more easily detoxified and released.

The Problem with Energetic Testing for Constitutional Remedies

Energetic testing can be helpful with case management, but terribly frustrating and unhelpful in determining the correct constitutional homeopathic simillimum. The reasons are threefold. For one, when a homeopath uses the Sankaran system, he opens up the possible remedies to consider in a patient's case to not just the known homeopathic remedies that are currently available (~3000), but to literally *any* substance (e.g., plant, animal, mineral, nosode, or imponderable) existing in the universe. This is a far cry from energetically testing for which of three different types of vitamin C is needed, or even which one of the thirty-eight Bach flower remedies resonates best in a patient. This infinite field of homeopathic remedies is hard for anyone to "own" during energetic testing—even for the most experienced homeopaths.

Additionally, it is only during an extensive and thorough case-taking process that the identity of the remedy fully emerges. In fact, in the majority of cases, patients are not aware of this chronic pattern, or "other song," that has been competing with their more "human song" and impeding the full expression of their physical, mental, emotional, and spiritual growth and realization. However, with a well-taken interview utilizing the Sankaran method, this plant, mineral, or animal pattern can clearly emerge to inform the homeopath of its level of desperation (which miasm), as well as the appropriate plant, mineral, or animal remedy (which kingdom and subkingdom) is needed. When energetic testers try to curtail or even skip this case-taking step (which often entails a two- to three-hour interview), they are then trying to test for a remedy that isn't apparent in the patient's awareness, and thus somewhat blindly searching for something that has no clear resonance in the patient's energetic field. In these cases, the tester cannot possibly determine that which has no discernible shape, form, presence, or even any perceptible conscious existence in the patient's consciousness.

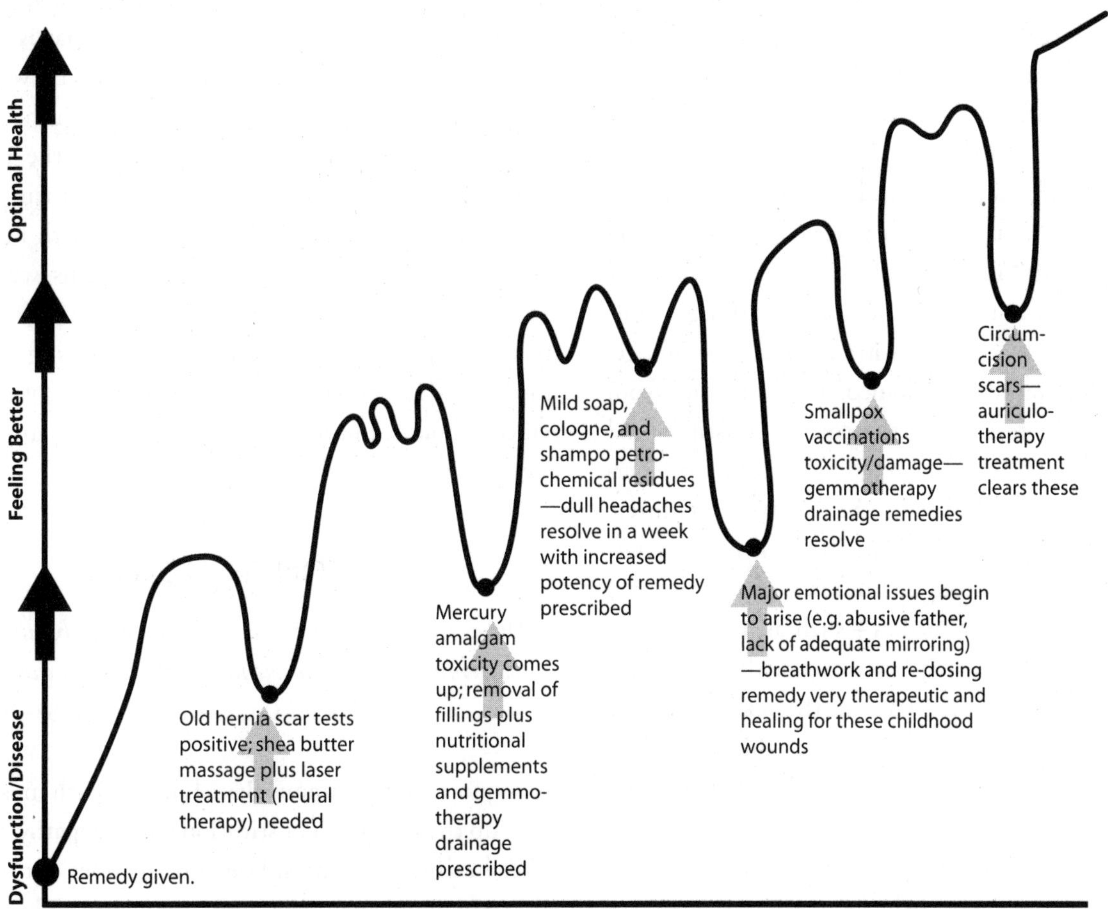

Figure 14.3. A graph depicting the typical highs (peaks of line graph) and lows (valleys of line graph) that arise when patients are on their correct homeopathic remedy

Thus, case taking is much more than a simple history-taking method; it is a dynamic unearthing of the chronically disturbing pattern tha has been deeply buried in the patient's unconscious. Sankaran-trained homeopaths are well aware of the transition that signals that this transformation is occurring during successful case taking. In fact, the energy in the room seems to imperceptibly shift when patients begin to speak not from a human level, but from the level of the plant, animal, or mineral pattern that has been coexisting in them for years, decades, or even their entire lifetime (or, perhaps, lifetimes). It is only through this integral dynamic process that a patient's underlying nonhuman pattern can be gently and patiently revealed, allowing the homeopath to then match the appropriate homeopathic simillimum.

A third challenge to energetically testing for the correct constitutional homeopathic remedy is that in the field of homeopathy there are many similar remedies with which a patient may resonate. An energetic tester can easily confuse these close, but not close enough, remedies with the most similar remedy, or simillimum. And although a close-but-not-quite-similar-enough remedy may alleviate some of the patient's symptoms temporarily, ultimately—after a few days, weeks, or months—it will prove to be insufficient. These similars can fool even the most precise and seemingly accurate energetic testing method, as those who practice honest testing will readily admit. Thus, based on these many similar remedies that can test falsely, the need for taking a thorough case in which the remedy itself will clearly emerge, and the infinite number of homeopathic remedies from which to choose, testing for the correct constitutional remedy—at this point in the ongoing evolution of energetic testing—has been found to be an abysmal failure.

However, when a homeopath has taken an extensive case, studied it thoroughly, and narrowed down the choices to two similar remedies—such as, for example, Crotalus horridus (North American rattlesnake) and Crotalus cascavella (Brazilian rattlesnake)—quality energetic testing can help determine which of these two reptile remedies best resonates and is therefore the needed simillimum.

Additionally, after the correct simillimum is chosen, energetic testing can also help facilitate case management. As discussed previously, it can assist in determining when a new issue is emerging, such as the need to replace toxic mercury amalgam fillings or treat a chronic scar interference field. Furthermore, guided by the homeopath's experience, energetic testing can help determine the needed potency of a remedy, as well as the dosage, and when it may be time to change the prescription to another potency and increase or reduce the dosage (e.g., liquid or pellets, taken one time only or more often). However, energetic testing in these cases should be attempted only by those who are skilled in both their particular method of energetic testing and in the field of homeopathy. Thus, energetic testing can be a valuable adjunct in the hands of a skillful tester who respects and follows the laws and principles of classical constitutional homeopathy.

It should be further noted that in the hands of a skilled craniopath, the homeopathic simillimum can be even more accurately determined. For example, after a two-hour case interview, a decision must be made between two very similar remedies. The correct remedy placed on the patient's energy field will stimulate dramatic change in craniosacral rhythms (CSR). (This is often in stark contrast to the remedy that is *not* the patient's simillimum.) Normally the CSR is between five and twelve cycles per minute. However, with the correct homeopathic remedy, I have experienced the rhythm slow to just two cycles per minute as the patient's body, mind, and spirit relaxed and communed with her most curative and healing remedy. Homeopaths who have training in craniosacral therapy may want to consider using this palpation method after case taking to diagnostically differentiate between two or more very close remedy choices. I have found it to be more accurate than energetic testing in these cases.

CONCLUSION

Drugs do not cure, popular opinion not withstanding.
Cure must come from within; or there is no cure.

Dr. Margaret Tyler (1857–1943)

This quote from a famous British homeopath most aptly sums up the genius of constitutional homeopathy. Unlike other healing modalities, homeopathy does not directly add to or supplement the body in any way. The correct homeopathic simillimum acts simply by resonating with a patient's "mistunement"—that is, the alteration or derangement of an individual's body, mind, and spirit caused from his or her pattern of chronic dysfunction or disease. This state of being out of tune—manifested by various physical, mental, and emotional symptoms—becomes in tune through its resonance with the constitutional remedy's similar but stronger frequency and vibration. Freed from the debilitating burden of this chronic "other song," an individual's true nature is enlivened and begins to more fully emerge and develop.

In this healthier body-mind environment, any major foci (dental or tonsil focal infections, scars, etc.) or areas of chronic toxicity (amalgam fillings, petrochemical-laden cosmetic use, intestinal dysbiosis, etc.) that cannot be completely ameliorated by the remedy will arise and may then be diagnosed through quality energetic testing and appropriately treated. When these "obstacles to cure" are cleared, and the constitutional homeopathic remedy is allowed to continue its healing action in the body, individuals experience increased levels of mental clarity, emotional stability, and a closer connection to their authentic true nature. Thus, real cure in constitutional homeopathy is achieved not only when individuals enjoy the freedom that optimal physical health renders but also when they can realize the fulfilling effects that profound psychospiritual healing bestows.

NOTES

1. J. Lazarou et al., "Incidence of Adverse Drug Reactions in Hospitalized Patients," *Journal of the American Medical Association* 279, no. 15 (April 15, 1998): 1200–1205.
2. S. Hahnemann, *Organon of the Medical Art,* ed. W. O'Reilly (Palo Alto, Calif.: Birdcage Books, 1996), 120–22.
3. Ibid.
4. Ibid., 122–23.
5. P. Gosch, *Vital Energy Medicine* (Provo, Utah: Chronicle Publishing Services, 2003), 55–56.
6. *Santa Rosa Press Democrat,* June 29, 2004, A2; www.biopharm-leeches.com; S. Finger, *Origins of Neuroscience* (New York: Oxford University Press, 1994), 430.
7. S. Hahnemann, *Organon of the Medical Art,* ed. W. O'Reilly (Palo Alto, Calif.: Birdcage Books, 1996), 120.
8. P. Bellavite and A. Signorini, *The Emerging Science of Homeopathy* (Berkeley, Calif.: North Atlantic Books, 2002), 13.
9. S. Hahnemann, *Organon of the Medical Art,* ed. W. O'Reilly (Palo Alto, Calif.: Birdcage Books, 1996), 228.
10. Ibid., xvi.
11. M. Wood, *Vitalism* (Berkeley, Calif.: North Atlantic Books, 2000), 37–39; R. Haehl, *Samuel Hahnemann: His Life and Work,* vol. 1 (New Delhi: B. Jain Publishers, 2001), 53, 69, 73; ibid., vol. 2, 47–48.
12. S. Hahnemann, *Organon of the Medical Art,* ed. W. O'Reilly (Palo Alto, Calif.: Birdcage Books, 1996), xv.
13. M. Wood, *Vitalism* (Berkeley, Calif.: North Atlantic Books, 2000), 40.
14. F. Vermeulen, *Prisma* (Haarlem, the Netherlands: Emryss, 2002), 442.
15. M. Wood, *Vitalism* (Berkeley, Calif.: North Atlantic Books, 2000), 54.
16. P. Bellavite and A. Signorini, *The Emerging Science of Homeopathy* (Berkeley, Calif.: North Atlantic Books, 2002), 13; V. McCabe, *Homeopathy, Healing, and You* (New York: St. Martin's Griffin, 1997), 60.
17. P. Bellavite and A. Signorini, *The Emerging Science of Homeopathy* (Berkeley, Calif.: North Atlantic Books, 2002), 13, 20.
18. S. Hahnemann, *Organon of the Medical Art,* ed. W. O'Reilly (Palo Alto, Calif.: Birdcage Books, 1996), 57; R. Haehl, *Samuel Hahnemann: His Life and Work,* vol. 1 (New Delhi: B. Jain Publishers, 2001), 57.
19. S. Hahnemann, *Organon of the Medical Art,* ed. W. O'Reilly (Palo Alto, Calif.: Birdcage Books, 1996), 57.
20. A. Lockie and N. Geddes, *Homeopathy: The Principles and Practice of Treatment* (London: Dorling Kindersley Limited, 1995), 10.
21. W. Heiby, *The Reverse Effect* (Deerfield, Ill.: MediScience Publishers, 1988), 70.
22. G. Vithoulkas, *The Science of Homeopathy* (New York: Grove Press, Inc., 1980), 94; R. Haehl *Samuel Hahnemann: His Life and Work,* vol. 1 (New Delhi: B. Jain Publishers, 2001), 81.
23. P. Bellavite and A. Signorini, *The Emerging Science of Homeopathy* (Berkeley, Calif.: North Atlantic Books, 2002), 21.
24. Ibid.
25. H. Coulter, *Divided Legacy* (Richmond, Calif.: North Atlantic Books, 1973), 101.
26. C. Hammond, *The Complete Family Guide to Homeopathy* (New York: Penguin, 1995), 20.
27. P. Bellavite and A. Signorini, *The Emerging Science of Homeopathy* (Berkeley, Calif.: North Atlantic Books,

2002), 21; H. Coulter, *Divided Legacy* (Richmond, Calif.: North Atlantic Books, 1973), 268.

28. Ibid., 439.
29. Ibid., 140.
30. Ibid., 241.
31. Ibid., 122–23.
32. Ibid., 181, 182; P. Bellavite and A. Signorini, *The Emerging Science of Homeopathy* (Berkeley, Calif.: North Atlantic Books, 2002), 22.
33. B. Gray, "Shaken, Not Stirred," *Health and Healing Wisdom* 24, nos. 3, 4 (2000): 12.
34. H. Coulter, *Divided Legacy* (Richmond, Calif.: North Atlantic Books, 1973), 181, 182, 199, 213.
35. Ibid., 213–14, 337, 439.
36. Ibid., 446.
37. R. Schoch, "A Conversation with Dana Ullman," *California Monthly,* February 1999, 27.
38. P. Bellavite and A. Signorini, *The Emerging Science of Homeopathy* (Berkeley, Calif.: North Atlantic Books, 2002), 22.
39. H. Coulter, *Divided Legacy* (Richmond, Calif.: North Atlantic Books, 1973), 449, 450.
40. Ibid., 37.
41. Ibid.
42. P. Bellavite and A. Signorini, *The Emerging Science of Homeopathy* (Berkeley, Calif.: North Atlantic Books, 2002), 33.
43. S. Hahnemann, *Organon of the Medical Art,* ed. W. O'Reilly (Palo Alto, Calif.: Birdcage Books, 1996), 4.
44. Ibid., 4, 68, 236.
45. Ibid., 58.
46. R. Sankaran, "The Sensation Method" (seminar, San Francisco, Calif., October 7–9, 2003).
47. D. Ewing, *Let the Tooth Be Known* (Houston: Holistic Health Alternatives, 1998), 131–32.
48. S. Hahnemann, *Organon of the Medical Art,* ed. W. O'Reilly (Palo Alto, Calif.: Birdcage Books, 1996), 77.
49. P. Bellavite and A. Signorini, *The Emerging Science of Homeopathy* (Berkeley, Calif.: North Atlantic Books, 2002), 9.
50. S. Hahnemann, *Organon of the Medical Art,* ed. W. O'Reilly (Palo Alto, Calif.: Birdcage Books, 1996), 144.
51. P. Bellavite and A. Signorini, *The Emerging Science of Homeopathy* (Berkeley, Calif.: North Atlantic Books, 2002), 64.
52. S. Hahnemann, *Organon of the Medical Art,* ed. W. O'Reilly (Palo Alto, Calif.: Birdcage Books, 1996), 153, 156, 158–59.
53. J. Yasgur, *Yasgur's Homeopathic Dictionary* (Greenville, Pa.: Van Hoy Publishers, 1998), 214.
54. V. McCabe, *Homeopathy, Healing, and You* (New York: St. Martin's Griffin, 1997), 72.
55. G. Vithoulkas, *The Science of Homeopathy* (New York: Grove Press, Inc., 1980), 101–2.
56. P. Bellavite and A. Signorini, *The Emerging Science of Homeopathy* (Berkeley, Calif.: North Atlantic Books, 2002), 11.
57. J. Yasgur, *Yasgur's Homeopathic Dictionary* (Greenville, Pa.: Van Hoy Publishers, 1998), 21.
58. W. Heiby, *The Reverse Effect* (Deerfield, Ill.: MediScience Publishers, 1988), 70.
59. R. Murphy, *Homeopathic Remedy Guide* (Blacksburg, Va.: H.A.N.A. Press, 2000), 176–82, 1147–54; R. Morrison, *Desktop Guide to Keynotes and Confirmatory Symptoms* (Albany, Calif.: Hahnemann Clinic Publishing, 1993), 39–44, 244–47.
60. R. Murphy, *Homeopathic Remedy Guide* (Blacksburg, Va.: H.A.N.A. Press, 2000), 244–47.
61. Ibid., 536, 538; R. Morrison, *Desktop Companion to Physical Pathology* (Nevada City, Calif.: Hahnemann Clinic Publishing, 1998), 571–79.
62. P. Bellavite and A. Signorini, *The Emerging Science of Homeopathy* (Berkeley, Calif.: North Atlantic Books, 2002), 11.
63. G. Vithoulkas, *The Science of Homeopathy* (New York: Grove Press, Inc., 1980), 101.
64. J. Yasgur, *Yasgur's Homeopathic Dictionary* (Greenville, Pa.: Van Hoy Publishers, 1998), 242.
65. S. Hahnemann, *Organon of the Medical Art,* ed. W. O'Reilly (Palo Alto, Calif.: Birdcage Books, 1996), 236–37.
66. G. Vithoulkas, *The Science of Homeopathy* (New York: Grove Press, Inc., 1980), 160.
67. S. Hahnemann, *Organon of the Medical Art,* ed. W. O'Reilly (Palo Alto, Calif.: Birdcage Books, 1996), 146.
68. W. Boericke and W. Dewey, *The Twelve Tissue Remedies of Schüssler* (Philadelphia: Hahnemann Publishing House, 1888), 16.
69. H. Coulter, *Homeopathic Science and Modern Medicine* (Richmond, Calif.: North Atlantic Books, 1980), 53; G. Vithoulkas, *The Science of Homeopathy* (New York: Grove Press, Inc., 1980), 166.
70. L. McTaggart, *The Field* (New York: HarperCollins Publishers, 2002), xiv, xvi.
71. Ibid., xv.
72. P. Bellavite and A. Signorini, *The Emerging Science of*

Homeopathy (Berkeley, Calif.: North Atlantic Books, 2002), 245, 266, 288, 293.
73. G. Vithoulkas, *The Science of Homeopathy* (New York: Grove Press, Inc., 1980), 166.
74. S. Hahnemann, *Organon of the Medical Art,* ed. W. O'Reilly (Palo Alto, Calif.: Birdcage Books, 1996), 240, 241.
75. J. Yasgur, *Yasgur's Homeopathic Dictionary* (Greenville, Pa.: Van Hoy Publishers, 1998), 196, 194.
76. D. Little, "Following in Hahnemann's Footsteps: The Definitive Years 1833–1843," www.simillimum.com/education/little-library/homeopathic-philosophy/fhf/article.php.
77. Ibid.
78. J. Yasgur, *Yasgur's Homeopathic Dictionary* (Greenville, Pa.: Van Hoy Publishers, 1998), 194.
79. G. Vithoulkas, *The Science of Homeopathy* (New York: Grove Press, Inc., 1980), 162.
80. S. Hahnemann, *Organon of the Medical Art,* ed. W. O'Reilly (Palo Alto, Calif.: Birdcage Books, 1996), 60.
81. H. Coulter, *Divided Legacy* (Richmond, Calif.: North Atlantic Books, 1973), 101.
82. I. Bell et al., "Translating a Nonlinear Systems Theory Model for Homeopathy into Empirical Tests," *Alternative Therapies* 8, no. 3 (May/June 2002): 58.
83. M. Wood, *Vitalism* (Berkeley, Calif.: North Atlantic Books, 2000), 146.
84. G. Vithoulkas, *The Science of Homeopathy* (New York: Grove Press, Inc., 1980), 231.
85. J. Yasgur, *Yasgur's Homeopathic Dictionary* (Greenville, Pa.: Van Hoy Publishers, 1998), 7.
86. A. Saine, "Hering's Law: Law, Rule or Dogma?" *Simillimum* 4, no. 4 (1991): 35.
87. A. Currim, "Hering's Law Revisited," *Simillimum* 16, no. 1 (Spring 2003): 55–56.
88. G. Null, *Germs, Biological Warfare, Vaccinations* (New York: Seven Stories Press, 2003), 145–46.
89. P. Bellavite and A. Signorini, *The Emerging Science of Homeopathy* (Berkeley, Calif.: North Atlantic Books, 2002), 2.
90. P. Lisa, *The Great Medical Monopoly Wars* (Newburyport, Mass.: Hampton Roads Publishing Co., 1994).
91. Ibid., 36.
92. J. Yasgur, *Yasgur's Homeopathic Dictionary* (Greenville, Pa.: Van Hoy Publishers, 1998), 98.
93. M. Dean, *The Trials of Homeopathy* (Essen, Germany: KVC Verlag, 2004), 170.
94. P. Bellavite and A. Signorini, *The Emerging Science of Homeopathy* (Berkeley, Calif: North Atlantic Books, 2002), 43, 44.
95. Ibid., 42, 43, 46, 49, 50, 282.
96. Ibid., 46–47.
97. Ibid., 62, 63.
98. Ibid., 39.
99. J. Pizzorno and M. Murray, "Placebo and Healing," *Textbook of Natural Medicine,* vol. 1 (New York: Churchill Livingstone, 1999, 2000), 53, 54.
100. H. Coulter, *Homeopathic Science and Modern Medicine* (Richmond, Calif.: North Atlantic Books, 1980), 57, 58.
101. P. Bellavite and A. Signorini, *The Emerging Science of Homeopathy* (Berkeley, Calif.: North Atlantic Books, 2002), 67.
102. P. Bellavite and A. Signorini, *The Emerging Science of Homeopathy* (Berkeley, Calif.: North Atlantic Books, 2002), 276, 293.
103. Ibid., 23.
104. G. Vithoulkas, *The Science of Homeopathy* (New York: Grove Press, Inc., 1980), 166.
105. V. McCabe, *Homeopathy, Healing, and You* (New York: St. Martin's Griffin, 1997), 70, 104–5.
106. Ibid., 68–70.
107. S. Lo, "Anomalous State of Ice," *Modern Physics Letters B* 10, no. 19 (1996): 909–19; S. Lo, "Physical Properties of Water with IE Structures," *Modern Physics Letters B* 10, no. 19 (1996): 921–30; V. Elia and M. Niccoli, "Thermodynamics of Extremely Diluted Aqueous Solutions," *Annals of the New York Academy of Sciences* no. 827 (June 1999): 241–48; M. Schiff, *The Memory of Water* (San Francisco: Thorsons, 1994), 21–30.
108. P. Bellavite and A. Signorini, *The Emerging Science of Homeopathy* (Berkeley, Calif: North Atlantic Books, 2002), 68.
109. Ibid., 288.
110. D. Ullman, "New Scientific Evidence for Homeopathic Microdoses," *Townsend Letter for Doctors and Patients,* October 1999, 17.
111. P. Bellavite and A. Signorini, *The Emerging Science of Homeopathy* (Berkeley, Calif.: North Atlantic Books, 2002), 85, 288.
112. L. McTaggart, *The Field* (New York: HarperCollins Publishers, 2002), 70; P. Bellavite and A. Signorini, *The Emerging Science of Homeopathy* (Berkeley, Calif.: North Atlantic Books, 2002), 265–75.
113. Ibid., 268–75.
114. L. McTaggart, *The Field* (New York: HarperCollins Publishers, 2002), xiii–xiv.
115. S. Hahnemann, *Organon of the Medical Art,* ed. W. O'Reilly (Palo Alto, Calif.: Birdcage Books, 1996), 66, 70.

116. J. Yasgur, *Yasgur's Homeopathic Dictionary* (Greenville, Pa: Van Hoy Publishers, 1998), 130.

117. V. McCabe, *Homeopathy, Healing, and You* (New York: St. Martin's Griffin, 1997), 71; J. Yasgur, *Homeopathic Dictionary* (Greenville, Pa.: Van Hoy Publishers, 1998), 244.

118. H. Coulter, *Homeopathic Science and Modern Medicine* (Richmond, Calif.: North Atlantic Books, 1980), 331.

119. Ibid., 334.

120. J. Kent, *Lectures on Homeopathic Philosophy* (Berkeley, Calif.: North Atlantic Books, 1979), ii.

121. H. Coulter, *Homeopathic Science and Modern Medicine* (Richmond, Calif.: North Atlantic Books, 1980), 335, 378–79.

122. Ibid., 363–64, 371–76.

123. Ibid., 382–83.

124. R. Haehl, *Samuel Hahnemann: His Life and Work,* vol. 2 (New Delhi: B. Jain Publishers, 2001), 419–20.

125. Ibid., 167.

126. Ibid., 267.

127. J. Yasgur, *Yasgur's Homeopathic Dictionary* (Greenville, Pa.: Van Hoy Publishers, 1998), 98.

128. H. Coulter, *Homeopathic Science and Modern Medicine* (Richmond, Calif.: North Atlantic Books, 1980), 268.

129. S. Hahnemann, *Organon of the Medical Art,* ed. W. O'Reilly (Palo Alto, Calif.: Birdcage Books, 1996), 118–20.

130. H. Coulter, *Homeopathic Science and Modern Medicine* (Richmond, Calif.: North Atlantic Books, 1980), 329–30.

131. C. Coulter, *Portraits of Homeopathic Medicines,* vol. 1 (St. Louis: Quality Medical Publishing, 1998), 326; ibid., vol. 2, 240; R. Sankaran, *An Insight into Plants,* vol. 1 (Mumbai, India: Homeopathic Medical Publishers, 2002), 222.

132. R. Sankaran, *The Spirit of Homoeopathy* (Mumbai, India: Homeopathic Medical Publishers, 1999), 21–102.

133. *The New Shorter Oxford English Dictionary,* vol. 2 (New York: Oxford University Press, 1993), 3591.

134. R. Sankaran, *The Spirit of Homoeopathy* (Mumbai, India: Homeopathic Medical Publishers, 1999), vi.

135. Ibid., vi, vii.

136. Ibid., viii.

137. R. Sankaran, *An Insight into Plants,* vol. 1 (Mumbai, India: Homeopathic Medical Publishers, 2002), 73–116.

138. J. Baker, "Sensations and Miasm: A Case, Illustrating Their Power and Potential," *Homeopathic Links* 16, no. 4 (Winter 2000): 254.

139. Ibid.

140. J. Lester, "Central Coast Homeopathy Course" (class taught in Watsonville, Calif., May 2001).

141. S. Hahnemann, *Organon of the Medical Art,* ed. W. O'Reilly (Palo Alto, Calif: Birdcage Books, 1996), 171, 252.

142. J. Lester, "Central Coast Homeopathy Course" (Watsonville, Calif.: September 2002).

143. H. Pscheidl, "Artificial versus Natural Diseases," *Homeopathic Links* 12, no. 1 (Spring 1999): 47.

144. S. Hahnemann, *Organon of the Medical Art,* ed. W. O'Reilly (Palo Alto, Calif.: Birdcage Books, 1996), 120.

145. H. Pscheidl, "Artificial versus Natural Diseases," *Homeopathic Links* 12, no. 1 (Spring 1999): 49.

146. E. Hubbard, *Homoeopathy as Art and Science* (Beaconsfield, England: Beaconsfield Publishers, Ltd., 1990), 332.

147. S. Hahnemann, *Organon of the Medical Art,* ed. W. O'Reilly (Palo Alto, Calif.: Birdcage Books, 1996), 2–3.

148. H. van Hootegem, "Current Topics: Limitations of Homeopathy," *Homeopathic Links* 7 (Winter 1994): 12–14.

149. J. Yasgur, *Yasgur's Homeopathic Dictionary* (Greenville, Pa.: Van Hoy Publishers, 1998), 125.

15

VACCINATIONS

The rather pejorative appellation "ugly twin" is used to describe vaccinations for two reasons—(1) homeopathic nosodes and vaccinations are somewhat "twinlike" in that they are superficially similar; and (2) if one truly reviews the scientific literature with an open mind, many experts agree that the negative and "ugly" effects of vaccinations greatly outweigh any possible benefits.

SIMILARITIES BETWEEN HOMEOPATHY AND VACCINATIONS

Both Originated in the Late Eighteenth Century

Although both had earlier origins in antiquity, homeopathy and vaccines both developed in the late 1700s.[1] The year 1789 marked the inchoate beginnings of homeopathy, in which Hahnemann conducted the first proving on himself. After taking bark from the Peruvian cinchona tree and experiencing its effects firsthand, Hahnemann noted in William Cullen's *Materia Medica* that this "quinine bark" cured malaria because it produced a fever similar to the disease of malaria itself. Dr. Hahnemann continued to experiment with and develop these two theories—the law of proving and the law of similars—until the year 1795, when they became firmly rooted as the "central guide for [his] medical practice."[2] The following year his findings were published in Christoph Hufeland's *Journal for Practical Medication Studies* in an article titled the "Law of Similars."[3]

It was in 1796 that British doctor Edward Jenner (1749–1823) first experimentally inoculated a young boy with live cowpox taken from the lesions of a young dairymaid in an attempt to protect him from smallpox.[4] Two years later, Jenner's theories were published in a book with the rather exhaustive title *An Inquiry into the Causes and Effects of the Variolae Vaccinae, a disease discovered in some of the western counties of England, particularly Gloucestershire, and known by the name of the Cow Pox.*[5] Although the use of various forms of vaccines has been traced as far back as 1000 CE in India, the origin of modern-day vaccines used in Western medicine is recorded in history as May 14, 1796, with Jenner's first experimental inoculation. In fact, the term *vaccine* derives from this first inoculation of a preparation derived from *vaccinia,* or cowpox (smallpox in cows).

Both Use Small Amounts of Diseased Tissue

In addition to having similar dates of origin, these two fields of medicine share several similar principles. As in homeopathic remedies, very small amounts of the original raw substance are used in vaccines. Furthermore, both homeopathic remedies and vaccines use diseased material to make remedies. The homeopathic remedies that utilize diseased tissue (e.g., Anthracinum is prepared from the spleen of cattle ill with anthrax) or the products of disease (e.g., Lyssin comes from the saliva of a rabid dog) are called *nosodes,* originating from the Greek terms *nosos,* meaning "disease," and *eidos,* meaning "from." Nosodes, although produced in the same manner as other homeopathic remedies, are prescribed on the principle not of similarity, but of *sameness.* In this isopathic branch of homeopathy, the raw material that is homeopathically diluted and potentized (e.g., Arsenicum or Diphtherinum) is identical to the illness being treated—that is, arsenic poisoning or diphtheria. Hahnemann has been credited with being the first individual to conceive that the products of disease could be used in the cure of disease. In fact, his nosode

Psorinum, made from excretions of diseased skin,* was designated as "the first vaccine ever made."[6]

> **isopathy:** The employment of homeopathically produced substances that are responsible for the disturbance or disease itself, including the use of nosodes from diseased tissues, as well as nondiseased tissues, such as in the case of *autohemotherapy,* when a drop of the patient's blood is used to make a remedy.

THE DIFFERENCES AND THE UGLY TWIN ASPECT

There is an exceptionally wide gulf, however, between vaccines and homeopathy in many other respects.

1. Genetic Mutations and Disease

The most significant of these differences is that homeopathic nosodes, primarily given in 30C potencies and above, do not contain live or attenuated (weakened) microbes that can cause chromosomal damage; vaccines do.

"Jumping Genes"

As early as the 1950s, Barbara McClintock, an American geneticist, reported that because viruses contain pure genetic material (DNA and RNA), they had the capability of "jumping genes." She contended that a virus living in a monkey, calf, or chick culture, in which most vaccine viruses are grown, readily enters into our human cells through the immediate transmission of injecting vaccines directly into the bloodstream. Within our cells, these foreign viruses are able to incorporate their (monkey, calf, or chick) DNA and RNA into our human DNA and RNA.[7] The genetic mutations and disorder that can ensue from an invasive virus "that has wrapped itself into [the] cellular genetic machinery" may manifest in various forms, including immunological impairment (chronic childhood ear and upper respiratory infections) or brain damage (learning disabilities, hyperactivity, social aggressiveness, seizures, and autism).[8]

There is a great difference between the action of a normally invasive virus—for example, the flu or the measles—and one that has been directly injected into the bloodstream through a vaccination. In the former case, the body senses the invading (influenza, measles, etc.) viruses that have replicated themselves in the cell's fluids and have flooded back into the bloodstream. When the immune system recognizes these newly produced viruses in the blood as foreign elements, it sends out natural killer (NK) cells to attack and destroy them. However, in the latter case, when the vaccine viruses are not making more viruses "but simply sitting in the cell's DNA, some scientists theorize it is possible that the detector antibodies may get befuddled." The immune system recognizes that there is a foreign element in the cell, but this element is tied in with the self-element (the human DNA). This can trigger the confused antibodies to send out NK cells to attack and destroy its own innocent cells, resulting in various autoimmune disorders. The particular tissues that are attacked are probably based on the predilection of the particular virus—for example, vaccination with the tetanus virus has been linked with an increase in allergies and asthma, while vaccination with the measles virus has been associated with an increase in ulcerative colitis and Crohn's disease—as well as the individual's specific miasm or reaction mode—for example, psorics would more likely succumb to skin diseases, and tuberculinics to respiratory illnesses.[9]

"Have We Traded Mumps and Measles for Cancer and Leukemia?"

Often, these vaccine viruses cause no immediate discernible outward symptoms. They simply remain as silent intracellular "time bombs" in our bodies that can trigger later autoimmune dysfunction (e.g., systemic lupus erythematosus, rheumatoid arthritis, celiac disease, pernicious anemia, schizophrenia,* Guillain-Barré† syndrome, and

*Psorinum was first made from the "sero-purulent matter contained in the scabies vesicle," but because this sample contained other microbes such as the acarus bacteria, it was later made from the "epidermoid efflorescence of pityriasis" (a common skin disease characterized by fine, branny scales). (F. Vermeulen, *Prisma* [Haarlem, the Netherlands: Emryss, 2002], 1101–2.)

*Current research indicates that at least one-third of all schizophrenia is autoimmune in nature. (R. McGuire, "Brain Antibodies in 33% of Schizophrenics," *Medical Tribune,* July 14, 1988, 6.)

†Guillain-Barré syndrome is "an acute, usually rapidly progressive form of polyneuropathy characterized by muscular weakness and mild distal sensory loss that about half the time begins five days to three weeks after a banal infectious disorder, surgery, or an immunization." (R. Berkow et al., *The Merck Manual,* 15th ed. [Rahway, N.J.: Merck Sharp and Dohme Research Laboratories, 1987], 1446.)

multiple sclerosis) or other "malfunction[s] in the genetic wiring" contributing to the future onset of cancer.[10] It is this mechanism—viral genes derived from vaccines hiding in our DNA for decades and later erupting into some form of immune disorder or disease—that prompted the late Dr. Robert Mendelsohn to ponder in regard to the subject of immunization, "Have we traded mumps and measles for cancer and leukemia?"[11]

VACCINES AND AUTOIMMUNE DYSFUNCTION

An article in *Science* described the autoimmune mechanism of vaccine injections in more detail: "The DNA vaccine gene may incorporate into and damage human chromosomes and the vaccines may prompt the body to make anti-DNA antibodies, which are found in people with autoimmune disorders such as lupus."[12]

2. *Immunological Bankruptcy?*

A further distinction between these two fields of medicine is that homeopathic nosodes do not reduce immune capacity by stimulating large numbers of antibodies to respond to a single given antigen (e.g., a pertussis bacterium or the measles virus); vaccines do.

Healthy Maturation through the Natural Immunity of Minor Illness

In the normal process of illness and recovery from infectious disease, the entire immune system is profoundly stimulated in an endeavor to clear foreign microbes from the body. This occurs through the action of the primary emunctories (liver, lungs, kidneys, skin, and intestines), manifested through numerous signs and symptoms such as fever, rashes, coughing, diarrhea, sweating, and so forth. These various reactions to infectious microorganisms, although unpleasant, are actually necessary for the maturation of a healthy immune system.[13] Thus, the relatively minor diseases of childhood—measles, mumps, rubella (German measles), flu, and chicken pox—that enter the body through the mucous membranes actually "season and strengthen" the body's immune system and ready it for future immunological challenges.[14]

"Deficit Spending" through the Artificial Immunity of Vaccines

In contrast, vaccines work through stimulating only one part of the immune system—the antibodies, which are proteins that defend the body from harmful germs known as antigens. However, once an antibody becomes committed to a given antigen, it becomes inert and incapable of responding to other antigens and challenges. Thus, giving children several (or many) vaccines can significantly reduce the number of antibodies they have available to defend against future microbial invasions and illnesses. In fact, it has been estimated that the artificial immunity conferred by multiple vaccines can commit an estimated 30 to 70 percent of the body's total antibody count. Dr. Harold Buttram, a prolific writer in the field of vaccines, has described this as a "form of deficit spending" that may lead heavily vaccinated individuals toward "immunological bankruptcy," when their few remaining antibodies left after childhood vaccinations are used up by antigenic challenges—influenza, herpes, mononucleosis, pneumonia, and so forth—incurred in their later teenage and adult years.[15] Furthermore, since vaccine injections that bypass the natural mucosal immune system do not confer lifelong immunity, this reduction of available antibodies can continue throughout life as patients comply with their allopathic physician's frequently recommended "booster" doses.[16]

In dramatic contrast, not only do children who recover from the normal spate of childhood illnesses have a lifelong immunity to them, but their more efficiently functioning immune systems have committed only an estimated 3 to 7 percent of their antibodies to this process, leaving them able to respond rapidly and effectively to future infections and challenges.[17]

3. *Toxic Preservatives, Foreign Proteins, and Viral Contaminants*

In further contrast, homeopathic remedies do not contain any other ingredients except the raw material used and pure water and alcohol; vaccines do.

The Mercury-Containing Thimerosal Preservative

The preservatives in vaccines include the widely used mercury-containing thimerosal, present in more than fifty licensed vaccines, as well as phenol (a coal tar derivative with a corrosive action on tissues), 2-phenoxyethanol (a toxic chemical comparable to antifreeze), formalin (a 37 percent solution of formaldehyde gas in water, used as a fixative and a preservative), and formaldehyde (a known cancer-causing agent).[18] Of all the various preservatives that have been used for almost a century in vaccines, none have been as controversial or wreaked as much havoc as the mercury-containing thimerosal.

History: From Merthiolate to Thimerosal. In 1929, Eli Lilly repackaged its popular topical antiseptic Merthiolate—the brand name for thimerosal—and formulated it for use as a preservative. Soon after, thimerosal began to be added to childhood vaccines, despite the fact that in 1935 it was reported to Eli Lilly that this mercury preservative was "unsatisfactory as a preservative for serum intended for use on dogs." Later, in the early 1990s, thimerosal was discontinued in vaccines for cattle. However, as of 1999, this mercury preservative was still being added to most infant vaccines, as well as many flu and booster shots. Other products that may contain thimerosal include immunoglobulins that can be administered during pregnancy (Rho[D] immunoglobuulin for Rh-negative mothers) and some eyedrops and eardrops prescribed for babies and young children.[19]

Thimerosal Preservative Not Even Very Effective. The use of toxic mercury in vaccines is even more insupportable in light of the fact that mercury hasn't even been found to be a reliable preservative. In 1982, an independent panel convened by the FDA reported that mercury was more bacteriostatic than bactericidal, meaning that although it slowed the growth of new bacteria it did not kill them altogether. In fact, in one study thimerosal was found to be "no better than water in protecting mice from fatal streptococcal infection." And even more offensive, although this panel ruled that all mercury-containing preservatives should be removed from all over-the-counter topical products such as Mercurochrome, skin bleaching agents, eardrops, eyedrops, and nasal sprays and be reclassified as "not generally recognized as safe and effective" in 1982, the FDA did nothing to reduce or remove thimerosal from vaccines—that are *injected* into the body—at this time.[20]

Thimerosal Still in Use Today in Some Vaccines. It wasn't until almost two decades later, on June 8, 1999, that the FDA "requested" that vaccine makers phase out vaccines that contain thimerosal.[21] A month later, in July 1999, the American Academy of Pediatrics and federal health officials announced that although "the current levels of thimerosal will not hurt children," this preservative would be phased out of children's vaccines.[22] However, since there was no ban enacted by the FDA or CDC, the July/August 2004 *Mothering* magazine reported that "thimerosal remains in vaccines five years after the FDA recommendation."[23] In fact, the 2003 and 2004 *Physicians' Desk Reference,* which lists the ingredients, indications, and contraindications for all currently used drugs, the DPT and DT shots, hepatitis B shot, the Hib (meningitis) shot, and the flu shot, which are all recommended for infants and children, still lists thimerosal in these vaccines. Furthermore, although in 2005 and 2006 the use of thimerosal was reportedly further reduced, it continues to be used in numerous vaccines.[24]

ELI LILLY AND THIMEROSAL

In 1991, Eli Lilly stopped manufacturing and selling thimerosal. However, licensing agreements demonstrate that sales of this product will continue until at least 2010 (to more than forty nations throughout the third world). In 1999, Lilly printed up a new Material Safety Data Sheet (MSDS) for laboratory workers on the proper procedures for handling thimerosal, stating that the preservative can cause:

> Nervous System and Reproduction Effects; Effects of exposure include fetal changes; Mercury poisoning may occur; Exposure in children may cause mild to severe mental retardation. . . .[25]

Autism "Exploding" in Third-World Countries. Sadly, rates of autism—an illness highly correlated to the use of thimerosal in vaccines—are now rising exponentially. At the turn of the twenty-first century in China, autism was virtually unknown. However, with the advent of thimerosal-laden vaccines being administered there, by 2005 1.8 million children in China had been diagnosed with autism. In other countries such as Argentina, Nigeria, and India, autism rates have been reported to be "exploding."[26]

Tiny Amounts of Thimerosal Cause Cell Death. In spite of the stance of vaccine advocates that "although mercury can be poisonous, the small amount in thiomersal [thimerosal] that is added to vaccines contains very little mercury, and there is no evidence that it has caused harm," current scientific evidence clearly reveals the falseness of this defense.[27] In fact, in a January 2005 report published in the journal *Neurotoxicology,* "very tiny" concentrations of thimerosal were reported to cause membrane damage and cell death, and this damage actually occurred after only a *three-hour* exposure.

Thimerosal Linked with Autism and Alzheimer's. Other studies have shown that individuals who had five consecutive flu shots between 1970 and 1980 had a *ten times* higher rate of developing Alzheimer's disease from the buildup of mercury and aluminum. Dr. Rashid Buttar testified to the U.S. Congress in May 2004 that at least 1,445 scientific papers have clearly demonstrated a link between mercury and neurodegenerative disease. Buttar stated that "mercury is the spark that ignites and re-ignites the fires" that causes autism in early life and Alzheimer's later in life. In his testimony, "Autism: The Misdiagnosis of Our Future Generation," Dr. Buttar warned that an entire generation of children is being damaged from the use of the mercury-containing thimerosal preservative.[28]

A recent study published in the journal *Acta Neurobiologiae Experimentalis* and conducted by researchers at the University of Pittsburgh found "remarkably similar brain changes" in infant monkeys given vaccines to those seen in the brains of autistic children. These changes took place in the amygdala—an important emotion-regulating center of the brain—and the abnormal growth and functioning appeared to be a direct result of the MMR (measles, mumps, rubella), DTaP (diphtheria, tetanus, acellular pertussis), and Hib (Haemophilus influenzae type B) booster vaccines.[29]

In this same primate model, researchers had already identified significantly delayed vital brain stem reflexes in infants receiving the thimerosal-containing hepatitis B vaccine on the first day of life. This vaccine is included in the CDC's recommended immunization schedule for newborns.[30]

The link between the use of thimerosal and autism is further strengthened by the fact that unvaccinated populations—the Amish, for example—have no incidence of autism. Furthermore, in a Chicago-based pediatric practice named Homefirst Health Services that has seen over 30,000 children and delivered 15,000 babies, pediatricians have seen no cases of autism in any of their unvaccinated patients.[31] However, in the general U.S. population, although the rate of autism was 1 in 10,000 children in the 1980s, it has now skyrocketed to 1 in 63 (160 per 10,000 children). And, if the child is a boy, more vulnerable to this devastating developmental disorder, the chances of being diagnosed with an autism spectrum disorder (ASD) rise to an astounding 1 in 38 (2.6 percent of all U.S. male children).[32]*

Children Exposed to Massive Amounts of Mercury in Multiple Vaccines. In fact, even the historically conservative FDA acknowledged in June 1999 that "infants who receive thimerosal injections may be exposed to more mercury than recommended by federal guidelines for total mercury exposure."[33] U.S. Congressman Dan Burton sponsored a bill in that same year to have thimerosal removed from vaccines. Sadly, Burton is all too familiar with the damaging effects of this widely used preservative. His grandson received vaccines for nine different diseases in one day, equaling an estimated 62.5 micrograms of mercury injected into this child's bloodstream—118 times the EPA's limit for daily exposure.[34] (According to his weight, Burton's grandson would only have been able to tolerate a level of 1.51 micrograms.) This child, who was in perfect health before he received the shots, is now autistic. The 1999 bill to remove thimerosal was never passed but was recently replaced with a new bill, the White House Conference on Autism Act of 2009 (HR 3703). However, this legislation that calls for a White House conference on addressing the increasing rate of Americans with autism spectrum disorder has been stuck in a subcommittee for health for over a year and is not expected to pass either.[35]

Thimerosal Exposure Linked to Neurological Damage. The relationship between autism and other types of neurological syndromes and mercury exposure has also been well documented in scientific literature. In

*Currently, one out of every six children has a developmental disorder or behavioral problem. (D. Kirby, *Evidence of Harm* [New York: St. Martin's Press, 2005], xiv.)

fact, a recent study found "statistically significant associations" between thimerosal-containing vaccines at two months of age and developmental delay; cumulative thimerosal exposure at age three months and tics (seen in Tourette's); cumulative exposure at one, three, and six months and neurodevelopmental delays; and cumulative exposure at six months of age and attention deficit disorder (ADD).[36]

A 2004 study published in *Neurology* linked the hepatitis B vaccine to a 310 percent increased risk of developing multiple sclerosis, clearly confirming the relationship between the vaccine and neurological damage.[37]

▶ For more information on this subject, go to the website of SafeMinds (Sensible Action For Ending Mercury-Induced Neurological Disorders) at www.SafeMinds.org.

Thimerosal Litigation Could Rival That of Asbestos and Tobacco. In 2002, after his son was diagnosed with autism spectrum disorder, Dr. Eric Colman, an FDA drug reviewer, commented, "The absence of appropriate preclinical testing of thimerosal is a staggering oversight." Later, in 2003, Representative Dan Weldon (R-Fla.), a conservative and a physician who sits on the Committee on Government Reform, stated, "If it is eventually determined that an entire generation of kids was essentially poisoned, a class-action suit against the federal government could be on the order of hundreds of billions of dollars, and so there's a very good reason for them [the CDC] to cover this up." In fact, one science writer has asserted that if vaccine manufacturers and government agencies are found liable for causing neurological damage to millions of infants, then the "TCV [thimerosal-containing vaccines] litigation could rival that of tobacco or asbestos." A comment made by Martha Herbert of Harvard University on the link between the current autism epidemic and thimerosal-containing vaccines best illustrates the reason for the major suppression underlying this inflammatory issue: "That human actions, rather than genes, might be responsible for compromising the health of a significant proportion of a whole generation is so painful as to be, for many, unthinkable."[38]

It's important to point out, however, that since Eli Lilly began adding thimerosal to vaccines in the early 1930s, this highly toxic preservative is not only currently damaging one generation, but has potentially caused some level—from mild learning disorders to severe autism—of neurodegenerative harm in at least *three generations* of children born in the twentieth and twenty-first centuries.

Adjuvant Heavy Metals and Solvents, Antibiotics, and Foreign Proteins

In addition, vaccines contain *adjuvant* (potentiating or additive) substances such as aluminum compounds (potent neurotoxins) and solvents like acetone (which can cause central nervous system depression).[39] Neomycin and streptomycin are also added to many vaccines, and these antibiotics can cause allergic reactions in susceptible individuals.[40] More serious allergic reactions, even death from anaphylaxis, can result from the injection of foreign animal proteins such as chick embryos, calf serum, dog kidneys, duck embryos, and monkey kidneys, in which most vaccine viruses and bacteria are cultured.[41] Chicken embryos are particularly susceptible to a whole host of avian (bird-related) viruses, which can be transferred to humans through the vaccine.[42] Other ingredients added to this veritable toxic soup include preservatives such as formaldehyde (a known carcinogen) and MSG (monosodium glutamate), a serious and highly allergenic neurotoxin.[43]

adjuvant: *Adjuvant* is used to describe a substance that heightens or stimulates the action of another substance. For example, when aluminum was added to the pertussis vaccine in 1943, fewer pertussis bacteria had to be included in the shot, which was believed to augment the safety of this vaccine.[44]

ALUMINUM IN VACCINES

While the use of mercury (thimerosal) has decreased in vaccines, the use of aluminum has greatly increased. Dr. David Ayoub, an expert on vaccine additives, has found a significant correlation between children diagnosed with ADHD and massive quantities of aluminum showing up in their toxicity profiles.[45]

One vaccine in particular, Pediatrix, a combination vaccine, has been identified by Ayoub as having excessively high amounts of aluminum—850 mcg compared to the average amount per shot of 200–400 mcg.[46]

In his popular holistic newsletter, Dr. Joseph Mercola states that not only is this metal toxic in and of itself, but aluminum impairs glutathione synthesis and the system's ability to excrete mercury, thus rendering any mercury stores even more of a toxic burden in the body.[47]

Monkey Virus Contaminants in Polio Vaccines

Foreign animal proteins also harbor their own viruses that may not be completely killed and made harmless by heat or formaldehyde. For example, in the case of both the injected Salk and oral Sabin (sugar cubes) polio vaccines that were grown on monkey kidneys, an estimated 30 to 100 million Americans and perhaps another 100 million or more other people throughout the world, between 1954 and 1963, were exposed to a simian virus (SV40) that has been confirmed as a catalyst for later brain, bone, and lung cancer and for leukemia.[48] In a study of 59,000 women, the children of mothers who received the Salk vaccine between 1959 and 1965 had brain tumors at a rate *thirteen* times greater than children of mothers who had not received these polio shots. One scientist, finding large cancer tumors growing on laboratory animals after they had been injected with polio vaccine growth medium, made the following prophetic statement to the U.S. Congress in 1972: "If you continue to allow these contaminated [polio] vaccines to go out, I guarantee you that over the next 20 years you will have epidemics of cancer unlike the world has ever seen."[49]

SALK'S ADMISSION

Dr. Jonas Salk himself acknowledged this tragic error:

> SV40 virus . . . was a contaminant in monkey kidney cell cultures. The last thing in the world one would want to do now is to make vaccines out of the tissues of monkeys that come from the jungle. That was a learning experience, you might say.[50]

The baby boomer generation is familiar with the term *learning experience*, but most of us did not know that these experiences began not during our "sex, drugs, and rock and roll" days, but actually when we were young children receiving contaminated vaccinations.

The African green monkey kidney tissues on which polioviruses were grown also harbored another dangerous contaminant—simian immunodeficiency virus (SIV), a virus closely associated with—and sometimes "virtually indistinguishable" from—human immunodeficiency virus (HIV). Based on this close similarity, many researchers have asserted that the SIV-contaminated polio vaccines probably later mutated into HIV and AIDS in more susceptible individuals.[51]

Parasites, Viruses, Possible BSE, and the Use of Aborted Human Fetuses

Fragments and antigens of the parasitic microorganism mycoplasma, presently implicated in the common upper respiratory infections seen in chronic fatigue and autoimmune disorders, have been identified as contaminants in both the polio and the MMR (measles, mumps, rubella) vaccines.[52] Furthermore, the fetal bovine (cow) serum contained in many vaccines carries the remote but possible risk of transmission of Creutzfeldt-Jakob disease—the human form of bovine spongiform encephalopathy (BSE), known as "mad cow" disease.[53] Additionally, the contamination and transfer of other microbes such as mycoplasma, bacteriophages, reoviruses, and parvoviruses have been linked to the addition of trypsin (used to disperse cells) and animal serum (used as a medium for cell growth) in various vaccines. Live vaccines produced from human serum have caused outbreaks of hepatitis B in some populations, due to the transference of this virus through direct injection of the vaccine.[54]

Finally, some individuals may object to the use of aborted human fetuses, referred to as *human fibroblasts* or *human diploid cells*, in which many of these viruses and bacteria are grown. (Many vaccines use both human and animal cultures.) The pharmaceutical companies' answer to this religiously controversial issue of using human embryos is to switch to vaccines made from genetically engineered (GE) viruses—a movement from bad to worse in many people's opinion.[55] However, these genetically modified organisms (GMO) or genetically engineered (GE) microorganisms are already in use in some animal vaccines.[56]

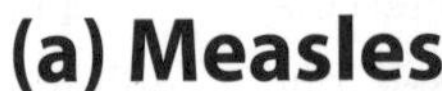

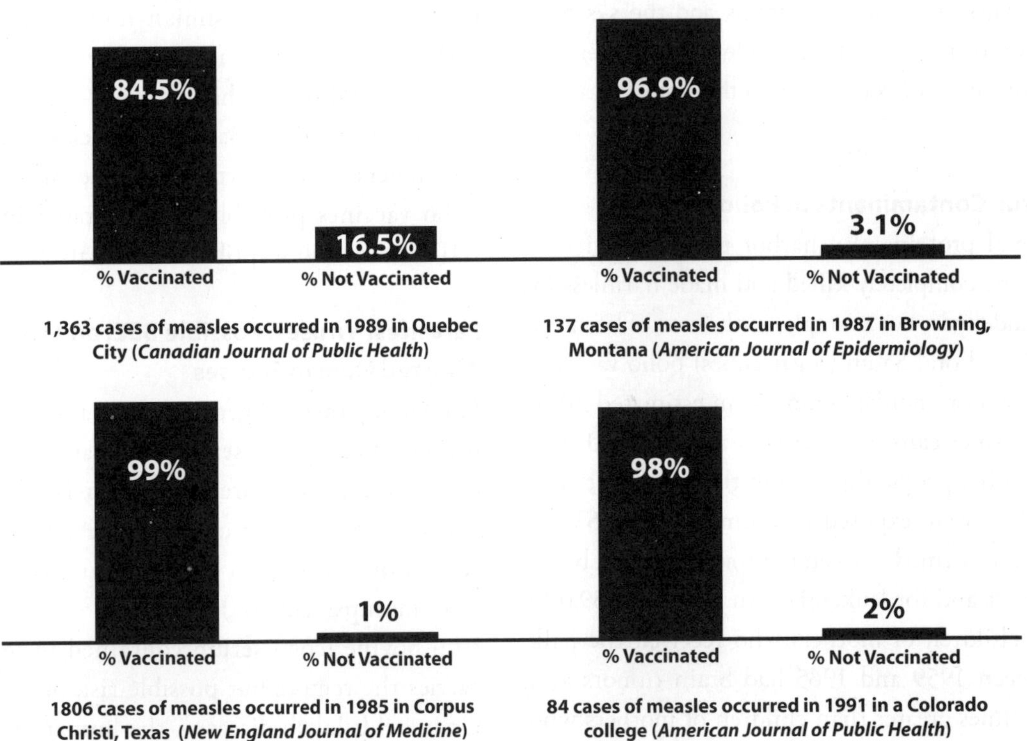

(b) Mumps

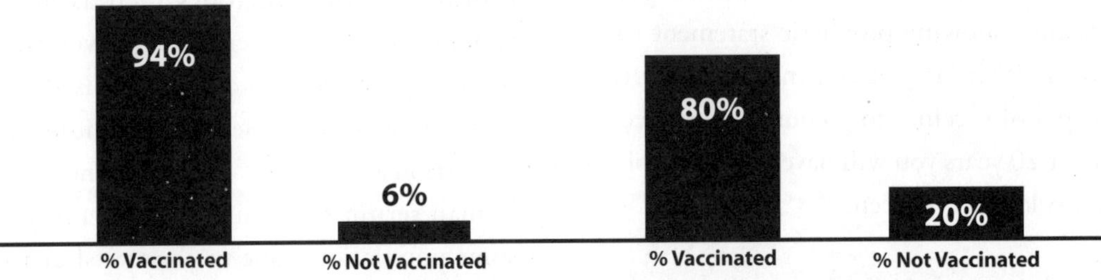

769 cases of mumps occurred in 1981 in Westwood, Massachusetts (*Morbidity & Mortality Weekly Report*)

2,300 cases of mumps occurred between December 2005 and April 2006 in the Midwest—more than half in Iowa (*Centers for Disease Control*)

Figure 15.1. In many cases, the measles (a) and mumps (b) vaccines have failed to confer immunity. (In fact, the vaccinated teens were more than twice as likely to contract the disease, as compared with their unvaccinated peers.)

4. Lack of Scientific Studies

As was previously described, respected and scientifically valid research must be conducted in a placebo-controlled, double-blind manner. This will probably strain the credulity of most readers, but unlike homeopathy, which has undergone numerous clinical research studies and a significant amount (although not nearly enough) of scientific laboratory investigation, vaccines have *never* been adequately scientifically researched.* In fact, many leading authorities categorically state

*The studies conducted in Finland and England that concluded there was no evidence for MMR-associated inflammatory bowel disease and autism were greatly flawed and made "crucial omissions," which were challenged even in the well-respected *Lancet* journal. For more information on these studies, see Neil Miller's book *Vaccines, Autism and Childhood Disorders* (Santa Fe: New Atlantean Press, 2003).

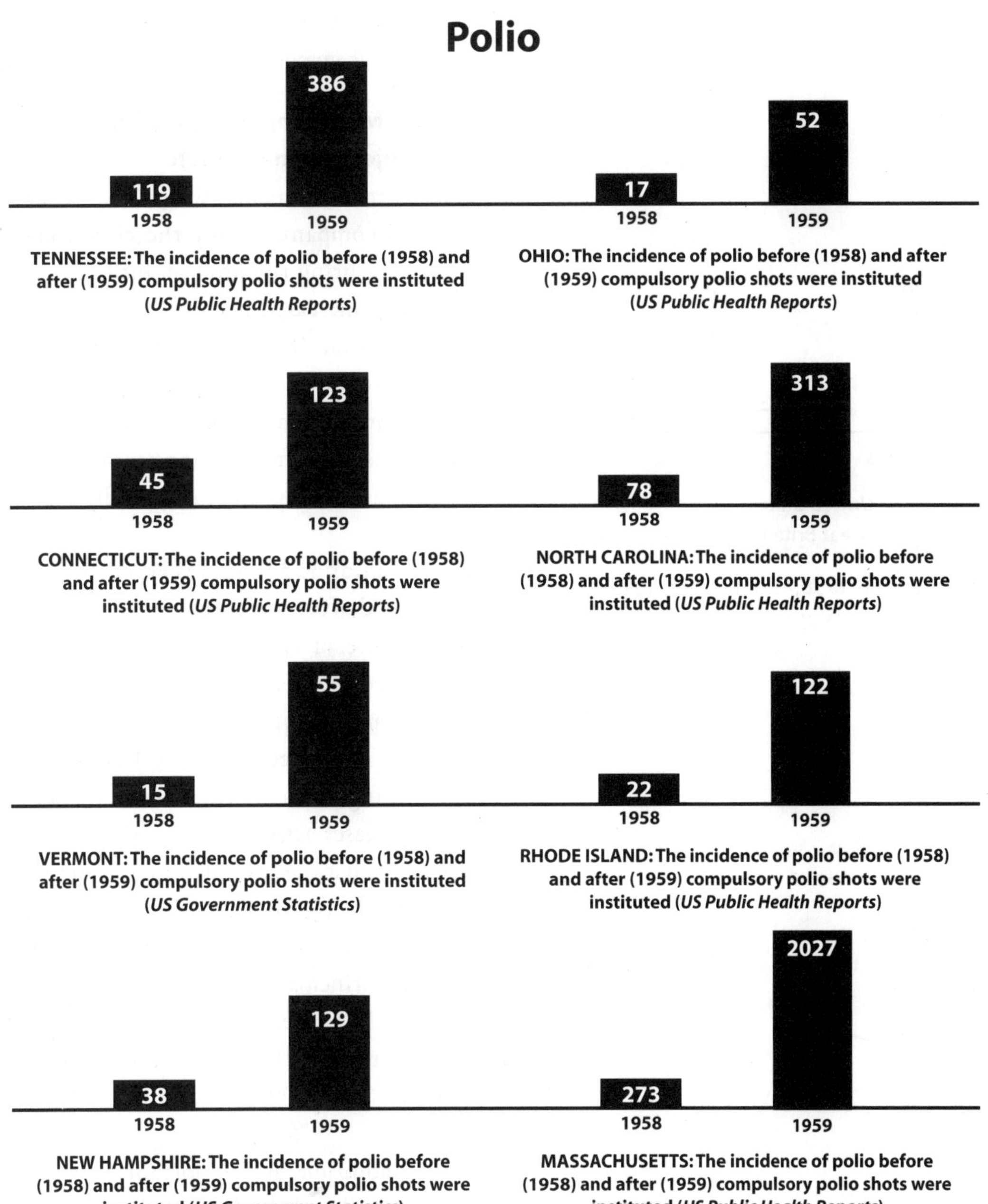

Figure 15.2. After polio vaccines were introduced the incidence of polio actually increased in many states.

that there have never been any double-blind, placebo-controlled research studies measuring the effectiveness of vaccinations, nor any long-term studies* to measure chronic clinical and subclinical side effects.[57] This dearth of quality scientific research is particularly alarming when one considers the billions of dollars spent by government agencies and pharmaceutical companies producing and promoting the use of vaccines, as compared with virtually no money given to the study of "alternative vaccinations" (homeopathic nosodes).

clinical/subclinical: Clinical side effects are symptoms or illnesses that obviously manifest such as autism or cancer; subclinical side effects are symptoms or illnesses that are not obviously

*For example, in one short-term test "adverse effects" were looked for three days following DPT inoculation and in another "systemic events" were analyzed within two days after pneumococcal inoculation (*Physician's Desk Reference,* 1556–57, 34579).

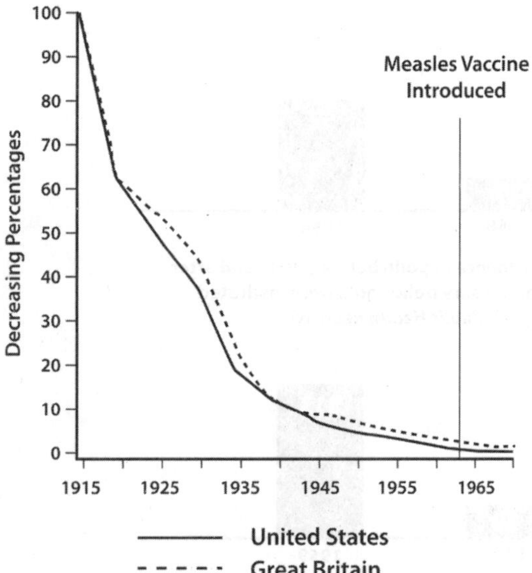

(a) Between 1915 and 1958, the measles death rate in the United States and the United Kingdom declined by 98 percent.

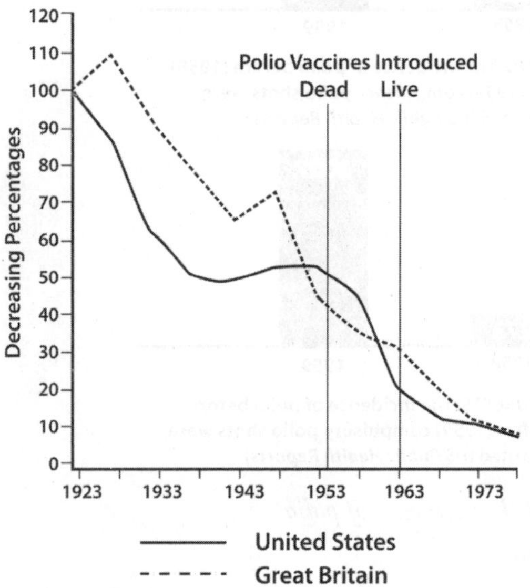

(b) Between 1923 and 1953, the polio death rate had declined in the United States by 47 percent and in England by 55 percent.

Figure 15.3. The measles (a) and polio (b) death rates were already decreasing on their own before the vaccines were introduced. (Reprinted with permission from N. Miller, Vaccines: Are They Really Safe and Effective? *[Santa Fe: New Atlantean Press, 2003].)*

apparent such as mild learning disabilities or chronic immune system impairment.

Simply Measuring Antibody Titers after Injection Inadequate

The primary means by which researchers and pharmaceutical companies study the effectiveness of vaccines is by measuring the level of antibody titers after injection (e.g., increased pertussis antibodies measured after a pertussis vaccination). However, the increased amount of antibodies circulating in the blood has never been proven an adequate and reliable indicator of improved immune system functioning against a particular illness. In fact, just the opposite is typically the case.

Some Childhood Illnesses Have Actually Increased after Vaccines

The failure of vaccines to confer immunity has been confirmed repeatedly, as illustrated by the outbreaks of measles and mumps in various populations in which the majority were vaccinated (see figure 15.1).[58] Even more astonishing, in many cases the outbreak of these childhood diseases actually *increased* after the institution of mass inoculations, as illustrated in the case of polio vaccinations in figure 15.2.[59] In 1976, Dr. Jonas Salk testified before Congress that the Sabin live-virus vaccine was the "principal if not sole cause" of all reported polio cases in the United States since its introduction in 1961. In fact, in 1992, the CDC acknowledged that *every* case of polio since 1979 was caused by the oral polio vaccine itself.

In addition, it's important to point out that for many childhood diseases, as depicted in figure 15.3 in the cases of measles and polio, the death rate from these diseases was already dramatically on the decline *before* the new vaccines were introduced, making the development of these new vaccines particularly counterintuitive.[60] For example, from 1923 to 1953, before the Salk and Sabin vaccines were introduced, polio death rates in the United States and England had already declined by 47 and 55 percent, respectively. However, after mass inoculations, the number of reported cases of polio almost doubled in the United States.[61]

Furthermore, from 1983 to 1991, not a single dose of oral polio vaccine (Sabin) met U.S. safety standards, which meant that those who received this live-virus vaccination had a greatly heightened risk of catching polio or diseases from its contaminated aspects.[62]

Microbes in Combination Vaccines Can Dangerously Potentiate Each Other

The adjuvant or additive effect of combining vaccinations into one shot as in the case of DPT (diphtheria, pertussis, and tetanus), MMR (measles, mumps, and rubella), or DPT with Hib (Haemophilus influenzae type B) has never been subjected to scientific scrutiny.[63] The primary reason these vaccines were initially combined was for the sake of convenience and to simplify the lives of children, their parents, and busy doctors—"not [for] safety and efficacy."[64] Moreover, several studies have shown that in many cases these combination vaccines not only confer "zero or very low immunity" but that three or more microbes can dangerously *potentiate* each other, resulting in a much more damaging shot than a single vaccine inoculation (not to mention the already described additive effect of mercury in the thimerosal preservative).[65] In addition, combination vaccines can unduly stress a child's immune system, as described by Dr. Gerald Poesnecker:

> Naturally acquired childhood diseases tend to automatically exclude others until the first disease is over, the immune system has recovered, and is prepared for the next onslaught. . . . On the other hand, if the body is injected with several vaccines at once (as *never* occurs in nature), the immune system has to call upon all its reserves immediately and, though it wins the battle, its forces are left battered, weakened, and decimated. The body's once proud army is now only a shell of itself and an easy prey to any other invader that may wander its way.[66]

THE "QUADRIGEN" SHOT

A four-in-one-shot combination vaccine, DPT plus polio, was instituted in 1959. However, this Quadrigen shot "evidently combined one too many vaccines" and was found to be highly reactive. It was withdrawn from the market in 1968 and several lawsuits were lodged against the Parke-Davis drug company by parents of children who had been damaged by it.[67]

If illnesses naturally occur in the body generally one at a time, as Hahnemann observed centuries before, it seems unnatural and counterintuitive to give three or more vaccines at once to a child.[68] Leading experts suspect that this "unwarranted coupling of more than one weakened pathogen per shot" can cause one virus (e.g., the mumps) to interrupt the immune system response to another (e.g., the measles or rubella in the case of the MMR vaccine).[69] For example, in 1995, the *New England Journal of Medicine* published a study showing that when children received an injection within one month of receiving a polio vaccine, they were eight times more likely to contract polio. In fact, *Lancet* and other respected medical publications have reported that when diphtheria and pertussis injections were introduced in the 1940s, cases of paralytic polio skyrocketed.[70]

BE INFORMED

All readers, and especially parents, should study both sides of the vaccine controversy before making the personal and often difficult decision of whether to vaccinate or not. There are many excellent books, websites, and journal articles on the subject of immunization. Six of the best of these sources have been heavily cited in this section: Neil Miller's *Vaccines: Are They Really Safe and Effective?* and *Vaccines, Autism and Childhood Disorders;* Gary Null's *Germs, Biological Warfare, Vaccinations;* Harris Coulter and Barbara Loe Fisher's *A Shot in the Dark;* Susan Curtis's *Homeopathic Alternatives to Immunisation*; and Jamie Murphy's *What Every Parent Should Know About Childhood Immunization*. Newer recommended publications on this subject include *Vaccination Is Not Immunization* by Tim O'Shea and *Saying No to Vaccines: A Resource Guide for All Ages* by Sherri Tenpenny; both are exceptionally clear and well documented and are available from the Price-Pottenger Nutrition Foundation (www.ppnf.org). Additionally, I also recommend one of the most "important and troubling" books perhaps ever written, *Evidence of Harm* by David Kirby. This thorough and well-referenced book published in 2005 details why autism grew from a relatively rare phenomenon in the 1980s (1 in 10,000) to the astounding level that it is at today, at the same time that the mercury exposure in infants and children from the preservative thimerosal in vaccines more than doubled.[71]

Readers and parents may also want to call the CDC immunization information hotline at (800) 232-4636, or go to the website www.cdc.gov/vaccines, for information about the purported advantages of vaccines that this government agency champions.

VACCINE REFERENCE GUIDE

In the interest of facilitating this information-gathering process, this section details those vaccinations commonly recommended in the United States and includes the possible components of each vaccine, the recommended ages of injection, and the reported adverse effects. This section can serve as a handy reference for parents and interested readers to quickly locate needed information on a specific vaccine.

Later in this chapter are suggested supportive and alternative treatments to vaccines—both childhood and travel—for those who choose not to vaccinate (or not to fully vaccinate). Treatment for older children, teenagers, and adults who have already received vaccinations and suspect they may be suffering from the clinical or subclinical (subtle) effects of vaccinosis* is also described. Additionally, the "No Shots, No School" compulsory aspect of vaccines is discussed, as well as legal avenues for those who choose not to vaccinate their children.[72] Finally, the potential adjuvant aspect of *all* our toxic challenges—that is, the intermixing and pathogenic potentiation of vaccine viruses and contaminants, toxic metals and chemicals, bacterial focal infections, chronic inflammatory scar interference fields, and so forth—is discussed after this section.

Because the number of and type of compulsory and recommended vaccines have varied over the decades, table 15.1 is included to give the adult reader an approximate idea of the vaccines he or she may have received as a child. Which vaccines were recommended, the ages at which they were given, and information on their exact ingredients before the 1980s is often difficult to ascertain. Before the 1980s, state

*As previously defined, the term *vaccinosis* describes the malaise or sequelae (aftereffects) caused by the administration of vaccines to healthy individuals. (J. Yasgur, *Homeopathic Dictionary* [Greenville, Pa.: Van Hoy Publishers, 1998], 272.)

TABLE 15.1. TIMELINE OF RECOMMENDED VACCINATIONS

Year Introduced	Vaccine, Number of Doses, and Age Range
1932–present	Diphtheria, usually given only after exposure
Pre-1940s	Smallpox, 1 dose before entering school
1940s–early 1970s	Smallpox, 3 doses between age five months and ten years
Late 1940s–1980s	DPT, 2 doses between age three months and three years ; DT, 2 booster doses between age five and ten years
1980s–present	DPT, 5 doses between age two months and six years; DT, 1 booster dose at age eleven or twelve years, and every ten years thereafter
1955–present	Polio, 4 doses between age two months and six years (or up to twenty-one years between 1955 and the 1980s)
1963–1967	Killed measles, 3 doses between age three months and six months
1963–1971	Live (attenuated) measles, 1 dose at nine months or twelve months
1971–present	MMR, 2 doses between age one year and six years
1985–1998	Hib, 1 dose at age two years
1988–present	Hib, 3 doses between age two months and twelve months
1991–present	Hepatitis B, 3 doses between birth and eighteen months
1996–present	Chicken pox, 1 dose at age one year
Oct. 1998–July 1999	Rotavirus, 3 doses before age one year
1999–present	Hepatitis A, 2 doses between age two years and eighteen years, for "high-risk groups"
2000–present	Pneumococcal, 4 doses between age two months and eighteen months
2002–present	Influenza, 1 dose annually from age six months to eighteen years (and thereafter as an adult)

laws on the compulsory nature of vaccines varied, and there was not a harmonized nationwide schedule for the immunization of children. Furthermore, mandatory vaccine requirements varied from state to state, as did the compliance of parents and doctors with these requirements.

► For a copy of the current vaccine schedule recommended by the CDC, the American Academy of Pediatrics, and the American Academy of Family Physicians, call (800) 232-4636 or download a schedule from www.cdc.gov/vaccines.

The possible components used in each vaccine as listed in the following sections are based on the 2003 *Physician's Desk Reference (PDR),* which was selected as the most representative year illustrative of early twenty-first-century vaccines. Parents who are trying to decide whether to vaccinate their children can consult the *PDR* in their doctor's office or the Institute for Vaccine Safety website (www.vaccinesafety.edu) for an updated list of vaccine ingredients.

Chicken Pox Vaccine (Varicella)[73]

Year Introduced: The vaccine was first developed in 1974, licensed in 1995, and routinely recommended beginning in 1996.

Ages Given: One dose at age one year (if child hasn't yet had chicken pox), and two doses at age thirteen years or older (if child hasn't yet had chicken pox).

Shot May Contain: Live, attenuated varicella virus grown on human embryonic lung cells, embryonic guinea pig cells, and human diploid cells (with residual DNA and proteins); sucrose; gelatin; monosodium L-glutamate (MSG); sodium phosphate monobasic; EDTA; neomycin; and fetal bovine serum.

For More Information: Contact Merck (Oka/Merck Varivax vaccine).

Reported Adverse Effects: Rash, herpes zoster (shingles), neurological disorders, brain inflammation, seizures, and death.

The Chicken Pox Illness: Chicken pox is considered by many experts to be a relatively harmless viral childhood disease, which includes symptoms of a fever, a runny nose, a sore throat, and an itchy skin rash. When the red lesions develop fluid vesicles (which look like dew drops), the illness is highly contagious and communicable. Only when the final lesions have crusted over is the child no longer contagious. The chicken pox disease confers permanent immunity.

Diphtheria Vaccine[74]

Year Introduced: In 1895, a diphtheria antitoxin was first developed; diphtheria toxoid was made in the 1920s and is still used today. Immunizations began between 1932 and 1935. Mass inoculations began around the late 1940s, when the diphtheria vaccine was combined with pertussis and tetanus vaccines to make the DPT shot.

Ages Given: Beginning in 1914, the diphtheria antitoxin or toxoid vaccine was administered generally only after exposure to the disease. Widespread use began in the late 1940s, when it was combined with pertussis and tetanus (see DPT section). After the DPT series in childhood, diphtheria/tetanus boosters are recommended every ten years from age eleven or twelve through adulthood.

Shot May Contain: See DPT.

For More Information: See DPT.

Reported Adverse Effects: See DPT. Since the diphtheria vaccine has been combined with tetanus (DT) as well as pertussis and tetanus (DPT) for decades, specific adverse side effects to this vaccine have not been well demonstrated. In fact, most of the side effects of the DPT vaccination have been attributed to the pertussis vaccine. However, in my clinical and energetic testing experience, the formation of a chronic tonsil focal infection, or the increased pathogenicity of an existing one, has often been traced to the diphtheria aspect of the DPT shot.

The Diphtheria Illness: Symptoms begin with a sore throat, coughing, headache, fever, and swollen cervical (neck) lymph nodes. In later stages, a thick grayish white membrane can cover the tonsils, which in severe cases can block the breathing passages and cause death. The incubation period (from the time of infection to when the first symptoms arise) usually ranges from one to five days. Transmission is from person to person, primarily through respiratory (breathing, coughing, sneezing, etc.) and physical contact (touching, kissing, etc.).

Diphtheria was a common contagious bacterial disease during the late nineteenth century. It was later conventionally treated with antibiotics. According to many authorities, improved hygiene has been the primary cause of its eradication in developed countries. In fact, the diphtheria death rate had plummeted long before the introduction of the vaccine. Currently in the United States, diphtheria has nearly disappeared.

DPT (Diphtheria, Pertussis, Tetanus) Vaccine[75]

Year Introduced: The vaccine was combined in the mid-1940s; mass inoculations began soon after.

Ages Given: Late 1940s: one dose between three and six months with a booster at two or three years of age; two DT (diphtheria/tetanus) boosters recommended at age five or six and again at nine or ten years of age.

In 1951, the American Academy of Pediatrics recommended the routine use of DPT inoculations in infancy.[76] In 1952, *Redbook* magazine published an article in which Dr. Edward Wilkes recommended a similar "new immunization schedule for infants," which more widely disseminated the DPT recommendation.[77]

1980s to present: Five doses, with the first three given at two months, four months, and six months; the fourth dose can be given at twelve months or between fifteen and eighteen months, and the fifth one between four and six years of age. A DT booster is recommended at age eleven or twelve, and after that once every ten years.

Shot May Contain: DPT shot: diphtheria and tetanus bacterial toxoids and acellular pertussis bacterial antigens; thimerosal; aluminum; formalin; formaldehyde; glutaraldehyde; 2-phenoxyethanol; barium chloride; ammonium sulfate; polysorbate 80; casamino acids (cow protein); bovine (cow) extract; and gelatin. DT shot: diphtheria and tetanus bacterial toxoids; formaldehyde; aluminum; and thimerosal.

For More Information: Contact Aventis Pasteur Inc. (distributor of Tripedia, Daptacel, and DT vaccines) or GlaxoSmithKline Biologicals (Infanrix).

Reported Adverse Effects: Primarily attributed to the pertussis aspect of the vaccine: *Acute*—autism;* fever (up to 106 degrees F); pain, swelling, and rash (around the area of the injection); projectile vomiting and diarrhea; excessive sleepiness; persistent inconsolable crying; cri encephalique (high-pitched screaming); seizures; anaphylactic shock, collapse, and death; brain damage; incoordination and loss of muscle control (hemiplegia or paraplegia); and SIDS (sudden infant death syndrome). *Chronic*—autism and minimal brain damage (MBD), learning disabilities, hyperactivity (ADHD, etc.); asthma; allergies and hypersensitivity; cough, runny nose, and ear infections; epilepsy; blood disorders (thrombocytopenia and anemia); diabetes and hypoglycemia; blindness; insomnia (reversal of sleep rhythms); and behavior disorders and aggressiveness.

*Autism may be acute (i.e., immediate) or chronic (i.e., not obviously showing up for months or years). For more information on the research studies and numerous actual cases linking autism and the pertussis vaccine, read *A Shot in the Dark* by Harris Coulter and Barbara Loe Fisher.

Hepatitis A Vaccine[78]

Year Introduced: Vaccine was licensed in 1995 and routinely recommended in 1999 to children and adolescents in high-risk groups and selected states and regions.

Ages Given: Two doses given at least six months apart, between the ages of two and eighteen years of age.

Shot May Contain: Inactivated hepatitis A viruses grown on human diploid cells; bovine (cow) albumin; formalin and formaldehyde; aluminum; 2-phenoxyethanol; polysorbate-20; thimerosal; neomycin; and yeast protein.

For More Information: Contact GlaxoSmithKline Biologicals (distributor of Havrix and Twinrix hepatitis A and B combined) or Merck (Vaqta).

Reported Adverse Effects: Anaphylaxis, Guillain-Barré syndrome, brachial plexus neuropathy, transverse myelitis, encephalopathy, meningitis, erythema multiforme, and multiple sclerosis.

The Hepatitis A Illness: Hepatitis A is a contagious liver disease associated with a flulike viral infection usually transmitted through contaminated (with fecal matter) food, drink, or water. The classic symptoms of fever, chills, diarrhea, and fatigue are usually self-limiting, however, and followed by a complete recovery. According to the CDC, the rate of hepatitis A has declined in the United States due to better hygienic and sanitary conditions.

The groups at highest risk for contracting hepatitis A are people traveling to countries where sanitation is poor, homosexual men, and intravenous drug users—not children. Nevertheless, the hepatitis A vaccine is recommended for children, for adolescents [and adults] in "selected states and regions," and for the aforementioned high-risk groups.[79]

Hepatitis B Vaccine[80]

Year Introduced: Vaccine was developed in 1981,* and then again developed, licensed, and recommended routinely in 1991.

Ages Given: Three shots—at birth, one to four months, and six months to eighteen months ("catch-up" vaccinations can be given from two years of age up to eighteen years if the first three shots were missed as an infant).

Shot May Contain: Hepatitis B viruses; aluminum; thimerosal; neomycin; formaldehyde; 2-phenoxyethanol; yeast; and soy.

For More Information: Contact Merck (distributor of Comvax [also contains haemophilus B and meningococcus] and RecombivaxHB) or GlaxoSmithKline (Twinrix [also contains hepatitis A] and Engerix-B).

Reported Adverse Effects: Diabetes, multiple sclerosis, Guillain-Barré syndrome, Bell's palsy, Rolf's palsy, ocular and brachial plexus neuropathy, optic neuritis and occlusion of the central retinal nerve and visual loss, central nervous system demyelinization, cerebral hemorrhage, autism, lumbar reticulopathy, transverse myelitis, autoimmune reactions, thrombocytopenic purpura, bleeding, pulmonary bleeding, bleeding diarrhea, anaphylaxis, rheumatoid arthritis, fever, headaches, pain, vomiting, vertigo, herpes zoster, convulsions, and hepatocellular carcinoma.

The Hepatitis B Illness: Hepatitis B is a flulike viral infection characterized by weakness, loss of appetite, diarrhea, pain in the upper right abdomen, and jaundice (yellowing of the eye and skin). It is contracted primarily through inadequately sterilized needles, poor surgical techniques, and sexual contact. In individuals with impaired immune systems, it can also be transmitted through sharing toothbrushes, razors, and washcloths and from eating contaminated shellfish. Acute hepatitis B usually runs its course within one year, but some chronic infections may progress to liver failure, coma, and death. High-risk groups identified by the CDC include intravenous drug users, prostitutes, those (straight or gay) with multiple sexual partners, children of immigrants from certain areas, healthcare workers, and newborns whose mothers are infected. Less than 1 percent of all cases occur in children younger than age fifteen, and in 90 percent of these cases the child experiences a mild flulike illness and recovers through the efforts of her immune system. Published studies in the *New England Journal of Medicine* as well as other respected journals have found that after four to five years, the hepatitis B vaccine no longer confers immunity to the disease. Surveys in medical journals (*Pediatrics* and *Journal of Family Practice*) indicate that up to 87 percent of pediatricians and family practitioners do not believe this vaccine is needed by their newborn patients.[81]

*In 1981, the FDA licensed a vaccine containing hepatitis B antigens (disease matter) from the blood of infected donors. However, the vaccine was later withdrawn from the market and several studies have suggested that this plasma-derived hepatitis B vaccine was contaminated with HIV, a precursor to AIDS. (N. Miller, *Vaccines: Are They Really Safe and Effective?* [Santa Fe: New Atlantean Press, 2003], 49.)

Hib (Haemophilus Influenzae Type B) Vaccine[82]

Year Introduced: The first polysaccharide vaccine, introduced in 1985, was taken off the market after a significant number of failures were reported in a large study of U.S. children.[83] From 1987 to 1990, several new vaccines were licensed; widespread use of this vaccine began in 1991.

Ages Given: From 1985 to 1988: a single dose of the polysaccharide vaccine was recommended at two years of age. From 1988 to present: three doses—two at two months, four months, or six months and a final dose at or after one year of age.

Shot May Contain: Haemophilus influenzae type B bacteria polysaccharides (and other microbes in these combination shots); bovine (cow) brain cells; aluminum; thimerosal; sucrose; dextrose; soy; yeast; chloride; phenol; formalin; and formaldehyde.

For More Information: All Hib are combination vaccines (with tetanus, hepatitis B, or diphtheria) and are often combined with the DPT vaccine as well: Aventis Pasteur Inc. (ActHIB [with tetanus]), Merck (Comvax [with hepatitis B] or Liquid PedvaxHIB [with meningitis*]), or Wyeth Lederle Laboratories (HibTITER [with diphtheria]).

**Neisseria meningitidis* bacteria are included in the shot.

Reported Adverse Effects: Meningitis,* Guillain-Barré syndrome, insulin-dependent diabetes, transverse myelitis, invasive pneumococcal disease, thrombocytopenia, erythema multiforme, fever, rash, hives, vomiting, diarrhea, seizures, and SIDS.

The Haemophilus Influenzae Type B (Hib) Illness: Hib infections, although they may sound like it, have no relation to the flu (influenza). Hib is a serious bacterial infection characterized by sudden symptoms of headache, high fever, shivering, vomiting, general malaise, photophobia (intolerance of light), drowsiness, and irritability. Hib infection can cause meningitis; pneumonia; hearing loss or neurological problems; epiglottitis (swelling of the throat); and death. Hib infection is spread by sneezing and coughing and through contact with other secretions from an infected person. Conventional treatment consists of intravenous antibiotics and oxygen therapy. Hib bacteria are normally present in the throats of approximately 30 percent of healthy individuals. Hib infections jumped 400 percent between 1946 and 1986, a period coinciding with mass DPT vaccinations. Rates have decreased greatly in recent years, with only 144 cases recorded in 1996 and 1997 combined. Seventy-five percent of all cases occur before age two—generally between six and eleven months of age. Children at risk are those from lower socioeconomic families; children in day care centers, particularly those who are not toilet-trained; and children who have received the Hib vaccine (due to an "increased susceptibility" to the disease during the first seven days after the vaccination).[84]

Influenza Vaccine[85]

Year Introduced: Licensed in 1936; recommended for children in 2002.

Ages Given: Annual doses from ages six months to eighteen years. The CDC also recommends that all adults who want to "reduce their risk of getting the flu" be vaccinated each fall, and that adults over age fifty receive annual flu shots, as well as pregnant women, adults and children six months and older with chronic heart or lung conditions, and people in close contact with high-risk groups—healthcare workers, nursing home workers, home care nurses and aides, etc.*

Shot May Contain: Three strains of influenza viruses; chick embryos; thimerosal; formaldehyde; polyethylene gly-

*The major side effect is what this vaccine is primarily supposed to protect against—meningitis. Several studies have found that Hib-vaccinated children are six times more likely to contract Hib meningitis during the first week after their Hib injection, and one study found that more than 70 percent would succumb to the disease three weeks after the shot. (N. Miller, *Vaccines, Autism and Childhood Disorders* [Santa Fe: New Atlantean Press, 2003], 56–57.)

*Currently, there is also a nasal-spray flu vaccine made up of live, weakened (attenuated) flu viruses approved for use in healthy people five to forty-nine years of age who are not pregnant. (See www.cdc.gov/flu/protect/keyfacts.htm for more information.)

THE HPV VACCINE

Another controversial vaccination has recently been perpetrated on the often too-trusting public: the human papilloma virus (HPV) vaccine. In 2007 Merck—the same company that made Vioxx, which has been linked to more than 60,000 deaths—began recommending its HPV vaccine, Gardasil, to girls between the ages of nine and twenty-six to purportedly protect them against future cervical cancer.[85] Despite the FDA's assertion that it causes no harm, Gardasil has caused numerous deaths from blood clots, respiratory failure, cardiac arrest, and sudden death due to "unknown causes."[86] Other side effects include miscarriages and spontaneous abortion, birth defects, paralysis, grand mal seizures, coma, and anaphylactic shock. Another disturbing statistic is that this vaccine has actually *induced* genital and facial wart outbreaks, even in patients who had tested negative for HPV prior to the vaccination.

Dr. Joseph Mercola has noted that when you compare the low chances of your daughter dying from cervical cancer with the ridiculously low possibility of Gardasil sparing her from cancer, "no reasonable person could argue for the use of this HPV vaccine." The Gardasil vaccine contains only four types of HPV out of the more than one hundred strains; it does not protect against the other ninety-six strains. Furthermore, in 90 percent of women infected, HPVs clear up on their own. It is only when the human papilloma virus lingers for many years in the cervix that abnormal cells could turn into cancer. Thus, the best way to protect yourself from cervical and other forms of cancer is clearly maintaining a healthy immune system through the "radical" (getting to the roots of disease) measures described in this book.[87]

col p-isooctylphenyl ether; tri(n)butylphosphate; polysorbate 80; and possible traces of gentamicin (antibiotic).

For More Information: Contact Aventis Pasteur (distributor of Fluzone) or Wyeth Lederle (Flushield).*

Reported Adverse Effects: Influenza (fever, chills, headache, muscle aches, and fatigue), Guillain-Barré syndrome, encephalopathy and brain stem encephalitis, arthritis, polyneuritis, thrombocytopenia, Alzheimer's, autism, and death.

In 1976, 565 people were stricken with paralysis (Guillain-Barré syndrome) and 10 died after receiving the swine flu vaccine.[89]

The Influenza Illness: The flu is a viral-caused contagious respiratory disease, typically accompanied by achiness and fever, as well as a sore throat, cough, and coryza (runny nose, weepy eyes, etc.). It is often epidemic in the fall and winter. Flu symptoms usually improve in two to three days in healthy individuals; in tuberculinic or luetic individuals, symptoms can linger for weeks or even months. Antibiotics are generally ineffective for this viral-caused illness. Doctors typically recommend bed rest and plenty of fluids. There are a whole host of homeopathic remedies that have proven effective in treating the flu.† The flu can lead to pneumonia and other complications in immune-compromised populations such as the elderly and in individuals with diabetes, anemia, and heart, lung, or kidney dysfunction. In 1918, the Spanish flu circled the globe within four short months and killed from 20 to 50 million people. If the annual flu vaccine contains the correct three strains of influenza virus, it has been found to be approximately 35 percent effective. When the strains don't correctly match the viral strains that are infecting people, the vaccine has been found to be completely ineffective, as

*The drug companies that supply the flu vaccine often change annually, primarily because of the high possibility of liability and the fact that vaccines are not big money-makers. For example, a year's worth of Lipitor, a cholesterol-lowering drug, costs $1,608 and a year's worth of Viagra costs $3,500. But a single dose of a vaccine that (supposedly) lasts for a year sells for around $7 to $10. ("The virus that strikes once a year," *The Week,* November 12, 2004, 17.)

†Homeopaths can refer to Sandra Perko's *The Homeopathic Treatment of Influenza* (extensive list) as well as Roger Morrison's *Desktop Companion to Physical Pathology* (briefer list, along with indicated remedies for other disorders and diseases).

THE GREAT "SWINE FLU" DEBACLE OF 2009

Swine flu is a respiratory illness in pigs caused by infection from the influenza A virus (SIV). These viruses normally very rarely infect humans. Symptoms typically range from a brief and mild respiratory infection to flulike symptoms with fever.

The misnomered "swine flu pandemic" of 2009 was caused by an H1N1 virus that was only *slightly* similar to the SIV virus found in pigs. For the 2009 flu season, for the first time in history, two flu vaccines were recommended by the Centers for Disease Control (CDC): the regular flu shot and the "swine flu" H1N1 vaccine. This recommendation pertained even to more vulnerable populations such as pregnant women and children six months of age and older.

However, what was not propagated by the CDC was that a Canadian study in September 2009 had already found that those who had received a regular seasonal flu shot were actually *twice* as likely to succumb to the swine flu.[90] Furthermore, although the World Health Organization (WHO) declared the swine flu a level 6 pandemic (the most serious level on a scale from 1 to 6) in June 2009, scientists specializing in virology had already found that the H1N1 virus was no more pathogenic than the regular seasonal flu—and in no way correlated with the extreme pathogenicity of the 1917–18 H1N1 virus.[91] In fact, 2009 ended up having lower death rates from influenza than ever in recorded history, despite two-thirds of the American public refusing the H1N1 vaccine. And although the CDC attempted to suppress the data (CBS News had to finally file a Freedom of Information request to obtain it), statistics revealed that there were actually very few cases of swine flu in 2009—for instance, only 2 percent of reported cases in California and 1 percent in Alaska were actually H1N1.[92]

Dr. Russell Blaylock, a board-certified neurologist who has extensively studied the vaccine issue, asserted in a Mercola.com article titled "Swine Flu—One of the Most Massive Cover-Ups in American History" that "we have all been hoodwinked by the governmental 'protection' agency called euphemistically, the Centers for Disease Control and Prevention." Blaylock charged that the CDC actually created this pandemic by "statistical sleight of hand," and that there is "no justification for the fear mongering" and "fueling this panic mentality."[93]

was the case in the 1997–1998 flu season.* Immunity from the flu shot is short-lived; antibody levels begin to decline within months. Permanent immunity to a particular strain of flu occurs only after contracting the disease naturally.

Measles Vaccine[94]

Year Introduced: Vaccines were developed in 1940 (the U.S. military conducted an experimental vaccination program with enlisted men, but the program was terminated after severe reactions occurred) and in the 1960s. Both a live and a killed measles vaccine were licensed in 1963.† In 1970, it was combined with mumps and rubella (MMR shot) and routinely recommended beginning in 1971.

Ages Given: From 1963 to 1967, three doses of the killed vaccine were given between three and six months of age. From 1963 to 1965, one dose of the live attenuated vaccine was given at nine months. From 1965 to 1971, one dose of the live attenuated vaccine was given at twelve months. From 1971 to the present, the MMR vaccine was given; see the MMR section.

Shot May Contain: See MMR.

For More Information: See MMR.

Reported Adverse Effects: Crohn's disease and ulcerative colitis,‡ encephalitis and subacute sclerosing panencephalitis (brain damage),§ Guillain-Barré syndrome, febrile and afebrile convulsions, ataxia (unsteady gait), ocular palsies, anaphylaxis, angioneurotic edema (hives), bronchial spasms, panniculitis (a form of lupus), vasculitis, atypical measles (a more severe form), Stevens-Johnson syndrome, erythema multiforme, deafness and otitis media (ear infection), retinitis and optic neuritis (including partial or total blindness), fever, dizziness, headaches, and death.

The Measles Illness: Measles is a common childhood contagious illness caused by a virus that affects the respiratory system, skin, and eyes. The incubation period (before symptoms appear) is about seven to fourteen days. Initial symptoms include a fever, cough, runny nose, conjunctivitis (red and watery eyes), and photophobia (sensitivity to light). Small spots on the gums (Koplik's spots) arise two to four days later, and one to two days after this the characteristic skin rash appears. Once the rash reaches the feet, the runny nose and cough disappear, the rash begins to fade, and the child feels better. Most children recover fully without treatment after about ten days. The disease confers permanent immunity. Measles can be dangerous in populations newly exposed to the virus, in malnourished children (especially those who are vitamin A deficient) living in undeveloped countries or in impoverished communities, in children with immune system deficiencies, when antipyretics (fever reducers such as aspirin) are used to control the rising temperature,* when the rash is suppressed by drugs,† and in those who have received a measles vaccination. According to the World Health Organization (WHO), those who have received the measles vaccine stand about a fifteen times greater chance of becoming infected with the measles virus than those who have not.[95]

MMR (Measles, Mumps, Rubella) Vaccine[96]

Year Introduced: The vaccine was combined in 1971.

Ages Given: Two doses—between twelve and fifteen months, and between four and six years.

Shot May Contain: Live attenuated measles, mumps, and rubella (German measles) viruses grown on chick embryos

*Similarly, the vaccine used for the December 2003 flu epidemic did not contain the most dangerous strain—the A/Fujian strain, which had surfaced in Australia and New Zealand earlier in the year. (Sandra Perko, *The Homeopathic Treatment of Influenza* [San Antonio, Tex.: Benchmark Homeopathic, 2005].)

†By the mid-1960s, these two vaccines had been given to millions of U.S. children. In 1967, the killed vaccine was removed from the market because it was causing "atypical" measles (a more severe form) and did not confer immunity. Between 1963 and 1967, an estimated 600,000 to 900,000 children had received the killed measles vaccine.

‡In 1994, an article in the *Lancet* journal (vol. 343, no. 105) found a link between the measles vaccine and bowel disease (three times the likelihood after vaccination). In 1995, this respected journal published another landmark study linking the measles vaccine with later inflammatory bowel disease. (S. Curtis, *Homoeopathic Alternatives to Immunisation* [Kent, England: Winter Press, 2002], 26; N. Miller, *Vaccines, Autism and Childhood Disorders* [Santa Fe: New Atlantean Press, 2003], 76–78.)

§Subacute sclerosing panencephalitis (SSPE) after the measles vaccination has been well documented (*Neurology*—1968, *JAMA*—1972 and 1973, *Journal of the Indian Medical Association*—1997). (N. Miller, *Vaccines, Autism and Childhood Disorders* [Santa Fe: New Atlantean Press, 2003], 74, 75.)

*In one study, children who received antipyretics had a five-times higher mortality rate than children who did not. (N. Miller, *Vaccines, Autism and Childhood Disorders* [Santa Fe: New Atlantean Press, 2003], 70–71.)

†Nonsuppressive relievers such as oatmeal baths are fine.

and human diploid cells; fetal bovine (cow) serum; gelatin; human albumin; neomycin; and sucrose.

For More Information: Contact Merck (distributor of M-M-R).

Reported Adverse Effects: Autism, meningitis, encephalitis, febrile seizures, subacute sclerosing panencephalitis (brain damage), transverse myelitis and other neurological disorders, nerve deafness, optic neuritis (including partial or total blindness), learning disabilities, diabetes, Guillain-Barré syndrome, muscle incoordination, fever, headache, joint pain, arthritis (acute and chronic), thrombocytopenia, anaphylaxis, allergies (chronic reaction), inflammatory bowel disease, Crohn's disease, ulcerative colitis, immune system disorders, and death.

Mumps Vaccine[97]

Year Introduced: The first vaccine originated in 1948 and was developed through the 1950s.* A later vaccine was licensed in 1967. The mumps vaccine was put into general use when it was included in the MMR vaccine in the mid-1970s.

Ages Given: See MMR vaccine.

Shot May Contain: See MMR.

For More Information: See MMR.

Reported Adverse Effects: Meningitis and encephalitis,† diabetes,‡ atypical mumps (more severe form), hearing loss, orchitis, anaphylaxis, and death.

The Mumps Illness: Mumps is a mild contagious disease caused by a virus. The primary characteristic symptom is swelling of one or both of the parotid salivary glands just in front of the ears and below the jaw. Other symptoms include fever, headache, muscle aches, and fatigue. In some cases, the testicles in males, and the ovaries and breasts in females, may swell. Because mumps is not a serious illness, the need for medical intervention is rare, and symptoms usually disappear within a week. The disease confers permanent immunity. When a teenager or adult is infected with mumps, complications are rare. However, mumps can potentially cause sterility in men, although this is also rare. Orchitis (inflammation of the testes) does occur in 20 percent of postpubescent males who succumb to the mumps, but nearly all of these cases clear up without sequelae (aftereffects). Furthermore, usually only one testicle is affected, leaving one functioning testicle that can still be sufficient for normal fertility.*

Pertussis (Whooping Cough) Vaccine[98]

Year Introduced: Vaccines were created in 1912 (France), 1925 (Denmark), and 1936 (United States). In the mid-1940s, the pertussis vaccine was combined with diphtheria and tetanus (DPT).

Ages Given: Before the late 1940s, the pertussis vaccine was usually administered only during whooping cough epidemics or after exposure to the disease. In the late 1940s, widespread use began when it was combined with diphtheria and tetanus. (See DPT section.)†

Shot May Contain: See DPT.

For More Information: See DPT.

Reported Adverse Effects: *Acute*—autism; fever (up to 106 degrees F); pain, swelling, and rash (around the area of the injection); projectile vomiting and diarrhea; excessive sleepiness; persistent inconsolable crying; cri encephalique (high-pitched screaming); seizures; anaphylactic

*In the 1950s, a mumps vaccine was tested on orphans and mentally disabled children. Researchers concluded that the test subjects did not sufficiently produce immunity from the illness and the vaccine was taken off the market.

†Numerous studies have found a link between the mumps vaccine and meningitis and other complications to the nervous system (*Lancet*—1989, 1992, and 1993, *British Medical Journal*—1987 and 1989, *Pediatric Infectious Disease Journal*—1989 and 1991, etc.). (N. Miller, *Vaccines, Autism and Childhood Disorders* [Santa Fe: New Atlantean Press, 2003], 94–95.)

‡The mumps vaccine has been associated with the later onset of diabetes (*Journal of Pediatrics*—1975, *Archives of Disease in Childhood*—1975, *Deutsche Medizinische Wochenschrift*—1991, etc.). (N. Miller, *Vaccines, Autism and Childhood Disorders* [Santa Fe: New Atlantean Press, 2003], 96.)

*Based on these facts, the late Dr. Robert Mendelsohn stated that the mumps vaccination should be administered only to males who haven't had the disease by the time they reach puberty. About 180 European medical doctors echoed this sentiment by stating that "there is no plausible reason . . . to immunize *girls* against mumps." (N. Miller, *Vaccines, Autism and Childhood Disorders* [Santa Fe: New Atlantean Press, 2003], 98.)

†In 1944, the American Academy of Pediatrics recommended routine tetanus inoculation in childhood; and in 1951, it recommended DPT inoculations in infancy and childhood. (S. Plotkin and E. Mortimer, *Vaccines* [Philadelphia: W. B. Saunders Company, 1994], 70.)

shock, collapse, and death; brain damage; incoordination and loss of muscle control (hemiplegia or paraplegia); and SIDS (sudden infant death syndrome). *Chronic*—autism and minimal brain damage (MBD), learning disabilities, hyperactivity (ADD, ADHD, etc.); asthma; allergies and hypersensitivity; cough, runny nose, and ear infections; epilepsy; blood disorders (thrombocytopenia and anemia); diabetes and hypoglycemia; blindness; insomnia (reversal of sleep rhythms); and behavior disorders and aggressiveness.

The Pertussis Illness: Whooping cough has plagued humankind since at least the sixteenth century, killing thousands of children in Europe, America, and other parts of the world. However, due to the vast improvements in living standards and sanitation, as well as a growing natural resistance to the disease, whooping cough deaths had *declined* by an estimated 79 to 90 percent (in England and the United States) by the time the pertussis vaccine was used on a widespread basis in the 1940s.[99] In fact, in 1998 it was reported that the pertussis vaccine was "out-killing" the disease by a ratio of ten to one. That is, although approximately ten people a year were dying from whooping cough, more than a hundred deaths per year were attributed to the pertussis vaccine.[100]

Whooping cough is a contagious bacterial disease that usually begins with symptoms typical of a common cold. However, after a week the child will begin to experience a violent, convulsive cough followed by a high-pitched "whooping" noise when trying to inhale between coughing attacks. In serious cases, inadequate oxygen can lead to convulsions and death. Although the disease is rarely fatal, when infants under six months contract pertussis, it can be serious and life-threatening, so professional advice should be sought at once. There is no specific allopathic treatment for pertussis; antibiotics and cough suppressants have had little effect. Full recovery often takes two to three months. The use of homeopathic remedies has been successful when the correct remedy has been chosen, as has been the use of the homeopathic nosode for pertussis (Pertussin or Pertussinum).[101]*

*Just before World War II, Dr. Dorothy Shepherd treated 250 cases of whooping cough in children with the nosode Pertussin 30C. One five-month-old baby died. Four other children did not continue treatment. In the remaining 245 cases, all recovered fully within two weeks.

Pneumococcal Vaccine[102]

Year Introduced: A vaccine was first developed in 1978. In 1983 and 2000, two new vaccines were licensed.* In 2000, this vaccine was routinely recommended.

Ages Given: Four doses—ages two months, four months, six months, and between twelve and eighteen months. (The CDC recommends that adults over sixty-five also get one dose.)

Shot May Contain: Pneumococcus and diphtheria combination shot—seven *Streptococcus pneumoniae* bacterial strains grown on soy; *Corynebacterium diphtheriae* grown on casamino acids (milk protein) and yeast; aluminum.

For More Information: Contact Wyeth-Lederle Laboratories (distributor of Prevnar).

Reported Adverse Effects: Wheezing and asthma, croup, seizures, vomiting, diarrhea, decreased appetite, rash or hives, ear infections, diabetes, autoimmune disease, thrombocytopenia, and SIDS (sudden infant death syndrome).

The Pneumococcal Disease: Pneumococcus (streptococcal pneumonia) is a serious bacterial disease that can cause meningitis, pneumonia, ear infections, sinusitis, and bacteremia (infection of the blood). About ninety strains of the bacteria have been identified as culpable in causing pneumococcus; the vaccine contains seven of these. Most healthy children are not at risk for this disease. In fact, pneumococci commonly inhabit the respiratory tract of about half the population, with no disturbance to the individual. The bacteria can be spread through droplets (coughing, sneezing, etc.), but true epidemics are rare. The patients most susceptible to pneumococcus bacteria are those with preexisting serious immune impairment including lymphoma, Hodgkin's disease, multiple myeloma, sickle cell disease, nephrotic syndrome (kidney dysfunction), spleen dysfunction (including individuals who have undergone a splenectomy), and AIDS and HIV infection, and those who

*A vaccine containing twenty-three strains of the pneumococcal bacteria was licensed in 1983 (Pneumovax 23 by Merck—contains phenol; and Pnu-Immune 23 by Wyeth—contains thimerosal) and is recommended for seniors and certain high-risk children over the age of two. In 2000, a new vaccine was approved (Prevnar by Wyeth) that has seven of the estimated ninety different pneumococcal strains. It is recommended for all children beginning at age two months. (N. Miller, *Vaccines: Are They Really Safe and Effective?* [Santa Fe: New Atlantean Press, 2003], 59.)

have had an organ transplant. Pneumococcal bacteria have been susceptible to and therefore treated with antibiotics; however, more and more strains have become resistant to antibiotics over the years.

Polio Vaccine[103]

Year Introduced: Salk's killed (inactivated) poliovirus vaccine was given as an injection from approximately 1955 to 1965.* Sabin's weakened live poliovirus vaccine was taken orally (e.g., as a sugar cube or in liquid) from approximately 1961 to the 1980s.†

Ages Given: Salk vaccine, 1955–1965. Sabin vaccine, 1961–1980s: four doses at approximately two months, five months, fifteen to eighteen months, and four to six years old or eighteen to twenty-one years. Present: four shots at approximately two months, four months, between six and eighteen months, and between four and six years.

Shot May Contain: 1955–1965 (Salk): killed (inactivated) polioviruses grown on monkey kidneys. 1961 to 1980s (Sabin): weakened live polioviruses grown on monkey kidneys. Present: three types of inactivated poliovirus grown on monkey kidney cells;‡ newborn calf serum; formalin and formaldehyde; 2-phenoxyethanol; and neomycin, streptomycin, and polymyxin B.

For More Information: Contact Aventis Pasteur (producer of IPOL).

Reported Adverse Effects: Polio, paralysis, and death; encephalitis; high fever; irritability; fatigue; vomiting and anorexia; Guillain-Barré syndrome; cancer (brain, bone, lung, leukemia); and possibly increased susceptibility to AIDS.

*After mass inoculations with the Salk vaccine greatly increased polio occurrences, it was considered by several authorities as "worthless as a preventive and dangerous to take." See the section "Monkey Virus Contaminants in Polio Vaccines" (page 453) for a discussion of the link between the Salk vaccine and the later development of cancer and AIDS.

†Just like the Salk vaccine, because the Sabin polio vaccine was also grown on the SV40- and SIV-contaminated kidneys of the African green monkey, it has also been implicated in the later causation of cancer and AIDS.

‡The CDC website states that the polio vaccines (still grown on monkey kidney tissue cultures) no longer contain SV40. (www.cdc.gov/nip/vacsafe/concerns/cancer/sv40-polio-cancer-facts.htm.)

The Polio Illness: Polio is a contagious disease purportedly caused by an intestinal virus* that can attack nerve cells in the brain and spinal cord. The incubation period is generally from seven to fourteen days but may be as long as thirty-five days. Ninety-five percent of individuals who are exposed to the poliovirus don't feel any symptoms, even during epidemics. In 5 percent of cases, polio is experienced as a mild flulike illness with symptoms of a slight fever, malaise, headache, sore throat, and stiffness of the neck and back. Most individuals fully recover within one to three days. In a small percentage of patients, paralysis sets in on approximately the fourth or fifth day, and muscle wasting occurs about three weeks later. Factors predisposing a patient to serious neurologic damage include increasing age (older children and adults), recent tonsillectomy, inoculation (DPT and polio),† pregnancy, and physical exertion concurrent with the onset of brain and spinal cord symptoms (bed rest with appropriate physical therapy is recommended). No polio cases have been reported since 1979 in the United States, *except by those who have received the vaccination.*

Rotavirus Vaccine[104]

Year Introduced: October 1998; removed in July 1999. RotaTeq approved in 2006.

Ages Given: Three doses given to infants under one year of age.

Shot May Contain: A new rotavirus vaccine, RotaTeq, was approved in 2006. Although it does not contain thimerosal, it does contain the following stabilizers: sucrose, sodium citrate, sodium phosphate monobasic mono hydrate, sodium hydroxide, polysorbate 80, cell culture media, and trace amounts of fetal bovine serum.

For More Information: Contact Wyeth-Lederle (Rotashield) or Merck (RotaTeq).

Reported Adverse Effects: Intussusception (bowel obstruction wherein one part of the intestine prolapses into another part of the intestine).

*The underlying cause of polio has also been linked to DDT and other pesticides (J. West, *Wise Traditions,* Fall 2002, 29–39), as well as streptococcus bacteria. (M. Fischer, *Death and Dentistry* [Springfield, Ill.: Charles C. Thomas, 1940], 36.)

†When diphtheria and pertussis vaccines were introduced in the 1940s, paralytic polio cases "skyrocketed." (N. Miller, *Vaccines: Are They Really Safe and Effective?* [Santa Fe: New Atlantean Press, 2003], 14–15.)

The Rotavirus Illness: Rotaviruses can cause serious diarrhea in susceptible individuals, especially infants and children under two years of age.

Rubella Vaccine[105]

Year Introduced: The first live (attenuated) rubella virus vaccine was licensed in 1969; it was combined into a single MMR shot in 1971. Mass inoculations with MMR began in the mid-1970s.

Ages Given: See MMR vaccine.

Shot May Contain: See MMR.

For More Information: See MMR.

Reported Adverse Effects: Arthritis; nerve pain, numbness, polyneuropathy, Guillain-Barré syndrome, transverse myelitis, and paralysis;* diabetes; and chronic fatigue syndrome (CFS).†

RUBELLA VACCINE AND ARTHRITIS

In 1971, the *American Journal of Diseases in Children* published a report that 10 percent of children developed arthritis after their rubella injection. In 1972, the *Journal of the American Medical Association* reported that 46 percent of women older than twenty-five years developed acute arthritis after their rubella vaccination. In 1986, the *Annals of the Rheumatic Diseases* reported that within four weeks of receiving the rubella vaccine, 55 percent of women develop arthritis. In 1991, the U.S. Vaccine Safety Committee acknowledged that the rubella vaccine causes both acute and long-term arthritis.[106]

RUBELLA VACCINE AND DIABETES

A 1978 *Lancet* report stated that "one virus consistently produces diabetes in man—the congenitally acquired rubella virus." Furthermore, the rubella virus can remain dormant for many years. For example, up to 20 percent of all individuals affected by congenital rubella virus succumb to type 1 diabetes *up to twenty years later.* In 1982, researchers documented that specific rubella immune complexes (rubella viruses combined with antibodies to them) attack the pancreas and were found in two-thirds of a rubella-vaccinated group. "These immune complexes were not found in persons who contracted rubella naturally or in those not infected by rubella."[107]

The Rubella Illness: Rubella, or "German measles,"* is a contagious viral disease that is relatively mild and harmless in children. Symptoms may include slight feverishness, a sore throat and runny nose, cervical (neck) gland swelling, and a rash that resembles measles and also tends to move down the body. The duration of illness is approximately three days. The disease confers permanent immunity. When a pregnant woman acquires rubella during the first trimester, there is an associated 10 percent risk that her baby may be born with congenital malformations (blindness, deafness, cleft palate, and heart or mental problems). This risk, termed congenital rubella syndrome (CRS), can be easily tested for through a blood test to determine if the woman has a natural immunity to rubella. Unfortunately, analysis of CDC data suggests that the rubella vaccine has not performed optimally in protecting unborn children from birth defects. In fact, there has been an *increase* in CRS-related birth defects since the introduction of the rubella vaccine. These statistics, as well as rubella "side effects," have not gone unnoticed by the medical profession. Although many hospitals require employees to be vaccinated against rubella, studies have revealed that from 78 to 81 percent of doctors, and 91 percent of obstetricians and gynecologists, refuse the shot.[108] Susan Curtis, a renowned British homeopath, suggests the use of the nosode Rubella 30C for any pregnant women who come in contact with the disease.

Smallpox (Variola) Vaccine[109]

Year Introduced: In 1796, Edward Jenner injected the first vaccine; in the early 1800s, smallpox vaccines became available; in the mid-1800s, smallpox vaccina-

*Reports on nervous system disorders following the rubella vaccine have been published in the *Journal of the American Medical Association* (1970), in the *Journal of Pediatrics* (1972), and by the U.S. Institute of Medicine. (N. Miller, *Vaccines, Autism and Childhood Disorders* [Santa Fe: New Atlantean Press, 2003], 101–2.)

†Articles in the 1982 *Lancet*, 1986 *Journal of Immuno-pharmacology*, 1988 *Medical Hypotheses*, and 1991 *Clinical Ecology* all reported links between the rubella vaccine and chronic fatigue syndrome (CFS). (N. Miller, *Vaccines, Autism and Childhood Disorders* [Santa Fe: New Atlantean Press, 2003], 103.)

*The first researchers to describe the rubella illness were German, thus, the common eponym.

tions were made compulsory for school attendance but the law was not widely enforced until the early 1900s; in the 1970s, U.S. doctors were advised to stop vaccinating with smallpox since the disease had been eradicated, and it was removed from the routine immunization schedule in 1972.

Ages Given: Pre-1940s, generally one shot was compulsory in order to attend school. In the 1940s through the early 1970s, three doses were given—at five months, five or six years, and nine or ten years of age.[110] In the 1970s, U.S. doctors were advised to stop vaccinating with smallpox since the disease had been eradicated. On May 8, 1980, the disease was officially declared eradicated from the planet by the World Health Organization (WHO). However, since the 9/11 terrorist attack, emergency-room medical personnel in many states are being asked to take smallpox vaccinations to (presumably) protect against future bioterrorist attack. Furthermore, the Model State Emergency Health Powers Act (MSEHPA) that gives public health officials the power to use state militia to enforce mandatory smallpox and anthrax mass vaccination campaigns during health emergencies has been passed in whole or in part by forty-four states.[111]

Shot May Contain: The smallpox injection is unusual in that it is given intradermally through five to fifteen sticks, with a needle that has been dipped into smallpox vaccine. Typically, a scab forms that leaves the characteristic smallpox vaccination scar, usually located on the left arm or buttock. Most vaccines currently available are grown on the skin of a calf and harvested after the sacrifice of the animal. The live variola viruses are then purified and attenuated through the addition of fluorocarbon and phenol. Variola viruses have also been grown on chick embryos, hen eggs, and rabbit kidney cells. Before the 1960s, the virus was passed through a variety of *vaccinifers* including cows, sheep, water buffalo, rabbits, horses, and even humans.[112]

> **vaccinifer:** *Vaccinifer* is the term for the source from which the smallpox vaccine is derived.

For More Information: Contact government agencies. Go to www.bt.cdc.gov/agent/smallpox/vaccination.

Reported Adverse Effects: General paralysis, eczema, encephalitis and encephalomyelitis, smallpox and death, cancer, and possibly AIDS.* Smallpox vaccine often fails to confer immunity and is even causative of the disease itself, as has been well documented throughout the world. Twenty years before the worst smallpox epidemics in Italy from 1887 to 1889, 98.5 percent of the Italian people had been vaccinated against the disease. In 1871, the most severe smallpox epidemic occurred in England and Wales after compulsory vaccination was enforced that year. In 1870 to 1871 in Germany, 124,948 deaths occurred from smallpox in a population that had a 96 percent smallpox vaccine compliancy. In England in the late 1800s, three hospitals recorded the following statistics: 145 out of 155 persons admitted with smallpox had been previously vaccinated, 870 out of 950 persons admitted with smallpox had been previously vaccinated, and 2,347 out of 2,965 persons admitted with smallpox had been previously vaccinated. Furthermore, in 1918 and 1919, after the United States took control of the Philippines and enforced mandatory smallpox vaccinations for the entire population, the worst epidemic of smallpox ever recorded occurred. After many people in the Philippines began refusing the vaccine, deaths from smallpox plummeted. Finally, in 1928, the *British Medical Journal* acknowledged that people vaccinated against smallpox were *five times* more likely to die from the disease, as compared to those who were not vaccinated.[113]

THE SMALLPOX-CANCER CONNECTION

Numerous doctors and scientists suspect that smallpox vaccines, as well as other vaccines, are causative of our present-day epidemic cancer rates:

> Vaccination does not stay the spread of smallpox, nor even modify it in those who get it after vaccination. It does introduce in the system contamination and, therefore, contributes to the spread of tuberculosis, cancer, and even leprosy. It tends to make more virulent epidemics and to make them more extensive.
>
> Dr. Walter M. James, Philadelphia practitioner

*In 1987, a WHO advisor was assigned to investigate whether the massive smallpox vaccination campaigns in Africa (Zaire, Zambia, Tanzania, Uganda, Malawi, Rwanda, and Burundi), Brazil, and Haiti may have triggered the AIDS epidemic. He, as well as Robert Gallo, a renowned authority on AIDS, concluded that the live virus used in the smallpox vaccine was a very possible activator of dormant HIV infections. (N. Miller, *Vaccines: Are They Really Safe and Effective?* [Santa Fe: New Atlantean Press, 2003], 80, 81.)

> Cancer was practically unknown until cowpox vaccination began to be introduced. I have had to deal with 200 cases of cancer and I never saw a case of cancer in an unvaccinated person.
>
> Dr. W. B. Clark, New York practitioner

> I am convinced that some 80 percent of these cancer deaths are caused by the [smallpox] vaccinations they have undergone. These are well known to cause grave and permanent disease of the heart also.
>
> Dr. Herbert Snow, surgeon,
> London Cancer Hospital

> I have no hesitation in stating that in my judgment the most frequent disposing condition for cancerous development is infused into the blood by vaccination and re-vaccination.
>
> Dr. Dennis Turnbull,
> thirty-year cancer researcher

Even more incriminating, malignant tumors at the exact site of the inoculation scar have been documented by numerous physicians and researchers, arising from three months to over forty years after the smallpox vaccination was given.[114]

The Smallpox Illness: Smallpox is a highly contagious disease caused by the variola major or minor virus. It is contracted by inhaling droplets from an infected person (coughing, sneezing, etc.). However, it can also be transmitted through *fomites*—that is, through infected linens, blankets, or clothing. The incubation period is twelve days, and symptoms include fever, nausea and vomiting, headache, backache, muscle pain, and prostration. A rash that can be confused with chicken pox covers the entire body. However, unlike the more superficial and not well-circumscribed chicken pox rash, smallpox skin lesions are round and well circumscribed, deep in the skin, and hard to the touch. The mortality rate of the more serious disease, variola major,* is 30 percent and higher. The mortality rate of the less serious disease, variola minor, is 15 percent or less. There is no antiviral or other drug that can treat smallpox once it is contracted. The disease confers permanent immunity. During the eighteenth century, smallpox epidemics were common throughout Europe. However, by the mid-1850s, it was no longer a major killer, and by 1967, the year that WHO initiated its worldwide vaccination campaign, smallpox had already stopped infecting people in more than eight out of ten countries in the world.[115] Better sanitation (clean streets and stables, trash removal, sewage systems, and drainage of swamps and marshes), nutritional reforms (improved roads so that food could be transported fresh to market), and water sanitation are credited by historians with reducing the incidence of contagious diseases such as smallpox, as well as scarlet fever and the plague (for which no vaccines were developed, yet they also disappeared). The use of smallpox inoculations in a targeted "ringlike" manner—that is, by quick identification and isolation of people with the disease and inoculation of their immediate contacts—versus "blanket" immunizations—that is, inoculating everyone in third-world countries where the disease was still occurring—is credited by many scholars as what finally "did the trick" in eradicating the disease.[116]

*An uncommon severe variant of variola major is hemorrhagic smallpox, characterized by extensive bleeding into the skin, mucous membranes, and gastrointestinal tract.

> **fomite:** A fomite is an object, such as a piece of clothing or a book, that is not in itself harmful, but that can harbor pathogenic organisms and thus serve as an agent of transmission of infection and disease.

Tetanus Vaccine[117]

Year Introduced: A tetanus toxoid became available in 1938 but was not widely used until 1941; later a tetanus antitoxin (immune globulin) became available; tetanus toxoids were combined with diphtheria and pertussis vaccines (DPT) in the mid-1940s.

Ages Given: Before the 1940s, the tetanus vaccine was usually only administered after the occurrence of a cut or injury. In 1941, the U.S. military began routine prophylactic inoculations on servicemen in World War II. In the late 1940s, widespread use began when the tetanus vaccine was combined with pertussis and diphtheria vaccines (see DPT section).* After the DPT series in childhood, diph-

*In 1944, the American Academy of Pediatrics recommended routine tetanus inoculation in childhood, and in 1951 it recommended DPT inoculations in infancy and childhood. (S. Plotkin and E. Mortimer, *Vaccines* [Philadelphia: W. B. Saunders Company, 1994], 70.)

theria/tetanus (DT) boosters are recommended every ten years from ages eleven or twelve through adulthood.

Shot May Contain: See DPT. Tetanus alone—tetanus immune globulin from the blood plasma of donors immunized with tetanus toxoid, tri-n-butyl phosphate, and detergent (sodium cholate). Thimerosal was removed in 1996.

For More Information: See DPT. For information about tetanus alone, contact Bayer Biological (producer of Baytet).

Reported Adverse Effects: Immune suppression;* Guillain-Barré syndrome, demyelinating diseases, arthritis and joint inflammation, asthma, and allergic reactions (anaphylaxis, increased food and environmental allergies, etc.).

The Tetanus Illness: Tetanus is unique among the childhood and adolescent vaccinations in that like many others, the illness (and the vaccine) does not confer immunity. Furthermore, tetanus is not contagious. Tetanus is caused by bacteria called *Clostridium tetani* that usually enter the body through a wound, especially deep penetrating wounds such as those caused by a nail. Dormant tetanus bacteria spores inhabit soil, dust, and animal manure and can grow and multiply only in anaerobic (oxygen-free) environments, such as those caused by puncture wounds. Tetanus may follow obviously contaminated wounds as well as trivial and small wounds. The incubation period (from the time of injury to when the symptoms first appear) usually ranges from five to ten days. The tetanus illness includes symptoms of restlessness, irritability, depression, headaches, a stiff neck, and muscular spasms that usually start in the jaw muscles (masseters) and prevent some victims from opening their mouths or swallowing (hence the common name *lockjaw*), and can thus interfere with breathing. In most cases, thorough wound hygiene eliminates the possibility of tetanus. Therefore, deep puncture wounds should be scrupulously cleaned as soon as possible (optimally within six hours) and not allowed to close until healing has occurred beneath the skin. After a wound is incurred, the tetanus vaccine is usually administered to unvaccinated individuals or those who have not had a recent booster.*

*A 1994 *New England Journal of Medicine* reported that the tetanus booster vaccine could cause a temporary "AIDS-like" drop in the ratio of helper-suppressor lymphocytes approximately three days to two weeks after the injection in *healthy* adults. The effect this vaccine has on the immature immune systems of children has not been measured. (N. Miller, *Vaccines: Are They Really Safe and Effective?* [Santa Fe: New Atlantean Press, 2003], 24–25; I. Golden, *Vaccination? A Review of Risks and Alternatives* [Daylesford, Victoria, Australia: self-published, 1998], 75.)

*In some doctors' opinions, "thorough wound toilet [cleaning] makes the use of either tetanus anti-toxin or prophylactic antibiotics undesirable." (I. Golden, *Vaccination? A Review of Risks and Alternatives* [Daylesford, Victoria, Australia: self-published, 1998], 76.)

THE DISEASE OF VACCINOSIS

The term *vaccinosis*—that is, the adverse sequelae (aftereffects) following vaccinations—was first coined in 1877 by Dr. Goullon from Weimar, Germany.[118] Later, James Compton Burnett (1840–1901), a famous and prolific British homeopathic physician who published twenty-seven books on homeopathy, noted that a vaccine virus frequently "rouses latent disease"—that is, miasms—most typically those of the sycotic or second reaction mode (see chapter 1).[119†] Dr. Burnett observed in the nineteenth century what modern homeopaths and other holistic physicians and practitioners are still seeing today: "Vaccinosis shews itself as a formidable acute disease that may terminate fatally, or it may manifest itself as a chronic affection."[120‡]

Reactions to the effects of vaccinations may display acutely, such as malaise (fatigue), rash, high fever, seizures, or even death immediately or soon after an injection (within the first few days or weeks), or chronically, through such symptoms as chronic intermittent ear infections, learning disorders and hyperactivity, autism, arthritis, or diabetes, which may not be evident for months or even years. In either case, all instances of injury after immunization—from mild to severe—should be reported to the Vaccine Adverse Event Reporting System.

▶ Go to http://vaers.hhs.gov, or call the Vaccine Adverse Event Reporting System (VAERS) at (800) 822-7967. Too many parents and adults, understandably angry at the government, fail to report damage from vaccines

†However, brain damage and autism following pertussis, for example, would fall into the most severely debilitating reaction mode—the luetic.

‡Of course, in the nineteenth century Burnett was only observing the effects of the smallpox vaccine; however, "modern homeopaths see similar cases of vaccinosis occurring after rabies, measles, polio, influenza, typhoid, paratyphoid, and even tetanus vaccines." (G. Vithoulkas, *The Science of Homeopathy* [New York: Grove Press, Inc., 1980], 115–16.)

in their children or themselves to this CDC- and FDA-cosponsored organization. However, the only way to make real change in the current system is for *everyone* to report every instance of vaccine injury.

Dramatic acute reactions such as anaphylactic shock, convulsions, or vomiting require immediate emergency treatment to mitigate the damaging effects of the vaccine. Similarly, subacute negative effects occurring hours, days, or even a few weeks later should serve as a signal to parents to seek help immediately. However, subtle adverse responses may be difficult to interpret. George Vithoulkas, one of the foremost homeopaths in the world, sheds light on interpreting the two basic responses that occur after vaccinations:

1. There is no reaction at all.
2. The vaccination may "take," indicating that some degree of reaction is produced.[121]

No Reaction at All: Can Be Very Positive or Very Negative

When an individual feels and displays no reactions at all from a vaccine, this can indicate that his or her system is quite healthy and not sensitive to—and therefore not disturbed by—the inoculation. However, it can also indicate exactly the opposite. That is, the individual's system is very weak and, therefore, incapable of mounting a defensive immune response. These latter depleted individuals are typically exhibiting existing or latent tuberculinic or luetic miasmic (third and fourth reaction modes) tendencies from a preexisting genetic or environmentally weakened constitution. Or in some cases, and especially when several vaccines are administered at the same time, these more serious reaction mode tendencies may manifest as a result of the severe toxic load (viruses, bacteria, heavy metals, chemical preservatives, etc.) injected into the bloodstream all at once, which would wreak havoc in almost anyone's body. Whichever the case, it is important to remember that no response does not always equate with a healthy infant or child.

A Reaction: Can Also Be Positive or Negative

In the second scenario, when the vaccination is said to "take," Vithoulkas has observed that there are basically three types of typical reactions:

1. A mild reaction
2. A strong reaction with associated fever, malaise, muscle aches, and so forth
3. A *very* strong reaction, with resulting complications such as encephalitis, paralysis, minimal brain damage (MBD), autism, chronic insomnia, and so forth[122]

Mild Reaction—Child Is Weakened

In the first case, a mild reaction reveals that the infant or child is indeed susceptible to the viral or bacterial disease against which he or she was vaccinated. This mild reaction indicates that the defense mechanism can react, with local symptoms around the site of injection (inflammation, itching, pain, or even a little pus), but is not strong enough to "fully deflect the effect of the vaccine." Thus, Vithoulkas has observed that the vaccine's "morbific influence then remains in the body, and the vibration rate of the entire organism is changed . . . [and may] become incapable of returning to the prevaccination level without the aid of homeopathic treatment."[123]

Strong Reaction—Healthy Immune Response

In the second case, a strong reaction indicates that this infant or child is sensitive to the viral or bacterial disease against which he or she has been vaccinated but *does* have the defensive capabilities to throw off the adverse effects of the vaccine.[124]

Very Strong Reaction—Negative Prognosis

In the third type of scenario, a *very* strong reaction indicates that the infant or child is quite susceptible to the viral or bacterial disease against which he or she has been vaccinated but is too weak to counteract the toxic effects, and subsequently, a deep illness is produced. In these "most tragic circumstances," Vithoulkas has found that "the weakening of the defense mechanism in such cases can be so severe that even careful homeopathic prescribing may require years to return the person to health."[125]

Emergency Treatments for Vaccinosis

When serious reactions to vaccines occur, or are suspected when the child exhibits no reaction at all, time is vital. In emergencies, contact the physician who administered the vaccine(s) or go to the emergency room. Additionally, contact your homeopath or other holistic practitioner for a post-vaccination assessment. Treatment can range from simply the need for algae (ProAlgen from Nordic Naturals) to bind residual mercury from the thimerosal preservative to the prescription of homeopathic *tautopathic* remedies (Pertussis Vaccine 200C, Measles Vaccine 200C, Tetanus Vaccine 200C, e.g.) or a classic homeopathic remedy that has historically been proven effective for vaccinosis (Thuja occidentalis, Malandrinum, or Silicea [three classic remedies for all types of vaccinosis], Ledum palustre [most specifically for tetanus], or Hypericum perforatum [for nerve injury and vital shock from the needle injection], etc.). When the infant or child (or adult) has received more than one vaccine, holistic practitioners who do quality energetic testing can often be invaluable in pinpointing the most damaging vaccine (or the particular damaging aspect of the vaccine—that is, mercury, formaldehyde, aluminum, viruses, etc.) and focus treatment primarily on it, thereby achieving more effective therapeutic results.

tautopathy: Tautopathy is a form of isotherapy (the law of sameness), in which allopathic medicines are homeopathically prepared to treat the adverse effects of such allopathic medicines.

However, perhaps the most valuable treatment of all is to re-dose your infant or child immediately after the inoculation with his or her constitutional remedy, prescribed according to the Sankaran system. If this remedy has not yet been determined, finding a skilled homeopath as soon as possible is essential.

▶ To find a homeopath near you, preferably utilizing the Sankaran system, contact the California Center for Homeopathic Education at (760) 466-7581, or go to www.cchomeopathic.com.

Subtle or Subclinical Responses

When prompt holistic treatment is not undertaken, or when the vaccine has severe effects, chronic symptoms and diseases can result. As listed previously in the "Vaccine Reference Guide" section, diseases such as diabetes, arthritis, and even cancer have the potential to arise years or even decades later as a result of vaccination. However, these clinically diagnosable illnesses may be only the tip of the iceberg. The growth and development of children can also be affected in much more subtle (i.e., subclinical) ways. In a 1982 television broadcast, *DPT: Vaccine Roulette,* the microbiologist Bobby Young asserted the following: "If the child is not frankly rendered a vegetable . . . how many infants that are receiving this [DPT] are in some way damaged by the vaccine, and how can you prove that they haven't been, or that they have been? All of them are vaccinated."[126]

Thus, children, teenagers, and adults who are plagued with mild learning disabilities, irritability, intermittent fatigue, and other more subtle symptoms may be suffering from a more subclinical form of vaccinosis. Unfortunately, until double-blind, placebo-controlled scientific studies are conducted comparing vaccinated individuals to unvaccinated individuals, no one can really know the extent of damage caused by early childhood vaccines. However, practitioners who use energetic testing "unearth" the subclinical effects of vaccinosis all the time, especially in their more "advanced" patients who are retracing childhood issues and injuries.

VACCINE STUDY FEASIBILITY

Vaccine proponents argue that a scientific study with a control group wouldn't be feasible since it would be unethical to deny vaccines to any portion of the population. However, there is a large and growing population of holistically oriented parents who would readily volunteer their children for the unvaccinated control group, from which a random sample could be made and matched with a group of children from pro-vaccine parents who have similar lifestyles (often eat organic foods, limit sugar, use nutritional supplements, etc.).

Thirty-six Doses of Vaccines Received before First Grade!

The need for scientifically conducted research has become even more crucial in recent years as the number of vaccines has dramatically increased. For example, those of us in the baby boomer generation received approximately six or seven vaccines (i.e., DPT, polio, and smallpox) before entering first grade, depending on the state in which we lived, the compliance of our parents, and the allopathic tendencies of the family doctor. In stark contrast, however, currently routinely vaccinated children receive a whopping *ten* to *twelve* vaccines before they're eighteen months old, and at least *twenty-eight* (and up to thirty-six) doses of vaccines before first grade.[127] (This breaks down to one chicken pox, five DPT, three hepatitis B, three Hib, six influenza, two MMR, four pneumococcus, and four polio. For children in "high-risk groups and selected states and regions" where the hepatitis A vaccine is administered, the number would rise to twenty-nine or thirty.) Dr. Russell Blaylock, an expert on impaired brain development and neurological damage from vaccines, has noted that with more recent additions to the CDC recommendations a child may now receive more than thirty-six injections before attending school. Blaylock has found that this excessive vaccination schedule increases the risk of not only autism but also neurodegenerative diseases and schizophrenia.[128]

The sheer toxic load (viruses, bacteria, chemical preservatives, toxic metals, and foreign protein antigens) contained in these vaccines that are injected directly into infants and toddlers is rather staggering to try to comprehend, especially in light of the fact that until age four or five, a child's brain is still "under construction" and has not completely developed. The authors of *Vaccine Roulette* comment on this disturbing issue: "Babies and infants are physically too immature to be able to cope with the toxic load of the vaccines. Their bodies, and especially their brains, have not finished developing and maturing."[129]

If even half of the existing research studies on the adverse effects of vaccines are correct, vaccinosis may well be the underlying reason why physicians are "being inundated by children with immune deficiency problems at an unprecedented rate," why developmental disabilities now plague one child in five, and perhaps even why incidents such as those at Columbine High School and other serious child and adolescent violence are increasing at such an alarming rate.[130]

developmental disabilities: Developmental disabilities include dyslexia, minimal brain damage (MBD), hyperactivity, functional enuresis, autism, and other appellations of dysfunction in infancy, childhood, or adolescence most often generated by encephalitis secondary to vaccinations.[131]

Vaccines Linked to Social Violence

In his book *Vaccination, Social Violence, and Criminality,* Harris Coulter concluded after an extensive review of the scientific literature and criminology statistics that "the so-called 'sociopathic personality' which is at the root of the enormous increase in crime over the past two to three decades, is also largely rooted in vaccine damage."[132] He further indicts the modern tendency of "success leading to excess," in regard to the use of multiple vaccines, as being severely disabling to our children and adolescents as well as to the fabric of our society itself:

> Thus the vaccination program has served to undermine the American school system—which is in collapse through inability to cope with the one-fifth or one-quarter of students who will never be able to read or to perform simple arithmetical calculations.
>
> And it has contributed to the wave of violent crime which is turning our cities into jungles where the strong and the vicious prey upon the weak and unprotected.
>
> The effects of vaccination have altered the very tone and atmosphere of modern society. Because the changes are so insidious and widespread, and because we lack perspective, they have been largely overlooked. It is not easy to discern the outlines of the incubus which the vaccination program has loosed upon us.[133]

VACCINES AND AGGRESSIVE ANIMALS

This tendency toward violence has been correlated with aggressive attacks by dogs that are vaccinated at an ever-increasing rate by allopathic veterinarians. Dr. Richard Pitcairn, a leading holistic veterinarian, has found over his many years of experience that this aggressive behavior is linked to rabies vaccinations. In fact, canine aggressive behavior—being suspicious, impulsive, and destructive and having an urge to wander—are actual symptoms of the rabies disease that Pitcairn has observed can be set off after receiving this vaccine. He cautions owners not to vaccinate these disturbed dogs again. However, the legal requirement for rabies vaccines—mandatory annually to every three years—can be hard to get around. Taking a blood sample to test for immunity to rabies (a rabies titer) can suffice in some counties as acceptable evidence for not needing another rabies shot. Dr. Pitcairn has not used vaccinations (other than the legally required rabies) in his practice for over twenty-five years, finding homeopathic nosodes (during times of likely exposure) not only safer, but actually more effective.[134]

More Vaccines Planned

Unfortunately, in our current capitalism-at-any-cost system that our forefathers (and mothers) never envisioned, the pharmaceutical companies that manufacture vaccines have an answer to these modern challenges—more drugs. In fact, an article in *U.S. News and World Report* lauded plans for new "miracle" vaccines for a whole host of diseases such as asthma, strep throat, hepatitis C, genital herpes, cancer, and AIDS*—illnesses that may have actually, in part or in whole, been *caused* by vaccines produced by these same companies.[135] This practice of prescribing more drugs to counteract the side effects of other drugs is not new, however, and is very well known to senior citizens and the seriously ill, who are often prescribed multiple medications, also known as *polypharmacy.*

Adults are not immune to the hazards of vaccines either, since they are urged to get diphtheria/tetanus boosters every ten years, flu shots annually, and those over sixty-five an annual pneumococcal vaccination.[136] One has to wonder, is increasing the numbers of vaccines moving in the right direction or the wrong one? Unfortunately, until well-designed scientific research studies are conducted consisting of control groups with unvaccinated individuals, society continues to remain in the dark.

CONTRAINDICATIONS TO RECEIVING VACCINATIONS

One important but not widely propagated fact about vaccines is that there are known contraindications to receiving them. A *contraindication* is a condition indicating that a vaccine or drug could be a possible danger to an individual. One classic contraindication is a history of severe allergies. For example, in a special immunization edition of *Mothering* magazine, contraindications to receiving the measles vaccine gleaned from the manufacturer's own package inserts include a hypersensitivity to neomycin or an allergy to eggs, chickens, or feathers.[137] However, although doctors are required by the National Childhood Vaccine Injury Act of 1986 to inform parents of these possible contraindications *prior* to administering vaccines, in reality this is the exception rather than the norm.[138]

In the book *A Shot in the Dark,* Coulter and Fisher commit a whole chapter to the serious issue of contraindications. In regard to the DPT shot, the authors list as contraindications a previously severe reaction to an earlier pertussis vaccination, a family history of convulsions or other central nervous system illnesses, a family predisposition to vaccine reactions (e.g., a sibling who has had a severe reaction), "cerebral irritation in the neonatal period," prematurity and low birth weight, and chronic illness or a recent severe illness.[139]

However, parents are rarely informed of these and other contraindications before their children receive vaccines in the doctor's office. Coulter and Fisher assert that this glaring form of malpractice has rendered the immunization program "intrinsically dangerous," and that it has been "implemented across the board in a careless way—without due concern for contraindications."[140]

Another major contraindication to receiving vaccinations is malnourishment. Giving medicine to undernourished and half-starved people has been characterized as *fruitless,* and an adequate diet deemed to be "the most effective 'vaccine' against most of the diarrhoeal, respiratory and other common infections" of the third world.[141] Thus, major philanthropic donations of hundreds of millions of dollars to help immunize children in developing countries may be misplaced, and this money might be better utilized in the form of food aid.[142] This is especially the case since many of these exported vaccines still contain the mercury-containing preservative thimerosal, which has been linked to autism and other neurological disorders.[143]

THE LEGAL ASPECTS OF VACCINATIONS

The fear generated by allopathic doctors and the popular press of playing the "risky game" of not getting

*In 1998 it was reported by the Associated Press that the developing AIDS vaccine had "suffered a serious setback" because tests revealed that the weakened virus that was employed was actually causing the disease in monkeys. (Associated Press, "Vaccine for AIDS May Cause Disease," *Marin Independent Journal,* July 3, 1998.) Despite more recent advances, an AIDS vaccine does not yet exist.

vaccinations is a powerful deterrent to thoughtful parents who might otherwise consider the decision more thoroughly.[144] Another major factor is that it's the law in most states, and disobeying this law has resulted in some cases of parents being charged with child abuse, or in the actual removal of children from their family and their forcible vaccination.[145]

Compulsory Vaccination Policies

Currently, forty-two states have mandatory vaccination policies. Many of these policies require by law that children have at least eighteen shots before entering first grade.[146] Furthermore, many colleges now require entering students to be fully vaccinated before admission,* and welfare benefits have been denied to families who refuse vaccinations. Authorities argue that these laws are necessary for the health of children, as well as to protect society as a whole from epidemics. However, if vaccines truly give immunity to disease, then only the small minority of unvaccinated individuals—currently estimated to be about 10 percent of the population†—would become ill with the diseases vaccinations are said to protect against, which is not the case, so the logic is specious.[147]

Exemptions from Immunization

Fortunately, *all* states currently provide exemptions for parents who choose not to vaccinate. Visit www.thinktwice.com/laws.htm for a copy of your particular state vaccination law and a sample exemption letter. Jamie Murphy's book *What Every Parent Should Know About Childhood Immunization* details how parents of both children and college students can oppose immunization on religious, medical, or philosophical grounds.[148]

Dr. Joseph Mercola notes that no one in the United States has the right to vaccinate you or your child against your will. If they attempt to do so, they can be legally charged with "assault with a deadly weapon." It is important to remember that no matter how the CDC, American Academy of Pediatrics, or local school districts word their immunization guidelines, due to the exemptions there are actually no compulsory immunization laws in the United States—complying is a personal decision and completely voluntary.[149]

- For more information on legally refusing immunizations, go to www.mercola.com/article/vaccines/legally_avoid_shots.htm.

Drug Company Liability: The Lilly Rider

Unfortunately, the constitutional right to seek justice for damages from vaccines was abridged by the Bush administration (George W.). In a move labeled by Senator John McCain as "the fix is in," a last-minute rider concerning the liability of pharmaceutical companies that produce vaccines was mysteriously inserted into the Homeland Security bill. As Neil Miller describes it:

> On November 13, 2002, lawmakers passed a Homeland Security bill that included a provision protecting drug companies from thimerosal lawsuits. "It looks like payback," a trial lawyer noted, considering "the industry [pharmaceutical companies] spent millions bankrolling [political] campaigns."[150]

This rider's net effect is to shield Eli Lilly and other pharmaceutical companies from paying out billions of dollars in anticipated lawsuits from mercury-induced vaccinosis—primarily autism and other neurological disorders—from the thimerosal preservative. The political machinations leading to the passage of this "Lilly Rider," championed by Senator Bill Frist (R-TN) and other Republican leaders, is thoroughly detailed in David Kirby's *Evidence of Harm: Mercury in Vaccines and the Autism Epidemic: A Medical Controversy.* The account of how this rider was successfully included and passed in this bill reads like a fascinating (albeit depressing) thriller, not unlike the Watergate conspiracy from the Nixon era.[151]

*Dr. Isadore Rosenfield, the allopathic columnist in *Parade* magazine, recommends the following shots for all college students: tetanus and diphtheria boosters (if it's been ten years since the last shot), annual flu shots, and meningitis, mumps (if there has been an outbreak nearby), and hepatitis B vaccines. All flu shots and many of the tetanus, diphtheria, meningitis, and hepatitis B vaccines still contain toxic thimerosal as a preservative. (I. Rosenfeld, "How to Stay Healthy at College," *Parade,* August 13, 2006, 12.)

†Although the figures will vary depending on how you define "unvaccinated" (many being partially vaccinated), the national goal is for 90 percent vaccination of young children, and the WHO-UNICEF estimates of immunization coverage indicate that this goal is being met for many of the vaccinations. (See www.cdc.gov/vaccines/stats-surv/imz-coverage.htm.)

MAKING A THOUGHTFUL, EDUCATED DECISION AND CARING FOR YOUR FAMILY

The decision of whether to vaccinate is an extremely important one that should not be entered into lightly. Parents should call the CDC hotline at (800) 232-4636 and consult the CDC website (www.cdc.gov/vaccines), as well as other resources, to familiarize themselves with the pro-vaccine stance. They should also read the books referred to previously in the "Be Informed" section (page 457) and visit the website www.thinktwice.com. In regard to the mercury preservative that is still in several vaccines, SafeMinds (www.safeminds.org) is an excellent nonprofit organization whose mission is to investigate and raise awareness of the risks to infants and children from exposure to mercury in vaccines. Parents may also want to consult with their allopathic physician, as well as their holistic practitioner, in order to make a well-considered final decision. Whatever the choice, the following treatment advice is suggested for everyone—to mitigate any deleterious effects of vaccinations for those who choose to get vaccines, or to holistically treat childhood illnesses for those who do not.

General Advice for All Parents

The following recommendations are important for keeping all families healthy, and they are relevant regardless of decisions made regarding vaccinations.

Prenatal Care

In many traditional cultures, pregnancy was sacred and women were revered and served by their family and community during this blessed time. Currently, however, women often continue full-time at stressful jobs and maintain hectic schedules throughout their pregnancy, with little support for their much-needed rest and contemplation during this yin period.* When women reduce their workload both at home and at the office, eat a healthy diet, avoid their primary food allergen(s), take quality supplements, are on their constitutional homeopathic remedy, have already removed and detoxified their amalgam fillings, and receive regular spinal adjustments, cranial manipulation, and/or massage, they are almost always rewarded with an easier labor* and a healthy and happy baby.

*In Chinese medicine, the *yin* aspect is the female principle, and the *yang* aspect is the male principle. Within these two complementary forces found in all things in the universe, yin embodies the principles most needed for a healthy pregnancy, including rest, passiveness, and introversion.

Breast-Feeding Infants

Antibodies to diseases that are transferred from mother to child during breast-feeding provide the child with the protection passive immunity confers. As the child matures, these antibodies mature and develop as diseases are contracted and overcome.[152] Research indicates that breast-fed babies are healthier than those who are bottle-fed.[153] If your child was bottle-fed with cow's or goat's milk (typically pasteurized and therefore lacking in many available nutrients plus often allergenic) or soy formulas (often allergenic, hormonally imbalancing, and possible containing toxic preservatives), his or her immune system has some serious "catching up" to do. Consult your holistic practitioner for appropriate treatment.

Shop at the Health Food Store

Unless money is a major issue, parents really can't afford *not* to shop at the local health food store.† The health benefits gained from avoiding foods laced with toxic and often carcinogenic chemicals and preservatives—as well as the reduction in future doctor's bills and prescription drugs—cannot be underestimated. Furthermore, shopping at quality health food stores ensures the reduction of devitalized, microwaved, sugary, hydrogenated, GE or GMO (genetically modified), and other forms of deadened foods that promote disease, and which children are currently inundated with at school, events, parties, and (nonholistic) friends' houses.

*A 1992 survey found that 81 percent of women in U.S. hospitals are given the drug Pitocin, either to induce labor or to augment the effects of labor. Pitocin has been linked with increased labor pain, fetal distress, neonatal jaundice, retained placenta, and possibly autism. (N. Griffin, "Let the Baby Decide: The Case Against Inducing Labor," *Mothering,* March/April 2001, 66.)

†And even if money is an issue, at least low-cost items should be purchased at health food stores, such as organic oat groats for morning porridges; organic rice, millet, and quinoa; and organic vegetables and fruit.

Avoid Primary Food Allergens

Continuously ingesting allergenic foods is exhausting to the immune system. Parents can utilize the elimination-challenge test directions described in chapter 6 to determine which foods may be primary allergens and then endeavor to eliminate or reduce these foods in their children's diet. (A good place to start is choosing the foods that the child's mother and father are most allergic to, since there is a major heredity component in allergies.) Studies in the United States and Europe show that elimination of gluten (primarily wheat, rye, oats, and barley) and casein (cow's milk, cheese, etc.) cause marked improvement in autistic children.[154] Children exhibiting other types of cognitive dysfunction such as MBD (minimal brain dysfunction), ADD (attention deficit disorder), ADHD (attention-deficit/hyperactivity disorder), Tourette's, epilepsy, or aggressiveness after vaccinations can also benefit from the avoidance of these disturbing foods.

General Nutritional Supplementation

Unfortunately, since ubiquitous modern-day toxins affect the air as well as food and water, in even the most conscientious environments, both children and adults need to supplement their diet with vitamins and minerals. This is especially true when children begin day care or school, where they are exposed to other children's germs, as well as the added stressors of learning to socialize and make good grades. A quality (sugar-free, binder-free, preservative-free) multivitamin such as the one from Thorne (Children's Basic Nutrients) is an excellent source of supplementation for children after they have stopped breast-feeding up to around ten years of age. Dosages can range from ⅛ capsule per day in infants to 1 capsule two or three times per day in children.

▶ Children's Basic Nutrients are available from Thorne at (800) 228-1966, or go to www.thorne.com.

If You Decide to Vaccinate: Specific Treatments for Vaccinosis in Children

If you suspect your infant or child has been damaged at any level after receiving a vaccine, the most effective treatment is a dose of his or her constitutional remedy.

Constitutional Homeopathic Remedy

As described previously, a constitutional homeopathic remedy prescribed according to the Sankaran system has been clinically found to be the most efficacious and curative. Therefore, if parents decide to vaccinate their child, the most important step they can take beforehand is to ascertain their child's constitutional remedy. Then, after vaccination, it can be re-dosed once, twice, or even more (depending on the severity of the reaction to the vaccine) to mitigate its damaging effects. During this time, stay in close contact with your homeopathic practitioner, as well as the allopathic physician who administered the vaccine, to make the most knowledgeable decisions possible in treating your child's potential symptoms of vaccinosis.

Plant Remedies for Excreting Toxic Metals and Chemicals

Despite the FDA's "request" that the mercury-containing preservative thimerosal be removed from vaccinations, it is still included in some vaccines.[155] Additionally, stores of vaccines in pharmacies and doctors' offices may not be used up for years in this country (and these mercury-containing vaccines are still being sold in other nations outside the United States). Furthermore, other toxic metals have been added to many vaccines; aluminum, for example, was added after it was discovered in 1943 that it has an adjuvant effect—that is, it strengthens the potency of the vaccine so that fewer bacteria or viruses (that in higher levels would be more dangerous) need to be included in the shot.[156] Herbal plant stem cell remedies such as Black Poplar have proven effective in chelating these toxic metals. In addition, vaccines contain chemical preservatives such as formaldehyde, formalin, and phenol, and the use of plant stem cell remedies such as Juniper and Rye can assist in furthering the excretion of these toxic chemicals. Therefore, after a vaccination, supplementation with these herbal remedies is highly recommended. Dosages can range from 1 drop one to three times a day in infants to 3 to 6 drops two or three times a day in children and adolescents.

Tautopathic Remedies

Tautopathy is the term for a homeopathic remedy made from an allopathic medicine, such as a vaccine, that is given to counteract the adverse effects of that medicine. For parents who choose to vaccinate, some homeopaths suggest taking a tautopathic remedy just after a vaccination is given to help mitigate any negative effects of that vaccine.* Because most tautopathic remedies are made from a drop of the vaccine itself, they can potentially treat not only the adverse effects of the particular virus or bacteria contained in the vaccine but also any preservatives (mercury, formaldehyde, etc.), adjuvants (aluminum), antibiotics (which may be allergenic), and foreign proteins (chicken, monkey, cow, etc.) included in the shot. Furthermore, because homeopathic remedies affect only the child's vital force and not the antibody titer like vaccines, knowledgeable homeopaths believe that these tautopathic vaccines will not interrupt any beneficial immunological actions of the vaccine.[157] For example, if parents choose to vaccinate their newborn child for hepatitis B, then giving Hepatitis B Vaccine 30C immediately afterward might reduce some or all of the common acute (e.g., diarrhea, fever, vomiting) and chronic (e.g., diabetes, multiple sclerosis, rheumatoid arthritis) adverse effects that have been attributed to this vaccine. This tautopathic remedy would especially be indicated if the child began to manifest these and other symptoms immediately after—or days or even weeks after—receiving the vaccine.

However, a strong caution needs to be added here that tautopathic remedies are not always effective and absolutely *should not* be counted on as a "safety valve" measure after each vaccination. The effects of vaccines can be so severe at times that even when the tautopathic remedy is given immediately afterward, it may have no beneficial effect. Thus, parents should make the decision of whether to vaccinate on the merits and drawbacks of the vaccine alone, without being influenced by any possible ameliorating aspects of tautopathic remedies.†

Dosage: Homeopaths generally advise administering tautopathic vaccines to infants by dissolving 2 pellets in a 4-ounce glass of water, and giving the baby a small amount of this mixture (e.g., ⅛ teaspoon) one, two, or more times after he or she has received the vaccination. If symptoms are moderate or severe, the infant can receive this dose more often, even hourly, *if* it appears to be helping. Toddlers and children can take 1 or 2 pellets orally, dissolved under the tongue. After the initial dose (or doses), parents should carefully observe their child's reaction, ideally in close contact with their homeopathic practitioner. If the infant or child improves with the tautopathic remedy but then later regresses (e.g., that night, the next day, or a few days later), then another dose, or several more doses, may be indicated. However, if there are no signs of improvement within a reasonable period of time (from hours to a day or two), the remedy should be stopped.

In the case of all symptoms—from mild to severe—always keep the allopathic physician who administered the vaccine informed. Furthermore, in the case of moderate to severe reactions, do not hesitate to go to the emergency room. The best outcomes are realized when the allopathic and the homeopathic physicians communicate and work together with the parents to serve the best interests of the child.

The following chart (table 15.2) lists the tautopathic remedies for each vaccine currently included on the U.S. immunization schedule for children and adolescents. Tautopathic remedies can be ordered from all major homeopathic pharmacies in the United States and abroad. A 200C or 1M potency may be indicated for moderate to severe symptoms of vaccinosis. Consult a knowledgeable homeopath for guidance.

► Two excellent homeopathic companies are Hahnemann Pharmacy in San Rafael, California, at (888) 427-6422 or www.hahnemannlabs.com, and Helios in England, at 011 44 1892 537254 or www.helios.co.uk.

TABLE 15.2. TAUTOPATHIC VACCINE REMEDIES

Vaccination	Tautopathic Remedy
Chicken pox	Varicella Vaccine 30C
Diphtheria/tetanus	DT Vaccine 30C
DPT	DPT Vaccine 30C
Hepatitis A	Hepatitis A Vaccine 30C
Hepatitis B	Hepatitis B Vaccine 30C
Hib	Hib Vaccine 30C
Influenza	Influenza Vaccine 30C
MMR	MMR Vaccine 30C
Polio	Polio Vaccine 30C*
Pneumococcal	Pneumococcal Vaccine 30C

*The Salk and Sabin tautopathic polio remedies can also be ordered for older patients who received these vaccines as children.

*Some homeopaths suggest taking the tautopathic remedy before receiving the vaccine.

†Furthermore, the child's personalized constitutional remedy most typically has stronger healing effects than tautopathic remedies.

Specific Nutritional Support

Proteolytic Enzymes. Due to the considerable amount of foreign proteins contained in most vaccines—from cows, chickens, monkeys, guinea pigs, and even aborted human fetuses (not quite so foreign but nevertheless different from one's own tissues), pancreatin with proteolytic enzymes can be a beneficial supplement. Proteolytic enzymes work somewhat like the PacMan video game, by stimulating the degradation and removal of these foreign microbes and tissues from the body. Dipan 9 from Thorne is one of the few lactose-free, preservative-free pancreatin formulas that is in the same dilution as our natural pancreatic enzyme output (9 or 10X), and therefore is readily absorbed and utilized within the body. Dosages can range from 1/16 teaspoon one to three times a day in infants to 2 capsules two or three times a day in adolescents.

▶ To order Dipan 9, contact Thorne at (800) 228-1966.

Vitamin A, Vitamin D, and Cod Liver Oil. In recent testimony to a Senate hearing on autism and vaccinations, Dr. Mary Megson, a pediatrician specializing in learning disabilities, ADHD, cerebral palsy, mental retardation, and autism, reported greatly improved results in children suffering from these developmental disabilities through the use of cod liver oil.[158] Other researchers have also reported cases of behavior and learning disorders favorably responding to the vitamin D component in cod liver oil.[159]* Therefore, in infants and children demonstrating developmental disabilities consistent with brain injury from vaccinosis, supplemental cod liver oil should be given for a trial period.† Dosages can range from 1/16 teaspoon per day in infants to 2 teaspoons per day in adolescents.

▶ A superior cod liver oil is Blue Ice Fermented Cod Liver Oil, available from Green Pasture (www.greenpasture.org or 402-858-4818). Fermented Skate Liver Oil is also a superior product available from this company; it often tests even better than the cod liver oil in both children and adults.

Vitamin B_6 and Magnesium. Eighteen studies conducted in six different countries have concluded that supplementation with high doses of vitamin B_6 and magnesium is effective in reducing the symptoms in autistic children and adults. Eleven of these studies were double-blind, placebo-controlled experiments. Dr. Bernard Rimlaud, director of the Autism Research Institute, testified before a congressional committee that "there is no drug that comes close to B_6/magnesium in terms of safety, efficacy, and positive research findings."[160] Therefore, in vaccine-damaged autistic children, as well as in those exhibiting more minor developmental disabilities, a trial supplementation with additional B_6 and magnesium should be considered with the family's holistic practitioner. Dosages can range from ⅛ capsule one to three times a day in infants to 2 capsules two or three times a day in adolescents.

▶ A quality B_6 supplement is B-Complex #6, and a good magnesium source is Magnesium Citramate; both are available from Thorne at (800) 228-1966.

Magnesium can also be supplemented through the Schuessler's cell salt (or tissue salt) Magnesium phosphoricum 6X. Cell salts have both homeopathic and biochemical effects in the body. They are successful in almost immediately alleviating muscle cramps and spasms because of their quick assimilation and utilization in the body. Dosages can range from ½ to 1 tablet (mashed up and dissolved in warm water) once a day for infants to 2 tablets one to three times a day in children and adolescents.

▶ Magnesium phosphoricum 6X is sold in health food stores and can also be ordered from Seroyal at (800) 263-5861.

Vitamin C and Other Antioxidants. As described earlier, vaccines contain toxic chemical preservatives. Extra vitamin C given along with the child's multivitamin can help reduce the damaging effects of this xenobiotic overload and is especially indicated when a child receives multiple vaccines. Dosages can range from 1/16 teaspoon per day in infants to 2 capsules two or three times a day in adolescents.

*Never supplement vitamin D without adequate calcium and magnesium supplementation at the same time. (The Children's Basic Nutrients supplement contains vitamins A and D, calcium, and magnesium.) Consider extra supplementation with cod or skate liver oil in children with developmental disorders or immune system deficiencies.

†After two and a half months of taking cod liver oil, Dr. Megson's gifted but dyslexic son exclaimed, "I can read now! The letters don't jump around on the page anymore!" (M. Megson, "Autism and Vaccinations," *Wise Traditions* 1, no. 3 [Fall 2000], 35.)

- Pure Radiance C is an excellent source of natural vitamin C derived solely from berries; contact the Synergy Company at (800) 723-0277.

When a combination antioxidant formula is needed, Triple Berry Probiotic Formula is an excellent product.

- To order Triple Berry Probiotic Formula, healthcare practitioners can contact BioImmersion at (425) 451-3112 or www.bioimmersion.com.

Spinal and Cranial Care

The mind of an infant or a child has difficulty distinguishing between an injection and being actually stabbed by a knife or a sword. Besides emotional comforting by the parents, quality chiropractic or osteopathic care is often needed to release the spinal and cranial misalignments that occur in response to the primal fear contraction pattern that is induced by the shock and pain of a needle piercing the skin.

If You Decide Not to Vaccinate: Prevention and Treatment of Childhood Illnesses

For parents who choose not to vaccinate their child, all the previously described recommendations such as good prenatal care, breast-feeding, shopping at the health food store, avoiding the child's primary food allergen, and taking a quality multivitamin/mineral supplement can assist in helping your child either not to succumb to a childhood illness or to recover from one quickly without any damaging aftereffects. Additionally, as elucidated in the previous chapter, a constitutional homeopathic remedy prescribed according to the Sankaran system has been clinically found to be superlative in helping children maintain good health and develop (physically, mentally, and emotionally) most optimally.

Nosode Remedies

Additionally, many homeopaths recommend the use of *homeopathic nosodes*—that is, remedies of diseased tissue or the products of disease—which have been used historically to prevent or mitigate childhood illnesses. For example, if measles is "going around" your child's class, the administration of Morbillinum 30C—the homeopathic nosode of a drop of blood taken from a child with measles—might prevent your child from getting it, or help mitigate the symptoms if she has already been infected.[161]* However, if your child is already on a well-acting constitutional remedy, the first step is usually to re-dose this remedy before going to a nosode. On the other hand, both might be used if necessary. Always consult with your homeopath if possible. Nosodes may be helpful for vaccinated as well as unvaccinated children, since many vaccines fail to confer permanent immunity.

Dosage: The dosage of nosodes for childhood illnesses is given in the same manner as described earlier in the tautopathic section. For infants, dissolve 2 pellets in a 4-ounce glass of water, and give them a small amount of this mixture (e.g., ⅛ teaspoon) one time if a childhood disease is going around or if the child is displaying symptoms of the illness. Toddlers and children can take 1 or 2 pellets orally, dissolved under the tongue. After the initial dose, parents should carefully observe their child's reaction. If the child improves with the nosode remedy but then later regresses (e.g., that night, the next day, or a few days later), then one or more additional doses may be indicated (e.g., 1 dose from one to three times a day for a few days to a week, depending on the severity of the illness). Consultation with an experienced homeopathic practitioner, as well as the child's pediatrician, is always optimum. If the child is battling an active infection such as the mumps, for example, he should receive several doses of Parotidinum 30C per day, reducing or stopping the dose as the child is getting well.

If the child shows no signs of improvement, stop the remedy and again consult your holistic/homeopathic and allopathic physicians. Either the diagnosis of the disease is incorrect (e.g., giving the chicken pox nosode for measles) or the child is not sensitive to, and therefore not responding to, the effects of the nosode remedy—another homeopathic remedy may be needed. In clinical homeopathic history, remedies such as Lathyrus sativus for polio or Arsenicum album or Baptisia tinctoria in the treatment of diphtheria and influenza have proven to be very effective.[162]

---

*The famous homeopath John H. Clarke, M.D., found that dissolving 8 or 10 globules of Morbillinum 30C in 6 ounces of water, and taking a small spoonful every two hours, along with alternate doses of Belladonna 30C, "was sufficient to carry through any uncomplicated case [of measles]." (R. Murphy, *Homeopathic Remedy Guide* (Blacksburg, Va.: H.A.N.A. Press, 2000], 1168.)

The following chart (table 15.3) lists nosodes for common childhood diseases. These remedies may be ordered from any major homeopathic pharmacy.* Nosodes for rare childhood illnesses such as hepatitis A and B and pneumococcus are not included in this list, but they are also available. In the case of severe illness, consider using 200C or 1M potencies.

TABLE 15.3. NOSODES FOR COMMON CHILDHOOD ILLNESSES

Illness	Nosode
Chicken pox	Varicellinum 30C
Diphtheria	Diphtherinum 30C
Influenza ("the flu")	Influenzinum 30C
Measles	Morbillinum 30C
Meningitis	Haemophilus influenza B 30C
Mumps	Parotidinum 30C
Pertussis (whooping cough)	Pertussin 30C
Polio	Polio 30C
Rubella (German measles)	Rubella 30C
Tetanus	Clostridium tetani 30C

Homeopathic Prophylaxis Is Questionable

Some homeopaths advocate "homeopathic prophylaxis" with nosodes. For example, they recommend giving infants and children childhood disease nosodes on a regular schedule, such as Pertussinum, to help prevent the childhood disease of pertussis, given at ages one month, two months, ten months, twenty-two months, and thirty-two months, or Morbillinum, to help ward off a bout of measles, at thirteen and twenty-five months.[163] Other homeopaths strenuously object to subjecting the child's vital force and immune system to strong nosode remedies *before* the onset of a childhood illness, when the child may not even be susceptible to that particular disease. Furthermore, given repeatedly (or even once in sensitive children), nosodes may have the potential to actually weaken a child and allow inherited dormant miasms (e.g., sycotic, tuberculinic, or luetic) to arise, which might not ever have manifested otherwise. George Vithoulkas, the world-renowned homeopath, echoes this anti-prophylactic sentiment by asserting that "a remedy given at an improper time either has no effect or creates actual damage."[164] However, most homeopaths agree that when there is an epidemic or even when your child (or your child's friends) are beginning to manifest symptoms of a particular childhood disease, giving a vaccine nosode (and/or re-dosing your child's constitutional remedy) at these "more acute" times can be quite appropriate.

Recommended Reading

An excellent book that is suitable for both parents and homeopaths is Susan Curtis's *Homoeopathic Alternatives to Immunisation.* Furthermore, homeopaths and parents may also want to read Dr. Dorothy Shepherd's *Homoeopathy in Epidemic Diseases,* a succinct hundred-page book that describes the homeopathic remedies she has successfully prescribed in the treatment of pertussis, mumps, measles, influenza, polio, and other contagious childhood illnesses. Additionally, Sandra J. Perko's book *The Homeopathic Treatment of Influenza* details the indications for the sixty-eight remedies that have been effective in treating this illness, as well as including a fascinating history of the major influenza epidemics and homeopathy's treatment successes during these periods. Finally, as described previously, it is essential never to hesitate to go to the emergency room if your child is seriously ill.

► All three recommended books are available at Minimum Price at (800) 663-8272, or other homeopathic bookstores.

Additional Support

Vitamin A, Vitamin D, and Cod Liver Oil. Several studies have confirmed that when vitamin A supplementation is given while a child is ill with measles, the complication rates and chances of dying are significantly reduced. In fact, as early as 1932, doctors who utilized cod liver oil (high in vitamins A and D) to treat measles lowered the mortality rate by 58 percent.[165] Therefore, when a child is exhibiting possible symptoms of the measles, or during an epidemic, cod or skate liver oil or supplementation with vitamin A is indicated.

► A superior oil is Blue Ice Fermented Cod or Skate Liver Oil, available from Green Pasture (www.greenpasture.org or 402-858-4818). If extra vitamin A

*See page 480 for the names of two recommended homeopathic companies.

is indicated in a severe case of measles, Thorne offers (unlike many manufacturers) a preservative-free vitamin A with beta-carotene and mixed carotenes, simply called Vitamin A. Contact Thorne at (800) 228-1966. However, please note that vitamin A supplementation can be toxic in megadoses and should not be given long-term in infants and children who do not have a continuing vitamin deficiency.

Vitamin C. Studies have shown that vitamin C is effective against whooping cough (pertussis) and tetanus.[166] Therefore, during suspected pertussis epidemics or after puncture wounds that might lead to tetanus, vitamin C supplementation is advised.

A 1954 study dramatically demonstrated the curative effect of megadoses of this vitamin. A group of children with tetanus who received daily intravenous administration of 1 gram (1,000 milligrams) of ascorbic acid had no fatalities, as compared with a 72 percent mortality rate in a comparable group of children with tetanus who did not receive vitamin C.[167] Dosages can range from ⅛ capsule one to three times a day in infants to 2 capsules two or three times a day in adolescents.

- Buffered C Powder or Vitamin C with Flavonoids from Thorne can be taken at high dosages. Contact Thorne at (800) 228-1966. However, oral administration of vitamin C at megadose levels can cause diarrhea. Therefore, if intravenous C is not available, monitor children carefully for signs of loose stools and diarrhea, in order not to induce prostration and dehydration.

Emotional Support. Parents are under considerable pressure to vaccinate their children—from government agencies, school administrators, and other parents in their community. The fear that pervades this allopathic thinking can have a negative placebo effect in and of itself. It is therefore important that parents who choose not to vaccinate have a holistically oriented support group in their doctor or practitioner, as well as in their friends and family. It is also extremely helpful that parents explain their decision to their child (if old enough), as well as the disease-preventing and immune system benefits of a natural lifestyle—clean water, organic food, reduced sugar, and no hydrogenated oils. The family's holistic practitioner can act as a positive force by prescribing appropriate nutritional supplements, herbs, homeopathic remedies, cranial and spinal adjustments, acupuncture or auriculotherapy, and other treatments that support and strengthen the child's body, mind, and spirit.

Parents can also take heart that many leading authorities are outspokenly against vaccines. Dr. Harold Buttram believes that vaccines are actually "stunting the development of the immune systems of children."[168] Dr. John Walker-Smith, an expert in intestinal diseases in children, which have sharply increased over the past decade, echoes this sentiment, stating that "the decline of many childhood infections might allow children in the West to grow up without the vigorous development of their immune system defenses that such infections would ordinarily promote."[169] Finally, the following quote from Dr. Phillip Incao is consistent with the well-known axiom in martial arts as well as in psychology that "the only way out, is the way through":

> There is no system of the human being, from mind to muscles to immune system, which gets stronger through avoiding challenges, but only through *overcoming* challenges.[170]

Travel Vaccines

For children, as well as adults, who are traveling out of the country, the decision on whether to take the recommended vaccines is always an important consideration.

Most Vacation Travel Vaccines Optional

With only one exception, no vaccine is actually mandatory for vacation travel anywhere in the world. That sole exception is the yellow fever vaccine when traveling to a South American or African country infected with yellow fever.[171]

Military or Work-Related Travel Vaccines Often Mandatory

However, in both the Peace Corps and the military, multiple vaccinations are often mandatory. Most recently, the vaccine Lariam that was given to many soldiers deployed in Afghanistan and Iraq has come under suspicion. This anti-malarial drug lists side effects ranging from dizziness to psychotic behavior. And although its manufacturer Hoffman-LaRoche, the Department of

Defense, and the Centers for Disease Control all claim that serious side effects are "rare," Dr. Joseph Habis, a tropical disease specialist, believes that neuropsychiatric symptoms show up in 15 to 30 percent of Lariam users. These neuropsychiatric or brain-damaging symptoms include rage, paranoia, homicidal and suicidal ideations, hallucinations, and grand mal seizures. And these symptoms are affecting soldiers who are in superb physical condition and in the prime of their life.[172] Much like the ongoing debacle of trying to diagnose and treat illnesses incurred during the Gulf War, the military has been less than forthcoming about the use of Lariam and slow in responding with adequate care.

▶ For more information on Lariam, go to www.lariaminfo.org; and for more information on Gulf War Syndrome, go to www.ngwrc.org.

A Protocol to Help Prevent Vaccinosis

Fortunately, when practitioners actively endeavor to "surround the dragon" of potential vaccinosis with holistic products, the negative impact of mandatory vaccines can often be greatly mitigated. In my practice, I have successfully used the following post-inoculation protocol for adults who had to be vaccinated prior to travel:

1. Re-dosing of the patient's constitutional remedy*
2. Taking 6 capsules of Pure Radiance C per day for five days
3. Rubbing 2 to 3 drops of Kombination Drops 4X into the injection site three times a day for two days

▶ Pure Radiance C can be ordered from the Synergy Company at (800) 723-0277 or through www.thesynergycompany.com.

▶ Kombination Drops 4X are available from BioResource at (800) 203-3775.

Tautopathic or Nosode Support

For individuals who are not on their constitutional remedy, tautopathic homeopathic remedies are an option. As with children's vaccinations, individuals who choose to take vaccines can help mitigate any potential vaccinosis effects through taking tautopathic remedies (or their constitutional remedy) afterward, as well as taking extra nutritional supplementation. Typhoid fever vaccine, Yellow fever vaccine, Malaria vaccine, and other tautopathic remedies can be ordered from most major homeopathic companies.* Furthermore, the homeopathic nosodes for these diseases—Salmonella typhi, Yellow fever, Malaria, China officinalis†—can also be ordered and carried throughout one's trip, to be taken either in epidemic areas or as soon as symptoms arise.

Recommended Reading

Two excellent resources for more information on travel vaccines are Susan Curtis's *Homoeopathic Alternatives to Immunisation* and Dr. Sherry Tenpenny's article "Far-Off Adventures: Vaccinations and Overseas Travel," in the September/October 2003 issue of *Mothering* magazine. Dr. Tenpenny, who has been a globetrotter for twenty-five years and has traveled to more than forty countries, has never personally felt the need to take any vaccines, even when traveling to more remote, exotic destinations. She advocates minimizing risks abroad by avoiding water, ice, and raw and undercooked foods, as well as using a natural mosquito repellent, rehydration in case of diarrhea (orally or intravenously if necessary), using a little-known remedy for malaria (artemisia, or wormwood), and other healthy tips for reducing the incidence of distress and disease while traveling.[173]

▶ Subscriptions or past copies of *Mothering* magazine can be ordered at (800) 984-8116. There is also an article in this edition about a woman's nineteen-year-old daughter who was sent to India armed with a homeopathic kit for any travel and illness emergencies. (Bonnie Price Lofton, "Backpack Homeopathy: Allison's Journey to India," *Mothering*, September/October 2003.)

▶ With more than 3,000 species of mosquitoes in the world, most capable of transferring diseases, defend-

*Every patient I treat is on his or her constitutional remedy as soon as energetic testing results reveal that it is appropriate to conduct a homeopathic interview.

See page 480 for the names of two recommended homeopathic companies.

†China officinalis is the homeopathic remedy made from Peruvian cinchona bark from which quinine used to be made (this drug is now synthetically derived). As discussed earlier, Dr. Hahnemann discovered that homeopathic Peruvian cinchona bark (China) was an excellent treatment for malaria.

ing yourself is essential. Citronella and neem oil have both been proven to repel insects naturally.

- Studies in China and Vietnam have found close to a 100 percent response rate with artemisia in the treatment of malaria. Thorne has a quality formulation of Chinese wormwood called Artecin; contact the company at (800) 228-1966.

Vaccinating Animals

Sadly, vaccinations for our beloved animal companions are just as controversial and potentially damaging as vaccines for humans. For example, independent researchers have found that the effectiveness of the feline leukemia virus vaccine for cats most typically falls within the 50 to 70 percent range, but can be as low as 17 percent. Another study found that 32 percent of cats died within twenty-four months following this vaccination.[174] Furthermore, the annual massive vaccination program instituted for canine parvovirus (panleukopenia virus) over thirty years ago has been linked with the increasing occurrence of inflammatory bowel disease and the heart muscle disease cardiomyopathy, which is often fatal in dogs. Finally, the established protocol of annual revaccinations for several types of animal vaccines, which yields tremendous revenue for veterinarians, has been called into question by holistic and conventional veterinary experts alike:

> A practice that was started many years ago and that *lacks scientific validity or verification* is annual revaccinations. Almost without exception, there is no immunologic requirement for annual revaccination. Immunity to viruses persists for years or for the life of the animal.[175]

Typical Vaccine Schedules

Typical vaccines currently recommended for kittens include FeBp (feline bordatella bacteria) at four weeks, FVRCP (panleukopenia virus or feline distemper, chlamydiosis or pneumonitis bacteria, calicivirus, and rhinotracheitis virus) at eight weeks, giardia parasite at eight weeks, FeLV (feline leukemia virus) at eight weeks, FIV (feline immunodeficiency virus) at eight weeks, FIP (feline infectious peritonitis virus) at sixteen weeks, and rabies virus at sixteen weeks.

BUILDING NATURAL IMMUNITY WITH RAW FOOD DIETS

Conventional cat and dog food is killing our beloved pets. Dr. Francis Pottenger's study of more than 900 cats proved the benefits of a raw meat diet and the detrimental effects of cooked and refined foods.*

For those with the time and energy, preparing your pet's raw food diet at home according to the protocol of holistic veterinarians such as Richard Pitcairn is an ideal choice. For those who don't have the extra time this takes, Rad Cat (www.radfood.com) and Answers Pet Food (www.answerspetfood.com) both make excellent products.

Fermented skate or cod liver oil (www.greenpasture.org) is beneficial to supplement a pet's diet from time to time and can reduce degenerative signs such as limping from arthritis and an unhealthy coat as well as anxiety and depression. Just smearing a fingerful of the oil on your pet's fur once or twice a week is usually sufficient, since it initiates an elaborate grooming ritual and the oil is thus ingested.

*See page 171 for more information on Pottenger's studies.

Typical vaccines currently recommended for puppies include DALP + Parvo (distemper virus, adenovirus/hepatitis or CAV-1 and CAV-2, parainfluenza virus, leptospirosis bacteria, parvovirus) at six weeks, coronavirus at six weeks, giardia parasite at eight weeks, bordatella bacteria (kennel cough) at eight weeks, Lyme disease bacteria at nine weeks, and rabies virus at sixteen weeks.

Further Reading

For more information on the important decision of whether or not to vaccinate, pet owners should read Dr. Don Hamilton's comprehensive and well-referenced book on holistic animal care, *Homeopathic Care for Cats and Dogs,* in which he addresses the issue of vaccinations from an experienced veterinarian's point of view. Catherine Diodati's book *Vaccine Guide for Dogs and Cats* is also an excellent resource. And finally, the leading holistic veterinarian in the United States, Richard Pitcairn, D.V.M., Ph.D., has recently come out with an exceptional book, *Dr. Pitcairn's Complete Guide to Natural Health for Dogs and Cats,* which discusses homeopathic nosode alternatives to vaccines, as well as a modified vaccine schedule if you feel compelled to immunize your pet.

Adult Vaccines and "The Damage Done"

Adults who choose to get vaccinations—whether they are diphtheria/tetanus boosters every ten years, annual flu vaccinations, or other recommended vaccines—may also choose the options of mitigating these with tautopathic remedies or stocking homeopathic nosodes in case of exposure. This is especially important for medical personnel in hospitals, medical centers, and nursing homes who are often required to take certain vaccines such as influenza,* hepatitis A and B, pneumococcal, and MMR.

Whether to Prescribe Nosodes for Chronic Vaccinosis

After reading this chapter, adults may wonder:

1. Has the damage already been done from my childhood vaccinations?
2. Can I just take a nosode remedy now to treat this suspected chronic vaccinosis?

The answer to this query is (1) possibly, and (2) absolutely not!

Although many adult illnesses such as chronic fatigue, depression, allergies, arthritis and back pain, asthma, ADD, irritable bowel symptoms, and even diabetes and cancer could have been initially precipitated, in part or in whole, by childhood vaccines (either from the microbes themselves or the contaminants, toxic metals, and chemicals), taking the nosode remedy now for the suspected vaccine is typically not effective, and, furthermore, it makes most individuals feel absolutely terrible.

The reason is multifaceted. For one thing, true healing occurs only through unlayering toxins and stressors in the order the body finds most efficacious, which is why quality energetic testing can be so valuable. It can "read" a patient's body to determine which treatment is needed next—mercury detoxification, drainage for dysfunctioning tissues and organs, auriculotherapy for that scar interference field, or other appropriate therapies. Furthermore, because damage from vaccinations usually occur at a young age, this injury—either the toxins themselves or the immune system's memory of these toxins—is often deeply buried in the individual's cells and tissues, as well as in the consciousness. In my experience, only advanced patients who have reasonably drained and detoxified their toxic metals and chemicals, had their foci treated at least once, and have received the stabilizing influence of their constitutional homeopathic remedy are good candidates for the treatment of vaccinosis through a short-term prescription of a homeopathic nosode.* However, in many cases, the patient's constitutional homeopathic remedy obviates the need for this intercurrent nosode prescription, as it typically can heal the damaging effects of vaccines even more effectively than the nosode.

Furthermore, because vaccinations can create an autoimmune-like mutation in susceptible individuals, giving a nosode for pertussis, polio (Salk or Sabin), or smallpox can actually stimulate an explosive immunological response when the body cannot differentiate its own tissues from the vaccine's microbes that have been coexisting together for decades. Additionally, many of these vaccine toxins are embedded in scar tissue—often in tonsil focal infections as well as in deep scar tissue in degenerated organs. Within these hidden scarified tissue stores, other "partners in crime" typically reside—most often mercury, pathogenic bacteria, and opportunistic fungus. In these cases, the vaccine nosode remedy is rarely able to completely clear the vaccine-related toxins or the imprinted contraction pattern on the vital force. Typically, it only impotently irritates and inflames these

*However, survey studies have revealed that doctors and nurses tend *not* to get their annual flu vaccines, at a rate of 70 percent. (N. Miller, *Vaccines: Are They Really Safe and Effective?* [Santa Fe: New Atlantean Press, 2003], 86–87.)

*Children and some "uncomplicated" teenage patients—that is, with no major history of excessive antibiotics and other pharmaceutical or street drugs; a reasonably clean diet; no major foci from surgeries, allopathic dental care, or chronic infections, etc.—can be exceptions to this rule and may be able to handle the detoxifying effects of a nosode. Furthermore, this vaccine nosode may be especially indicated and beneficial when parents have tracked the demise of their child's health beginning from the date of being immunized. In homeopathic nomenclature, this decline is referred to as the "never well since" syndrome. However, once again, the child or teen's constitutional remedy is typically superior to the nosode remedy for healing the effects of chronic vaccinosis.

focal areas and their related disturbed fields, creating more by-products of incomplete metabolism to add to the already burdened body of toxins. The exception is when the nosode remedy is actually also the patient's constitutional remedy, such as when a patient needs Diphtherinum constitutionally, and also has never been well since receiving a DPT shot. Doctors and practitioners can learn how to determine this from seminars teaching the Sankaran system of homeopathy.

Treating Chronic Vaccinosis Requires Clearing All Negative Effects in the Body

Therefore, the most effective way to treat symptoms suspected to arise from chronic vaccinosis is to follow the recommendations outlined in this book: clean up your diet, take quality nutritional supplements, and replace your cosmetic and personal care items with chemical-free ones. Furthermore, it is imperative to find a good holistic practitioner and dentist to guide you through mercury and other heavy metal detoxification, drainage for congested tissues and organs, auriculotherapy or neural therapy for your chronic focal infections and scar interference fields, and, most essentially, constitutional homeopathy for the deepest healing of the mind, body, and spirit. Armed with these effective treatments, when nosode remedies for any vaccine toxins (or the immunological memory of these toxins) are indicated, although healing responses may still come up, they will not be crises, and the patient's stronger and healthier vital force will finally be able to throw off any negative effects of these early childhood vaccinations.*

CONCLUSION

"Show Us the Science"

On September 8, 2000, five hundred representatives from thirty-seven states and thirty distinguished scientists gathered in Arlington, Virginia, at the Second International Public Conference of the National Vaccine Information Center (NVIC).* The conference chair, Barbara Loe Fisher, an authority on the subject of immunization, made the following opening remarks:

> The purpose of this conference is . . . to provide a forum for an open discussion and debate about the science, policies, and ethics of vaccination. . . . We believe that a child who dies from a vaccine is just as important as a child who dies from an infectious disease. We believe that a humane society will place equal emphasis on preventing both kinds of deaths and injuries. We support the rights of all health-care consumers to know what is and is not known about vaccines. We are not antivaccine. We are pro-education.[176]

During this international conference—about which *Mothering* magazine published an exclusive report titled "Show Us the Science"—"nearly every presenter concluded with a call for government-funded research on the reported links between vaccines and neurological and autoimmune disorders, including learning disabilities, attention deficit disorder, autism, asthma, diabetes, otitis media, multiple sclerosis, lupus, Crohn's disease (intestinal disorders), chronic fatigue syndrome, rheumatoid arthritis, Alzheimer's, cancer, AIDS, Gulf War syndrome, and personality disorders."[177] Unfortunately, although this fall 2000 conference was considered a resounding success, it has yet to accomplish its primary goal, which scientists and educators have been entreating the U.S. government to do for decades: the conduction of well-designed, double-blind, and *longitudinal* (long-term) studies that compare vaccines in groups of vaccinated children with control groups of unvaccinated children.

The Tipping Point for Change

However, it is important that readers aren't discouraged by the lack of response to this conference's report or by the growing mass of literature in magazines, books, and websites questioning the wisdom of vaccinations. According to Malcolm Gladwell's book *The Tipping Point,* at heart we are all "gradualists"—that is, our

*In some cases, I have found that a homeochord potency—30C/200C/1M—of the particular vaccine nosode is the most efficacious. This is often followed ten minutes later by 2 tablets of the Schuessler cell salt Silicea 6X. The patient dissolves 2 tablets in his or her mouth, either one time only or a few more times after that. This Silicea remedy helps attract the healing of the nosode to scar tissue, which the Silicea can then help break down.

*Although representatives from the CDC and the NIH were in attendance, they did not make any presentations.

knowledge and expectations are acquired over the steady passage of time.[178] Furthermore, at a certain point—*the tipping point*—a change is realized and the unexpected can become the expected.

Even more heartening, Gladwell emphasizes that this transformation can be accomplished though the "law of the few." In other words, all that is really required to catalyze major change in our culture—whether it is in sales, fashion, crime waves, or society as a whole—is the action of a dedicated, knowledgeable, and influential few. Thus, a small minority can effect widespread change, much like an epidemic itself. In the right context and favorable environment, news from an individual or a small group of individuals can spread like a virus, "infecting" a larger group of people with new information and ideas.[179]*

In regards to the vaccine controversy, there are signs that this revolutionary change has already begun. In the town of Ashland, in southwestern Oregon, there is now a "28 percent and rising" vaccine exemption rate in kindergartens, compared with a rate of about 4 percent statewide.[180] At one alternative school in this progressive town of 20,000, the parents who have refused to vaccinate their children are actually in the majority—a full 67 percent of children in this school have not received vaccinations.[181] Instead, these parents rely on the traditional wisdom of our foremothers and forefathers to build natural immunity in their children with a nutrient-dense organic diet, healthy exercise, and a loving and supportive home environment. A Pediatric Academic Societies meeting in Vancouver, Canada, in May 2010 revealed that in 2008 39 percent of parents either refused or delayed vaccinations for their children, compared to 22 percent in 2003.[182] These significant statistical changes show that more and more courageous and enlightened parents are refusing to blindly follow the dictates of their conventional allopathic doctors, and that real change is occurring.

*The "staying power" of new information or behavior change, what Gladwell refers to as the *stickiness factor,* is further enhanced by the veracity of the message. In this regard, the validity of the vast number of scientific research studies detailing the adverse effects of vaccinations, as well as the hundreds of reported clinical cases of damaged children, can no longer be denied. Furthermore, this mass of disturbing literature calls for—literally cries out for—more thorough scientific investigation conducted by independent and unbiased researchers.

Never Doubt

It is hoped that this chapter on the adverse effects of vaccinations will add to the already massive amount of accumulated evidence and help provide the tipping point to contagiously spread this knowledge throughout the U.S. population, as well as the world. It is only through the dissemination of facts and knowledge in a conscientious population that appropriate pressure can be brought to bear on our government agencies, and through this, the routine requirement of childhood (as well as adult) vaccines thoroughly reconsidered and reevaluated. Margaret Mead's famous quote most succinctly underscores this time-honored principle:

> Never doubt that a small group of thoughtful, committed citizens can change the world. Indeed, it is the only thing that ever has.[183]

NOTES

1. P. Gosch, "A Brief History of Bacterial and Fungal Isopathic-Homeopathic Remedies," *BioMed Report,* Winter 2002, 7.
2. M. Wood, *Vitalism* (Berkeley, Calif.: North Atlantic Books, 2000), 40.
3. P. Gosch, "A Brief History of Bacterial and Fungal Isopathic-Homeopathic Remedies," *BioMed Report,* Winter 2002, 7.
4. Ibid.; G. Null, *Germs, Biological Warfare, Vaccinations* (New York: Seven Stories Press, 2003), 132–33; J. Yasgur, *Yasgur's Homeopathic Dictionary* (Greenville, Pa.: Van Hoy Publishers, 1998), 272.
5. J. Yasgur, *Yasgur's Homeopathic Dictionary* (Greenville, Pa.: Van Hoy Publishers, 1998), 272.
6. Ibid., 164.
7. N. Miller, *Vaccines: Are They Really Safe and Effective?* (Santa Fe: New Atlantean Press, 2003), 90–91.
8. G. Null, *Germs, Biological Warfare, Vaccinations* (New York: Seven Stories Press, 2003), 159–66; H. Coulter and B. Fisher, *A Shot in the Dark* (Garden City Park, N.Y.: Avery Publishing Group, Inc., 1991), 22–82; H. Coulter, *Vaccination, Social Violence and Criminality* (Berkeley, Calif.: North Atlantic Books, 1990).
9. G. Null, *Germs, Biological Warfare, Vaccinations* (New York: Seven Stories Press, 2003), 161; N. Miller, *Vaccines: Are They Really Safe and Effective?* (Santa Fe: New Atlantean Press, 2003), 26, 29.

10. G. Null, *Germs, Biological Warfare, Vaccinations* (New York: Seven Stories Press, 2003), 159–66; H. Coulter and B. Fisher, *A Shot in the Dark* (Garden City Park, N.Y.: Avery Publishing Group, Inc., 1991), 22–82; H. Coulter, *Vaccination, Social Violence and Criminality* (Berkeley, Calif.: North Atlantic Books, 1990).

11. G. Null, *Germs, Biological Warfare, Vaccinations* (New York: Seven Stories Press, 2003), 161.

12. Ibid.

13. S. Curtis, *Homoeopathic Alternatives to Immunisation* (Kent, England: Winter Press, 2002), 6.

14. H. Buttram and J. Hoffman, *Vaccinations and Immune Malfunction* (Quakertown, Pa.: The Humanitarian Publishing Company, 1985), 54; G. Null, *Germs, Biological Warfare, Vaccinations* (New York: Seven Stories Press, 2003), 151.

15. H. Buttram and J. Hoffman, *Vaccinations and Immune Malfunction* (Quakertown, Pa.: The Humanitarian Publishing Company, 1985), 6.

16. G. Null, *Germs, Biological Warfare, Vaccinations* (New York: Seven Stories Press, 2003), 133.

17. H. Buttram and J. Hoffman, *Vaccinations and Immune Malfunction* (Quakertown, Pa.: The Humanitarian Publishing Company, 1985), 6; S. Curtis, *Homoeopathic Alternatives to Immunisation* (Kent, England: Winter Press, 2002), 6.

18. H. Coulter and B. Fisher, *A Shot in the Dark* (Garden City Park, N.Y.: Avery Publishing Group, Inc., 1991), 9; N. Miller, *Vaccines: Are They Really Safe and Effective?* (Santa Fe: New Atlantean Press, 2003), 40, 64; C. Horowitz, "Immunizations and Informed Consent," *Mothering,* no. 26 (Winter 1983): 27; E. Davis, "Health Hazards of Mercury," *Wise Traditions* 4, no. 2 (Summer 2003): 27.

19. A. Rock, "Toxic Tipping Point," *Mother Jones,* March–April 2004, 71–73.

20. D. Kirby, *Evidence of Harm* (New York: St. Martin's Press, 2005), 83.

21. M. Tucker, "Vaccines Under Fire," *Pediatric News* 8, no. 33 (1999): 1, 7.

22. A. Rock, "Toxic Tipping Point," *Mother Jones,* March–April 2004, 77.

23. P. O'Mara, "A Quiet Place: Mercury Must Be Removed from Childhood Vaccines–NOW!" *Mothering,* no. 125 (July/August 2004): 10.

24. Institute for Vaccine Safety: Johns Hopkins Bloomberg School of Public Health, "Thimerosal Content in Some US Licensed Vaccines" (updated February 2005), www.vaccinesafety.edu; "Vaccine and Thimerosal," www.thimerosal-news.com/html/vaccine.html.

25. D. Kirby, *Evidence of Harm* (New York: St. Martin's Press, 2005), 209.

26. M. Sircus, "The Vaccine Industry vs Robert F. Kennedy Jr." http://educate-yourself.org/cn/thimerosalpoisoning22jun05.shtml.

27. G. Null, *Germs, Biological Warfare, Vaccinations* (New York: Seven Stories Press, 2003), 143.

28. J. Koster, "Are Autism and Alzheimer's Disease Really New?" *Health and Healing Wisdom* 29, no. 1 (Spring 2005): 19.

29. L. Hewitson et al., "Influence of Pediatric Vaccines on Amygdala Growth and Opioid Ligand Binding in Rhesus Macaque Infants: A Pilot Study," *Acta Neurobiologiae Experimentalis* 70 (2010): 147–64.

30. SafeMinds, "Ground-Breaking Monkey Study: Mercury-Containing Hepatitis B Vaccine Causes Brain Damage," September 30, 2009, www.safeminds.org/news/wakefield-hewitson-mercury-hepB-vaccine.html.

31. M. Kennedy, "Autism Not Prevalent in Unvaccinated Children," *Naturopathic Doctor News and Review,* March 2006, 23.

32. D. Kirby, "Autism Rate Now at One Percent of All U.S. Children?" August 11, 2009, www.huffingtonpost.com.

33. G. Null, *Germs, Biological Warfare, Vaccinations* (New York: Seven Stories Press, 2003), 145.

34. L. Reagan, "What About Mercury? Getting Thimerosal Out of Vaccines," *Mothering,* no. 5 (March/April 2001): 55.

35. J. Donnelly, "Legislation Seeks to Convene Conference Before 2011, Explore Federal Policy Options," October 6, 2009, http://burton.house.gov/posts?tag=Autism.

36. L. Redwood et al., "Predicted Mercury Concentrations in Hair from Infant Immunizations: Cause for Concern," *Neurotoxicology* 22 (2001): 691–97.

37. M. Hermán et al., "Does the Hepatitis B Vaccine Cause Multiple Sclerosis?" *Neurology* 63 (September 14, 2004): 772–73.

38. A. Rock, "Toxic Tipping Point," *Mother Jones,* March–April 2004, 71, 72, 77.

39. H. Coulter and B. Fisher, *A Shot in the Dark* (Garden City Park, N.Y.: Avery Publishing Group, Inc., 1991), 9; C. Horowitz, "Immunizations and Informed Consent," *Mothering* no. 26 (Winter 1983): 27.

40. N. Miller, *Vaccines: Are They Really Safe and Effective?* (Santa Fe: New Atlantean Press, 2003), 23–25, 29, 32, 34, 41, 50, 64.

41. G. Null, *Germs, Biological Warfare, Vaccinations* (New York: Seven Stories Press, 2003), 151; N. Miller, *Vaccines, Autism and Childhood Disorders* (Santa Fe: New Atlantean Press, 2003), 14, 73, 78, 94, 95, 100, 101.
42. J. Murphy, *What Every Parent Should Know About Childhood Immunization* (Boston: Earth Healing Products, 1993), 36.
43. CDC, "Ingredients of Vaccines—Fact Sheet," www.cdc.gov/vaccines/vac-gen/additives.htm.
44. H. Coulter and B. Fisher, *A Shot in the Dark* (Garden City Park, N.Y.: Avery Publishing Group, Inc., 1991), 9.
45. J. Mercola, "New Warning About Everyday Poison Linked to Alzheimer's, ADHD, and Autism," March 20, 2010, Mercola.com.
46. Ibid.
47. Ibid.
48. N. Miller, *Vaccines: Are They Really Safe and Effective?* (Santa Fe: New Atlantean Press, 2003), 20–22; G. Null, *Germs, Biological Warfare, Vaccinations* (New York: Seven Stories Press, 2003), 146–48.
49. J. Roberts, "Polio: The Virus and the Vaccine," National Health Federation, www.thcnhf.com/article.php?id=1767.
50. G. Null, *Germs, Biological Warfare, Vaccinations* (New York: Seven Stories Press, 2003), 146–47.
51. N. Miller, *Vaccines: Are They Really Safe and Effective?* (Santa Fe: New Atlantean Press, 2003), 22–23.
52. G. Null, *Germs, Biological Warfare, Vaccinations* (New York: Seven Stories Press, 2003), 145–46.
53. S. Curtis, *Homoeopathic Alternatives to Immunisation* (Kent, England: Winter Press, 2002), 7, 22; *Physicians' Desk Reference* (Montvale, N.J.: Thomson PDR, 2003), 2022, 2023.
54. J. Murphy, *What Every Parent Should Know About Childhood Immunization* (Boston: Earth Healing Products, 1993), 36.
55. B. Norberg and B. Rose, "Foes of GMO Ban Redo Fliers to Fix Error," *The Press Democrat,* November 2, 2005, 1.
56. B. Rose, "County's Veterinarians Oppose Ban on GMOs," *The Press Democrat,* October 12, 2005, A1.
57. G. Null, *Germs, Biological Warfare, Vaccinations* (New York: Seven Stories Press, 2003), 141; H. Coulter and B. Fisher, *A Shot in the Dark* (Garden City Park, N.Y.: Avery Publishing Group, Inc., 1991), 13, 23; I. Golden, *Vaccination? A Review of Risks and Alternatives* (Daylesford, Victoria, Australia: self-published, 1998), 4; R. Moreau-Horwin and M. Horwin, "Link Between Increasing Rate of Pediatric Cancers and Childhood Vaccines," *Townsend Letter for Doctors and Patients,* December 1999, 75; S. Plotkin and E. Mortimer, *Vaccines,* 2nd. ed. (Philadelphia: W. B. Saunders Company, 1994), 51.
58. N. Boulianne et al., "Major Measles Epidemic in the Region of Quebec Despite a 99% Vaccine Coverage," *Canadian Journal of Public Health* 3, no. 82 (1991): 189–90; R. Davis et al., "A Persistent Outbreak of Measles Despite Appropriate Prevention and Control Measures," *American Journal of Epidemiology* 3, no. 126 (1987): 438–39; T. Gustafson, "Measles Outbreak in a Fully Immunized Secondary-School Population," *New England Journal of Medicine* 13, no. 316 (March 1987): 771–74; B. Hersh et al., "A Measles Outbreak at a College with a Prematriculation Immunization Requirement," *American Journal of Public Health* 3, no. 81 (1991): 360–64; N. Miller, *Vaccines, Autism and Childhood Disorders* (Santa Fe: New Atlantean Press, 2003), 96; K. Santich, "A Swelling Problem," *Orlando Sentinel,* May 9, 2006, 1.
59. "Polio Increased 300% in States Which Had Compulsory Vaccination," www.health.org.nz/polio.html; N. Miller, "The Polio Vaccine: A Critical Assessment of Its Arcane History, Efficacy, and Long-Term Health-Related Consequences," *Medical Veritas* 1 (2004): 241.
60. N. Miller, *Vaccines: Are They Really Safe and Effective?* (Santa Fe: New Atlantean Press, 2003), 16, 28.
61. Ibid., 14–17.
62. D. Shaw, "Government Repeatedly Approved Substandard Polio Vaccine," *The Seattle Times,* June 19, 1993, A1, A7.
63. G. Null, *Germs, Biological Warfare, Vaccinations* (New York: Seven Stories Press, 2003), 149–50; N. Miller, *Vaccines, Autism and Childhood Disorders* (Santa Fe: New Atlantean Press, 2003), 13; P. Kidd, "Autism, An Extreme Challenge to Integrative Medicine, Part I: The Knowledge Base," *Alternative Medicine Review* 7, no. 4 (2002): 308–9.
64. N. Miller, *Vaccines, Autism and Childhood Disorders* (Santa Fe: New Atlantean Press, 2003), 13; G. Null, *Germs, Biological Warfare, Vaccinations* (New York: Seven Stories Press, 2003), 9.
65. G. Null, *Germs, Biological Warfare, Vaccinations* (New York: Seven Stories Press, 2003), 68, 149–50.
66. H. Buttram and J. Hoffman, *Vaccinations and Immune Malfunction* (Quakertown, Pa.: The Humanitarian Publishing Company, 1985), 54–55.
67. H. Coulter and B. Fisher, *A Shot in the Dark* (Garden City Park, N.Y.: Avery Publishing Group, Inc., 1991), 9.
68. S. Hahnemann, *Organon of the Medical Art,* ed. W. O'Reilly (Palo Alto, Calif.: Birdcage Books, 1996), 81.

69. G. Null, *Germs, Biological Warfare, Vaccinations* (New York: Seven Stories Press, 2003), 149–50.
70. N. Miller, *Vaccines: Are They Really Safe and Effective?* (Santa Fe: New Atlantean Press, 2003), 14.
71. D. Kirby, *Evidence of Harm* (New York: St. Martin's Press, 2005), xiv.
72. H. Buttram and J. Hoffman, *Vaccinations and Immune Malfunction* (Quakertown, Pa: The Humanitarian Publishing Company, 1985), 56.
73. N. Miller, *Vaccines: Are They Really Safe and Effective?* (Santa Fe: New Atlantean Press, 2003), 52–55; S. Plotkin and E. Mortimer, *Vaccines,* 2nd ed. (Philadelphia: W. B. Saunders Company, 1994), 395; CDC, "Recommended Childhood and Adolescent Immunization Schedule" (January–June 2004), www.cdc.gov/nip; *Physicians' Desk Reference,* 57th ed. (Montvale, N.J.: Thomson PDR, 2003), 2108; *The Merck Manual,* 15th ed. (Rahway, N.J.: Merck Sharp and Dohme Research Laboratories, 1987), 2030.
74. N. Miller, *Vaccines: Are They Really Safe and Effective?* (Santa Fe: New Atlantean Press, 2003), 37–39; S. Plotkin and E. Mortimer, *Vaccines,* 2nd ed. (Philadelphia: W. B. Saunders Company, 1994), 42, 45, 49, 50; C. L. Daenell, "Childhood Vaccination," *Townsend Letter for Doctors and Patients,* May 1997, 79; S. Curtis, *Homoeopathic Alternatives to Immunisation* (Kent, England: Winter Press, 2002), 21.
75. N. Miller, *Vaccines: Are They Really Safe and Effective?* (Santa Fe: New Atlantean Press, 2003), 40–42; S. Curtis, *Homoeopathic Alternatives to Immunisation* (Kent, England: Winter Press, 2002), 22; CDC, "Recommended Childhood and Adolescent Immunization Schedule" (January–June 2004), www.cdc.gov/nip; *Physicians' Desk Reference,* 57th ed. (Montvale, N.J.: Thomson PDR, 2003), 790, 809, 811, 1554; H. Shelton, *Vaccine and Serum Evils* (San Antonio: American Natural Hygiene Press, 1951), 28; H. Coulter and B. Fisher, *A Shot in the Dark* (Garden City Park, N.Y.: Avery Publishing Group, Inc., 1991), 22–82.
76. S. Plotkin and E. Mortimer, *Vaccines,* 2nd ed. (Philadelphia: W. B. Saunders Company, 1994), 70.
77. H. Shelton, *Vaccine and Serum Evils* (San Antonio: American Natural Hygiene Press, 1951), 28.
78. N. Miller, *Vaccines: Are They Really Safe and Effective?* (Santa Fe: New Atlantean Press, 2003), 64–65; CDC, "Recommended Childhood and Adolescent Immunization Schedule" (January–June 2004), www.cdc.gov/nip; *Physicians' Desk Reference,* 57th ed. (Montvale, N.J.: Thomson PDR, 2003), 1536, 1669, 2105.
79. CDC, "Recommended Childhood and Adolescent Immunization Schedule" (January–June 2004), www.cdc.gov/nip.
80. N. Miller, *Vaccines: Are They Really Safe and Effective?* (Santa Fe: New Atlantean Press, 2003), 49–52; G. Null, *Germs, Biological Warfare, Vaccinations* (New York: Seven Stories Press, 2003); CDC, "Recommended Childhood and Adolescent Immunization Schedule" (January–June 2004), www.cdc.gov/nip; R. Moreau-Horwin and M. Horwin, "Link between Increasing Rate of Pediatric Cancers and Childhood Vaccines," *Townsend Letter for Doctors and Patients,* December 1999; *Physicians' Desk Reference,* 57th ed. (Montvale, N.J.: Thomson PDR, 2003), 898, 2212.
81. N. Miller, *Vaccines: Are They Really Safe and Effective?* (Santa Fe: New Atlantean Press, 2003), 49–52.
82. N. Miller, *Vaccines: Are They Really Safe and Effective?* (Santa Fe: New Atlantean Press, 2003), 56–59; S. Plotkin and E. Mortimer, *Vaccines,* 2nd ed. (Philadelphia: W. B. Saunders Company, 1994), 337–38; CDC, "Recommended Childhood and Adolescent Immunization Schedule" (January–June 2004), www.cdc.gov/nip; S. Curtis, *Homoeopathic Alternatives to Immunisation* (Kent, England: Winter Press, 2002), 28; I. Golden, *Vaccination? A Review of Risks and Alternatives* (Daylesford, Victoria, Australia: self-published, 1998), 84; *Physicians' Desk Reference,* 57th ed. (Montvale, N.J.: Thomson PDR, 2003), 786, 1958, 2052, 3402.
83. W. Atkinson, J. Hamborsky, L. McIntyre, and S. Wolfe, eds., *Epidemiology and Prevention of Vaccine-Preventable Diseases,* 9th ed. (Washington, D.C.: Public Health Foundation, 2006).
84. Ibid.
85. N. Miller, *Vaccines: Are They Really Safe and Effective?* (Santa Fe: New Atlantean Press, 2003), 83–88; S. Plotkin and E. Mortimer, *Vaccines,* 2nd ed. (Philadelphia: W. B. Saunders Company, 1994), 5; S. Perko, *The Homeopathic Treatment of Influenza* (San Antonio: Benchmark Homeopathic Publishers, 2005), 45; CDC, "Recommended Childhood and Adolescent Immunization Schedule" (January–June 2004), www.cdc.gov/nip; S. Curtis, *Homoeopathic Alternatives to Immunisation* (Kent, England: Winter Press, 2002), 24; *Physicians' Desk Reference,* 57th ed. (Montvale, N.J.: Thomson PDR, 2003), 795, 3406.
86. Mercola, "HPV Vaccine Blamed for Teen's Paralysis," http://articles.mercola.com/sites/articles/archive/2008/08/02/hpv-vaccine-blamed-for-teens-paralysis.

87. J. H. Tanne, "Questions over Human Papillomavirus Vaccine in the U.S. and Australia," *British Medical Journal* 334 (June 7, 2007): 1182–83.
88. Mercola, "HPV Vaccine Blamed for Teen's Paralysis," http://articles.mercola.com/sites/articles/archive/2008/08/02/hpv-vaccine-blamed-for-teens-paralysis.
89. R. Mendelsohn, "The Truth About Immunizations," *The People's Doctor* 2, no. 4 (April 1978): 3.
90. J. Mercola, "Regular Flu Vaccine Actually INCREASES Risk of Swine Flu," May 1, 2010, www.mercola.com.
91. R. Blaylock, "Swine Flu—One of the Most Massive Cover-ups in American History," November 3, 2009, www.mercola.com.
92. Ibid.
93. Ibid.
94. N. Miller, *Vaccines, Autism and Childhood Disorders* (Santa Fe: New Atlantean Press, 2003), 69–72; S. Plotkin and E. Mortimer, *Vaccines,* 2nd ed. (Philadelphia: W. B. Saunders Company, 1994), 237–38; CDC, "Recommended Childhood and Adolescent Immunization Schedule" (January–June 2004), www.cdc.gov/nip; S. Curtis, *Homoeopathic Alternatives to Immunisation* (Kent, England: Winter Press, 2002), 26; I. Golden, *Vaccination? A Review of Risks and Alternatives* (Daylesford, Victoria, Australia: self-published, 1998), 56; *The Merck Manual,* 15th ed. (Rahway, N.J.: Merck Sharp and Dohme Research Laboratories, 1987), 2022–23; "Current Status of Measles Immunization," *Journal of the American Medical Association* 194 (1965): 1237–38.
95. N. Miller, *Vaccines, Autism and Childhood Disorders* (Santa Fe: New Atlantean Press, 2003), 81.
96. N. Miller, *Vaccines, Autism and Childhood Disorders* (Santa Fe: New Atlantean Press, 2003), 3–14; CDC, "Recommended Childhood and Adolescent Immunization Schedule" (January–June 2004), www.cdc.gov/nip; S. Curtis, *Homoeopathic Alternatives to Immunisation* (Kent, England: Winter Press, 2002), 31; *Physicians' Desk Reference,* 57th ed. (Montvale, N.J.: Thomson PDR, 2003), 2022.
97. N. Miller, *Vaccines, Autism and Childhood Disorders* (Santa Fe: New Atlantean Press, 2003), 93–98; CDC, "Recommended Childhood and Adolescent Immunization Schedule" (January–June 2004), www.cdc.gov/nip; S. Curtis, *Homoeopathic Alternatives to Immunisation* (Kent, England: Winter Press, 2002), 31.
98. N. Miller, *Vaccines: Are They Really Safe and Effective?* (Santa Fe: New Atlantean Press, 2003), 93–98; S. Curtis, *Homoeopathic Alternatives to Immunisation* (Kent, England: Winter Press, 2002), 39; G. Null, *Germs, Biological Warfare, Vaccinations* (New York: Seven Stories Press, 2003), 153; H. Coulter and B. Fisher, *A Shot in the Dark* (Garden City Park, N.Y.: Avery Publishing Group, Inc., 1991), 4–8.
99. H. Coulter and B. Fisher, *A Shot in the Dark* (Garden City Park, N.Y.: Avery Publishing Group, Inc., 1991), 6; N. Miller, *Vaccines: Are They Really Safe and Effective?* (Santa Fe: New Atlantean Press, 2003), 40, 41.
100. G. Null, *Germs, Biological Warfare, Vaccinations* (New York: Seven Stories Press, 2003), 153.
101. D. Shepherd, *Homeopathy in Epidemic Diseases* (Essex, England: The C. W. Daniel Company Limited, 1996), 64–68.
102. N. Miller, *Vaccines: Are They Really Safe and Effective?* (Santa Fe: New Atlantean Press, 2003), 59–61; CDC, "Recommended Childhood and Adolescent Immunization Schedule" (January–June 2004), www.cdc.gov/nip; *Physicians' Desk Reference,* 57th ed. (Montvale, N.J.: Thomson PDR, 2003), 3455.
103. N. Miller, *Vaccines: Are They Really Safe and Effective?* (Santa Fe: New Atlantean Press, 2003), 13–23; S. Plotkin and E. Mortimer, *Vaccines,* 2nd ed. (Philadelphia: W. B. Saunders Company, 1994), 166; S. Curtis, *Homoeopathic Alternatives to Immunisation* (Kent, England: Winter Press, 2002), 32–33; *Physicians' Desk Reference,* 57th ed. (Montvale, N.J.: Thomson PDR, 2003), 802–4; *The Merck Manual,* 11th ed. (Rahway, N.J.: Merck Sharp and Dohme Research Laboratories, 1966), 1714–1715, and *The Merck Manual,* 15th ed. (Rahway, N.J.: Merck Sharp and Dohme Research Laboratories, 1987), 2036–39.
104. National Immunization Hotline at (800) 232-2522; the CDC National Immunization Program website at www.cdc.gov./nip/publications/fs/rotavirus.htm; *Physicians' Desk Reference,* 53rd ed. (Montvale, N.J.: Thomson PDR, 1999); N. Vitaro, "Vaccine Spotlight," *Naturopathic Doctor News & Review,* September 2006, 18.
105. N. Miller, *Vaccines, Autism and Childhood Disorders* (Santa Fe: New Atlantean Press, 2003), 99–110; S. Plotkin and E. Mortimer, *Vaccines,* 2nd ed. (Philadelphia: W. B. Saunders Company, 1994), 303; CDC, "Recommended Childhood and Adolescent Immunization Schedule" (January–June 2004), www.cdc.gov/nip; S. Curtis, *Homoeopathic Alternatives to Immunisation* (Kent, England: Winter Press, 2002), 34; *The Merck Manual,* 15th ed. (Rahway, N.J.: Merck Sharp and Dohme Research Laboratories, 1987), 2027.
106. N. Miller, *Vaccines, Autism and Childhood Disorders* (Santa Fe: New Atlantean Press, 2003), 101.
107. Ibid., 102.

108. Ibid., 104–10.

109. N. Miller, *Vaccines: Are They Really Safe and Effective?* (Santa Fe: New Atlantean Press, 2003), 74–82; S. Plotkin and E. Mortimer, *Vaccines,* 2nd ed. (Philadelphia: W. B. Saunders Company, 1994), 20–21; G. Null, *Germs, Biological Warfare, Vaccinations* (New York: Seven Stories Press, 2003), 45–48, 132–36; www.909shot.com/Action-Alerts/what you need to know.htm; "Hospital Staffs Consider Smallpox Vaccinations," *Marin Independent Journal,* December 1, 2002, A5; I. Golden, *Vaccination? A Review of Risks and Alternatives* (Daylesford, Victoria, Australia: self-published, 1998), 88, 89.

110. H. Shelton, *Vaccine and Serum Evils* (San Antonio: American Natural Hygiene Press, 1951), 28.

111. The Centers for Law and the Public's Health: A Collaborative at Johns Hopkins and Georgetown Universities, "The Model State Emergency Health Powers Act (MSEHPA)," www.publichealthlaw.net/ModelLaws/MSEHPA.php.

112. S. Plotkin and E. Mortimer, *Vaccines,* 2nd ed. (Philadelphia: W. B. Saunders Company, 1994), 20–21.

113. I. Golden, *Vaccination? A Review of Risks and Alternatives* (Daylesford, Victoria, Australia: self-published, 1998), 88, 89; N. Miller, *Vaccines: Are They Really Safe and Effective?* (Santa Fe: New Atlantean Press, 2003), 76, 77, 80.

114. G. Wilde, "Vaccine Production and Contamination as Contributing Etiologic Factors in Neoplastic Disease and Allergy," *Journal of Naturopathic Medicine* 5, no. 1 (December 29, 2001): 9, 10.

115. N. Miller, *Vaccines: Are They Really Safe and Effective?* (Santa Fe: New Atlantean Press, 2003), 74.

116. G. Null, *Germs, Biological Warfare, Vaccinations* (New York: Seven Stories Press, 2003), 134–35.

117. N. Miller, *Vaccines: Are They Really Safe and Effective?* (Santa Fe: New Atlantean Press, 2003), 23–59; S. Plotkin and E. Mortimer, *Vaccines,* 2nd ed. (Philadelphia: W. B. Saunders Company, 1994), 68–71; CDC, "Recommended Childhood and Adolescent Immunization Schedule" (January–June 2004), www.cdc.gov/nip; S. Curtis, *Homoeopathic Alternatives to Immunisation* (Kent, England: Winter Press, 2002), 35; I. Golden, *Vaccination? A Review of Risks and Alternatives* (Daylesford, Victoria, Australia: self-published, 1998), 73–78; *Physicians' Desk Reference,* 57th ed. (Montvale, N.J.: Thomson PDR, 2003), 907; *The Merck Manual,* 15th ed. (Rahway, N.J.: Merck Sharp and Dohme Research Laboratories, 1987), 98–99.

118. J. Yasgur, *Yasgur's Homeopathic Dictionary* (Greenville, Pa: Van Hoy Publishers, 1998), 272–73.

119. H. Chitkara, *Best of Burnett* (New Delhi: B. Jain Publishers, 1995), 146–47.

120. Ibid., 147.

121. G. Vithoulkas, *The Science of Homeopathy* (New York: Grove Press, Inc., 1980), 113.

122. Ibid., 114.

123. Ibid.

124. Ibid., 114–15.

125. Ibid., 115.

126. H. Coulter and B. Fisher, *A Shot in the Dark* (Garden City Park, N.Y.: Avery Publishing Group, Inc., 1991), 27.

127. J. Murphy, *What Every Parent Should Know About Childhood Immunizations* (Boston: Earth Healing Products, 1993), 39; N. Miller, *Vaccines, Autism and Childhood Disorders* (Santa Fe: New Atlantean Press, 2003), 45.

128. R. Blaylock, "The Dangers of Excessive Childhood Vaccinations," April 1, 2008, www.mercola.com.

129. G. Null, *Germs, Biological Warfare, Vaccinations* (New York: Seven Stories Press, 2003), 173–74.

130. H. Buttram and J. Hoffman, *Vaccinations and Immune Malfunction* (Quakertown, Pa.: The Humanitarian Publishing Company, 1985), 53; H. Coulter, *Vaccination, Social Violence, and Criminality* (Berkeley, Calif.: North Atlantic Books, 1990), xiii.

131. H. Coulter, *Vaccination, Social Violence, and Criminality* (Berkeley, Calif.: North Atlantic Books, 1990), xiii–xiv.

132. Ibid., ix, xiv.

133. Ibid.

134. R. Pitcairn, *Dr. Pitcairn's Complete Guide to Natural Health for Dogs and Cats* (Emmaus, Pa.: Rodale, Inc., 2005), 203, 414.

135. J. Schrof, "Miracle Vaccines," *U.S. News and World Report* (November 23, 1998): 57–67.

136. T. Mitchell, "Health Advice: Advice That Won't Hurt a Bit," *USA Weekend,* October 12–14, 2001; CDC, "Recommended Childhood and Adolescent Immunization Schedule" (January–June 2004), www.cdc.gov/nip.

137. "Be Cautious with Vaccines," in *Immunizations,* special issue, *Mothering* (1987): 29.

138. N. Miller, *Vaccines: Are They Really Safe and Effective?* (Santa Fe: New Atlantean Press, 2003), 97.

139. H. Coulter and B. Fisher, *A Shot in the Dark* (Garden City Park, N.Y.: Avery Publishing Group, Inc., 1991), 110–11, 115, 123–25, 129, 130–31.

140. Ibid., 259.

141. G. Null, *Germs, Biological Warfare, Vaccinations* (New York: Seven Stories Press, 2003), 139–40.

142. Associated Press, "Gates Helps Build Immunization Fund," *Marin Independent Journal,* December 3, 1998, B8.
143. L. Redwood et al., "Predicted Mercury Concentrations in Hair from Infant Immunizations: Cause for Concern," *Neurotoxicology* 22 (2001): 691–97.
144. S. Schultz, "Parents Who Don't Vaccinate Play a Risky Game," *U.S. News and World Report,* November 23, 1998, 65.
145. N. Miller, *Vaccines: Are They Really Safe and Effective?* (Santa Fe: New Atlantean Press, 2003), 103; H. Coulter and B. Fisher, *A Shot in the Dark* (Garden City Park, N.Y.: Avery Publishing Group, Inc., 1991), 201–2.
146. M. Faria, "Mandatory Vaccination Programs and Medical Ethics," www.heartland.org/policybot/results/702/Mandatory_Vaccination_Programs_and_Medical_Ethics.html.
147. N. Miller, *Vaccines: Are They Really Safe and Effective?* (Santa Fe: New Atlantean Press, 2003), 102–3.
148. J. Murphy, *What Every Parent Should Know About Childhood Immunization* (Boston: Earth Healing Products, 1993), 109.
149. J. Mercola, "How to Legally Avoid Unwanted Immunizations of All Kinds," www.mercola.com/article/vaccines/legally_avoid_shots.htm.
150. N. Miller, *Vaccines, Autism and Childhood Disorders* (Santa Fe: New Atlantean Press, 2003), 52.
151. D. Kirby, *Evidence of Harm* (New York: St. Martin's Press, 2005), 232–69.
152. G. Null, *Germs, Biological Warfare, Vaccinations* (New York: Seven Stories Press, 2003), 163–64.
153. N. Miller, *Vaccines: Are They Really Safe and Effective?* (Santa Fe: New Atlantean Press, 2003), 104.
154. G. Null, *Germs, Biological Warfare, Vaccinations* (New York: Seven Stories Press, 2003), 45.
155. Associated Press, "FDA Wants Mercury Preservative Taken Out of Vaccines," *Marin Independent Journal,* July 8, 1999; "Vaccine and Thimerosal," www.thimerosal-news.com/html/vaccine.html.
156. H. Coulter and B. Fisher, *A Shot in the Dark* (Garden City Park, N.Y.: Avery Publishing Group, Inc., 1991), 9.
157. I. Golden, *Vaccination? A Review of Risks and Alternatives* (Daylesford, Victoria, Australia: self-published, 1998), 157.
158. M. Megson, "Autism and Vaccinations," *Wise Traditions* 1, no. 3 (Fall 2000): 33–35.
159. K. Sullivan, "The Miracle of Vitamin D," *Wise Traditions* 1, no. 3 (Fall 2000): 14.
160. N. Miller, *Vaccines, Autism and Childhood Disorders* (Santa Fe: New Atlantean Press, 2003), 45.
161. R. Murphy, *Homeopathic Remedy Guide* (Blacksburg, Va.: H.A.N.A. Press, 2000), 615, 877, 1168, 1319.
162. D. Shepherd, *Homoeopathy in Epidemic Diseases* (Essex, England: The C. W. Daniel Company Limited, 1996), 31, 78; S. Curtis, *Homoeopathic Alternatives to Immunisation* (Kent, England: Winter Press, 2002), 24; R. Murphy, *Homeopathic Remedy Guide* (Blacksburg, Va.: H.A.N.A. Press, 2000), 616.
163. N. Miller, *Vaccines, Autism and Childhood Disorders* (Santa Fe: New Atlantean Press, 2003), 156.
164. G. Vithoulkas, *The Science of Homeopathy* (New York: Grove Press, Inc., 1980), 134.
165. N. Miller, *Vaccines, Autism and Childhood Disorders* (Santa Fe: New Atlantean Press, 2003), 70.
166. G. Null, *Germs, Biological Warfare, Vaccinations* (New York: Seven Stories Press, 2003), 257–58; I. Golden, *Vaccination? A Review of Risks and Alternatives* (Daylesford, Victoria, Australia: self-published, 1998), 77.
167. Ibid.
168. N. Miller, *Vaccines: Are They Really Safe and Effective?* (Santa Fe: New Atlantean Press, 2003), 9.
169. Ibid., 9–10.
170. G. Null, *Germs, Biological Warfare, Vaccinations* (New York: Seven Stories Press, 2003), 165.
171. S. Tenpenny, "Far-off Adventures: Vaccinations and Overseas Travel," *Mothering,* September/October 2003, 32.
172. J. Kramer, "Dangerous Side Effects," *Pacific Sun,* August 25–31, 2004, 12, 15.
173. Ibid., 30–33.
174. D. Hamilton, *Homeopathic Care for Cats and Dogs* (Berkeley, Calif.: North Atlantic Books, 1999), 360.
175. Ibid.
176. L. Reagan, "Show Us the Science," *Mothering,* March/April, 2001, 40.
177. Ibid.
178. M. Gladwell, *The Tipping Point* (Boston: Little, Brown and Company, 2000), 13–14.
179. Ibid., 1–14, 19–22, 92.
180. Jeff Barnard, "Don't Vaccinate? Doctors Paying to Hear Views," www.msnbc.msn.com/id/28581743.
181. Ibid.
182. J. Mercola, "You ARE Making a Difference! Many More Parents Are Refusing Vaccines!!" www.lewrockwell.com/orig10/mercola41.1.html.
183. A. Hochschild, "Against All Odds," *Mother Jones,* January/February 2004, 73.

PART SIX

THE STRUCTURAL COMPONENT

ꕥ

Structural therapies are placed toward the end of *Radical Medicine* because—with two notable exceptions—these treatments are typically most effective *after* the issues in the other chapters have been addressed. For example, a person receives little long-term benefit from spinal adjustments for low back pain when the true cause of this pain is chronic intestinal dysbiosis secondary to an undiagnosed gluten allergy. Nor is chronic fatigue and muscular pain (diagnosed as fibromyalgia) ameliorated by massage therapy when the primary cause is systemic mercury poisoning from a mouthful of amalgam fillings. Finally, lifelong feelings of anxiety and low self-esteem that trigger chronic bruxism (grinding of the teeth) are often most effectively addressed through the prescription of the correct constitutional homeopathic remedy as well as quality psychospiritual work (see chapter 18) before, or at least in tandem with, the fitting of a dental appliance.*

In my experience, the cause of chronic structural symptoms in most patients is rarely simply structural. Only when this actual cause is specifically addressed—be it a focus, mercury toxicity, or chronic anxiety—can the secondary structural pain and dysfunction be most effectively treated. However, the *two chief exceptions* to this rule are when the structural issues are truly causative and primary: acute trauma and major dental malocclusions (and/or jaw joint or temporomandibular dysfunction—TMD).

1. **Acute Trauma.** In the case of sudden trauma, a patient's structural injuries should be addressed first, and furthermore, these injuries should be treated as soon as possible. For example, if an individual has a traumatic accident such as being rear-ended in a car, then her injuries should be addressed promptly through appropriate structural care (e.g., spinal adjustments, craniosacral therapy, and massage) as well as supportive homeopathic and nutritional supplementation.* In fact, in these acute trauma cases, *time* is vital. Treatments are most effective when given immediately after the accident—or at least as soon as possible. In contrast with long-term structural care for chronic problems, intense D.C., D.O., and L.M.P. acute-care treatment schedules are entirely appropriate in these situations. Thus, after a motor vehicle accident, it is often essential to initially schedule structural therapies daily for the first week, and then three times a week or so for the next couple of months depending on the severity of the accident, and finally tapering down as healing occurs to help restore proper structural integrity and optimal neurological functioning.

D.C., D.O., and **L.M.P.:** *D.C.* stands for Doctor of Chiropractic Medicine, *D.O.* stands for Doctor of Osteopathic Medicine, and *L.M.P.* stands for licensed massage practitioner (or *L.M.T.* in some states for a licensed massage therapist).

2. **Malocclusions and TMD Syndrome.** Another exception to this "secondary structural rule" is the presence of significant dental malocclusions (bad bites) and/or temporomandibular joint (jaw joint or TMJ) pain and dysfunction. A classic signal of malocclusion is when patients' teeth are so misaligned that they can't find a comfortable bite when bringing their teeth together. An example of TMD syndrome or temporomandibular joint dysfunction is the inability of a patient to open or close his mouth fully without pain. In both these cases, the

*A dental appliance or splint can restore normal functioning to the bite or occlusion (the way the teeth fit together) and the jaw joint (also known as the temporomandibular joint, or TMJ).

*For example, Arnica montana 30C prescribed acutely (e.g., 2 pellets, three times a day for three days) can be exceptionally healing, as can quality vitamin C for soft tissue support and fish oil to reduce inflammation.

chronic structural and neurological instability of not having a functional bite or jaw joint, sometimes intensified by chronic pain in and around the head and neck, can be extremely debilitating and limit the effectiveness of other treatments. Therefore, in these cases it is quite appropriate, and even essential, to first refer these patients to a qualified holistic dentist who specializes in treating malocclusions of the teeth and TMD before commencing other treatments. Additionally, if the patient is damaging his or her teeth through chronically grinding and clenching them, a protective appliance is entirely appropriate. (For more information on effective appliances, see the "Orthopedic Treatment" section on page 524.)

STRUCTURAL PROBLEMS USUALLY THE RESULT, NOT THE CAUSE

With the exception of acute trauma and moderate to severe dental malocclusions and TMD, structural problems are rarely the underlying cause of chronic pain or dysfunction—in fact, typically they are the result. That is, neck and back pain, tension headaches, and stiff shoulder and hip joints are most often *secondary* to more serious and even life-threatening dysfunction in the body. For example, asthma that is secondary to the long-term use of toxic paints and solvents by artists often causes chronic neck and upper back pain and tension. Alternatively, an abscessed—but often silent—tooth (dental focus) typically triggers chronic ipsilateral shoulder or hip pain. In these common scenarios, massage or adjustments of these painful joint and muscle areas does little good in the long run, and thus is rarely curative.

This assertion does not diminish the great work done by chiropractic and osteopathic physicians or massage therapists. However, it is important to illustrate that, in most cases, structural therapies are most valuable to the patient *after* addressing the primary issues—for example, a dental focus, toxic metals, or other "obstacles to cure." Once the underlying causes of a patient's chronic symptoms have been treated (or reasonably ameliorated), then structural repair and regeneration is greatly beneficial and longer lasting.

ACCURATE DIAGNOSIS SAVES TIME, MONEY, AND EMOTIONAL STRESS

Careful and accurate diagnosis of the true cause of a patient's structural or dental dysfunction greatly saves the patient time and money. For example, spending hundreds of dollars on osteopathic cranial manipulation when a patient has a major malocclusion does little for that patient. Alternatively, seeing a chiropractor for years is only mildly ameliorative and never truly curative for long-term low back pain when the pain is actually secondary to a major food allergy that triggers gas and bloating and chronically refers pain to the low back area.

Additionally, the clarification of *why* patients have suffered from pain or other dysfunction for years can be greatly relieving and lift their spirits—and therefore their immune system functioning—immeasurably. For instance, in the previously described example, the diagnosis of fibromyalgia does little practical good except to put a medical term to a set of symptoms. It does not tell the patient why she is sick, nor does it lead her to any appropriate action except suppressive drugs to reduce the pain. However, when that same patient receives a second opinion from a holistic practitioner versed in amalgam filling toxicity, she can then go home and search the Internet for the key words *fibromyalgia* with *mercury amalgam* and read hundreds of pages from referenced sources on this subject.* Furthermore, when her amalgam fillings are then carefully removed by a holistic (or biological) dentist with appropriate supportive remedies and nutritional products, she can begin to experience firsthand the pain relief that detoxification of this poisonous metal bestows.†

---

*Toxic mercury increases glutamate (or aspartate, an excitatory neurotransmitter) in the central nervous system, resulting in an excess of free radicals (xanthine oxidase, oxygen radicals, etc.), which causes increased sensitivity to pain as seen in chronic fatigue syndrome (CFS) and fibromyalgia.

†Severe and long-term muscular pain, fatigue, and other chronic flulike symptoms—often labeled fibromyalgia—often require other treatments as well, including strict avoidance of the patient's food allergen(s), prescription of the correct homeopathic constitutional remedy, and the clearing of focal infections and scar interference fields.

STRUCTURAL THERAPIES
True *Chirurgery* in Appropriate Patients

In appropriate patients—that is, those who have cleared much of their toxicity and foci and are on the correct constitutional remedy—structural therapies can be *exceptionally* effective. In fact, in these cleaner and clearer "advanced" patients, chiropractic and osteopathic manipulation as well as deep tissue massage can be likened to surgery, or *chirurgery*. This latter term from the French is the origin of the modern-day term *surgery* and may be considered rather synonymous with the little-known but first definition of *surgery* in *Oxford's Dictionary*: "The branch of medical practice which treats injuries, deformities, and other bodily disorders by physical operation or manipulation."[1]

In appropriate patients, the results of quality structural therapies can be as dramatic as the amazing results late-nineteenth- and early-twentieth-century D.C.s and D.O.s experienced, such as curing migraine headaches with one adjustment or clearing chronic constipation simply through craniosacral manipulation. Indeed, before the debilitating mid-twentieth-century onslaught of toxins and allopathic medical and dental care that has weakened so many individuals, results like these were common. In contrast, today even "functional" disturbances such as migraines and constipation often require considerable detoxification before structural intervention can be effective.

Structural therapies are also often indispensable in releasing the chronic myofascial and skeletal distortion patterns that are secondary to longstanding dysfunction in the body. For example, although low back pain for twenty years that is secondary to intestinal dysbiosis can be relieved with dietary changes, herbal drainage remedies, and enzymes, effective treatment often requires structural intervention at some point to heal and repair the chronically impaired nerves, muscles, and vertebrae in the lumbosacral area. Furthermore, although the removal of a major left-sided dental focus can greatly ameliorate chronic left shoulder pain, structural therapy is essential after cavitation surgery to restore normal functioning and the full range of motion to this joint. Thus, in patients in which the primary toxic issues have been addressed, effective chirurgery through manipulation and massage is truly essential and can be quite curative when administered at the appropriate time.

myofascial: *Myofascial* refers to muscle and connective, or soft, tissue in the body.

In chapter 16, the diagnosis and treatment of dental malocclusions and TMD syndrome will be described. Chapter 17 will cover musculoskeletal dysfunction and holistic structural treatments such as spinal adjustments, craniosacral therapy, and massage as well as provide a definition of a truly holistic chiropractic or osteopathic physician.

NOTES

1. L. Brown, ed., *The New Shorter Oxford English Dictionary* (Oxford: Clarendon Press, 1993), 3158.

16

DENTAL MALOCCLUSIONS AND TMD SYNDROME

Structural dysfunction in the teeth and jaws comprises two closely interrelated syndromes: dental malocclusions and temporomandibular joint (jaw joint) dysfunction or TMD syndrome (see figure 16.1).

MALOCCLUSION CAN TRIGGER TMD

Your *occlusion* is the way that your upper and lower teeth fit together. A *malocclusion,* often referred to as a bad bite, is when the teeth do not occlude—that is, do not fit together properly—upon closing. When the occlusion is faulty—which can be due to myriad causes from inadequate breast-feeding to numerous ill-fitting fillings and crowns—the teeth don't fit together harmoniously when they meet. In these cases, as the late Dr. Jerome Mittelman, a holistic dentist specializing in treating malocclusions, described, "the jaws are then inclined to search for a convenient and comfortable place to close so that the hills and valleys of the opposing teeth do not interfere with one another."[1] When the mandible (lower jawbone) eventually finds a more comfortable but out-of-normal-alignment position, the jaw joint or

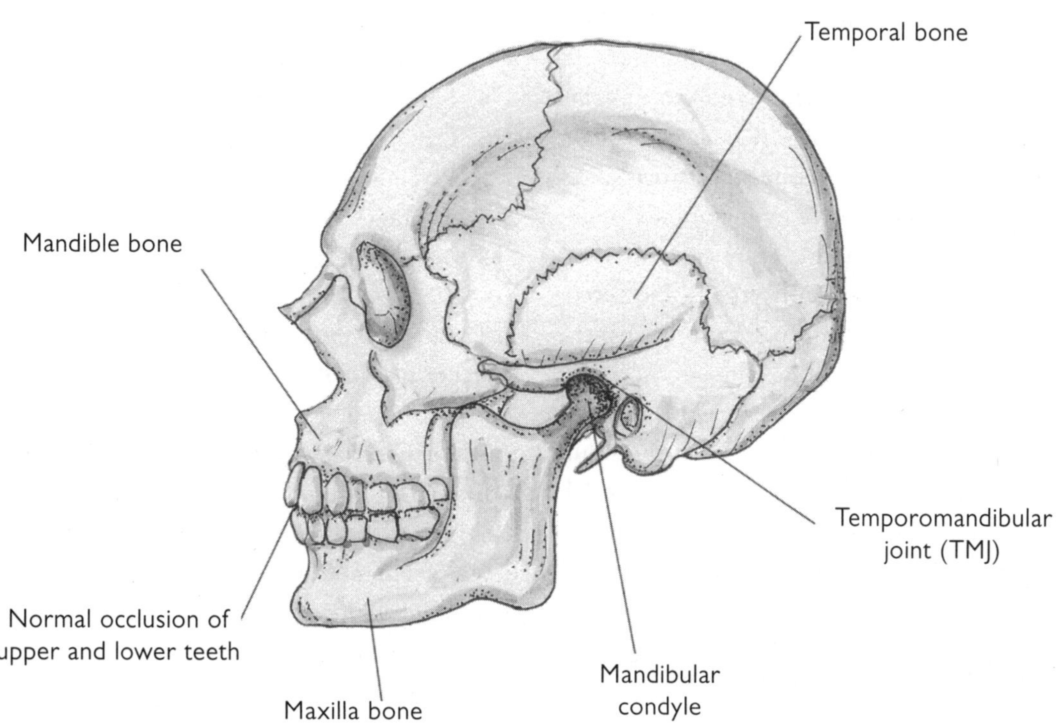

Figure 16.1. The occlusion is the way the upper and lower teeth fit together. The temporomandibular joint (TMJ), or jaw joint, is a ball (mandibular condyle) and socket (temporal bone cavity) hingelike joint. Dysfunction in the TMJ can trigger a wide range of symptoms.

temporomandibular joint is then pulled out of its normal position or alignment, resulting in chronic (mild to major) dysfunction.

CRITERIA FOR PROPER OCCLUSION

According to dental textbooks, proper occlusion occurs when three criteria are met: "(1) All teeth touch at the same time on closing with a cusp tip point contact to a flat surface; (2) During movement of the teeth to the side, guidance comes from the cuspid (eye) tooth. Guidance is transferred to the front teeth in extreme side movements or when moving the jaw forward; and, (3) The posterior (back) teeth should not bump or drag on one another during side or forward motions."[2]

This same phenomenon can occur in any joint in the body. Take, for example, another ball-and-socket joint in the body, such as the hips. When individuals sit cross-legged for extended periods, this joint signals its distress through pain. Over time, and especially in the extreme case of certain Indian yogis who meditate most of the day, hip joints can become severely misaligned and even deformed. In this same way, a chronic malocclusion of the teeth can eventually trigger full-fledged temporomandibular joint dysfunction syndrome, as the jaw joint becomes progressively more deranged through damage to the supporting soft tissue structures (disk, ligaments, and muscles) and the bony mandibular condyle (the ball part of the mandible bone that fits into the temporal bone socket) eventually erodes. However, the temporomandibular joints are particularly vulnerable to derangement because of all the joints in the body, they have the most freedom of movement.[3] This flexible design bestows upon this hinge joint between the skull and the jaw the ability to accomplish myriad essential movements—chewing, talking, shouting, kissing, and so forth—but also renders it somewhat fragile.

TMD CAN TRIGGER MALOCCLUSION

TMD syndrome does not develop only from malocclusion of the teeth; it can also be caused by trauma. For example, head injuries or "whiplash" (cervical hyperextension/ flexion) can overstretch and tear the delicately balanced ligaments and disks in the temporomandibular joints. Without prompt and appropriate treatment, normal TMJ alignment is deranged and jaw joint functioning can become significantly impaired. In fact, if not treated promptly, damaged temporomandibular joints over time initiate malocclusion of the teeth, when the torqued jaw forces the teeth into an unnatural occlusion. Of course, if the trauma is severe enough, the teeth can also become chipped or fractured, initiating an immediate malocclusion problem too. *Thus, dental malocclusion can trigger TMJ dysfunction, and TMJ dysfunction can trigger dental malocclusion.* Furthermore, after a significant amount of time, these two misalignments potentiate each other, escalating the severity and dysfunction of the other.

CAUSES OF DENTAL MALOCCLUSION AND TMD SYNDROME

In this section, the most common causes of malocclusion and TMD are briefly summarized. They fall under the following eight general categories:

1. Lack of breast-feeding and maternal nutrition
2. Excessive thumb sucking and pacifier use
3. Inadequate nutrition
4. Fungicides and other toxic chemicals
5. Cavities, extractions, and premature equilibration
6. Psychological stress and bruxism
7. Trauma
8. Neighboring foci and ganglia

1. Lack of Breast-Feeding and Maternal Nutrition

Nearly everyone in the holistic community is aware of the health advantages of breast-feeding, such as providing ideal infant nutrition, better absorption and assimilation, fewer food allergies, better immunological development, and more stable and healthy psychological maturation.[4] However, few are aware of another compelling benefit of breast-feeding—the proper development of an infant's hard palate for the optimal growth and alignment of the teeth and jaws. Although scientific literature has documented the fact that infants who are breast-fed have significantly fewer malocclusions than children who are bottle-fed, few parents seem to be aware of this benefit, as well as the substantial savings in later orthodontic bills.[5]

> **hard palate/soft palate:** The hard palate is the hard, bony anterior (forward) part of the roof of the mouth. The soft palate is the soft and fleshy part behind it.

Bottle-Fed Infants Twice as Likely to Develop Malocclusions

In one 1987 study that reviewed nearly 10,000 children between three and seventeen years old, bottle-fed children were almost two times more likely to have malocclusions than those who had been breast-fed. Among the breast-fed children in this study, those who had been breast-fed for three months or less had a malocclusion rate of 32.5 percent, whereas those who had been breast-fed for more than twelve months had a malocclusion rate of only 15.9 percent.[6] Furthermore, bottle-feeding has been found to increase the risk of otitis media (ear infections) in infants and children at least fivefold.[7]

FORMULA NUTRITION

A small informal survey of Weston A. Price Foundation (WAPF) members found that bottle-fed children who were given a homemade formula of raw whole milk from cows that graze on green grass or raw goat milk with added organic liver developed naturally straight teeth. Sally Fallon notes that it is impossible to determine the effects of bottle-feeding without accounting for possible nutritional deficiencies in the formula being fed to the child. Clearly more research is needed to compare the effects of bottle-feeding with nutrient-dense versus nutrient-deficient formulas. For mothers who can't breast-feed, substituting an appropriate formula "does not necessarily condemn a child to having a narrow palate—nor does breast-feeding guarantee normal development."[8]

▶ If mothers can't breast-feed, they should refer to the "Feeding Babies" chapter in the second edition of Sally Fallon's book *Nourishing Traditions.* (Order from your local bookstore or from Radiant Life at 888-593-9595.)

Breast-Feeding and Palate Development

The primary difference on a simply structural and mechanical basis between breast- and bottle-feeding is in the muscular action of the tongue. When a baby is breast-fed, the infant obtains milk by a natural peristaltic, or wavelike, motion of the tongue in order to compress the soft breast nipple against the hard palate. It's important to remember here that in the case of an infant, this upper palate (known as the hard palate) is almost as malleable as softened wax. Therefore, when this natural tongue-rolling movement that occurs during breast-feeding comes in contact with the infant's very supple "hard" palate, the palate is slowly and gently molded into a "U" shape.[9] This U-shaped hard palate allows the teeth to develop properly in the jaw and erupt in correct alignment.

In contrast, the bottle-fed infant must employ a more forceful squeezing or "pistonlike" tongue movement to obtain cow's (or goat's or soy) milk or formula from an artificial nipple, leading to a narrow and unnatural "V"-shaped hard palate. This more narrow palate, along with a more narrow face, nasal cavity, and cheekbones, has been significantly linked with an increased incidence of dental malocclusion in the scientific literature.[10]

Bottle-Feeding and Abnormal Swallowing

In addition to properly molding the hard palate, breast-feeding also greatly augments a normal swallowing habit. A normal swallow is initiated when the tip of the tongue braces itself *just above the upper front teeth* while the bolus of food or saliva is dumped toward the back of the throat and swallowed. In an abnormal swallow, the tongue muscles push *against the front teeth themselves* in what is termed a "tongue thrust." This abnormal tongue thrust movement develops from the unnatural piston-style tongue motion during bottle-feeding, as well as from a related but somewhat opposite problem referred to as "fast-flow."[11]

Fast-flow is the term used when the milk or formula flows too quickly from an artificial nipple (with a large hole in the tip), forcing infants to hold their tongue up against the hole to keep from choking. This fast-flow problem, which, incidentally, also occurs in 10 percent of nursing mothers, triggers a faulty pattern termed *reverse swallow* or *traumatic swallow,* as infants are forced to reject the too-abundant flow of milk or formula.[12*] Without treatment, this traumatic swallowing habit will remain with the individual throughout his or her life, and also greatly contributes to the faulty development of the palate and future malocclusion.

V-Shaped Palate Linked to Mouth-Breathing

When the roof of the mouth is pushed up in a sharp V-shaped angle, the floor of the nasal cavity rises as well. This creates a narrower nasal chamber, which can have a significant effect on breathing efficiency. In one 1997 study published in the *Annals of Internal Medicine,* a high palate and narrow arch were both shown to be notable predictors of snoring and obstructive sleep apnea.[13]

A narrow nasal cavity forces children (and adults) to open their mouths at night when they sleep to receive more oxygen. This altered mode of breathing also leads to a lowered tongue position, or tongue thrust, and abnormal muscular movements and pressure. These chronic mouth-breathing children typically exhibit narrow faces, a high palate, and various dental malocclusions (crossbite, overbite, and the maxillary and mandibular incisors projecting backward).[14]

Mouth-Breathing Generates More Cavities

This nocturnal mouth-breathing habit dries out the saliva, rendering it more "ropey and dessicated instead of detergent and cleansing." This can lead to a greater amount of plaque formation (the germ colonies that lie around the necks of the teeth that cause decay and gum disease), eventually creating cavities that must be filled or crowned.[15] Furthermore, the resulting numerous fillings and crowns erode the normal height of the natural tooth, which over time can further impair the bite or occlusion.

Mouth-Breathing Creates Sugar Craving and Reduces Assimilation

Finally, the dry mouth that chronic mouth-breathing creates can stimulate cravings for sweets to combat this parched feeling, which also leads in the same domino fashion to more cavities, reduced tooth height, and worsening malocclusions. Additionally, the need to drink abnormal amounts of water during meals due to this dry mouth dilutes the stomach and intestinal acid, which reduces nutrient assimilation and further feeds the craving/cavity/malocclusion cycle.[16] Thus, a narrow nasal chamber and obstructed airway can influence the formation of a malocclusion in a secondary manner through plaque aggregation, sugar cravings, and excessive thirst.

Systemic Effects of Mouth-Breathing

In an article in *Wise Traditions* journal, Raymond Silkman, D.D.S., detailed the systemic effects of mouth-breathing—that is, the effects occurring throughout the body. These effects include a chronic lack of sufficient oxygenation in the cardiovascular system, or the lungs and heart, due to the dry, unhumidified, unfiltered, and nitric oxide–deficient* air that is continuously inhaled through the mouth instead of through the nasal passages. This insufficient oxygen in the cardiovascular system also triggers anoxia (lack of oxygen) systemically, since the lungs are constantly receiving poorly oxygenated air and the heart must pump this deficient and abnormal mixture of gases throughout the body. Dr. Silkman illustrates the effect this chronic anoxia has on the nervous system as a subconscious feeling "akin to a hand or choker around the neck.[17] He further describes this chronic distress signal to the sympathetic nervous system† as "a kind of tightness, a kind of permanent tension, which can be very stressful and depleting to the body." Silkman has found that individuals who are mouth-breathers are therefore on "high alert" all the time due to their "amped-up sympathetic nervous systems."[18]

This resulting chronic, mild to major systemic anoxia has a negative effect on every cell in the body because they are subsequently deprived of sufficient oxygen, which could contribute to the future onset of cancer, since cancer cells are anaerobic (lacking oxygen) by nature. Mouth-breathing and reduced oxygenation throughout the body also give rise to some types of headaches, hypertension, reduced heart output, blood-clotting dysregulation, enuresis (bed-wetting), and chronic ear or sinus infections.[19]

*Do you have trouble swallowing pills? If so, you may have a malocclusion.

*Nitric oxide is a potent vasodilator produced in the nasal sinuses that enhances the uptake of oxygen in the lungs.

†As described previously, the sympathetic system is that part of the autonomic nervous system that is triggered under stress and increases heart rate, breathing, and muscle strength.

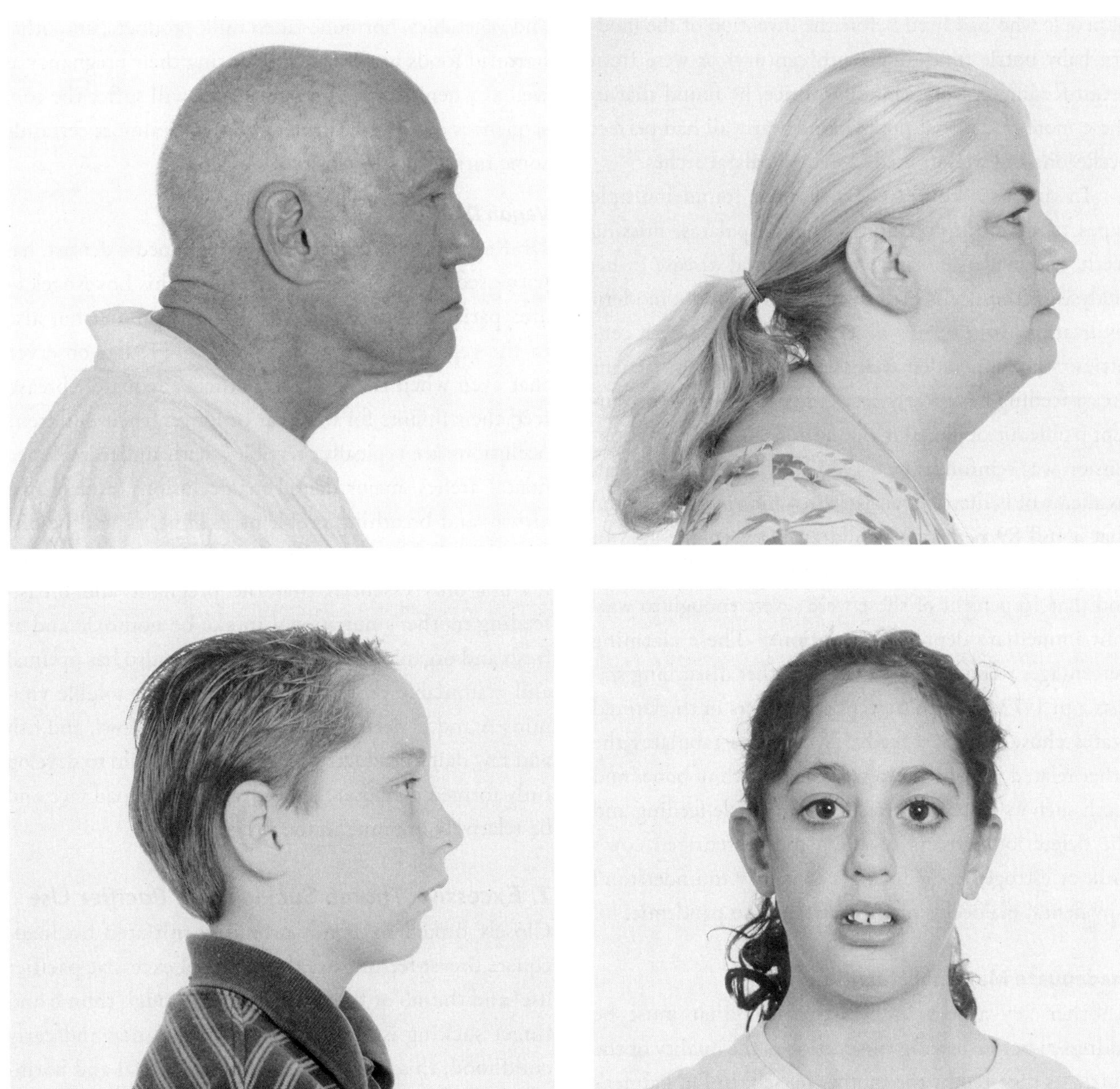

Figure 16.2. Indications of chronic mouth-breathing and associated poor dental and facial development include forward head tilt, postural abnormalities, weak chins, narrow faces, and circles under the eyes. (Reprinted here with permission from Dr. Raymond Silkman.)

As many holistic dentists and chiropractors are aware, mouth-breathers typically compensate by tilting their heads forward to receive more air (figure 16.2). Other signs of mouth-breathing and associated poor dental and facial development include narrow faces, a weak chin, chronically chapped lips, the sclera (white part) showing under the irises, circles under the eyes, a tendency for the face to sag, and a nose bump.[20]

Historical Evidence of the Benefits of Breast-Feeding

Dr. Brian Palmer, a holistic Kansas City dentist who can be likened to a modern-day Weston Price based on his extensive (and self-financed) anthropological research, has specialized for over twenty years in the diagnosis and treatment of snoring, sleep apnea, and infant nutrition. In one study, Dr. Palmer evaluated approximately 600 skulls of people who had lived before the invention of the modern baby bottle (mid-nineteenth century) or were from breast-feeding cultures. Like Dr. Price, he found that in these more traditional populations nearly all had perfect occlusions and well-formed U-shaped palatal arches.[21]

In dramatic contrast, Dr. Palmer found multiple types of malocclusion and V-shaped palates, missing teeth, and evidence of severe periodontal disease in his analysis of the skulls of individuals from more modern civilizations in the later nineteenth and twentieth centuries.[22] He concluded that the lack of or insufficient breast-feeding has greatly accelerated the rise of the current pandemic of dental malocclusions. Dr. Palmer's conclusion was reinforced by a 1973 study by the American Academy of Pediatric Dentistry in which it was reported that a full 89 percent of children between the ages of twelve and seventeen had some form of malocclusion, and that 16 percent of these were severe enough to warrant immediate dental intervention.[23] These alarming percentages were consistent with another disturbing statistic: in 1973, only 26 percent of mothers in the United States chose to breast-feed.[24] When one tabulates the other related factors that retard the growth of bones and teeth such as reduced nutrients from bottle-feeding and the deleterious effects of allergenic pasteurized cow's milk or estrogenic soy formula, it is easy to understand why dental malocclusions are currently so pandemic.

Inadequate Maternal Nutrition

Another key aspect to breast-feeding that must be addressed before leaving this section is the quality of the nutrients ingested by the mother herself. In Dr. Palmer's research, it is important to note that not only did he study the skulls of people from breast-feeding cultures but that these people lived in the 1800s—a century before the onslaught of processed and refined foods.

Toxic Refined Foods

Unfortunately, today, with toxic foods sold in every conventional grocery store, breast-feeding alone cannot ensure a healthy baby. Many modern holistic dentists have observed this fact and concluded that adequate breast-feeding and adequate maternal nutrition must both be met to ensure that infants and children fully grow and develop their cranial and facial bones. Mothers who mindlessly eat junk foods, pesticide-ridden fruits and vegetables, hormone-laden milk products, and other harmful foods just before and during their pregnancy as well as when they are breast-feeding, will suffer the consequences of an unhealthier child with almost certainly some form of malocclusion.

Vegan Diet

Dr. Raymond Silkman, a holistic orthopedic dentist, has witnessed this phenomenon not only in his Los Angeles–area patients who eat a refined and toxic diet but also in the vegan mothers in his practice. He has observed that even when these vegan mothers adequately breast-feed their infants for one year or longer, their children's occlusions are typically "terrible," with underdeveloped dental arches, major dental malocclusions, and related airway and breathing problems.[25] Thus, as will be discussed in the upcoming "Inadequate Nutrition" section, it's not only essential that the pregnant and breast-feeding mother's nutritional intake be nontoxic and as fresh and organic as possible, but that it also has optimal and assimilable protein, minerals, and fat-soluble vitamins A and D derived from organic meat, fowl, and fish and raw dairy products* in order for her child to develop fully formed dental arches and a healthy broad face and be relatively immune to tooth decay.

2. Excessive Thumb Sucking and Pacifier Use

Closely linked to, if not primarily initiated by, inadequate breast-feeding are the habits of excessive pacifier use† and thumb or finger sucking. Although thumb and finger sucking is a normal stage in infancy and early childhood, this habit can become abnormal and harmful when it becomes excessive. Orofacial myologists—therapists who specialize in treating disturbed muscle patterns in the head and face—define "excessive" by three factors: (1) intensity—how hard is the suck-

*As discussed in chapter 5, raw (unpasteurized) dairy products can be beneficial for those whose ancestral heritage included these foods (e.g., many Western and Eastern Europeans, Russians, etc.), but they are often allergenic for those without that background (e.g., Hawaiians and other Pacific Islanders, many Africans, many Asians, etc.) as well as those who have simply developed a major dairy allergy by overeating pasteurized cow's milk products in their childhood.

†Pacifiers should be made out of less toxic silicone or latex, which are free of the harmful chemical phthalates found in soft plastic pacifiers. However, some infants may be allergic to latex. (L. Berkson, *Hormone Deception* [Contemporary Books, 2000], 98.)

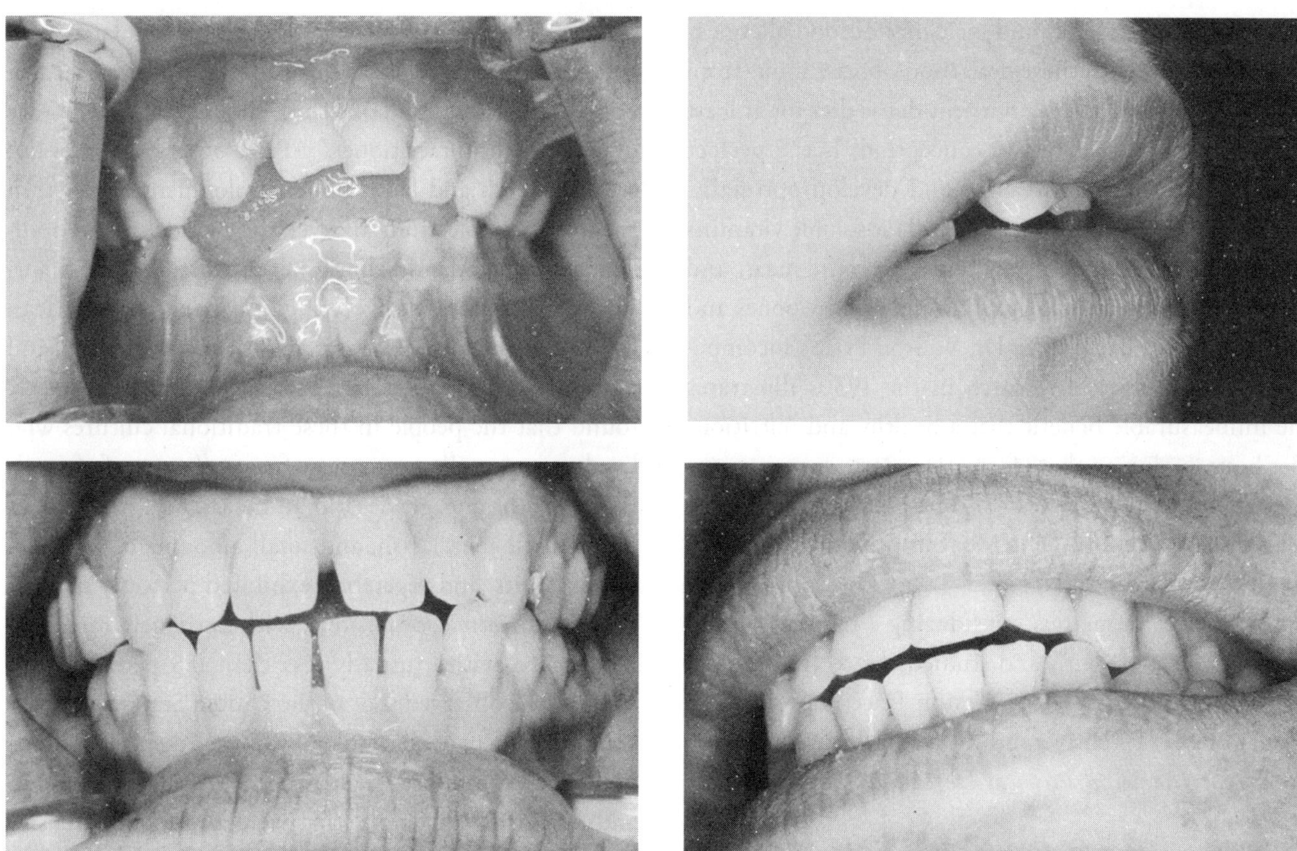

Figure 16.3. Malocclusions from long-term thumb sucking and pacifier use. The upper two photos demonstrate an abnormal forward thrust of the tongue upon swallowing, protruding teeth, and an open bite in a child. The lower two photos show the typical flaring teeth and open bites in two adults. (Reprinted here with permission from Jerome Mittelman, D.D.S., and Beverly Mittelman, B.S., C.N.C.)

ing?; (2) frequency—how often does it occur?; and (3) duration—how many months or years has the habit persisted? When thumb sucking and pacifier use are excessive—that is, persisting for years—malformation of the teeth and jaws is almost inevitable. The resulting malocclusions that commonly occur from these oral habits include "anterior open bites," where the front teeth do not meet upon closing; "overbites" and "overjets," where the upper jaw teeth become displaced forward; and "crossbites," where the lower teeth are abnormally positioned outside of the upper teeth due to a too narrow upper arch (see figure 16.3).[26]

▶ For more information on the Mittelmans' pediatric work with malocclusions and how best to take care of your child's teeth and gums, order their book *Healthy Teeth for Kids: A Preventive Program, Prenatal through the Teens* from the Price-Pottenger Nutrition Foundation at (800) 366-3748.

Furthermore, because pacifier use and thumb sucking put strong and continuous pressure on the TMJ, inflammation in the jaw joints and neighboring ears is common. Studies have shown that pacifier use *doubles* the chance of developing otitis media (ear infections) in children under twelve months of age and is responsible for at least one-fourth of all acute otitis media in children under three years of age.[27]

3. Inadequate Nutrition

Damages Children's Immune and Digestive Systems

From estrogenic soy-based infant formulas to sugary cereals made with high fructose corn syrup, children are inundated with profoundly toxic foods (see chapter 5). These so-called foods pack the triple punch of giving no nutritive benefits, damaging organ systems through disruption of normal hormonal development and exhaustion of the digestive and immune systems, and augmenting the severity and incidence of food allergies.

In contrast with these dead foods, breast milk (from mothers who have eaten a nutrient-dense diet for at least six months to a year before conception) is the perfect food to allow infants to grow and develop optimally. Children need utilizable protein and fat-soluble vitamins A and D in the form of raw butter, organic meat, and (non-farm-raised) fish to grow strong, healthy bones and fully developed occlusions. Dr. Weston Price's incomparable anthropological research in the 1930s illustrates the immeasurable benefit that a healthy and nutritious diet bestows during these formative years.

Weston A. Price and "The Most Important Health Book Ever Written"

In 1939, after numerous trips during a ten-year period in which he lived with and studied the teeth and jaws of "primitive" peoples, Dr. Weston Price published the results of this extensive anthropological odyssey in his book *Nutrition and Physical Degeneration*.[28] Dr. A. C. Fonder, also a giant in the dental profession, later characterized Price's book as "the most important health book ever written" and one that "should be in the library of every health practitioner."[29] Price observed and evaluated the teeth and facial bone development of fourteen groups of people from all over the world—isolated villagers in Switzerland, Aborigines in Australia, the Maori in New Zealand, native tribes in Canada, American Indians in the Florida Everglades, the Incas in Peru, and numerous tribes in Africa.[30] He and his wife consistently found that the people in these traditional cultures who lived on raw milk, eggs, meat from *all parts* of animals (bone broths and gravies, organ meats, etc., rather than only muscle meat), fish, and small amounts of (organic) grains, fruits, and vegetables exhibited perfectly straight teeth and normal occlusions, with extremely rare incidences of cavities (usually less than 0.5 percent).[31] In contrast, he observed that in the United States and other countries where people ate many of the "displacing foods of modern commerce" such as refined sugar, white flour, and rancid vegetable oils (that were already in extensive use in the early 1900s—although *not* as extensive as today), there was a 25 to 75 percent incidence of "facial and dental arch deformities"* and numerous dental cavities.[32] (See figures 16.5 through 16.8.)

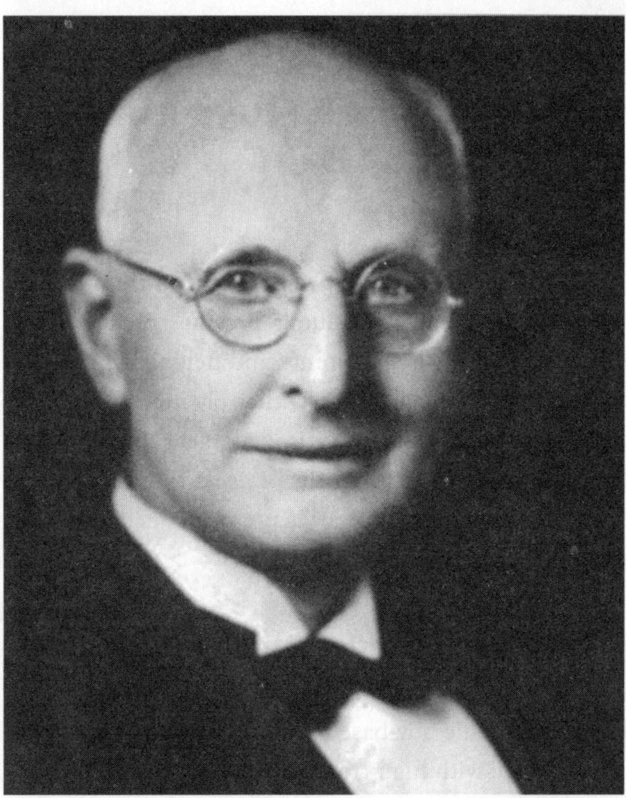

Figure 16.4. Dr. Weston A. Price was a brilliant researcher and pioneer in the fields of holistic dentistry, nutrition, and diet. (Reprinted with permission from the Price-Pottenger Nutrition Foundation.)

Price's Observations Verified by Other Researchers

Huge U.S. Survey Confirms Price's Assertions

In 1938, Dr. Thomas Parran (1892–1968), Surgeon General of the U.S. Public Health Service, reported the same results as Price after sampling 2,660,000 Americans from various communities and from different economic levels:

> With the adoption of our white bread and sugar the nutritional elements were not present to build sturdy bodies. The face became narrow, teeth were crowded, decay became a problem for the first time, the younger children were smaller. Tuberculosis and arthritis rapidly became problems when before they were nonexistent. The

*These deformities included overbites ("buckteeth"), narrowed faces, underdevelopment of the nose, pinched nostrils, and the lack of well-defined cheekbones.

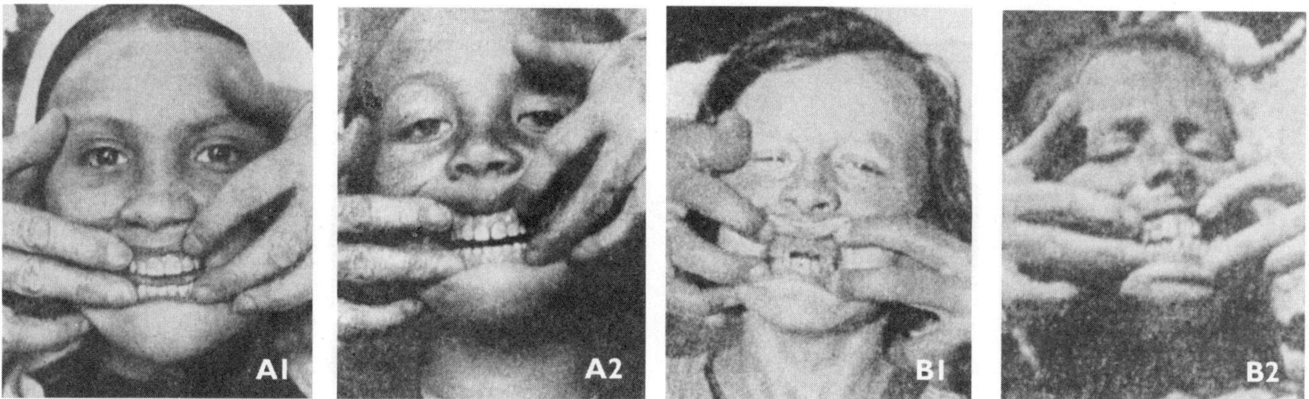

Figure 16.5. (A) Normal tooth and bone development in people from a Swiss village with a diet of whole milk, meat, and rye (appropriately wide facial and dental arches with well-formed nostrils, and only 2 percent with any tooth decay), as compared with (B) those in a modernized Swiss district who ate a more refined diet (narrower faces, badly formed dental arches, slow eruption of teeth, crowding, and almost 30 percent tooth decay). (Photos reprinted here with permission from the Price-Pottenger Nutrition Foundation.)

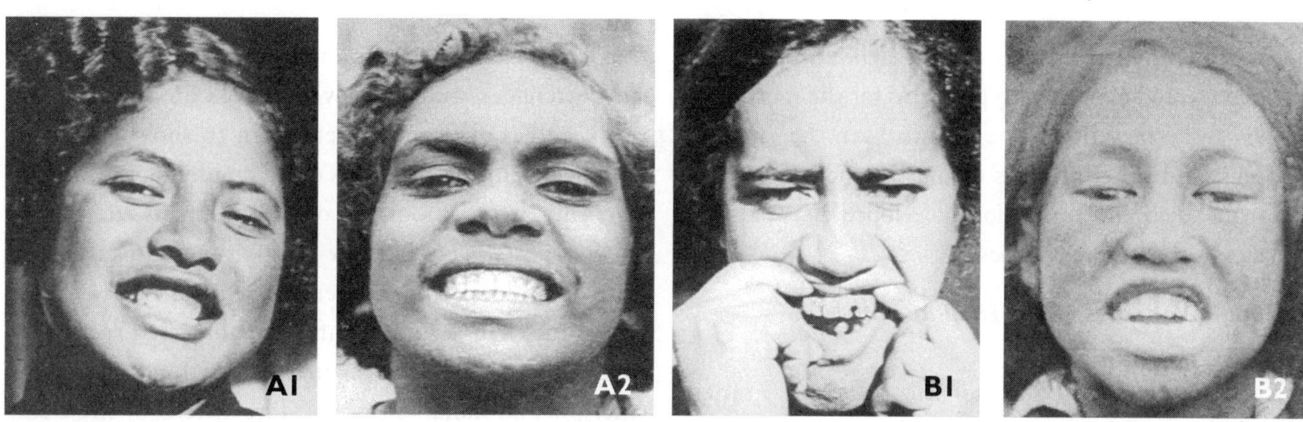

Figure 16.6. (A) "Splendid" tooth and facial bone development in the Maori of New Zealand (only about one tooth in one thousand had tooth decay), as compared with (B) rampant tooth decay and narrow facial bone development after the adoption of a modern diet. (The B2 girl has such badly developed dental arches that she cannot close her front teeth together, which is known in dentistry as an "open bite" deformity.) (Photos reprinted with permission from the Price-Pottenger Nutrition Foundation.)

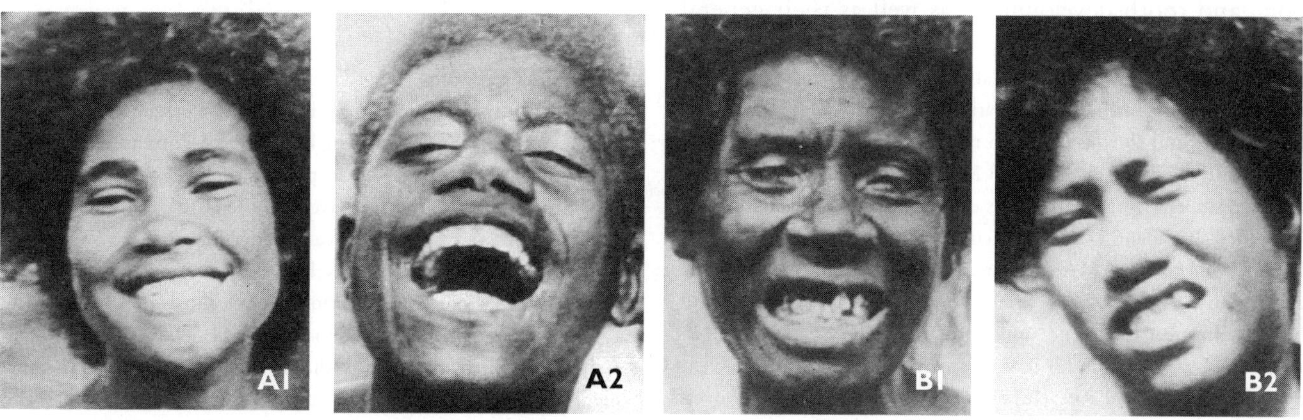

Figure 16.7. (A) These photographs show the full development of the facial bones and teeth in South Sea Islanders with a diet consisting of seafood, plants, and fruit, as compared with (B) the next generation born after the parents had adopted imported modern foods in their diet. Note the marked tooth decay in the B1 woman, and the narrowed facial features of the B2 girl. (Photos reprinted with permission from the Price-Pottenger Nutrition Foundation.)

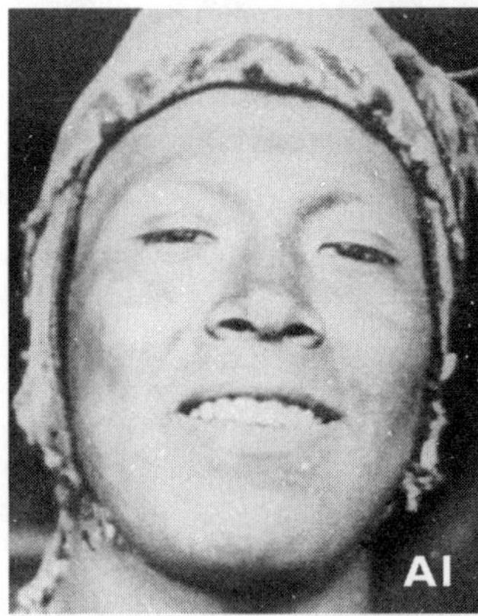

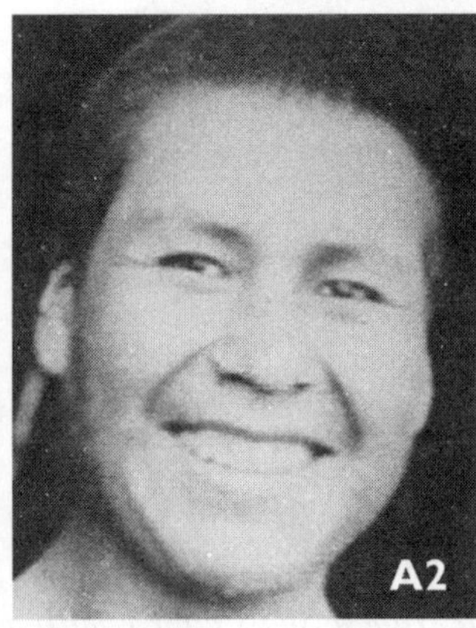

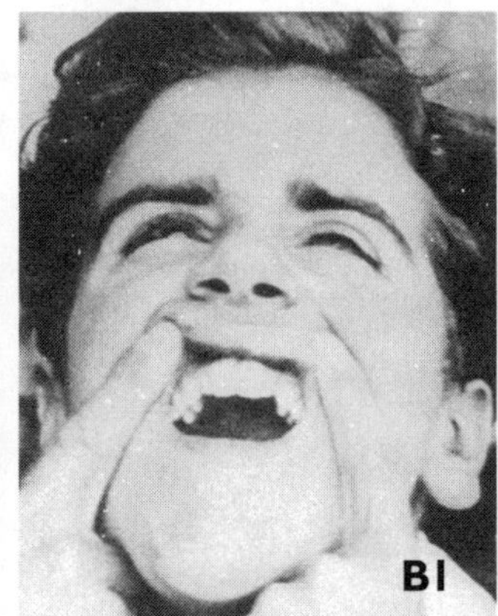

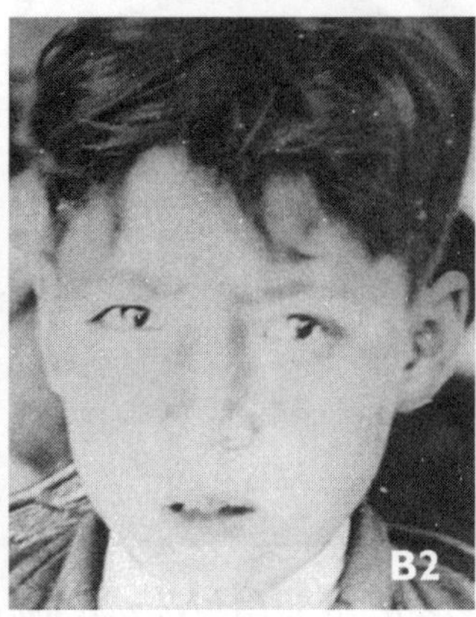

Figure 16.8. (A) Note the "magnificent physiques" and excellent facial and dental arch development on these young men raised on their native Incan diet in Peru, as compared with (B) these Peruvian boys whose parents adopted the "foods of modern commerce." The B2 boy is a mouth-breather due to insufficient nasal bone development, and thus, inadequate airway passages. (Photos reprinted with permission from the Price-Pottenger Nutrition Foundation.)

> narrowing of the pelvis causing delayed births had created many health problems for the mothers and especially for the infants. Even the cats, pigs, and other animals eating the food scraps from sugar and white flour developed cleft palates and deformed bodies.[33]*

Pottenger Validates Price's Findings with Studies on Cats

Price's contemporary and holistic colleague Francis Pottenger, M.D. (1901–1967), observed the same debilitating effects from refined foods through a ten-year study (1932–1942) utilizing cats. This well-controlled and longitudinal study yielded the same results as Price's study with humans—that is, when cats, who thrive best on raw meat, ate refined foods, their bone and tooth development, as well as their general health, seriously deteriorated. In fact, the adult cats in Pottenger's study that were placed on a pasteurized milk and cooked meat diet began to show unhealthy conditions in their mouths quite rapidly—often within just three to six months. Long-term effects, after three to five years, were chronic gingivitis, incrustations of salivary calculi, and numerous cavities. Furthermore, these cats had seriously infected, abscessed teeth that over time decayed and crumbled, leaving most of the incisors and molars missing.* The kittens of these cats also exhibited considerably narrowed malar and orbital arches (cheek and eye bones), maxillas (upper jawbones), and mandibles (lower jawbone), leaving insufficient room for a complete set of teeth to develop and descend. Nor did the genetic damage from these processed foods stop with this first generation. The third

*Unfortunately Dr. Parran, who also worked hard to sway public opinion away from the condemnation of syphilis and other venereal diseases and to consider them more as medical conditions, was attacked in 1948 by the American Medical Association by its head, Morris Fishbein, while Parran was campaigning for national health insurance. President Truman's decision not to reappoint Parran is believed due to the AMA's censure. Morris Fishbein, editor of the AMA journal from 1924 to 1949, also attacked Harry Hoxsey and his herbal cancer treatment, suing the Dallas pioneer a total of 125 times and harassing him for more than 25 years. Fishbein also went after Royal Raymond Rife (1888–1971), who invented the Universal Microscope and had also documented the cure of cancer patients with his frequency instrument. Fishbein further attacked Max Gerson, the German physician who first successfully instituted nutritional approaches for treating cancer.

*Interestingly, the cats' "fangs," or canine teeth, proved to be exceptionally resistant to abscesses and decay. (F. Pottenger, *Pottenger's Cats: A Study in Nutrition* [San Diego: Price-Pottenger Nutrition Foundation, 1995], 22). This exception is probably secondary to the body's instinctual desire to survive, and the biting, and thus protective effects, these canine teeth can render in animals also persists in the human body and psyche. However, another benefit is that these teeth relate to liver function, as was illustrated in the dental relationship chart discussed in chapter 11. Thus, the liver—one of the most ill-treated organs thanks to toxic diets, metals, and chemicals—is unusual in that it rarely reflexively damages the canine teeth as the other organs do the molars and incisors. Furthermore, in my clinical experience, when the canine teeth are impaired—that is, abscessed or root-canalled—the patients are almost invariably seriously ill.

generation of kittens exhibited small and irregular teeth, lack of eruption of teeth, and failure of the posterior molars to erupt—mirroring the current near-universal problem of impacted wisdom teeth in humans.[34] Price, finding the same thing in primitive tribes that Pottenger found in his cat studies, commented on this modern-day problem in his book:

> Two serious defects from which many individuals in our modernized civilization suffer are impacted teeth and the absence of teeth due to their failure to develop. It is significant that in the arches of the primitive races practically all teeth form and erupt normally, including the third molars.[35]

Sadly, when we consider the progress the big food and agricultural industries have made in the last century in refining the U.S. diet, it is understandable why the need for braces is currently pandemic in our youth. Poor diet is also the major reason why it is the rare individual nowadays who still has enough room for the proper eruption and development of the wisdom teeth.

Pottenger's study is the origin of the expression, "We're third-generation cats," often referred to among holistic practitioners. That is, in the case of many of the baby boomers—and certainly for younger generations—their grandparents and parents ingested a very refined and devitalized diet before their conception, and this diet rendered them considerably weaker genetically at birth. By appreciating this triple genetic threat, we can also see why degenerative diseases are currently epidemic, and why even top-quality holistic therapeutic protocols often require several years to restore optimal health. However, as Sally Fallon points out in her book *Nourishing Traditions,* these weaknesses of nature can be greatly mitigated through adequate nurture—that is, the use of bone broths and organic organ meats, free-range eggs, raw organic butter, and other whole foods in your diet. Additionally, removing toxic chemicals and metals from the body, treating dominant foci, receiving the correct constitutional homeopathic simillimum, and, finally, having the courage to face your fears and egoic defenses through quality psychospiritual work can also greatly mitigate, and even reverse, these genetic limitations.

4. Fungicides and Other Toxic Chemicals

Another pernicious effect on normal teeth and bone development in industrialized cultures is the extensive use of fungicides, pesticides, insecticides, herbicides, and other toxic chemicals after World War II.

Minimal Research

Because the effect of these toxins can be insidious and costly longitudinal studies are required to truly measure their full effect, the research on the retarded development of tooth and bone growth caused by chemicals has been minimal. However, the human and animal studies that have been published document such a dramatic and destructive relationship that further research, and appropriate corrective action, seems essential to our very survival as a species.

Links to Bone and Teeth Deformities

One study in Ireland linked the use of fungicide to combat potato blight in the 1980s to a high incidence of various physical malformations, including bone and facial deformities in babies. In a six-year investigation in the United States beginning in 1996, herbicides and fungicides were found to be culpable in causing severe bone and dental abnormalities in horses, deer, elk, antelopes, birds, and other animals. Astonishingly, this study, which identified numerous malformations including overbites ("bucked teeth"), underbites ("bulldog appearance," where the lower mandible protrudes out farther than the upper maxilla), crooked teeth, and cleft palates (underdevelopment of the upper maxilla), was conducted in Bitterroot Valley, Montana—ironically advertised as the "Last Best Place" on earth due to the purported clean air and water. Even more alarming, these abnormalities were linked not only to the direct spraying of herbicides by trucks and helicopters along roads and forest and pastureland but also to the wind drift of fungicides carried from Idaho, Washington, Oregon, California, and even as far away as Asia.[36]

5. Cavities, Extractions, and Premature Equilibration

When a cavity is detected in a tooth, dentists repair this hole with an appropriate restoration—a filling, inlay, onlay, or crown. Because it is difficult to emulate the exact height of a natural tooth, the restoration often ends up too high or too low.

HOLISTIC VS. ALLOPATHIC DENTAL RESTORATION

As discussed in chapter 11, holistic dentists place the most conservative restoration possible in order to preserve as much of the natural tooth as they can. Thus, they utilize larger fillings, inlays, or onlays for larger cavities, whereas their allopathic colleagues tend to jump from fillings to crowns. Crowns drill away from 40 to 75 percent of the original tooth structure, greatly increasing the risk that the tooth may die.[37] Three major reasons why allopathic dentists recommend inlays or onlays less often than their holistic colleagues is because: (1) they take more time to make and to fit; (2) they require more skill and training on the part of the dentist; and (3) they receive lower reimbursement coverage from insurance companies than for crowns.[38]

Effects of Improper Restoration Height

A dental restoration that is too high can create interference with the rest of the occlusion, or bite—and in the densely innervated region of the oral cavity a "molehill" of a couple of millimeters truly does feel like a "mountain" to the patient. This interference can result in the tooth hitting its opposing tooth prematurely and too hard, and thus, over time, bruising the nerves, periodontal ligament, and gum tissue of both teeth. It is therefore important that the patient returns to the dentist as soon as possible to have the interfering surfaces filed down (equilibrated), so that the tooth (as well as the opposing tooth) doesn't undergo irreparable damage and die.[39]

The opposite problem—when a restoration is placed too low—is also a common occurrence. Because dentists have been more aware of the problem of interference from too high a restoration for decades, they are currently taught in many dental schools to "dish out" the filling. Although this solves the problem of interference, after the placement of several fillings the patient's original tooth height is significantly reduced from these "too low" fillings, and the teeth no longer fit well together. This iatrogenic (doctor-induced) malocclusion typically stimulates clenching and grinding (bruxism) in a vain attempt to find a comfortable resting place for the teeth and the jaws. However, chronic bruxism only compounds the problem by further eroding the height of the teeth, resulting in a common syndrome that dentists refer to as "a loss of vertical dimension." This erosion of the tooth's filling is especially pronounced (and hazardous) in mercury amalgam, which is particularly sensitive to grinding stresses.[40]

Extractions and the Loss of Vertical Dimension

Having teeth pulled without proper replacements such as bridgework or a removable partial also creates malocclusions.* Not only does the bite suffer from a loss of normal height or decreased vertical dimension, but the two neighboring teeth often start leaning into the empty space created by the extraction. Over time, these two neighboring teeth will suffer the effects of abnormal shearing forces from chewing, clenching, and grinding and become inflamed and even infected. When these structurally induced dental focal infections undergo enough damage and devitalization, their extraction leaves an even larger hole in the patient's occlusion and further reduces the patient's chewing ability and the absorption of essential nutrients.

A common cause of reduced vertical dimension and the resulting malocclusion is the accepted but injurious practice of the extraction of the four first bicuspid teeth before orthodontia. Many patients experience TMD and malocclusion-related symptoms after orthodontia work (braces and retainers) because the majority of orthodontists myopically concentrate on improving the bite for aesthetic—versus healthful—purposes.† Another unacceptable practice is pulling teeth simply due to decay as is sometimes the case in rural areas, third-world countries, or by military dentists, rather than treating them with a filling or other appropriate restoration.

Equilibration Is a Double-Edged Sword

The term *equilibration* is defined as the "adjustive grinding of an interfering tooth structure" or the grinding of many teeth in order "to equalize occlusal stress, to produce simultaneous occlusal contacts, or to achieve harmonious occlusion."[41] The former definition—the grinding away of an area of interference from a recently placed restoration (a filling, inlay, onlay, or crown, as pre-

*However, it's important to point out that not all extractions require replacement bridges. For example, sometimes the last molars in the mouth (second or third) do not need a bridge or partial.

†For more information on the harm done by the orthodontic protocol of four bicuspid extractions, see the upcoming "Orthodontic Treatment" section.

viously described)—is often necessary and appropriate.

However, the latter definition of equilibration—the grinding down of numerous tooth surfaces for (usually short-term) symptomatic relief—is what gives the term *equilibration* a negative connotation in the field of holistic dentistry. Whole-mouth equilibration is appropriate only *after* a patient's condition is stable—that is, after his or her symptoms (both dental and in the rest of the body) have been diagnosed and treated. The reason is that a patient's seemingly occlusal-related symptoms may not be due to his or her bite but can be primarily caused by other contributing causes. These causes include dental foci (impacted wisdom teeth, abscessed teeth, failed root canals, etc.), malnutrition, anxiety, toxic mercury amalgam fillings, and so forth. Thus, *only* when the underlying causes of the malocclusion are addressed and treated can the bite be appropriately equilibrated. Additionally, when the patient's malocclusion itself is indeed the major disturbance, the bite should not be equilibrated until after holistic orthopedic dental work (functional appliances sometimes followed by braces) is completed.

Appropriate Equilibration Necessitates Clinical Expertise

Final occlusal equilibration requires great technical expertise and training on the part of the dentist, acquired in dental school as well as in postgraduate continuing education courses. David Walther, D.C., addresses this issue in his book on the stomatognathic system (the mouth and jaws):

> [Equilibration] is a procedure requiring great skill and knowledge, and it must be correlated with the total stomatognathic system rather than simply tooth-to-tooth contact. In no case should it be taken lightly, especially when the natural dentition is involved, because selective grinding is an irreversible loss of tooth enamel.[42]

Unfortunately, in nonholistic dental offices, full-mouth equilibration is common and the whole-body ramifications of this procedure are rarely taken fully into account. Furthermore, this practice of premature equilibration affords the patient only temporary relief in the majority of cases.[43] Additionally, it typically "locks in" the underlying causes of the bad bite and misaligned TMJ, triggering more serious adaptation on the part of the patient. For example, undiagnosed dental foci may continue to flourish unimpeded in their production of pathogenic bacteria, depression and anxiety may escalate, and pain syndromes may (sooner or later) intensify.

Thus, equilibration is a double-edged sword: very beneficial to fine-tune the height of a filling, inlay, onlay, or crown but harmful when done prematurely to try to balance a bad occlusion. Therefore, most holistic orthopedic or TMD dental specialists who treat patients with major malocclusions often use a team approach with other practitioners—chiropractors, osteopaths, naturopaths, massage therapists, and physical therapists—to adequately address all the issues underlying a bad bite, and to treat these problems effectively before completing their work with a final equilibration. Additionally, Dr. Fonder, an orthopedic TMD dentist, cautions that dentists may need to gently equilibrate periodically for a certain amount of time while carefully observing the results after each session, "until all musculature has settled into a completely compatible physiological relationship throughout the head, neck and body."[44] Finally, it is essential to mention here that the final equilibration of a bite may require building up the height of some of the teeth that have lost their vertical dimension through wear, grinding and clenching, and inadequate restorations (fillings, inlays, crowns, etc.).

6. *Psychological Stress and Bruxism*

The causes of *bruxism*—chronic grinding of the teeth—are numerous. Any of the aforementioned or upcoming factors that cause an unnatural and abnormal occlusion—from lack of breast-feeding to toxic ganglia—can trigger bruxism.

Bruxism Perpetuates and Worsens Malocclusions

In most cases, bruxism is simply an unconscious habit pattern that is an attempt to adapt to the existing malocclusion—through clenching and grinding—in order to find a more comfortable "home position" of the teeth and jaws. However, this habit has serious consequences. By slowly eroding the normal height of the teeth, bruxism further damages and perpetuates the malocclusion of the teeth and TMD.

Nocturnal Bruxism Is Common

Many patients are unaware that they clench and grind their teeth. That is because most people grind their teeth at night, referred to as *nocturnal bruxism*. It is often their mate who is disturbed by the noisy grating sounds at night or their dentist who recognizes the erosion patterns of bruxism who first informs them that they grind their teeth.

Psychological Stress Is a Major Contributor to Chronic Bruxism

Another classic causation of bruxism, not necessarily dependent on an existing malocclusion, is chronic psychological tension and stress. Often overlooked by doctors and dentists, chronic anxiety, depression, insecurity, and other mental and emotional symptoms can trigger unconscious clenching and grinding, as well as other negative oral habits such as fingernail biting. In fact, the anger that usually underlies chronic depression can often be physically demonstrated by palpating the strongest muscle in our bodies—the masseter.[45] This powerful jaw muscle that runs from the cheekbone (zygomatic arch) to the lower surface of the jaw (mandible) often has painful "trigger points"—little nodules of degenerated muscle tissue and inflamed nerves—in patients who clench and grind their teeth. Unfortunately, this chronic clenching only "exercises" and strengthens this muscle more—much like weightlifting does when building up one's bicep muscles—thus rendering the masseter even more shortened and contracted over time. (See figure 16.9.)

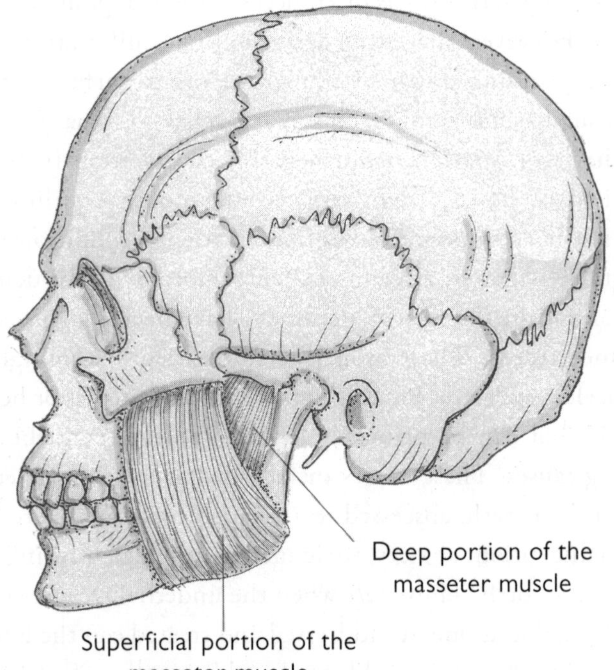

Figure 16.9. Exquisitely painful trigger points in the masseter jaw muscle are often an indication of bruxism secondary to psychological stress and/or a malocclusion.

JAW TRIGGER POINTS AND TOOTH PAIN

Active trigger points in the masseter muscle—as well as other craniofacial jaw muscles such as the pterygoids and the temporalis—can refer pain into the teeth themselves. Dr. Felix Liao, a biological dentist in the Washington D.C. area, recommends that not only patients diagnosed with a malocclusion but also those who have been told they need a root canal should have their trigger points evaluated. Practitioners looking for more information on trigger point therapy should consult *Travell & Simons' Myofascial Pain and Dysfunction: The Trigger Point Manual*, volume 1.

Effective Treatments: Psychological Work and Homeopathy

Effective psychological work can greatly reduce bruxism and engender more relaxation in the minds and bodies of patients. Jungian and rebirthing (breathwork) therapies that reach the deep unconscious levels that primarily drive the bruxing habit are especially efficacious. Several (or a typical series of ten) rebirthing sessions prescribed near the end of orthopedic dental treatment for patients with major malocclusions and TMD can be particularly useful to find the most relaxed and balanced bite before final equilibration. Additionally, the prescription of a patient's correct homeopathic constitutional remedy can be incredibly transformative in relieving chronic stress from both genetic and environmental miasmic tendencies. In the case of a patient without an obvious malocclusion, I would prescribe a constitutional remedy before referring her to a holistic dentist for orthopedic appliance therapy.

Bruxism Signaled Poor Health Even in Ancient Times

It is interesting to note that bruxism has been recognized since ancient times "as a sign of poor health and even impending death." Several references to bruxism were found on Sumerian clay tablets dating back from 3500 to 3000 BCE, including the following: "If he grinds his teeth the disease will last a long time." Furthermore, around 1000 BCE, healthy teeth among the Hebrews was so revered that it was listed as an essential physical requirement for high priests.[46]

7. Trauma

Direct Blows

As actor Burt Reynolds is intimately familiar with, trauma to the teeth or jaws can initiate an immediate misalignment of the teeth and/or jaw joint. And as was the case with this famous movie star, an injury-induced malocclusion/TMD can become seriously debilitating over time. Reynolds developed his chronic TMD after being hit in the jaw while filming *City Heat*. When he finally received a correct diagnosis and appropriate treatment—after years of suffering and even rumors that he had AIDS—Reynolds's TMD-induced headaches, fatigue, and visual problems resolved.[47]

"TMJ-lash" Injuries from Car Accidents

Both direct and indirect blows (elsewhere on the head or body) can misalign the TMJ by dislodging the disk (the fibrous pad that cushions the joint), straining the jaw and neck muscles, and spraining the surrounding ligaments that help anchor the jaw joint in its proper position. Forces of noncontact to the body such as the common whiplash injury incurred from car accidents can displace the jaw joint as well as cause maloccluded teeth. Upon rear-end impact by another car, the neck is first hyperextended backward (acceleration phase), which strains both the cervical muscles by stretching them beyond their normal range of motion and the jaw muscles by forcing the mouth open excessively wide (see figure 16.10A). This excessive mouth opening displaces the jaw joint from its normal position and propels the TMJ disk forward. This anterior displacement of the TMJ disk can be significantly damaging to the joint and can be the primary etiology underlying later arthritic deterioration of the temporomandibular joint.[48]

In the next moment, when the eight- to fourteen-pound head is thrust forward into hyperflexion (the deceleration phase), the teeth slam together, which can cause micro-fractures, or even chipped teeth if the impact is forceful enough (see figure 16.10B). The mandible is forced backward during this hyperflexion stage, and this abnormal stretch often damages the TMJ disk, joint capsule, and supporting ligaments, thus further deranging their natural functional position in the jaw joint. This pattern of jaw-joint injury from car accidents is commonly referred to as "TMJ-lash."

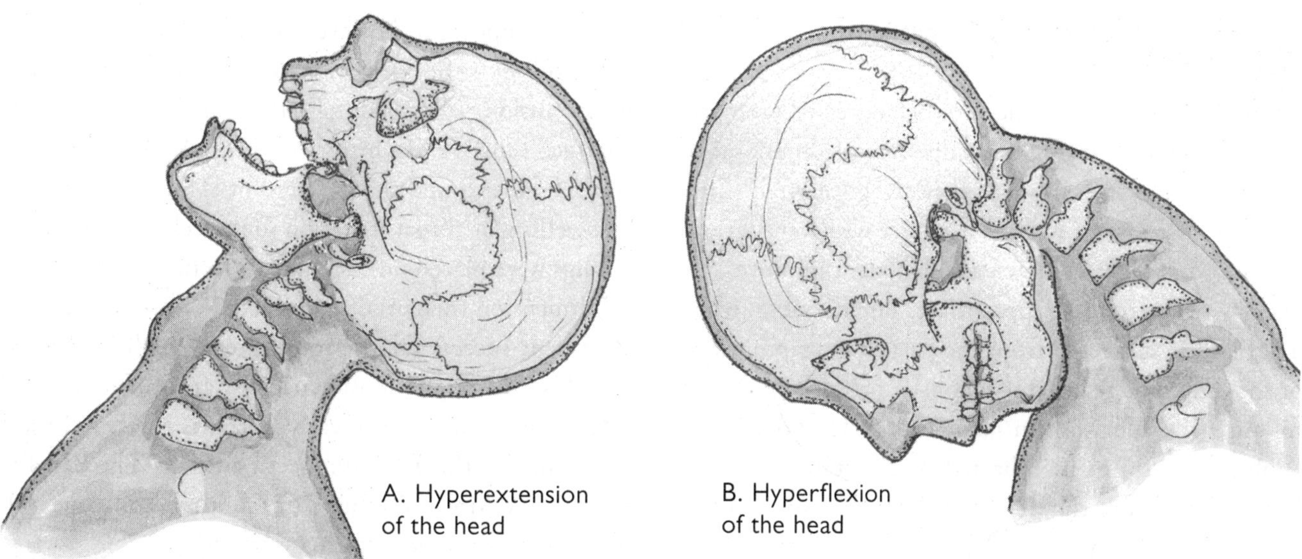

Figure 16.10. Hyperextension (A) and hyperflexion (B) injuries such as whiplash from rear-end collisions cause not only neck pain but also TMJ-lash injuries to the jaw.

Even Minor Accidents Can Cause Significant Injury

Although many people are aware of neck injuries (cervical sprains and strains) occurring from whiplash accidents, few are aware of the serious "TMJ-lash" injuries that can occur in the jaw joint. Even minor car accidents—that is, when the rear-ending car at fault is traveling at slow speed—can be significantly damaging. As Dr. Dennis Steigerwald, a San Diego TMD specialist, states in his book *Whiplash and Temporomandibular Disorders,* "Abnormal muscular forces generated during the collision are capable of producing injurious forces within the joint which are disproportionate to the force of the impact of the collision." Furthermore, the degree of injury received from whiplash accidents is often compounded in individuals with predisposing weaknesses, such as mild to major malocclusions, TMD, and chronically strained cervicothoracic (neck and shoulder) muscles. Finally, although lap belts and shoulder harnesses have significantly reduced ejection injuries (where victims are thrown through the windshield), as well as chest and facial traumas (through contact with the dashboard, steering wheel, etc.), cervical and thoracic spine injuries have increased. The reason is that the shoulder harness actually strengthens the cervical hyperflexion forces by acting as an anchor stabilizing the shoulders and trunk to the car seat, while the head continues its forward motion unrestrained, with even more velocity and force.[49]

Prompt and Comprehensive Treatment Essential

Acute structural injuries need to be addressed promptly and comprehensively. Spinal adjustments, craniosacral manipulation, and massage therapy given frequently over the first several weeks (or longer with very serious injuries), and tapering down as the patient improves, are entirely necessary and appropriate. Furthermore, when TMJ-lash is suspected from the patient's symptoms, he or she should be referred to a holistic orthopedic dentist for further evaluation. In many cases a temporary oral appliance or splint is indicated to facilitate soft-tissue healing, recapture the displaced TMJ disk (or disks, if both sides were affected), and restore normal occlusal and TM joint function.

8. Neighboring Foci and Ganglia

Any chronic infection in the head and neck can retard the growth and development of the teeth and jaws. Chronic sinus and ear infections secondary to food allergies are classic culprits. Furthermore—although they aren't as common in children as in adults—major dental focal infections also retard normal jawbone development. However, the worst offender in this category of truncated growth, and certainly the most common, is the tonsil focus.

The Relationship between Tonsil Foci and Dental Malocclusions

Hypertrophic (enlarged) tonsils and adenoids have been correlated in the research literature to the development of posterior crossbites (lower teeth wrongly positioned outside of the upper teeth in the back molars), crooked teeth and jaws, and other forms of malocclusion.[50] Additionally, these large and "chronically smoldering" (inflamed) masses of lymphatic tissue in the throat, in concert with the developing malocclusion, further reduce breathing capacity and contribute to snoring, sleep apnea, various forms of insomnia, and chronic fatigue.[51] Typically, children who suffer from chronic ENT (ear, nose, and throat) infections are often mouth-breathers. As discussed previously, mouth-breathing leads to malocclusions from a lowered tongue position that pushes on the front teeth, as well as from abnormal lip and cheek muscle movements.[52]

It is important, however, to also address the opposite etiology—the formation of a tonsil focus from a malocclusion. In a study of fifty children with grossly enlarged tonsils and a history of recurrent tonsillitis, Dr. A. C. Fonder found that 96 percent exhibited no tonsillar swelling or throat irritation four weeks after occlusal fillings were placed on back molars to increase the vertical dimension (height) of their teeth.[53] This outstanding treatment success for the tonsil area, which is unquestionably one of the most tenacious and difficult focal infections in the body, greatly warrants further clinical research. (See the upcoming section titled "The Benefits of Primary Molar Buildups in Children" on page 530 for more information on this subject.)

Neck and Head Ganglia: Storage Centers for Toxins

Another subject elaborated on in chapter 9 was the role of the autonomic ganglia. These clusters of nerve cell bodies distributed throughout the body direct autonomic nerve flow like "little brains" outside of the central nervous system, regulating function in various parts of the body. However, these ganglia also serve an important secondary purpose as storage centers for microbes, heavy metals, and other toxins—and nowhere is this storage function more apparent than in the head and neck ganglia.

Excess Toxins Diffuse Out into Surrounding Muscles and Tissues

The craniofacial (head/face) and cervical (neck) ganglia, in an effort to maintain normal function, store excess toxins generated in the region. These can include bacteria from chronic focal infections (dental, tonsil, ear, and sinus), heavy metals (mercury amalgam fillings, nickel- and aluminum-containing crowns, etc.), and toxic chemicals (makeup, petroleum-laden shampoos, and coloring agents, etc.). However, when these ganglia eventually become overloaded, the toxins tend to diffuse out into the neighboring tissue. This eventually triggers congestion and tension in the surrounding muscles and fascia, causing them to contract and spasm.

The Vagal Ganglia and TMD

Nowhere has this protective and sacrificial role been more apparent than in the vagal ganglia, located bilaterally (on either side of the cranium) just under the jugular foramina (two holes in the skull where the jugular veins exit), and anterior to the mastoid processes (the bones just behind the ears). Because toxic metals and microbial excretion products from the oral cavity as well as the digestive system often overload these ganglia, the facial and cervical muscles surrounding the vagal ganglia can become quite congested with toxins over time. These toxic and contracted muscles and fascia then exert a subtly disturbing pulling and pressure on the jaw joint, which greatly contributes to chronic jaw joint tension, pain, and dysfunction.

Dr. Klinghardt and Dr. Williams have found that when these vagal ganglia test positive energetically and are treated with neural therapy, the surrounding neck and jaw muscle tension can be so greatly reduced that the patient's chronic TMJ pain significantly subsides. After witnessing this phenomenon on numerous occasions, they coined this effect "false TMD syndrome." In this syndrome, the TMJ dysfunction is not primary but secondary to the congested and strained muscles pulling on the joint structures from the overloaded neighboring vagal ganglia. Due to this experience, Klinghardt and Williams teach holistic dentists to include assessment of the vagal ganglia in every TMD diagnostic workup. They also teach that it is essential for the holistic dentist to be aware that simply treating the vagal ganglia will result in only temporary relief if the actual causes underlying the congestion of the ganglia are not simultaneously addressed. These include any toxins axonally transported into the ganglia from the mouth, including mercury from amalgam fillings and bacteria from dental foci, as well as toxins from the gut, such as by-products of maldigestion from undiagnosed food allergies, the ingestion of refined and preservative-laden foods, and bacteria and yeast from chronic intestinal dysbiosis.

Other Ganglia Contributing to TMD

Other commonly overloaded and toxic craniofacial and cervical ganglia include the sphenopalatine (receives toxins from the nasal cavity, sinuses, upper teeth, and tonsils), the otic/gasserian (receives toxins from the teeth and salivary glands), and the superior cervical (receives toxins from the tonsils and teeth). Cutting-edge and knowledgeable holistic TMD (or orthopedic) dentists always make sure that their patients' mouths are free of foci and heavy metals, and that these neighboring congested ganglia are cleared (using laser therapy, needles, auriculotherapy, etc.), before fashioning a therapeutic oral appliance or finally equilibrating their patients' occlusions.

As many readers may have personally identified with while reading this section, most malocclusions and TMJ dysfunction are multifactorial and arise from a combination of several predisposing factors. Furthermore, other factors not described can also play a contributing role, such as birth trauma (especially if forceps were used), size differences between the parents, and significant inherited tendencies such as one or both parents having major malocclusions or other significant pathology.[54] Additionally, although there is no specific research in this area, vaccinations likely have a significant adverse effect on the normal growth and development of the teeth and jaws, especially since modern children receive as many as *thirty-six* vaccines before even entering first grade. Thankfully, much of this early damage done in infancy and childhood—and even genetically—can be greatly mitigated through proper diet, nutritional supplementation, drainage and detoxification, homeopathy, and holistic TMD (orthopedic) dentistry.

SYMPTOMS

Because jaw joint and related malocclusion symptoms can be so variable, temporomandibular dysfunction (TMD) has been labeled "The Great Imposter" because of the way it often mimics other disorders.[55] Additionally, because maloccluded teeth and TMJ dysfunction can affect every other system in the body, the more distal and remote symptoms are often not recognized by practitioners as being dentally related. Thus, patients often waste valuable time and money on various tests and specialists before receiving a correct diagnosis and effective treatment. To understand how dental malocclusions and TMD syndrome could cause such diverse symptoms throughout the body, a basic understanding of the neurological factors is essential.

Neurological Factors: The Trigeminal, or Fifth Cranial, Nerve

Although other nerves innervate the teeth and TMJ, the primary nerve that controls function in this region is the trigeminal. This nerve, the largest of the twelve cranial nerves, is often referred to as the "trigeminal nervous system" because of its vast anatomy and extensive connections in the body.[56] The trigeminal nerve, also referred to as the fifth cranial nerve, receives sensory information from the teeth, mouth, nasal cavity, face, and scalp. It also has a motor division that controls function in the muscles of mastication (TMJ muscles).[57] Additionally, the trigeminal system can affect the rest of the body through its connection with nerve tracks that traverse the entire spinal cord (the substantia gelatinosa, the tract of Lissauer, and the spinothalamic tract).

What is rarely taught in neurology in medical schools, or even in the holistic medical school curricula taught in chiropractic and naturopathic colleges, is that the trigeminal nervous system is not only richly endowed with these general sensory and motor nerves—the *somesthetic* nerves—but also densely innervated with *sympathetic* nerves of the autonomic nervous system.[58] This important point can be illustrated by the fact that the nerves from these two systems respond differently to pain.

Somesthetic vs. Sympathetic Nerve Pain

Pain experienced through the somesthetic nerves is generally sharp and discrete—that is, easily localized. But pain felt through the sympathetic nerves is of a dull and diffuse nature, and therefore not easily localized. Furthermore, the sympathetic nerves are primarily responsible for referred pain of a dull, burning, or cramping nature, through stimulation of *wide dynamic range* (WDR) nerve cells that can affect several levels in the spinal cord simultaneously.[59] Therefore, an infection in a tooth or TMJ pain can result in the classic localized and sharp pains indicative of a toothache through the sensory somesthetic trigeminal nerves, as well as dull and achy referred sympathetic nerve pain to the neck and shoulder muscles, or elsewhere in the body. In the latter case, it is understandable why a chronic dental focus, TMD, or a malocclusion can trigger throughout the body subtle and nonspecific symptoms that are rarely diagnosed as arising from the mouth or jaw.

Additionally, sympathetically mediated pain has a strong emotional effect, due to the direct connection between these phylogenetically oldest autonomic nerves and the "emotional brain," or limbic system (primarily the amygdala, hippocampus, and cerebral cortex), which mediates emotional expression and experience.[60] Thus, a new ill-fitting filling or crown can engender emotional disturbance ranging from a sense of simply "feeling off" to more serious feelings of chronic anxiety or irritability, if this acute dental malocclusion is not remedied in a timely manner.

Research Study: Induced Malocclusions Cause Autonomic Failure

In an animal laboratory study performed in Japan, the vast influence of the trigeminal nerves was particularly shown to be dramatic. Dogs that had their teeth maloccluded on one side of their mouths (ground down 3 millimeters) soon exhibited weight loss, postural imbalances, and jaw deviations (the mandible shifting to the right side, where the teeth had been ground down). Furthermore, symptoms of autonomic failure included hair loss and loss of luster, salivation, lacrimation (tearing), resting tremors, and muscle weakness. These signs and symptoms were clearly a direct result of the connection between the inflamed trigeminal nerves from the maloccluded teeth and misaligned jaw and the areas of the brain that the trigeminal nerves innervate: the striatum and substantia nigra, which affect muscle strength and proprioception, and the amygdala, which is a primary central nervous system regulator of autonomic function.[61]*

proprioception: Proprioception is the felt sense of one's posture and position in space, sensed by the nerves in the joints and muscle tendons and interpreted and regulated by structures in the brain (cerebellum, substantia nigra, etc.).

Thus, because the trigeminal nerve directly connects to every part of the brain (the reticular system, cerebellum, thalamus, hypothalamus, limbic system, and cerebral cortex), as well as with nerve tracts that traverse the entire spinal cord, it is understandable why the effects of teeth and jaw problems can be so extensive and widespread. Furthermore, because the trigeminal nerve carries somesthetic (general sensory and motor) as well as sympathetic nerves, even a minor malocclusion or TMD can have a chronically disturbing effect anywhere in the body and cause a wide array of diverse symptoms.[62]

Common Head, Neck, and Face Symptoms

Lawrence Funt, D.D.S., and Bruce Kinnie, D.D.S., two TMD specialists, have charted a multitude of symptoms in the head, neck, and face based on their years of experience in treating thousands of patients with TMJ dysfunction. These include eye symptoms—pain and/or pressure, blurring of vision, photophobia (light sensitivity), excess lacrimation (watering of the eyes) and bloodshot eyes; head pain and dysfunction (migraine, tension or cluster headaches, scalp sensitivity, jaw pain, tension and clicking/cracking, and sinus pain and pressure); ear-related problems—ringing, diminished hearing, frequent ear infections, stuffy or itchy ears, balance problems and vertigo; and neck and shoulder symptoms—reduced range of motion, stiffness and pain, and arm/finger tingling or numbness.[63]

Respiratory and Circulatory Symptoms

Respiratory and breathing problems secondary to a compromised airway are also a major symptom of a lack of adequate development in the teeth and jaws. Dr. David Page, an orthopedic/TMD dentist, comments on the essential role the mouth and TMJ play in healthy breathing and sleep functions:

> Teeth act like pillars to keep upper and lower jaws apart. Premature tooth loss can cause jaws to collapse.[64] If jaws collapse, tongue and airway space is lost. A tongue can become a deadly choker. The jaws and tongue can drip into the throat and block the airway when sleeping on the back. Snoring may signal a dangerously blocked airway.

In fact, studies have shown that there is a direct relationship between small upper airway size and asthma, respiratory disorders, obstructive sleep disorders, hypertension, and heart disease.[65]

Back Pain, Scoliosis, Bed-Wetting, and Hormonal Dysfunction

Musculoskeletal pain and tension—from the neck to the low back to the legs and feet—have also been greatly alleviated through addressing causal occlusive and jaw joint dysfunction.[66] Various forms of scoliosis—curvature of the spine—have also been dramatically reduced with the appropriate treatment (appliances or molar buildups) for patients' malocclusions.[67] Additionally, TMD and malocclusions have generated bladder irritation (bed-wetting, urgency, urinary frequency) as well

*Although the emotional effects of this experimentally induced malocclusion on these caged dogs were not discussed here, based on the symptoms reported they were certainly not good. Once again, like the rabbits used by Dr. Weston Price described in chapter 8, the doubly compounding tragedy about animal experimentation is that not only did these beagles experience pain and suffering, but that their great contribution to dental science has not been widely disseminated or even recognized by the great majority of dentists and orthodontists.

as menstrual dysfunction (premenstrual tension and depression, water retention, menstrual cramps).[68] Other reported endocrine dysfunctions linked—at least in part—to chronic jaw muscle tension associated with TMD and malocclusions are hyper- and hypothyroidism, hyperparathyroidism and osteomalacia (softening of the bones), adrenal insufficiency, diabetes mellitus, and testosterone deficiency.[69]

Chronic Digestive Dysfunction

Because maloccluded teeth as well as TMD greatly reduce chewing efficiency, these syndromes typically cause mild to major forms of maldigestion. This chronic dysfunction pattern initially arises in the mouth itself, where chewing generates the production of saliva that contains amylase, an enzyme for splitting carbohydrates. When this first process of carbohydrate digestion is impaired due to the reduced chewing efficiency from a malocclusion or TMD, as clinical nutritionist Elizabeth Lipski asserts, "the stomach receives chunks of food instead of mush."[70] When this occurs, the stomach and intestine must then bear the burden of producing extra enzymes to make up for the oral deficit of amylase, which can be another factor—along with psychological stress and toxic foods—in the depletion and eventual exhaustion of these digestive organs. Thus, chronic fatigue, irritable bowel syndrome, chronic constipation or diarrhea, and all the other myriad symptoms secondary to chronic maldigestion can be linked—in whole or in part—to compromised occlusal and TMJ functioning.

Disturbed Immune System Functioning

Stimulation of the parotid glands through chewing not only produces amylase enzymes but also releases hormones that stimulate the thymus to produce T-cells.[71] Thus, good TMJ function and balanced occlusions also help promote a healthy and protective immune system, and dysfunction in this oral area can be a detriment.

Careful Diagnosis Essential

It is important to be aware that such a wide range of symptoms can be indicative of mild to major TMD and malocclusions. However, because these diverse symptoms can so greatly mimic other disorders (e.g., candida overgrowth, food allergies, or amalgam toxicity), positive physical examination findings are essential in the accurate diagnosis of a truly significant malocclusion of the teeth and/or TMJ dysfunction.

DIAGNOSIS

Although a definitive diagnosis of TMD and dental malocclusions can only be made by a specially trained TMD dentist (and a few holistic practitioners), fortunately many of the positive signs can be assessed at home before making an appointment.

Patient Assessment of Possible Malocclusion/TMJ Dysfunction

Dr. A. C. Fonder (1916–2003), often referred to as the father of holistic orthopedic dentistry, clearly elucidated the deleterious effects of malocclusions and TMD in what may be referred to not as the "ABCs" but the "SBCs"—that is, difficulty in *swallowing, breathing,* and *chewing.*[72] For example, individuals with malocclusions often have difficulty swallowing pills, problems breathing including sleep apnea and insomnia, and impaired chewing ability that limits the nutrients they can absorb and assimilate from food. Besides these three major areas of dysfunction, Dr. Fonder and other holistic dentists became aware of other signs and symptoms typical of malocclusions and TMD:

1. Suffering from any of the previously described symptoms in the "Symptoms" section, especially just after dental work or injury to the jaw, can be a strong indicator.
2. A "noisy jaw"—that is, popping, clicking, cracking, or crepitus (grating sound) upon opening or closing the jaw—is also a positive indicator. This sign, however, should not be too heavily weighted, since the vast majority of individuals (estimated to be from 60 to 80 percent of the population) have some kind of noise upon jaw opening or closing.[73] Thus, almost all of us have some kind of minor malocclusion, but we adapt to it. However, excessive and loud jaw joint noises should be counted as a strong indicator.
3. Pain upon opening or closing the jaw is a major indicator of TMD. (Pain upon opening usually indicates an anteriorly displaced—or prolapsed forward—TMJ disk.)

4. A reduced TMJ range of motion is another positive indicator. According to Dr. Janet Travell, originator of trigger point therapy, as well as the renowned orthopedist Stanley Hoppenfeld, an individual should be able to comfortably insert the knuckles of three fingers between the upper and lower teeth.[74] However, many TMD dentists feel that the ability to place the knuckles of two fingers comfortably in the mouth is a sufficiently healthy jaw-opening range of motion. The inability to place three (or even two) knuckles in the mouth without pain or tension is a positive indicator of TMD.
5. When looking in the mirror, the observance of the jaw noticeably deviating to one side, or both sides in an "S-shaped" opening or closing pattern, is another positive indicator of TMJ dysfunction.
6. A history of ever having the jaw locked in a "stuck open" or "stuck closed" position is a pathognomonic (extremely characteristic; a diagnostic symptom) of TMD.
7. Not being able to find your bite when closing the teeth together is a near-pathognomonic symptom of TMD and malocclusion. This sign is most characteristic of a functional versus a dysfunctional occlusion—that is, whether you are comfortable with the way your teeth fit together.

Practitioner Assessment of Malocclusion/ TMJ Dysfunction

In order to refer a patient to a TMD dental specialist, practitioners should be reasonably familiar with normal versus abnormal occlusions and the cardinal signs and symptoms of TMJ dysfunction.

Holistic Dental Seminars

Attending holistic dental meetings is an excellent way to become not only acquainted with TMD (orthopedic) dentists and how they diagnose and treat occlusal and jaw joint dysfunction, but also how dentists assess and treat mercury amalgam toxicity and dental focal infections. The three top associations in the United States that specialize in all aspects of holistic dentistry are the International Academy of Biological Dentistry and Medicine (IABDM), the International Academy of Oral Medicine and Toxicology (IAOMT), and the Holistic Dental Association (HDA). There are five major dental associations that specifically address the treatment of malocclusions and TMD: the American Academy of Craniofacial Pain (AACP), the American Academy of Gnathologic Orthopedics (AAGO), the American Association for Functional Orthodontics (AAFO), the International Association of Facial Growth Guidance (IAFGG), and the Facial Development/OrthoSmile organization. Developing a close relationship with a TMD dentist in your area is also essential in order to refer patients for appropriate diagnosis and treatment.

▸ IABDM: (281) 651-1745 or www.iabdm.org
IAOMT: (863) 420-6373 or www.iaomt.org
HDA: (305) 356-7338 or www.holisticdental.org
AACP: (800) 322-8651 or www.aacfp.org
AAGO: (800) 510-AAGO or www.aago.com
AAFO: (800) 441-3850 or www.aafo.org
IAFGG: (888) 404-3223 or www.orthotropics.com
OrthoSmile Inc.: (518) 943-7703 or www.facialdevelopment.com

Physical Examination

The following signs during physical examination should be noted as indicators of possible or probable TMJ/ malocclusion issues in your patients.

1. If any of the symptoms and signs listed under the preceding seven patient self-assessments is significant, they should be charted. It is also helpful to incorporate these signs into your physical exam (e.g., "Can you find your bite?" "Swallow—easy or difficult?" "Open wide, and now close," etc.). Note any trembling or other discomfiture of the jaw muscles if the patient cannot find his or her bite, or is in obvious distress with a bite position that appears strained or abnormal.
2. Upon visual inspection, it is helpful to record whether the patient has an obvious Class I (crowded, rotated teeth), Class II (overbite: a Class II type or division 1 is an overjet of the maxillary teeth, and a Class II type or division 2 is when the mandibular teeth are trapped by the maxillary teeth tipping backward), or Class III (underbite) malocclusion.* Also note any facial asymmetry,

*These classifications of malocclusions can facilitate good communication between dentists and doctors and can be learned at holistic dental seminars.

indicating abnormal growth and development of the craniofacial bones.

3. During this inspection of the patient's teeth, notice other signs contributing to a possible malocclusion—missing teeth, exceptional wear and erosion of the teeth, and bridges, crowns, or dentures that don't appear or "feel" functional or properly balanced.
4. Placing the tips of your little fingers within the patient's external ear canal with gentle pressure forward while the patient slowly opens and closes his or her mouth can allow you to palpate uneven opening and closure of the jaw. A traumatic closure with probable anterior displacement of the TMJ disk can also be ascertained, through feeling the too-hard (and often one-sided) pressure of the patient's mandibular condyle hitting your finger pads.
5. A hypertonic (+++) jaw jerk response is indicative of trigeminal nerve dysfunction in the brain centers (upper motor neurons); and an absent (0) or diminished (+) reflex may indicate some level of dysfunction along the course of the trigeminal nerve peripherally (or nervousness on the part of the patient).*
6. If the patient has a past or present history of wearing a "night guard" or bridgework across the upper central incisors, this oral splint or bridge can lock up and therefore distort the maxillary craniosacral micromotion or rhythm. Night guards and other hard plastic upper appliances (not split down the middle) can aggravate existing malocclusions and TMJ dysfunction, after the typical brief initial honeymoon period—that is, the first few weeks of temporary relief from the increased vertical dimension—after they have been placed in the mouth. (See "Craniosacral Movement: Locking Up the Maxillary Suture" in the "Orthopedic Treatment" section.)
7. Energetic testing is a well-recognized way to determine malocclusions and TMJ dysfunction. In Applied Kinesiology, weak cervical muscles (e.g., neck flexors) can be positive indicators of tooth and jaw disturbances. The weakening of a strong indicator muscle when the patient clenches the teeth together (or retrudes, protrudes, laterally deviates, or opens the jaw wide) is also a positive indicator of a minor to major problem in the occlusion and TMJ.[75] In the Matrix Reflex Testing (MRT) method, these same tests can be performed using the arm length measurement as an indicator.

*To perform the jaw jerk test, have the patient relax his or her mouth, so that it is partially open, and place two fingers side by side over the chin. Then tap your fingers with the reflex hammer (Hoppenfeld). The Chvostek reflex over the masseter muscles, although classically indicative of a calcium (or magnesium) deficiency through the seventh (facial) cranial nerve, can also signal TMJ dysfunction.

Referral to an Orthopedic (TMD) Dentist

If enough of these physical exam findings are positive, and if the patient has a history indicative of a malocclusion or jaw joint dysfunction, he or she should be referred to a TMD (orthopedic) dental specialist. However, as described previously, only patients with major malocclusions or TMD should be referred immediately. Those with minor or moderate dysfunction should be observed carefully during treatment. As mercury amalgam fillings are removed; dental, tonsil, sinus and other focal infections are cleared; and constitutional homeopathy, drainage, cell (tissue) salts, and nutritional supplements are prescribed, these earlier positive examination findings are greatly reduced, and sometimes even completely remedied, over time.

Furthermore, treatment of a malocclusion and TMJ dysfunction—even by the most ethical holistic TMD dentist—is almost always a lengthy and costly process. Therefore, it should be reserved for only those patients who truly need it and *will not* be able to benefit from other treatments until their jaw and bite are stable. Others—the great majority of individuals with minor malocclusions—can often be treated through addressing the other contributing disturbances outlined in this book, until a final equilibration of the teeth (and therefore jaw) by a holistic dentist is appropriately made near the end of patients' course of treatment. Patients who still have moderate, or significant, malocclusions at the end of treatment can benefit by the fact that their bite can be more reliably measured—since all the contributing factors (dental foci, vagal ganglia toxicity, mercury fillings, food allergies, etc.) have been addressed and treated—and now a more curative oral appliance (and possibly braces) can be made to finally rebalance their occlusion and jaw joints.

ORTHOPEDIC VS. ORTHODONTIC DENTAL THERAPY

There are two primary dental treatments for malocclusions and TMJ dysfunction: *orthopedic* and *orthodontic.*

Many holistic TMD dentists use the term *orthopedic* to describe the various treatments that they offer, in contrast with the practices utilized by *orthodontic* dentists. *Orthopedic* refers to the treatment of disorders affecting *all* the bones and joints in the body, whereas *orthodontic* more narrowly refers to simply "serving to correct irregularities of the teeth and jaws."[76] The differences in therapy between a holistically oriented orthopedic dentist and a conventionally trained orthodontist are great and can have a profound impact on an individual's structural growth, nutritional assimilation, immune system functioning, and central nervous system development (mentally, emotionally, and even as it relates to IQ).

ORTHODONTIC TREATMENT

The typical orthodontist straightens teeth with little regard to the effect on the rest of the patient's body. The most odious example of this attitude began in the early twentieth century and remains the standard of care in the orthodontic profession: the extraction of the four first bicuspid (premolar) teeth followed by the placement of braces and then retainers (see figure 16.11).[77*]

Extraction of the Bicuspids

This sacrifice of these four healthy teeth is done to alleviate the common problem of dental crowding—that is, too many teeth in too small a space due to jawbone underdevelopment (as a result of the lack of breast-feeding, poor nutrition, etc.). Unfortunately, this practice often causes rather disturbing negative consequences to a patient's health as well as appearance. Two notable orthopedic dentists, John Witzig and Terrance Spahl, describe the devastating results of this orthodontic practice:

> The therapeutic mechanics that follow bicuspid extractions often leave the patients with dished-in faces, flattened smiles, unstable occlusions, and retracted maxillary anteriors [front teeth point backward], all of which cause the mandibular arc of closure to be retruded [lower jaw pushed backward], often to the point of causing severe TMJ problems.[78]

*Sometimes orthodontists pull the second bicuspids instead.

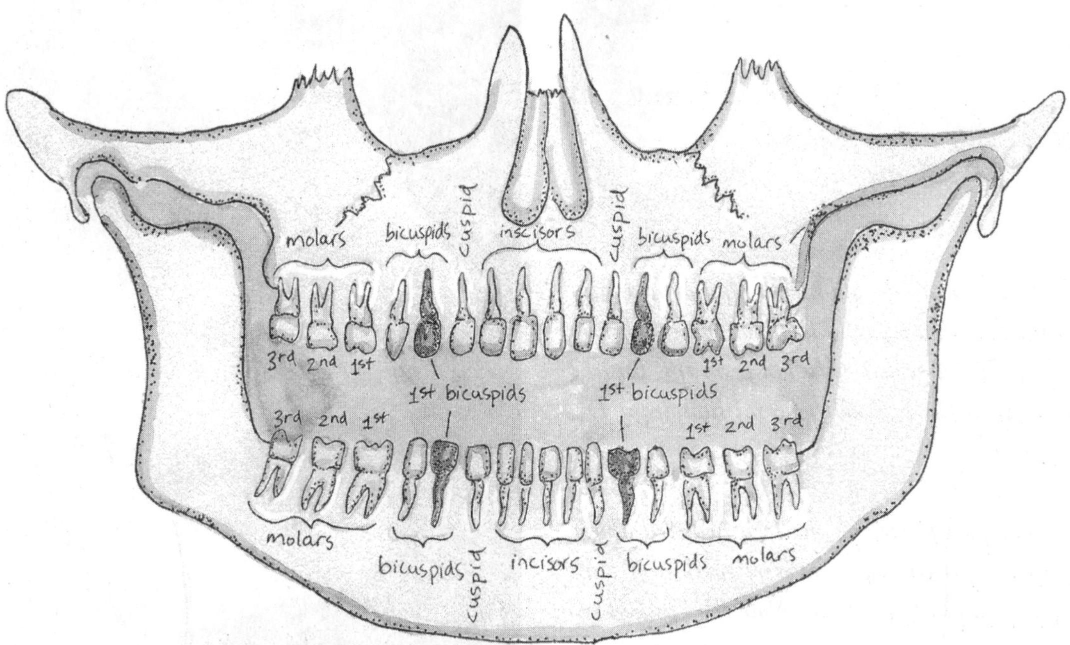

Figure 16.11. The four first bicuspid teeth (in gray) that are typically extracted before braces are just behind the cuspids, or canines (eye teeth), and in front of the second bicuspids. Next come the three molar teeth (the third molars are the "wisdom teeth").

Bicuspid Extraction Generates Chronic TMD and Facial Deformity

These unfortunate aftereffects of orthodontic treatment are graphically illustrated by Witzig and Spahl in *The Clinical Management of Basic Maxillofacial Orthopedic Appliances,* which has stood the test of time as one of the bibles of orthopedic dentistry. For example, the occlusion of a sixteen-year-old girl in figure 16.12 after a four-bicuspid extraction and braces looks perfectly normal from the frontal view. However, from the side in figure 16.13, the retruded (pushed back) position of the maxilla (upper jaw), and even more severe retrusion in the mandible (lower jaw), is apparent. This retrusion of the lower face is not only unattractive but also jams the mandibular condyle (jawbone) into the temporal bone fossa, resulting in some level of chronic TMJ dysfunction throughout one's life.

The Dramatic Identical Twin Study

An example of the negative consequences of orthodontia was even more vividly demonstrated in a case of identical twins who had (identical) Class I malocclusions, or overcrowding of their teeth. One twin, "OE," (standing for "orthodontic extraction") was treated in the conventional orthodontic way, with extraction of her four bicuspid teeth followed by braces.* The other twin, "OF," ("orthodontic functional") was treated orthopedically with no extractions and fitted for a functional appliance (Fraenkel) to expand and develop her arches (teeth and jawbones).[79] Treatment lasted two and a half years for both twins. As can be seen in the before (figure 16.14) and after (figure 16.15) photos, the results were dramatic.

*This twin had already had her deciduous (baby teeth) canines extracted by her family dentist in anticipation of the customary later removal of her first bicuspids and fitting for braces, before presenting to Dr. Eirew, the orthopedic dentist who conducted the study. Thus, Dr. Eirew did not arbitrarily decide which twin should receive (what he considered as a holistic dentist) the more beneficial treatment.

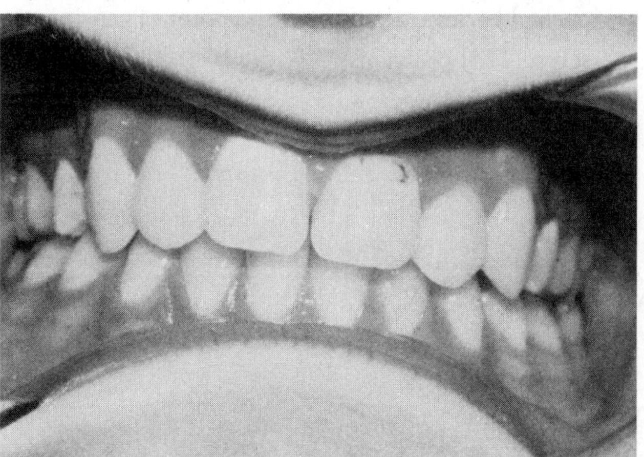

Figure 16.12. This sixteen-year-old's teeth after orthodontia (extraction of the four first bicuspid teeth followed by braces and retainers) appear in perfect occlusion from this limited frontal view. (Reprinted here with permission from Dr. Terrance J. Spahl.)

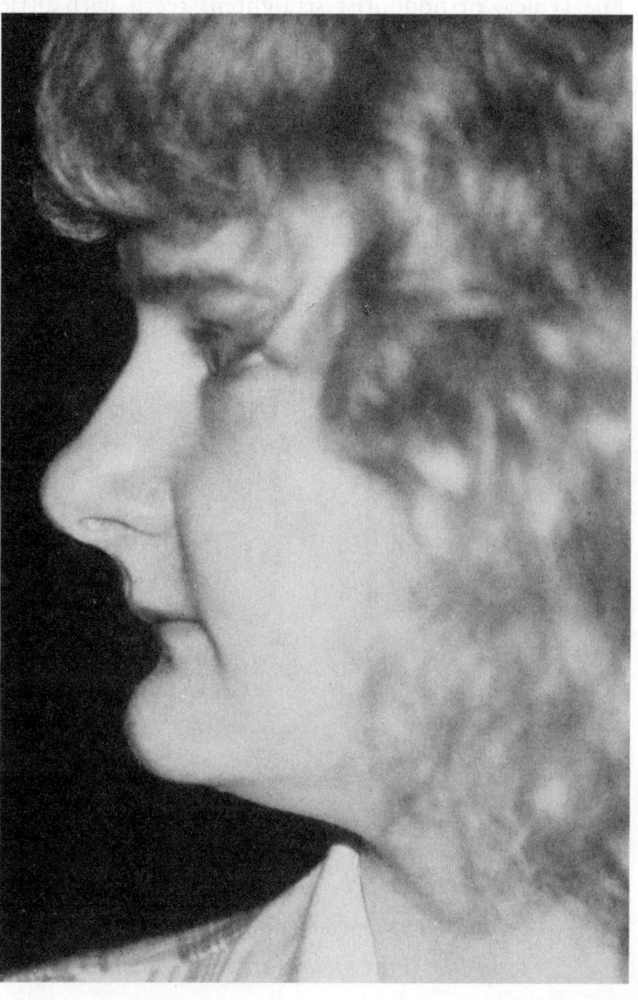

Figure 16.13. The profile view of the teen depicted above in figure 16.12 reveals the severe over-retraction of both the maxillary and mandibular teeth. Note the "dished-in" appearance of the lower third of her face, the retruded (pushed back) maxilla (upper jaw), and the severely retruded mandible (lower jaw). (Reprinted with permission from Dr. Terrance J. Spahl.)

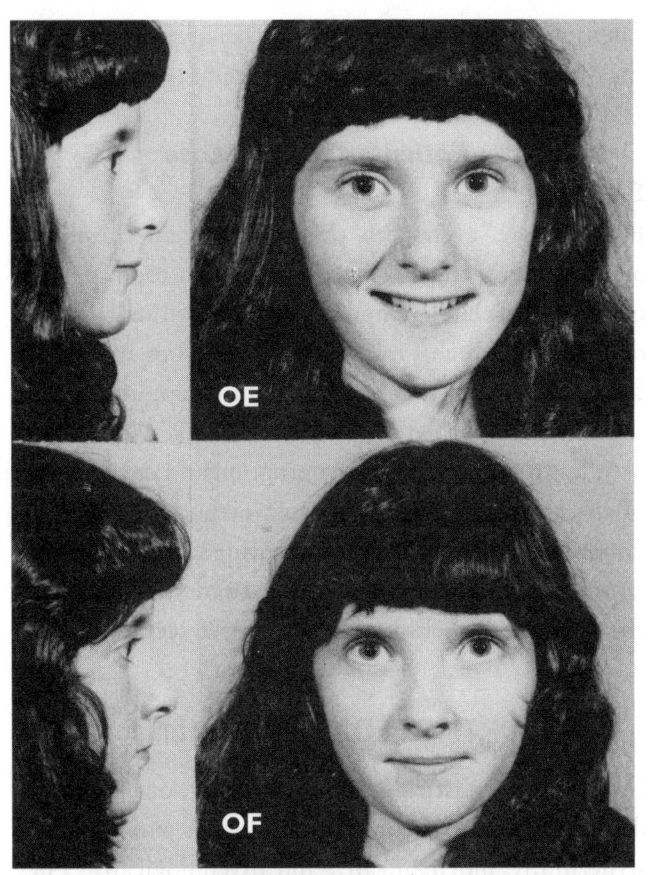

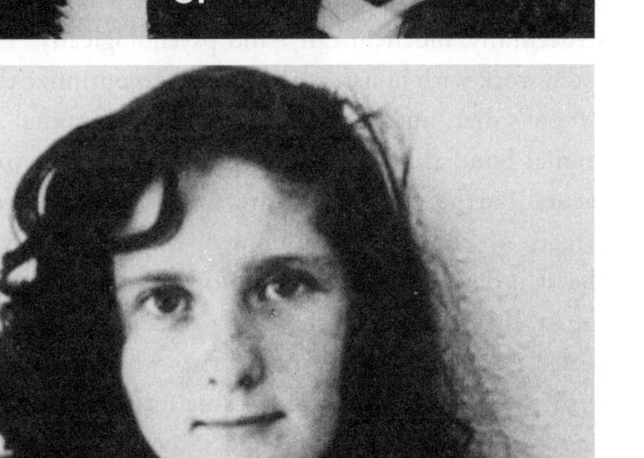

Figure 16.14. Before treatment: the appearance of identical twins prior to orthodontic ("OE") and orthopedic ("OF") treatments. (Reprinted here with permission from Dr. Terrance J. Spahl.)

Figure 16.15. After treatment: post-treatment comparison of the faces of twin "OE" (orthodontic extraction and braces) and twin "OF" (orthopedic functional appliance). Dr. Spahl commented on these before and after pictures that "res ipsa loquitur" *("the thing speaks for itself"). (Reprinted with permission from Dr. Terrance J. Spahl.)*

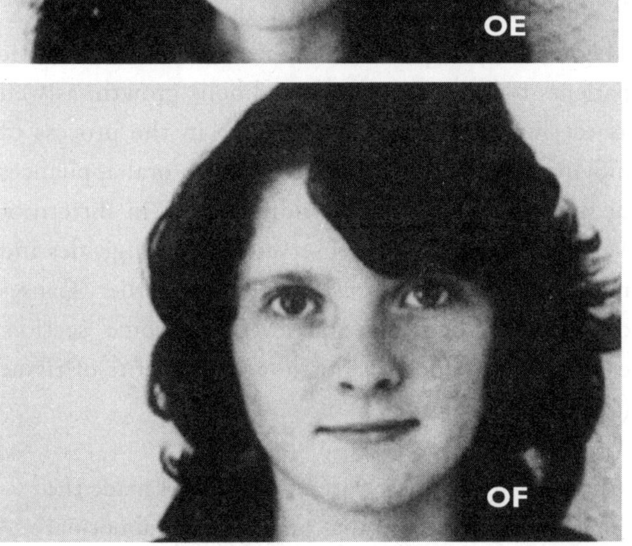

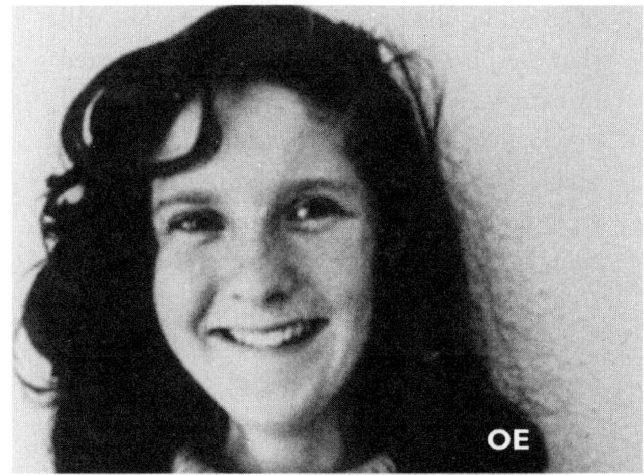

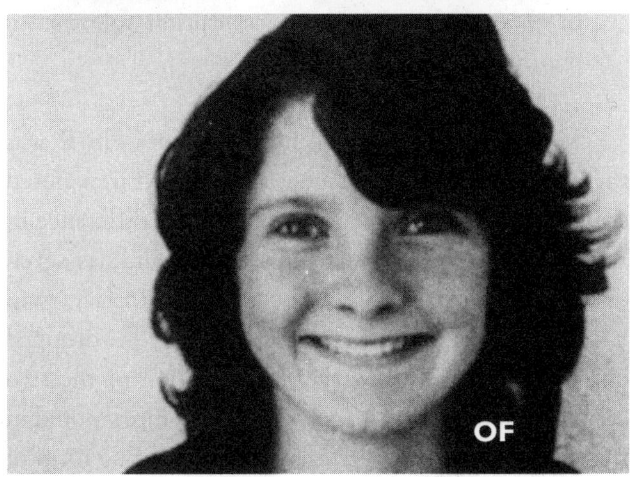

Dr. H. L. Eirew, who published this clinical study in the *International Journal of Orthodontics,* made the following observations about the orthopedic treatment of twin "F" ("OF") and the resulting effects:

> Twin F, treated by the Fraenkel appliance, shows a pleasing round arch form. The upper dental arch was widened by 4–5 mm between the first premolars [bicuspids] and by 2 mm between the first molars. Lower arch development was similar. . . . Facially the girl is good looking, with a rounded facial form matching her attractive rounded dental arch. She is happy with the result of her orthodontic treatment and considers the effort to wear the appliance well rewarded.[80]

In regard to twin "E" ("OE"), who received the classical orthodontic treatment of extractions and braces, Dr. Eirew noted the following:

> Twin E, treated by extractions, shows some relief of crowding and of incisal irregularity. She still [however] has a tapering arch form accentuated by narrow arch width. There has been no lateral development. Residual extraction spaces are still visible after more than three years. The cheek teeth have slipped out of correct occlusion and contact on both sides. The deep bite persists. Dental arch appearance is poor. . . .
>
> Her facial deterioration has been *quite disastrous.* In the years from [age] 12 to 14 she has become a "little old woman" in relation to her sister. The changes shown resemble those seen in the elderly when bone resorption follows multiple tooth loss.[81]

Most distressing of all, however, for twin E was the emotional effect orthodontia had. Dr. Eirew noted that she was "acutely aware of the marked difference in appearance between herself and her sister and has developed a considerable inferiority complex."[82] In fact, twin E was so distraught as the "ugly sister," that she dropped out of the study and further investigation of the two cases had to be discontinued.[83] Sadly, Dr. Eirew noted in the conclusion of his study that at this point no form of functional orthopedic appliance therapy could remedy the "skeletal and facial damage" done to twin E.[84]

Orthodontic Patients Typically Lose Eight Teeth

Furthermore, even with the extraction of these four bicuspid teeth, there is often not enough room posteriorly to allow the development of the third molars (wisdom teeth), which typically begin to erupt in the late teens and twenties.[85] This problem is amplified when the teeth are pushed backward by braces, which leaves even less room for the proper eruption and development of the third molars. Thus, most orthodontic patients also lose their wisdom teeth, resulting in the net loss of *eight* teeth, leaving them with only twenty-four teeth for chewing out of their original thirty-two teeth.

ORTHOPEDIC TREATMENT

In contrast, holistically oriented TMD, or *orthopedic,* dentists take into account their patient's whole body—structurally, biochemically, and psychologically. They often work with holistic practitioners to optimize their patient's diet, nutritional supplements, and spinal and cranial bone alignment before and after dental treatments. Furthermore, many are aware of the dramatic effects of constitutional homeopathy, especially in the still-developing infant, child, or adolescent, and use it themselves or refer their patients to homeopaths. Additionally, holistic dentists who are familiar with the dramatic effects of tissue (cell) salts readily prescribe these well-assimilated mineral supplements (Calcarea phosphoricum 6X, Calcarea fluoricum 6X, Magnesium phosphoricum 6X, etc.) to their pediatric patients to encourage tooth and bone growth, as well as to their adult patients who are in the process of moving teeth and facial bones through oral appliances or splints. Judy Hoy, the wildlife expert in Bitterroot Valley, Montana, whose observations on fungicides and malocclusions were discussed under the earlier "Causes of Dental Malocclusion and TMD Syndrome" section, confirms the superlative orthopedic benefits of tissue (cell) salts:

> In caring for these pathetic animals, I made the amazing discovery that prognathism [abnormal

protrusion of the jaws—underbites or overbites] exhibited at birth could be remedied in many individuals by administering homeopathic cell salts orally, provided that the jaws were not twisted or malformed. . . . Giving the cell salts resulted in the upper face developing to a normal size and length so the maxilla and mandible matched in a perfect bite.[86]

Assisting Mother Nature with Functional Appliances

In another striking contrast to their orthodontic colleagues, orthopedic dentists try hard to avoid pulling healthy teeth. If the patient's dentition is crowded due to underdeveloped and narrow dental arches (the maxillary and mandibular bones), they often opt to assist Mother Nature through the use of expansion appliances. These aptly named *functional appliances,* also known as *splints* or *orthotics* or *biteplates* (but *not* night guards),* encourage the growth of underdeveloped dental arches both anteriorly and posteriorly (i.e., forward and backward) as well as expansion laterally (i.e., sideways). These appliances are numerous, but some of the most commonly used are the Bionator, Schwartz-Sagittal, ALF, and Crozat. Over time, these orthopedic functional appliances gently move and expand both the upper and lower arches, allowing the bones to grow according to—or at least more closely approximating—their original genetic blueprint of development.

The making of and the subsequent adjusting of these functional appliances requires great skill. Holistic orthopedic dentists learn the complicated art and physics required to treat malocclusions and TMD in postgraduate courses. Besides initial panoramic X-rays (panellipse, panorex, panograph, etc.) that allow the full picture of the teeth and the bilateral joints to be seen clearly, tomography studies that show slices of the TMJ further facilitate accurate diagnosis and guide appropriate treatment.[87] Effective articulator instruments are also essential. These instruments, in which the plastic models of the patient's teeth are mounted, are necessary to diagnose the exact degree of malocclusion and TMJ dysfunction, and to determine the specific shape and dimensions of the needed functional appliance (or for final equilibration). Dr. A. C. Fonder was a master at treating with these functional appliances and found over many years of clinical experience that they accomplished the following:

> Functional appliances . . . allow balanced, functional distress-free tooth and "jaw" relationships to more correctly develop. TMJ remodeling, head bone adaptation, and facial form normalization can occur simultaneously during the repositioning of the mandible, the arch expansion, the aligning of the dental arches, and the eruption of teeth to physiologic vertical and a flattened plane of occlusion [that is, to their appropriate height and position in the mouth].[88]

▶ The AccuLiner instrument is lauded by many orthopedic dentists as the best articulator made. For more information call (800) 458-6627, e-mail info@acculiner.com, or visit the website at www.acculiner.com.

Reducing Time in Braces

If braces are required at some point to more completely straighten the teeth into a more harmonious occlusion, the time required to wear these braces can be greatly reduced with the prior use of functional appliances. In contrast to orthodontics that can require years of braces followed by rigid retainers to hold the (often disturbed) new bite in place, orthopedic dentists may need to utilize braces only short term—from several months to a single year, for example—after the functional appliance has already greatly reshaped the jawbones and repositioned misaligned teeth. This reduced time in braces has many benefits, because there are many health concerns associated with braces.

Braces Increase Exposure to Toxic Nickel and Chromium. First, braces are made up of stainless-steel wires that contain nickel and chromium, both of which, as described in chapter 3, are clearly carcinogenic.[89] Furthermore, there is a significant percentage of the population—14 percent of women and 6 percent of men—who are hypersensitive to nickel, in which one of the main symptomatic manifestations is depression.[90] Thus, it is not out of the question that braces in

*For information on the negative consequences of most mouth guards, see the upcoming "Craniosacral Movement: Locking Up the Maxillary Suture" section (page 532).

adolescents, who are already dealing with a tremendous number of hormonally induced mood changes, could contribute to suicidal ideations and/or attempts.[91] The longer-term use of oral appliances to restore more normal functioning, followed by, if necessary, the short-term use of braces, can greatly reduce this toxic metal insult. Due to this nickel toxicity, many orthopedic dentists use wires with a lowered nickel, or even nickel-free, content.* Some also prescribe nutrients to their patients during this necessary but somewhat stressful period of wearing braces. For example, supplementation with Black Poplar, Mountain Pine, or Juniper plant stem cell remedies at a gentle dose (e.g., 1–2 drops three times a week) while braces are being worn can greatly mitigate the short-term effects of nickel-bearing braces, as well as the other heavy metals that make up stainless steel (chromium, molybdenum, iron, etc.).

Braces Reduce Normal Cranial Motion. Braces also cause harm by reducing the normal cranial movement (or rhythm) in the maxillary suture when they are worn on the upper teeth. Locking up this maxillary joint can contribute to muscle pain and tension, headaches, and mood disturbances. However, the chainlike aspect of braces does not jam this suture quite as firmly as a rigid upper appliance (not split down the midline) or fixed bridges that span the upper front teeth (central incisors) do, and therefore patients can usually deal with this less-fixed biomechanical stress for short-term periods.†

Braces Can Potentially Induce Dental Focal Infections. The long-term use of braces has the potential to cause irreparable harm to teeth, such as pulp degeneration from the often extreme orthodontic pressures placed on the roots of the teeth.[92] Thus, lengthy and aggressively made adjustments to the wires used in braces can potentially result in later dental focal infections (see chapter 11) and the possible subsequent loss of teeth. In contrast, braces worn for shorter periods and placed by orthopedic dentists have a less deleterious impact on individual teeth. Furthermore, the initial use of a functional appliance that more favorably balances the occlusion and makes significant positive changes in the position of the teeth can reduce the need for extreme pressure from wires on the teeth.

Braces Can Cause Long-Term Gingivitis. Braces require a high level of oral cleanliness because chronic food impaction between the teeth—especially from stringy meats and fibrous foods—is common. In fact, long-term gum problems (gingivitis and periodontitis) and tooth decay can occur within a few months if careful dental hygiene is not performed assiduously.[93] Short-term use—as well as an emphasis on educating teens on the importance of oral hygiene—can obviate this additional adverse effect of braces.

Invisible Aligners: Good Substitute for Braces in Milder Malocclusions

Thankfully, an increasing number of orthopedic and orthodontic dentists are using the recently developed positioning-type appliances that can straighten teeth, similar to braces. With the initial help of functional appliances, these positioning appliances, or *aligners,* can be used later in place of braces. When patients have relatively mild malocclusions, such as an uncomplicated Class I, these clear aligner appliances are ideal. Because these aligners are relatively invisible, they are a much more pleasing alternative than the more unsightly metal braces for both teenage and adult patients.

▶ For more information about these aligners, contact Invisalign at www.invisalign.com or (800) INVISIBLE.

The Benefits of Functional Appliances

For the health of the teeth and jaws as well as the whole body, the most optimal treatment of malocclusions in the vast majority of cases in both pediatric and adult populations is through functional appliance therapy by a well-trained holistic or orthopedic dentist.

*Unfortunately, and quite strangely, wires with less nickel in them (noninium wire, nickel lite, menzanium, etc.), have not tested better than regular nickel-containing stainless-steel wires in my energetic testing experience. Furthermore, the "clear" wires have proved to be difficult to work with, and many dentists and orthodontists have stopped using them. Newer porcelain brackets, although they still require nickel-containing wires, do cut down on the toxic metal load considerably and have proven to be functional and easy to use. Additionally, for those who are not sensitive to titanium, wires made from this less disturbing metal are available.

†Many holistic practitioners caution that metal crossing the midline, such as in the case of braces or the use of metal glasses, can cause brain disturbance and "switching." I have not found this in itself to be significant, however, probably because people have become well adapted over time to metal glasses, zippers, the snap on their jeans, etc.

Enhancing Hormonal Functioning

Functional orthopedic appliances encourage not only the appropriate expansion and development of the craniofacial bones but also the organs they support. For example, the size of the cup-shaped sella turcica bone in which the pituitary snugly fits is also enlarged with the expansion of the palate, allowing for more appropriate release of essential hormones to the body. Both clinical practice and two documented research studies show that orthopedic expansion appliances have positive benefits on various premenstrual and menstrual disorders.[94]

Reducing Delinquency

As discussed in chapter 5, in the early twentieth century Dr. Weston Price was keenly aware of the negative effects nutritionally inadequate modern diets had on the brain as well as on body functioning. He posited that severe malocclusions often resulted in "mental backwardness, pre-delinquency and criminality."[95] In fact, in one study at a state penitentiary, Price was unable to find one inmate with normal facial development and in many he witnessed major dental malocclusions and severely truncated craniofacial bone growth. It is not coincidental that violence and the incidence of malocclusions have both skyrocketed since the early twentieth century. Correcting these dental deformities with expansion appliances and a nutrient-dense diet would certainly have a tremendous impact in our institutions housing juvenile delinquents.

Transforming Down Syndrome and Cranial Underdevelopment

Price noted in his book *Nutrition and Physical Degeneration* that a "striking" example of the relationship between cranial development and intelligence can be demonstrated in individuals with Down syndrome. He noted that in moderately to severely impaired individuals, the middle third of the face is markedly underdeveloped, resulting in a nose with a flat bridge, narrow nostrils, and a narrow and retruded (pushed back) upper dental arch (~ Class III malocclusion).[96] Price was aware of previous research studies that had correlated palatal abnormalities with lowered IQ. In 1891, Clouston had noted that although deformed palates occur in normal individuals, they are much more frequent in "psychopaths and the mentally defective." His research found that deformed palates were present in approximately 19 percent of normal individuals, 33 percent of those with mental disorders, 55 percent of criminals, and 61 percent of those with Down syndrome. Later, in 1904, Petersen validated Clouston's research, finding palatal deformities in 82 percent of the mentally impaired population, in 76 percent of epileptics, and in 80 percent of those with mental disorders.[97]

In one dramatic case of a sixteen-year-old with Down syndrome who had an IQ measured to be approximately that of a four-year-old, Price widened his narrowed upper arch about ½ inch with a palatal expansion rod located between his upper teeth (new maxillary bone filled in rapidly). This space was later maintained with a fixed bridge carrying two additional teeth. The results were striking. The patient grew 3 inches in four months and developed whiskers, and his genitals developed from those of a child to those of a man. These hormonal maturation changes were the direct result of the stimulation of the pituitary gland through the expansion of the sella turcica. The failure of development of the pituitary, or *hypopituitarism,* has been well documented in Down syndrome populations. Furthermore, this sixteen-year-old's IQ increased markedly. Although previously he was so seriously physically and mentally impaired that he typically played with blocks on the floor, after six months of palatal expansion he was able to go to the grocery store and bring back correct change to his mother, change trains and make transfers on streetcars accurately and safely, and read children's stories and newspaper headlines. Another benefit was that his previously completely occluded left nostril opened up, and he was no longer troubled with severe sleep apnea. Finally, his physical appearance changed dramatically—from infantile to a more normal-looking adolescent (see figure 16.16).[98]*

*Unfortunately, this patient later had to be institutionalized for sexual perversion. This lack of concomitant moral and emotional development along with the sexual maturation occurring was probably due to many factors. First, perhaps the maxillary expansion was not gradual enough—even ½ inch in six months is an enormous change to the body. This movement stimulated positive pituitary hormonal changes, but they were probably too fast for the body and mind to regulate and normalize. Another possible problem was that the palatal expansion bar was *rigidly* attached to this patient's right and left maxillary teeth, and the fixed bridge used later to maintain the ½-inch expansion was also rigid and immovable—both interfering with normal craniosacral motion. (More information on this

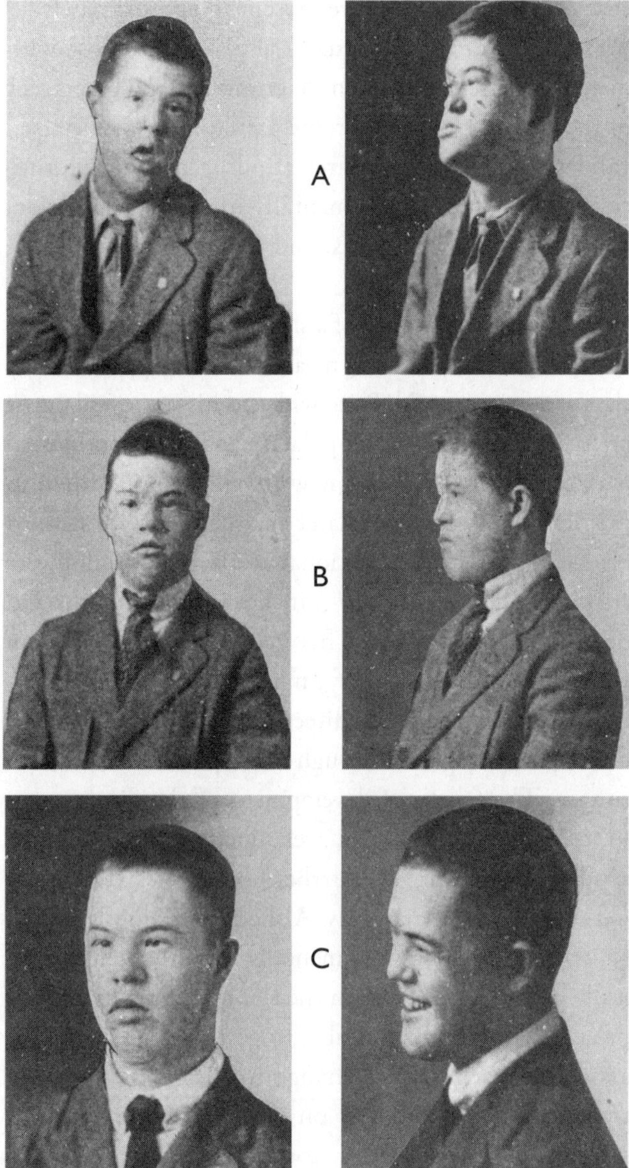

Figure 16.16. The remarkable changes in appearance in a sixteen-year-old with Down syndrome—from infantile (A) to less infantile (B) (after thirty days) to adolescent (C)—in six months with maxillary expansion

Further Support for the Link between Malocclusions and IQ

In a larger study of 100 schoolchildren, Dr. A. C. Fonder found dramatically similar results to Price in regard to the influence of dental malocclusions on intelligence. Out of a group of forty-seven "remedial" students who scored below average on IQ and achievement tests, Fonder found that 100 percent had "minor" (17 percent) to "severe" (83 percent) dental malocclusions. This was in striking contrast to the fifty-three above-average students who had only one "severe" (2 percent) and forty-three "minor" (81 percent) malocclusions, and nine "ideal" occlusions (17 percent).[99]

Psychological Health and Hearing Ability

The psychological differences between these two groups were just as revealing. The remedial students with minor to severe malocclusions all had "some" (68.1 percent) psychological problems, while 31.9 percent had serious issues. The advanced students with mostly minor to no malocclusions had no "serious" psychological problems, and the majority (77.4 percent) demonstrated no psychological issues at all. Knowing that hearing capacity is greatly correlated to intelligence as well as closely associated with proper functioning of the neighboring jaw joint, Fonder also measured the audiometric, or hearing acuity, of these two groups. The results were again striking: 83 percent (thirteen out of fifteen) of the remedial group possessing serious psychological problems had 15 to 40 percent loss of their overall hearing acuity, while 100 percent of the advanced students with ideal occlusions (nine children) had *above*-normal hearing acuity.[100]

Enhancing Normal Structure and Function: Vertical Dimension

Another benefit of functional appliances is the ability to increase the vertical dimension at the same time lateral and sagittal expansion of the jaws is occurring. Reduced height of the teeth, known as the "loss of vertical dimension," can be generated by any of the previously described causes of malocclusions (lack of breast-feeding, insufficient nutrition, bruxism, etc.). Fortunately, the appropriate functional appliance can dramatically reverse this loss of vertical dimension, thereby allowing the teeth over time to erupt to their more natural height. This

---

(*continued from page 527*) problem is described in the upcoming section titled "Craniosacral Movement: Locking Up the Maxillary Suture.") And finally, this boy had an invalid mother and a father who had suffered an injury working on the railroad, and they were probably not able to render him the amount of care and nurturing that he required during this major transition in his life. Nor was he, of course, privy to the behavioral and developmental teaching that modern-day Down syndrome children receive in special classes and schools.

eruption, termed *superextrusion,* is encouraged by orthopedic dentists by various means (e.g., pivot points over one molar to allow the two neighboring molars to superextrude over time).*

Restoring Normal Sleep

Through this normalization of the height of the teeth and therefore their occlusion, combined with the adequate expansion of the dental arches, functional appliances balance and augment the normal development of the craniofacial bones. These more normal—and therefore more functional—mouth, jaw, neck, and chest structural relationships often resolve commonly associated respiratory symptoms (snoring, sleep apnea, etc.) from a previously diminished airway space.[101] In a 1975 study where 310 "mouth-breather" patients received functional oral appliances to expand their palate, 80 percent became nasal breathers after only one to three months of treatment. Functional appliances have also been a positive alternative to CPAP pumps† for the 5 to 20 percent of the population who suffer from significant sleep disorders (snoring, obstructive sleep disorder, chronic insomnia, etc.). Another more recent research study demonstrated that oral appliances can be effective not only for mild or moderate sleep disorders but also even for patients requiring CPAPs who suffer from sleep apnea.[102] Furthermore, as was the case with Dr. Price's patient, individuals with mental impairments and neuromuscular disabilities (Down syndrome, cerebral palsy, etc.) who are particularly susceptible to obstructive sleep apnea can be greatly improved through the use of appropriate oral appliances.[103]

> **obstructive sleep apnea:** Obstructive sleep apnea syndrome is characterized by the cessation of breath for brief periods intermittently during sleep due to some type of airway obstruction (large tonsils, tongue, etc.).

Reducing Muscle Tension

Functional appliances can also provide dramatic relief from chronic muscle tension, pain, and spasm not only in the jaw muscles but throughout the patient's musculoskeletal system.[104] For example, the common problem of forward head posture and loss of the normal cervical lordotic curve ("military spine" in the neck), which often results from a reduced vertical dimension in the mouth, can be completely cleared, or at least greatly diminished, with appliance therapy.[105] Chronic tension headaches caused from jaw and cervicothoracic (neck and upper back) muscle tension also greatly reduce, or even completely subside, with the placement of the appropriate functional appliance.[106] Furthermore, because it is a "fundamental biological fact that the relation of the head to the neck is the primary relationship to be established in all proper positioning and movement of the body," orthopedic dentistry can have profound effects on the musculoskeletal system in the entire body.[107]

Releasing Negative Malocclusion Engrams

Oral appliances exert a curative effect in the neuromuscular system through the more functional occlusion and balanced muscle tone that gradually feedbacks into the negatively habituated brain memory (engram). Over time, the newly forming memory of a more balanced occlusion replaces the negative engram of chronic neuromuscular tension from the malocclusion. After the appliance is no longer needed and the patient receives a final equilibration of the teeth and bite, the body and brain can then continue to function in this newly conditioned and more harmonious occlusal and jaw joint position. Dr. David Walther, author of *Applied Kinesiology,* volume 2: *Head, Neck, and Jaw Pain and Dysfunction—The Stomatognathic System,* comments on this positive neurological patterning as a result of functional appliances:

> With a bite plane [functional appliance], the mandible no longer maintains a specific position during occlusion; there is freedom for it to move with the muscular change that develops

---

*These pivot points need to be rotated frequently or they can cause the iatrogenic problem of *superintrusion*—the tooth directly under the pivot point reducing in height with increasing pressure at its root, which can cause possible damage to the tooth and symptoms in the tooth's corresponding organs and tissues that are on the same meridian. See chapter 11 for more information on the five-element meridian relationships between the teeth and the body.

†Continuous positive air pressure (CPAP) pumps are the gold standard for obstructive sleep apnea. However, compliance with the use of these pumps is low because a face mask must be worn the entire night and the pump is noisy, and since the CPAP is not curative, it is required during the entire lifetime of sleep apnea patients—a rather bleak prescription.

> as a result of the engram breakdown. . . . With the abolition of the proprioceptive stimulation in the periodontal ligament [respite to the teeth and muscles from aberrant neurological signals], the muscles relax to allow the mandible to move into a position of physiologic centric relation [normal occlusion] in harmony with relaxed muscles.[108]

Increasing Muscle Strength and Coordination

Another benefit of functional appliances was first discovered in the field of athletics. Athletes have worn mouth guards* for decades for the same reasons many dental patients receive appliances for their chronic bruxism—to protect their teeth and jaws from trauma. However, it wasn't until the Notre Dame football team dentist, John Stenger, published his original research in the 1970s that the idea surfaced that these same mouth guards "could also provide some increment of increased muscle balance, strength and/or coordination."[109] Since then, numerous scientific studies have confirmed Stenger's assertion that mouth guards and other oral appliances significantly increase isometric muscle strength and efficiency, as well as balance and coordination, when compared with control groups.[110] This same phenomena has been observed clinically in hundreds of physicians' offices with Applied Kinesiology methods, when a wax buildup or two tongue depressors placed between the teeth renders a previously weak indicator muscle dramatically strong.[111]

Can Augment Normal Growth and Development of the Wisdom Teeth

Functional expansion appliances can also assist in providing adequate room for the eruption and normal growth of the third molars, or wisdom teeth, which typically occurs in the late teens and early twenties. This possibility is especially augmented if orthopedic dentists are allowed to intervene early enough during a patient's childhood and adolescence, as will be discussed in the next section.

*These athletic mouth guards are usually made of plastic that has a bit of "give." Thus, they don't lock up the maxillary suture or reduce the craniosacral rhythm as most conventional mouth guards worn overnight do.

The Benefits of Primary Molar Buildups in Children

Another intervention that is similar to functional appliances but can be instituted even earlier in childhood is the primary molar buildup, also known as the "occlusal filling" method. This procedure involves the placement of plastic composite material (filling material) over the tops of the first and second primary molar teeth to raise the height of these teeth and therefore increase the vertical dimension of the child's bite. Since potential Class II malocclusions (overbites) can be detected as early as age five or six, a simple buildup of plastic composite material on the child's primary (deciduous or baby) lower molars encourages over time a more normal occlusion, or at least greatly minimizes the need for later expansion appliances and (possibly) braces.[112] Dr. Merle Loudon, a Washington State dentist, enumerates the advantages of this simple method in his study published in *The Functional Orthodontist* journal:

> Primary crown buildups can result in many added benefits for a young, overclosed patient. Early treatment can save months of later orthodontic vertical treatment. Temporomandibular condylar position may be greatly enhanced. The return to a normal tongue position will allow for normal growth of the mandible.[113]

Automatic Compliance

This technique has the additional benefit of compliance. Young children, for whom this method is best suited, can resist wearing appliances, and often lose them. However, plastic composite buildups on the molars, when properly fitted and appropriately equilibrated, do not require any effort or willpower on the part of the child. Furthermore, this procedure hastens the eruption of the permanent first molars, as well as the other adult teeth, into a more functional and healthy occlusion.

Can Reduce Chronic Ear Infections

Another orthopedically oriented dentist, Dr. David Page, advocates the use of plastic composite buildups (and even functional appliances) for even younger children—as early as age two. In fact, he asserts that 90 percent of the head growth and approximately 80 percent of jaw development has already occurred by age six, so intervention before this age is actually optimal. Dr. Page has had success in treating persistent ear infections—the most frequent diagnosis made in physicians' offices in patients under age fifteen. In fact, children with deep dental overbites (Class II) are almost three times more likely to have ear tubes placed or recommended by a pediatrician.[114] Dr. Page cites the following case of his own son that was published in *The Functional Orthodontist:*

> After 20 ear problems in 2½ years, I put plastic dental composites on my son's lower back baby molar teeth to open the deep bite. His lower jaw moved down and forward away from his ears. He has not had ear problems since.[115]

Thus, in a classic "structure determining function" relationship, the abnormal anatomical pressure that the mandibular condyle of the jaw joint from a deep bite (malocclusion) exerts on the neighboring ear tissues creates chronic inflammation over time. Eventually, this inflammation can trigger in a domino manner chronic ear infections by serving as a breeding ground for bacterial growth. Other causes of pressure-induced otitis media include the long-term use of pacifiers and thumb sucking.[116] Food allergies (especially dairy), the ingestion of refined sugar, and neighboring focal infections (dental, tonsil, and sinus) are also major factors in the etiology of this persistent illness for which antibiotics are prescribed more often than for any other illness.[117]

☙

Unfortunately, the majority of children—whether age two or twelve—never experience the benefits of seeing a holistic dentist or physician during these formative years. Therefore, it has become increasingly rare for individuals to receive the necessary effective orthopedic dentistry (as well as sufficient breast-feeding, nutrition, and so forth) that will later facilitate the complete and full eruption of all thirty-two teeth—even with the help of later expansion appliances. This rather depressing fact is underlined by a previously noted study conducted over twenty years ago in which the American Academy of Pediatric Dentistry found that nearly 90 percent of children between the ages of twelve and seventeen had some form of malocclusion.[118] In the cases of these teenagers (and young adults) who did not receive early enough intervention such as functional appliances or the primary molar buildup, the sacrifice of the second molars has proved superior to the extraction of the first bicuspids or the third molars.

When Teeth Must Be Sacrificed: Second Molar vs. First Bicuspid Extraction

A sizable percentage of patients—notwithstanding the best efforts with plastic buildups or functional appliances—cannot expand their jawbones sufficiently to accommodate all thirty-two teeth. Furthermore, as discussed in the last section, many children are simply not afforded the benefits of a holistic orthopedic dentist during these formative years of bone growth and development. Thus, whether these children or teens have major malocclusions and TMJ dysfunction or just not enough room for the eruption and normal growth of their third molar (wisdom) teeth, teeth must be sacrificed in order to clear the existing—or potential—malocclusion issues. These necessary extractions can also eliminate the potential for the development of future focal infections in one or more of the misaligned or impacted wisdom tooth sites.

In these cases, most orthopedic dentists (and a few knowledgeable orthodontists) opt to extract the second molars instead of the first bicuspids, if the child or teen is evaluated early enough. The decision to sacrifice these molar teeth rather than the bicuspids first evolved in the 1950s with Dr. H. E. Wilson.[119] As a specialist in temporomandibular dysfunction (TMD), this London dentist observed that many of his patients who had previously had the classic four-bicuspid extraction type of orthodontics displayed a variety of significant disturbances. These problems included major TMJ dysfunction, deep overbites (Class II malocclusions), distally tilted canines and lower anteriors (the four canines and the lower front teeth were tilted backward), mesially tilted posterior teeth (back molars were tilted inward toward the tongue), and, finally—a complication known firsthand by an estimated 50 percent of all patients treated orthodontically—the problem of relapsing cases, where the teeth drift out of the (abnormal) position in which the braces had placed them. In an effort to obviate these problems, Wilson sought an alternative to the four-bicuspid extraction method, eventually leading to the second molar extraction solution.

Second Molar Extraction Can Allow Full Eruption of the Wisdom Teeth

The extraction of these next-to-last back molars has many significant benefits. (The third molars, or wisdom teeth, are the teeth farthest back in the mouth.) Front teeth do not need to be retracted (pushed back) because there are no bicuspid spaces to close (remember, the bicuspid teeth are between the front teeth and the back molars). Furthermore, with this method the normal anterior development (forward and down) of the face and jaws is encouraged, which protects the TMJ from harm. And finally, the removal of the second molars encourages the normal eruption and development of the third molars. In fact, in a sizable study of 500 cases, Wilson found that the wisdom teeth in an extremely high percentage (87 percent) of patients who had had second molar extractions were able to fully erupt in the appropriate position in the mouth. This result is in direct contrast to the "four-bi" extraction orthodontic method that Witzig and Spahl greatly discourage in their book, *The Clinical Management of Basic Maxillofacial Orthopedic Appliance,* because extraction of the bicuspids doesn't benefit the eruption of the third molars: "The third molar, however, is often unaffected by the gain of arch length of the other teeth in the anterior segments [by the bicuspid extraction] and is still left on its own, unaided, to shift for itself."[120]

Small Window of Opportunity for Second Molar Extraction

However, the window for this more therapeutic second molar extraction method is not wide, so timing is critical. In fact, a holistically oriented oral surgeon, Dr. John Austin from St. Paul, Minnesota, advocates "the evaluation radiographically of every 11- to 12-year-old, regardless of his or her need for orthodontics, to determine whether second molars should be extracted . . . for the advantage of the avoidance of the impacted third-molar situation." Witzig and Spahl recommend the following guidelines: "Second-molar extraction is best between the ages of 10 or 11 up to 15 years in the lower arch or even as late as age 20 years for the uppers. The actual limiting factor for successful eruption to take place seems to be at around the time the bifurcation of the roots of the third molar begin to be clearly seen (when the dividing of the roots of the wisdom teeth is clearly seen on X-ray)."[121] In conclusion, Witzig and Spahl sum up the importance of considering this highly beneficial orthopedic procedure in children and teens with present or potentially future malocclusions, who are also at risk for future third molar focal infections:

> [T]o avoid dished-in faces, flattened smiles, unstable occlusions, and compromised temporomandibular joints, for the patient needing orthodontic treatment accompanied by dental extractions, *there is no alternative* to second-molar extraction; *there is no debate.*
>
> The second molar replacement technique becomes both for the patient and the treating clinician a therapeutic mandate![122]

Craniosacral Movement: Locking Up the Maxillary Suture

Before leaving the subject of treatment, one admonition should be made that even holistic orthopedic dentists are rarely cognizant of—that it's essential not to restrict the motion that exists within the maxillary suture (the joint between the two front teeth). Unfortunately, commonly used rigid plastic appliances spanning the upper palate, as well as fixed bridges between the upper front teeth, do precisely this, which in turn restricts at some level normal cranial movement in the skull and even throughout the rest of the body. Although U.S. dental and medical schools teach that in adults there is absolutely no motion in this cranial bone joint, or anywhere else in the skull for that matter, this dogma flies in the face of current research. In fact, there are currently more than three hundred documented references that confirm the existence of a subtle but perceptible micro motion in the cranium.[123] Further evidence of this motion has been supplied by the internationally known anatomist Marc Pick, D.C., whose dissection of over 150 craniums has unequivocally proven that the sutures (joints in the skull) have hingelike and sliding movements that allow for micro motion in the skull (see figure 16.17).[124]

maxillary suture: The maxillary suture is also known as the mid-palatine or cruciate suture.

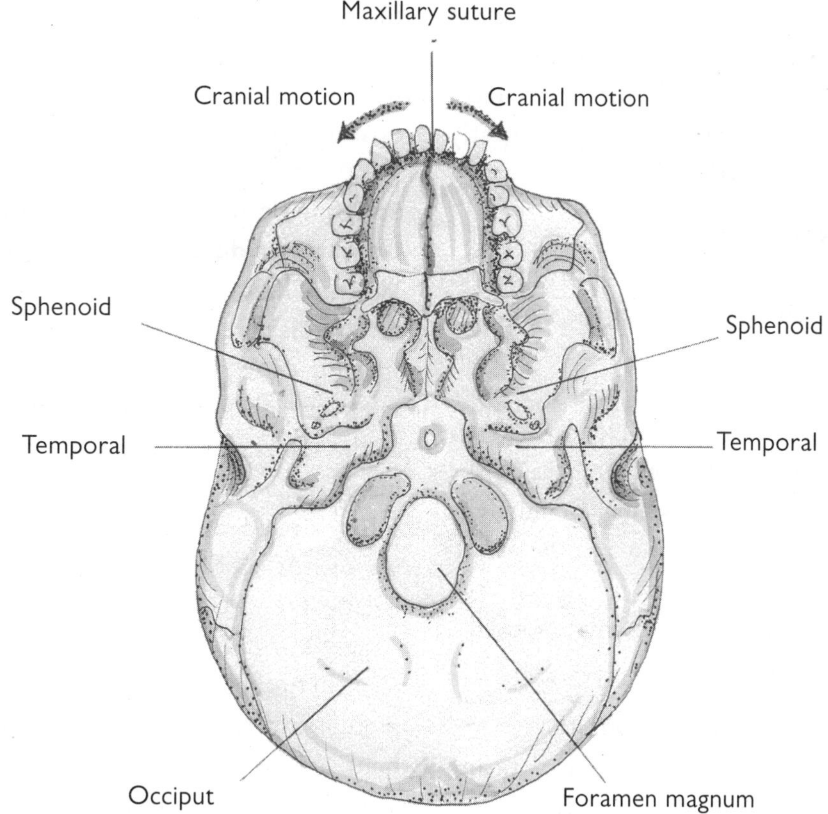

Figure 16.17. The maxillary suture (inferior view here) allows for motion between the two halves of the maxillae bones. Fixed bridges and hard plastic appliances (not split down the middle) such as night guards and retainers can restrict this important cranial micro motion.

Suture is the term used for a type of serrated-like joint in which the two opposing surfaces are closely interdigitating or interlocking, such as in the skull or cranium. Cranial sutures contain connective tissue, blood vessels, and nerves.[125]

Cerebrospinal Fluid Circulation Moves the Cranial Bones

This cranial movement is primarily due to the circulation of the cerebrospinal fluid (CSF) that flows within the dura mater—the "tough mother" or external fascial (tissue) sheath that surrounds and protects the entire central nervous system (CNS). The CSF circulates within this CNS and "bathes" these brain and spinal cord tissues continuously from head (the cranium) to "tail" (the sacrum), typically at a rate of about eight to twelve cycles per minute. These circulatory cycles, known as the *craniosacral rhythm,* circulate at a slightly slower rate than the normal respiratory rhythm of the lungs (twelve to twenty breaths per minute).[126] Craniopaths—primarily osteopaths, chiropractors, and some massage therapists—are trained to perceive this subtle craniosacral rhythm and to treat fixated areas and other distortion patterns within this system through gentle manipulative pressure and intention.

Hard Plastic Appliances Restrict Craniosacral Motion

In the mouth, hard plastic immobile appliances covering the upper teeth and palate that cross the maxillary suture can greatly diminish this craniosacral motion.[127] Dr. Fonder was well aware of the so-called functional appliances (e.g., the Farrar splint) that "tend to lock the cranial bones" and cause the "cerebral spinal fluid flow and blood circulation to the head and brain [to be] restricted." He therefore advocated appliances that allow full movement of the cranial bones, "so necessary for cranial breathing and the circulation thereby produced."[128] The commonly prescribed night guards that fit over both the upper and lower teeth and hold them rigidly in position to reduce nocturnal bruxism are the most typical offenders. The hard plastic retainers that teens often have to suffer with for years after their braces are removed also lock up this maxillary joint and greatly restrict normal craniosacral rhythm.

Braces and Dentures Not So Restrictive

Although braces can diminish maxillary suture motion, this restriction is less than expected since the wires run from tooth to tooth. In contrast, appliances and retainers arc over the entire upper palate, which is a more constrictive architectural formation. Dentures don't strongly restrict this cranial motion either, because the teeth are absent and the dentures simply fit snugly—but not rigidly—in the palatal arch and over the maxillary bone. Furthermore, because dentures are removed at night, any stress they put on this normal motion is relieved for at least eight hours per day.

Bridges Restrict the Maxillary Suture Motion

Fixed bridges that cross this maxillary cranial suture due to the loss of one or both of the upper front teeth (central incisors) are particularly notorious for creating symptoms in the head and neck. Dr. Gerry Smith, a Pennsylvania holistic orthopedic dentist who has lectured on the problem of upper bridgework for decades, describes the serious implications of this dental-induced disturbance:

> One of the most frequently violated areas of the cranium occurs when conventional dental techniques restrict cranial bone motion by crossing the maxillary midline with fixed bridgework. Because the maxilla articulates the nine other cranial bones (malar, frontal, ethmoid, vomer, palatine, lacrimal, sphenoid, inferior nasal concha, and other half of the maxilla) it represents direct contact with 45 percent of the cranium. In essence, locking the maxillae will restrict to varying degrees the entire craniosacral mechanism.[129]

Dr. Smith has recorded numerous cases of severe headaches, facial pain, chronic fatigue, mental confusion, eye pain, irritability, and disequilibrium that have resolved rapidly simply after the removal of this fixed bridgework. This innovative dentist has also originated the use of a piston-cylinder (male-female) attachment that can be used between the front teeth when bridgework is required, which allows more normal motion to exist between the maxillary bones.[130]

Splitting Hard Plastic Appliances Down the Middle

When a hard upper plastic appliance is required in orthopedic dentistry (and hard is often better than soft), splitting this appliance down the center and installing screws usually allows enough "play" within the midline of the appliance to permit full movement between the maxillary bones. This split-down-the-middle upper oral splint is referred to as a *sagittal* appliance and is often used when lateral expansion is indicated in the upper palate.* However, whether maxillary bone expansion is required or not, sagittal appliances have enough "give" in them to allow for relatively normal craniosacral micro motion. Alternatively, because the mandible is a single bone and has no suture, the placing of hard plastic appliances over the lower teeth causes no real interruption or disturbance in the craniosacral rhythm.

Dural Torque Compensatory Patterns

In kinesiological testing, the locking-up of this maxillary suture can be determined by the weakening of a strong indicator muscle upon therapy localization (intentionally touching this joint just between and above the two front teeth). Furthermore, Klinghardt and Williams have observed a common torquing type of pattern that often occurs in adaptation to the jamming of this maxillary suture through appliances, retainers, or bridgework.[131] Dura mater torquing patterns are well known to craniopaths, who palpate the cranial and spinal bones that

*Patients are given a tiny screwdriver that allows them to intermittently turn the screws in the sagittal splint at home (e.g., once every week or two weeks turn the screws a quarter turn or less) in order to expand this appliance laterally, so that it can further laterally expand their too-narrow palate and maxillary arch. Unfortunately, overly enthusiastic dentists often instruct their patients to turn the screw more often and more than a quarter turn at a time. This causes unnecessary pain and can even truncate the movement of the maxillary bones. Orthopedically oriented dentists are typically more aware of the Arndt-Schulz law that states that a "small stimulus enhances growth, a medium stimulus impedes it or maintains normality and a strong stimulus inhibits, or destroys, activity." (J. Yasgur, *Yasgur's Homeopathic Dictionary* [Greenville, Pa.: Van Hoy Publishers, 1998], 214.)

lie just over this continuous sheath of fascia.[132] However, the disturbing effects of this dural torque pattern in response to sutural restrictions have not been confined to clinical observation by craniopaths. In human and primate cadaver studies, abnormal fibrous changes—that is, scar tissue—have also been documented in areas of significant structural tension in the dural membrane.[133]

Because this tough dural sheath that surrounds the brain and spinal cord is continuous with the other fascia throughout the body, compensatory torquing due to midline restriction (the maxillary suture) is transmitted systemically. Dr. John Upledger, a renowned craniopath, describes the ubiquitous nature of fascia in his book *Craniosacral Therapy:*

> The fascia of the human body is continuous from head to toe. You can travel from the top of your head to your liver, spleen or right medial malleolus [ankle] without ever leaving fascia.[134]

Therefore, locking up the maxillary suture causes fascial strain not only in the dural membrane of the craniosacral system but also in the peripheral fascia and in the muscles that this fascia surrounds. The specific torquing pattern, demonstrated by a "crisscrossing" of muscle weakness, mirrors the adaptive twisting pattern of the dura mater membrane in response to the midline (maxillary suture) restriction. This compensatory myofascial (muscle and fascia) weakness results from the body's attempt to maintain postural stability and balance while standing or walking, as well as to preserve normal function in underlying organs and tissues, despite this abnormal midline restriction. Figure 16.18 illustrates a classic myofascial weakness pattern often seen clinically. In this example, the kinesiologist would find the following weak muscles: the right neck flexor muscles, the left arm and shoulder muscles, the right hip and low back muscles, and the left ankle and foot muscles.[135] (Of course, the reverse of this pattern is also commonly found: the left neck flexor muscles, the right arm and shoulder muscles, the left hip and low back muscles, and the right ankle and foot muscles.)

Most people never connect their recent reduced cervical (neck) range of motion or their right hip pain with the fact that they have just received a new bridge across their upper front teeth (or an appliance, a retainer, etc.).

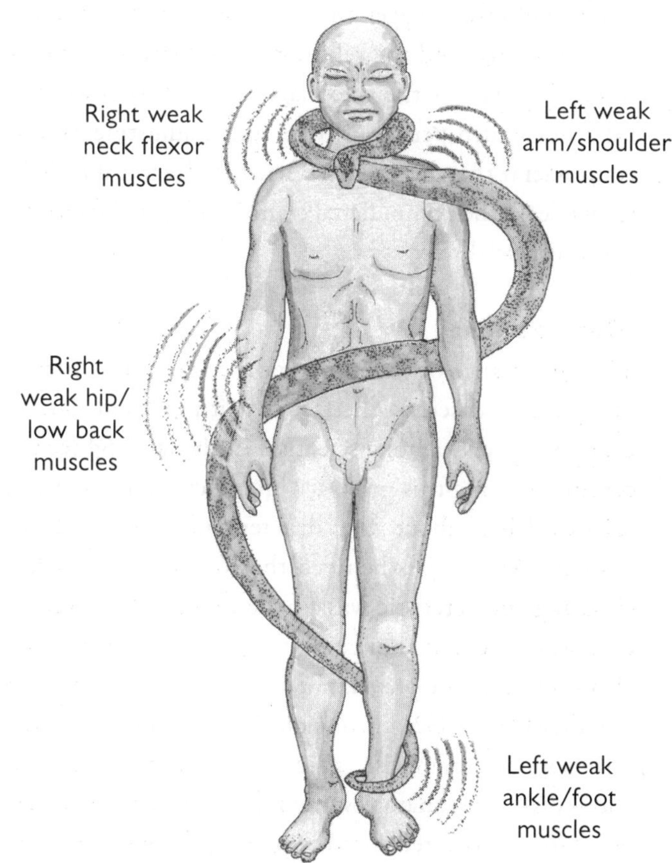

Figure 16.18. A typical myofascial weakness pattern mirroring the dural torquing response to the locking-up of the maxillary suture with a bridge, retainer, appliance, or night guard

This link is often especially difficult to make because the resulting decreased range of motion or joint pain can take weeks or months to manifest. Furthermore, the majority of us are already in adaptation daily anyway, compensating for mild to major torsional twists of the muscles, fascia, and spine due to overuse of the dominant hand, poor sedentary and postural habits, and compensation for a host of stressors (psychological issues, chronic foci, toxic metals and chemicals, etc.).[136] However, for a certain percentage of sensitive individuals, the locking-up of the maxillary suture is (consciously or unconsciously) intolerable and creates many symptoms. For these individuals, as well as for the symptomless who are experiencing the more silent but nevertheless adverse effects, removing the offending appliance or having the fixed bridge midline connection cut in two by a holistic dentist (if enough signs and symptoms warrant this emergency step that will require new bridgework at some point) will often trigger an immediate muscle strengthening response and the release of this dural torque pattern. However, if the maxillary suture was restricted for an extended period of time, spinal adjustments and craniosacral therapy are often needed afterward to help fully release the accumulated cranial and spinal fixations and myofascial restrictions.

"Goethe's Bone"

The importance of this region of the cranium is particularly underscored by the fact that it provoked significant controversy among scientists in the late eighteenth century. During this pre-Darwinian period, there was a spirited debate about what differentiated humans from animals. Anatomists believed that one primary differentiating characteristic was a bone found in all animals that was absent in humans—the *intermaxillary bone,* also known as the *premaxilla.*[137] Johann Wolfgang von Goethe (1749–1832), the famous German novelist, poet, philosopher, dramatist, painter, scientist, politician, and—yes—even anatomist, found this theory preposterous. Goethe asserted that the premaxilla bone must be present in humans as well because "each creature, human or animal, is just one little piece of a unique wholeness intertwined, [and that] each little bone is to be found in either human or animal alike."[138] His philosophy, whose work later influenced Charles Darwin, was that "diversity in form springs from a preponderance of one part over the others" in each particular mammal, and that is what primarily differentiates humans from animals. Thus, in humans, the preeminence of the head and the highly developed human brain, as Rudolf Steiner elucidated in his text *Nature's Open Secret,* "[Goethe believed] places the human being at the pinnacle of creation, [and] creates the possibility of such high perfection in the human being."[139]

Goethe therefore set out to disprove this "error" that seemed to be a "tear in nature's web," by examining and comparing various human and animal skulls. In 1784, he succeeded in his venture and announced the discovery of "something that gives me unspeakable joy—the human *ossis intermaxillaris*!" He further commented that this bone, coined "Goethe's bone," was "like the keystone to the human being."[140] More recent research in the *Anatomy and Embryology* journal similarly describes this bone in structural terms "as a stabilizing element within the facial skeleton similar to a keystone of a Roman arch."[141] Although after the third month in utero there exists no facial evidence of this bone, because it fuses with the maxilla, the palatal sign of separation—that is, a suture—between the premaxilla and the rest of the maxilla can persist until middle age.[142]

Thus, the intermaxillary or premaxilla bone is an important region of the body that should be recognized as a crucial joint in the body not only by dentists but all practitioners as well. Furthermore, this important "keystone" of the cranium is an area that every holistic dentist should endeavor to keep mobile, and not lock up with a fixed bridge or hard plastic appliance.*

CONCLUSION

Prevention Is Optimal

The most important lesson from this chapter is that the prevention of malocclusions and temporomandibular joint (TMJ) dysfunction in infants and children is the most effective way to preserve and maintain optimal health in the teeth and jaws, as well as in the rest of the body. The first step in healthy tooth and jaw development is breast-feeding and a nutritious diet. If that step is suboptimal, or if other factors contribute such as pesticide use or tonsil foci, then the next step is finding a qualified *orthopedic* dentist—in contrast to an *orthodontist*†—to fashion a functional expansion appliance or build up the child's primary teeth with composite material. If this step is not sufficient to clear an existing malocclusion or TMD, or if there is simply not enough room in the adolescent's mouth to accommodate all thirty-two teeth, then it is better in most cases to extract the second molar teeth if this can be done in a timely fashion. This extraction can obviate later potential third molar focal infections as well as the stress and dysfunction generated by their related disturbed fields and neighboring toxic ganglia.

---

*This knowledge inspired Darick Nordstrom, D.D.S., of Hollister, California, to develop the ALF—Advanced Lightwire Functional—appliance in the early 1980s in order to correct the alignment of and expand the maxillary bone and suture, as well as the rest of the cranial bones and sutures.

†Fortunately, there is a growing number of holistically oriented orthodontists as the advantages of whole body, or orthopedically oriented, dentistry becomes more widespread.

Adults Can Also Benefit from Functional Appliances

Orthopedic appliances can also be extremely helpful for adults who suffer from a major malocclusion or TMD, and even dramatically so when used in conjunction with other holistic therapies. In fact, finding a healthy bite that allows relaxation of the body and normal functioning in chewing and swallowing is necessary at some point for everyone who truly desires optimal health.

Jaw and tooth development continues approximately to age thirty. Therefore, adults younger than thirty years of age more quickly respond to functional orthopedic appliance therapy. Adults older than thirty can also greatly benefit from orthopedic appliances, although expansion and other tooth and jaw movement will be slower.

Appropriate Referral

Your practitioner, if he or she is truly holistic, should know an orthopedic or TMJ dentist (or one of the growing number of holistic orthodontists) to refer to locally, or at least in a nearby city. Recommendations from friends who have gone through orthopedic treatment are also often reliable. Other helpful sources include contacting holistic dental organizations that specialize in treating malocclusions and TMD:

- AAGO: (800) 510-AAGO or www.aago.com
  AACP: (800) 322-8651 or www.aacfp.org
  AAFO: (800) 441-3850 or www.aafo.org
  IAFGG: (888) 404-3223 or www.orthotropics.com
  OrthoSmile Inc.: (518) 943-7703 or
  www.facialdevelopment.com

Finally, as was discussed previously, unless you have a major malocclusion and/or TMD that necessitates stabilizing the bite before other therapies can have any real positive effect, it is best to wait before treating mild to moderate jaw and teeth misalignments.* That is, only after mercury amalgams and toxic metal crowns have been removed, personal care products are petroleum-free, dominant foci have been treated, gemmotherapy herbals have drained toxins and tonified organs and tissues, and the homeopathic simillimum has significantly improved your constitution can a holistic dentist most knowledgeably design the most appropriate functional appliance for treatment of moderate malocclusions and TMD, or most skillfully equilibrate the bite in the case of more minor dysfunction.

This therapeutic holistic physician/orthopedic dentist plan has two positive effects. For one, many of the treatments that clear toxins and chronic muscle spasms actually favorably alter the position of the jaw joint or the bite (e.g., "false TMD syndrome," dental and tonsil focal infections, mercury in the jaw tissues, dental galvanism, etc.), thus reducing both the time needed for future functional appliance therapy and the amount of drilling required during equilibration. Second, only when these interfering factors are cleared as much as possible can the orthopedic dentist then determine the most favorable oral appliance, or simply the most beneficial final equilibration position, to best facilitate optimal occlusion and TMJ function.

*Unless, of course, as previously mentioned, the moderate occlusal dysfunction is causing significant damage through chronic bruxism. In these cases, an appliance is appropriate to reduce the wear and tear to the teeth. However, it should not lock up the motion of the maxillary suture, as described previously.

NOTES

1. J. Mittelman, "It's the Bite That Counts," *PPNF Journal* 26, no. 3 (Fall 2002): 8.
2. B. Palmer, "The Influence of Breastfeeding on the Development of the Oral Cavity: A Commentary," *PPNF Journal* 23, no. 4 (Winter 1999): 21.
3. R. Mittelman, "Temporomandibular Joint Dysfunction," *Journal of the American Society of Psychosomatic Dentistry and Medicine* 19, no. 1 (1972): 15.
4. B. Palmer, "The Influence of Breastfeeding on the Development of the Oral Cavity: A Commentary," *PPNF Journal* 23, no. 4 (Winter 1999): 4; F. Pottenger, "The Relative Influence of the Activity of Artificial and Breast Feeding on Facial Development," *PPNF Journal* 23, no. 4 (Winter 1999): 6.
5. B. Palmer, "The Influence of Breastfeeding on the Development of the Oral Cavity: A Commentary," *PPNF Journal* 23, no. 4 (Winter 1999): 5; B. Palmer, "Breastfeeding: Reducing the Risk for Obstructive Sleep Apnea," *PPNF Journal* 24, no. 1 (Spring 2000): 12.
6. B. Palmer, "The Influence of Breastfeeding on the Development of the Oral Cavity: A Commentary," *PPNF Journal* 23, no. 4 (Winter 1999): 5.

7. D. Page, *Your Jaws, Your Life* (Baltimore: SmilePage Publishing, 2003), 61.
8. L. Williams, "From Attention Deficit to Sleep Apnea: The Serious Consequences of Dental Deformities," *Wise Traditions* 10, no. 3 (Fall 2009): 20.
9. B. Palmer, "The Influence of Breastfeeding on the Development of the Oral Cavity: A Commentary," *PPNF Journal* 23, no. 4 (Winter 1999): 5.
10. Ibid.; F. Pottenger, "The Relative Influence of the Activity of Artificial and Breast Feeding on Facial Development," *PPNF Journal* 23, no. 4 (Winter 1999): 6–8.
11. J. Mittelman, "It's the Bite That Counts," *PPNF Journal* 26, no. 3 (Fall 2002): 8.
12. B. Palmer, "The Influence of Breastfeeding on the Development of the Oral Cavity: A Commentary," *PPNF Journal* 23, no. 4 (Winter 1999): 4; J. Mittelman, "It's the Bite That Counts," *PPNF Journal* 26, no. 3 (Fall 2002): 8.
13. B. Palmer, "The Influence of Breastfeeding on the Development of the Oral Cavity: A Commentary," *PPNF Journal* 23, no. 4 (Winter 1999): 21.
14. J. Ahlin et al., *Maxillofacial Orthopedics* (Longwood, Fla.: Xulon Press, 2004), 58–59.
15. J. Mittelman, "It's the Bite That Counts," *PPNF Journal* 26, no. 3 (Fall 2002): 8.
16. Ibid.
17. Ibid., 19, 20, 23.
18. R. Silkman, "Is It Mental or Is It Dental? Cranial and Dental Impacts on Total Health," *Wise Traditions* 7, no. 1 (Winter 2005/Spring 2006): 19, 23.
19. Ibid., 19.
20. Ibid., 19–23.
21. B. Palmer, "The Influence of Breastfeeding on the Development of the Oral Cavity: A Commentary," *PPNF Journal* 23, no. 4 (Winter 1999): 5, 20.
22. Ibid.
23. B. Palmer, "Breastfeeding: Reducing the Risk for Obstructive Sleep Apnea," *PPNF Journal* 24, no. 1 (Spring 2000): 12.
24. D. Page, *Your Jaws, Your Life* (Baltimore: SmilePage Publishing, 2003), 47.
25. Personal communication with Dr. Raymond Silkman, September 2006.
26. D. Zimmerman and J. Zimmerman, "Thumb and Finger Sucking: Questions and Answers" (self-published pamphlet, 1987); J. Ahlin et al., *Maxillofacial Orthopedics* (Longwood, Fla.: Xulon Press, 2004), 62–65.
27. D. Page, *Your Jaws, Your Life* (Baltimore: SmilePage Publishing, 2003), 60–61.
28. W. Price, *Nutrition and Physical Degeneration* (Los Angeles: The American Academy of Applied Nutrition, 1948), 1–4.
29. A. Fonder, *The Dental Physician* (Rock Falls, Ill.: Medical-Dental Arts, 1985), 25–26.
30. S. Fallon, "Nasty, Brutish and Short?" *The Ecologist* 29, no. 1 (January/February 1999): 22.
31. S. Fallon and M. Enig, "Out of Africa: What Dr. Price and Dr. Burkitt Discovered in Their Studies of Sub-Saharan Tribes," *PPNF Health Journal* 21, no. 1 (Spring 1997): 1.
32. S. Fallon, "Nasty, Brutish and Short?" *The Ecologist* 29, no. 1 (January/February 1999): 22; W. Price, *Nutrition and Physical Degeneration* (Los Angeles: The American Academy of Applied Nutrition, 1948), 1, 2.
33. A. Fonder, *The Dental Physician* (Rock Falls, Ill.: Medical-Dental Arts, 1985), 27–28.
34. F. Pottenger, *Pottenger's Cats: A Study in Nutrition* (San Diego: Price-Pottenger Nutrition Foundation, 1995), 1, 21–26.
35. W. Price, *Nutrition and Physical Degeneration* (Los Angeles: The American Academy of Applied Nutrition, 1948), 325.
36. J. Hoy, "Clouds of Death: Catastrophic Effects of Wind-Drift Chemicals and Locally Sprayed Pesticides on Western Montana Fauna," *Wise Traditions* 3, no. 3 (Fall 2002): 12–24.
37. F. Jerome, *Tooth Truth* (San Diego: ProMotion Publishing, 1995), 235.
38. D. Ewing, *Let the TOOTH Be Known,* 2nd ed. (Houston: Holistic Health Alternatives, 2002), 81, 82.
39. Ibid., 92.
40. L. Williams, "Craniomandibular Syndrome: The Chiropractic-Dental Connection," *The New Times,* June 1987, 19.
41. *Dorland's Illustrated Medical Dictionary,* 26th ed. (Philadelphia: W. B. Saunders Company, 1981), 457.
42. D. Walther, *Applied Kinesiology,* vol. 2 (Pueblo, Colo.: Systems DC, 1983), 375.
43. L. Mittelman, "It's the Bite That Counts," *PPNF Journal* 26, no. 3 (Fall 2002): 9.
44. A. Fonder, *The Dental Physician* (Rock Falls, Ill.: Medical-Dental Arts, 1985), 105–6.
45. P. Rowan, *Some Body* (New York: Alfred A. Knopf, 1995), 32.
46. D. Page, *Your Jaws, Your Life* (Baltimore: SmilePage Publishing, 2003), 24–25.
47. N. Collins, "Here He Goes Again After Too Long an Absence, One of Hollywood's Favorite Sons Is Back on

the Screen—And He's Looking Better Than Ever," *ELLE Magazine,* April 1987.

48. O. Rogal, *Mandibular Whiplash* (seminar manual) (Philadelphia: self-published, 1988), 12–13.
49. D. Steigerwald et al., *Whiplash and Temporomandibular Disorders* (San Diego: Keiser Publishing, 1992), 19, 25, 27, 52.
50. C. Oulis et al., "The Effect of Hypertrophic Adenoids and Tonsils on the Development of Posterior Crossbite and Oral Habits," *Journal of Clinical Pediatric Dentistry* 18, no. 3 (Spring 1994): 197–201.
51. Ibid.; O. Brown et al., "Cor Pulmonale Secondary to Tonsillar and Adenoidal Hypertrophy: Management Considerations," *International Journal of Pediatric Otorhinolaryngology* 16 (1988): 131–39; D. Page, *Your Jaws, Your Life* (Baltimore: SmilePage Publishing, 2003), 84–85.
52. J. Ahlin et al., *Maxillofacial Orthopedics* (Longwood, Fla.: Xulon Press, 2004), 58–59.
53. A. Fonder, *The Dental Physician* (Rock Falls, Ill.: Medical-Dental Arts, 1985), 166–68.
54. B. Palmer, "Breastfeeding: Reducing the Risk for Obstructive Sleep Apnea," *PPNF Journal* 24, no. 1 (Spring 2000): 12–13.
55. M. Tasner, "TMJ: A Minor Misalignment of the Jaw Can Produce an Astonishing Variety of Chronic Pains," *Medical Self-Care,* November–December 1986, 19.
56. H. Hooshmand, *Chronic Pain: Reflex Sympathetic Dystrophy Prevention and Management* (Boca Raton, Fla.: CRC Press, 1993), 74.
57. D. Walther, *Applied Kinesiology,* vol. 2 (Pueblo, Colo.: Systems DC, 1983), 116.
58. H. Hooshmand, *Chronic Pain: Reflex Sympathetic Dystrophy Prevention and Management* (Boca Raton, Fla.: CRC Press, 1993), 74.
59. Ibid., 37, 44.
60. Ibid., 35, 37; P. Williams, *Gray's Anatomy* (New York: Churchill Livingstone, 1995), 1121–22.
61. T. Sumioka, "Systemic Effects of the Peripheral Disturbance of the Trigeminal System: Influences of the Occlusal Destruction in Dogs," *Journal of Kyoto Prefectural University of Medicine* 10, no. 98: 1077–79, 1081.
62. H. Hooshmand, *Chronic Pain: Reflex Sympathetic Dystrophy Prevention and Management* (Boca Raton, Fla.: CRC Press, 1993), 52; P. Williams, *Gray's Anatomy* (New York: Churchill Livingstone, 1995), 980.
63. L. Funt and B. Kinnie, *Anatomy of a Headache* (St. Paul, Minn.: European Orthodontic Products, 1985), 5–14.
64. E. Ohm and J. Silness, "Size of the Mandibular Jaw Angle Related to Age, Tooth Retention and Gender," *Journal of Oral Rehabilitation* 11, no. 26 (November 1999): 883–91.
65. D. Page, *Your Jaws, Your Life* (Baltimore: SmilePage Publishing, 2003), 29, 33.
66. H. Gelb, *Killing Pain without Prescription* (New York: Harper and Row, 1982), 6.
67. A. Fonder, "Gynecological Problems and the Dental Distress Syndrome," *Basal Facts* 4, no. 4 (1981): 105–26.
68. G. Olson et al., "The Incidence and Severity of Premenstrual Syndrome among Female Craniomandibular Pain Patients," *The Journal of Craniomandibular Practice* 6, no. 4 (October 1988): 330–37; A. Fonder, "Gynecological Problems and the Dental Distress Syndrome," *Basal Facts* 4, no. 4 (1981): 123–32; D. Mahony, Academy of General Dentistry annual meeting, Nashville, July 17–20, 2003; D. Page, *Your Jaws, Your Life* (Baltimore: SmilePage Publishing, 2003), 40–46; A. Fonder, *The Dental Physician* (Rock Falls, Ill.: Medical-Dental Arts, 1985), 204–7.
69. H. Gelb, *Clinical Management of Head, Neck and TMJ Pain and Dysfunction* (Philadelphia: W. B. Saunders Company, 1985), 137–57; A. Fonder, *The Dental Physician* (Rock Falls, Ill.: Medical-Dental Arts, 1985), 88–91.
70. E. Lipski, *Digestive Wellness* (Los Angeles: Keats Publishing, 2000), 45.
71. Ibid.
72. A. Fonder, *The Dental Physician* (Rock Falls, Ill.: Medical-Dental Arts, 1985), 93.
73. J. Witzig and T. Spahl, *The Clinical Management of Basic Maxillofacial Orthopedic Appliances,* vol. 1, *Mechanics* (Littletown, Mass.: PSG Publishing Company, 1987), 186.
74. H. Gelb, *Clinical Management of Head, Neck and TMJ Pain and Dysfunction* (Philadelphia: W. B. Saunders Company, 1985), 519–20; S. Hoppenfeld, *Physical Examination of the Spine and Extremities* (New York: Appleton-Century-Crofts, 1976), 132.
75. Ibid., 478, 479.
76. L. Brown, ed., *The New Shorter Oxford English Dictionary* (Oxford: Clarendon Press, 1993), 2025.
77. J. Witzig and T. Spahl, *The Clinical Management of Basic Maxillofacial Orthopedic Appliances,* vol. 1, *Mechanics* (Littletown, Mass.: PSG Publishing Company, 1987), 155–60.
78. Ibid., 212.
79. H. Eirew, "An Orthodontic Challenge," *International Journal of Orthodontics* 14 (1976): 21–25.

80. Ibid., 22–23.
81. Ibid., 23.
82. Ibid.
83. J. Witzig and T. Spahl, *The Clinical Management of Basic Maxillofacial Orthopedic Appliances,* vol. 1, *Mechanics* (Littletown, Mass.: PSG Publishing Company, 1987), 162–66.
84. H. Eirew, "An Orthodontic Challenge," *International Journal of Orthodontics* 14 (1976): 24.
85. J. Witzig and T. Spahl, *The Clinical Management of Basic Maxillofacial Orthopedic Appliances,* vol. 1, *Mechanics* (Littletown, Mass.: PSG Publishing Company, 1987), 162–66.
86. J. Hoy, "Clouds of Death: Catostrophic Effects of Wind-Drift Chemicals and Locally Sprayed Pesticides on Western Montana Fauna," *Wise Traditions* 3, no. 3 (Fall 2002): 15.
87. D. Curl, *The Chiropractic Approach to Temporomandibular Disorders* (Baltimore: Williams and Wilkins, 1991), 106–7.
88. A. Fonder, *The Dental Physician* (Rock Falls, Ill.: Medical-Dental Arts, 1985), 273–74.
89. F. Jerome, *Tooth Truth* (San Diego: ProMotion Publishing, 1995), 297.
90. D. Ewing, *Let the TOOTH Be Known,* 2nd ed. (Houston: Holistic Health Alternatives, 2002), 78.
91. F. Jerome, *Tooth Truth* (San Diego: ProMotion Publishing, 1995), 297, 298.
92. J. Witzig and T. Spahl, *The Clinical Management of Basic Maxillofacial Orthopedic Appliances,* vol. 1, *Mechanics* (Littletown, Mass.: PSG Publishing Company, 1987), 193.
93. Ibid.; F. Jerome, *Tooth Truth* (San Diego: ProMotion Publishing, 1995), 296.
94. G. Olson et al., "The Incidence and Severity of Premenstrual Syndrome among Female Craniomandibular Pain Patients," *The Journal of Craniomandibular Practice* 6, no. 4 (October 1988): 330–37; A. Fonder, "Gynecological Problems and the Dental Distress Syndrome," *Basal Facts* 4, no. 4 (1981): 123–32.
95. W. Price, *Nutrition and Physical Degeneration* (Los Angeles: The American Academy of Applied Nutrition, 1945), 357–59.
96. Ibid., 366–67.
97. A. Tredgold, *A Textbook of Mental Deficiency* (Baltimore: The Williams & Wilkens Company, 1947), 122.
98. W. Price, *Nutrition and Physical Degeneration* (Los Angeles: The American Academy of Applied Nutrition, 1945), 367, 368, 370–71.
99. A. Fonder, *The Dental Physician* (Rock Falls, Ill.: Medical-Dental Arts, 1985), 339–50.
100. Ibid.
101. M. Urbanowicz, "Alteration of Vertical Dimension and Its Effect on Head and Neck Posture," *The Journal of Craniomandibular Practice* 9, no. 2 (April 1991): 177; J. Ferguson et al., "A Short Term Controlled Trial of an Adjustable Oral Appliance for the Treatment of Mild to Moderate Obstructive Sleep Apnea," *Thorax* 52 (1997): 362–68.
102. D. Page, *Your Jaws, Your Life* (Baltimore: SmilePage Publishing, 2003), 38, 79, 81.
103. Ibid., 86–87; G. Schuster and R. Giese, "Retrospective Clinical Investigation of the Impact of Early Treatment of Children with Down's Syndrome According to Castillo-Morales," *Journal of Orofacial Orthopedics* 62, no. 4: 255–63.
104. D. Walther, *Applied Kinesiology,* vol. 2 (Pueblo, Colo.: Systems DC, 1983), 366.
105. H. Gonzalez and A. Manns, "Forward Head Posture: Its Structural and Functional Influence on the Stomatognathic System: A Conceptual Study," *The Journal of Craniomandibular Practice* 14, no. 1 (January 1996): 72.
106. H. Gelb, *Clinical Management of Head, Neck and TMJ Pain and Dysfunction* (Philadelphia: W. B. Saunders Company, 1985), 126–29.
107. R. Dart, "The Postural Aspect of Malocclusion," *The Official Journal of the D.A.S.A.* 1, no. 1 (September 1946): 14.
108. D. Walther, *Applied Kinesiology,* vol. 2 (Pueblo, Colo.: Systems DC, 1983), 367.
109. H. Gelb et al., "Relationship of Muscular Strength to Jaw Posture in Sports Dentistry," *New York State Dental Journal,* November 1995, 58–59.
110. Ibid., 59–60; A. Forgione et al., "Strength and Bite, Part I: An Analytical Review," *The Journal of Craniomandibular Practice* 9, no. 4 (October 1991): 305–15; A. Forgione et al., "Strength and Bite, Part II: Testing Isometric Strength Using a Mora Set to a Functional Criterion," *The Journal of Craniomandibular Practice* 10, no. 1 (October 1991): 13–20.
111. H. Gelb, *Clinical Management of Head, Neck and TMJ Pain and Dysfunction* (Philadelphia: W. B. Saunders Company, 1985), 475–79.
112. M. Loudon, "Vertical Dimension—Primary Molar Buildup," *The Functional Orthodontist,* May/June 1987, 38–39.
113. Ibid., 39.
114. D. Page, *Your Jaws, Your Life* (Baltimore: SmilePage Publishing, 2003), 55, 60, 63, 65.
115. Ibid.

116. Ibid., 61.
117. W. Li et al., "Pathogens in the Middle Ear Effusion of Children with Persistent Otitis Media: Implications of Drug Resistance and Complications," *Journal of Microbiology, Immunology and Infections* 34, no. 3 (September 2001): 190–94.
118. B. Palmer, "Breastfeeding: Reducing the Risk for Obstructive Sleep Apnea," *PPNF Journal* 24, no. 1 (Spring 2000): 12.
119. J. Witzig and T. Spahl, *The Clinical Management of Basic Maxillofacial Orthopedic Appliances,* vol. 1, *Mechanics* (Littletown, Mass.: PSG Publishing Company, 1987), 167.
120. Ibid., 185.
121. Ibid., 212, 213.
122. Ibid.
123. G. Smith, "Evaluating Craniomandibular Somatic Dysfunction (CSD) Patient Utilizing the Physiologic Adaptive Range (PAR) Philosophy," *Basal Facts* 5, no. 2 (1985): 36; J. Upledger and J. Vredevoogd, *Craniosacral Therapy* (Chicago: Eastland Press, 1983), 273–358.
124. G. Smith, "Craniodontics," www.drfarid.com/cranio.html.
125. J. Upledger and J. Vredevoogd, *Craniosacral Therapy* (Chicago: Eastland Press, 1983), 152.
126. Ibid., 277.
127. G. Smith, "Dental Bridgework May Be the Source of Your Patient's Headaches, Neck Aches and Facial Pain," *The Source* 3, no. 3 (Summer 1985): 10.
128. A. Fonder, *The Dental Physician* (Rock Falls, Ill.: Medical-Dental Arts, 1985), 283–84.
129. G. Smith, "Dental Bridgework May Be the Source of Your Patient's Headaches, Neck Aches and Facial Pain," *The Source* 3, no. 3 (Summer 1985): 10.
130. Ibid., 11.
131. D. Klinghardt and L. Williams, *Neural Kinesiology I* (Seattle: AANT, 1994), 75.
132. D. Denton, *Craniopathy and Dentistry* (Los Angeles: self-published, 1979), 10–11.
133. J. Upledger and J. Vredevoogd, *Craniosacral Therapy* (Chicago: Eastland Press, 1983), 60.
134. Ibid., 247.
135. D. Klinghardt and L. Williams, *Neural Kinesiology I* (Seattle: AANT, 1994), 75.
136. R. Dart, "Voluntary Musculature in the Human Body: The Double Spiral Arrangement," *British Journal of Physical Medicine* 13 (1950): 265–68.
137. R. Steiner, *Nature's Open Secret* (Herndon, Va..: Anthroposophic Press, 2000), 29.
138. J. Goethe, *Goethes Sämtliche Werke: Schriften zur Naturwissenschaft I* (Stuttgart and Berlin: J. G. Gotta'sche Buchhandlung Nachfolger, 1910–1920), xx. Translation of Goethe's text provided by Tina Cash-Woebling.
139. R. Steiner, *Nature's Open Secret* (Herndon, Va.: Anthroposophic Press, 2000), 23, 27.
140. Ibid., 29–30, 31.
141. K. Barteczko and M. Jacob, "A Reevaluation of the Premaxillary Bone in Humans," *Anatomy and Embryology* 207, no. 6 (March 2004): 417–37.
142. P. Williams, *Gray's Anatomy* (New York: Churchill Livingstone, 1995), 602.

17

MUSCULOSKELETAL DYSFUNCTION

It should be clear, simply through a perusal of the eight common factors that cause malocclusions and TMD outlined in the previous chapter, that the majority of the current population has some form of bite or jaw joint dysfunction. For many, mild dysfunction can be ameliorated during the course of holistic therapies (rebirthing, cavitation surgery, amalgam removal, etc.). Others with more moderate to major jaw and bite dysfunction may require functional appliances, second molar extractions, and/or short-term braces.

Depending on the degree of dysfunction, malocclusions and TMD can cause stress and subsequent adaptation in the rest of the body. These various adaptive mechanisms are particularly common structurally. In fact, the pain patients present with in chiropractic and osteopathic doctors' offices is often referred—in whole or in part—from dysfunction in their teeth and jaws. This is caused by the major neurological influence that the trigeminal nerve (discussed in the previous chapter) has over the rest of the body through its extensive connections throughout the entire spinal cord (e.g., the substantia gelatinosa).[1]

CONTRIBUTING FACTORS TO MUSCULOSKELETAL ADAPTATION

The Direct Jaw-Neck Relationship

Sir Charles Sherrington (1857–1952), a Nobel Prize–winning British neurologist, was the first to elucidate in his research the systemic effects nerves have in the body. His experiments demonstrated that sensory neuron information can vertically overlap several segments in the spinal cord, and that this overlapping occurs in the substantia gelatinosa region. This effect, termed the Sherrington phenomenon, explains why appendicitis pain is often felt in the left side or upper (epigastric) regions of the abdomen, rather than being localized over the inflamed appendix itself (in the lower right abdominal area). This phenomenon occurs because the inflamed sensory nerves from the appendix area that innervate (connect with) the upper lumbar regions of the spinal cord also affect—through the vertical communication up and down the substantia gelatinosa—adjacent areas of the spinal cord (the lower thoracic and lower lumbar) that innervate other parts of the abdomen.[2] This overlapping and relay of referred pain information that occurs in the substantia gelatinosa, which directly connects with the trigeminal spinal nucleus and nerves, is one reason why the jaws and teeth can so greatly affect the cervical spine. In fact, chronic neck pain has been greatly alleviated in many patients, and sometimes even completely cured, with a functional appliance that rebalances their bite and stabilizes their temporomandibular joint (TMJ).

Gravity: Another Major Factor

Another factor greatly contributing to the major influence the jaws and teeth have on the body is gravity. Any disturbed and aberrant postural forces of the jaw and teeth, such as a protruded (too far forward) or retruded (too far backward) jaw, must be continually adapted for posturally by the rest of the body for an individual to stand reasonably erect and to walk straight without listing to one side or the other. All of these various musculoskeletal effects that are primarily initiated by jaw (TMD) and bite (malocclusion) dysfunction are referred to as *stomatognathicsomatic* reflexes, since "stomatognathic" refers to the teeth and jaws collectively.[3*]

Structural Tissues Will "Sacrifice" for Visceral Organ Tissues

As discussed in chapter 16, with the exception of acute trauma and some malocclusions and TMD, joint and muscle pain is characteristically secondary to other factors. These chronic structural symptoms compensate for not only major malocclusions and TMD but also for tonsil and dental focal infections, mercury amalgam toxicity, petroleum chemical poisoning, and other modern insults to the body. The reason is that bones, muscles, and ligaments serve a dual protective function in our bodies. First, these more sturdy tissues house and protect our more delicate and vulnerable internal organs. Second, bones and soft tissues easily adapt, or compensate, to preserve normal function in these vital organs. This latter protective function is unfortunately unfamiliar to many modern osteopaths and chiropractors.

All the structural tissues in the body—bones, muscles, tendons, ligaments, fascia, and teeth—adapt for or "sacrifice" themselves to help preserve function in the more vital organs. For example, the body's innate intelligence will induce a chronic sacroiliac sprain pattern with accompanying low back pain over time to save further degeneration of a dysbiotic and toxic gut (small and large intestine). This chronic referred pain (non-accident-induced) in the sacroiliac region not only is caused by the gut and sacroiliac joint sharing the same (inflamed and disturbed) sympathetic nerve supply but also is induced for the sake of a greater wisdom operating in the body—the preservation of life. This shunting of disturbance from the more-essential-to-life gut to the less-essential-to-life sacroiliac joint is mediated through both higher central nervous system (brain) centers and the enteric nervous system, recently termed the "second brain."[4] Thus, because the assimilation of vital nutrients in the gut is a more important function to the preservation of life than reducing pain in the sacroiliac joints and muscles, these musculoskeletal structures bear the greater burden of stress.

The sacrificial nature of another hard and protective tissue in the body—the teeth—was discussed in chapter 11. The decay and eventual loss of teeth is analogous to the loss of function and resulting pain that also occurs in our hard bones, firm muscles, and sinewy ligaments. Thus, all of these more sturdy and protective structural tissues sacrifice themselves, to a certain degree, to allow more optimal functioning in the underlying vital organs and tissues.* This sacrificial function is further illustrated simply through reviewing the numbers of each of these tissues. That is, humans have only *one* heart, *one* liver, and *two* kidneys. In dramatic contrast, however, they have *32* teeth, about *206* bones, and approximately *639* muscles.[5] The body can much more easily afford to lose function in one or more of these much more numerous structural tissues, as compared with the vital organs that number in the single digits. (See the preference pyramid, figure 11.8, on page 335.)

HOLISTIC CHIROPRACTORS AND OSTEOPATHS MUST BE SUPERIOR DIAGNOSTICIANS

It is imperative that chiropractors, osteopaths, and other structurally oriented physicians be capable of diagnostically differentiating between *primary* joint pain due to the specific misalignment and degeneration of that joint and *secondary* joint pain due to other factors. It is not appropriate, nor even ethical, for that matter, to prescribe ongoing spinal adjustments for months or even years in a patient with chronic back pain that is caused by major temporomandibular joint dysfunction (TMD). Nor is it helpful to a patient in terms of time or money to do lengthy craniosacral therapy over an extended period of time when his tension headaches are secondary to a major Class II (overbite) malocclusion. In fact, these patients will lose much of the healing benefits of their adjustment or craniosacral treatment within hours after the appointment, as soon as they eat their next meal. The aberrant forces from chewing with an abnormal bite or jaw exert such an

**Stomatognathic* is pronounced stow-mah-tog-nath'-ik.

*When one considers the growing number of hip, knee, and other joint replacements, the analogy between sacrificial teeth and joints becomes even more appropriate in these modern times of surgical intervention.

extreme pressure into the bones, fascia, and muscles that much (or all) of the old adapted structural distortion pattern is quickly reinstated. Thus, it is essential that osteopathic and chiropractic physicians be reasonably versed in the signs and symptoms of major bite and jaw dysfunction to guide patients in the correct—and most efficient—direction of healing.

Because teeth, bones, and muscles help protect us from external harm not only through their firm and stabilizing structural makeup but also by sacrificing their integrity and functioning to help preserve the functioning of damaged vital organs, it is again clear why holistic practitioners trained in structural therapies must be the *least myopic* of any of their colleagues in regard to diagnosis and treatment. That is, it is much more probable that the chronic joint or muscle pain with which a patient of a chiropractor or osteopath is presenting is due *not* to primary musculoskeletal dysfunction, but to a secondary organ (or focus) etiology. Thus, due to this typical adaptation pattern, the burden of accurate and precise diagnosis weighs on the chiropractic and osteopathic practitioner's shoulders more heavily than on any other physician specializing in holistic medicine. Unfortunately, as will be discussed in more detail in the later section "What Is a Holistic Chiropractor or Osteopath?" both of these professions have lost much of their holistic roots, and therefore a more comprehensive understanding of how the body works, over the past few decades. However, with a little research and help from appropriate referral sources, prospective patients should be able to find a practitioner who is truly practicing according to his or her holistic origins.

In the following pages, the benefits of accurate diagnosis and appropriate treatment for musculoskeletal symptoms will be thoroughly covered. The first sections will describe the difference between secondary musculoskeletal pain and dysfunction versus primary musculoskeletal pain and dysfunction. The benefits of spinal manipulation, craniosacral therapy, and massage will also be explained. Finally, the tumultuous histories of chiropractors and osteopaths will be briefly outlined, and the definition of a truly holistic practitioner will be proposed.

SECONDARY MUSCULOSKELETAL PAIN AND DYSFUNCTION

As previously discussed, with the exception of acute trauma, most chronic musculoskeletal pain or dysfunction has a deeper underlying cause. The following list summarizes the most common causes of secondary referred pain in the musculoskeletal system:

1. Stomatognathicsomatic referral—secondary musculoskeletal pain or dysfunction referred from a primary malocclusion or TMD
2. Focalsomatic referral—secondary musculoskeletal pain or dysfunction referred from a primary focal infection or scar interference field
3. Gangliosomatic referral—secondary musculoskeletal pain or dysfunction referred from a primary toxic and congested ganglion
4. Viscerosomatic referral—secondary musculoskeletal pain or dysfunction referred from primary organ dysfunction or organ degeneration
5. Psychosomatic referral—secondary musculoskeletal pain or dysfunction referred from primary psychological stress

Stomatognathicsomatic Referral (Secondary Dysfunction from Malocclusion or TMD)

As described previously, because TMD (jaw joint dysfunction) and malocclusions (bad bites) are structural issues themselves, they are included with acute trauma as primary causes of musculoskeletal pain and dysfunction. This primary musculoskeletal dysfunction refers to pain in the *local* jaw and facial muscles and joints induced by the jaw or bite. However, when TMD or a malocclusion induces pain in *distal* tissues—such as in the neck or low back—this pain is secondary to the jaw or bite dysfunction. Thus, any attempt to treat the back pain itself, instead of noticing the primary causative factor (the jaw or bite), would result in not only an incorrect diagnosis but an incorrect (and futile) treatment plan because the back is not causing the back pain. Thus, when back pain is caused by a bad bite or jaw, it is secondary to (or the result of) this bad bite or jaw dysfunction.

As strongly recommended in the previous chapter, it is essential that holistic practitioners be at least reasonably familiar with the signs and symptoms of malocclusions and TMD to appropriately refer to a holistic dentist in these cases. Otherwise an underlying stomatognathicsomatic complaint such as chronic (non-accident-induced) back pain may be misdiagnosed as a primary musculoskeletal symptom for years—or even a lifetime. In these misdiagnosed cases, patients may spend thousands of dollars and hours of their time receiving spinal adjustments and massage, when a functional appliance—in conjunction with these realigning and rebalancing structural therapies—could have greatly reduced (or even cleared) the symptoms within a much shorter time period.

Focalsomatic Referral

(Secondary Dysfunction from Scar Interference Field or Focal Infection)

Scar Interference Fields

In chapter 9, an example of a *focalsomatic* pattern emanating from a scar interference field was described. This example, also referred to as a *cutaneosomatic* reflex, was that of tension headaches (-somatic) arising soon after a bike accident that created a scar interference field (cutaneo-). Untreated scar interference fields—that is, disturbing wrinkles in our sheet of skin—always cause some kind of mild to major musculoskeletal adaptation and dysfunction. These problems can include headaches, joint and muscle pain and tension, decreased range of motion and stiffness, and an abnormal gait (imbalanced walking or running, limping, etc.).

Focal Infections

In the same way, focal infections generate similar musculoskeletal dysfunction patterns. In part 4, it was explained that the particular pattern of musculoskeletal pain or dysfunction can even help identify the exact location of the suspected focal infection. For example, *bilateral* (both right- and left-sided) hip or shoulder pain is often caused by impacted wisdom teeth on *both sides* of the oral cavity, while unilateral hip or shoulder pain is more often secondary to a *single* dental focal infection that is *ipsilateral* (same side) to the pain. For example, right hip pain originating from a (#30) right lower first molar failed root canal is a common focalsomatic relationship. Additionally, systemic joint pain, as is often seen in rheumatoid arthritis or degenerative arthritis, is often secondary to the migration of streptococcus bacteria harbored for decades in a (bilateral) tonsil focal infection.

Structural Therapies Are Effective Once the Focus Is Addressed

When these scar interference fields and focal infections are appropriately diagnosed and reasonably cleared through the effective treatments outlined in chapter 10, then later spinal adjustments, craniosacral therapy, and massage are entirely appropriate and quite effective.

Gangliosomatic Referral

(Secondary Dysfunction from Congested and Toxic Ganglia)

The gangliosomatic relationship refers to musculoskeletal pain and dysfunction secondary to a toxic or congested ganglia (autonomic nerve control centers located throughout the body). In chapter 16, the term *false TMD syndrome* described how chronically contracted and tense jaw muscles (-somatic) adversely affecting the TMJ and occlusion could be generated—in whole or in part—by a toxic and congested (with heavy metals, bacteria, etc.) neighboring vagal ganglion. Other examples of toxic ganglia affecting nearby structural tissues are the sphenopalatine ganglia (under the temple area) triggering headaches, the superior cervical ganglia (upper front of the neck region) contributing to chronic neck and muscle tension, the celiac ganglia (upper abdominal area) affecting the thoracic vertebrae and causing mid-back pain, and the Frankenhäuser's or inferior hypogastric ganglia (surrounding the uterus or prostate) initiating low back and hip pain.

Through manuals and courses such as "Neural Therapy without Needles," holistic practitioners can learn the location of autonomic ganglia and how to appropriately treat them (see chapter 10). Again, it is only after these toxic ganglia are addressed that structural therapies to the symptomatic areas of pain and tension can be truly lasting and effective.

Viscerosomatic Referral
(Secondary Dysfunction from a Disturbed Organ)

Viscerosomatic reflex pathways were also described in chapter 9. *Viscero-* refers to the referred pain (or other symptoms) that can be generated from a primary *visceral,* or organ, dysfunction. This pain is then transferred to a secondary *somatic* tissue, such as the skin, muscles, joints (spinal or extremity), ligaments, or fascia (connective tissue). The corollary to the viscerosomatic referral—that is, a damaged joint (somatic) causing pathology of one form or another in its related organ—is termed a *somatovisceral* reflex.

A holistic chiropractor or osteopath will often suspect a probable viscerosomatic issue from the patient's history. For example, if an individual has eaten a fast-food diet for years, it is likely that his acute low back pain that occurred "from just leaning over to pick up the newspaper" is probably due not to this activity, but to chronically congested and weakened digestive organs. In hindsight, it is simply not logical or reasonable that after twenty years of leaning over to pick up the morning paper this normally benign movement would suddenly trigger severe low back pain. However, what does make sense (physiologically and neurologically) is that the fries and milkshake he ate for dinner the night before overburdened his already burdened pancreas and small intestine so greatly that leaning over the next day triggered this "accident waiting to happen" referred pain pathway—from the gut to the low back.

Brown's and Teale's Research in the Early 1800s

The viscerosomatic connection is the most widely studied of all the various somatic relationships discussed in this section and was first described in 1828 by Dr. Thomas Brown of Scotland.* Dr. Brown's research mostly concentrated on the somatovisceral relationship—that is, joint dysfunction affecting a related organ—but he also observed the reverse of this relationship: "on some occasions, the affection of the spine disorders the digestion, but that, in other instances, indigestion is the primary disease, and the spine merely sympathizes with it."[6]

*However, it should be noted that years earlier, in 1821, through a letter to the editor in the *Quarterly Journal of Science* (vol. 12, pp. 428–30), an English surgeon, Dr. Richard Player, briefly described both the somatovisceral and viscerosomatic referrals.

Later that same year, Dr. Thomas Pridgin Teale elaborated on the viscerosomatic reflex in a 120-page monograph.* The British surgeon noted many associations between spinal pain and the viscera in his research practice, as well as the need for treating not the peripheral (spinal irritation) but the central "more remote and less obvious seat of the disease." Dr. Teale was also aware of the autonomic controlling influence of viscerosomatic referred pain. He observed that various heart and digestive organ disturbances, including palpitations, dyspnea (difficulty breathing), pyrosis (heartburn), gastrodynia (stomach pain), dyspepsia (stomach acidity), and extreme flatulence, could be observed segmentally through the "irritation of the ganglia of the [related] sympathetic nerve."[7] One of his colleagues commented that in regard to these viscerosomatic relationships, "prejudice sometimes operates against the idea of connexions [sic] so remote."[8] It is interesting to note that this prejudice and skeptical attitude—for example, that heart disease is the underlying cause of upper thoracic pain and disturbance, or that an irritable bowel generates chronic low back pain and weakness—is still operant even today.

"Head Zones" in the Late 1800s: Sir Henry Head Documents the Viscerosomatic Reflex

It wasn't until later in the century that another British physician, Sir Henry Head (1861–1940), clinically researched and documented viscerosomatic referred pain and dysfunction.† This renowned late-nineteenth-century neurologist identified through his laborious clinical research the typical cutaneous (skin) areas that were affected (with increased pain and sensitivity) by visceral disease, via sensory sympathetic nerve pathways. Head mapped out these "areas of tenderness in visceral disease" on the body, which are still referred to as "Head zones"

*Dr. Teale asserted, however, that he was the first to name the viscerosomatic, as well as the somatovisceral, referral pathways in the body. Teale's assertion was backed by a colleague who stated that the British surgeon had first described these phenomena as early as 1821. (F. Schiller, "Spinal Irritation and Osteopathy," *Bulletin of the History of Medicine* 45 [1971]: 254.)

†Head was a contemporary of another great neurologist and physiologist, Sir Charles Sherrington, who first studied the *dermatomes* in the body—the areas of the skin supplied by each spinal sensory nerve. In 1900, Head mapped out these specific dermatomal areas on the body based on his research studying the disturbed cutaneous areas caused by shingles (herpes zoster).

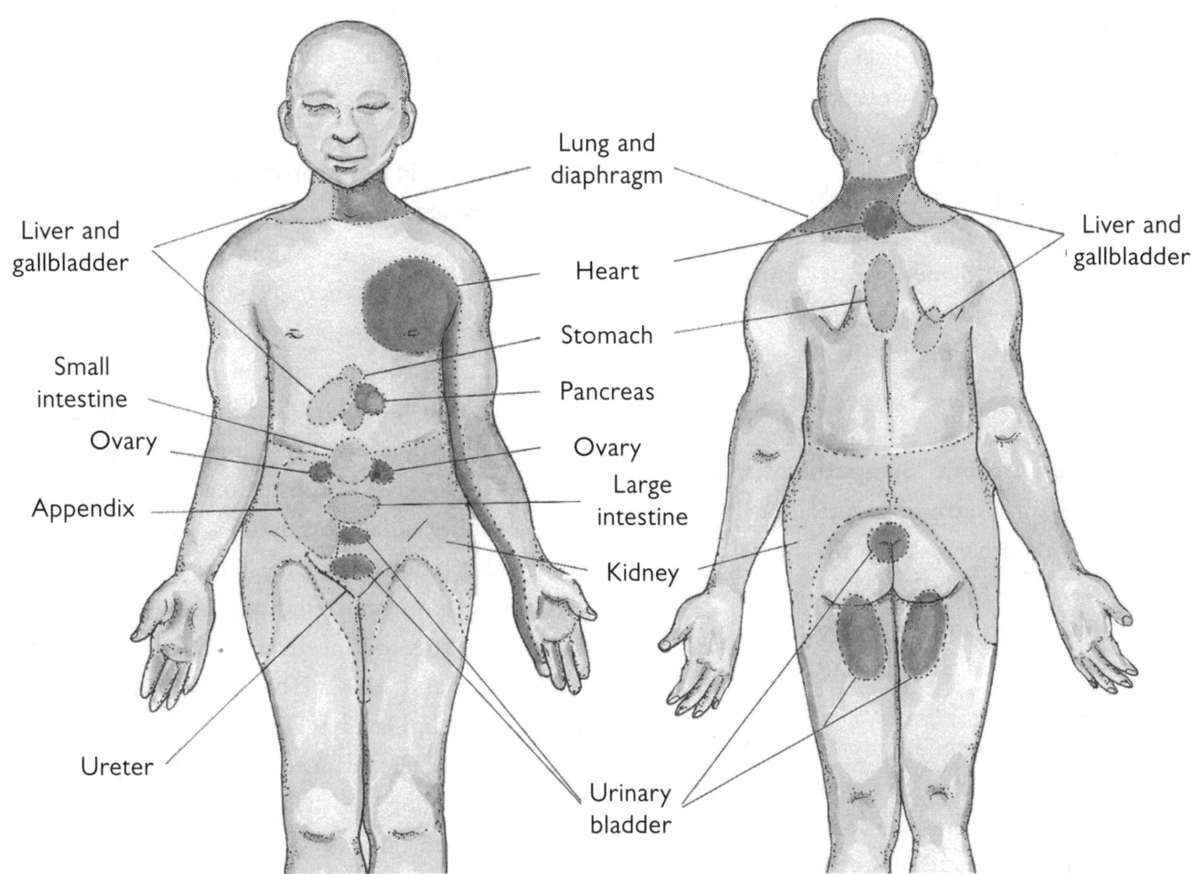

Figure 17.1. The areas of referred pain, also known as "Head zones," are generated from chronic visceral (organ) dysfunction and disease. (See plate 9 for a color version of this figure.)

in European countries and termed "areas of referred pain" in the United States.[9] Head was the first to scientifically prove the viscerosomatic reflex—that is, that sensory impulses from a distressed internal organ can create a disturbance in other tissues that are innervated by the same inflamed nerves.[10] Later researchers such as Jonas H. Kellgren (1938), David Sinclair (1948), and J. M. Hockaday and C. W. M. Whitty (1967) validated Head's findings and mapped out the distal referred pain sites that were consistently triggered after stimulation (injection of salt solutions or scratching the bone with a needle) of various parts of the spine.[11] Other clinical researchers who contributed to the viscerosomatic literature include osteopath Louisa Burns and chiropractor Carl Cleveland, Jr.

Common Viscerosomatic Relationships

Heart Attack Triggers Left Neck and Arm Pain

A well-known example of these viscerosomatic relationships is left chest, neck, and arm referred pain triggered by the inflamed nerves of the heart from an impending myocardial infarction (heart attack). Pain results from inflamed sensory nerve signals from the heart (which lies centrally and slightly to the left in the chest cavity) converging on the C3 through T5 (lower cervical and upper thoracic) spinal segments, which also innervate and therefore inflame the structural tissues (muscles, joints, skin, etc.) of the chest, neck, and arm (see figure 17.1).[12]*

Liver and Gallbladder Dysfunction Generates Right Neck and Shoulder Pain

Another well-known visceromatic referral is right neck, right shoulder, and the tip of the right scapula (shoulder blade) pain secondary to liver and gallbladder dysfunction

*Although burning, crushing, and cutting of the skin and deeper tissues (muscles, tendons, ligaments, etc.) cause severe pain, the noxious stimuli that trigger visceral pain are different. Visceral pain, often dull but sometimes sharp, is primarily caused by distention (bloating), anoxia (lack of oxygen), and acidity (pH imbalance). (H. Hooshmand, *Chronic Pain: Reflex Sympathetic Dystrophy Prevention and Management* [Boca Raton, Fla.: CRC Press, 1993], 83.)

and disease. Additionally, subclinical kidney infections often manifest as chronic low back, hip, or groin and inner thigh pain (or numbness, weakness, rashes, etc.).

Other Common Connections

Other typical referred pain connections are stomach problems referring to the muscles and spinal vertebrae between the shoulder blades, throat inflammation or infection triggering ear pain, and diaphragmatic (breathing) restrictions being felt in the shoulder and neck areas.[13]

Korr's Research on Chronic "Sympathicotonia"

These Head zones, or viscerosomatic relationships, were later confirmed by another visionary in the field of neurophysiology, Irvin Korr, Ph.D. (1909–2004). Dr. Korr was renowned in the osteopathic profession for his innovative research methods demonstrating that chronically "facilitated segments" in the spine can cause visceral pathology through autonomic sympathetic nerve pathways (a somatovisceral reflex). However, he also validated the existence of viscerosomatic pathways—that is, abnormal sympathetic nerve activity in organs can trigger pathology in related tissues innervated by these same nerves. Using an instrument to measure skin resistance (dermometer), Korr consistently found areas of positive sympathetic nerve activity in patients with a history of myocardial infarcts, which Head had originally identified as areas of referred pain (or other sensation) secondary to chronic heart disease.[14] In fact, in one dramatic case, Korr found high sympathetic nerve readings over the chest and scapula heart-reflex areas three weeks before one of his research subjects suffered a heart attack. He noted, however, that the serious effects of this "sustained sympathicotonia"—that is, chronic sympathetic nerve hyperactivity and dysregulation—were often overlooked in standard medical diagnosis.[15] Sadly, it is true that few physicians, with the exception of holistic chiropractors and osteopaths, are clinically knowledgeable about viscerosomatic referred pain and dysfunction, and its major value in accurate differential diagnosis.

> **dermometer:** A dermometer is a device that measures skin resistance. Areas of chronically low skin resistance have been correlated to high underlying sympathetic nerve activity (think more sweaty skin due to increased sympathetic sudomotor activity equals low resistance) caused by chronic visceral (and other) dysfunction in the body.

Viscerosomatic Relationships and Applied Kinesiology

George Goodheart, D.C., and his Applied Kinesiology (AK) colleagues, further advanced the research on these classic viscerosomatic, as well as somatovisceral, reflexes by correlating specific muscles in the body to specific organ relationships. Dr. Goodheart (1918–2008), who originated Applied Kinesiology in 1964, originally derived these relationships primarily through acupuncture organ-meridian correlations. These and other neurological relationships were later augmented through AK clinical research findings using techniques such as positive therapy localizations and "two-pointing."* Goodheart and his AK colleagues, including Walter Schmitt, D.C.; David Walther, D.C.; David Leaf, D.C.; and many others, further correlated specific muscle weakness to congested lymphatic areas (neurolymphatic reflexes) based on the work of Frank Chapman, D.O., as well as to ischemic (blocked) vascular regions (neurovascular reflexes) based on the work of Terence Bennett, D.C.[16]

Through these and other viscerosomatic relationships, Applied Kinesiologists are able to demonstrate clinically, in vivo, to their patients that their chronic muscle and joint pain is often secondary to toxic and dysfunctioning organs. And, for example, an athlete who is "hooked" on sugar is much more motivated to

*A positive therapy localization (TL) is determined when an indicator muscle responds with a change in muscle tone to a challenge that has a significant connection with that TL. For example, when a weak psoas muscle responds to a TL over a kidney, this response is called a positive therapy localization. In AK, the psoas muscles have been correlated clinically to the kidneys. The positive TLs (as well as the weak muscles related to the dysfunctioning viscera) in AK often correspond to Head's original reflex zones that were researched almost a century ago, as well as to Korr's areas of low skin resistance, indicative of (abnormally) high sympathetic nerve activity. A "two-point" is the phenomenon wherein one area correlates to another area or product through a change in muscle strength. For example, when a strong indicator muscle weakens from a TL over the small intestine (a "one-point") but then strengthens when the patient holds a digestive enzyme in his or her mouth, which is a "two-point," this indicates the probable need for this patient to take digestive enzymes to supplement impaired intestinal digestion.

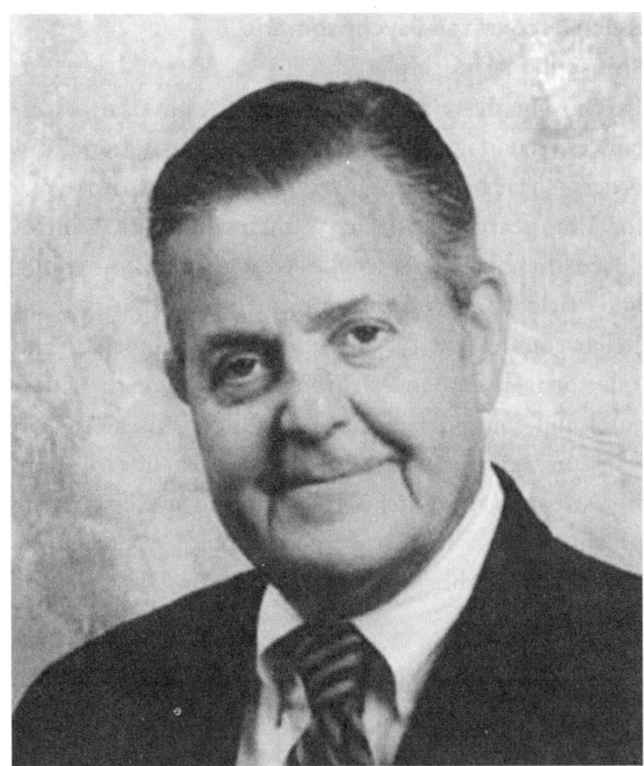

Figure 17.2. George Goodheart, D.C., was the founder of Applied Kinesiology—a muscle testing method that diagnoses and treats viscerosomatic and somatovisceral reflex dysfunction.

give up his toxic habit when an AK physician demonstrates that a dysbiotic small intestine can chronically weaken the quadriceps muscle (the muscle group on the front of the thighs). Applied Kinesiology treatment for this exhausted small intestine, as well as other organs, can then be made through various therapies to the meridian, lymphatic, and vascular related points, as well as through nutritional support, dietary changes, and craniosacral and spinal manipulation. Over time, clinical success can be demonstrated by the strengthening of this quadriceps muscle, as well as enhanced athletic performance and a healthier body and mind. Although more research is needed in this exciting field of clinical science, a significant number of studies attesting to the efficacy of AK diagnosis and treatment have been published in the scientific literature.[17]

- For licensed physicians who are interested in learning Applied Kinesiology, contact the International College of Applied Kinesiology (ICAK) at (913) 384-5336 or visit the website at www.icakusa.com.
- For practitioners without a doctorate degree (e.g., acupuncturists, physical therapists, nutritionists, etc.), another AK physician, John Thie, D.C., later originated the Touch for Health (TFH) Foundation, which teaches many similar concepts. For TFH classes near you, visit the website www.touch4health.com.

Clinical Kinesiology

Later a protégé of Dr. Goodheart's, Alan Beardall, D.C. (1938–1987), further illuminated the viscerosomatic relationship with his exhaustive and painstakingly precise clinical research. By identifying functional divisions within existing muscles and then isolating their specific reflexes, Beardall expanded Goodheart's original 54 muscles into more than 250 muscle relationships. Through this innovative research, as well as other clinical investigations including the use of specific finger positions known as *hand modes* or *mudras* to further the specificity of diagnosis and treatment, Beardall originated in 1975 his own form of advanced muscle testing, called Clinical Kinesiology (CK).[18]

In particular, Beardall emphasized the importance of

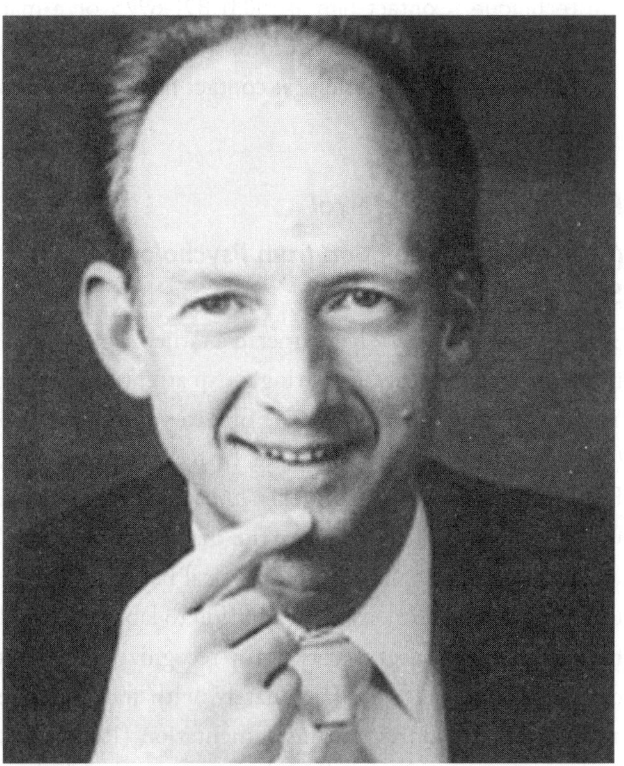

Figure 17.3. Alan Beardall, D.C., originated Clinical Kinesiology and greatly expanded diagnostic testing in the field of muscle testing through the use of hand modes.

the viscerosomatic relationship in Clinical Kinesiology. For example, he often discussed the adaptive nature of the first vertebra in the spine, termed the *atlas.* This ringlike bone, the only one in the spinal column without a vertebral body, constantly adapts (shifts positions) to maintain the sensitive and crucial balance between the head and the neck. Dr. Beardall often taught that because of the direct relationship with the vagus nerve that provides parasympathetic innervation to the digestive organs (viscera), anyone who continually eats his or her primary allergenic foods will *never* maintain a stable atlas (somatic). Thus, patients who must continually get chiropractic cervical adjustments should consider trying the two-week elimination-challenge test (discussed in chapter 6) to determine whether the underlying cause of their chronic upper neck pain is from a viscero- (stomach and intestines) -somatic (atlas) origin. It is interesting to note that almost a century earlier, Dr. Head had also observed that "organs innervated by the vagus nerve would often refer pain to cutaneous zones related to cervical spinal nerves."[19]

▶ For those interested in learning Clinical Kinesiology, Dr. Beardall's son, Dr. Chris Beardall, teaches this technique. Contact him at (503) 891-6925 or e-mail him at beardall@hotmail.com. Robert Shane also teaches Clinical Kinesiology; contact him at shanebob @msn.com.

Psychosomatic Referral (Secondary Dysfunction from Psychological Stress)

The term *psychosomatic* has garnered a rather negative connotation over the years, conjuring up an attention-seeking and emotionally dependent type of patient with no real (or at least discernible) problems. In many cases, as Dr. Hooshmand states in his book *Chronic Pain,* this term was too often applied "to cover the diagnostic shortfall" when the doctor could find no physical basis for disease using limited physical exam, in addition to laboratory and radiographic measures that typically recognize only gross disease and pathology.[20] Fortunately, with more precise and subtle procedures and instrumentation (PET scans, brain mapping, etc.), as well as the exponential growth of psychoneuroimmunological research in recent years, psychosomatic illnesses are recognized today as real syndromes that have a significant impact on the physical body.

Reich Recognized Psychosomatic "Muscular Armoring"

Psychosomatic relationships—that is, physical disturbances secondary to primary mental or emotional disorders—have been recognized in the field of psychology for almost a century. Dr. Wilhelm Reich first introduced these concepts to the West through his mind-body field of specialization termed *character analysis.* Reich could identify patients' particular mental and emotional disturbances through analysis of their postural and "muscular armoring." One of his most brilliant protégés (as well as patients), Alexander Lowen, M.D., expanded Reich's research and understanding of chronically held and unconscious psychosomatic tension by establishing the Institute for Bioenergetic Analysis in 1956.[21]

Lowen Correlated Abnormal Postures to Negative Emotions

Lowen identified many aberrant body postures and correlated them to various suppressed negative thoughts and feelings. For example, individuals with psychosomatically caused low back pain are often suppressing feelings of inferiority and unworthiness by adapting a locked-knees and slumped-shoulders postural habit. Over time, this abnormal and stressful body position exerts undue pressure on the sacroiliac joints and excessive wear and tear on the lumbosacral muscles and ligaments, resulting in low back pain and tension. Additionally, the expression of chronic fear is often seen in a "coat-hanger" posture: shoulders raised and somewhat squared off, head and neck inclined forward, chest raised, and the arms hanging loosely from their joints. Dr. Lowen comments on the insidious nature of this classic musculoskeletal holding pattern that often contributes to chronic neck and shoulder pain and tension, as well as headaches:

> Habitually raised shoulders reveal that the person is locked in an attitude of fear he cannot shrug off, since he is unaware of being frightened. Generally, the situation that caused the fear is forgotten and the emotion itself has been suppressed. Such habitual postures do not develop from a single experience but represent a continued exposure to a fright-

> ening situation. For example, this could be the experience of a boy who was long afraid of his father.[22]

While Lowen most typically observed the coat-hanger posture in males, in older females he more often witnessed the "meat-hook" posture signaled by a prominent "dowager's hump" (upper thoracic kyphosis),* developed over time by feelings of unexpressed anger (see figure 17.4):

> In animals, a cat or a dog, the feeling of anger is manifested by the erection of hair along the spine and by the arching of the back. Darwin pointed this out in *The Expression of the Emotions in Man and Animals.* My reading of the body tells me the hump is produced by the pileup of blocked anger. Its occurrence in older women indicates that it represents the gradual piling up of unexpressed anger as a result of a lifetime's frustration.[23]

*A dowager's hump occurs through osteoporosis of the spine, which allows a prominent bowing in the upper thoracic region (upper back area) and a rounding forward of the shoulders.

Knowledgeable Practitioners Refer Appropriately

Once again, in these cases, it is often up to the holistic chiropractic or osteopathic physician to recognize a patient suffering from psychosomatically induced musculoskeletal pain and tension, and to refer appropriately. In these cases, the combination of appropriate structural therapies (spinal adjustments, craniosacral therapy, or massage) with experiential psychological approaches such as rebirthing that allow the patient to fully relive and release buried emotions, physical sensations, and vivid sensory data is often superlative to conventional talk therapies.* (See chapter 18 for more information on rebirthing or breath therapy.) Additionally, Lowen's bioenergetic exercises, the Feldenkrais method, and many other mind-body balancing techniques (tai chi, yoga, chi kung, Pilates, etc.) can be extremely effective in the understanding and release of chronically held body-mind painful patterns. As summarized here by Alexander Lowen:

*However, gentle counseling techniques are most appropriate for patients who have repressed great stores of painful memories, especially initially, or are not emotionally stable enough for the often strong releases that rebirthing and other experiential techniques can produce. Again, it is up to the referring physician and the therapist (or psychologist or psychiatrist) to make this clinical decision.

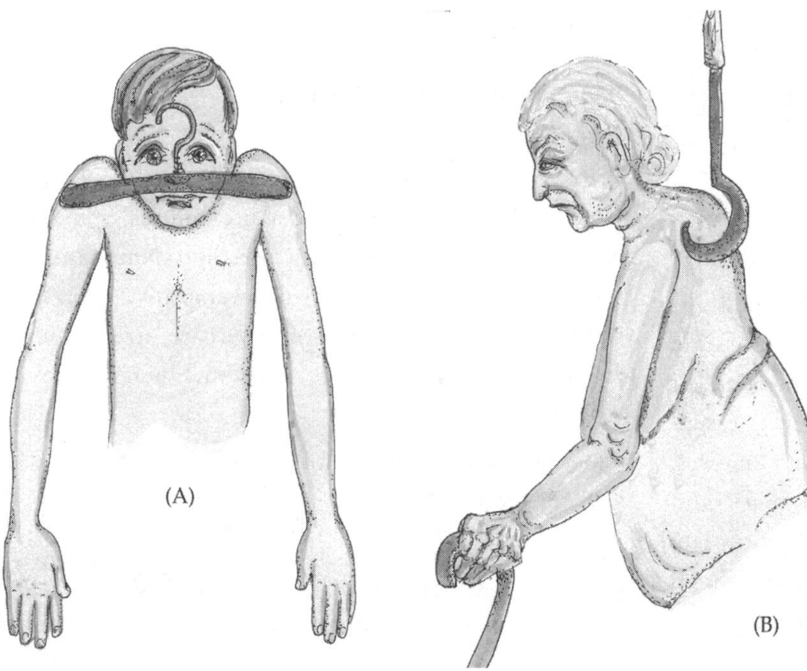

Figure 17.4. Abnormal postural habit patterns associated with unconscious chronic fear—the "coat-hanger" (A)—and chronic anger—the "meat hook" (B)

> Rigidity or chronic tension diminishes one's aliveness and decreases one's energy. At birth, an organism is in its most alive, most fluid state; at death, rigidity is total, rigor mortis. We cannot avoid the rigidity that comes with age. What we can avoid is the rigidity due to chronic muscular tensions resulting from unresolved emotional conflicts.[24]

- ▶ For information about bioenergetic analysis, visit www.bioenergetic-therapy.org or www.bioenergeticspress.com.
- ▶ For information about the Feldenkrais method, call (866) 333-6248 or visit the website www.feldenkrais.com.
- ▶ For nearby yoga, tai chi, chi kung, or Pilates classes, consult your yellow pages or the holistic directory in weekly magazines or other local publications.

PRIMARY MUSCULOSKELETAL PAIN AND DYSFUNCTION

When one is injured in an accident, fight, or other trauma, the pain and dysfunction are due to the primary effect of the specifically strained or crushed muscles, injured nerves, sprained or torn ligaments, broken skin, or fractured bones.

"Macrotrauma" or Acute Trauma

As discussed previously, acute (recent) trauma, also referred to as *macrotrauma,* is one of the major exceptions to the typical secondary aspects of most musculoskeletal pain.

Prompt and Appropriate Structural Therapies Are Essential

With these acute injuries, time is vital. An accurate diagnosis by a chiropractic or osteopathic physician, or in the emergency room by a medical doctor, is essential, especially in the case of moderate to severe injuries. If necessary, fractures must be diagnosed and set, and larger wounds sutured together promptly. Appropriate structural therapies—spinal adjustments, craniosacral manipulation, or massage—and acute homeopathic remedies should also be rendered as soon as possible. These remedies include Arnica montana for muscle strain, bruising, and bleeding; Cantharis vesicatoria for serious burns; Hypericum perforatum for injury to the nerves or the spinal cord; and Symphytum officinale, or "boneknit," to heal fractures.* Additionally, in contrast to the care of chronic musculoskeletal pain, it is essential in the case of acute injury that patients receive several, or even daily, treatments for the first week or two, tapering off after a few weeks or months (depending on the severity) as signs and symptoms improve. Finally, in the case of major injuries with lasting repercussions, longer-term physical therapy and occupational therapy sessions to retrain functioning (walking, range of motion, prosthetic use, etc.) are essential.

Unhealed Acute Trauma Injuries Generate Somatovisceral Reflexes

If these acute macrotrauma injuries are serious and are not treated, or are not treated adequately, then deeper manifestations from these injured joints and tissues can arise over time. In these cases, the damaged joints and muscles eventually cause some form of dysfunction in their related target organs, resulting in a chronic somatovisceral disturbance. Unfortunately, few physicians have the training and knowledge to diagnose these long-standing somatovisceral reflex patterns, when their patients present with seemingly unrelated chronic heart disease, bladder dysfunction, or asthma.

"Microtrauma" or Chronic Repetitive Trauma

Primary somatovisceral referrals do not arise simply from neglected or maltreated acute injuries. Spinal and extremity subluxations (joint misalignments) and persistent muscle strain can also develop over time from the chronic *microtrauma* of repetitive stress injuries from typing (carpal tunnel syndrome); bending, twist-

*However, it should be mentioned that Symphytum acts *so* quickly in mending broken bones that it should not be administered if the fracture is compound (bone is sticking out of the skin) or comminuted (splintered or crushed bone), until the bone has been surgically set. Otherwise, it can potentially heal the misaligned bone or bony fragments in the wrong position.

ing, or lifting in jobs requiring heavy labor; overtraining athletically (stress fractures, shin splints); extensive sitting (grad student syndrome or truck driving); or standing on hard floors all day (sales clerks). Over time, these structurally induced wear-and-tear injuries damage joints so significantly that they may then begin to initiate more serious visceral dysfunction and disease in the related organs. In fact, it has been proposed that one of the primary reasons that many chiropractors and dentists finally succumb to heart disease is that the bending over required in the manipulation of the spine and in detailed dental work strains the cervical and upper thoracic spinal muscles, which share the same sympathetic nerves that innervate the heart (T1 though T4).

The Somatovisceral Reflex (Spinal-Organ Referrals)

Thus, serious acute joint injuries that do not heal, repetitive strain injuries (gardening, physical labor, athletics, etc.), and congenital bony malformations (scoliosis, dislocation of the hips, club foot, etc.) are all examples of chronic *primary* structural dysfunction that can *secondarily* adversely affect visceral organs and generate a long-term somatovisceral reflex. These spinal-organ somatovisceral relationships, primarily triggered by chronic vertebral joint fixations in the spine, are mediated through autonomic nerve pathways. The reverse pathway of viscerosomatic reflexes—that is, impaired organs that generate joint and muscle pain in the spine—is also transmitted by these same autonomic nerves. An example of both these reflexes is illustrated in figure 17.5.

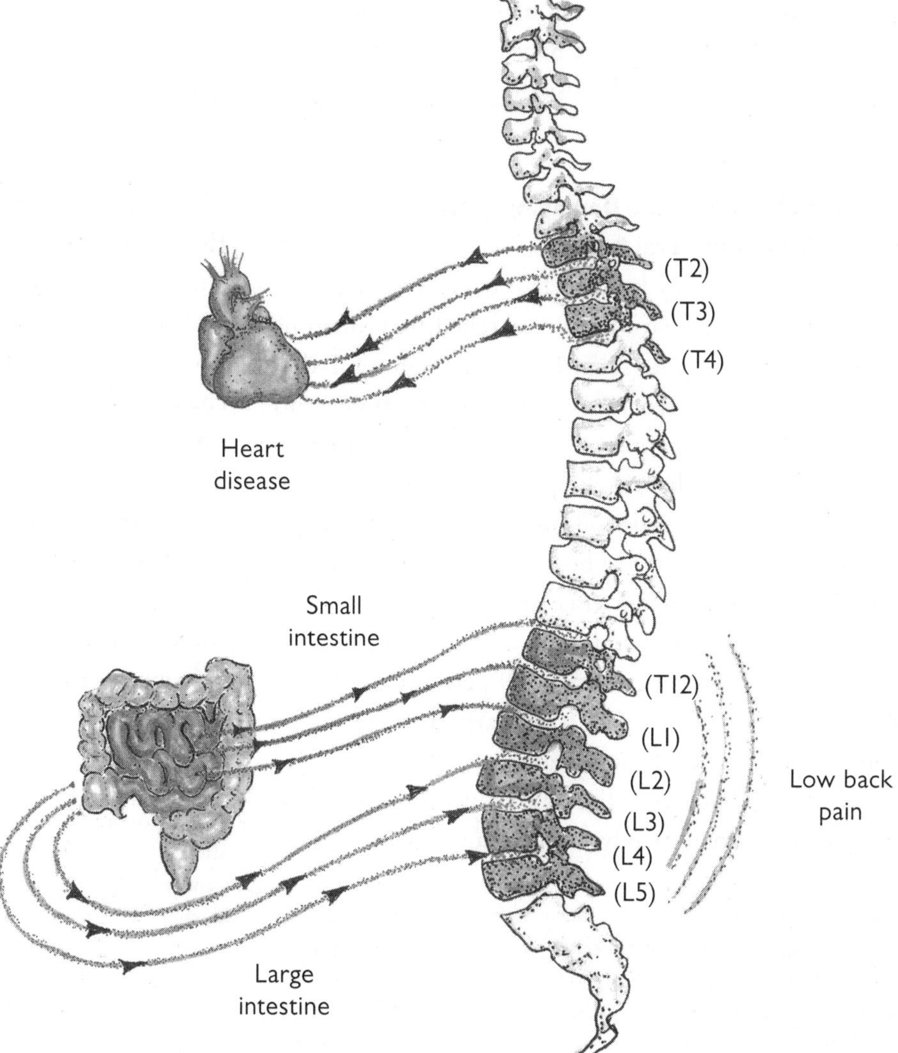

Figure 17.5. Dentists who chronically strain their neck and upper back leaning over at work for years may eventually experience heart problems, through inflamed autonomic somatovisceral (spinal-heart) nerve pathways. An individual who eats sugar and junk food may over time experience chronic low back pain through inflamed autonomic viscerosomatic (intestinal-spinal) nerve pathways. (See plate 10 for a color rendition of this figure.)

Origins of the Somatovisceral Referral Theory

Dr. Thomas Brown of Scotland originally described these somatovisceral referrals, as well as viscerosomatic relationships. In fact, Brown was also the first physician to introduce the term *spinal irritation,* a concept that later greatly influenced early chiropractors and osteopaths.[25] In the 1828 *Glasgow Medical Journal,* he reported on his observation of the parts of the spinal cord affecting the organs, such as the dorsal spine (thoracic) affecting thoracic organs (stomach, pancreas, heart, etc.) and the lumbar spine's nerve connections to the abdominal and pelvic organs.[26] He further recorded his success from the treatment of the painful spinal area, stating that the somatovisceral disturbance "yields, if the irritation of the spine is removed, and returns whenever this irritation is renewed."[27]* As described previously, Dr. Thomas Pridgin Teale of England later published a monograph detailing twenty-two cases that illustrated the somatovisceral referral, and he identified the spinal irritation through autonomic nerve signals such as "perverted or impaired" skin "sensibility" and muscle tremors or spasms.[28]

Research Validates the Damaging Effects of the Somatovisceral Reflex

Since their discovery by Brown and Teale, somatovisceral relationships have been researched by numerous other physicians and scientists. Such common disturbances as impaired heart and lung function[29] and various digestive disorders[30] have been correlated to cervical (neck) or thoracic (upper and mid-back) spinal injuries. Noncongenital scoliosis (curvature of the spine not apparent at birth) has been particularly researched and linked to subsequent visceral disease. In fact, three separate studies—two on cadavers and one on live animals—revealed a better than 99 percent correlation between the scoliotic apex (the sharpest angle in the spinal vertebrae) and the diseased organ.[31] In another study of fifty cadavers, disease that was observed histologically (through study of the tissues) in 139 organs was correlated to the spinal curvatures and deformities that shared the same sympathetic nerve innervation 128 times, resulting in a dramatic 92 percent positive somatovisceral correlation.[32]* In related research studies, sudden infant death syndrome (SIDS or crib death) has been correlated to latent (undetected) upper cervical spinal cord injuries as a result of traumatic births (especially breech and forceps deliveries).[33]

OTHER SOMATIC DISTURBANCES SECONDARY TO MUSCULOSKELETAL DYSFUNCTION

The viscera or organs are not the only targets from somatic disturbance. Although it is a less common scenario, the jaws and dental occlusion (somatostomatognathic referral), focal areas (somatofocal referral), the ganglia (somatoganglionic referral), and an individual's mental and emotional state (somatopsychic referral) can all be affected and secondary to chronic spinal subluxations, cranial bone misalignments, muscle tension and spasm, and aberrant postural habits.

The Viscerosomatic Reflex More Common than the Somatovisceral

The viscerosomatic referral is typically more common and more pathological than the somatovisceral reflex because the *less essential* musculoskeletal structures characteristically adapt in response to the *more essential* vital organs, or viscera. (See "Structural Tissues Will 'Sacrifice' for Visceral Organ Tissues" earlier in this chapter.) However, unhealed acute macrotrauma or repetitive microtrauma, as described in this section, although not as common, certainly do occur. Therefore, these somatovisceral reflexes must also be recognized and appropriately diagnosed and treated.

*The principal treatments for pain or irritation at this time were leeches, cupping, or counter irritation by blisters to the spine. Although "bonesetters" who performed various manipulations of the spine were extant in Europe, physicians did not use these methods until the late nineteenth century when osteopathic and chiropractic medicine originated in the United States.

*Furthermore, in ten of eleven subjects in which the curvatures did not correlate, the curvatures were found in vertebrae just adjacent to the curve. Because nerve fibers pass up three segments and down two segments when entering or leaving a segment in the spinal cord, these adjacent segments could also have contributed to visceral disease. Thus, by including adjacent vertebral segments, this study found a 99 percent (138 out of 139) correlation between spinal curvatures and the visceral organs that shared the same sympathetic nerve outflow.

That "Old Whiplash" Rarely the Primary Problem

However, although significant somatovisceral derangements can continue from unhealed *major* injuries, minor to moderate accidents rarely induce significant long-term organ dysfunction, or even, for that matter, joint or muscle pain. For example, although many patients present with neck or back pain because of "a whiplash accident that occurred ten years ago," these injuries rarely cause significant long-standing tissue damage. Although post-injury soft-tissue damage and abnormal structural patterns can remain for months, and even years, without adequate treatment, they rarely remain as the primary disturbing effect in the body. Nor are they usually consequential enough (in the case of these mild to moderate injuries) to continue to generate significant dysfunction in related target organs (somatovisceral referral). Muscles, ligaments, and joints heal over time a lot more effectively than impaired visceral digestive organs, which are typically subjected to a more serious injury—the daily bombardment of toxic and allergenic foods. Although there can certainly be subtle (or worse) *somatovisceral* dysfunction from an old injury, in most cases the daily stress of life on the vital organs is much more enervating, and this resulting ever-present *viscerosomatic* pattern is typically more serious. For example, a patient's chronic neck pain is more likely to be secondary to her allergy to dairy, which she unknowingly eats daily. Over time, this daily milk ingestion creates a chronic viscerosomatic reflex, inflaming the parasympathetic nerves (vagus) that run from her stomach and intestine to her cervical (neck) area. Thus, the more injurious assaults to survival—organ disease and degeneration, toxic diets and allergenic foods, mercury amalgam fillings and chronic focal infections—affect the body more strongly than mild to moderate musculoskeletal injuries, and therefore typically trigger more viscerosomatic referrals.

A Vicious Reflex Cycle

It often can be difficult differentiating between "the chicken and the egg"—that is, between a primary viscerosomatic and a primary somatovisceral reflex. For example, it is not easy to determine whether a patient's heart disease came first and is the primary factor underlying his chronic upper thoracic subluxations (a viscerosomatic referral) *or* if the heart disease is actually secondary to major repetitive stress to the upper spinal area caused by years of heavy lifting at his job.[34] Furthermore, after a certain amount of time, these diagnostic distinctions blur because both the musculoskeletal areas of dysfunction and the viscera eventually become seriously damaged and degenerated without effective intervention. Thus, each pathology potentiates the other, resulting in a chronic cycle of inflammation and dysfunction between the spine and its target organ.

Treat Both the Spine and the Organ

In these chronic cyclical pathologies, it is most efficacious to simultaneously treat the major joint and muscle areas along with the related visceral dysfunction. Thus, in the office of a holistic Applied Kinesiologist, when the heart region and the upper thoracic (upper back) vertebrae both test positive and are consistent with the patient's history, physical exam, and laboratory findings, this strongly indicates a treatment plan that should include spinal adjustments for the somatovisceral (thoracic/heart) reflex, as well as nutritional and dietary support for the chronic viscerosomatic (heart/thoracic) referral.* *Radical Medicine*–oriented physicians† would also rule out other pathology such as heart-damaging foci (dental and tonsil bacterial focal infections), toxic ganglia (vagal, upper thoracic sympathetic, cardiac plexus, etc.), and heavy metal intoxication (amalgam fillings, nickel crowns, and dental galvanism).

TREATMENT: SPINAL MANIPULATION

The manual correction of spinal misalignments, or *subluxations,* is primarily performed by chiropractors and a small number of osteopaths. A *subluxation* is simply a disturbed joint created by the deranged positioning or motion of one bone in relation to another.[35] This (immobile or hypermobile) misalignment compresses and inflames the nerve roots exiting the spinal cord through

*Applied Kinesiology protocols also include the treatment of neurovascular, neurolymphatic, and acupuncture points; craniosacral therapy; herbal and drainage remedies; assessment of related emotional issues; and other holistic therapies. See appendix 3, "Energetic Testing Explained" for more information on Applied Kinesiology.

†This also may include Applied Kinesiology physicians.

the bony holes between the vertebrae (intervertebral foramina).* Subluxations cause (mild to major) pain, numbness, muscle weakness or spasm, and over time some level of dysfunction in the target organs that are served by the same autonomic nerves (the viscerosomatic pathway). Subluxations, also known as *fixations,* can be located anywhere in the body but are most typically diagnosed in the spinal vertebrae. The nerve interference caused from a fixated joint can cause *hypo*-sympathetic effects (vasodilation, immunosuppression, reduced muscle tone, etc.) as well as *hyper*-sympathetic neurological effects (pain, visceral dysfunction, muscle spasm, etc.).[36] Spinal fixations, although a chiropractic and osteopathic specialty, are a well-known pathology among all disciplines.[37]

subluxation: *Sub*-luxation was originally coined to indicate a minor displacement or partial malpositioning of a joint, as opposed to *luxation,* which refers to the complete malposition, or dislocation, of a joint.

fixation: A fixation is defined as a loss of normal motion and function between *two* or more adjacent vertebrae, as opposed to the malposition of *one* vertebra in relation to another in subluxations.

JOINT MANIPULATION AND ORTHOPEDIC TRAINING

In a study published in 1991 in the *American Journal of Public Health,* joint manipulation was done 94 percent of the time by chiropractors, 4 percent of the time by osteopaths, and 2 percent of the time by medical doctors (e.g., orthopedists and physiatrists). In a more recent 2004 review published in *Physician and Sportsmedicine,* it was revealed that the "average time spent in rotations or courses devoted to orthopedics during medical school was only 2.1 weeks. One third of these examinees graduated without *any* formal training in orthopedics."[38]

---

*Only three of the thirty-one pairs of nerve roots do not exit the spinal column through the intervertebral foramina. These are the first cervical roots, which exit between the atlas (first vertebra) and the occiput (back of the head), and the last sacral roots and the coccygeal nerves (there is only one pair of coccygeal nerve roots), which exit through the sacral hiatus. (J. Dvorak and V. Dvorak, *Manual Medicine* [New York: Georg Thieme Verlag, 1984], 28.)

History of Spinal Manipulation

The treatment of spinal fixations through various manipulative therapies has been recorded for millennia. Ancient China, Japan, Tibet, India, Babylonia (Iraq), Polynesia, and Central America all utilized manipulative therapies.[39] Many years before Christ, ancient Egyptians practiced the "replacing of displaced vertebra," and early Greek physicians used spinal manipulation to cure disease.[40] In fact, the father of medicine himself, Hippocrates, instructed other physicians in a manipulative technique for treating vertebral fixations that is strikingly similar to the modern-day chiropractic recoil-adjusting method:

> [T]he physician or anyone else who is strong and not ignorant should place the thenar [palm] of the one hand upon the protuberance and the thenar of the other hand upon the former, to force the particular vertebra, by a quick jerk, to slip back into its former proper place.[41]

However, it wasn't until the late nineteenth century that the art and science of manipulative healing was formalized into the two fields of healing known today as osteopathy and chiropractic.

The Origins of Osteopathy

Osteopathy's founder, Andrew Taylor Still (1828–1917), was the son of a Methodist preacher who supported his family at the time of Andrew's birth by farming and practicing medicine. As an adult, Dr. Still* practiced conventional medicine for a period but was also strongly influenced by the tenets of magnetic healing, which emphasized "the metaphor of man as a divinely ordained machine." Magnetic healers in the United States such as Andrew Jackson Davis (1826–1910) and Edwin Dwight Babbitt (1828–1905) espoused the use of spinal treatments more so than their European colleagues in the treatment of many illnesses including asthma, headache, muscular complaints, and convulsions. At some point during the late 1870s, Still also became interested in bonesetting, an ancient form of

*Still's medical education was typical of that of a self-taught country doctor. Before the opening of his practice in 1854, it consisted of work performed at his father's side and the study of texts in anatomy, physiology, surgery, and materia medica (book of remedies).

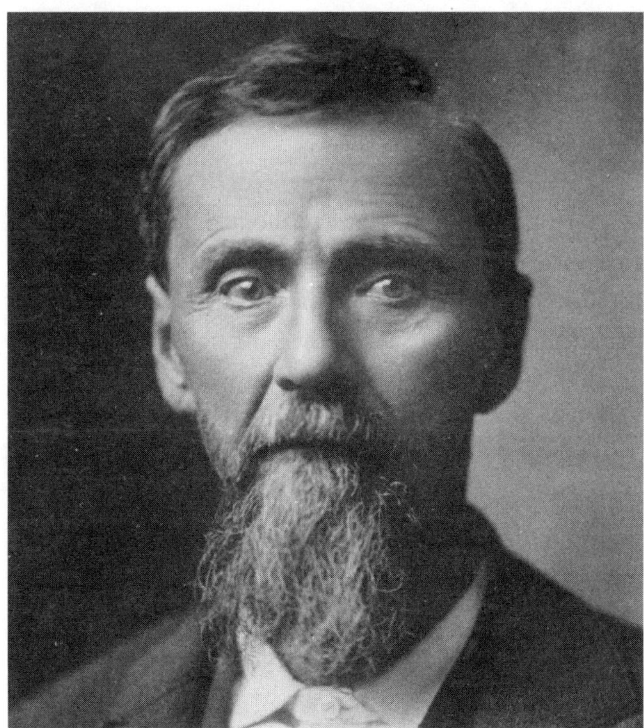

Figure 17.6. Dr. Andrew Taylor Still, the founder of osteopathy (photograph courtesy of the Still National Osteopathic Museum and National Center for Osteopathic History)

manipulative practice, and began to advertise himself as the "lightning bonesetter." Through his skillful manipulation of the spinal vertebra back into their "proper position," Still gained renown throughout Missouri by curing many patients.[42] He became particularly well respected in Kirksville, where the paralyzed daughter of the town's minister regained the ability to walk after his spinal treatments.

MAGNETIC HEALING AND BONESETTING

The field of magnetic healing was founded by Austrian physician Franz Mesmer (1734–1815). Dr. Mesmer postulated that an invisible and universal magnetic fluid or spirit flowed throughout the body, and that too much or not enough of this energy was the cause of disease, particularly nervous disorders. Mesmer's early cures attracted patients from all across Austria; however, pressure from the Vienna medical doctors' association forced his departure to Paris. Although Mesmer was not the first physician to heal through the use of touch, "he was the first to fashion this approach into a coherent system of medical practice."[43] In America, many lay healers and physicians practiced magnetic therapy, which is similar to the current techniques of Reiki and Therapeutic Touch, as well as the more energetic forms of spinal manipulation such as Network Chiropractic, Logan Basic, and Spinal Touch.[44]

Bonesetters were so successful in manipulating painful and diseased joints that they not only treated the poor who could not afford a regular physician but also had the patronage of the upper classes, including many of the royalty in Europe. Bonesetters were active in the United States since the colonial era. In 1884, it was estimated that in every city in the United States "may be found individuals claiming mysterious and magical powers of curing disease, setting bones, and relieving pain by the immediate application of their hands."[45]

Later, in 1892, Still opened the American School of Osteopathy in this small Missouri town, in which he charged the first eighteen students $500 for several months of his personal instruction.* Based on the great healing successes of the school's infirmary and the later expansion of its faculty and curriculum—and despite the attempts of the Missouri state medical association to stop them—osteopaths were licensed to practice in the state of Missouri in 1897.[46] This legislative triumph was celebrated by students and townspeople alike as they marched down the streets cheering:

Rah! Rah! Rah!
Missouri passed the bill
For AT Still
Goodbye Pill†

*Osteopathic college currently consists of a four-year curriculum with completion of pre-med undergraduate courses required before entering—the same as for chiropractic, naturopathic, and medical schools. (See appendix 1 for more information on the training of D.O.s.) Medical education in the late nineteenth and early twentieth centuries was also "hopelessly inadequate" and did not improve until after the findings of the Flexner Report were published in 1910. (H. Coulter, *Divided Legacy: The Conflict between Homoeopathy and the American Medical Association* [Berkeley, Calif.: North Atlantic Books, 1982], 215, 446.)

†Dr. Still greatly eschewed the use of allopathic "fatal drugs" and even homeopathy, stating, "No homeopathic practice with its sugar coated pills, must be allowed to stain or pollute our spotless name." (N. Gevitz, *The DOs* [Baltimore: The Johns Hopkins University Press, 1982], 23.)

We are the people
Of Kirksville.[47]

▶ For more detailed information of the history of osteopathic medicine, read *The DOs: Osteopathic Medicine in America* by Norman Gevitz, published by the Johns Hopkins University Press.

The Origins of Chiropractic

Just a few years later, in 1895, Daniel David Palmer (1845–1913) founded the field of chiropractic, which also centered on healing through spinal manipulation.[48] Dr. D. D. Palmer was also a magnetic healer who practiced in Davenport, Iowa. Like Still, Palmer was inspired to teach his method after a miraculous cure. One day a janitor who worked in Palmer's office building told him that he had gone deaf seventeen years earlier after something "gave way" in his back. Palmer, reasoning that a displaced vertebra was the cause, manipulated the man's fourth thoracic (T4) spinal segment and the astonished janitor then announced that his hearing had fully returned.* After this and other successes, Palmer began to teach his adjusting technique in 1898 in Davenport, Iowa, in a school that was later named Palmer Chiropractic College.[49]

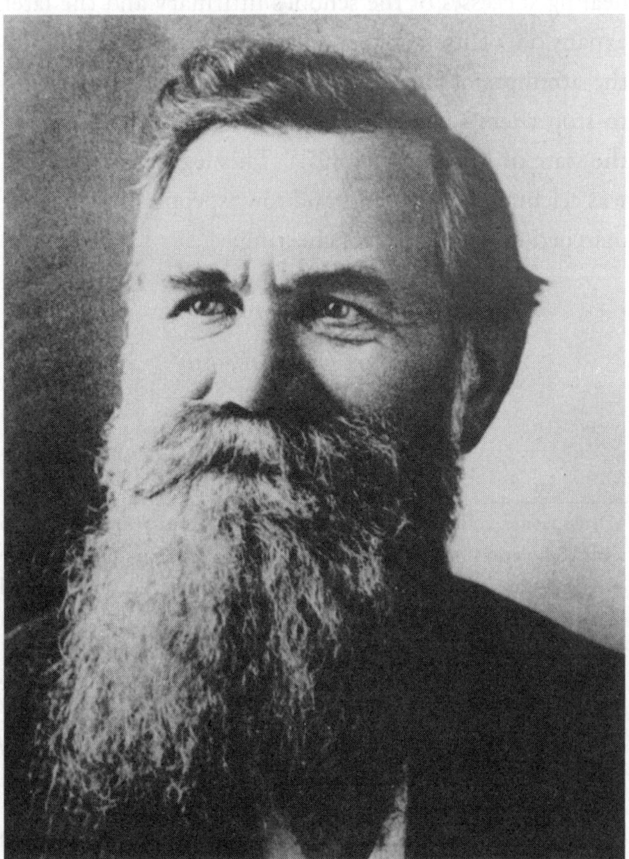

Figure 17.7. Dr. Daniel David Palmer, the founder of chiropractic (photograph courtesy of the Archive Division of the Palmer College of Chiropractic)

In 1906, Dr. Palmer was sentenced to six months in jail for practicing medicine without a license.[50] During this incarceration, his son, B. J. Palmer (1881–1961), took over the operation of the college, which created a contentious rift between father and son that only widened through the years. The younger Palmer was an enthusiastic promoter of chiropractic, and by 1916 the campus had more than 1,400 students who received their D.C. degree—doctorate in chiropractic—after one year's training.[51]† As the Davenport college flourished, other chiropractic colleges were established across the country. In 1913, despite the lobbying efforts of M.D.s and D.O.s, Kansas and Arkansas became the first two states to legalize chiropractic. By 1922, twenty other states had followed suit.[52] Much later, Mississippi (1973) and Louisiana (1974) became the last two states in the United States to grant chiropractic licensing.[53]

Early Controversy

The close similarities as well as the almost parallel origins of these two fields of manipulative healing caused much interprofessional controversy and enmity. The osteopaths claimed that the chiropractors were infringing on their turf, while the chiropractors asserted that their two methods were distinctly different.

Different Philosophies of Health

The chiropractors argued that while Still believed that the "free flow of blood . . . constituted the key to health,"

*Although detractors have ridiculed this story, it is important to note two facts. First, in the early part of the twentieth century (and earlier), before the widespread use of prescription drugs, amalgam fillings, and other toxic metals and chemicals, miraculous cures such as this were not so uncommon. Second, in modern clinical research the resolution of hearing loss through spinal manipulation has also been reported, even in one case through the specific manipulation of the fourth thoracic vertebrae. (C. Masarsky and M. Todres-Masarsky, *Somatovisceral Aspects of Chiropractic* [New York: Churchill Livingstone, 2001], 183–86.)

†Chiropractic college currently consists of a four-year curriculum with completion of pre-med undergraduate courses required before entering—the same as for osteopathic, naturopathic, and medical schools. (See appendix 1 for more information on the training of D.C.s.)

Palmer believed in the supremacy of the nervous system in regulating normal function in the body.[54] Dr. Still's deep feelings about the importance of blood circulation is evidenced in his later writing:

> I proclaimed that a disturbed artery marked the beginning to an hour and a minute when disease began to sow its seeds of destruction in the human body. That in no case could this be done without a broken or suspended current of arterial blood, which by nature was intended to supply and nourish every nerve, ligament, muscle, skin, bone, and the artery itself. He who wished to successfully solve the problem of disease or deformity of any kind in every case without exception would find one or more obstructions in some artery or vein.[55]

In contrast, Palmer emphasized the primary role of the nervous system in regulating normal function in the body:

> Life is the expression of tone. In that sentence is the basic principle of chiropractic. Tone is the normal degree of nerve tension. Tone is expressed in functions by normal elasticity, activity, strength and excitability of the various organs, as observed in a state of health. Consequently, the cause of disease is any variation in tone.[56]

Thus, this difference in philosophy—the fact that "osteopathy attempts to restore health by following the *rule of the artery,* [while] chiropractic has always recognized the primacy of the nervous system"—was, and remains today, one of the primary distinguishing philosophical factors between these two healing professions.[57]

Different Manipulative Techniques

Chiropractors also argued that the chiropractic vertebral adjustment was unique and distinctly different from the osteopathic manipulation of the spinal segments. For example, while osteopaths generally mobilize more than one vertebral segment to treat a given area, chiropractors typically manipulate a specific segment to treat a particular disturbance. Furthermore, osteopathic manipulations were based on the lever principle, where the vertebrae were often held while the osteopath twisted the patient's torso in various directions to overcome resistance in the spinal fixation area. In contrast, chiropractors thrust directly over a specific area of the subluxated vertebra (e.g., one of the vertebral transverse processes) to release the fixated joint.[58]

Same Spiritual Beliefs

Whatever differences the practitioners of these two holistic pioneering fields had, they both, like Hahnemann, recognized "the healing powers of nature" or the body's "vital force." Dr. Still referred to this healing and regulating energy that was fully enlivened through manual manipulation as "divine essence," while Dr. Palmer referred to it as "innate intelligence."[59]

Clinical Research

The late nineteenth and early to mid-twentieth century could be referred to as the "renaissance" period of osteopathy and chiropractic. In these less-toxic pre–World War II years, manipulation of the spine often yielded what would be considered astounding results, especially in contrast to our current more mechanistic model.

Early Osteopathic Research

In 1925, a study involving the osteopathic manipulation of the thoracic spine (T4 and T5) found that it yielded not only significant relief but even complete cessation of asthma in the majority of subjects.[60] In a 1946 study, osteopathic physicians proved the essential relationship between the spine and the immune system by showing that spinal manipulation could restore normal autonomic tone, reduce or clear chronic systemic infections, and increase white blood cell count.[61]

Early Chiropractic Research

Chiropractic physicians also documented similar and often dramatic successes. For example, in one 1949 national survey of "350 nervous and mental cases," a majority (95 percent) reported improvement in mental symptoms after chiropractic care, as opposed to no change or worsening (91 percent) from previous medical and psychiatric treatments.[62] In fact, evidence of this dramatic somatopsychic healing had been witnessed for almost forty years in Davenport, Iowa, where the chiropractic profession maintained two major mental hospitals—Forest Park Sanitarium (1922–1950)* and Clear View Sanitarium (1926–1961). At Clear View Sanitarium, the initial patient evaluation consisted of physical examination, X-rays, blood work, urinalysis, and assessment with a neurocalograph (heart reading) instrument that assisted the subsequent chiropractic adjustment.[63] Dr. W. H. Quigley describes the amazing results he observed as director of Clear View, in which chiropractic adjustments could "break the cyclic reverberations of ANS [autonomic system] imbalance":

> I frequently saw agitated schizophrenics, dangerous to themselves and others, arrive at Clear View in straitjackets, completely out of contact with the world of reality. They were not responsive to words, care, or any type of ministration. However, after chiropractic adjustments a dramatic change occurred, in which the patient began to orient himself by asking questions as to who we were, where he was, what had happened to him. Soon he was released from restraints, had freedom of the ward and was eventually released from the Sanitarium.[64]

In one longitudinal study in which schizophrenic patients were monitored for seven years after discharge, Quigley documented that 70 percent remained "socially restored" and were back to normal mental health and functioning.[65] Although Quigley himself admitted the deficiencies of this and other studies due to being "plagued by the inability to have a control population for study," the outstanding results certainly warrant further research on the subject of the effects of spinal adjusting on mental health.†

*In 1950, a fire swept through all three floors of Forest Park Sanitarium. It was later sold in 1959 and became a nursing and retirement facility.

†In one interview I had with Dr. Quigley in Los Angeles in 1981, he confessed that the period in which he was director of Clear View was the most exciting of his life. He even met one of his colleagues and most famous mentors there: Dr. Hans Selye. Selye toured Quigley's phenomenally successful sanitarium, and there they discussed the beneficial effects chiropractic was having on mental and emotional stress. Dr. Selye, the renowned author of *The Stress of Life,* defined *stress* as the abnormal autonomic tone and resulting organ degeneration that manifests from chronic chemical, physical, or psychological damaging agents.

Current Research

More recent scientific studies have confirmed the effectiveness of manual manipulation. However, this modern research is primarily limited to the treatment of musculoskeletal disorders such as cervical tension headaches and back pain.[66] One reason is that patients intoxicated from heavy metals, petroleum chemicals, and pharmaceutical medications that came into widespread usage after World War II do not respond as quickly or as successfully to manipulation now as they did in these less-toxic pre-war years. The second reason is the narrowing of scope in both the chiropractic and osteopathic professions as a result of harassment by allopathic medicine.

TREATMENT: CRANIOSACRAL THERAPY

As previously described in the "Craniosacral Movement: Locking Up the Maxillary Suture" section in chapter 16, *craniopathy* or *craniosacral therapy* or *craniosacral manipulation* is the treatment of restrictions of movement in the bones that surround either end of the central nervous system—the cranium (skull bones) and the sacroiliac (pelvis). Craniopaths spend many years training to feel the subtle yet perceptible rhythmic movement arising from the circulation of the cerebrospinal fluid within the surrounding fascial membranes (e.g., dura mater) that surround the spinal cord and cranium. In fact, this pulsation—varying from approximately six to twelve times per minute—can be felt throughout the body by a skilled craniopath. Aberrations of this movement—too slow, too fast, or various patterns of torsion, strain, or compression—are treated through gentle fingertip pressure in an indirect fashion. Craniopaths generally use a *very* gentle cranial hold with less than an ounce of pressure—almost undetectable by the patient.

In contrast to spinal manipulation that is a *direct* adjustment of a misaligned or fixated joint, craniopathic manipulation is *indirect.* Craniopaths gently encourage the distortion pattern of the patient (i.e., subtly *increase* the imbalance) until the body recognizes its error and readjusts itself. Thus, craniopathy is similar to the indirect methodology underlying homeopathy, where the energies of a plant, animal, or mineral resonate with the disturbed pattern in the patient and gently influence this pattern to dissipate over time. Spinal manipulation, on the other hand, is more comparable to nutritional or herbal supplementation, which treats (and supplements) the pathology *more directly*. The former is more yin; the latter is more yang.

History of Craniosacral Therapy

Although spinal manipulation can definitely claim ancient origins, craniopathy has no real historic roots before the nineteenth century.[67] During the latter part of this century and the early twentieth century, it was both a chiropractor and an osteopath who almost concurrently discovered and developed the art and science of craniosacral manipulation.[68]

Chiropractic Roots

After having only palliative results with two previous spinal adjustments on an "insane and raving" patient, Nephi Cottam, D.C. (1883–1996), "was guided" to release the jammed coronal suture between the frontal (forehead bone) and the parietal bones (uppermost side bones of the skull). The results were phenomenal; the patient's former agonizing head pain that had stimulated her "crazy" and agitated behavior was immediately relieved.* After similar successful responses on other patients and examining the "dovetailing" configuration of the cranial sutures on many skulls, Cottam "became convinced that cranial bones do move [and] soon derived adjustments for the opening of all the sutures."[69]

In 1928, he applied for a patent on an intraoral form of craniopathy (the manipulation of the cranium through the mouth), and one month later he reported his findings on the "adjustment of cranial bones" to the "largest group of chiropractors ever assembled in Utah."[70] The Salt Lake City *Deseret News* reported on January 28, 1929, Cottam's demonstration of "removal of brain pressure by adjustment of the bones of the head": "This method of adjustment is a discovery made by Dr. Cottam which, he explains, will greatly extend the province of chiropractic in cases of mental derangements, subnormal mentality of children and adults, epilepsy and paralysis."[71]

Later, in 1936, Cottam founded the Cottam School of Craniopathy in Los Angeles and published his book, *The Story of Craniopathy*.[72]

Osteopathic Roots

Around this same period, William Garner Sutherland (1873–1954) was also studying the bones of the skull while he was a student at Dr. Still's school of osteopathy in Kirksville, Missouri.[73] He began teaching "his personal hobby—the theory of cranial articular mobility" in September 1929. Later, in 1939, Sutherland published his book on his theories of the cranium and his system of cranial manipulation, titled *The Cranial Bowl*.[74]

Sutherland's insights and system of cranial manipulation have remained the cornerstone of craniosacral therapy to this day. Not only did he espouse and teach the mobility of the cranial sutures, but he also identified the "primary respiratory mechanism" (or craniosacral rhythm)—that is, the involuntary and rhythmic fluctuation of the cerebrospinal fluid (continuously filtered out from the blood) that circulates throughout the central nervous system (the brain and spinal cord). Furthermore, Sutherland also realized the importance of the intracranial fascia or the "reciprocal tension membranes."[75] These three membranes—the dura mater, arachnoid membrane, and pia mater—contain and circulate the cerebrospinal fluid as it continuously circulates from the cranium down to the sacrum and back up to the cranium in a rhythmic cycle of approximately six to twelve times per minute.*

The Adaptive Nature of the Cranium, Compensating for the Body Below

Sutherland taught that the "cranio-sacral mechanism is the master adaptation process available to the body to accommodate stresses and strains until the cerebrospinal fluid is able to lubricate and clear the stress."[76] This understanding of cranial adaptation—that is, that the top of the body (roof of the house) often adapts to problems below (in the basement)—is a key point of

*John Upledger, D.O., later reported excellent results in a child with cerebral palsy through mobilization of the coronal suture. (J. Upledger and J. Vredevoogd, *Craniosacral Therapy* [Chicago: Eastland Press, 1983], 262.)

*The primary respiratory cyclic rhythm of six to twelve times per minute is actually created by four factors: (1) the fluctuation of the cerebrospinal fluid; (2) the reciprocal tension membranes (dura, arachnoid, and pia); (3) the inherent motility of the brain and spinal cord; and (4) the mobility of the twenty-two cranial bones and the sacrum between the ilia (pelvic bones). (R. Holding, *Craniosacral Therapy in the Context of Clinical Kinesiology* [London: self-published, October 1988], 4.)

understanding that is often missed by even the most adept craniopath.

Discerning between a Still Point and a Crash

Dr. Richard Holding, an osteopath and master craniopath, teaches the importance of being aware of this common form of adaptation in the body in the Clinical Kinesiology energetic testing method.[77] He and his colleague, Dr. Ashley Robinson, have observed specific kinesiological clues to confirm a skilled craniopath's perception of the "subtle quiet feel" of a still point, in contrast to the "subtle deadening feel" of a "crash."

The induction of a *still point* by a craniopath is the underlying treatment mode for all cranial corrections. A still point occurs when the craniosacral rhythm pauses, and during this period of deep relaxation spontaneous corrections can occur primarily through the pooling and "bathing" of cerebrospinal fluid into tissues that were deficient in this rhythm and flow.

A "crash" occurs when the autonomic nervous system becomes so overloaded by the discordant and aberrant signals arising in a patient's consciousness from a disturbing area in the body that these nerves reach a level of chaos where they simply can no longer clearly respond to muscle testing.[78]* This crash of the sympathetic nervous system can actually be measured using a galvanic skin response meter. When these "autonomic crashes" occur, the more holistically oriented and aware craniopath will search for the source of this lack of neurological and energetic response in the patient's body. Skilled and experienced craniopaths can actually perceive the location of the disturbance (even though their hands remain on the cranium) simply by projecting their awareness into the patient's body and sensing the area(s) of dysfunction—signaled by a reduced craniosacral (flexion or extension) rhythm, tissue congestion and torsion, or other types of distortion pattern.*

Often the cause is a disturbed or degenerated organ, a focal infection or scar interference field, a toxic and congested ganglion, or the emergence of a previously suppressed psychological issue. After the craniopath addresses and treats this arising issue (e.g., drainage remedies for a dysbiotic small intestine or auriculotherapy for a tonsil focus), then craniosacral therapy may be resumed. At this point, typically many craniosacral distortion patterns spontaneously clear, the patient's cerebrospinal rhythm and vitality are greatly enhanced, and a much more profound and long-lasting healing effect occurs than would ever be possible with conventional craniosacral therapy alone.

Craniopathy Wasted on Patients with Major Malocclusions or TMD

Dental malocclusions and jaw joint dysfunction, quite understandably so, have a primary impact on the rest of the cranium. As described earlier, craniopaths (typically D.O.s and D.C.s) must be skilled in diagnosing major dental malocclusions and TMJ dysfunction and their stomatognathicsomatic effects in the cranium, spinal vertebrae, and sacrum. At the very least, craniopaths should include an examination of the jaw and teeth in the initial office visit and appropriately refer to a holistic dentist those patients who exhibit any obvious pathology (mercury amalgam fillings, mixed metals, fixed bridges or hard plastic appliances crossing the maxillary midline, signs of impacted wisdom teeth, widespread decay and gum disease, serious TMJ dysfunction, and major malocclusions—Class II or buckteeth, open bites, Class III or underbites, etc.). To not do so and to treat a patient for months and years with only craniosacral therapy borders on malpractice. Dr. David Walther, a foremost Applied Kinesiologist, comments on the futility of cranial manipulation in the face of a major malocclusion:

> The muscles of mastication pull with a great amount of leverage into the cranium. . . . [The cranial correction is often] temporary, especially

*Dr. Ashley Robinson discovered in the Clinical Kinesiology technique that the loss of a positive hand chakra—analogous to a computer screen going black—indicated a "crash." Likewise, after the issue that has caused this "biocomputer crash" is found and treated, the patient's hand chakra will then test positive once again, indicating the "biocomputer" (the autonomic nervous system) is now back "online" and functioning. For more information on CK and other methods, see appendix 3, "Energetic Testing Explained."

*Craniopaths who utilize energetic testing methods (Clinical Kinesiology, Neural Kinesiology, and the MRT method) can back up their perceptions through testing for the loss of a hand chakra in the patient's dominant hand (signaling a crash) and therapy-localizing the suspected area of dysfunction.

> when the malocclusion is present . . . the temporary correction will most often be immediately lost as soon as the individual bites down or swallows.[79]

Accurate Diagnosis Essential for Craniopaths

Thus, just as with spinal manipulation, accurate diagnosis is essential. Furthermore, when the same spinal or cranial distortion patterns (e.g., patient continues to display the same short leg year after year) continue to show up visit after visit, practitioners must exercise their logical mind and realize that they must be missing something. In the case of a major malocclusion, only after the patient receives effective treatment (an orthopedic appliance, new dentures, conservative equilibration, etc.) can cranial manipulative therapy be truly efficacious and lasting. Treatment is particularly beneficial when craniopaths and orthopedic dentists work in cooperation in the rebalancing and restoration of a patient's normal bite and cranium.[80] Finally, it is important to note that in cases of mild malocclusions or minor TMJ dysfunction, craniosacral therapy can be effective alone, or with only a minimum of additional dental intervention.

Craniosacral Therapy for All Ages

Cranial Distortions Common after Birth

Cranial manipulation of infants and children can be particularly effective. The importance of early craniosacral treatments has been particularly evidenced in the cranial osteopathic research literature. In one landmark study, Dr. Viola Frymann, a master cranial osteopath, evaluated 1,250 infants just after ("normal" vaginal) birth for cranial distortion patterns. A highly significant number of these infants, 1,105 or 88 percent, exhibited mild to major cranial strain and compression patterns. Through correlating infant symptoms with these cranial bone distortions, Frymann concluded that these abnormal cranial bone patterns were of "considerable significance in the production of nervous symptoms, namely vomiting, hyperactive peristalsis [diarrhea], hypertonicity, tremor and irritability," as well as respiratory and circulatory symptoms.[81]

Babies who are birthed through cesarean section have another set of problems. In utero, the skull bones slightly overlap each other. The pressure of a vaginal birth naturally decompresses and then expands these cranial bones as the infant exits the vagina.[82] In the absence of this vaginal pressure, the craniums of C-section infants are characteristically too tightly compressed, with multiple fixated sutures and reduced cerebrospinal fluid motion. These babies' seemingly healthy-appearing heads are typically inaccurately praised for being so "perfectly well-rounded and well-shaped."[83]

Craniosacral Manipulation Greatly Beneficial after Birth

Gentle craniosacral manipulation in infants born through C-sections or even vaginal births is very healing and, in fact, can be clinically dramatic. For example, craniopathy has been proven to be significantly effective in reducing hyperirritability of the nervous system, crying to excess, poor muscle tonus ("floppy baby" syndrome), excessive regurgitation and bowel dysfunction, breathing difficulties, and other signs of respiratory distress.[84] Additionally, as infants mature, so do their craniums, reaching 90 percent of their fully developed size by age five.[85] Thus, just as with quality nutrition and a loving environment, these first few formative years of childhood are an especially important time to receive skilled craniosacral care. Typical childhood conditions such as chronic otitis media (recurring ear infections), brain dysfunction (autism, dyslexia, hyperactivity, and cerebral palsy), strabismus (deviation of the eye), asthma, sleep apnea, and other syndromes have also been shown to respond beneficially to cranial manipulation.[86]

Craniopathy Beneficial in Adults Too

Craniosacral therapy has also been shown to be effective in adults, ameliorating or clearing diverse issues such as chronic pain, acute sprains and strains, infections (local and systemic), Raynaud's disease, bowel dysfunction, rheumatoid arthritis, headaches, and emotional disorders (anxiety and depression).[87] In these adult cases, however, ancillary care is often needed, such as treatment of chronic foci, careful removal of toxic amalgam fillings, psychological therapy (rebirthing, Jungian, etc.), and stabilization of a significant malocclusion or TMD syndrome.

Finding a Craniopath

Osteopaths and chiropractors are the primary physicians who specialize in craniosacral therapy. Dr. John

Upledger, a renowned cranial osteopath and author, has also taught therapists (massage, physical, and occupational), nurses, and laypersons (e.g., parents) cranial manipulation. Although criticized for teaching nonphysicians, Upledger found that therapists, with their already well-developed sense of touch, learned quickly.[88] Furthermore, when frequent manipulation is required, such as in the cases of children with cerebral palsy, seizures, and learning disorders, he often found it necessary to teach the parents. Finally, because the majority of modern-day osteopaths have lost much of their holistic structural orientation and beliefs, Upledger's widespread influence has had the additional benefit of attracting more D.O.s to learn craniosacral therapy—a major aspect of their educational roots in the early twentieth century.*

The best referral is word of mouth from satisfied former patients of craniopaths. Additionally, one can contact the Upledger Institute, the Cranial Academy, SORSI (primarily chiropractors trained in craniopathy), and ICAK (for kinesiologists who practice craniopathy) to find a qualified craniopath.

▶ To contact the Upledger Institute, go to www.upledger.com. To locate an osteopathic physician who utilizes craniosacral manipulation, go to www.cranialacademy.org. To contact SORSI, go to www.sorsi.com or www.soto-usa.org. To contact ICAK, go to www.icakusa.com.

TREATMENT: MASSAGE THERAPY

For many, the terms *bodywork, therapeutic touch,* or *massage*—generally defined as the systematic and therapeutic rubbing, friction, or kneading of the body—conjure up a pleasant experience that helps reduce muscle soreness and calm the mind. However, for those who have experienced the profound effects of a highly skilled and intuitive body worker, massage evokes a great deal more.

*At the time that Upledger began teaching, there were only three qualified colleagues of his practicing in the entire state of Michigan. Furthermore, in the 1980s, typical of most osteopathic schools at the time, the Texas College of Osteopathic Medicine in Fort Worth had only one cranial manipulation course, which was offered as an elective.

Ancient Origins and Present-Day Resources

The benefits of massage and other forms of therapeutic touch have been known since antiquity. From the instruction of the Yellow Emperor in China (~2550 BCE) to the Greek father of medicine Hippocrates (460–377 BCE) to the great Swiss physician and alchemist Paracelsus (1493–1541), massage has been regarded as a principal and indispensable therapeutic modality.[89] In the latter part of the twentieth century, there was a renaissance of this therapeutic tool concurrent with the growth of holistic medicine, evidenced by both the great increase of practitioners as well as the explosion of new—and rediscovered—massage techniques. Patients may currently choose from a vast array of different massage methods, ranging from the most gentle and energetic such as Reiki to stronger techniques such as Rolfing, shiatsu, Anatomy Trains, and Tui-Na. Choosing a massage therapist (LMT) or practitioner (LMP)* can be as individual as choosing the right psychotherapist. Some individuals respond better to gentle touch and energetic practices, while others require stronger manipulation. One of the best resources is word of mouth from friends who have had good experiences and can often describe in detail the exact style and technique that the massage practitioner utilizes. Other resources include local magazines, weekly newspapers, or holistic catalogs that list practitioners along with a description of their particular type of massage modality.

A FEW BODYWORK TECHNIQUES DEFINED

- *Reiki* is a subtle form of bodywork in which the practitioner's hands direct healing energy through the patient's closest energy field—the *wei qi* or electromagnetic field (EMF) located next to (within millimeters of) the patient's physical body.
- *Rolfing,* originated by Ida Rolf, involves deep muscle and connective tissue manipulation to balance, reorient, and reeducate chronic musculoskeletal holding patterns and adhesions.
- *Shiatsu* is a traditional Japanese approach that uses concentrated finger pressure on acupressure points in a particular sequence to release chronic areas of

*Some states license massage practitioners as "Licensed Massage Therapists" or "LMTs," and others use the term "Licensed Massage Practitioners" or "LMPs."

spasm and pain and restore harmonious circulation of the meridian chi throughout the body.

- *Anatomy Trains* is a method whereby strains and tension in the myofascial meridians, or "tracks" of muscle and connective tissue distortion patterns in the body (laterally, vertically, and spiraling), are diagnosed and released through deep tissue therapy.
- *Tui-Na* is an ancient Chinese practice that utilizes deep pressure and rhythmic motions to realign muscles, balance the spine and nervous system, and restore chi (vital energy or life force).

▶ For information on Rolfing, go to www.rolf.org. For information on Anatomy Trains, go to www.anatomytrains.com. For information on Tui-Na, go to www.tui-na.com.

Massage Essential after Acute Injuries

In the same manner as scheduling for spinal or cranial manipulation, frequent massage therapy is necessary and entirely appropriate after acute injuries. In fact, massage (as well as spinal manipulation) has been proven to be so valuable in the scientific literature that even conservative insurance companies provide full coverage and reimbursement after most car accidents or other personal injury cases.

Most Effective after "Obstacles to Cure" Have Been Addressed

However, in the case of treatment for chronic symptoms—and once again, analogous to spinal and cranial manipulation—massage therapy is most efficacious when the major blocks to healing have been cleared. That is, only when major focal infections, toxic metals and chemicals, intestinal dysbiosis, and other "obstacles to cure" have been appropriately treated can massage therapy be most beneficial. In fact, in a "cleaner" and clearer patient who is without amalgam fillings, focal infections, and scar interference fields and is on his or her correct constitutional homeopathic remedy, Rolfing, Anatomy Trains, and Tui-Na can have a significantly stronger and even curative impact in the body. Furthermore, these transformative therapies can also be instrumental in treating structurally induced foci—that is, after injuries or accidents that were significant enough to generate a chronic distortion pattern in the body and the mind (negative engram), as well as a chronic somatovisceral referral.

Restoring Normal Movement and Function: The "Thixotropic," or Melting, Effect

Deane Juhan, in *Job's Body: A Handbook for Bodywork,* describes another benefit of massage—the *thixotropic* effect. Just like common gelatin that solidifies when sitting in the refrigerator but melts when it is whipped up or heated, our gel-like connective tissues become more fluid and less viscous when they are stirred up through massage. This thixotropic effect is induced in the same way by the pressure, stretching, and heat of manual manipulation that restores more fluidity to injured tissues and thus, over time, imparts more normal function in the area.[90] Juhan summarizes the effects of this thixotropic principle in his book:

> The hands of the therapist can literally supply the mechanical activity which a sluggish limb fails to produce, raising the metabolic rate and restoring some of the fluidity of its connective tissues. [Thus] . . . bodywork accomplishes its ends in an utterly different fashion than do the additive and subtractive means of pharmaceuticals and surgery. Skillful manipulation simply raises energy levels and creates a greater degree of sol (fluidity) in organic systems that are already there, but are behaving sluggishly.[91]

Significantly Detoxifying in "Advanced" Patients

This liquefying effect created through the friction and heat generated by skillful manual manipulation not only restores more normal mechanical function in the joints and muscles but also releases any stored toxins in these tissues. This is why deep massage can have curative effects in "advanced" patients who have already removed their petroleum-chemical-laden soaps and shampoos, replaced their amalgam fillings, and had their bacterial focal infections treated. In this group of "cleaner" and clearer individuals, deep tissue manipulation encourages the remaining embedded stores of toxic metals, chemicals, and microbes to be released into the general circulation, where they can be effectively excreted out of the body. Furthermore, it is the reason these patients can experience and recognize these detoxifying effects better than new patients (who have not begun the detox process) yet also can more quickly and efficiently release these toxins through a more functional and less burdened body.

Releasing Chronic Psychosomatic Patterns

Massage therapy, in the hands of a master practitioner, has the curative potential of releasing all forms of chronic and habituated negative patterns—physically, emotionally, and mentally. Physically massage can release and elongate stiff, shortened, and thickened muscles and connective tissue caused from disuse, overuse, injury, or illness. Emotionally, bodywork often liberates chronically held muscular armoring and defensive postural attitudes devolved from unresolved feelings of fear, sorrow, and anger. Additionally, over time massage can help free patients from the many habitual negative thought patterns that limit life in every respect. A quote from one of the geniuses of bodywork, Dr. Milton Trager, best expresses this mind/body relationship:

> The mind is the whole thing. That is all that I am interested in. I am convinced that for every physical non-yielding condition there is a psychic counterpart in the unconscious mind, corresponding exactly to the degree of the physical manifestation. . . . These patterns often develop in response to adverse circumstances such as accidents, surgery, illness, poor posture, emotional trauma, stresses of daily living, or poor movement habits. The purpose of my work is to break up these sensory and mental patterns which inhibit free movement and cause pain and disruption of normal function.[92]

WHAT IS A HOLISTIC CHIROPRACTOR OR OSTEOPATH?

In the early and mid-part of the twentieth century, using the word *holistic* as an adjective for a chiropractic (D.C.) or osteopathic physician (D.O.) would have been absurdly redundant. Both these schools of healing have strong roots in holistically oriented philosophy, and chiropractic and osteopathic physicians have been using natural therapies for over a century now. Sadly, however, this is no longer always the case. In the following pages, the medical persecution and slow infringement of more allopathically oriented beliefs into chiropractic and osteopathy will be thoroughly covered. At the conclusion of this section, the physicians who still honor their holistic origins will be described, as will how best to locate one nearby for treatment.

The Chiropractic Saga: Persecution by Allopaths

It would be a spirited discussion indeed to determine which group in U.S. history was more persecuted by the American Medical Association—homeopaths or chiropractors. The account of the nineteenth-century suppression of homeopathy and the eventual extinction of all the homeopathic colleges in the United States in the early twentieth century was detailed in chapter 14. How the chiropractic profession survived the destructive machinations of allopathic medicine is briefly outlined here.

► For more information on the history of chiropractic and the roots of the somatovisceral and viscerosomatic concepts, read the excellent book *Somatovisceral Aspects of Chiropractic* by Dr. Charles Masarsky and Dr. Marion Todres-Masarky, published in 2001 by Churchill Livingstone.

Chiropractic Treatment of Disease and Dysfunction Angered Medical Doctors

D. D. Palmer was not the only chiropractor imprisoned for "practicing medicine without a license." Many other early and even mid-twentieth-century chiropractors were also arrested. The charges were primarily based on prevailing state medical practice acts that specified "all healing is the practice of medicine."[93] In these early days, chiropractors treated all manner of disease and dysfunction through spinal manipulation, as well as "proper diet and balanced and properly-timed rest and exercise, pure air, [and] sunlight."[94] Palmer and his early colleagues were greatly influenced by European research on "spinal irritation" by Dr. Thomas Brown, Dr. Thomas Pridgin Teale, and later Sir Henry Head, which validated both the somatovisceral and viscerosomatic theories of healing though spinal autonomic nerve reflex pathways.[95]* Like the osteopaths, chiropractors had remarkable success in treating through spinal manipulation and other therapies a wide range of maladies that encompassed menstrual disorders, asthma, cystitis (bladder inflammation), constipation, heart disease, mental illness, and even various forms of paralysis—all of which the allopathic doctors believed belonged solely in their domain.[96] However, despite the vigorous opposition of many medical boards, as well as some osteopathic state boards, chiropractors became licensed in the great majority of states by the early 1930s, and in all fifty states by 1974.[97]

"GO TO JAIL FOR CHIROPRACTIC"

In Alameda County, California, the slogan "Go to jail for chiropractic" was adopted in 1917, requiring its members to go to prison rather than paying fines. In one infamous year, 450 D.C.s went to jail, singing "Onward Christian Soldiers" on the way. Once there, they would set up their portable adjusting tables and treat inmates. As a result, public opinion began to turn against the medical practice acts, and in 1923 the governor pardoned all chiropractors, feeling that they had been unjustly accused by the more powerful and influential California Medical Association (CMA).[98]

The AMA Conspired to "Exterminate" Chiropractic

Unfortunately, this medical subversion was not simply limited to the issue of chiropractic licensing. Similar to the attacks on homeopathic physicians, defamation of character by labeling chiropractors as "quacks" and an "unscientific cult" was allopathic medicine's second line of defense against this encroaching economic threat.[99] In fact, as early as 1922, officials of the American Medical Association "met in secret conclave in Chicago and adopted the slogan, 'Chiropractic must die,' [and] . . . they gave themselves ten years in which to exterminate it."[100]

The "Chicago Five's" Lawsuit against the AMA

These and other libelous statements as well as nefarious tactics by the AMA were made dramatically evident in a class-action lawsuit filed by five D.C.s, known as the "Chicago Five," in the mid-1970s. In this case, Dr. Chester Wilk and four other Chicago D.C.s charged that the AMA and fourteen other medical groups conspired to violate the U.S. Sherman Antitrust Act "by conducting an illegal boycott in restraint of trade directed at chiropractors in an effort to contain and destroy the profession."[101] Dr. Chester Wilk was not simply "fishing in the dark" here. In the early 1970s, William Trever's book *In the Public Interest* contained evidence that the AMA's "Committee on Quackery," which was established in 1963, was really a front to destroy the chiropractic profession.[102] The source of the information contained in this book came from thousands of internal AMA documents that were smuggled out by an anonymous individual who came to be known as "Sore Throat" (after the infamous "Deep Throat" of Watergate fame).[103] Additionally, "Sore Throat," whom we now know as P. Joseph Lisa, who later wrote *The Assault on Medical Freedom,* also sent copies of internal AMA documents to most of the major newspapers, with many of these documents identical to those that had been revealed in *In the Public Interest*.[104] The following is from of one of these documents, a memo sent on January 4, 1971, from the AMA's Committee on Quackery to the AMA's Board of Trustees, that characterizes the AMA's animosity toward the field of chiropractic:

> Since the AMA Board of Trustees' decision at its meeting of November 2–3, 1963, to establish a Committee on Quackery, your Committee has considered its prime mission to be, first, the containment of chiropractic and, ultimately, the elimination of chiropractic.[105]

These and other leaks slowly revealed the pattern of underhanded tactics that the AMA's Committee on

*An example of the great influence of the theory of "spinal irritation," first elucidated in the early 1800s, is exemplified by this quote from a leading chiropractic teacher and writer, Dr. John Howard, in his book *Encyclopedia of Chiropractic,* published a century later: "We have not maintained that all diseases have their origin from subluxation of the spinal column, or compression and shock to the spinal cord, yet we do contend that in the majority of diseases, spinal irritation is present, and that contractions of the spinal muscle and ligaments result as a consequence, and these irritations and contractions, when permitted to continue for any length of time, produce subluxated vertebrae." (J. Howard, *Encyclopedia of Chiropractic* [Chicago: National School of Chiropractic, n.d.], xxix–xxx.)

Quackery had engaged in for decades, as described in the following passage from John Robbins's book *Reclaiming Our Health:*

> Soon, Taylor* [head of the "Quackery" committee] was contacting hundreds of medical groups and societies, encouraging them to deem it unethical for a physician to refer patients to chiropractors or to consult with chiropractors professionally or personally. In order to further sabotage and undermine chiropractors' activities, Taylor created a team of agents who took assumed names, pretended to be chiropractors, spied on chiropractic conventions, and did what they could to generate divisiveness and dissension.[106]

Additionally, it was revealed during the courtroom drama that medical doctors were also persuaded to label D.C.s as "quacks," and not to refer patients to them.

> AMA physicians were encouraged to give patients referred to them by chiropractors a "quack pack," which was used to discourage the patient from returning to the chiropractor. These clearly anti-competitive activities successfully denied patients both chiropractic services and the advantage of a team containing both medical and chiropractic physicians.[107]

Furthermore, the AMA worked hard to eliminate insurance coverage for chiropractic care:

> [During 1963–1975] the AMA effectively and adversely influences private insurance companies and Medicare against chiropractic coverage. It "fixes" a so-called independent study commissioned by the Department of Health, Education and Welfare, done by Stanford Research Institute, to determine whether or not chiropractic services should be paid for by Medicare. It also works to influence Blue Cross/Blue Shield and other insurers against chiropractic.[108]

In fact, during the discovery process of this trial, plaintiffs learned that just about *every* anti-chiropractic statement coming from the media and organizations such as unions or senior citizen groups had been spread through the AMA's systematic plan to destroy chiropractic.[109] These deceptive tactics surfaced during the trial:

> Evidence at the trial showed that the defendants took active steps, often covert, to undermine chiropractic educational institutions, conceal evidence of the usefulness of chiropractic care, undercut insurance programs for patients of chiropractors, subvert government inquiries into the efficacy of chiropractic, engage in a massive disinformation campaign to discredit and destabilize the chiropractic profession, and engaged in numerous other activities to maintain a medical physician monopoly over health care in this country.[110]

After sixteen years of litigation, Wilk and the Chicago Five finally won the case in 1987,* based on the numerous trial testimonies and evidence demonstrating that the AMA had clearly "conspired to undermine both the public's confidence in chiropractic and proper doctor-patient relationships."[111] In this verdict for the plaintiffs, the court required the AMA and the other medical defendants to reverse their anti-chiropractic policies and to "implement new policies that did not discourage professional association with members of the chiropractic profession."[112] Furthermore, the AMA was ordered to make a $3.5 million payment to cover the chiropractors' legal costs.[113]

---

*The AMA's general counsel, Robert B. Throckmorton, hired Iowa attorney Doyle Taylor to head the Committee on Quackery campaign. In 1963, Taylor and Throckmorton coauthored the AMA's position "that chiropractic is an unscientific cult whose practitioners . . . constitute a hazard to health care in the United States." Realizing, however, that it would not look good if this campaign became known to the public, Throckmorton repeatedly emphasized that the AMA's actions should be covert, and "behind the scenes whenever possible." (J. Robbins, *Reclaiming Our Health* [Tiburon, Calif.: H. J. Kramer, 1996], 186–87.)

*In 1990, on appeal, the Illinois Court of Appeals again found the AMA guilty. Later that year, the U.S. Supreme Court upheld the trial court and the Court of Appeals' rulings. Finally, in January 1992, the case was finally settled for the plaintiffs, thus ending one of the longest antitrust legal battles in U.S. history.

Lasting Effects of the AMA's Smear Campaign: Prejudice and Defamation against D.C.s Still Extant

Although this favorable verdict did make some positive changes, it is debatable how much of a lasting and real effect this lawsuit has had on medical-chiropractic relations. For one, although the results of this trial were ordered to be propagated to the public, few newspapers carried the article, and hardly any deemed it front-page news. Furthermore, even today it is rare for an M.D. to refer his patients, even with back pain, to a D.C. Additionally, although the Wilk verdict mandated that the (AMA-controlled) Joint Commission on the Accreditation of Hospitals can no longer force hospitals (through loss of accreditation) to exclude chiropractors from having staff privileges, the number of chiropractors who are allowed to treat patients in hospitals, or even to consult with orthopedists and neurologists in hospitals, is still extremely small.[114] P. Joseph Lisa, or "Sore Throat," who went undercover at the AMA headquarters and was privy to "thousands of documents" from their files on "quackery," corroborated this observation in his 1994 book, *The Assault on Medical Freedom.* Lisa revealed that after the Wilk case, the war against chiropractic simply went underground, along with the AMA's propaganda campaigns against "psychic healing, faith healing, acupuncture, cancer and arthritis 'cures,' . . . homeopathy, naturopathy, vitamins, herbs, and more."[115] In fact, in 1993 the AMA self-published a book titled *Alternative Health Methods,* which described holistic medicine as "a mélange of banalities, truisms, exaggerations, and falsehoods, overlaid with disparagement . . . of logical reasoning itself."[116]

Thus, despite the triumphant verdict of the Chicago Five, as well as later successful lawsuits, the AMA's smear campaign had already successfully stigmatized the chiropractic profession's reputation. This continuous type of overt as well as covert discrimination can be quite effective when waged long enough, hard enough, and by a ruling class of people. Unfortunately, for over a century chiropractors have endured the negative professional and personal effects of the AMA's attempt to destroy, or at the very least discredit, them.

The Loss of Chiropractors' Holistic Roots—Narrowing Their Scope of Practice

One of the most common defense mechanisms against continuous defamation is for a minority group to hide or at least to become a smaller target. In the case of health professions, this tactic can be accomplished through greatly reducing one's scope of practice. In many cases, chiropractic physicians themselves chose this path of least resistance, while in other situations D.C.s had no real choice. For example, in Canada, Australia, and several U.S. states, chiropractors were forced to narrow their focus to only the treatment of musculoskeletal pain—with no mention of the beneficial effects on organs or disease—in order to become licensed. The ordeal British chiropractors endured in their efforts to obtain legitimacy, after chiropractic was introduced in 1908 from the United States, illustrates this point:

> Like chiropractic in other countries, British chiropractic has evolved from a heterodox health system that claimed to be a complete alternative to biomedicine [allopathic medical care], to one that has increasing come to accept a more limited niche in health care as a manual musculoskeletal specialty. Some, if not many, chiropractors lament this development, but an increasing number of chiropractors view it as the trajectory which is most likely to grant them legitimacy.[117]

Chiropractors in the United States were under this same pressure, particularly in the 1960s and 1970s, to maintain a low profile as holistic physicians. Dr. Fred Barge, a holistically oriented chiropractor, describes the pressure coming from his own colleagues to reduce the chiropractic scope of practice in an article titled "Chiropractic's Greatest Tactical Error":

> I can so clearly remember being told by the Wisconsin Chiropractic Association (in the late 1960s) to stop lecturing on the chiropractic care of infectious conditions. . . . The WCA [Wisconsin Chiropractic Association] told me to be silent on controversial subjects, to stick to back pain and the musculoskeletal domain. They said we need to get a "foot in the door," so

> to speak; we need to be included in Medicare, worker's compensation, and other third-party plans. . . . Today, the majority of chiropractors see very few disease problems, they have been relegated to the aches, pains, cricks, and strains of an orthopedic type practice.[118]

Thus, many chiropractic leaders themselves, in an effort to survive in the competitive healthcare industry, chose to impose on their profession a more limited, but more acceptable, scope of practice. With this self-imposed involution, educational institutions in the 1960s and 1970s soon followed suit and were constrained against teaching the positive effects of manipulation on internal organs (viscerosomatic referrals) and illness. A former president of the American Chiropractic Association (ACA) describes this process:

> [At] least two chiropractic college presidents, whom I will never name, confided in me. They told me that it was now an unwritten rule that the profession from an educational standpoint would make no reference to chiropractic treatment of internal disease.[119]

These changes in a chiropractor's individual practice as well as in education led the Panel on Chiropractic History, after reviewing the field of chiropractic since its inception in the 1890s, to issue the following statement in the early 1990s:

> For the first 75 years of its history, chiropractic emphasized the visceral importance of the spinal adjustment. About 1975, following the NINCDS Conference in Bethesda, MD, the emphasis changed to biomechanical problems with emphasis on back pain. [Thus,] at least one generation of chiropractors has been educated in the musculo-skeletal format with inadequate exposure to the importance of the autonomic nervous system [the viscerosomatic and somatovisceral reflexes].[120]

By relegating chiropractic to the manual manipulation "corner" for only the treatment of pain, medicine significantly reduced D.C.s' ability to diagnose and treat other illnesses. Furthermore, allopathic medical doctors (and pharmaceutical companies) greatly benefited financially by claiming more of a share of the economic healthcare pie in the treatment of illness and disease.

The Chiropractic Profession Survives . . . at a Cost

Through limiting themselves, chiropractic survived as a profession, and even thrived economically over time. However, this survival was not without its costs. The crucial concepts that laid the foundation of chiropractic medicine—the viscerosomatic referral (i.e., disturbed organs can cause structural pain) and the somatovisceral referral (i.e., structural disturbance can cause organ dysfunction) were slowly lost to the next generation of D.C.s. Due to this shift away from their holistic roots, many D.C.s lost their standing as holistic physicians—an especially unfortunate phenomenon because the alternative medicine movement was gaining momentum and power during this same period.

This narrowed scope greatly reduced the holistic diagnostic skills of many D.C.s. Thus, too many modern "straight" chiropractors, although still well schooled in the differential diagnosis of pathology in their colleges, often continue to adjust the same spinal segments in patients, without consideration of other underlying viscerosomatic causes (or gangliosomatic causes, psychosomatic causes, general toxemia from heavy metals or chemicals, etc.) in their differential diagnosis. These D.C.s, who often run a financially successful factory-like practice, are typically the butt of jokes regarding the excessive frequency of office visits that they commonly prescribe (e.g., three times a week for months). Whereas the therapeutic successes of holistic D.C.s who carefully diagnose and are aware of the role of the autonomic nervous system in both musculoskeletal and visceral disease (such as Applied Kinesiologists) are not well known, nor are they well propagated to the general public.

The Osteopathic Odyssey

Early osteopaths also recognized the holistic role of manual manipulation of the spine to effect positive changes in the organs, to reduce or even cure infections, and to strengthen the immune system. Dr. Still and his colleagues at the Kirksville school proved this through their success with all manner of disease, including paralysis (facial, arm, and leg), headaches, heart disease, arthritis, varicose veins, and mental illness.[121] Dr. Still was also aware of the disturbing effects of fixated vertebrae on the function of internal organs (the somatovisceral referral). Furthermore, two of his students and later osteopathic colleagues, Charles Hazzard and J. Martin Littlejohn, argued that the reverse could also occur—that is, disturbed and diseased organs could cause structural pain and disturbance through sympathetic nerve reflex pathways (the viscerosomatic referral). These early osteopaths were greatly influenced, like the chiropractors, by the previous neurophysiology research emanating from Europe, particularly that of Thomas Brown's "spinal irritation" theory in 1828, as well as John Hilton's writing on visceral pain and its segmentally related vertebrae in 1863.[122]

Allopaths Label Osteopathy a "Cult"

The successful cures occurring in Kirksville, Missouri, propagated by Still's monthly magazine, the *Journal of Osteopathy,* as well as neighboring Midwestern newspapers, did not escape the attention of the M.D.s. As early as 1889, the Missouri state medical association tried to debunk osteopathic theory and pass laws through the state legislature to stop osteopaths from practicing. Later, other state medical boards continued to label osteopathy as a "cult system of healing" and to declare that "all professional associations with him [an osteopath] are unethical."[123] When these measures and libelous accusations failed to stop the tide of osteopathic medicine in Missouri and other states, medical doctors tried another tactic—*amalgamation.*

California Osteopaths "Sell Out"

In the 1940s, the California Medical Association (CMA), after decades of failing to eliminate the osteopathic profession, decided that the only viable strategy left "was through the absorption of the D.O.s, much as the homeopaths and the eclectics [herbal doctors] had been swallowed up early in the century."[124] In 1943, the CMA offered a proposal to the California osteopaths for amalgamation—having them included and combined with M.D.s—by granting them medical degrees. Although this measure failed, primarily through the efforts of Morris Fishbein (editor of *JAMA*),* who was notorious for opposing any association between "physicians and cultists," it was later adopted by the California Osteopathic Association (COA) in 1961. In exchange for the removal of the cultist label as well as being able to be licensed as an "M.D.," the California osteopaths passed the measure, by a margin of one hundred to ten votes, agreeing to change the name of their college from the College of Osteopathic Physicians and Surgeons to the California College of Medicine, to cease to identify themselves as osteopathic practitioners, and that there would be no future licensing of D.O.s in the state.[125]

AOA Resists Becoming "Little M.D.s"

Fortunately, the American Osteopathic Association (AOA), as well as many osteopathic state boards, resisted "all efforts to be absorbed, amalgamated, or destroyed," and the major AOA publications wrote stinging editorials criticizing "the little M.D." in California and in other states where amalgamation was occurring.[126] Additionally, through the united efforts of the U.S. osteopaths who wanted to maintain autonomy, D.O.s were granted equivalent status to M.D.s as military physicians and were also given accrediting agency status over their hospitals' eligibility for Medicare reimbursement in the latter part of the 1960s. In response to these osteopathic lobbying efforts, the AMA again tried to adopt a resolution to convert osteopathic schools to "orthodox medical institutions." However, the AOA, as well as the majority of individual osteopathic physicians and colleges, once more resisted these efforts and supported an anti-merger professional policy. This progress by the anti-merger D.O.s also had a positive influence on the California osteopaths who had almost completely dissolved their professional autonomy. In 1974, a state Supreme Court ruling overturned the 1961 amalgamation law barring new osteopathic licensing in California as well as the establishment of new

*Morris Fishbein was editor of the *Journal of the American Medical Association* for many years. During his tenure, he also criticized the American father of naturopathy, Benedict Lust, as well as the American founder of scientific naturopathy, Henry Lindlahr, characterizing their treatments as "strange diets, air baths, water cures, light treatments, chiropractic, osteopathy, homeopathy, herbals, psychoanalysis, and other monkey business that any strange healer might bring temporarily into the limelight." (F. Kirchfeld and W. Boyle, *Nature Doctors* [Portland, Ore.: Medicina Biologica, 1994], 196, 248.)

osteopathic colleges in the state. Soon after, the College of Osteopathic Medicine of the Pacific opened in Pomona, California.[127]

A Pyrrhic Victory: The Loss of Osteopaths' Holistic Roots

Although D.O.s won the battle to establish their autonomy, it was a Pyrrhic victory, because much of Dr. Still's original philosophy and teaching was subsequently lost to the profession. As the osteopaths worked to remain a viable and independent healing profession, they had to initiate changes in their colleges, hospitals, and office practices in order to achieve a status equal to, or at least parallel with, that of the M.D.s. Unfortunately, these more allopathically oriented changes were often at the expense of their commitment to holistic medicine and manual manipulation. Thus, beginning in the 1930s, the teaching and practice of osteopathic manipulative therapy began to wane.[128]

Allopaths Try to Co-opt Manual Medicine

Furthermore, through their goal of eliminating osteopathic as well as chiropractic competition, medical schools soon began to capitalize on osteopathy's reduced emphasis on manual manipulation by teaching this subject in their own orthopedic and physiatry departments beginning in the mid-1950s.[129] This movement of co-opting manual manipulation was most dramatically illustrated in the mid-1980s by the arrogance of a group of Australian medical doctors who first instituted a *correspondence* course on manipulation for M.D.s. Later, this group offered a *single-weekend* course titled "Back Pain and Spinal Manipulation for [Medical] Doctors," despite intense protestations from chiropractors and osteopaths worldwide.[130]*

A "Precarious Position": Distinguishing Osteopaths from M.D.s

Based on these and other factors, by the end of the 1950s articles in the most respected osteopathic journal failed to include manual manipulation, or if so, only briefly and as an adjunctive therapy.[131] By 1974, a survey carried out by the National Center for Health Statistics estimated that fewer than 17 percent of osteopathic physicians practiced manual manipulation.[132] A recent study revealed that this relatively low percentage had dropped even more precipitously, when it was found that currently only 6.2 percent of osteopaths practice manipulation on their patients.[133] In an accompanying editorial to this study, Joel Howell, M.D., Ph.D., commented that the osteopathic practice is in a "precarious position":

> Today, osteopathic medicine has moved close to the mainstream—close enough that in general it is no longer considered alternative medicine. The long-term survival of osteopathic medicine will depend on its ability to define itself as distinct from and yet still equivalent [to allopathic medicine practiced by M.D.s.][134]

Finding a Holistic Chiropractic or Osteopathic Physician Today

Fortunately, with the growing interest in holistic medicine in the past few decades, there has been a concomitant expansion of holistically oriented osteopaths and chiropractors.

Holistic Osteopathic Physicians

Many osteopathic colleges are now teaching manual manipulation during at least three out of four years of their students' curriculum.[135] Furthermore, a small but growing group of osteopaths, primarily influenced by Upledger's teachings and the expansion of holistic health care, are providing craniosacral manipulation in their offices. To find an osteopath who utilizes manual manipulation, go to www.osteopathic.org and search for "Osteo Manipulative Medicine" to view the list of D.O.s practicing in the United States. To find an osteopathic physician who specializes in craniosacral therapy, go to www.cranialacademy.org.

Holistic Chiropractic Physicians

Many D.C.s are also currently re-embracing their holistic roots, primarily through various chiropractic techniques. Applied Kinesiologists who utilize the triad of health model—that is, that disease can be caused by structural, psychological, and biochemical imbalances—are often the best holistic physicians in their community. To find

*Despite these efforts, manual manipulation by medical doctors is still exceedingly rare, especially when compared with the large number of chiropractic physicians who specialize in spinal adjusting.

an Applied Kinesiologist near you (the great majority are chiropractors), go to www.icakusa.com, or call (913) 384-5336. To find other (nonkinesiologist) holistic chiropractors who utilize nutrition and other natural medicines and therapies along with their specialty of manual manipulation, word of mouth from satisfied friends and family is often the best referral.

In conclusion, the modern holistic D.C. or D.O. recognizes that many factors cause back pain, and that simply adjusting an area of the spine because it is painful or has limited motion is not acceptable. He or she is well versed in somatovisceral as well as viscerosomatic relationships, through the study of older research literature, as well as current neurological and physiological findings. Based on the patient's history, examination findings, laboratory and radiographic findings, and, for a certain percentage, energetic testing methods, the holistic physician first diagnoses the cause of the spinal fixation and then chooses (or tests for) the most appropriate treatment. This treatment typically includes spinal manipulation, craniopathy, and other supportive natural therapies (nutritional supplementation, homeopathy, drainage, auriculotherapy, etc.). If he or she is not well versed in one of these holistic modalities that seems necessary for the patient, then a referral to another holistic physician is made.

Holistic D.C.s and D.O.s further realize the importance of referring to holistic dentists to remove significant "obstacles to cure" in their patients. They are well aware that spinal fixations and muscle pain are often secondary to the obstacles of mercury amalgam toxicity, dental focal infections, and major malocclusions and TMD. If a patient's history and tests indicate serious disease such as cancer or an impending heart attack, the holistic physician *and* the patient will discuss working in conjunction with an allopathic oncologist or heart specialist. Holistic D.C.s and D.O.s—as well as N.D.s and nonallopathic holistic M.D.s—all recognize that patient education and communication are just as essential to healing as an accurate diagnosis and the skillful application of their natural therapies.

CONCLUSION

Because structural problems so often signal deeper pathology, the burden of skillful and accurate differential diagnosis falls heavily on the shoulders of those doctors who most often serve as the initial portal of entry for sufferers of back pain—chiropractic and osteopathic physicians. Through both conventional methods (a thorough history and physical exam, lab work, X-rays, etc.), as well as holistic measures such as energetic testing, the holistic D.O. or D.C. can arrive at a well-considered diagnosis and proposed treatment plan. In chronic cases, patients often need to be first referred to a holistic dentist (amalgam removal, cavitation surgery, a functional orthopedic appliance, etc.), or to a good psychotherapist (rebirthing, Jungian therapy, etc.), or simply to go home and avoid their primary food allergen for a few weeks. In the vast majority of cases, these initial measures render subsequent manipulative treatments more effective and lasting.

Holistic dentists also shoulder the heavy responsibility of making thoughtful and accurate differential diagnoses, especially concerning preventive dental medicine. The signs of moderate to major malocclusions can be observed quite early, and treating young children in a timely fashion can reduce and even prevent more challenging teeth and jaw problems later. The placement of primary molar buildups ("occlusal fillings") or functional orthopedic appliances can make dramatic changes in young children, as well as in adults who are burdened with bad bites and TMD. Additionally, conscientious dentists also utilize dietary counseling, nutritional supplementation, or cell (tissue) salts, or refer out to holistic practitioners who can render these treatments. Dentists who treat the whole body not only rightfully serve their patients but also fulfill the promise of their trailblazing forefathers Weston A. Price and A. C. Fonder, in appropriately functioning as invaluable holistic physicians and clinical researchers in the field of dental medicine.

NOTES

1. H. Hooshmand, *Chronic Pain: Reflex Sympathetic Dystrophy Prevention and Management* (Boca Raton, Fla.: CRC Press, 1993), 52; P. Williams, *Gray's Anatomy* (New York: Churchill Livingstone, 1995), 980.
2. H. Hooshmand, *Chronic Pain: Reflex Sympathetic*

Dystrophy Prevention and Management (Boca Raton, Fla.: CRC Press, 1993), 51–52.

3. *Dorland's Illustrated Medical Dictionary,* 26th ed. (Philadelphia: W. B. Saunders Company, 1981), 1305.
4. M. Gershon, *The Second Brain* (New York: HarperPerennial, 1999), xi–xvi.
5. P. Rowan, *Some Body* (New York: Alfred A. Knopf, 1995), 30, 32.
6. T. Brown, "On Irritation of the Spinal Nerves," *Glasgow Medical Journal,* May 1828, 147.
7. F. Schiller, "Spinal Irritation and Osteopathy," *Bulletin of the History of Medicine* 45 (1971): 254–55.
8. R. Player, "On Irritation of the Spinal Nerves," *Quarterly Journal of Science* 12 (1821): 429.
9. H. Head, "On Disturbances of Sensation with Especial Reference to the Pain of Visceral Disease," *Brain* XVI (1893): 1–131; S. Finger, *Origins of Neuroscience* (New York: Oxford University Press, 1994), 138–39.
10. C. Masarsky and M. Todres-Masarsky, *Somatovisceral Aspects of Chiropractic* (New York: Churchill Livingstone, 2001), 51–52.
11. H. Head, "On Disturbances of Sensation with Especial Reference to the Pain of Visceral Disease," *Brain* XVI (1893): 3.
12. Ibid., 52–53.
13. "Referred Pain," Healthcaps, www.icakusa.com.
14. Ibid.
15. AAOM, *The Collected Papers of Irvin M. Korr* (Indianapolis: American Academy of Osteopathy, 1993), 77.
16. D. Walther, *Applied Kinesiology Synopsis* (Pueblo, Colo.: Systems DC, 1988), 2, 46–49.
17. M. Rosen, "Research Status of Applied Kinesiology, Part I," *Applied Kinesiology Review* 1, no. 1 (Fall 1990): 42–54; M. Rosen and L. Williams, "Research Status of Applied Kinesiology, Part II," *Applied Kinesiology Review* 1, no. 2 (Spring 1991): 34–47.
18. S. Levy and C. Lehr, *Your Body Can Talk* (Prescott, Ariz.: Hohm Press, 1996), 5.
19. C. Masarsky and M. Todres-Masarky, *Somatovisceral Aspects of Chiropractic* (New York: Churchill Livingstone, 2001), 51.
20. H. Hooshmand, *Chronic Pain: Reflex Sympathetic Dystrophy Prevention and Management* (Boca Raton, Fla.: CRC Press, 1993), 121.
21. A. Lowen, *Bioenergetics* (New York: Penguin Books, 1975), 13, 38.
22. Ibid., 186–87, 237.
23. Ibid., 190.
24. A. Lowen and L. Lowen, *The Way to Vibrant Health* (New York: Harper Colophon Books, 1977), 4.
25. F. Schiller, "Spinal Irritation and Osteopathy," *Bulletin of the History of Medicine* 45 (1971): 252–54.
26. T. Brown, "On Irritation of the Spinal Nerves," *Glasgow Medical Journal,* May 1828, 131–41.
27. F. Schiller, "Spinal Irritation and Osteopathy," *Bulletin of the History of Medicine* 45 (1971): 254.
28. Ibid., 255
29. J. Greenhoot, "The Effect of Cervical Cord Injury on Cardiac Rhythm and Conduction," *American Heart Journal* 83 (1972): 659–62; D. Davis, "Respiratory Manifestations of Dorsal Spine Radiculitis Simulating Symptoms of Cardiac Asthma," *Annals of Internal Medicine* 32 (1950): 954–59; M. Eadie, "Paroxysmal Positional Giddiness," *Medical Journal of Australia* (1967): 1169–73; P. Sherwood, "Effective Prevention of Coronary Heart Attacks," *Digest of Chiropractic Economics,* November/December 1985, 54–57, 122–23.
30. J. Carnett, "The Simulation of Gall Bladder Disease by Intercostal Neuralgia of the Abdominal Wall," *Annals of Surgery* 86: 747–57; R. Gilsdorf et al., "Central Nervous System Influence on Experimentally Induced Pancreatitis," *Journal of the American Medical Association* 5, no. 192 (1965): 134–37.
31. N. Ussher, "The Viscerospinal Syndrome," *Annals of Internal Medicine* (May 1940): 205–9.
32. H. Winsor, "The Evidences of the Association, in Dissected Cadavers, of Visceral Disease with Vertebral Deformities of the Same Sympathetic Segments," *The Medical Times* 49 (November 1921): 267–71.
33. A. Towbin, "Latent Spinal Cord and Brain Stem Injury in Newborn Infants," *Development Medicine and Child Neurology* 11 (1969): 54–68.
34. M. Beal, "Palpatory Testing for Somatic Dysfunction in Patients with Cardiovascular Disease," *Journal of the American Osteopathic Association* 82 (1983): 73–74.
35. C. Masarsky and M. Todres-Masarky, *Somatovisceral Aspects of Chiropractic* (New York: Churchill Livingstone, 2001), 12.
36. J. Dvorak and V. Dvorak, *Manual Medicine* (New York: Georg Thieme Verlag, 1984), 29.
37. S. Haldeman, "The Compression Subluxation," *Journal of Clinical Chiropractic* 7 (1971): 10–21; L. Ely, "Subluxation of the Atlas," *Annals of Surgery,* no. 54 (1911): 20–29.
38. A. Vasquez, "Allopathic Usurpation of Natural Medicine:

The Blind Leading the Sighted," *Naturopathy Digest* 1, no. 2 (February 2006): 14.

39. C. Masarsky and M. Todres-Masarky, *Somatovisceral Aspects of Chiropractic* (New York: Churchill Livingstone, 2001), 12; M. Gatterman, *Chiropractic Management of Spine Related Disorders* (Baltimore: Williams and Wilkins, 1990), xv.
40. C. Masarsky and M. Todres-Masarky, *Somatovisceral Aspects of Chiropractic* (New York: Churchill Livingstone, 2001), 12.
41. K. Ligeros, *How Ancient Healing Governs Modern Therapeutics* (New York: G. P. Putnam's Sons, 1937), 465–66.
42. N. Gevitz, *The DOs* (Baltimore: The Johns Hopkins University Press, 1982), 1, 12–13, 15–18.
43. Ibid., 12.
44. C. Masarsky and M. Todres-Masarsky, *Somatovisceral Aspects of Chiropractic* (New York: Churchill Livingstone, 2001), 12.
45. N. Gevitz, *The DOs* (Baltimore: The Johns Hopkins University Press, 1982), 16.
46. Ibid., 19, 26–29.
47. Ibid., 29.
48. A. Homewood, *The Neurodynamics of the Vertebral Subluxation* (St. Petersburg, Fla.: Valkyrie Press, 1962), 16.
49. N. Gevitz, *The DOs* (Baltimore: The Johns Hopkins University Press, 1982), 58–59.
50. Ibid., 58.
51. Ibid., 58–59; C. Masarsky and M. Todres-Masarky, *Somatovisceral Aspects of Chiropractic* (New York: Churchill Livingstone, 2001), 13.
52. N. Gevitz, *The DOs* (Baltimore: The Johns Hopkins University Press, 1982), 59.
53. C. Masarsky and M. Todres-Masarsky, *Somatovisceral Aspects of Chiropractic* (New York: Churchill Livingstone, 2001), 29.
54. N. Gevitz, *The DOs* (Baltimore: The Johns Hopkins University Press, 1982), 58.
55. Ibid., 14.
56. C. Masarsky and M. Todres-Masarsky, *Somatovisceral Aspects of Chiropractic* (New York: Churchill Livingstone, 2001), 3.
57. Ibid., 12.
58. N. Gevitz, *The DOs* (Baltimore: The Johns Hopkins University Press, 1982), 59.
59. Ibid., 90.
60. N. Ussher, "The Viscerospinal Syndrome—A New Concept of Visceromotor and Sensory Changes in Relation to Deranged Spinal Structures," *Annals of Internal Medicine* (May 1940): 2069–70.
61. R. Tilley, "Practical Aspects of the Treatment of Chronic Systemic Infections," *Journal of the American Osteopathic Association,* May 1946, 391–95.
62. G. Hartmann, "An Analysis of 350 Emotionally Maladjusted Individuals Under Chiropractic Care," *NCA Journal of Chiropractic,* November 1949, 14.
63. C. Masarsky and M. Todres-Masarsky, *Somatovisceral Aspects of Chiropractic* (New York: Churchill Livingstone, 2001), 234.
64. H. Schwartz, ed., and W. Quigley, *Mental Health and Chiropractic* (New York: Sessions Publishers, 1973), 115.
65. Ibid., 115–16.
66. W. Kirkaldy-Willis and J. Cassidy, "Spinal Manipulation in the Treatment of Low Back Pain," *Canadian Family Physician* 31 (1985): 535–40; J. Cox, "Chiropractic Statistical Survey of 100 Consecutive Low Back Pain Patients," *Journal of Manipulative Physiological Therapeutics* 6, no. 3 (1983): 117–28.
67. C. Cottam, "The Roots of Cranial Manipulation: Nephi Cottam and 'Craniopathy,'" *Chiropractic History* 1, no. 1 (1981): 31.
68. J. McParland and E. Mein, "Entrainment and the Cranial Rhythmic Impulse," *Alternative Therapies* 3, no. 1 (January 1997): 40.
69. N. Cottam, *The Story of Craniopathy* (Los Angeles: self-published, 1936).
70. C. Cottam, "The Roots of Cranial Manipulation: Nephi Cottam and 'Craniopathy,'" *Chiropractic History* 1, no. 1 (1981): 31–32.
71. Ibid., 32.
72. Ibid.
73. W. Sutherland, *The Cranial Bowl* (Mankato, Minn.: Free Press Co., 1939), 1.
74. J. McParland and E. Mein, "Entrainment and the Cranial Rhythmic Impulse," *Alternative Therapies* 3, no. 1 (January 1997): 40.
75. Ibid., 40–41.
76. R. Holding, *Craniosacral Therapy in the Context of Clinical Kinesiology* (London: self-published, October 1988), 2.
77. Ibid., 11.
78. D. Klinghardt and L. Williams, *Neural Kinesiology II* (Seattle: AANT, 1994), 32–33; L. Williams, *Basic and Advanced AM/FM Manual, Part II* (San Anselmo, Calif.: AANK, 1999), 32–33.

79. D. Walther, *Applied Kinesiology Synopsis* (Pueblo, Colo.: Systems DC, 1988), 368.
80. S. Blood, "The Craniosacral Mechanism and the Temporomandibular Joint," *Journal of the American Osteopathic Association* 86, no. 8: 85–92; E. Baker, "Alteration in Width of Maxillary Arch and Its Relation to Sutural Movement of Cranial Bones," *Journal of the American Osteopathic Association* 70 (February 1971): 559–64.
81. V. Frymann, "Relation of Disturbances of Craniosacral Mechanisms to Symptomatology of the Newborn," *Journal of the American Osteopathic Association* 65: 1059–75.
82. R. van Assche, "Visceral Manipulation" seminar (notes), Hawaii (October 1997).
83. R. Holding, "Craniosacral Therapy in the Context of Clinical Kinesiology" seminar (notes), Santa Fe (October 1988).
84. P. Manley, "Cranial Osteopathy and the Infantile Craniopathies," *Frontier Perspectives,* Fall/Winter 1991, 31–33; J. Upledger and J. Vredevoogd, *Craniosacral Therapy* (Chicago: Eastland Press, 1983), 260.
85. G. Smith, *Cranial Dental Sacral Complex* (Newtown, Pa.: self-published, 1983), 13.
86. J. Upledger and J. Vredevoogd, *Craniosacral Therapy* (Chicago: Eastland Press, 1983), 260, 262–64, 269; J. Upledger, "Craniosacral Function in Brain Dysfunction," *Osteopathic Annals* 11, no. 7 (July 1983): 57–64; P. Manley, "Cranial Osteopathy and the Infantile Craniopathies," *Frontier Perspectives,* Fall/Winter 1991, 31–33; F. Marasa and B. Ham, "Case Reports Involving the Treatment of Children with Chronic Otitis Media with Effusion via Craniomandibular Methods," *The Journal of Craniomandibular Practice* 6, no. 3 (July 1988): 256–70.
87. J. Upledger and J. Vredevoogd, *Craniosacral Therapy* (Chicago: Eastland Press, 1983), 267–68, 291.
88. C. Reuben, "Craniosacral Therapy," *East West,* October 1987, 23.
89. D. Juhan, *Job's Body* (Barrytown, N.Y.: Station Hill, 1998), xx, xxi, xxv.
90. Ibid., 68–69.
91. Ibid., 69–70.
92. Ibid., xxv.
93. C. Masarsky and M. Todres-Masarky, *Somatovisceral Aspects of Chiropractic* (New York: Churchill Livingstone, 2001), 23.
94. J. Howard, *Encyclopedia of Chiropractic* (Chicago: National School of Chiropractic, n.d.), xxix.
95. Ibid.; F. Schiller, "Spinal Irritation and Osteopathy," *Bulletin of the History of Medicine* 45 (1971): 252–54.
96. D. Palmer, *The Chiropractor* (Los Angeles: Press of Beacon Light Printing Company, 1914), 3, 4, 67–71, 76–77; N. Gevitz, ed., *Other Healers: Unorthodox Medicine in America* (Baltimore: The Johns Hopkins University Press, 1988), 158–59, 162–65; H. Schwartz, ed., and W. Quigley, *Mental Health and Chiropractic* (New York: Sessions Publishers, 1973); C. Masarsky and M. Todres-Masarky, *Somatovisceral Aspects of Chiropractic* (New York: Churchill Livingstone, 2001), 109.
97. P. Lisa, *The Assault on Medical Freedom* (Norfolk, Va.: Hampton Roads Publishing Company, 1994), 206–7.
98. N. Gevitz, ed., *Other Healers: Unorthodox Medicine in America* (Baltimore: The Johns Hopkins University Press, 1988), 165.
99. C. Masarsky and M. Todres-Masarky, *Somatovisceral Aspects of Chiropractic* (New York: Churchill Livingstone, 2001), 30, 31.
100. N. Gevitz, ed., *Other Healers: Unorthodox Medicine in America* (Baltimore: The Johns Hopkins University Press, 1988), 174.
101. C. Masarsky and M. Todres-Masarky, *Somatovisceral Aspects of Chiropractic* (New York: Churchill Livingstone, 2001), 30.
102. J. Robbins, *Reclaiming Our Health* (Tiburon, Calif.: H. J. Kramer, 1996), 189–90.
103. P. Lisa, *The Assault on Medical Freedom* (Norfolk, Va.: Hampton Roads Publishing Company, 1994), 17.
104. J. Robbins, *Reclaiming Our Health* (Tiburon, Calif.: H. J. Kramer, 1996), 190.
105. P. Lisa, *The Assault on Medical Freedom* (Norfolk, Va.: Hampton Roads Publishing Company, 1994), 207.
106. J. Robbins, *Reclaiming Our Health* (Tiburon, Calif.: H. J. Kramer, 1996), 188.
107. C. Masarsky and M. Todres-Masarky, *Somatovisceral Aspects of Chiropractic* (New York: Churchill Livingstone, 2001), 31.
108. P. Lisa, *The Assault on Medical Freedom* (Norfolk, Va.: Hampton Roads Publishing Company, 1994), 237.
109. M. Pedigo, "Wilk vs. AMA: Was It Worth the Fight?" www.chiroweb.com/archives/16/15/14.
110. Ibid.
111. C. Masarsky and M. Todres-Masarky, *Somatovisceral Aspects of Chiropractic* (New York: Churchill Livingstone, 2001), 30.
112. Ibid., 31.

113. J. Robbins, *Reclaiming Our Health* (Tiburon, Calif.: H. J. Kramer, 1996), 193.

114. C. Masarsky and M. Todres-Masarky, *Somatovisceral Aspects of Chiropractic* (New York: Churchill Livingstone, 2001), 31.

115. J. Robbins, *Reclaiming Our Health* (Tiburon, Calif.: H. J. Kramer, 1996), 195–96.

116. Ibid.

117. H. Baer, "The Sociopolitical Development of British Chiropractic," *Journal of Manipulative and Physiological Therapeutics* 14, no. 1 (January 1991): 44.

118. F. Barge, "Chiropractic's Greatest Tactical Error," *Dynamic Chiropractic* 18 (1993): 45.

119. C. Masarsky and M. Todres-Masarky, *Somatovisceral Aspects of Chiropractic* (New York: Churchill Livingstone, 2001), 2.

120. Ibid.

121. Ibid., 17, 18.

122. Ibid.; J. Howard, *Encyclopedia of Chiropractic* (Chicago: National School of Chiropractic, n.d.), xxix–xxx.

123. N. Gevitz, *The DOs* (Baltimore: The Johns Hopkins University Press, 1982), 23–29, 102, 118.

124. Ibid., 101.

125. Ibid., 101–2, 114–15.

126. N. Gevitz, ed., *Other Healers: Unorthodox Medicine in America* (Baltimore: The Johns Hopkins University Press, 1988), 149; N. Gevitz, *The DOs* (Baltimore: The Johns Hopkins University Press, 1982), 119, 122.

127. Ibid., 124–25, 135.

128. Ibid., 89.

129. Ibid., 110.

130. D. Chapman-Smith, "Weekend Manipulation for MDs," *The Chiropractic Report* 3, no. 6 (September 1989): 1.

131. N. Gevitz, *The DOs* (Baltimore: The Johns Hopkins University Press, 1982), 93.

132. N. Gevitz ed., *Other Healers: Unorthodox Medicine in America* (Baltimore: The Johns Hopkins University Press, 1988), 154.

133. WebMD, "Total Body Medicine," www.webmd.com/balance/features/total-body-medicine.

134. Ibid.

135. Texas College of Osteopathic Medicine, curriculum, www.hsc.unt.edu/education/tcom/courses.cfm.

PART SEVEN

MENTAL AND EMOTIONAL FACTORS

Consciousness is a funny thing. Once you become conscious, you can't just regress. In fact, the opposite happens: you find yourself becoming conscious of more and more. And consciousness is the predecessor of transformation.

PATRICIA IRELAND

The term *holistic medicine* was first used by Russian physiologist and psychologist Dr. Ivan Pavlov (1849–1936).[1]* In contrast to the reductionistic approach of allopathic medicine, holistic medicine recognizes the interconnectedness of the whole being. Thus, whereas conventional allopathic medicine typically reduces psychological problems to a biochemical level and prescribes drugs to sufficiently suppress the symptoms, holistic medicine takes into account every *possible* aspect of the human being that could contribute to mental and emotional disturbance.

In many cases, these symptoms derive primarily from psychological issues themselves, such as when a woman struggles with chronic depression from not being valued as a child, or when a man consistently reacts with inappropriate anger that was learned from an abusive father.

In other cases, the primary etiology of mental and emotional pain can be far afield from classic psychological origins. These can include chronic irritability and anger secondary to mercury intoxication from amalgam fillings, obsessive-compulsive symptoms manifesting from a dominant tonsil focus, and intermittent anxiety or depression triggered by the daily use of conventional and toxic soaps, shampoos, and other personal care products. Although the prescription of an antidepressant may give short-term (real or placebo) relief for some of these symptoms, in the long term it only intoxicates the body even more. Additionally, these synthetic medications can significantly muddy the diagnostic waters, reducing the chance of the patient ever receiving a clear and accurate assessment that can lead to effective treatment.

TREATING MAJOR ISSUES AT ALL LEVELS

This interconnected body-mind relationship is exemplified by the fact that astute holistic physicians are aware that invariably almost every major symptom, or "chief complaint," that a patient experiences needs to be addressed at *every* level.

For example, chronic heart disease can never be entirely healed without treatment of the underlying emotional pain that typically originated in early childhood. Although identification and treatment of a culpable dental focal infection, auriculotherapy of related (bypass surgery) scar interference fields, gemmotherapy remedies to drain toxins from the cardiac muscle,* and nutritional supplementation to strengthen and restore cardiac muscle function (coenzyme Q-10, magnesium, taurine, etc.) are all superlative and essential treatments, they are rarely sufficient to achieve a complete cure. In fact, even the near-miraculous effects of the most perfectly fitting constitutional homeopathic simillimum

*In 1904, Ivan Petrovich Pavlov received the Nobel Prize for observing that dogs salivated before eating simply through anticipation of their meal that was signaled by a stimulus—a bell, whistle, metronome, tuning fork, and various visual stimuli. Pavlov termed this stimulus-response phenomenon a *conditional reflex,* and it later greatly influenced the development of the psychology of behavior modification.

*Hawthorn (*Crataegus oxyacantha*), a gemmotherapy drainage remedy made from the young shoots of the hawthorn tree, is often indicated for patients with various forms of cardiovascular disease. However, almost equally as often, Crataegus comes up positive in energetic testing for patients with no physical heart-related history but with unresolved past emotional pain and trauma.

(according to the Sankaran system), which can heal deeply at every level, still cannot replace the insight, self-understanding, and true maturity that quality psychospiritual work bestows. Thus, an individual needs to heal not only the body but also the mind and spirit to fully release the deep feelings of grief that "broke the heart" and weakened the cardiac muscle in the first place.*

psychospiritual: The term *psychospiritual* refers to therapies, schools, or paths that meld modern Western psychology with Eastern spiritual traditions.

ACCURATE DIAGNOSIS AND APPROPRIATE REFERRAL

Based on these observations, psychotherapists and psychiatrists should be aware of the toxic, microbial, and focal origins of mental and emotional disturbances and appropriately refer patients to practitioners who treat these conditions. Conversely, practitioners must be cognizant of and able to diagnose issues that are arising primarily from mental and emotional disorders and readily refer patients for competent psychological help. It is necessary that both professions realize that patients require treatment at *both* levels—the psychological and the physical—to fully heal all of the ramifications arising from a major life "wound."

Therapeutic Healing Field Is Essential

Some doctors attempt to clear the emerging psychological issues a patient is experiencing themselves. If the practitioner has a sufficient background in psychology, this decision may be appropriate. However, this therapeutic work must be conducted in a supportive environment. Testing a root-canal dental focal infection in one moment, and then later in the same appointment inquiring into a patient's relationship with an abusive parent, rarely supports a therapeutic field of deep awareness and insight that is imperative for real healing. In fact, this changing of "hats" from doctor to therapist can be not only confusing to a patient but often counterproductive and sometimes quite harmful.

Identification and Mitigation of the Core Issue

When psychological issues come up during energetic testing, I choose to gently discern the particular limiting belief or emotion and mitigate its acute impact through essential oils, flower remedies,* or NET—percussion (sympathetic nerve stimulation) of the area of the spine that reflexes (psychosomatically) with the organ associated with the core disturbing emotion. If the issue is significant (and it usually is), the patient is then referred to a psychotherapist, psychologist, psychiatrist, or teacher† who can more deeply assess and inquire into these arising issues. Knowledgeable practitioners—who have some training in psychology as well as personal experience in healing their own wounds—can make the most insightful referrals to the appropriate therapist.

► For more information about NET, or Neuro Emotional Technique, visit the website www.netmindbody.com.

Psychospiritual Work: "Grow Up" as well as "Wake Up"

Some patients, especially those with significant anxiety or disabling depression,‡ require long-term counseling or psychotherapy through more gentle cognitive and behavioral psychology approaches to slowly reduce the damage done to their young ego structure incurred from major abuse (physically, sexually, or verbally) or neglect during the early stages of development. Others who have sufficient ego stability to handle the deconstruction of the egoic self—concomitant with the arising of one's more authentic or true self—can be referred to psychospiritually oriented therapists (transpersonal psychologists, Jungian therapists, rebirthing therapists, etc.) or paths (Ridhwan or Diamond Heart) from the outset. These

*A February 2005 article in the *Washington Post* on the findings of a study in the *New England Journal of Medicine* confirmed the damaging psychophysical effects of a broken heart: "A traumatic breakup, the death of a loved one or even the shock of a surprise party can unleash a flood of stress hormones that can stun the heart, causing sudden, life-threatening heart spasms in otherwise healthy people." (R. Stein, "A Broken Heart Can Kill," *The Press Democrat,* February 10, 2005, A-1, A-9.)

*Typically, flower remedies are given to newer patients. In advanced patients who are already on their constitutional remedy, the re-dosing of this remedy is typically indicated.

†In the transpersonal school of psychospiritual healing called Ridhwan or Diamond Heart, therapists are referred to as "teachers."

‡For example, patients with major mental or emotional disorders, neuroses, or borderline personality tendencies.

particular psychospiritual approaches, which John Welwood, Ph.D., characterizes as those that help us both "*grow up*—to ripen into a mature, fully developed person," as well as "*waking up* to our ultimate spiritual nature," are essential in healing and transcending the deepest wounds to our body, mind, and spirit.[2]

Time, Energy, and Commitment to Truth

Typically, the more "advanced" patients—those who have cleared the bulk of their toxins and foci and are on their appropriate constitutional homeopathic remedy—have the most profound commitment to truth. Therefore, they more often have the inner strength and courage to investigate a particular referral to see if the therapist or work truly serves their growth. Additionally, because these individuals have also progressed further away from their initial "survival mode" existence (e.g., the tuberculinic and luetic miasmic levels), they now have the time, energy, and capacity to focus on their unique psychological and spiritual growth.* Furthermore, as their physical body becomes healthier and thus energetically (and sometimes physically) lighter, the weight of any remaining unresolved psychological issues begins to emerge into the foreground of their consciousness. In these more "advanced" patients, the strong will that first guided them to reject the suppressive effects of allopathic drugs and seek alternatives in holistic medicine also animates their movement toward effective psychospiritual healing.

NOTES

1. P. Dosch, *Manual of Neural Therapy* (Heidelberg: Haug, 1984), 25.
2. J. Welwood, *Toward a Psychology of Awakening* (Boston: Shambhala, 2000), xviii.

*This natural evolution from matter to spirit was well elucidated by the founder of humanistic psychology, Abraham Maslow (1908–1970). In Maslow's hierarchy of needs, survival and safety must be met before individuals can become self-actualized and realize their maximum potential.

18

ADVANCED APPROACHES TO PSYCHOSPIRITUAL HEALING

True healing must take place at the physical, psychological, and spiritual levels. So far, this book has covered the optimum holistic practices and modalities for physical recovery. Now we will look at the interrelationship of psychology and spirituality for psychospiritual healing. This newer term, *psychospiritual,* can be best explained by reviewing the history of psychology itself.

THE DEVOLUTION OF THE FIELD OF PSYCHOLOGY

The twentieth century saw a push for all disciplines to achieve a more scientific respectability. Unfortunately, the field of psychology was one of the foremost victims of the widespread reductionism that was the chief side effect inherent in this movement. Over time, the inclination to compartmentalize and explain psychology in merely mechanistic terms became predominant. This modern trend is particularly underscored by the current definition of the term *psychology* in the Oxford English dictionary, where the word *mind* has been inserted in place of the former term *soul:*

> [Psychology is] the science of the nature, functioning, and development of the human mind (formerly of the human soul).[1]

Psyche and Spirit Originally Inseparable

Ken Wilber, a leader in the field of transpersonal psychology, clearly elucidates the modern devolution of psychology from "soul and spirit" to "matter and mind" in his book *Integral Psychology.* Wilber makes the point that not only did the term *psychology* originally refer to the study of *both* the mind and the spirit but that Sigmund Freud (1856–1939), the father of psychoanalysis, actually used concepts from Eastern spiritual traditions in formulating his theories.[2]

> **transpersonal psychology:** Transpersonal psychology incorporates the insights gained in Western psychology of the personal and interpersonal, along with the illumination of the spiritual *suprapersonal* aspects of human nature.[3] Thus, this holistic field of psychology encompasses the knowledge of both the East and the West to facilitate the healing of the mind and emotions, as well as the spirit. Well-known modern transpersonal psychologists include Jack Kornfield, Michael Murphy, John Welwood, and Ken Wilber. (Transpersonal psychology, relatively synonymous with the term *psychospiritual,* will be discussed in more detail later in this chapter.)

Freud's Use of Concepts from Eastern Traditions

Freud's concept of the *id*—the term describing the unconscious and instinctive mind—was taken from Georg Groddeck's *The Book of the It,* which was based on "the existence of a cosmic Tao or organic universal spirit."[4] This understanding of the human spirit in association with the unconscious mind had actually been popularized thirty years before Freud through von Hartmann's book *Philosophy of the Unconscious,* which was largely derived from the German philosopher Arthur Schopenhauer through his extensive study of Eastern mysticism, Buddhism, and the Upanishads.[5*]

THE UPANISHADS

The Upanishads is a collection of 108 texts that makes up the second part of India's scriptures, known as the Vedas. The first part of the Vedas, which later became the central core of Hindu philosophy, is made up of hymns and poetry worshipping the natural forces and elements in life and explanations of ritual and symbolic sacrifices. However, the second part, the Upanishads, conveys the first comprehensive and universal spiritual teachings ever spoken (~3000 BCE) and recorded (~1500–500 BCE). The word *upanishad,* meaning "sitting down near," indicates the source of these teachings—that is, at the feet of an illumined teacher. From this spiritual instruction, the emphasis shifted in spirituality and religion from invoking external gods to realizing the god within, or "the sacred force (*brahman*) that lives in all things." Thus, the Upanishads teach what Aldous Huxley later termed the Perennial Philosophy, namely that "oneness can be realized directly, without the mediation of priests or rituals or any of the structures of organized religion, not after death but in this life, and that this is the purpose for which each of us has been born and the goal toward which evolution moves." The Upanishads view ultimate reality from different levels of spiritual awareness and define these central ideas as the following: "*Brahman,* the Godhead; *Atman,* the divine core of personality; *dharma,* the law that expresses and maintains the unity of creation; *karma,* the web of cause and effect; *samsara,* the cycle of birth and death; *moksha,* the spiritual liberation that is life's supreme goal."[6]

*German philosopher Arthur Schopenhauer (1788–1860) was the first Western philosopher to have access to—and to be profoundly affected by—the Vedic and Buddhist teachings of the East. In *Memories, Dreams, Reflections,* Carl Jung was impressed that Schopenhauer "was the first to speak of the suffering of the world" and further that "here at last was a philosopher who had the courage to see that all was not for the best in the fundaments of the universe." (C. Jung, *Memories, Dreams, Reflections* [New York: Vintage, 1989], 39.)

Jung Integrated Eastern Philosophy into Western Psychology

The Swiss psychiatrist Carl Gustav Jung (1875–1961), who was a colleague of Freud's, greatly elaborated the interconnectedness of Eastern and Western thought. Because he was also influenced by Schopenhauer, Jung felt a strong bond with the spirit of the East, which was exemplified through his writings on the emphasis of one's inner experience and the belief that self-understanding went beyond the "narrow confines of the conscious ego."[7] Through his friendship with Richard Wilhelm, Jung helped propagate the Chinese philosophy of the I Ching* and integrated many Taoist concepts into his psychological body of work. An understanding of yin and yang gained from Taoism also influenced Jung in the development of his theory of the collective unconscious and the concepts of the *animus*—the male side in each female—and the *anima*—the female side in each male. Other influences from his Eastern studies included the identification of the *shadow*—the violent and animalistic impulses he witnessed arising from dreams—and *archetypal* memories—the set of images originating from mythology, art, and religion that are purportedly stored in the unconscious of every human being.[8] Jung's study of Eastern spiritual traditions further shaped his concept of *individuation,* which he defined as the soul's journey toward realization—a journey he believed began in the heart chakra.[9]

Origins of the Term *Therapist*

This original inseparable linkage of psyche and spirit is further exemplified in the word *therapy* itself, which comes from the Greek word *therapeia,* meaning "serving the gods" or "doing the gods' work." Additionally, the root word for therapist, *therapeutikos,* translates to "servant." Thus, most ideally, a knowledgeable and conscious psychotherapist or psychologist, as Socrates declared, could be said to be one who is in service to, and doing, "God's work."[10†]

*Jung wrote the introduction to Wilhelm's translated book, *I Ching: The Book of Changes.* Jung also coined the term *synchronicity,* which correlated with the I Ching belief that events occur in life more than through mere chance but through a "marvelous, fluid, interconnected system of relations." (R. Wing, *The I Ching Workbook* [St. Charles, Mo.: Main Street Books, 1978], 8.)

†In Plato's works, he quoted Socrates as saying the term *therapy* refers to "service to the gods." (T. Moore, *Care of the Soul* [New York: Harper Perennial, 1992], xvii.)

Psychospiritual Work Is Most Transformative

Despite having holistic roots that were originally inclusive of both Eastern and Western philosophy and spiritual traditions, the field of orthodox psychology has narrowed so greatly that it presently is considered rather "soul-less," in that it primarily concentrates on the study of the human mind (brain) and the dissecting of human behavior. Therefore, the term *psychospiritual* has been employed in this chapter to more accurately describe the original roots of psychology, and so that it is not confused with modern approaches such as behavioral psychology, experimental psychology, neuropsychology, developmental psychology, and cognitive psychology. This usage does not negate the great body of valuable information that has developed from these various disciplines but simply clarifies that these more behaviorist and cognitive approaches do not encompass the entire field of psychology. Furthermore, because the psychospiritual approaches have been the most effective and transformative both in my practice (especially for the more "advanced" patients for whom this book was primarily written) and personally, they will be highlighted and described most fully in this chapter.

THE BENEFITS OF LIVING NOW
Easy Access to Psychospiritual Work

Although there are countless negative aspects of this modern world—pandemic petroleum chemicals, toxic metals, devitalized foods, and the widespread use of suppressive pharmaceutical drugs—one of the major positive aspects of living now (besides flush toilets and modern sanitation) is both the acceptance of and the easy access to psychospiritual literature, therapists, and pathways.

The Taboo Has Shifted

For the first time in history, the onus of what Alan Watts referred to as "the taboo against knowing who you are" has shifted, at least in many parts of the United States and the rest of the world.[11] In fact, in those areas with a more progressive populace, *not* engaging in a certain amount of psychospiritual healing—especially in those individuals with obvious signs of unresolved grief, fear, or anger—is looked on with as much disdain as refusing to seek medical attention when bleeding from a wound. (As those who have undergone effective psychospiritual healing are well aware, there is little difference in intensity between the pain of untreated physical wounds and the pain of acute or chronically suppressed emotional wounds.) Unfortunately, the level of denial about a psychological wound even existing is still relatively high in the general population, as exemplified by the numerous "numbing out" behaviors of overeating and excessive television watching in our culture.*

Eastern Spirituality Augments Psychospiritual Approaches

The revolutionary spirit of the 1960s and 1970s that stimulated the rise of holistic medicine also augmented the emergence of its corollary—psychospiritual healing. As more and more baby boomers began to investigate the traditions and practices of Eastern religions, centers for studying Hinduism (Transcendental Meditation, hatha yoga, Hare Krishnas, etc.), Buddhism (Mahayana, Vajrayana, Zen, etc.), and Sufism began to spring up all over the West. Correspondingly, nontraditional Western modes of psychotherapy—greatly influenced by the philosophy of these Eastern religions—flourished as the benefits of their more holistic psychological approach were proven effective.

Acknowledging Abuse of Power in Some Cases

Of course, not all of these approaches were valid and effective, and in some instances they were harmful. Just as physicians can abuse their power, so too can therapists and spiritual teachers. Additionally, many paths did not adequately screen their incoming students, and

*The results of a mental health study that is conducted every ten years were published in the June 2005 *Archives of General Psychiatry.* This study, based on interviews of 10,000 individuals, found that approximately half of all people in the United States will develop a mental disorder at some point in their lives—with half of these cases beginning by age fourteen and three-quarters by age twenty-four. Most of these individuals take years—nine to twenty-three years for anxiety disorders—to seek treatment, and only about one in three receives treatment that meets the minimum standards of care. (A. Barnum, "Mental Illness Will Hit Half in U.S., Study Says," *San Francisco Chronicle,* June 7, 2005, www.sfgate.com/cgi-bin/article.cgi?f=/c/a/2005/06/07/MNGB3D4N3K1.DTL.)

individuals with too-fragile ego boundaries often inappropriately engaged in strong egoic-annihilating therapies or paths to their detriment. In other cases, severely narcissistic individuals who were drawn to psychospiritual groups or paths for the primary purpose of seeking attention rather than for real healing wasted other students' time through continually dramatizing their issues childishly.

Furthermore, in the popular press, the good work performed by these psychological approaches and paths was often drowned out by the more widely publicized drama of their more sensational failures.

Knowledge and Freedom to Choose

However, in the twenty-first century, many teachers, therapists, and psychospiritual paths have learned from the naïveté and mistakes that undermined some aspects of the personal growth and consciousness-raising movements of the 1960s and 1970s. For example, many psychospiritual schools and spiritual paths now require extensive initial interviews and testing before admitting students. Furthermore, due to the growth and popularity of nontraditional psychology, there is presently an abundance of psychological professionals (with master's and doctorate degrees) in these schools, as well as in every major city and even in many smaller towns. Thus, potential clients or students currently have the freedom to choose from several different therapists, teachers, or psychospiritual paths to find the most suitable match.

Additionally, the literal explosion of interest in psychology and spirituality that has been extensively covered in the media over the past forty-plus years has spawned a much more educated populace. Individuals can currently investigate each type of therapy or tradition through the Internet, books, videos, magazines, and journal articles before deciding whether to approach a therapist or group personally. Finally, one of the most valuable referral sources—just as with finding a good holistic practitioner—is a friend or other acquaintance who has had firsthand knowledge of a therapist, teacher, or group.

THREE RADICAL PSYCHOSPIRITUAL APPROACHES

In keeping with the cutting-edge treatments as well as the title and theme of this book, three "radical" psychospiritual therapies are discussed in detail in this chapter. These three approaches all fit the dictionary definitions of the term *radical,* meaning "going to the root or origin" and "pertaining to what is fundamental, far-reaching, and thorough."[12] Furthermore, these more in-depth approaches truly recognize the injury—or at least the lost opportunity—that quick-fix therapies offer, as stated in the book *Care of the Soul* by Thomas Moore:

> Care of the soul, looking back with special regard to ancient psychologies for insight and guidance, goes beyond the secular mythology of the self and recovers a sense of the sacredness of each individual life. This sacred quality is not just value—all lives are important. It is the unfathomable mystery that is the very seed and heart of each individual. Shallow therapeutic manipulations aimed at restoring normality or tuning a life according to standards reduces—shrinks—that profound mystery to the pale dimensions of a social common denominator referred to as the adjusted personality.[13]

In contrast to more superficial approaches, effective psychospiritual therapists and teachers are aware that the most powerful self-negating thoughts and emotional wounds will quietly smolder in one's subconscious ad infinitum without effective intervention. Thus, unlike many conventional psychotherapy and spiritual paths that try simply to help the individual adapt around the painful issue, advanced psychospiritual approaches realize that these wounds act as "both obstacles and doorways to self-realization."[14] Thus, only through the process of *deeply reconnecting* with as well as *thoroughly understanding* the roots and origins of these original traumas can an individual be truly free from the dictates of these prisons of past experience. Furthermore, as the false egoic patterns constructed on these unconscious memories slowly deconstruct, the more fully human and authentic self begins to emerge.

The first of these approaches, *transpersonal psychology,* uses the insights of Western psychology to help individuals recognize their chronic negative egoic patterns, and the wisdom inherent in Eastern religions to assist them in releasing and transcending them. The second approach, termed *rebirthing* or *breathwork*, centers on the letting go of chronic psychophysically held traumatic memories, suppressed painful emotions, and negative beliefs through a conscious breathing process. The final method, the *Ridhwan* or *Diamond Approach*—perhaps the most comprehensive of the three in that it includes the tenets of transpersonal psychology as well as breathwork—is a unique system based on the most in-depth forms of Western psychology synthesized with the wisdom of George Ivanovich Gurdjieff, Sri Aurobindo, Sufism, Buddhism, and others, along with the direct experience of its founder, Hameed Ali.

In the following sections you may find yourself drawn to one or more of these approaches. Readers are encouraged to follow up on their feelings and instincts with further research through the Internet, books, and friends or acquaintances who have had personal experience with one or more of them. It is important to stress that the choice of a particular approach is a deeply personal one and most appropriately made by informed individuals who have the maturity to trust their heart impulse to guide them to the path that most fully serves their growth. Furthermore, it is essential for those who have in their lives significant psychological issues that have required them to be hospitalized or undergo extended therapy to consult with their psychotherapists, psychologists, or psychiatrists before entering into a particular path or seeing a new therapist.*

1. TRANSPERSONAL PSYCHOLOGY

Abraham Maslow and Anthony Sutich formally founded the field of transpersonal psychology in 1969 with the first edition of their publication, *Journal of Transpersonal Psychology*.[15]* John Welwood, Ph.D., a psychologist in San Francisco and associate editor of this journal, explains the need for the development of this field of psychology that brings together the philosophies of the East and the West:

> While the traditional spiritual cultures of the East have specialized in illuminating the timeless, *suprapersonal* ground of being—the "heaven" side of human nature—Western psychology has focused on the earthly half—the *personal* and the *interpersonal*. We need a new vision that embraces all three domains of human existence—the suprapersonal, the personal, and the interpersonal—which no single tradition, East or West, has ever fully addressed within a single framework of understanding and practice.[16]

The term *transpersonal* means to go beyond or transcend the limitations of the individual ego. Transpersonal psychology requires insight and understanding in each of these aspects of being: the *suprapersonal* (spiritual practice), the *personal* (individual psychological work), and the *interpersonal* (psychological work on one's relationships or sociological). Dr. Welwood describes the inherent value of this holistic approach:

> My particular approach to the psychology of awakening emphasizes *practice* in these three domains—meditation for the suprapersonal dimension, psychological work for the personal, and conscious relationship practice for the interpersonal—and how these three can work together and enhance one another. Each of these practices also has ramifications for the other two domains. Meditation can have a profound influence on

*In general, most transpersonal professionals have a master's degree (psychotherapist), a Ph.D. (psychologist), or an M.D. (psychiatrist). In the Ridhwan, or Diamond Heart, approach there is extensive screening conducted before a new student is allowed to join the school. Furthermore, Ridhwan teachers study and train for decades in numerous fields of Western psychology and Eastern spiritual and religious traditions. Rebirthing is less regulated and can be performed by professionals as well as those who become certified after participating in a series of courses. Never hesitate to thoroughly check out the credentials of a prospective therapist or teacher before embarking on this very personal and very sacred journey.

*The fact that some authors consider Carl Jung's work to be the first model for the later development of the field of transpersonal psychology has great validity. (B. Cortright, *Psychotherapy and Spirit* [Albany, N.Y.: State University of New York Press, 1997], 82.) The only reason Jung was not included in this section is that his work is truly so immense and far-reaching that briefly summarizing it here seemed impossible. Readers are referred to the many books written on Carl Jung for insight into this brilliant thinker, as well as to searching online for "Jungian therapists" to help locate a therapist nearby.

how we treat ourselves and others. Psychological work can promote spiritual deepening as well as greater interpersonal sensitivity. And conscious relationship work can help us both awaken from our conditioned patterns and become a more authentic person.[17]

Ken Wilber further defines the term *transpersonal:*

> The soul is without persons, and the soul is grounded in God. "Impersonal," however, is not quite right, because it tends to imply a complete negation of the personal, whereas in higher development the personal is negated and preserved, or transcended and included: hence, "transpersonal."[18]

Or as Alan Watts wrote more than fifty years ago in *Psychotherapy East and West:*

> [T]he aim of a way of liberation is not destruction of *maya* [the illusion of the world and this conditional realm] but seeing it for what it is, or seeing through it. . . . For when a man no longer confuses himself with the definition of himself that others have given him, he is at once universal and unique.[19]

Thus, the transpersonal approach allows individuals to awaken to their deeper nonseparative self, through the inclusion—*not the rejection*—of their unique nature and present embodiment. The success of this more integrated and holistic psychospiritual approach is reflected by its continued growth since the late 1960s, as well as its widespread influence in both classical psychology and some spiritual traditions.

- ▶ Although transpersonal psychologists practice throughout the United States, most of their organizations and colleges are located in northern California. Individuals interested in locating a therapist in their area should call the Association for Transpersonal Psychology at (650) 424-8764, or visit the website at www.atpweb.org.
- ▶ For individuals who would like to train in transpersonal psychology, the Institute of Transpersonal Psychology (ITP) in Palo Alto, at (650) 493-4430 or www.itp.edu, and the California Institute of Integral Studies (CIIS) in San Francisco, at (415) 575-6150 or www.ciis.edu, are both excellent and internationally renowned. Dr. John Welwood, a member of the CIIS faculty, also holds workshops and training in transpersonal psychology and can be reached at (415) 381-6077.
- ▶ To study the work and teachings of Ken Wilber, contact the Integral Institute at (866) 483-0168, or go to www.integralinstitute.org.

2. REBIRTHING AND BREATHWORK

One could almost say that the root of all anguish is an unconscious memory of birth and its terrors.

FREDERICK LEBOYER

Although this quote from the "father of non-traumatic births," Frederick Leboyer, M.D.,[20] may sound rather far-reaching, a number of perinatal research studies have observed a disturbing link between birth trauma and future psychological disorders. In a dramatic study published in *Lancet* in 1985, Lee Salk and four other psychiatrists and psychologists at Cornell University Medical College found a significant correlation between birth trauma and teenage suicide. These researchers were investigating the results from an earlier study that had found suicide rates steadily rose in the young in the United States during the period from 1949 to 1974, and further that this tendency implied "an *early* and *lasting* influence [toward committing suicide]."[21] For their study, Dr. Salk and his colleagues matched each of the fifty-two teenage subjects who had committed suicide with two controls. Blind analysis* of the data revealed three specific risk factors had a "powerful capacity" in contributing to a later inclination to suicide:

1. Mothers who were sick during their pregnancy (including chronic anemia, previous rheumatic fever with a residual heart murmur and arthritis,† chronic

*The investigators did not know who they were analyzing—a control or a suicide subject in the study.

†As described in chapter 12, this can indicate the presence of a chronic focal infection—commonly the tonsils and/or the teeth.

anxiety with treatment, asthma, high blood pressure, multiple surgeries, extreme obesity, etc.)

2. Mothers who had inadequate prenatal care for the first five months of their pregnancy
3. Infant respiratory distress for more than one hour at birth[22]

Although Dr. Salk cautioned that *perinatal* (before, during, and after birth) problems could not be directly correlated to future suicide and that further research was greatly needed, he did assert the following: "What it suggests is that kids who have problems at birth or even before are more vulnerable to the stresses of life later on, to the point of taking their own life."[23]

Physical and Emotional Problems and the Perinatal Imprint

The crucial nature of the positive or negative perinatal imprint between mother and child has been borne out in other studies. In one 1970s analysis by Dr. Dennis Stott, ten out of fourteen women undergoing long-term personal stress during pregnancy bore children with subsequent chronic physical or emotional problems. Two other studies—in Germany involving 2,000 women and another in Austria with 141 subjects—concurred with Stott's findings: the attitude of mothers toward their unborn children—accepting or rejecting—was the most significant factor in the future emotional and physical health of their offspring.[24] In one extraordinary case, a young French child astounded her parents by understanding English perfectly although she had never had a lesson in it. The only possible exposure the parents later reasoned with her doctor was that the mother had worked as an English translator during the child's pregnancy.[25]

The Father's Influence

This prenatal influence is not confined only to the obvious symbiotic closeness between mother and fetus. New research reveals that the father's attitude toward his wife and the expectant child is one of the single most important factors in determining a healthy pregnancy. In one study of more than 1,300 children, a mother in a bad marriage ran a *237 percent* greater risk of bearing a physically or psychologically damaged child than a woman in a secure and nurturing relationship.[26] Other studies have also illustrated how the developing fetus is directly impacted by the positive or negative influence of the presence of the father. For example, in one study newborns significantly responded positively to their father's voices within the first hour or two of life (e.g., stopped crying), when these fathers had talked to their child in utero throughout the pregnancy using short soothing words.[27]

Oxytocin Reduces Painful Birth Memories

Prenatal memory flies in the face of conventional medical science as well as psychiatric opinion, which have both maintained that children prior to the age of two cannot remember anything. More current research indicates that during the third trimester, however, and especially from the eighth month, the child's brain and nervous system are operating at near normal adult levels. The reason that few of us readily recall prenatal events and birth is primarily due to the hormone oxytocin. This posterior pituitary hormone that controls the rate of labor contractions and stimulates the ejection of milk for breast-feeding also has a third function—amnesia-type effects in both the mother and fetus when labor begins.[28] This short-term reduction in recall is probably nature's way of lessening the trauma of the painful birth process.

ACTH Helps Retain Painful Birth Memories

However, another hormone from the anterior portion of the pituitary, adrenocorticotropic hormone (ACTH), which is secreted during stress, has the opposite effect of oxytocin—that is, ACTH augments the *retention of memory.* Thus, when a pregnant or birthing woman (or anyone) is tense or fearful, her body automatically releases ACTH, which floods the fetus's system as well.[29] This deluge of ACTH can explain why some individuals recollect their birth—or at least some images and vivid emotions about their birth—more than others, especially if it was a difficult one. In one study by David Chamberlain, Ph.D., author of *Babies Remember Birth,* children (from ages nine to twenty-three) were able to accurately describe even minor details about their birth. Dr. Chamberlain wrote that in some cases the dovetailing of the two independent narratives from mother and child were "uncanny," and included the child's accurate description of the time of day, the persons present, the instruments used (suction,

ANESTHESIA'S EFFECTS ON MOTHER-CHILD BONDING

Unfortunately, partial or full anesthesia is commonly used during labor (and, of course, in C-sections) to reduce pain. Although few are aware of the carcinogenic effects of anesthesia, as discussed in chapter 4, even fewer are aware that anesthesia may have deleterious effects on mother-child bonding. In several fascinating animal research studies, the experience of maternal pain was found to be a *significant* factor in a mother's love for her offspring. For example, several studies have shown that when given full anesthesia, animal subjects completely reject their offspring. Furthermore, even with partial anesthesia, animal mothers were typically in great doubt as to whether to accept or reject their offspring. From these experiments, Eugène Marais, a South African scientist, concluded that "birth pain is the key which unlocks the doors to mother love . . . where pain is negligible, mother love and care are feeble."[30]

These animal studies raise serious questions about the widespread use of anesthesia, especially in planned cesarean sections (C-sections) where the mother experiences none to little labor pain. Additionally, it was recently reported in one study that because epidurals have not been shown to increase the chance of C-section and can make a mother's time in labor ninety minutes shorter, they are now recommended early in labor, which according to Marais can reduce the mother-child bonding even further.[31]

Obviously, more research on this subject is needed. However, the strong effect of anesthesia on the child has already been dramatically observed by hundreds of rebirthers and their clients, when the room actually starts smelling like anesthesia as the client is deeply breathing and reexperiencing the trauma of birth. Furthermore, in the majority of these cases, clients report an extreme level of fatigue and dizziness during the session, and often a sense of living their life in a "fog" and feeling very disconnected at times. Often these clients "go unconscious" during rebirthing—their minds blank out and they cannot think well—which is a theme commonly mirrored in their relationships and in their work.[32]

Dr. Thomas Verny, a psychiatrist and author of *The Secret Life of the Unborn Child,* writes that infants whose mothers had general anesthesia during delivery tend to be more sluggish initially and have less motor coordination. Furthermore, he advises that "drugs, forceps, fetal monitors, cesarean sections and the other elaborate technology" were specifically designed for emergencies. He cites that their present widespread use—80 percent of women receive at least one drug during birth, 30 percent of infants "are dragged into the world with forceps," and 15 percent of deliveries are C-sections—has a significant effect on the mental and emotional health of the infant.[33] (Currently, C-sections range from 15 to 25 percent of births in the United States, varying according to the particular proclivity of the doctor or hospital toward recommending these surgical births.)

forceps, incubator), and in two cases even the mother's specific hairstyle.[34]

The memory-retaining effects of this hormone are not simply limited to birth trauma. In fact, ACTH, which stimulates the release of hormones from the adrenal glands, is a primary factor underlying the retention of memory of *every* trauma, whether a painful and terrifying birth or later life events—that first day of school, divorce (your parents' or your own), death (family, friend, or spouse), and so forth. The human automatic reaction to stress, also known as the fight-or-flight response, is mediated by the sympathetic nervous system. This sympathetic response to overwhelming stress, whether being chased by a lion in the jungle or being fired from one's job, produces the same effects in the body: the eyes dilate, muscles tense, digestion slows or stops, and heart rate and breathing speed up. In fact, if the trauma is major enough, the well-known "gasp"—that is, the sudden inhalation and complete cessation of breath for a few moments—commonly occurs.* These characteristic effects of stress do not

*It is interesting to note that the adjective *breathtaking*—surprising, astonishing, and that which takes the breath away—can refer to beautiful sunsets as well as shocking and frightening events.

always resolve after the traumatic event is over. In fact, as psychologists who specialize in post-traumatic stress disorder (PTSD) can verify, the imprint of major emotional, mental, and physical trauma can remain in the body indefinitely. Freud was aware of this even in the late nineteenth century, half a century before Selye led the way in researching and propagating the damaging effects of chronically high levels of ACTH and cortisol triggered by chronic stress:

> The mortification suffered thirty years ago operates, after having gained access to the unconscious sources of affect [emotions], during all these thirty years as though it were a recent experience. Whenever its memory is touched, it revives, and shows itself to be cathected [connected] with excitation which procures a motor discharge for itself in an attack [fight-or-flight sympathetic response].[35]

Fortunately, experiential therapies such as rebirthing are effective in reducing the lasting mental, emotional, and physical (subtle or not-so-subtle) hypervigilance associated with these repressed and unprocessed memories, as well as helping to resolve the associated life-negating chronic feelings and tendencies.

Advantages of Rebirthing

During *rebirthing,* also known as *conscious breathing* or *breathwork,* traumatic perinatal memories and sensations—as well as other life traumas—typically arise.

Releasing "Psychological Birthmarks"

Through the process of relaxing and breathing deeply while in the presence of a skillful and supportive therapist, repressed and unresolved painful memories are not only remembered but also reexperienced in a healing environment. It's important to point out here that normal breathing circulates oxygen to sustain life and removes waste products of internal cellular processes (carbon dioxide, water, and volatile organic chemicals). However, when this normally automatic and unconscious process is brought into one's conscious awareness and magnified, the traumatic "waste products" in our memories are also awakened. Thus, conscious and connected breathing can oxygenate and enliven areas of suppressed sorrow, fear, and anger and initiate the removal of the toxic waste of these painful "psychological birthmarks" from the body. Individuals who "breathe through" and release these distressing memories and their associated bodily contraction patterns experience greater awareness, clarity, and presence in their lives.

STORAGE OF MEMORY THROUGHOUT THE BODY

The late anthropologist Gregory Bateson concluded, "It is not only legitimate, but logically inevitable to assume the existence of mental processes on all the levels of natural phenomena of sufficient complexity—cells, organs, tissues, (and) organisms."[36] Thus, as many rebirthers and body workers have observed, painful memories are literally stored and remembered not just in the brain but *throughout* the body. Holistic physicians who treat scar interference fields with neural therapy and auriculotherapy have also witnessed this phenomenon. For example, memories of past rape, incest, or traumatic delivery arise vividly (and often unexpectedly if the patient has already done psychotherapeutic work on these issues) when hysterectomy or episiotomy scars are treated. Thus, when emotional traumas are significant enough, they seem to be stored in the DNA of the locally damaged cells (as well as firmly embedded as central nervous system engrams), and they require both effective psychological work as well as holistic therapies for their complete resolution.

Shallow Breathing a Defense against Underlying Anxiety

Breathwork therapies are based on what the pioneer of psychosomatic medicine, Wilhelm Reich, M.D. (1897–1957), discovered in the early and mid-1900s—that shallow breathing is a chronic body defense used to reduce subconscious anxiety. Through extensive clinical research with hundreds of patients, Dr. Reich found that breath therapy could not only cure certain neurotic symptoms but, through the "liberation of powerful suppressed emotions," also "produce a condition of joyous inner freedom."[37]

Breathwork Loosens Psychological Defenses

Another pioneer in this field, Stanislav Grof, a psychiatrist who has done extensive clinical research in

Big Sur and the San Francisco Bay area, found that by encouraging both the depth and the rate of breathing, breathwork most effectively "loosens the psychological defenses and leads to release and emergence of the unconscious (and superconscious)* material." The majority of participants in Grof's seminars and workshops reported that this powerful healing tool was "far superior" to other forms of verbal therapy that they had experienced in the past such as counseling, psychoanalysis, or traditional psychotherapy.[38] Dr. Grof elaborates on the advantages of breathwork over conventional "talk" therapies:

> One condition necessary for the emergence of the memory is that the issue be of sufficient emotional relevance. Here lies one great advantage of experiential psychotherapy in comparison with verbal approaches. The techniques that can directly activate the unconscious seem to reinforce selectively the most relevant emotional material and facilitate its emergence into consciousness. They thus provide a kind of inner radar that scans the system and detects material with the strongest charge and emotional significance.[39]

Parasympathetic Deep Breathing Reduces Sympathetic Stress

These charged and significant memories that do not heal over time simply remain. Initially, they are laid down in the body by the flooding of the ACTH hormone. However, they continue to exist in the psyche through the strong neuromusculoskeletal freeze response and chronic holding pattern that was established in reaction to the original shock of the trauma and overwhelming threat. Without significant therapeutic intervention, these memories remain for the most part just below conscious awareness, intermittently exacerbated by life's inevitable struggles. However, during breathwork, this overlay of chronic sympathetic nerve stress can be brought to one's attention by the opposite action—the parasympathetic action of breathing deeply. In fact, Wilhelm Reich believed so fully in the healing effects of this "rest and relax" portion of the autonomic nervous system (as opposed to the fight-or-flight sympathetic nervous system) that he even asserted that "the Unconscious is located in the para-sympathetic nervous system."[40] In her book *Breath & Spirit,* Gunnel Minett elaborates on this rebalancing effect on the autonomic nervous system through breathwork:

> The parasympathetic system contributes . . . a passive, immobile, energy-saving reaction. It thereby calms the body's vital functions, makes the muscles relax, lowers the voice, and slows movement (as in a state of sleep or deep relaxation). Since the tension of the muscles is lowered, breathing becomes deeper and more open. The body opens up, facilitating circulation. This is also a signal for the brain to start the "replay mechanism" for processing and integrating impressions.[41]

Reliving and Releasing the Deepest Sensations of Trauma

This replay mechanism is the most significant benefit of all forms of body-mind therapies (e.g., hypnosis, Janov's primal therapy, Levine's Somatic Experiencing, Gestalt therapy, etc.), in that it stimulates the vivid recollection and actual reexperiencing of chronically held traumatic memories, resulting in their more complete psychological and physical release. Thus, it is not uncommon for a client to feel painful emotions (e.g., crying, expressions of anger and fear, etc.), physical sensations (e.g., the cold and clammy feelings of fear, sweat, shaking, muscle twitching, etc.), as well as mental insights ("This stomach nausea is the same that I felt during my parent's divorce" or "My legs feel as weak as when we moved to a new town," etc.). Dr. Grof describes this process more clearly:

> In deep experiential psychotherapy, biographical data is not [simply] remembered or recon-

*Through his extensive clinical research, Grof concluded that the "perinatal process transcends biology," based on the numerous *superconscious* memories that were reported—and convincingly relived—by hundreds of his patients in deep states of consciousness. These superconscious states included the reliving of incarnation memories (past lives) as well as many archetypal themes from Jung's concept of the *collective unconscious,* for example, vivid identification with animal spirits—birds, wolves, reptiles, etc.; a sense of nonduality or union with Mother Earth, or the Divine; and even extraterrestrial experiences. (S. Grof, *The Adventures of Self-Discovery* [Albany, N.Y.: State University of New York Press, 1988], 46, 52–58, 67–68.)

> structed; it can actually be fully relived. This involves not only the emotions, but also physical sensations, visual perceptions, as well as vivid data from other senses.[42]

Grof and his colleagues have observed this reexperiencing and age regression to be so real in breathwork and other experiential psychotherapy sessions that they have documented positive neurological responses (e.g., sucking reflex, Babinski's reflex, etc.)* during these sessions that are characteristic *only* for an infant—not an adult client.[43] These clinical regressions are consistent with a report in 1976 by the neurologist Wilder Penfield that it was indeed possible to trigger photographic memories (often quite remote) simply by touching various areas of the brain with an electrode during brain surgery.[44] More recent research in the field of cognitive neuroscience through the use of PET scans (positron emission tomography), and more recently fMRIs (functional magnetic resonance imaging), which trace blood flow associated with neuronal activity, has enabled researchers to confirm Penfield's original assertion that the memory of past trauma is stored—for years, decades, or even a lifetime—in various parts of the brain.

Therapist Provides a Supportive Holding Field

Some of these recollected experiences can be seen—once they are fully released—as harmless childhood memories from one's present adult perspective.[45] However, when more intense and frightening experiences are provoked, the therapist can gently encourage clients to continue breathing while also continuing to deeply feel their fearful and painful memories without dissociating out of the body. When the experiences are particularly traumatic, the empathetic therapist can remind the client that these feelings are just memories, and not the client's present reality. Dr. Grof further delineates the role of the therapist:

> The task of the facilitator or *therapist* (the term is used here in the original Greek sense of assisting to heal) is then to support the experiential process with full trust in its healing nature, without trying to change it.[46]*

This support is greatly influenced by what quantum scientists refer to as "the field" or "morphogenetic field" that surrounds and subtly influences every living thing. Thus, it is extremely important (if not essential) that rebirthers themselves have reached a level of self-understanding and inner development in which they can fully understand and "hold" in a safe and supportive environment any issues—negative or positive—that their clients may bring up during a session.

morphogenetic field: The term *morphic field* or *morphogenetic field* was originated by Rupert Sheldrake while on an inspirational retreat in an ashram in India. Morphogenetic fields surround everything—from molecules to mountains—and have a deep and subconscious influence on humans through their subtle emissions.[47]

holding: The term *holding* primarily derives from the field of object-relations psychology and describes an empathetic and supportive holding environment on the part of the therapist, which is essential when clients process deep grief and emotional pain.

Releasing Negative Imprints from Physical Trauma

The psychosomatic healing effects of breathwork can also be physically transformative. For example, many holistic practitioners who use energetic testing have observed that even with the best post-injury care (homeopathy, structural therapy, support from friends and family, etc.), often the deep psychic memory of coming very close to death or disability can subtly remain in the body.† Dr. Grof has also seen physical trauma—especially injuries and accidents

---

*Babinski's reflex—dorsiflexion of the big toe and fanning of the other toes when the sole of the foot is stroked—is normal in early infancy but disappears soon after birth. Additionally, the sucking reflex—sweeping a tongue depressor lightly across the lips stimulating a puckering and protrusion of the lips—is normal in early infancy but not in later life.

*This more "client-centered" and "organic" form of therapy in which the client's breath itself activates relevant memories removes any bias or controlling tendencies on the therapist's part based on his or her training, particular philosophy, or personal beliefs.

†One energetic test is to have the patient remember the traumatic event. If the patient can recall the event without the weakening of a strong indicator muscle or previously even arms now going uneven, then he or she has relatively cleared all the disturbing memories associated with this trauma. If not, more work is indicated.

that threatened the survival or the "integrity of the organism"—"leave permanent traces in the system and contribute significantly to the development of emotional and psychosomatic problems" (depression, suicidal tendencies, sadomasochistic inclinations, sexual dysfunction, migraine headaches, asthma, etc.).[48] It is often *only* by reliving these traumatic memories through rebirthing (or other effective experiential psychotherapeutic methods such as the more recent Somatic Experiencing technique) that these negative imprints in the body-mind can be fully felt and understood, and the associated post-traumatic stress fully released in the presence of a well-trained and trusted therapist.

History of Rebirthing

Eastern Origins

Specific techniques involving breathing to evoke deeper levels of consciousness have been known for millennia. Various breath exercises and practices have been utilized in kundalini, hatha, raja, and siddha yoga; the Tibetan Vajrayana; Sufism; Burmese Buddhist and Taoist meditation; Chinese chi kung; Soto Zen Buddhism, and in some Taoist and Christian traditions.[49]

Western Origins

Among Western psychologists, Otto Rank (1884–1939), a friend and contemporary of Freud's, believed that traumatic birth experiences were pivotal in influencing emotions and behavior later in life.[50] However, Wilhelm Reich, considered to be "Freud's most radical disciple," is credited with originating modern-day breathwork.[51]

Synthesis of Eastern and Western Therapies

Similar to transpersonal psychology and Ridhwan (discussed in the next section), breath therapies are a synthesis of Eastern breathing practices, such as *pranayama,* combined with Western psychotherapy. That is, through various modifications of the breath techniques taught for centuries in India, Tibet, China, Burma, and elsewhere in Asia and the Middle East, the client's unconscious memories arise to present consciousness. During this process of breathwork or rebirthing, therapists trained in Western psychology can support and further their clients' understanding of the experience of uncovering and fully feeling past traumatic memories.

pranayama: Pranayama is a yogic system of breathing for calming and balancing the mind in order to ultimately most fully receive what is called the "Divine siddhi," or spirit current, from God. For more information on this subject, go to www.pranayama.org.

Types of Breathwork

Currently, individuals can choose between three major schools of rebirthing.

Reichian Therapy

Some psychiatrists and psychologists use a more Reichian approach, in which the client is instructed to breathe deeply, with an emphasis on fully exhaling. Since Reich found that breathing troubles and muscular tension were closely interwoven, those who use his approach encourage their clients to breathe deeply while intermittently drawing their attention to areas in the body that appear contracted and tense.[52] Alexander Lowen, M.D., Reich's foremost disciple, described his first session:

> I was told to relax and breathe with my mouth open and my jaw relaxed. . . . After some time Reich said, "Lowen, you're not breathing." I answered, "Of course I'm breathing; otherwise I'd be dead." He then remarked, "Your chest isn't moving. Feel my chest." I placed my hand on his chest and noticed that it was rising and falling with each breath. Mine clearly was not.
>
> I lay back down and resumed breathing, this time with my chest moving outward on inspiration and inward on expiration. Nothing happened. After a while Reich said, "Lowen, drop your head back and open your eyes wide." I did as I was told and . . . a scream burst from my throat. . . . [Later in the session] Dr. Reich asked me to repeat the procedure. . . . Again the scream came out. . . . The scream happened to me. Again I was detached from it, but I left the session with the feeling that I was not as all right as I thought. There were "things" (images, emotions) in my personality that were hidden from consciousness, and I knew then that they would have to come out.[53]

Orr's Rebirthing

The other two principle schools of breathwork were developed in the 1970s. Leonard Orr, a San Francisco metaphysical teacher, discovered the transformative power of conscious and connected breathing through the experience of his own birth memories in the 1960s in his bathtub. Later, in collaboration with others, he found breathing "in the dry" could also be effective. Orr originated the term *rebirthing,* as well as the particular style of breathing advocated: a rhythmic and connected breathing in which there is no pause at the end of the inhalation or the exhalation.[54]* The recommended course of sessions is twenty—ten with a female rebirther and ten with a male rebirther (in no particular order, although some recommend working with someone of your own gender first). Other certified teachers utilizing this method include Bob Mandel, Fred Lehrman, Sondra Ray, Jim Leonard, and Phil Laut, who have widely propagated rebirthing through individual and group sessions, teacher trainings, and books.

Grof's Holotropic Breathwork

In 1976, Stanislav Grof, with his wife, created *holotropic* breathwork, after years of experience in treating clients in "nonordinary" states of consciousness. After concluding that a specific technique of breathing is less important than simply breathing faster and more effectively than usual, Grof trusted "the intrinsic wisdom of the body" and simply instructed clients during sessions to increase their rate of breathing. The chief aim of this more intensive breathing, or *pneumocatharsis,* is to free clients from "old stresses and traumatic imprints" and at the same time allow the unfolding of "one's true identity" and connection with the universal consciousness.[55]

holotropic: The word *holotropic* derives from the Greek *holos,* meaning "whole," and *trepein,* meaning "moving in the direction of."

*Although clients can hyperventilate, especially during the initial sessions, as long as the relaxed exhale is maintained despite the speed and intensity of the breathing, hyperventilation will gradually diminish or not occur at all. (G. Minett, *Breath and Spirit* [San Francisco: The Aquarian Press, 1994], 65.)

Cautions and Suggestions

Before referring readers to particular breathwork and rebirthing therapists and schools, a few points must be made.

Suitable for More "Advanced" Individuals

First, rebirthing is a powerful tool best utilized by more "advanced" clients—that is, those who have gained a certain level of insight and self-understanding, typically from previous psychotherapy and personal growth work. It is not recommended for individuals with significant neurotic symptoms, borderline tendencies, or fragile ego development—at least not initially. These latter individuals are best served by establishing a relationship with a psychotherapist, psychologist, or psychiatrist (with a master's or Ph.D. in psychology, or an M.D. who is board-certified in psychiatry) to engage in long-term therapy in order to help establish a more stable self.

Certified Practitioners Should Work with a Professional Therapist

Furthermore, many rebirthing and breathwork practitioners are certified by various schools but may not have a formal psychology background. Many of these certified practitioners are very well trained, quite naturally intuitive, and excellent rebirthers. Nevertheless, because of the intense emotions and sensations that arise during breath sessions, it is recommended that these practitioners have a relationship with a professionally trained therapist, whom they confer with, or refer clients to, when necessary.

Skip the Superficial Affirmations

Finally, in some schools of rebirthing, positive affirmations are used at the end of the session. In my opinion, this practice seems to be an unfortunate juxtaposition of one of the most in-depth and effective treatments (rebirthing) with one of the more superficial and ineffective methods of behavior modification (affirmations). Although affirmations that use the creative power of the mind have their place in certain situations, at the end of a breathwork session they can thrust clients back into their heads and often evoke negative thought forms ("But I don't really feel that 'I always receive what I need' or 'I deserve love.'") Although noting the negative responses to these positive affirmations can be helpful, ruminating on these contradictions is rarely therapeutic at the end of a breath session, when many clients are in a more vulnerable and unguarded state while deeply processing the feelings and sensations they have just experienced.

Nonverbal Therapy Allows for the Most Effective Integration

In my experience, when there is time at the end of a breath session, Jungian art therapy is one of the most healing and nondirective things one can do. This therapy can include writing haiku poetry, drawing or painting, or modeling with clay. These nonverbal forms of therapy allow the unconscious to more fully integrate the most recent and fledgling deeper understanding it has just gained during rebirthing. Furthermore, expressive art therapy can be very grounding without reducing or disturbing the blissful feelings that can arise in a higher state of consciousness. A simple walk—especially one that is slow and focused—can also help one to integrate thoughts and feelings and better assimilate the mental, emotional, and physical experiences and insights gained during the session.

- Two of the most well-written and thorough books on the subject of rebirthing and breathwork are *The Adventure of Self-Discovery* by Dr. Stanislav Grof and *Breath & Spirit* by Gunnel Minett.
- To locate a Reichian-oriented therapist, go to the Radix Institute website at www.radix.org. For rebirthers utilizing the Orr method, consult the www.rebirthing-breathwork.com website. To locate a holotropic-certified practitioner (Grof), call (415) 383-8779, or go to www.holotropic.com.

3. THE DIAMOND APPROACH OR RIDHWAN PATH

I myself can recommend the Diamond Approach as probably the most balanced of the widely available spiritual psychologies/therapies.

Ken Wilber

The Diamond Approach is a contemporary psychospiritual teaching that has been developed by A. Hameed Ali* over the past twenty-five years. Its educational branch, the Diamond Heart Institute, is taught through the Ridhwan Foundation. Students in the school commonly refer to this path as Ridhwan or Diamond Heart.

> **ridhwan:** *Ridhwan* is a Sufi term that translates rather awkwardly to mean "contentment" or "happily contenting." It refers to the generous and genuine feeling of real contentment that is possible only in an individual who can experience his or her true self, unfettered by the constraints of the ego personality.

Ridhwan is a "psychologically sophisticated spiritual system" that has been referred to as possibly the most comprehensive psychospiritual path currently available in the world.[56] However, far from being simply a combining of Eastern and Western thinking, the Diamond Approach is its own system, arising from the influence of Gurdjieff, Sufism, Vajrayana, and Zen Buddhism and modern psychological theory (Freud, Jung, Kohut, Kernberg, Mahler, etc.), as well as utilizing the unique insights derived from the direct experience of Hameed Ali, other Ridhwan teachers,† and his students.

Psychological Pain Derives Most Fundamentally from Spiritual Angst

Because Ridhwan teaching falls within the transpersonal psychology genre, it shares many concepts with the approaches previously described. For example, although Ali acknowledges that numerous psychotherapeutic approaches and self-improvement techniques can help us become more satisfied and effective in our lives, he

*A. Hameed Ali was born in Kuwait in 1944. At the age of eighteen, he moved to the United States to study at the University of California at Berkeley. While Hameed was working on his Ph.D. in physics, he reached a turning point in his life that began his inquiry into the psychological and spiritual aspects of human nature. (For more information on Ali, go to www.ahalmaas.com and click on "Bio.")

†Hameed was the original thinker and innovator of the Diamond Approach, with significant contributions from Karen Johnson and Faisal Muqaddam. Karen Johnson continues to function as the most senior teacher in the Ridhwan school. However, in the early 1980s, Muqaddam left the Ridhwan work to start his own psychospiritually oriented approach (see www.diamondlogos.com).

teaches that without exploring our deeper nature and spiritual truth they are all inherently limited.[57]

> Human beings typically live in a state of arrested development in which the psychological domain rules our consciousness. Reaching the fullness of our potential entails resuming our development, which leads beyond the psychological to the realm of Being or spirit.[58]

Thus, a chief limitation in Western traditional psychotherapy is that it does not take into consideration *spiritual* angst. Anxiety, depression, and other painful psychological states are generated not simply from painful personal and interpersonal issues but most fundamentally from the loss of contact with Being,* or Divine Consciousness.[59]

Many Spiritual Traditions Avoid or Deny the Self

In direct correlation to the common lack of understanding of spiritual suffering in modern psychology is the very common lack of understanding of psychological suffering typical of most Eastern spiritual traditions. In fact, Ali has found that many spiritual teachings even negate "the possibility of being a person and being real" in their members and devotees.[60] In the following quote Ali (pen name A. H. Almaas) explains that often "the man of spirit" relegates the individual human experience to being *all* egoic:

> To be free from ego means to the man of spirit the realization of Being, and Being is almost always taken to be impersonal. For them it is not possible to experience oneself as a person without identifying with ego. Being a person is for them a clear indication that one is not free. It is also an indication that one is not experiencing Being, but only identifying with a self-image.[61]

*Ali capitalizes *Being* in order to differentiate it from the ordinary definition meaning simply the sense of existence. In his teaching, Being is defined as the direct experience of the presence of God in one's life.

Tibetan Buddhists have traditionally given prominence to this "no self" perspective in their teaching, as the (14th) Dalai Lama has written:

> As I may well emphasize again, the teachings of no-self-soul is upheld by all schools of Buddhist thought since all alike recognize the atman-view* that is adhering to belief in some permanent soul-entity, as the root of all trouble.[62†]

This belief has been reiterated by Nisargadatta Maharaj, one of the most profound Hindu Vedanta teachers in India: "There is no such thing as a person. There are only restrictions and limitations. The sum total of these defines the person."[63]

Thus, since in many Eastern religions and spiritual paths experiencing oneself as a person is *always* a manifestation of the ego and seen to be false, any arising psychological issues are rarely, if ever, addressed. From this perspective Ali states, "It is not only that there is no person; there is also no life and no humanity. All are concepts, appearance, the dance of Maya‡ or the dream of God.[64]

Spiritual Bypassing

Other transpersonal-oriented teachers and authors have noted this self-negating tendency in various religious and spiritual traditions. Beginning in the 1970s, John Welwood began to notice a disturbing trend among members of spiritual communities. This San Francisco psychologist found that many of these individuals were using their spiritual practice as a way to avoid, or bypass, dealing with their emotional and personal issues.

*In the Hindu religion, the term *atman* refers to the soul in every being and *Brahman* refers to God, or the Absolute. The mantra *Tat tvam asi,* or "Thou art that," in the Upanishads teaches that atman and Brahman are one. However, Ali contends that in Hinduism atman is considered to be not personal but infinite and boundless, and it is therefore not synonymous with his definition of the soul, or the Personal Essence. (A. Almaas, *The Pearl Beyond Price* [Berkeley: Diamond Books, 1990], 15.)

†However, in other Buddhist traditions, there is recognition of "the pristine existential experience of Being (Dharmakaya)," referred to as "Buddha nature" or "Bodhicitta." (A. Almaas, *The Void* [Boston: Shambhala, 2000], 73.)

‡*Maya* refers to the perspective that this world, this "conditional realm," is all just an illusion, or the dream of God.

Welwood coined the term *spiritual bypassing* for this phenomenon.

> While still struggling to find themselves, many people are introduced to spiritual teachings and practices that urge them to give themselves up. As a result, they wind up using spiritual practices to create a new "spiritual" identity, which is actually an old dysfunctional identity—based on avoidance of unresolved psychological issues—repackaged in a new guise.[65]

The tendency to "avoid facing the unresolved issues of the conditioned personality," Welwood observed, "only keeps us caught in their grip."[66] This common pitfall among spiritual aspirants was also underscored by Steven Hedlin, Ph.D., in a paper titled "Pernicious Oneness and Premature Disidentification," in the classic text *Chop Wood, Carry Water:*

> [T]oo often people try to lose their "ego," or sense of self, before they have actually worked through their own personal psychological material, and established a healthy sense of self—one which allows them to live effectively in the world.

"Put simply," Dr. Hedlin asserted, "you have to be somebody before you can be nobody."[67]

PHYSICAL BYPASSING

In *Leaving My Father's House,* feminist and Jungian analyst Marion Woodman echoes this same sentiment. In a chapter by one of the contributing authors, Mary Hamilton, active dialoguing with Hamilton's inner voice revealed the following:

> Spirituality can only be lived within a body that is aware of its human dimension, both positive and negative. If the awareness is not there, spirituality becomes a self-centered path of self-aggrandizement.

And on the related subject that could be termed *physical bypassing,* which is encouraged in some renunciate traditional paths, Hamilton wrote:

> Many people on the spiritual path believe that the physical body is less sacred than the spirit of the Self. Your body is crucial for your work on the planet. Honor her; treat her with the greatest respect and love. She is your responsibility. Great music requires a finely tuned instrument. Spirituality requires a finely tuned body and mind capable of aligning itself with the Self.[68]

Satprem, who chronicled the life of Sri Aurobindo, one of the few Eastern gurus who was not satisfied with "impersonal states of enlightenment" and who "worked toward the actualization of a liberated human life," expressed a similar belief: [69]

> On the other hand, if we exclude everything to arrive at so-called spiritual goals, it is very difficult afterwards to retrace our steps, to descend from our fragile heights . . . we are far too comfortable up there to stir up all that mud, and, to tell the truth, we can *no longer* do it. In fact, we don't even think about it, for how could we even conceive of undertaking such an enormous task if, from the start, we consider the mind, the vital and the body perishable, and aim only at escaping from life and gaining our salvation?[70]

Through this (subtle or not-so-subtle) repression of thoughts and feelings, strictly religious or spiritual devotees can become stuck over time in their own destructive psychological patterns. Thus, long-term spiritual practitioners who do not continue to examine their repressed feelings can find it particularly difficult to reach them over years of habitually detaching from the self. In rebirthing circles, for example, it is well known that devotees of spiritual masters, or gurus, typically tend to dissociate out of themselves into blissful states (co-opted from their spiritual teacher) during the initial (or even later) breathwork sessions, rather than accessing their more uncomfortable unresolved emotional conflicts and wounds. Hameed Ali has observed this spiritual bypassing tendency in the Ridhwan school:

> Emotional freedom and maturity are important for self-realization; disconnection from

emotions will cause narcissistic disturbance even for those with a degree of self-realization. We sometimes encounter this situation in our work, when a student has done a great deal of spiritual practice but no work on the emotions. Since spiritual work exposes and intensifies both pathological and fundamental narcissistic issues, these issues generally distort or limit the person's self-realization unless they are worked through. Without psychological understanding they are not easy to deal with.[71]

ACKNOWLEDGING PARTIAL REALIZATION

A common misperception is that spiritual realization is fully integrated in all aspects of one's experience and functioning. In actuality, this is rarely the case. Hameed Ali explains how realizing a certain state does not mean that this level of understanding is integrated throughout one's being, as many spiritual books and teachings characterize it:

> They give the impression that realization is always complete and absolute. The fact is that things are not like that most of the time. Realization can be partial. In fact, realization is partial in most instances for most people, which means that a persona can have Brilliancy in a certain area but not in others. So a scientist can be brilliant in his field and not be brilliant when it comes to his or her emotional makeup.[72]

Ken Wilber has described this phenomenon in detail, through his paradigm of the lines of human development, or the evolution of consciousness, which he has written about extensively.[73]

The Ultimate Dimension Is Not the Only Dimension

Ali explains in his book *The Pearl Beyond Price* that one reason for the widespread denigration of the personal in spiritual paths is that the experience of oneness with the Absolute Dimension, or God, feels "so real, so profound, and so comprehensive that it has a flavor of finality to it."[74]

> This is a very profound dimension, which shows us our ultimate nature. This level of realization is required for complete freedom from ego identifications. It is, nevertheless, only a part of the true potential of the human being. In a sense it is the ultimate dimension, but it is not the only dimension.[75]

To reiterate, Ali is asserting that the experience of the Ultimate Dimension and realization of God "is required for complete freedom from ego identifications." That is, only through the experience of this most profound and ultimate realization—communion with God or Divine Consciousness—is ego dissolution possible. *However,* it is not the only dimension. The realized Being must also be aware of and fully in contact with his or her human dimension.

Thomas Keating, a Trappist monk and author, also recognized this concomitant need for ongoing psychological work when entering into spiritual life, where he found "Grace is there, but so is the false self":[76]

> A lot of emptying and healing has to take place if we are to be responsive to the sublime communications of God. The full transmission of divine life cannot come through and be fully heard if the static of the false self is too loud.[77]

Personal Essence—The Experience of Being and a Human Being

Most modern-day conventional psychological approaches as well as ancient spiritual traditions, therefore, have one thing in common: they both tend to ignore the fully developed human dimension—that is, the recognition of the individual soul. Ali has termed this dimension of the true human being—the one the Sufis characterize as being "in the world but not of it"—Essence or Personal Essence.[78] Ali described this state as follows:

> The Personal Essence is the true integration of the ideals of both the man of spirit and the man of the world. It is Being, but it is also a person. It is a person that is completely spiritual, made out of spiritual substance, but at the same time living in the world a personal life. He is Being, and he is a human being.[79]

Personal Essence: The term *Personal Essence,* as well as *Being, Essence, Self, true self, essential self, true nature,* and *soul,* are all utilized in this chapter to refer to the "you" who is not defined by your parents, your history, your mind or body, or your personality. Byron Brown, in *Soul without Shame,* most eloquently describes this fundamental nature of our being: "The closer you are to sensing your own immediate aliveness, the closer you are to soul. The soul is the substance of living consciousness. To feel it is to recognize the miraculous and mysterious quality of what you are—a flowing presence, dynamic, alive and ever-changing. To feel you are a soul is to know the unboundedness of life . . . the soul is better felt, sensed, and known in the heart than it is through the structures and perceptions of the mind."[80]

Thus, as he has written and taught for over twenty-five years, Ali realized that "psychological processes and spiritual perceptions are inextricably linked as parts of the same spiritual domain," and are not separate dimensions at all.[81]

The Incompleteness of One Dimension

In fact, as Ali clarified, this sense of self or essence is "clearly a greater development than either living a life solely as a man of spirit or solely as a man of the world":[82]

> The human being is incomplete if he identifies with one dimension, regardless of how "high," to the exclusion of others. The complete man is the integration of all dimensions of reality. . . . One who has integrated the Personal Essence completely is able to experience any dimension of reality, depending on the requirement of the moment.[83]

Moreover, to live in only one dimension—an impersonal spiritual existence or an egoically identified worldly existence—is not, by the fullest definition, really living at all. Ali elaborates further on this subject:

> For human life to be complete and balanced, it must consist of the harmony of all dimensions of reality, from the ultimate non-conceptual source to the various dimensions of manifest existence. It must integrate in a harmonious whole the universe of the man of spirit and the universe of the man of the world. Otherwise there is either no life or a fake life.[84]

Personal Essence—The Bridge Across

Not only is the development of the Personal Essence in one's life a more complete realization than existing *only* in the egoic worldly pattern or *only* in a monklike spiritual realm, but it is the *bridge across* these two different experiences. As Ali has explained, the difference in consciousness between the egoically identified personality and spiritual realization is otherwise simply too wide a river to ford:

> [I]t is very difficult for most individuals to let go of the separateness of their individuality, a condition necessary for the realization of the unbounded aspects of Being. However, the Personal Essence makes this transition much easier and more natural.[85]

Thus, through a growing awareness of one's true self, or Personal Essence, one can more easily sense and experience the impersonal and timeless reality of the Divine, or the ultimate Reality. Through this awareness, one can begin to simultaneously experience the impersonal and unbounded sense of Divine Consciousness, therefore, without the exclusion of, or the loss of, one's sense of self.

Individuals Must Successfully Navigate Each Developmental Stage

Ken Wilber has also emphasized the need to not "repress, exclude, alienate, [or] dissociate" the personal self, or any stage of consciousness, for another.[86] In fact, Wilber asserts that it is only through fully integrating each level of development that the higher stages of consciousness, which, by definition, will include the components of earlier stages, can be reached. In the foreword of Wilber's book *A Brief History of Everything,* Tony Schwartz described this need:

> Wilber wrote . . . that human development unfolds in waves or stages that extend beyond those ordinarily recognized by Western psychology. Only by successfully navigating each developmental wave, Wilber argued, is it possible first to develop a healthy sense of individuality, and then ultimately to experience a broader identity that transcends—and includes—the personal self.[87]

Ego as the Window into the Personal Essence

In the Diamond Approach, an individual's egoic pattern, or the "outer shell" of the superficial personality, is not rejected or ignored but actually seen as the *key* to unlocking the individual's sense of Self, or Personal Essence. Hameed Ali expounds on this subject:

> The ego is a reflection of this true element of Being, the Personal Essence, and exploring the characteristics of the reflection can lead us to the reality being reflected. By isolating and understanding the elements of the false, we can begin to approach the elements of the real.[88]

In fact, in the Ridhwan school, Ali has likened the ego to "a surface membrane over the reality of Being."[89] When this membrane is particularly thick and solid, no amount of meditation, spiritual practice, or even the grace of a purportedly realized master, or guru, can penetrate it (for long) without a concomitant deep level of self-understanding and a growing sense of one's true nature. However, when a student is committed to the realization of truth and deep self-understanding, this egoic membrane can thin and become more permeable to Being.

Methods for Accessing Personal Essence

In the Diamond Approach, a number of practices are used to achieve this aim of accessing Personal Essence, including daily meditation and various focusing and awareness exercises. Four other methods—inquiry, breathwork, superego work, and the enneagram—are specifically described in the following sections.

Inquiry: The Allowing of Experience to Unfold

Inquiry is a psychospiritual method of exploration of whatever is arising in one's mind and body, where one allows the experience to unfold in whatever direction it wants to go. It is open-ended and goal-less and generally leads to a shift in one's experience through insight, emotional release, or a sense of greater spaciousness and awareness.[90] In his book *The Diamond Approach* John Davis, a Ridhwan teacher and professor of psychology, describes inquiry in further detail:

> Any experience can be the starting point for your search. From here, it proceeds in an integrated way that includes perceptions, memories, insights, emotions, body sensations, intuitions, and awareness of subtle energies such as chi. As this exploration proceeds from one experience to another, your awareness opens to deeper levels of experience and, eventually, to Essence. As the Inquiry continues, deeper levels and dimensions of Essence are revealed and integrated. In this way, Inquiry leads to growth, healing, release, and fulfillment.[91]

Inquiry is conducted in several ways: among two or three students during a large group meeting, in small groups (e.g., eight to twelve students) where a teacher works directly with a student, and between a student and teacher in individual sessions. Various formats of inquiry are used, rather than relying on an explicit technique or specific strategy. This is because the Ridhwan approach "recognizes that Being itself can direct the process of Inquiry." That is, at some point, the student often begins to feel guided by Essence, which is often characterized by a sense of flow, insight, and greater clarity and understanding.[92]

RIDHWAN TEACHERS

In Ridhwan, the facilitators are referred to as "teachers" to distinguish the Ridhwan teacher from a "therapist" in the classic psychotherapeutic approach. Ridhwan teachers are rigorously trained and highly experienced. Their basic instruction includes at least seven years of study of vast amounts of psychological, spiritual, and religious teachings, as well as the experiential understanding gained in teacher workshops and the continuing experience of being a student in the school. After this period, they spend two years supervised as a teacher, while still continuing advanced training courses. This extensive training, however, does not guarantee the automatic bestowal of teacher status. These teachers-in-training must also demonstrate a genuine grasp of the work and manifest it personally through their growing sense of self, before qualifying for certification as a Ridhwan teacher.

Ego Not the Barrier but the Doorway

Thus, in contrast to many psychological approaches and spiritual traditions where egoic tendencies (chronic anger, fear, hurt, arrogance, sorrow, resentment, etc.) are treated as a problem, in the Ridhwan school they are seen as a doorway—and in fact the only effective doorway—into the deeper dimensions of one's Personal Essence, or Self. Again, Davis illustrates this philosophy in more depth:

> Rather than suggesting we fight against these obstacles to find fulfillment and contentment, the Diamond Approach invites us to understand them from a radically different perspective. In this view, they are not merely barriers; they are doorways, too. Hurt is not simply a block to genuine compassion. It is also the access to compassion. Anger or the desire to inflict hurt is not just a shallow and frustrating substitute for authentic strength. Experienced and understood deeply, it is the key to unlocking the treasure of expansion, capacity and vitality that is our birthright. . . . The Diamond Approach shows us the precise relationship between these counterfeit qualities, their attendant difficulties, and the more real aspects of our nature and our potential.[93]

Egoic Tendencies Are a "Distortion of the Real Thing"

Thus, our egoic tendencies are not unrelated aspects of our defensive outer personality shell but actually a "distortion of the real thing."[94] For example, typically the mirror image of chronic anger and irritability is real strength, the flip side of constant confusion and a lack of clarity in one's life is keen insight and perceptiveness, and often those who are most compassionate have most deeply felt the hurt of a lack of compassion in their lives. These qualities of genuine strength, insight, perception, and compassion are aspects of our sense of self, or Personal Essence. However, through the experience of intense fear or outright abuse in infancy or childhood, or due to a lack of mirroring from our parents who were unable to see or hear us (and thus allow our essential development), false egoic patterns developed to cover and defend where we were most vulnerable and aware. John Welwood, who writes that these traumas are a kind of shock to our soul, quotes a stanza from one of Emily Dickinson's poems that most poignantly describes this shattering of self:

> *There is a pain so utter*
> *It swallows Being up.*[95]

False Will Develops through Loss of the Essential Will

In his book *The Pearl Beyond Price,* Ali describes how false ego structures develop in life through the example of one of the qualities of our Personal Essence, the *Will.*

> Will is one of the aspects of Essence, an element of the true human potential. In childhood it can be cut off and lost from one's sense of who one is. The absence of this aspect will be felt as a sense of castration, of a lack of inner support and a lack of personal confidence. This deficiency is then usually defended against by creating a false will.
>
> The false will is a willfulness, a hard and rigid kind of determination, a stubbornness. . . . The essential Will, on the other hand, is an aspect of Being, an existential presence, an actuality in the present. It is flexible and realistic, and does not have the hardness of the ego will. It manifests as a natural, spontaneous and implicit sense of inner support and confidence.[96]

An individual with an overriding false will may act out rebelliously, depend on others for support, go from one menial job to another, or even turn to crime—and may never manifest the will, determination, and strength to confront his fears. Or she may do the opposite and demonstrate an "iron will," rigidly moving through an unexamined life and projecting an outward grandiose self-image that only appears to be successful and fulfilling. Or the individual may collapse with a sense of "no legs" or "no grounding," which a lack of essential will commonly conveys, and live an aimless and anxiety-ridden life, chronically procrastinating and engaging in magical thinking (searching for a "prince charming," winning the lottery, etc.) in the futile hope that things will eventually change. Thus, these individuals spend their life shielding their pain through the adoption of a false persona and continually fantasizing for a more hopeful future.

The "Empty Hole" or Deep Wound of Deficiency

In Ridhwan, the various egoic personas that represent a thwarted will are utilized as valuable *doorways of inquiry.* Through continued inquiry (a repeating question to another person, telling about how one's false will has manifested in one's life to two other students, working on this issue in a small group with a Ridhwan teacher, or feeling one's false will during breathwork in an individual session), the student often reaches a block or a sense of emptiness, in which deeper feelings of deficiency are experienced. This underlying feeling of emptiness that lies at the root of the formation of the false will (as well as all other defensive postures including false strength, compassion, love, power, joy, etc.) sheds light on why effective psychospiritual work (with the ultimate aim of ego dissolution) is often greatly resisted. No one enjoys experiencing the excruciating pain of the "empty hole" or the deep wound of deficiency that can be felt beneath the defensive strategies overlying false states of being.[97] Kahlil Gibran (1883–1931), a Lebanese poet, philosopher, and artist, expressed this most perfectly in his masterpiece, *The Prophet*:

> *And a woman spoke, saying, Tell us*
> *of Pain.*
> *And he said:*
> *Your pain is the breaking of*
> *the shell that encloses your*
> *understanding.*[98]

In reality, however, most individuals spend a majority of their time vigorously defending their egoic personality shell and *guarding against* pain by trying to fill the hole with food, drugs, acquisition of money or relationships, and so forth. Ali describes this hole, or sense of deep deficiency, further:

> A hole refers to any part of you that has been lost, meaning any part of you that you have lost consciousness of. What is left is a hole, a deficiency in a certain sense. And what we have lost awareness of, is of course, our essence. . . . It could be the loss of love, loss of value, loss of capacity for contact, loss of strength, loss of will, loss of clarity, loss of pleasure, any of those qualities of essence. There are many of them. But when they are lost, they are not gone forever; they are never gone forever. You are simply cut off from them.[99]

Experiencing Essence through Inquiry into the "Hole"

This movement that commonly occurs during inquiry—from a defensive egoic position to feeling the emptiness and deficiency inside—is not only necessary but crucial to the Ridhwan process. In fact, it is only through awareness and understanding of one's deep sense of deficiency that the true self can emerge.[100] Through this retracing process, as well as a deep commitment to the truth on the part of the student, "what's false arises," and what remains afterward is one's true nature, or Essence:

> When we experience a block deeply, it leads to that which the block was covering. This brings a painful experience of deficient emptiness, followed by a sense of presence and the direct experience of Essence.[101]

Thus, the abandonment of the "false gold"—that is, inquiry into the egoic reflection of the true dimensions of being—although painful, inexorably leads over time to a sense of fullness and deeper understanding of one's true nature. Once tasted, this authentic sense of self, informed by the Divine, is truly a "pearl beyond price" and worth all the time, dedication, and even "conscious suffering"* that the student undergoes to realize the alchemy of ego into Essence.

THE "PEARL BEYOND PRICE"

The experience of the Personal Essence is so unusual that some Sufis refer to it as the "rare Mohammedan pearl." The late Indian Guru Baba Muktananda described the experience of "his inner nature as a person of consciousness," not identified with the ego, as the "blue pearl." Krishna, considered to be a god himself in personal form—that is, an incarnation of God on earth—is almost always represented in pictures ornamented with many pearls over his body. Thus, Ali refers to the experience of realizing one's Personal Essence, or true Self, as a "pearl beyond price."[102]

Open-Ended Inquiry: The Central Practice of Ridhwan

Pure and open-ended inquiry is the central method employed in the Diamond Approach, and one that primarily distinguishes it from other paths or approaches. For example, the majority of paths and practices have an underlying agenda to influence their students into a particular state or to encourage them to have a specific experience that is considered "spiritual," or clearer and more realized. In contrast, the aim in Ridhwan is to be free from any particular orientation or mind-set. Ali explains this approach more fully:

> So true meditation, true practice, according to the Diamond Approach, consists of following your thread, which means being where you are and continuing to be where you are without trying to make your experience go in any particular way. This requires practice because most of the time, you do not know where you are, you do not understand where you are, or you are fighting and rejecting where you are.[103]

Ali explains that this sensation of not knowing where you are is the typical state of the ego, which is constantly trying to get someplace as well as judging and rejecting what is actually arising. Only through this true and open-ended inquiry can one become aware of one's real and authentic nature versus continuing to remain trapped in the ego-self. However, since the ego-self is typically so vigorously defended against its own dissolution, other methods that help support deep inquiry are also utilized in the Ridhwan school, including the use of breathwork.

Breathwork or "Body-Centered Inquiry"

Ridhwan teachers use a Reichian-type style of breathwork in their individual sessions with students. Through this psychophysical-oriented therapy, students can more fully integrate and embody the inchoate experience of their developing sense of Self, or Personal Essence. In Ridhwan breathwork, students are encouraged to breathe fully into their abdomens, while the teacher observes and supports inquiry into any arising feelings or phenomena. Similar to Dr. Reich's approach, when the student reports—or the teacher senses—any tension or contraction in the body, the teacher gently encourages the student to continue feeling into this area. Through this body-centered inquiry, these areas of chronic tension as well as the unresolved issues underlying their presence begin to dissolve. Often the sense of peace and a quieter mind and body that can arise after the release of these chronic contractions is a profound experience, as Ali describes:

> Awareness of the body completely without mental representation is profoundly surprising. It moves to dimensions beyond those encountered in bioenergetics analysis, or in any body-centered therapy.
>
> In full self-realization we experience the body as a transparent, diaphanous form of presence. . . . This experience of body is not easy to access; it involves a leap of consciousness that generally requires a great deal of inner work, such as decades of intense meditation practice.[104]

As discussed in the previous "2. Rebirthing and Breathwork" section, breathwork augments a palpable

*The great Russian mystic and teacher Gurdjieff used the term *conscious suffering* to describe an individual's willingness to inquire into and feel the pain of his or her core wounds and inner obstacles in order to overcome them. (J. Welwood, *Love and Awakening* [New York: Harper Perennial, 1977], 8.)

release of the chronic contraction patterns generated from past mental, emotional, and physical anxiety and trauma. Within the context of the Diamond Approach teaching, and with the support of the community of students, these reexperienced emotions, mental constructs, and even bodily pain perceived in the presence of a Ridhwan teacher are often more effectively discharged, metabolized, and integrated than they are for individuals undergoing rebirthing or other forms of breathwork alone.

Superego Work: Disengaging from Self-Judgment

Disengaging from self-judgment, often referred to as the "internal critic" or the superego, is another core teaching in the Ridhwan work. In fact, when one begins to fully open up to and hear the sheer number of negative and judgmental thoughts that occur in one's mind daily (or even hourly), it can be a bit like awakening in the middle of a nightmare. This emerging recognition of the prevalence and resulting pain of one's superego is also one of the primary motivators of many individuals who first enter the work. Hameed Ali has found the superego to be so universal and debilitating that this work makes up a large part of the Ridhwan core teaching during the first two years, and even intermittently thereafter. In the following passage, he describes the sabotaging effect of this internal judge:

> Invalidating your essence is an aspect of your ego and superego. From what I have observed, people often do not acknowledge what's really happening, or what the force is that's operating in them precisely because there is something in them that resists seeing and experiencing essence. It's not just a mistake in judgment; there is an active motivation behind it. It is a defensive function of the superego itself.[105]

A Defense against Feeling the "Empty Hole" or Deficiency

This defensive function of the superego is most vigilant in resisting the sense of deficient emptiness, or the "empty hole" described previously. Again, Ali expounds on this subject:

> A typical reaction to this deficient emptiness comes in the form of superego attacks. One feels worthless, not important, not good enough, or perhaps fake. The deficient emptiness is the feeling of having no self, which feels like a lack of center or orientation. When this emptiness is arising, superego reactions—self-attacks, such as feeling one is worthless, not important, or not good enough—might arise as resistances to directly experiencing the deficiency.[106]

Inquiry and Present-Centered Awareness Disengage the Superego

At this point, what is most needed is not continued defense but inquiry into and awareness of one's sense of worthlessness or deficient emptiness. Through the acceptance and "holding field" of the Ridhwan teaching, individuals are most fully supported into deeply inquiring into their feelings of deficiency. Through this process, students begin to sense and feel the falseness of their superegoic attacks and defensive egoic patterns. A growing sense of aliveness and presence emerges through this most artful disengagement from—and not suppression of—one's harsh and judgmental inner critic.

"HOLDING" AND THE "NARCISSISTIC WOUND"

In the Ridhwan practice, an empathetic and kind *holding* environment on the part of the therapist is required when clients process deep grief and emotional pain. Ali has recognized that this empathic understanding must not simply mirror the sense of one's conventional self but also allow the student to open up to his or her deeper essential nature:

> When the teacher can empathetically support the student as she is feeling the narcissistic wound, and the student is able to tolerate it and feel it fully, it will deepen and expand, until the rip is complete and the cut becomes a total dissolution of the shell. The wound then becomes a window which can open up to a vast emptiness. This emptiness is the specific place of no self. This is what makes it so vulnerable. . . .
>
> The dissolution of the shell is actually a surrender of the self, letting go of the concept of self. The opening can then become an entrance into vastness, and into the fundamental presence and truth of the self.[107]

Working on the "narcissistic wound"—the sense of existential dread and often bottomless grief experienced from inadequate mirroring (not being seen and heard) in childhood, and the resulting disconnection from one's true self—is indeed a *very* profound experience. It requires the presence of an advanced teacher, as well as a committed and advanced student who has experienced and developed a sense of his or her own Personal Essence through the years. Because of the intensity of this potential experience, the Ridhwan school carefully screens all incoming students to make sure that they have enough ego development to undergo the dissolution of the false ego shell, and to endure and feel through the profound sense of hurt and loss that eventually arises in this course of inquiry.

In his book *Soul without Shame,* a senior Ridhwan teacher, Byron Brown, points out that present-centered awareness is one of the most effective ways to defend against superegoic attacks because "the judge gets all its juice from directing your attention toward the past and the future."[108] As students learn to become more and more in touch with their conscious awareness of present experience and develop the strength to stay with this experience for longer periods, the self develops:

> Your awareness is not only useful, it is valuable to experience as the ground of your essential nature. . . . Awareness has a sense of no boundaries, an openness from which nothing is excluded and in which things are not separate. It has no opinions, priorities, or values about what it is aware of. When you are aware, you feel awake, attentive and attuned, clear and spacious. Awareness can begin with your own breathing and the hairs on the back of your hand, and extend deep into your most hidden feelings, and wide into the hearts and minds of others.[109]

Thus, although these superego judgments are universal and deeply embedded in everyone's psyche, with enough inquiry and support they become increasingly easier to access over time. Moreover, the study of the enneagram—an ancient paradigm of nine typical egoic types—can greatly refine this exploration and therefore quicken students' understanding and eventual disengagement from their chronic underlying false personality patterns.

RECOGNIZING THE SUPEREGO

In general, it takes approximately one to two years of Ridhwan work for most students to consistently recognize their superego judgments and attacks. However, even then, more subtle and insidious internal criticisms can intermittently arise. For example, what Ali refers to as the *spiritual superego*—"You should meditate longer than that," "After all these years of quality psychospiritual work you should be more realized by now," and so forth—can continue to block deeper understanding. Again, through inquiry and present-centered awareness, even these more insidious "whispers" in the mind can be revealed and sensed more clearly, which gradually removes their charge and eventually even their presence.

The Enneagram

The word *enneagram* derives from the Greek word *ennea,* meaning "nine," and *grammos,* meaning "points" or "graph."[110] This nine-pointed symbol is more than 2,000 years old, evolving from a secret school in the Middle East, and it is intrinsic to Sufi mysticism.[111] However, underlining the universality of this ancient model, the enneagram also closely parallels and even overlaps the Kabbalistic teaching from the esoteric and mystical Jewish tradition.[112]

In the West, a form of the enneagram was taught at the turn of the twentieth century by Russian spiritual teacher and mystic George Ivanovitch Gurdjieff (1867–1949)* as a device to help his students in their inner life training. Much of what they learned about this subject was nonverbal, however, as he had his students perform elaborate movement patterns on an enneagram model marked on the floor of his hall, the Institute for the Harmonious Development of Man. Gurdjieff believed that through participating in these movement exercises his students could begin to shift their attention away

*Gurdjieff was born in Alexandropol in the Russian Caucasus region to a Greek father and an Armenian mother. His exact date of birth is unknown. The birthdate on his passport was November 28, 1877, but historians believe he was probably born five or six years earlier than that. (S. Zannos, *Human Types: Essence and the Enneagram* [York Beach, Maine: Samuel Weiser, Inc., 1997], 6.)

from chronic thinking patterns and truly inculcate a sense of the energetic forces and rhythms embodied in this ancient archetypal enneagram symbol.[113]

GURDJIEFF'S DISTINCTION BETWEEN ESSENCE AND PERSONALITY

Gurdjieff not only engaged in nonverbal teaching in other related psychospiritual matters but also wrote and lectured extensively. In particular, he taught his students attention practices—called self-observation and self-remembering—in order to see through "the distorting glasses of our personality." Helen Palmer noted in her book *The Enneagram* that *personality, ego,* and *"false" personality* "are simply terms that make the distinction between what Gurdjieff called our essential nature and the personality that we acquire during the course of our lives."[114] In the following paragraphs, Gurdjieff clearly differentiated between personality and essence:

> Essence is the truth in man; personality is the false. But in proportion as personality grows, essence manifests itself more and more rarely, and more and more feebly and it very often happens that essence stops in its growth at a very early age and grows no further. It happens very often that the essence of a grown-up man, even that of a very intellectual and, in the accepted meaning of the word, highly "educated" man, stops on the level of a child of five or six. . . .
>
> A very important moment in the work on oneself is when a man begins to distinguish between his personality and his essence. A man's real I, his individuality, can grow only from his essence.[115]

In the early 1970s, the enneagram was further developed and taught by another mystic and spiritual teacher, Oscar Ichazo, to a group of followers in Arica, Chile.* One of his students, the Chilean psychiatrist Claudio Naranjo, introduced this enneagram teaching to a small group in Berkeley in 1971, which included Hameed Ali as well as Helen Palmer, now a renowned enneagram teacher and author.* Most of the modern versions of the enneagram today emanate from this original teaching by Ichazo, which has been elaborated on by Naranjo, Palmer, Ali, and others.[116]

Distinguishing between One's Personality Fixation and Essence

Typically, the enneagram is used to identify one's personality tendencies, and through recognition of these tendencies, one becomes less fixated and stuck in their particular psychological pattern. However, in more progressive schools, this ancient system is used to aid spiritual aspirants at a more profound level in differentiating between their acquired personality and their essential nature. Like his predecessors Gurdjieff and Ichazo, Ali imparts a much deeper understanding of the enneagram through teaching that the ennea-type fixations arise because of the loss of Essence, or one's true nature:

> Working with the enneagram only on the psychological level leaves us stuck on the psychological level. Working with the enneagram as part of a larger spiritual work, however, leads to a much deeper realization of truth and thus, a freedom from personality patterns that is literally unimaginable from the perspective of ego.[117]

Helen Palmer echoes Ali's teaching through her recognition that the mirror image of one's personality fixation is the loss or absence of the related essential quality:

> The search for a particular aspect of essence is motivated by the fact that you suffer from its absence. For example, if you are chronically afraid, then you have suffered the loss of the child's essential trust, in the environment and in others; therefore the search for courage will be a motive in your life.[118]

*In 1970, fifty-four North Americans, most of them Californians from the Esalen Institute in Big Sur, met in Arica, Chile, for ten months of intensive training by Ichazo. This group included Dr. Claudio Naranjo from Chile and Dr. John C. Lilly—a well-known author, psychoanalyst, and associate-in-residence at Esalen.

*This group also included Sandra Maitri, who is a senior Ridhwan teacher and the author of two books on the enneagram: *The Spiritual Dimension of the Enneagram: Nine Faces of the Soul* and *The Enneagram of Passions and Virtues: Finding the Way Home.* Learn moe about her at www.sandramaitri.com.

Ichazo called this essential quality a *Holy Idea*. He viewed the Holy Ideas as necessary "psycho-catalyzers" required for the work of "psycho-alchemy" on the ego, as he elaborates below:

> When we turn away from our primal perfection, our completeness, our unity with the world and God, we create the illusion that we need something exterior to ourselves for our completion. This dependency on what is exterior is what makes man's ego.[119]

In Ali's book on the enneagram, *Facets of Unity,* he elaborates on Ichazo's concept of the Holy Ideas:

> The transmitted view of the Enneagram is that each ennea-type fixation is the expression of a limited mental perspective on reality, and that each of the nine egoic perspectives is the direct result of the loss or absence of the enlightened perception of one of the Holy Ideas.[120]

Thus, through the loss of wisdom—that is, Ichazo's Holy Idea—each ennea type constructs a particular egoic personality in compensation for this particular loss. In human nature, nine of these personality types have been identified, and this number continues to "hold up" over time as consistent with reality, as well as perfectly fitting the constructs and relationships within the ancient nine-pointed enneagram symbol. Finally, since the term *Holy Idea* itself can sound a bit confusing, it is defined more clearly here by Sandra Maitri from her book *The Spiritual Dimension of the Enneagram:*

> The nine Holy Ideas are nine different direct perceptions of reality, when it is perceived without the filter of the personality, so they are nine different enlightened perspectives. The use of the word *idea* may be misleading here, since we usually think of an idea as a mental concept. In the language of the enneagram, however, idea refers to a particular perception of reality, a vantage point from which it is seen, experienced, and understood. It is important to clearly grasp that the Holy Ideas are not particular spiritual experiences or states of consciousness but rather are views of reality freed from the prejudices of the personality.[121]

Examples of Ennea-Type Fixations and the Loss of the Holy Idea

Thus, the case of the chronic fear type referred to in Palmer's previous example—that is, the central fixation of the enneagram number six—is based on this ennea type's loss of the Holy Ideas of faith and trust. The "six fixation" can be obvious in someone who is chronically fearful and anxious, but it can be more subtle when it manifests in what is termed a *counter-phobic* manner. In this latter case, an ennea-type six masks his or her fears by engaging in risky or daredevil-like activities.

Another example is the ennea-type one, who deeply feels the disconnection with the genuine perfection embodied in his or her true nature. These types try to inexpertly re-create this perfection artificially in their own lives, by taking the moral high ground, being judgmental and critical of imperfections, and always trying to improve themselves and others.[122]

The ennea-type seven has lost the Holy Idea of a "Holy Plan," which is the perception that the universe is not arbitrary but unfolds according to a kind of "cosmic blueprint" or divine plan.[123] The Holy Plan, therefore, can be defined as the innate knowing and understanding that there is a plan or pattern of development for each soul, which can only be revealed to us when we are fully present and open to its wisdom and revelations. When the ennea-type seven loses contact with this Holy Idea, he or she compensates through the related, but distorted, personality fixation of obsessively planning. Sandra Maitri elaborated on this subject:

> A Seven feels that he has lost his place in the vast pattern of unfoldment in the universe, and as he matures, the more he loses trust in his soul's capacity to unfold naturally. With this blind spot, it seems to him that reality does not support him in naturally developing and fulfilling his potential. His solution is to take matters in his own hands and to try and figure out how things work—what the plan is—and to try to make his process fit into it. Mapping and planning for the future, then, become his personal-

ity's imitation of Holy Plan, and become a substitute for full engagement in the present.[124]

As a defensive strategy for the loss of essential understanding of the "meaningful design and pattern of how things unfold," ennea-type sevens constantly try to imitate this state egoically. Therefore, sevens are typically obsessive planners, focusing on future possibilities to escape the pain of their present disconnection from their essential nature. Other typical personality fixations sevens use to avoid feeling this pain are addictive-type behaviors (gluttony), intellectualizing and giving advice, and appearing cheerful and carefree through always trying to give everything a positive spin.[125]

Personality Fixation Is the Doorway of Inquiry

In Ali's experience, these personality fixations, or false egoic tendencies, of the ennea types are actually the perfect (and truly only) doorways to uncovering and revealing an individual's lost essential state. Therefore, the study of the enneagram is an excellent fit to the core Ridhwan work of inquiry, allowing students to further and deepen their self-understanding and connection to Being. For example, only by sincerely inquiring into his constant planning and future-oriented behavior can a seven begin to feel the deep loss of the aspect of his essential nature in which he felt the most connected—the divine unfolding of the universe, or the Holy Plan. Furthermore, only through inquiring into and really feeling her anger and perfectionist tendencies can an ennea-type one begin to experience the loss and disconnection from the genuine perfection of the divine, or Holy Perfection. And finally, only when a six can face the fear and doubt that drive her personality and pattern her false egoic states can she recognize the loss of Holy Faith, for which she most yearns. Thus, through the enneagram the flip side of egoic functioning is once again revealed. That is, individuals tend to act out in an egoically distorted and effortful manner the loss of the very essence in which their Being was originally most intimate with and connected to—their Holy Idea.

The Enneagram Symbol

The enneagram symbol is depicted in figure 18.1, along with a list of several of the personality tendencies, termed *fixations,* of each of the nine types. The first two words in bold in each list refer to the ennea type's "chief feature" (primary weakness) and "chief passion" (major emotional tendency), respectively, according to Dr. Palmer's book *The Enneagram.* The remaining terms help further define each ennea type and are taken from several different sources. The Holy Idea associated with each ennea type is listed after the fixations in italics and is derived from A. H. Almaas's (Hameed Ali's) book *Facets of Unity.*

It is important to once again remind the reader that these rather harsh-sounding personality descriptions are not truly who you are but characteristic of your false self or "ego shell." These egoic tendencies are what you have assumed over time in order to survive in the world when your true nature was not mirrored—that is, seen, heard, and allowed to fully develop in childhood. Unless awareness brings them to the fore, these personality fixations tend to operate unconsciously for years, or even for your entire lifetime. The purpose is not to become identified with your specific ennea type but, with study and over time, to be able to better witness and naturally move away from these fixations that continually truncate your growth. Thus, the knowledge contained within this ancient teaching symbol is not designed to box you in but, as Don Riso, a prominent enneagram author, states, "to show you what boxes *to get out of.*"[126]

- ▶ The sacred psychology taught through the enneagram is not a quick study, as anyone who engages in any form of in-depth psychospiritual work is well aware. For those readers new to the concepts embodied in the enneagram and who want to begin to learn more about this fascinating system, Helen Palmer's *The Enneagram* is an excellent basic text. Additionally, for busy readers, Dr. Palmer has a CD set titled *The Enneagram Workshop* (published by Sounds True in Boulder, Colorado), which can be listened to in the car.

- ▶ For more in-depth information on this system, I recommend the following books: *Facets of Unity,* by A. H. Almaas; *The Spiritual Dimension of the Enneagram* and *The Enneagram of Passions and Virtues: Finding the Way Home,* by Sandra Maitri; "The Arica Training" chapter by John C. Lilly and Joseph E. Hart in the book *Transpersonal Psychologies,* edited by Charles Tart; and *The*

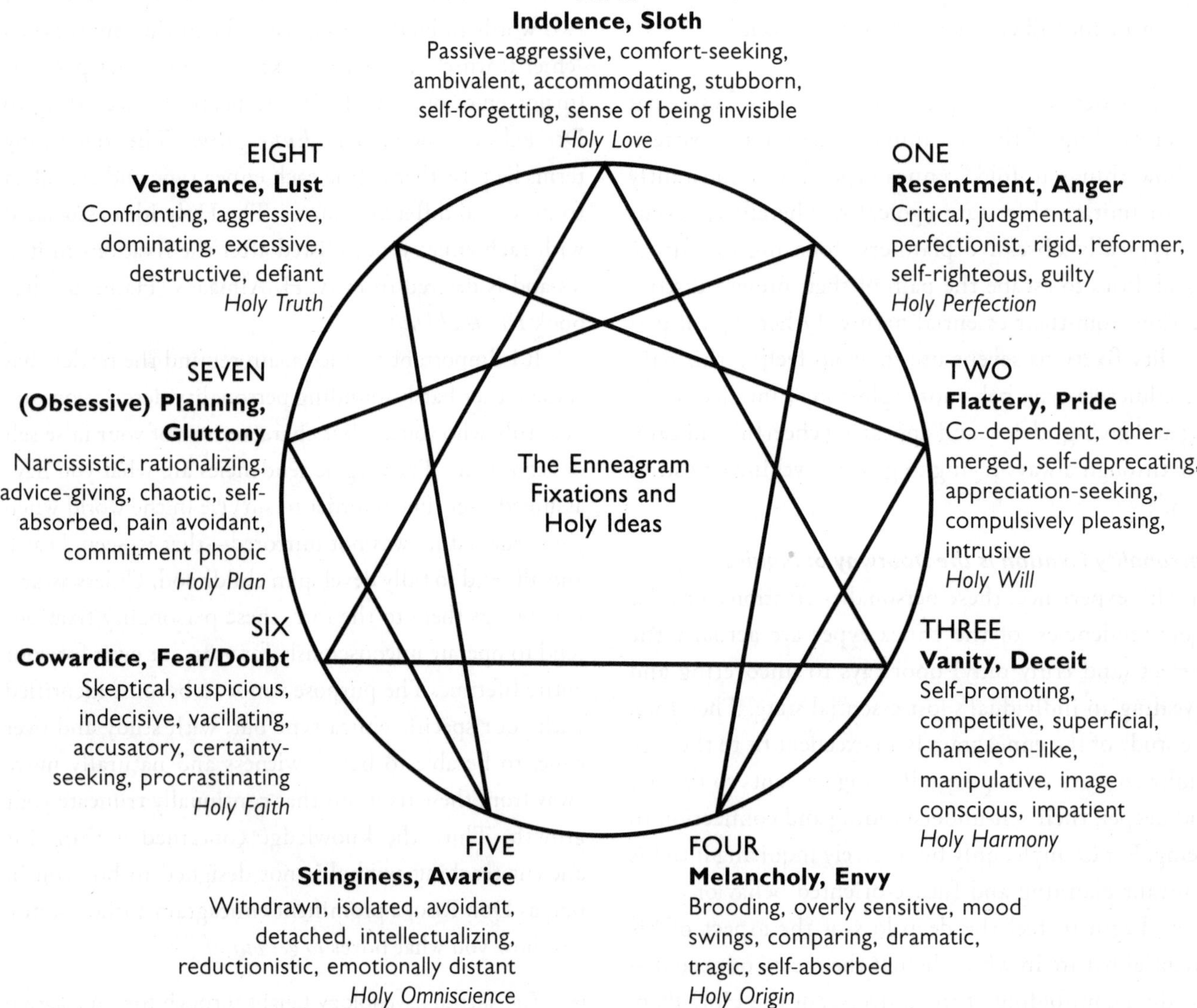

Figure 18.1. The nine enneagram fixations (the egoic tendencies) that manifest from the loss of the associated "Holy Ideas" (the enlightened perceptions of reality).

Wisdom of the Enneagram: The Complete Guide to Psychological and Spiritual Growth for the Nine Personality Types by Don Richard Riso and Russ Hudson.

- Individuals who are interested in further study on the enneagram can contact Helen Palmer at (866) 366-8973 or go to www.enneagramworldwide.com.

ℛ

In Ridhwan, psychological growth is not just an aspect of spiritual growth but considered *inseparable* from it. Thus, the perception, awareness, and ultimate dissolution of the false personality is worked on *simultaneously* with the perception, awareness, and ultimate development of one's essential nature.[127] Through this synthesis of Western and Eastern approaches, students have the potential of experiencing their genuine humanity or Being, inseparable from Divine Consciousness. As Ali states in the epilogue to his book *Essence:*

> The desire for freedom, liberation, enlightenment, self-realization, inner development, or whatever it is called is not a response to a call from outside you. . . . It is not a desire for self-improvement. . . . It is a response deep within

you. The quest does not bring about improvement or perfection. It brings about a maturity, a humanity, and a wisdom.[128]

▶ For more information on the Diamond Approach, go to www.ahalmaas.com or www.ridhwan.org or call (510) 841-7683. Additionally, the book *The Diamond Approach* by John Davis provides a good overview of the Ridhwan work. Other excellent introductory books are *Elements of the Real in Man* (book I in the *Diamond Heart* series) and *Spacecruiser Inquiry,* both written under Ali's pen name, A. H. Almaas. For more in-depth information, readers should refer to Almaas's two classic texts, *The Pearl Beyond Price* and *The Point of Existence.*

CONCLUSION
Healing All Aspects of Our Nature

Authentic healing requires addressing all aspects of our nature—the physical, psychological, and spiritual. The mentally and emotionally healing benefits embodied in holistic medicine through drainage, detoxification, healing foci, and constitutional homeopathy are truly immeasurable, and every holistic psychological practice should be aware of these benefits. However, it's just as vital that holistic practitioners recognize the need for deeper self-understanding arising in their patients and refer them to appropriate therapists or teachers.

Cognitive and behavioral psychological approaches can be beneficial for those new to self-exploration or those with emotional instabilities and weak ego development. However, because these modern psychological schools rarely address the spiritual aspect of the individual, they cannot reach the depths of self-understanding and awareness that psychospiritual approaches embody. In contrast, religious and devotional paths that ignore the human dimension, or the soul, can be just as limiting. For those individuals who are truly committed to the realization of their authentic Self and true nature, therefore, it is necessary to address both the psychological and spiritual aspects of Being. To be truly human requires accessing the spiritual dimension, and to be truly spiritual requires addressing the human dimension.

NOTES

1. L. Brown, *The New Shorter Oxford English Dictionary* (New York: Oxford University Press, 1993), 2402.
2. K. Wilber, *Integral Psychology* (Boston: Shambhala, 2000), ix.
3. J. Welwood, *Toward a Psychology of Awakening* (Boston: Shambhala, 2000), xi.
4. K. Wilber, *Integral Psychology* (Boston: Shambhala, 2000), ix.
5. Ibid.
6. E. Easwaran, *The Upanishads* (Tomales, Calif.: Nilgiri Press, 1993), 10–14; E. Easwaran, *The Bhagavad Gita* (Tomales, Calif.: Nilgiri Press, 2007), 9.
7. J. Clarke, *Jung and Eastern Thought* (New York: Routledge, 1994), 5–6.
8. E. Hoffman, *The Wisdom of Carl Jung* (New York: Citadel Press, 2003), 23.
9. A. Judith, *Eastern Body, Western Mind: Psychology and the Chakra System as a Path to the Self* (Berkeley, Calif.: Celestial Arts Publishing, 1997), 179.
10. J. Kottler, "Magical Mystery Tour," *Ode,* December 2004, 45.
11. A. Watts, *The Book* (New York: Vintage Books, 1966), ix–x.
12. L. Brown, *The New Shorter Oxford English Dictionary* (New York: Oxford University Press, 1993), 2462.
13. T. Moore, *Care of the Soul* (New York: Harper Perennial, 1992), 19–20.
14. J. Davis, *The Diamond Approach* (Boston: Shambhala, 1999), 8.
15. Association for Transpersonal Psychology, "Welcome to ATP," www.atpweb.org/index.html.
16. J. Welwood, *Toward a Psychology of Awakening* (Boston: Shambhala, 2000), xi.
17. Ibid., xvii.
18. K. Wilber, *The Essential Ken Wilber* (Boston: Shambhala, 1998), 9.
19. A. Watts, *Psychotherapy East and West* (New York: Ballantine Books, 1961), 21.
20. F. Leboyer, *Birth without Violence* (Rochester, Vt.: Healing Arts Press, 2002).
21. G. Murphy and R. Wetzel, "Suicide Risk by Birth Cohort in the United States, 1949 to 1974," *Archives of General Psychiatry* 37 (May 1980): 523.
22. L. Salk et al., "Relationship of Maternal and Perinatal

Conditions to Eventual Adolescent Suicide," *Lancet* (March 16, 1985): 624–27.

23. S. Ray and B. Mandel, *Birth & Relationships* (Berkeley, Calif.: Celestial Arts, 1987), 161.
24. T. Verny, with J. Kelly, *The Secret Life of the Unborn Child* (New York: Dell Publishing, 1981), 45–46, 47–50.
25. A. Tomatis, *The Conscious Ear* (Barrytown, N.Y.: Station Hill Press, 1991), 145, 146.
26. T. Verny, with J. Kelly, *The Secret Life of the Unborn Child* (New York: Dell Publishing, 1981), 49–50.
27. Ibid., 31.
28. Ibid., 184, 186, 187.
29. T. Verny, with J. Kelly, *The Secret Life of the Unborn Child* (New York: Dell Publishing Co., Inc., 1981), 186–87.
30. E. Marais, *The Soul of the White Ant* (London: Jonathan Cape Ltd. and Anthony Blond Ltd., 1971), 90–91.
31. B. Williams, *NBC Nightly News,* February 16, 2005.
32. S. Ray and B. Mandel, *Birth and Relationships* (Berkeley, Calif.: Celestial Arts, 1987), 93–97.
33. T. Verny, with J. Kelly, *The Secret Life of the Unborn Child* (New York: Dell Publishing Co., Inc., 1981), 108–9.
34. D. Chamberlain, *Babies Remember Birth* (New York: Ballantine Books, 1988), 105–20.
35. A. Schore, *Affect Regulation and the Origin of the Self* (Hillsdale, N.J.: Lawrence Erlbaum Associates, Publishers, 1994), 443.
36. S. Grof, *The Adventure of Self-Discovery* (Albany, N.Y.: State University of New York Press, 1988), 66.
37. E. Chesser, *Salvation through Sex* (New York: William Morrow & Company, 1973), 63–65.
38. S. Grof, *The Adventure of Self-Discovery* (Albany, N.Y.: State University of New York Press, 1988), 171.
39. Ibid., 4.
40. E. Chesser, *Salvation through Sex* (New York: William Morrow & Company, 1973), 62.
41. G. Minett, *Breath & Spirit* (San Francisco: The Aquarian Press, 1994), 97.
42. S. Grof, *The Adventure of Self-Discovery* (Albany, N.Y.: State University of New York Press, 1988), 4.
43. Ibid.
44. G. Minett, *Breath & Spirit* (San Francisco: The Aquarian Press, 1994), 118.
45. Ibid., 20.
46. S. Grof, *The Adventure of Self-Discovery* (Albany, N.Y.: State University of New York Press, 1988), 167.
47. L. McTaggart, *The Field* (New York: Harper, 2003), 47.
48. S. Grof, *The Adventure of Self-Discovery* (Albany, N.Y.: State University of New York Press, 1988), 6.
49. Ibid., 170.
50. O. Rank, *The Trauma of Birth* (New York: Dover Publications, 1993), 187–91.
51. E. Chesser, *Salvation through Sex* (New York: William Morrow & Company, 1973), 63–64 and jacket summary.
52. Ibid., 64.
53. A. Lowen, *Bioenergetics* (New York: Penguin Books, 1975), 17–18.
54. C. Retzler, "Rebirthing," www.positivehealth.com.
55. S. Grof, *The Adventure of Self-Discovery* (Albany, N.Y.: State University of New York Press, 1988), 166, 171.
56. J. Davis, *The Diamond Approach* (Boston: Shambhala, 1999), 7.
57. A. Almaas, *The Point of Existence* (Berkeley, Calif.: Diamond Books, 1996), 7.
58. A. Almaas, *Facets of Unity* (Berkeley, Calif.: Diamond Books, 1998), x.
59. A. Almaas, *The Pearl Beyond Price* (Berkeley, Calif.: Diamond Books, 1990), 140.
60. Ibid., 110.
61. Ibid., 109.
62. Ibid., 14.
63. Ibid.
64. A. Almaas, *The Pearl Beyond Price* (Berkeley, Calif.: Diamond Books, 1996), 111.
65. J. Welwood, *Toward a Psychology of Awakening* (Boston: Shambhala, 2000), 12.
66. Ibid., 13.
67. R. Fields et al., *Chop Wood, Carry Water* (Los Angeles: Jeremy P. Tarcher, 1984), 11.
68. M. Woodman, *Leaving My Father's House* (London: Rider & Co., 1993), 170.
69. A. Almaas, *The Pearl Beyond Price* (Berkeley, Calif.: Diamond Books, 1990), 121, 122.
70. Satprem, *Sri Aurobindo or the Adventure of Consciousness* (New York: Institute for Evolutionary Research, 1984), 108.
71. A. Almaas, *The Point of Existence* (Berkeley, Calif.: Diamond Books, 1996), 72.
72. A. Almaas, *Brilliancy* (Boston: Shambhala, 2006), 36–37.
73. K. Wilber, *A Brief History of Everything* (Boston: Shambhala, 2000).
74. A. Almaas, *The Pearl Beyond Price* (Berkeley, Calif.: Diamond Books, 1996), 11, 110, 111.
75. Ibid., 111.

76. F. Halligan, *Listening Deeply to God* (Mystic, Conn.: Twenty-Third Publications, 2003), 75.
77. T. Keating, *Invitation to Love* (New York: Continuum, 2004), 17.
78. A. Almaas, *The Pearl Beyond Price* (Berkeley, Calif.: Diamond Books, 1990), 123.
79. B. Brown, *Soul without Shame* (Boston: Shambhala, 1999), 112.
80. Ibid., 4.
81. A. Almaas, *Brilliancy* (Boston: Shambhala, 2006), 26.
82. A. Almaas, *The Pearl Beyond Price* (Berkeley, Calif.: Diamond Books, 1990), 113.
83. Ibid., 111.
84. Ibid., 29.
85. Ibid., 120–21.
86. K. Wilber, *A Brief History of Everything* (Boston: Shambhala, 2000), 61.
87. Ibid., xi.
88. A. Almaas, *The Pearl Beyond Price* (Berkeley, Calif.: Diamond Books, 1990), 32.
89. Ibid., 142.
90. J. Davis, *The Diamond Approach* (Boston: Shambhala, 1999), 27.
91. Ibid., 25.
92. Ibid., 30, 31.
93. Ibid., 5.
94. A. Almaas, *Diamond Heart,* book 1, *Elements of the Real in Man* (Berkeley, Calif.: Diamond Books, 1998), 7.
95. J. Welwood, *Love and Awakening* (New York: Harper Perennial, 1997), 12.
96. A. Almaas, *The Pearl Beyond Price* (Berkeley, Calif.: Diamond Books, 1990), 96.
97. A. Almaas, *Diamond Heart,* book 1, *Elements of the Real in Man* (Berkeley, Calif.: Diamond Books, 1998), 17.
98. K. Gibran, *The Prophet* (New York: Alfred A. Knopf, 2005), 52.
99. A. Almaas, *Diamond Heart,* book 1, *Elements of the Real in Man* (Berkeley, Calif.: Diamond Books, 1998), 17, 18.
100. A. Almaas, *The Pearl Beyond Price* (Berkeley, Calif.: Diamond Books, 1990), 134–35.
101. J. Davis, *The Diamond Approach* (Boston: Shambhala, 1999), 7.
102. A. Almaas, *The Pearl Beyond Price* (Berkeley, Calif.: Diamond Books, 1990), 110, 119, 123.
103. A. Almaas, *Spacecruiser Inquiry* (Boston: Shambhala, 2002), 185–86.
104. A. Almaas, *The Point of Existence* (Berkeley, Calif.: Diamond Books, 1996), 75.
105. A. Almaas, *Diamond Heart,* book 1, *Elements of the Real in Man* (Berkeley, Calif.: Diamond Books, 1998), 15–16.
106. A. Almaas, *The Point of Existence* (Berkeley, Calif.: Diamond Books, 1996), 217.
107. Ibid., 315–316.
108. B. Brown, *Soul without Shame* (Boston: Shambhala, 1999), 67.
109. Ibid., 67, 68.
110. H. Palmer, *The Enneagram* (San Francisco: Harper, 1991), 10.
111. Ibid.; A. Almaas, *Facets of Unity* (Berkeley, Calif.: Diamond Books, 1998), 3.
112. H. Palmer, *The Enneagram* (San Francisco: Harper, 1991), 10.
113. Ibid., 10, 11.
114. Ibid., 17.
115. P. Ouspensky, *In Search of the Miraculous* (Boston: Houghton Mifflin Harcourt, 2003), 162, 163.
116. S. Maitri, *The Spiritual Dimension of the Enneagram* (New York: Jeremy P. Tarcher/Putnam, 2000), 5, 6, 7.
117. A. Almaas, *Facets of Unity* (Berkeley, Calif.: Diamond Books, 1998), 6, 7.
118. H. Palmer, *The Enneagram* (San Francisco: Harper, 1991), 18–19.
119. A. Almaas, *Facets of Unity* (Berkeley, Calif.: Diamond Books, 1998), 7.
120. Ibid., 6.
121. S. Maitri, *The Spiritual Dimension of the Enneagram* (New York: Jeremy P. Tarcher/Putnam, 2000), 10.
122. Ibid., 110, 111.
123. S. Maitri, *The Spiritual Dimension of the Enneagram* (New York: Jeremy P. Tarcher/Putnam, 2000), 226.
124. Ibid., 229.
125. Ibid., 226, 230.
126. "Enneagram Introduction, Theory and Research," www.9types.com/writeup/enneagram.html.
127. J. Davis, *The Diamond Approach* (Boston: Shambhala, 1999), 7, 22.
128. A. Almaas, *Essence* (York Beach, Maine: Samuel Weiser, 1986), 181–82.

FINAL WORDS

TO ALL READERS

The fact that you are reading this book (and have reached these final paragraphs!) places you in that special group of discriminating individuals whose internal compass is magnetically attuned to what feels true and genuine—no matter how unorthodox or "radical." I am honored that you have read my book, and hope that the serendipity that led you to *Radical Medicine* was perfectly synchronous with your needs, and that it has quickened and furthered your own personal journey toward optimal health.

For readers who have been through a lot of personal pain and healing—physically and emotionally—the following quote from the poet Kahlil Gibran is a fitting tribute to your courage and determination, as well as an appropriate conclusion to this book:

> *Then a woman said, Speak to us of Joy*
> *and Sorrow.*
> *And he answered:*
> *Your joy is your sorrow unmasked.*
> *And the selfsame well from which your*
> *laughter rises was oftentimes filled*
> *with your tears.*
> *And how else can it be?*
> *The deeper that sorrow carves into*
> *your being, the more joy you can*
> *contain.*[1]

TO HOLISTIC DOCTORS AND PRACTITIONERS

The counseling of a patient on the toxicity of amalgam fillings, focal infections, chronic food allergies, and so forth, when we ourselves have not addressed these issues, is not conducive to an honest doctor-patient relationship. It not only imparts a subtle sense of (conscious or unconscious) distrust in patients but also wears on the practitioner over time, and greatly contributes to eventual burnout in one's practice.

The following story about Gandhi illustrates the importance for healers—and actually for all those who advise and teach—to be consistent with the truth:

> One day a mother brought her young son to Gandhi and asked him to tell the boy to stop eating sugar. Gandhi told them both to come back in three weeks.
>
> Three weeks later the mother returned with her son. Gandhi then told the boy to stop eating sugar. The mother asked Gandhi why he waited to tell her son something he could have said three weeks ago, and he replied, "Because three weeks ago I was still eating sugar."

In the same way, as a holistic practitioner, you yourself should endeavor to stop consuming refined sugar and eat a healthy diet in order to have a truly authentic impact when counseling patients to do the same. Additionally, when you are strong enough, replacing your amalgam fillings or any nickel/palladium-containing crowns with less toxic alternatives is essential. Suspected focal infections and scar interference fields should also be assessed and treated if they test positive. Finding a Sankaran-trained homeopath and receiving your deepest constitutional remedy is probably the most effective healing modality presently known. Additionally, you may need to stabilize a chronic malocclusion with an orthopedic appliance or simply build up or lightly equilibrate a mildly disturbing bite. Replacing toxic cosmetics and soaps with petroleum-free alternatives is perhaps the simplest step, and can be done immediately.

Finally, since ignoring any aspect of our being is always "inevitably one-sided" and will eventually truncate our development, if you are not actively involved in some form of psychospiritual work, you may want to consider investigating one of these advanced approaches.[2]

When you treat not only your patients but yourself, according to the guidelines described in *Radical Medicine,* your practice will profoundly change. The communication of the truth that you have directly experienced will create a pure and more consistent energetic field between practitioner and patient. Furthermore, through the psychophysical effects of having a clearer mind and body, you will sharpen your diagnostic skills and be more effective in your treatments. Finally, through a "cleaner" and more transparent self, you can more fully experience your true nature, which has profound effects in every aspect of your life.

NOTES

1. K. Gibran, *The Prophet* (New York: Alfred A. Knopf, 2005), 29.
2. G. Gurdjieff, *Life Is Real Only Then, When "I Am"* (New York: Penguin, 1978), x.

Appendix 1

DESCRIPTION OF HOLISTIC PRACTITIONERS

The following pages provide a brief description of the five types of primary care physicians—N.D., D.C., D.O., M.D., and D.D.S.—and the chief acupuncture practitioners (L.Ac.) licensed in the United States. However, every doctor and practitioner is unique, so healing techniques and philosophies within each profession can vary widely. Thus, the summary description of each profession is a *general* characterization of the majority—but not all—of the doctors and practitioners in each group.

NATUROPATHIC DOCTORS (N.D.) The Consummate Holistic Physicians

More than any other practitioner, N.D.s are taught and practice the widest range of holistic therapies in natural medicine. Naturopathic doctors are the *only* physicians who are taught homeopathy and botanical (herbal) medicine as part of their college curriculum. Furthermore, they receive more hours in nutrition than any other practitioner.

FINDING A "HOMEOPATHIC DOCTOR"

Individuals often ask where they can find a "homeopathic doctor." The answer to this question is threefold: First, as was discussed in chapter 14, because all homeopathic colleges were closed down in the early and mid-twentieth century through the successful efforts of the American Medical Association, there are no "Doctors of Homeopathy" licensed in this country anymore. Second, since naturopaths are the only healthcare professionals who are taught homeopathy in their medical school curriculum, naturopathic physicians (who specialize in homeopathy) come closest to fulfilling this former "Doctor of Homeopathy" role. (There is, however, a homeopathic college opening in Arizona. Go to www.amcofh.org for more information.) And third, naturopaths as well as other physicians (D.C.s, D.O.s, M.D.s, and D.D.S.s), practitioners (L.Ac.s), and many talented laypeople study homeopathy in courses and seminars offered after graduation and can become certified in homeopathy through various postgraduate groups and institutions. As discussed in chapter 14, I strongly recommend doctors and practitioners who have studied and are proficient in the new and revolutionary work of Dr. Rajan Sankaran and his Mumbai, India, colleagues, because it is the most accurate means of determining the deepest constitutional homeopathic remedy.

Naturopathic Medical Education

Like other doctors, naturopaths must satisfy premed science requirements in their undergraduate education, before admission into a naturopathic medical school. Students then attend a four-year naturopathic college or university where the curriculum includes basic science courses (anatomy with human dissection, pathology, biochemistry, immunology, histology, etc.), as well as comprehensive training in natural therapies (botanical medicine, homeopathy, therapeutic nutrition, counseling, manipulation, hydrotherapy, environmental medicine, physical therapy, natural childbirth, etc.), physical and clinical diagnosis, pharmacology, clinical ecology, and minor surgery (suturing, wound infection and burn management, use of local anesthetics, etc.). Like other doctors, naturopathic students also receive extensive clinical experience and training through treating patients under the supervision of naturopathic

EDUCATIONAL COMPARISON OF THE SIX MAJOR HEALING PROFESSIONS

Profession	Undergraduate Requirements	Graduate School Requirements	National Licensing Exams	Postgraduate Requirements
N.D. (Naturopathic Doctor)	4 years (including science courses)	4 years (naturopathic medical school, N.D. degree)	NPlex Parts I & II (licensed to practice as an N.D.)	Continuing education credits required annually. One-year residencies in general medicine are available postgraduation. Many N.D.s also continue to take courses in their field of specialty postgrad (e.g., botanical medicine, homeopathy, nutrition, etc.).
D.C. (Doctor of Chiropractic)	3–4 years (including science courses)	4 years (chiropractic college, D.C. degree)	NBCE Parts I, II, III, IV & PT (licensed to practice as a D.C.)	Continuing education credits required annually. Many D.C.s also continue to take courses in their field of specialty postgrad (spinal adjusting, craniopathy, nutrition, Applied Kinesiology, etc.).
D.O. (Doctor of Osteopathy)	4 years (including science courses)	4 years (osteopathic medical school, D.O. degree)	NBOME Parts I, II & III (licensed to practice as a D.O.)	Continuing education credits required annually. Osteopaths who want to specialize in a particular field enter a 2- to 3-year postgrad residency program (e.g., dermatology, gynecology, neurology, etc.).
M.D. (Medical Doctor)	4 years (including science courses)	4 years (medical school, M.D. degree)	USMLE Parts I & II (licensed to practice as an M.D.)	Continuing education credits required annually. M.D.s who want to specialize in a particular field (e.g., pediatrics, radiology, obstetrics, etc.) enter a 2- to 3-year (or longer) residency program.
D.D.S. (Doctor of Dental Surgery)	3–4 years (including science courses)	4 years (dental school, D.D.S. degree)	JCNDE Parts I & II and state dental boards (AADD) (licensed to practice as a D.D.S.)	Continuing education credits required annually. Many holistic D.D.S.s continue to take courses in their field of specialty postgrad (e.g., cavitation surgery, mercury amalgam removal, TMD, etc.).
L.Ac. (Licensed Acupuncturist)	2 years (including science courses)	3 years (acupuncture college, L.Ac. degree)	NCCAOM (licensed to practice as an acupuncturist)	Continuing education credits required annually. Many acupuncturists continue to take courses in their field of specialty postgrad (e.g., Chinese herbal medicine, electroacupuncture, etc.).

Requirements can vary slightly from school to school. Contact the college you are interested in for more specific information.

physicians in their college clinics, as well as in preceptorship programs while interning with naturopathic physicians in their private clinics.

Currently, there are six fully accredited naturopathic medical schools in North America: Bastyr University (Kenmore, WA), Boucher Institute of Naturopathic Medicine (New Westminster, BC), Canadian College of Naturopathic Medicine (Ontario, Canada), National College of Natural Medicine (Portland, OR), Southwest College of Naturopathic Medicine (Tempe, AZ), and the University of Bridgeport College of Naturopathic Medicine (Bridgeport, CT). The National University of Health Sciences in Lombard, IL, was granted candidacy status from the Council on Naturopathic Medical Education (CNME) in 2008. Also, Bastyr University is in the process of establishing a campus in California, scheduled to open in 2011. After graduation, N.D.s must pass national boards recognized by the U.S. Department of Education (NPLEX Parts I and II) in order to be licensed to practice naturopathic medicine.

Licensing

Due to the successful lobbying efforts of competing professions (primarily M.D.s), naturopathic doctors are currently licensed to practice in only fifteen states—Alaska, Arizona, California, Connecticut, Hawaii, Idaho, Kansas, Maine, Minnesota, Montana, New Hampshire, Oregon, Utah, Vermont, and Washington, as well as the District of Columbia and the U.S. territories of Puerto Rico and the Virgin Islands.

"Doctors" as Compared to "Practitioners"

Some schools and institutes offer very brief or even mail-order programs that allow their graduates to use "N.D." after their name. This practice is understandably disturbing to the N.D.s who have satisfied premed undergraduate requirements, graduated from four-year fully accredited naturopathic medical schools, and passed national boards recognized by the U.S. government. Furthermore, it is extremely confusing to the general public.

Until this practice is changed, naturopathic doctors might want to utilize in smaller subscript the particular naturopathic medical school that they have graduated from after their "N.D." title.* Thus, patients who are seeking a naturopathic physician† would look for the following after their prospective doctor's name:

John Doe, $N.D._{Bastyr}$
Jane Doe, $N.D._{Boucher}$
John Doe, $N.D._{CCNM}$
Jane Doe, $N.D._{NCNM}$
John Doe, $N.D._{SWCNM}$
Jane Doe, $N.D._{UBCNM}$

This in no way would limit the practice of those individuals graduated from mail-order or brief programs, but it would simply clearly differentiate between naturopathic *practitioners,* or perhaps *counselors* or *educators,* and naturopathic *doctors* or *physicians.** Hopefully, through these more descriptive "N.D." appellations, the public can make a more informed choice when determining its healthcare providers.

▶ To locate a naturopathic physician or find more information on naturopathic medicine, contact:

The American Association of Naturopathic Physicians (AANP)
3201 New Mexico Avenue NW, Suite 350, Washington, DC 20016
phone (866) 538-2267 or (202) 895-1392
or fax (202) 274-1992
www.naturopathic.org

CHIROPRACTIC DOCTORS (D.C.) Musculoskeletal Experts and Master Energetic Testers

D.C.s are well known for being the most knowledgeable primary care physicians† for the treatment of muscle and joint pain and dysfunction. This recognition is well deserved, because chiropractic colleges require more hours in neuromusculoskeletal diagnosis and treatment than any other programs. In addition, chiropractic physicians receive extensive training in clinical nutrition—both in the classroom and in their college outpatient clinics.

*In the state of Arizona naturopaths use the title "NMD" after their name—Naturopathic Medical Doctor.

†The terms *doctor* and *physician* are synonymous. However, legally in some states N.D.s are only allowed to use the term *doctor,* due to the lobbying efforts of the medical doctors in that state.

*In fact, a "health freedom" bill (SB 577) that passed in California in 2003 allows all (non-physician) health practitioners to utilize natural modalities—nutrition, herbs, homeopathy, light, air, and water—without fear of prosecution simply for using "alternative" forms of healing.

Naturopathic doctors were licensed under the Naturopathic Doctors Act (SB 907) in California in 2004 to diagnose and treat disease and practice as primary care physicians. SB 907 allows other practitioners to use the terms *naturopathy, naturopath, traditional naturopath,* and *naturopathic practitioner* to describe their practice. However, it reserves the following titles and professional abbreviations for N.D.s who have graduated from fully accredited naturopathic medical schools and passed state and national board requirements: N.D., Doctor of Naturopathy, Doctor of Naturopathic Medicine, and Licensed Naturopathic Doctor.

†The terms *doctor* and *physician* are synonymous. However, legally in some states D.C.s are only allowed to use the term *doctor,* due to the lobbying efforts of the medical doctors in that state.

Many D.C.s facilitate their standard diagnostic assessment methods (history, exam, laboratory, and X-ray findings) with energetic testing techniques. Although not all D.C.s use a form of energetic testing, as a group they have a much larger number of practitioners who specialize in this esoteric diagnostic skill than any of the other healing professions. Many use kinesiology techniques such as Applied Kinesiology (AK), Clinical Kinesiology (CK), Autonomic Response Testing (ART), and so forth. However, several arm- and leg-length measurement indicator methods are also widely utilized, including the Matrix Reflex Testing technique (MRT), Directional Non-Force Technique (DNFT), Derifield, Activator Technique, and others. Finally, some D.C.s—as well as a number of other holistic practitioners—use electroacupuncture techniques that originated in Germany with Dr. Voll and Dr. Vega. Chiropractors who use energetic testing not only study these methods during college but also train in postgraduate courses extensively, continually learning and improving their technique throughout their professional lives. As discussed throughout *Radical Medicine,* effective energetic testing techniques allow practitioners to more precisely determine the cause of a particular dysfunction or illness, as well as to assess the most appropriate treatments. (For more information on energetic testing, see appendix 3, "Energetic Testing Explained.")

Chiropractic Education

Like other doctors, chiropractors must satisfy premed science requirements in their undergraduate education. They then attend four-year postgraduate chiropractic colleges whose curriculum is composed of basic and clinical sciences including anatomy with human dissection, neurophysiology, radiology, histology, cellular physiology, immunology, pathology, clinical psychology, biochemistry, pharmacology, and so forth. Additionally, D.C.s receive over 550 hours in spinal analysis and adjusting techniques, as well as extensive training in differential diagnosis that greatly augments their clinical expertise in distinguishing between somatovisceral (primary musculoskeletal dysfunction that secondarily adversely affects an organ) and viscerosomatic (primary organ dysfunction that secondarily adversely affects the muscles and joints) relationships, as discussed in part 6. Chiropractic students also gain valuable clinical experience and training through treating patients under the supervision of chiropractic physicians in their college clinics, as well as in preceptorship programs with chiropractic physicians in their private clinics.

Currently, there are seventeen fully accredited chiropractic colleges in North America. Go to www.cce-usa.org for their names and locations, or call the Council on Chiropractic Education (CCE) at (480) 443-8877.

After graduation, D.C.s must pass national board exams recognized by the U.S. Department of Education (NBCE Parts I, II, III, IV, and PT) to be licensed to practice chiropractic.

Licensing

Chiropractic doctors are licensed to practice in all fifty states, Puerto Rico, and the U.S. Virgin Islands (as well as in other parts of the world).

► To locate a chiropractic physician, or to find out more information about the chiropractic profession, contact:

The American Chiropractic Association (ACA)
1701 Clarendon Boulevard, Arlington, VA 22209
phone (703) 243-2593 or fax (703) 276-8800
memberinfo@acatoday.org
www.acatoday.org

OSTEOPATHIC DOCTORS (D.O.) Master Allopaths and Some Musculoskeletal Experts

As was discussed in part 6, due to considerable harassment and persecution in the early and mid-twentieth century from the allopathic medical profession, osteopathic colleges reduced much of their emphasis on manual manipulation in order to survive as a profession. However, over the last few decades with the rise of holistic medicine, the number of osteopaths practicing spinal manipulation and craniosacral therapy has been increasing. Therefore, newer graduates—as well as older D.O.s who attended osteopathic college in the mid-twentieth century when spinal manipulation was more respected as a healing art—are more likely to utilize these hands-on healing approaches.

In most cases, however, the majority of osteopaths currently practice almost identically to M.D.s, primarily utilizing the allopathic tools of prescription drugs and surgery as their basic healing modalities.

Osteopathic Medical Education

Much like other physicians, osteopaths must satisfy premed admission requirements before attending four-year osteopathic medical colleges and universities. And like other physicians, an osteopath's medical education includes the basic and clinical sciences (anatomy with human dissection, pathology, histology, radiology, biochemistry, pharmacology, physical and clinical diagnosis, etc.), as well as extensive hands-on training through treating patients under the supervision of osteopathic physicians in osteopathic college clinics and hospitals.

Additionally, in the curriculum of the Kirksville College of Osteopathic Medicine—the original osteopathic school (founded by A. T. Still)—students currently receive 196 hours in osteopathic theory and methods (including manual manipulation), as well as four weeks of clinical rotation on this subject during their last two years. One course in craniosacral manipulation is offered as an elective.

Currently, there are twenty-six fully accredited osteopathic colleges in thirty-four locations in the United States. Go to www.aacom.org to view a list of these colleges.

After graduation, osteopaths must pass national boards recognized by the U.S. Department of Education (NBOME Parts I, II, and III) in order to be licensed to practice osteopathic medicine.

D.O.s, like M.D.s, can practice as general practitioners at this point, or they can go on to specialize in a particular field (e.g., dermatology, gynecology, neurology, etc.), generally through a three-year* postgraduate residency program.

Licensing

Osteopathic physicians are licensed to practice in all fifty states (as well as in other parts of the world).

- ▶ To locate an osteopathic physician, or to find more information about the osteopathic profession, contact:

*Some residency programs are shorter (e.g., two years), while some are longer (e.g., seven years).

The American Osteopathic Association (AOA)
142 East Ontario, Chicago, IL 60611-2864
phone (800) 621-1773
info@osteopathic.org
www.osteopathic.org

To locate an osteopathic physician who utilizes craniosacral manipulation, go to www.cranialacademy.org

MEDICAL DOCTORS (M.D.) Master Allopaths and Some Holistic Physicians

Due to the major influence pharmaceutical companies have had on modern medical teaching, medical schools have offered no courses in botanical (herbal) medicine or homeopathy and have averaged only two hours of course work in nutrition throughout most of the twentieth century.[1] Based on this strong allopathic orientation, the vast majority of medical doctors utilize two major methods of healing—prescription drugs and surgery. However, due to the increasing popularity of alternative medicine in the past few decades, some M.D.s have endeavored to remedy their lack of holistic medical training by taking postgraduate seminars after their medical school education. These courageous few—often attacked by their allopathic colleagues and state boards—are fortunately growing in number. Additionally, a number of medical schools are now offering nutrition, botanical medicine, massage, and acupuncture both online and residentially in integrative medicine programs designed to be complementary to mainstream medical care.*

NUTRITIONAL EDUCATION

Currently, only 30 percent of medical schools have a required nutrition course, and 25 percent of schools do not require or could not quantify nutritional education in their programs. This has been the case for decades at even the best institutions, as exemplified by Andrew Weil's disclosure during a Larry King interview that at

*These schools include the University of Arizona (Dr. Andrew Weil), the University of Maryland, and the M. D. Anderson Cancer Center (Web-based teaching for patients and physicians).

Harvard he received only about *thirty minutes* of training in nutrition! Even in the 1990s, according to a National Academy of Sciences study, two-thirds of medical schools still offered no required nutrition courses, and the typical graduating M.D. had an average of only about twenty classroom hours in nutrition. Compare this to N.D.s, who receive approximately 200 hours of classroom training in clinical nutrition, and another 1,200 hours in clinical education in which nutritional therapy is an important diagnostic consideration in treatment.[2] Recently, however, due to the rising influence of natural medicine and the efforts of holistic physicians such as Dr. Weil, more colleges have begun to offer hours in nutrition (through either elective or required courses) during the four-year medical school curriculum. Additionally, since one of the chief barriers to incorporating nutrition into medical schools is that often no faculty members are specifically trained in clinical nutrition, home study through computer technology is being proposed at many colleges.[3]

Medical School Education

As with the other physicians described in this section, prospective medical students must satisfy premed requirements in undergraduate colleges and universities, before being accepted into four-year medical schools. An M.D.'s education is similar to that of other physicians and includes the basic and clinical sciences (anatomy with human dissection, pathology, histology, biochemistry, pharmacology, physical and clinical diagnosis, etc.), as well as extensive clinical training through treating patients under the supervision of medical doctors in medical school clinics and hospitals.

There are numerous fully accredited medical schools in the United States. Contact the specific college or university you are interested in to find out more information.

After graduation, M.D.s must pass national boards recognized by the U.S. Department of Education (USMLE Parts I and II) to be licensed to practice medicine.

M.D.s may then work as general practitioners or go on to specialize in a particular field (e.g., pediatrics, psychiatry, orthopedics, etc.), generally through a three-year* postgraduate residency program.

*Some residency programs are shorter (e.g., two years), while some are longer (e.g., seven years or more).

Licensing

Medical doctors are licensed to practice in all fifty states (and every other country in the world).

► To locate a medical doctor or to find more information on the medical profession, contact:

The American Medical Association (AMA)
515 N. State Street, Chicago, IL 60610
phone (312) 464-5000
www.ama-assn.org

To locate an M.D. utilizing a more holistic approach, contact:

American Holistic Medicine Association (AHMA)
www.holisticmedicine.org

DOCTORS OF DENTAL SURGERY (D.D.S.)
Holistic and Nonholistic Dentists

The Good, the Bad, and the Ugly

Presently, three types of dental physicians exist in the world: the *good*—those who keep abreast of the current research that incontrovertibly proves the toxic and debilitating effects of mercury amalgam fillings and therefore no longer use it; the *bad*—those who don't keep up with the current research or continue to believe the American Dental Association's (ADA) unscientific stance that mercury is stable and nontoxic once it is placed in the mouth;* and the *ugly*—those dentists who are aware of the current research and yet continue (out of fear of reprisal from the ADA or just a general lack of caring) to place it in their patients' mouths.

Furthermore, because the curriculum at dental schools is still guided by the ADA's untenable stance on mercury, the majority of newly graduated dentists continue to use mercury amalgam fillings, as they were trained in college.† And, although some are aware of the amalgam controversy, very few are cognizant of the toxic potentiating effects of *dental galvanism,* when gold or other metal crowns are placed on or next to amalgam fillings.

*This assertion has been proven as completely false in multiple well-conducted scientific research studies (see chapter 3).

†The placement of composite fillings is also taught in dental schools. However, the use of these "white" fillings is primarily explained as being necessary only for cosmetic purposes (e.g., in front teeth), while amalgam fillings remain the standard in the back molars.

Similar to holistic M.D.s, holistic or "biological" dentists are frequently attacked by their nonholistic colleagues and state boards and risk losing their license and even their livelihood, simply for practicing based on the prevailing scientific evidence on the toxicity of mercury amalgam, as well as their own courage and integrity. Fortunately, a growing percentage of dentists are becoming educated about nontoxic dentistry through postgraduate courses sponsored by holistic dental associations. At these biological dental association meetings, dentists can learn about the most cutting-edge and nontoxic methods of replacing amalgam fillings and the devastating effects of dental galvanism (chapter 3), be trained in the diagnosis of dental focal infections and their removal through appropriate cavitation surgery techniques (chapter 11), and study the most effective treatments for malocclusions and temporomandibular joint dysfunction (chapter 16).*

Dental Schools

Like other physicians, prospective dental students must satisfy basic science or premed requirements in undergraduate colleges and universities before being accepted into four-year dental schools. Furthermore, similar to other doctors, a dentist's education includes the basic and clinical sciences (anatomy with human dissection,† pathology, histology, biochemistry, pharmacology, physical and clinical diagnosis, etc.), as well as extensive clinical training through treating patients (fillings, crowns, surgery, etc.) under the supervision of dental physicians in dental school clinics.

There are numerous dental schools in the United States and Canada. Contact the American Dental Education Association (ADEA) at (202) 289-7201 or go to www.adea.org for a list of fully accredited colleges.

After graduation, dentists must pass written national boards (JCNDE) recognized by the U.S. Department of Education and clinical exams given in the state in which they are planning to practice (AAOD) to be licensed to practice dentistry.

Dentists may then work as general practitioners or specialize in a particular field (e.g., oral and maxillofacial surgery, orthodontics, pediatrics, periodontology, etc.) through continuing their training in two- to six-year postgraduate residency programs.

Licensing

Dentists are licensed to practice in all fifty states and throughout the world.

- To locate a conventional dentist or find out more information about the dental profession, contact:

The American Dental Association (ADA)
1111 14th Street NW, Suite 1100, Washington, DC 20005
phone (202) 898-2400 or fax (202) 898-2437
www.ada.org

- To locate a holistic dentist, contact one of the three major biological dental associations in the U.S.:

Holistic Dental Association
P.O. Box 151444, San Diego, CA 92175
phone (619) 923-3120 or fax (619) 615-2228
info@holisticdental.org
www.holisticdental.org

International Academy of Biological Dentistry and Medicine (IABDM)
17222 Red Oak Drive, Suite 101, Houston, TX 77090
phone (281) 651-1745 or fax (281) 440-1258
drdawn@drdawn.net
www.iabdm.org

*Because dentists hold the degree of Doctors of Dental Surgery (D.D.S.), they are licensed to perform surgery. And since general dentists are typically more holistically oriented, they attend postgraduate courses on cavitation surgery and specialize in this biological dental method in greater numbers than oral surgeons. Therefore, it's important to ensure that a particular dentist is skilled and experienced in cavitation surgery and has a successful track record among patients, rather than simply deciding on the basis of whether he or she is an oral surgeon versus a general dentist. However, when a particular surgery is complicated, dentists often refer patients to oral surgeons (and when these surgeons have studied cavitation techniques they can be particularly valuable).

The same is true when comparing general dentists trained in "orthopedic" techniques to orthodontists. As discussed in chapter 16, orthopedic dentists tend to consider the structure and function of the *whole* body and make use of functional appliances more often than orthodontists. Therefore, when deciding on a doctor to treat a malocclusion or TMD, don't simply choose between an orthodontist and a general dentist, but take into mind both professionals' postgraduate training as well as their success with former patients.

†Dissection of the entire body with an emphasis on the head and neck.

International Academy of Oral Medicine and Toxicology (IAOMT)
8297 Champions Gate Blvd., Suite 193, Champions Gate, FL 33896
phone (863) 420-6373 or fax (863) 419-8136
info@iaomt.org
www.iaomt.org

- The holistic organization dedicated to informing patients about toxic versus nontoxic dentistry, DAMS, is also an excellent resource:

Dental Amalgam Mercury Solutions
1043 Grand Ave., #317, St. Paul, MN 55105
phone: (800) 311-6265 or (651) 644-4572
dams@unsfamily.net

ACUPUNCTURISTS (L.Ac.) Chinese Medicine Experts

Acupuncture practitioners learn and practice all aspects of Chinese medicine but are most well known for treating acupuncture points with needles and prescribing Chinese herbal medicines. In the past few decades, scientific studies have proven what acupuncturists have known for millennia—that Chinese medicine can be effective in the treatment of all types of disease and dysfunction. Chinese medicine, and Ayurvedic medicine from India can be considered the two original systems of holistic medicine because they both view patients' symptoms in relationship to their whole body functioning, and furthermore, they use natural nonsynthetic medicines and healing techniques.

Acupuncture Education

Acupuncture and Oriental medicine colleges require a minimum of two years in undergraduate school before admission into their three-year program. An acupuncturist's education consists of studying Western medicine (anatomy and physiology, biology, pathophysiology, etc.) as well as Chinese medicine (Oriental medicine diagnosis, five-element diagnosis, acupuncture meridians, Chinese herbal medicines, Qigong energetics, etc.). Additionally, students receive supervised clinical instruction in needling techniques, using moxibustion, prescribing Chinese herbs, and so forth, in their college clinics and in preceptorship programs with licensed acupuncture practitioners.

After graduation, acupuncturists must pass national board exams (NCCAOM) to be licensed to practice Chinese medicine.

Licensing

Currently, acupuncturists are licensed in thirty-nine states.

- To locate a licensed acupuncturist or to find more information about acupuncture and Oriental medicine, contact:

American Association of Acupuncture and Oriental Medicine (AAAOM)
P.O. Box 162340, Sacramento, CA 95816
phone (866) 455-7999 or (916) 443-4770
www.aaaomonline.org
info@aaaomonline.org

NOTES

1. J. Robbins, *Reclaiming Our Health* (Tiburon, Calif.: H. J. Kramer, 1998), 3–4.
2. P. Bergner, "Nutrition Education in US Medical Schools," *The Naturopathic Physician,* Fall 1992, 26–27.
3. K. Cooksey et al., "Getting Nutrition Education into Medical Schools: A Computer-Based Approach," *American Journal of Clinical Nutrition* 72, no. 3 (September 2000): 868.

Appendix 2

SEVEN PATIENT EXAMPLES

A true diagnosis should not only define the symptoms of a particular disease or syndrome but also indicate the cause. Most medical diagnoses currently describe only the symptoms, which allopathic physicians usually try to suppress with prescription drugs. This typical protocol of "dead-end" diagnoses and the chronic use of toxic and suppressive prescription drugs leave little hope for cure. The following seven case studies highlight the differences between an allopathic diagnosis and a holistic diagnosis. Each case includes the treatment protocol that I prescribed for the patient.

This appendix includes four recent patient examples (2007–2010) as well as three cases from earlier years (2003–2006). Although the latter three examples do not include some of the newer herbal and nutritional supplements described in this book, they demonstrate that drainage, detoxification, homeopathy, auriculotherapy, and other natural healing modalities are effective therapies even when utilizing "older" products. Including cases from the past several years also allows the reader to see the progression of therapeutic protocols over the last decade.

1. THE "CRAMPING" OF SUPPRESSED EMOTIONS

Allopathic Diagnosis: Irritable bowel syndrome (IBS)
Holistic Diagnosis: IBS and achalasia (esophageal spasm) secondary to childhood abuse, mercury toxicity, and a scar interference field
Treatment: Constitutional homeopathy, drainage, mercury amalgam removal and detoxification, nutritional supplementation, and auriculotherapy

Symptoms

Barbara C.,* a thirty-six-year-old white female, initially presented on 2/12/03 with symptoms of a spastic throat and esophagus, which caused great difficulty in swallowing and pain. In fact, she had never been able to swallow pills and had to eat soft foods and chew very slowly to avoid getting the food caught in her throat and choking, which naturally caused her great anxiety. Barbara's throat pain and constriction were most prominent on the left. She was also prone to IBS—alternating diarrhea and constipation, with often a sense of incomplete evacuation of the stool (tenesmus). Hormonally, Barbara suffered from moderately severe menstrual cramps and premenstrual feelings of anxiety and grief that "felt like a wave" in the stomach area.

Additionally, Barbara's left second and third fingers were scarred and quite sensitive from a childhood injury, and she would experience sharp nerve pain if they were ever accidentally hit.

Significant History

1. A nervous stomach and frequent vomiting as a child, including the first day of school every year through high school.
2. Alternating loose stools and constipation intermittently; diagnosed with IBS at age twenty.
3. At age two, her left second and third fingers were almost completely cut off. She was taken to the emergency room, where they reattached the bone, nerves, and soft tissues.
4. Abuse—physically from her "rage-aholic" mother and angry brother, and sexually from her maternal grandfather.
5. Six mercury amalgam fillings.

*Patient names have been changed to protect privacy.

Significant Exam Findings

Barbara's tongue was pale with a fine white coat. Her reflexes were globally hyperactive (+++) and her ankle clonus test was moderate (++) bilaterally, suggestive of heavy metal toxicity.* She had visible scars on her left second and third fingers. Her ileocecal valve (right lower quadrant), splenic flexure (left upper quadrant), and sigmoid (left lower quadrant) abdominal regions were tender on palpation.

Energetic Testing

Barbara initially presented with "sympathicotonia"—a hypertonic (too strong) defensive muscle strength. Only the prescription of a constitutional homeopathic remedy would be able to get through this strongly defensive initial presentation, so no further energetic testing was attempted at this point and the patient's case was then taken.

Treatment

Initial Visit, 2/12/03

After a homeopathic interview, it was clear that the chronic spasmodic tendency in her body (throat, esophagus, stomach burps, intestinal tenesmus, and menstrual cramps), as well as her chronic underlying grief from an abusive childhood, strongly indicated the remedy Ignatia amara.† I prescribed for her a 200K potency one time only, a daily dose of a 12C potency once a week, and a booster dose of an LM1 potency once every two weeks.

Second Visit, 3/24/03

Barbara reported excitedly that she felt much better and that she was rarely choking now, although some stringy foods could still cause problems. Her bowel movements were more normal and her PMS emotional symptoms were reduced. She still experienced some menstrual cramps but was able to avoid taking ibuprofen.

Barbara presented clear on energetic testing, with even arms and legs and normal muscle tonus. Testing indicated that she should continue taking the same potencies of Ignatia, and also a multiple vitamin-mineral (Nutri-Fem from Thorne) as well as enzymes for a sensitive gut mucosa (Gastric Comfort, aka #601)—now that she could better swallow pills.

Third Visit, 4/15/03

Barbara reported that she had experienced a scary five-minute episode of severe pain in her splenic flexure region (where the large intestine turns in the left upper abdominal region), along with nausea, sweating, and cramping in her calves. She remembered that she had had this occur one time before.

Energetic testing of the mucosa of her entire large intestine produced a positive TL (therapy localization). The gemmotherapy remedy *Vaccinium vitis-idaea* was prescribed to drain and tonify the large intestine. Additionally, an anti-ulcer formula with bismuth and licorice root (Formula SF734) was prescribed to heal and soothe Barbara's inflamed intestinal mucosa.

She further tested as needing to take a higher potency of the Ignatia now, in the form of LM3 taken once a week.

Fourth Visit, 6/5/03

Barbara reported that her digestion was still improving but that recently she had experienced intermittent dizziness, nausea, and a sense of "hot, prickly heat shooting up from my stomach to my face."

On examination with energetic testing, Barbara's arm length test indicated oscillation secondary to mercury amalgam toxicity. I prescribed three additional supplements to help detoxify the suspected mercury poisoning (ProAlgen, Heavy Metal Support, and Thiocid) and referred her to a holistic dentist for appropriate removal. During the Five Dental Detox Days,* she was instructed to double the dose of these three supplements.

---

*Ankle clonus is a neurological test used by Dr. Dietrich Klinghardt to indicate upper motor neuron (brain) disturbance, often secondary to mercury toxicity from amalgam fillings.

†"The spasms of Ignatia" is a common saying among homeopaths, because this remedy can be so effective at treating spasms, cramping, tics, etc.

*The Five Dental Detox Days include the day of and the four days after the removal of toxic metals from the mouth. European studies have found that this period is the most critical time for significant detoxification measures because mercury levels greatly increase in the body, especially on the second and third days after amalgam removal.

Her home urinalysis test (without provocation) was a "milkish white-gray," indicating a light contamination of toxic metals.*

Fifth Visit, 11/6/03

Because of the financial constraints of being a grad student, Barbara had not yet been able to remove her amalgam fillings as of her fifth visit.

Sixth Visit, 4/7/04

Finally, in March and April of 2004, Barbara had her amalgam fillings removed. She returned on 4/7/04 reporting happily that her digestion improved markedly as each quadrant of mercury amalgam fillings was removed. However, she still felt intermittently a sense of pressure and discomfort in the upper left abdominal region.

She tested as needing to retake her Ignatia 200K potency one more time, and to continue taking her LM3 potency once a week to further assist mercury detoxification. She also tested for the need for intestinal probiotics (HMF Neogen)† and to continue her ProAlgen, Heavy Metal Support, and Thiocid for at least three more months. Her Nutri-Fem multiple vitamin and Gastric Comfort enzymes also tested positive.

Seventh Visit, 10/8/04

Barbara reported feeling very good and able to eat almost everything. However, two weeks prior she had experienced a sharp, stabbing pain in her left second and third fingers. She said that she had not felt this pain for eleven years.

On energetic testing, the scars on her left second and third fingers tested positive as scar interference fields, and they further tested as affecting her emotionally as well as chronically disturbing her small intestine through the blockage of an acupuncture point (the "disturbed field"). She was treated with auriculotherapy for the skin scars (a phase 3 ectodermal point), the emotional unbalancing effects (the Shen Men point), and the blocked small intestine meridian (the Small Intestine 15 point on the ear).

Her Ignatia potencies stayed the same, and she tested as needing to continue on the Nutri-Fem multiple and the #601 enzymes.

Eighth Visit, 10/29/04

Barbara reported that she had felt grief-stricken all week, and that she couldn't stop crying although no particular issue was arising. She was reassured that this type of spasmodic-like sobbing was a typical (and healthy) sign of the releasing of deep grief classically seen in patients who need Ignatia. Furthermore, this response was probably secondary to the emotionally freeing effects of the treatment of her left finger scar interference fields during the last visit. She did not need to be referred for psychological work because her Ph.D. was in that field and she was already processing with a psychospiritually oriented therapist. Barbara presented as clear energetically (even arms and legs, good energy field, and normal tonus in her muscles). Her nutritional supplement dosages remained the same, and I told her to re-dose her Ignatia only as needed for major stress (or to call me).

Ninth Visit, 9/8/05

Barbara reported some left foot pain that had improved with several massages as well a gum infection over her upper left canine tooth. She also reported some bloating and gas after eating. On this visit she presented in oscillation and tested energetically with chronic vaccinosis from a childhood mumps vaccine. She further tested positive for a dairy allergy (and admitted that she had begun drinking raw milk lately). I gave her a nosode to take two times (Mumps vaccine 30C) and told her to re-dose her Ignatia 200K a few hours after taking the nosode. I also prescribed coenzyme Q10 and two cell salts (Calc phos and Kali phos) to help heal her gum infection. Additionally, she tested for the need for bitters before meals (dandelion, yarrow, prickly ash, and goldenseal) as well as continuing Gastric Comfort to support digestion. I also instructed her on the elimination-challenge test for dairy products.

*Without provocation from drugs (DMPS or DMSA, e.g.)—which are themselves relatively toxic to the body—a positive laboratory test for toxic metals is hard to obtain. See chapter 3 for more discussion on those who don't excrete toxins well, and are therefore most prone to mercury intoxication and subsequent illness; these are the same patients who usually give false-negative lab results (i.e., the lab work looks good not because of low mercury levels but because of an inability to excrete mercury in the urine or feces, where it can be measured).

†HMF Neogen, classically for infants, was prescribed because at the time it was the only Seroyal product not containing the sugar FOS (fructooligosaccharide), which is too disturbing to a chronically dysbiotic gut. However, recently Seroyal has made available the product HMF Capsules, which is FOS sugar free.

Phone Check-in

In October, Barbara reported that her gum infection and left foot pain had cleared up. Furthermore, the added bitters as well as avoiding dairy greatly reduced her bloating and gas symptoms.*

Tenth Visit, 3/14/06

Barbara reported feeling "really good," with no problems swallowing and excellent digestion. She was quite active in her work and excited about her career goals since her completion of graduate school. She has only needed to re-dose her Ignatia remedy when she was under significant stress on two occasions, and she could occasionally eat dairy products (e.g., raw butter and goat/sheep cheese) without any ill effects. On examination she tested completely clear (strong muscles, even arms and legs, good energy field) and no longer needed the coenzyme Q10 and cell salts. She did test as needing to continue the Gastric Comfort enzymes and bitters as needed for digestion and was further prescribed the Basic PreNatal multivitamin/mineral since she and her husband had decided to begin trying to have their first child.

► Nutri-Fem, Formula SF734, and the Basic PreNatal multiple vitamin-mineral supplements are available from Thorne at (800) 228-1966. Heavy Metal Support, which contains essential minerals and antioxidants to help replace the minerals that mercury and other toxic metals have displaced in the body, and Thiocid, which contains alpha-lipoic acid, which has an antioxidant effect in both water- and fat-soluble tissues and thus is especially efficacious in detoxifying the (fatty) nerves in the central nervous system (brain and spinal cord), are also available from Thorne.

For Gastric Comfort, contact Enzymes, Inc., at (800) 637-7893. Gemmotherapy remedies are available from Seroyal at (800) 263-5861. ProAlgen is no longer available, but the same formulation, Alginate Plus, is available from Rx Vitamins at (800) 792-2222.

*These left-sided symptoms likely arose from her small intestine disturbed field (lingering from her left finger scar interference fields), which was acutely inflamed along with the liver (related to the canine tooth) from drinking too much raw milk—her primary allergenic food.

Discussion

This case exemplifies a saying used throughout this book: "What's false arises." Four months after Barbara began taking her correct constitutional remedy of Ignatia, the toxic mercury that had infiltrated her digestive mucosa as well as the rest of her body arose and tested positive energetically. After that, the next major block to healing came up over a year later—the scar interference field on her left fingers (mother side)* from a serious injury at age two.

Barbara had the will and courage to do a significant amount of psychospiritual healing in her adult years to heal her devastatingly abusive childhood. However, as a child no such avenue was available to her. Therefore, as children will do out of love for even the toughest parents, Barbara tried to keep silent and control her grief. But these suppressed feelings had to be expressed in some way and they seeped out in the classic cramping and spasmodic Ignatia-like manner in her throat and esophagus, her stomach and intestine, and her uterus. It is further interesting to note that despite her years of quality psychospiritual work, Barbara still experienced a strong spasmodic bodily emotional release from the Ignatia, as well as after her major left finger scar interference fields had been treated, demonstrating the profound and deeply emotionally healing effects of the combination of constitutional homeopathy and auriculotherapy.

Finally, Barbara's case is an example of the common mistake many health-minded individuals make in indulging in raw milk. Although this is the best and most mineral-rich milk we can drink, a significant percentage of the population is allergic to dairy—raw or pasteurized—and this is especially true when there is a history of severely compromised digestion.

2. THE MIRACLE OF ELIMINATING A MAJOR FOOD ALLERGY

Allopathic Diagnosis: Oral herpes, tension headaches, and bipolar disorder

Holistic Diagnosis: Oral herpes, tension headaches,

*It is interesting to note that Barbara broke her *left* wrist at age nine and then her *left* elbow at age fifteen. Furthermore, her throat was primarily constricted and painful on the *left*. This pattern indicates a major break from and sense of betrayal with her mother, who not only didn't protect her child but violently beat her.

and a bipolar tendency secondary to gluten intolerance, mercury toxicity, and a major malocclusion

Treatment: Avoiding gluten, amalgam removal, drainage, nutritional supplementation, and functional expansion appliances

Symptoms

Karel H., a thirty-one-year-old white male, initially presented in May 2004 with the following chief complaints:

1. Oral herpes since age three, with his whole mouth covered with "really bad" sores approximately six times per year. Both his parents and two siblings also get cold sores frequently.
2. Emotionally unstable, diagnosed as bipolar in his late twenties, often "funnels his emotions through anger and paranoia," and can "cycle really quickly" between mania and depression, but he generally "keeps it in check" and is not on medication.
3. Difficulty falling asleep and "shutting his 'Type A' brain off."
4. Tension headaches since his late twenties that occur about once a week.

Significant History

Karel grew up on a farm in Holland and was a very healthy child except for the intermittent outbreaks of oral herpes that ran in his family. He received his first mercury amalgam filling at age twelve, and later received three more. At age fourteen, his left upper second bicuspid tooth (#13) was extracted due to crowding before he had braces put on to straighten his (crowded) crooked teeth. At age twenty-six all four of his wisdom teeth were removed due to growing pressure and pain in the lower two, which were erupting sideways and pushing against the other teeth. Karel needs to eat a lot to maintain a stable blood sugar and mood but never seems to gain weight, which he attributes to his "Type A" metabolism. He works out four or five times a week and takes walks at least twice a week to help balance his tendency toward more manic moods. He also reported significant emotional problems growing up around his father, whom he also suspects of having bipolar tendencies.

Karel takes Acyclovir intermittently to help suppress his oral herpes outbreaks when they arise, which was originally prescribed four years ago when the herpes lesions started becoming so extensive that they went into his throat. He also takes aspirin and other NSAIDS weekly for his tension headaches.

Karel smoked cigarettes from age nineteen to age twenty-four.

Significant Exam Findings

Karel had the following positive exam findings linked with heavy metal toxicity:

1. Hyperactive deep tendon reflexes (+++)
2. Significant tremor in both hands with finger extension
3. Moderate ankle clonus test

Additionally, Karel had a right bicuspid crossbite (teeth #4 and #5 were abnormally positioned behind teeth #28 and #29 below).

Energetic Testing

Karel presented with the following positive findings:

1. Sympathicotonia (hypertonic muscles systemically) secondary to a gluten (wheat) allergy
2. Mercury amalgam toxicity

Treatment

Initial Visit, 2004

Karel was instructed on how to do the home elimination-challenge test to ascertain if the suspected gluten sensitivity was truly significant. I prescribed the following gemmotherapy drainage remedies: *Juniperus communis* (liver), *Juglans regia* (stomach, pancreas, and intestine) and *Lonicera nigra* (intestine). He also needed to supplement with Gastric Comfort (aka #601)* enzymes to aid digestion and ProAlgen to help bind and chelate out mercury.

Second Visit, 2005

Karel did not return for a follow-up visit for a year. However, on this visit he happily reported that all of his

*Karel was prescribed this enzyme formula without protease because I suspected that areas of his intestinal mucosa were probably eroded and inflamed after years of taking aspirin and other anti-inflammatory medications for his tension headaches.

symptoms had cleared up through avoiding gluten. He no longer had weekly tension headaches, he was not as hyper and had no paranoid symptoms, and he fell asleep relatively easily now and slept deeply through the night. He further stated that he had much better bowel movements now and no stomachaches—he had forgotten to mention during the initial visit that he had occasional stomachaches and diarrhea.

Karel additionally said that his oral herpes outbreaks had reduced from approximately six a year to about two a year, and that now the blisters were "much smaller and not as rampant." During the past year, Karel also had his four mercury amalgams removed by a holistic dentist, against the advice of his allopathic dentist.

However, Karel reported that he had a new set of symptoms occurring for approximately one month: mild to moderate right shoulder pain, intermittent numbness in his right lower back, his right leg sometimes falling asleep, and dry eyes—worse on the right. Additionally, he had begun to notice that some of his right-sided teeth would catch on his lip from time to time and cut his gums slightly.

On energetic testing, Karel presented in oscillation (neurological disorganization), with right-sided muscle weakness. This weakness correlated to his right-sided dental crossbite, or malocclusion, as evidenced by a positive tongue depressor test—that is, placing tongue depressors between the teeth strengthened all the previously weak right-sided muscles and stopped the oscillation pattern. I referred Karel to an orthopedic dentist to assess the need for functional appliances to treat his malocclusion.

Third Visit, 2006

Karel returned in the spring of 2006 wearing upper and lower Crozat (wire expansion) appliances. He reported that all of his previous right-sided symptoms had cleared up. This was confirmed on examination, where he exhibited no oscillation, he had even arm and leg measurements, and his muscles bilaterally tested strong. He also reported that as long as he avoided gluten he felt fine. Karel further stated that he had had no oral herpes outbreaks for one year.

During this visit, Karel tested for the need for HMF capsules to help restore normal flora in his intestines. He no longer needed to supplement with Gastric Comfort or ProAlgen. Since he had no current symptoms and felt "really good," he was not rescheduled for another visit but told to return if any future symptoms arose.

Phone Check-in

In October 2006, Karel reported by phone that he was still feeling very good and emotionally stable, and that he had had no oral herpes outbreaks the entire year. He and his dentist both reported that his teeth were also stabilizing into a more balanced occlusion through the use of the Crozat appliances.

► Gemmotherapy remedies are available from Seroyal at (800) 263-5861 and Gastric Comfort is available from Enzymes, Inc., at (800) 637-7893. Although ProAlgen is no longer available, the same formulation, Alginate Plus, is available from Rx Vitamins at (800) 792-2222.

Discussion

This case is an excellent example of the unwinding process that occurs in energetic testing. Although Karel displayed a significant dental malocclusion (crossbite) on the initial examination, this issue did not test positive until the two more critical issues in his body were addressed—a major gluten sensitivity and mercury amalgam toxicity. However, when these two initial issues were cleared, the malocclusion then presented with a vengeance—with the patient experiencing significant symptoms acutely for one month and the entire system displaying positive signs (right-sided weak muscles and oscillation) on energetic testing.*

Karel's case further exemplifies the significant effects a gluten allergy can have in the body, and the dramatic relief of emotional as well as physical symptoms that can occur when a patient eliminates allergenic foods from his diet. The removal of the amalgam fillings certainly also had an impact, probably most significantly in the further reduction of his serious oral herpes outbreaks.

---

*In fact, I was so worried about the trauma to his teeth from these dramatically positive tests that I urged him several times by phone to see a holistic orthopedic dentist *soon*. I explained to him that if his malocclusion wasn't treated in a reasonable time, he might be dealing with a dental focal infection in the near future and the possible loss of one or more of his teeth involved in his (recently arising) traumatic crossbite pattern.

3. WORKING LIKE A DOG

Allopathic Diagnosis: None; patient had not consulted an allopath

Holistic Diagnosis: Moderate fatigue, constipation, migraine headaches, sinusitis, and hay fever secondary to a primary dairy allergy, mercury toxicity, and constitutional feelings of deficiency

Treatment: Nutritional supplementation, cell salts, isopathy, and constitutional homeopathy

Symptoms

Dorothy P., a thirty-seven-year-old white female, presented on 12/29/05 with the following chief complaints:

1. Intermittent exhaustion since age nineteen after mononucleosis
2. Migraine headaches approximately two times a week
3. Constipation approximately two times a week
4. Seasonal hay fever (can be really bad in summer)
5. Chronic sinusitis and drainage in the mornings
6. Intermittent anxiety

Significant History

Dorothy received many doses of antibiotics as a child for chronic tonsillitis, as well as at age nineteen when she had high fever (104°F) and mononucleosis. She was born through C-section and was not breast-fed, and her mother had had nine miscarriages prior to her birth. In high school, she was treated several times for hyperventilation secondary to anxiety. Furthermore, she said she was traumatized as a child from a significant amount of corporal punishment (slapped and spanked) by both of her parents, as well as from a move to a new town away from her extended family at age seven.

Dorothy has five amalgam fillings. From ages fifteen to seventeen she had braces and then a retainer. At age twenty, she had all four of her wisdom teeth pulled under general anesthesia.

Significant Exam Findings

1. Hypertrophied (enlarged) left tonsil
2. Bilateral moderate hand tremors on extension*
3. Moderate ankle clonus test

*This indicates possible mercury toxicity.

Energetic Testing

Dorothy presented in level one oscillation (mild neurological disorganization) secondary to a major dairy allergy. She tested for the need for digestive enzymes, but since she was already taking a product from the health food store, I told her she could continue on this enzyme formula until the bottle was empty. Dorothy also tested positive for the need for the (nonconstipating) cell salt Ferrum phosphoricum 6X to treat iron deficiency and related fatigue, as well as ProAlgen and Pure Radiance C to help mitigate the mercury toxicity from her amalgam fillings.

Treatment

Initial Visit, 12/29/05

In addition to the energetic testing and prescriptions described above, I instructed Dorothy on the home elimination-challenge test for dairy (milk) products during her initial visit.

Second Visit, 5/16/06

Dorothy enthusiastically reported that all her digestive issues were virtually gone. She no longer had constipation or migraine headaches. She had even lost eight pounds and felt "way better" emotionally. Although she had had a lot of drainage initially from her sinuses, she reported that they had now cleared up considerably. Dorothy was also happy that she could eat small amounts of dairy with no ill effects.

During this visit, she was energetically tested for the most inert dental composite materials to use when replacing her five amalgam fillings. These materials were recorded and sent to the holistic dentist she had chosen. She additionally tested for the need for Calcarea phosphoricum 6X to take after amalgam removal, to help remineralize the teeth and surrounding bone and gum tissues after drilling. Finally, I instructed her on the Five Dental Detox Days Protocol.

Phone Call

In June, Dorothy called and said that she was concerned about having continuing pain in her left ear one week after the removal of the last (left-sided) fillings. I told her that this could indicate some nerve damage in one or more of the teeth that were recently filled, and that she should come pick up the laser and some Notatum 4X drops that day to treat the teeth and the ear.*

Third Visit, 6/18/06

Dorothy happily reported that she didn't even bother using the laser because the Notatum drops took the pain away almost immediately.

During a two-hour homeopathic interview on this visit, Dorothy stated that her chief complaint was a sense of an overall compromised immune system. She said she was tired of being "so sensitive" and never being able to fight off infections well. She further said that she felt "low, tired, and lethargic" most of the time. Going deeper into these issues, Dorothy revealed that her core belief was that "you weren't acceptable unless you worked like a dog." She added that often at work she felt "blamed, criticized, manipulated, and overcontrolled." She further disclosed that at work she felt like she was often treated like "a small child, scolded, and at the bottom of the pile—like the dog who is the least liked and needs the most control."

Based on these and other thoughts and sensations, utilizing the Sankaran system, I prescribed the remedy Lac caninum 200C and LM2. She additionally tested as needing to continue her ProAlgen and Pure Radiance C, and to continue her Calcarea phosphoricum 6X cell salts for just two more weeks. Dorothy also tested as needing to begin HMF capsules in about ten days, to help replenish her healthy intestinal flora.

Phone Call

In August, Dorothy reported that she had been feeling much better on the remedy until just the past week. She said that she had experienced a real shift in her behavioral patterns and that she could "actually fully express myself now." She further stated that she was able to stand up to bullying coworkers and that although she was still working hard, it was at a much more relaxed and steady pace where she was actually even more productive and effective.

She said, however, that after an acupuncture session, her constipation had returned along with significant abdominal cramping that radiated down to her perineum. She further stated that she had also begun to experience some of the old stress she had felt at work before she had taken the remedy. I explained to Dorothy that sometimes acupuncture needles can interrupt the action of the homeopathic remedy and told her to re-dose her Lac caninum 200C one time a day for the next two days.

By phone a week later, she reported that all her symptoms had cleared up after re-dosing the remedy.

Fourth Visit, 9/16/06

Dorothy again reported that although she had been feeling exceptionally better on the remedy, she had had significant abdominal pain, gas, and general malaise for the past week. When queried about her general state, she said that at work she was expressing herself more and receiving validation from her boss and coworkers. Additionally, she said that she no longer experienced the other sensations of feeling "brainwashed, trapped at work" or "like an outcast dog that gets kicked."

On examination, Dorothy presented in distortion (short right leg and short left arm) with the stomach area isolated as the chief disturbed tissue. Energetic testing revealed that her digestive enzyme product with hydrochloric acid and proteolytic enzymes was too strong and probably further eroding her already-damaged stomach and intestinal mucosa. I told her to stop taking this product and prescribed the gentle digestive formula Gastric Comfort (aka #601). During this visit, she further tested for the need for a multiple vitamin-mineral formula for women under forty (Nutri-Fem). Additionally, Dorothy tested as no longer needing to take her ProAlgen because her mercury levels were no longer detectable. Finally, since she said she had to dose the 200C potency more frequently during stressful weeks at work, I prescribed the higher potency of Lac caninum 1M.

Phone Call

In October, Dorothy said that she had had no stomach discomfort since switching to the hydrochloric-acid-free, protease-free Gastric Comfort formula. Furthermore, she reported that she continued to "stand her ground" more now and that she saw "the power, honesty, and attractiveness of self-expression." I told her to continue the same protocol.

*I was out of town; otherwise, I would have had her come in for an appointment.

Fifth Visit, 11/18/06

Dorothy reported continued progress. She said she was happy and enjoying her work and felt more in control and valued. When asked about the sensations of being "small, low," and "at the bottom of the pile," she said she rarely felt that way anymore and could hardly remember that state clearly now. She further stated that she was amazed at the power of the remedy, and now she really believed in homeopathy.

Dorothy tested clear energetically (even arms and legs, good energy field) and had no "files" (issues) testing positive. At this point, she tested as needing to continue her Nutri-Fem, Pure Radiance C, and Gastric Comfort. However, I told her to re-dose her Lac caninum 1M only as needed, when she felt the old feelings arise under significant stress. I rescheduled her for a check-up four months later.

▶ ProAlgen is no longer available, but the same formulation, Alginate Plus, is available from Rx Vitamins at (800) 792-2222. Ferrum phos 6X and Calc phos 6X are both available from most health food stores or from Seroyal at (800) 263-5861. HMF Capsules are also available from Seroyal. Pure Radiance C is available from the Synergy Company at (800) 723-0277. For Notatum 4X drops, contact BioResource at (800) 203-3775. Gastric Comfort, or #601, is available from Enzymes, Inc., at (800) 637-7893. Nutri-Fem, as well as Meta-Fem for women over forty, have tested well for years and are available from Thorne at (800) 228-1966.

Discussion

This case presented a number of excellent examples:

1. Once again, simply the avoidance of a major food allergen such as dairy yielded significant results in ameliorating chronic symptoms. Furthermore, this patient's chronic allergy symptoms were completely understandable and consistent with her history of not being breast-fed and having a mother with significantly weakened kidney and spleen chi energy (so many miscarriages).
2. The effects of Notatum 4X in clearing ear pain referred from teeth with new fillings demonstrated the remarkable ability of these isopathic drops to treat acute nerve injury. Although intermittent ear pain is a common symptom after cavitation surgery (and quite disturbing if it lingers), it is not common after the placement of fillings, and that is why I urged this patient to treat her teeth and ear with the Notatum drops and laser as soon as possible.
3. This was also a good example of when the patient is so identified with the state of the remedy that she actually names the remedy source during the interview. Lac caninum is a remedy made from dog's milk, and patients who need it typically experience the sensations of feeling "low, small, and controlled like a dog."
4. In my experience, it is quite common that patients (who almost all universally present) with significant intestinal dysbiosis do not typically test for the need to supplement with acidophilus and bifidus until the major causes for their toxic gut are removed—in this case, the allergenic dairy products and mercury amalgam fillings. It is hard to plant seeds and grow good flora in poor soil (a dysbiotic intestinal terrain).
5. This case demonstrated that sometimes acupuncture needles can antidote the action of a constitutional remedy. This is especially true when the patient has only been on the homeopathic remedy for a few months.*
6. Finally, this case was an excellent example of the hazards of taking a regular digestive formula when one has a history of gastritis, ulcers, or just intermittent but significant abdominal pain. Because Dorothy didn't report this symptom initially, I simply suggested that, to save money, she could continue on her own enzyme formula for a while. However, when the problem with this formula was revealed, the Gastric Comfort (#601) formula tested as ideal for her since it has enough enzymes to support digestion (amylase, lactase, lipase, sucrase, papaya, etc.), but no protease and hydrochloric acid, which can be quite inflaming to an already compromised and inflamed stomach and intestinal mucosal lining.†

---

*If patients are seeing an acupuncturist, they should be instructed to call, or simply re-dose the remedy, if they feel "off" after an acupuncture treatment.

†The use of bismuth, licorice root, and natural antibiotic herbs (Oregon grape root), such as in Thorne's product Formula SF734, is also helpful to supplement if the abdominal pain is significant, as it was in Barbara's case.

4. TREATING LYME DISEASE WITH THE SANKARAN SYSTEM

Allopathic Diagnosis: Lyme disease with neuropathy, arrhythmia, and hypertension
Holistic Diagnosis: Lyme disease with neuropathy, arrhythmia, and hypertension secondary to the patient's constitutional homeopathic pattern
Treatment: Constitutional homeopathy according to the Sankaran system, scar interference field protocol, plant stem cell remedies, MSM sulfur, and Quinton marine plasma

Symptoms

Marilyn M., a forty-one-year-old white female, initially presented on 10/7/09. She had tested positive for Lyme (IGeneX) at age thirty-seven and was being treated by several holistic M.D.s for the following symptoms:

1. Right-sided neuropathy (hand, arm, neck, hip, and leg) characterized by tingling, numbness, and a heavy sensation
2. Hypertension with heart arrhythmia (intermittent premature ventricular contractions, or PVCs, and premature atrial contractions, or PACs) diagnosed by EKG

Significant History

At age thirty-seven various antibiotics such as Doxycycline were prescribed orally for Marilyn's neuropathy symptoms, but the side effect of sun sensitivity was so extreme that she had to go off the medication. Injections of Bacillin were then prescribed. These were taken once a week from age thirty-eight until a few months ago, when the injections were reduced to every two weeks. Without this antibiotic injection Marilyn's neuropathy symptoms would worsen considerably.

The blood pressure medication Diovan had also been prescribed since age thirty-seven at a dosage of 8 mg daily.

At age thirty-five Marilyn had a right breast lump "blow up like a third breast" and was subsequently diagnosed as infected with *Staphylococcus* bacteria; a lumpectomy was performed.

Marilyn reported that her holistic M.D.s had prescribed numerous nutritional supplements including a multiple vitamin-mineral, probiotics, fish oil, potassium magnesium aspartate, 5 HTP, a mushroom formula, vitamin D, and half an aspirin.

Significant Exam Findings

Because this patient had already covered so many bases with other doctors—that is, she had a "clean" mouth (amalgam fillings removed at age thirty-two) and no significant dental foci (one root canal on #18 had been redone with Endocal by a holistic dentist at age thirty-two; since this tooth was on the left side of the mouth it was most likely not contributing to the right-sided neuropathy, according to the ipsilateral rule)—and was on a lot of nutritional supplements, we decided to do only a brief initial exam and then begin with the homeopathic interview according to Sankaran right away.

During the initial exam, Marilyn's blood pressure tested at 136/90.

Energetic Testing

The brief MRT (Matrix Reflex Testing) exam revealed oscillation (a pattern indicating neurological disorganization and connective tissue stress in the body), a Lesser Yin display (the deepest and most adaptive of the six coupled meridians in the six-channel Chinese theory), and parasympathicotonia (all muscles tested weak).

Treatment

Initial Homeopathic Interview, 10/7/09

In the Sankaran system of homeopathy, the correct remedy is ascertained through the patient's chief complaint. Marilyn had three of these.

First, she complained of heart arrhythmia, describing it as "this big rush into my head and neck of pressure and fullness." Marilyn said that this "upward rush" was "like a whoosh feeling" and always came after the arrhythmia sensation of a premature beat in the heart that "felt like a butterfly in my throat." She said that this upward rushing movement would cause dizziness, shortness of breath, and a "foggy" head feeling—"like when you have taken a bike pump and blown up a tire—all this pressure." If a lot of these missed beats and then upward-rush sensations came in a row, she felt "very ungrounded" and anxious, and even had the fear that she could actually die.

Marilyn's second chief complaint was the right-sided

numbness, tingling, and heaviness she attributed to the Lyme disease. She described these symptoms as feeling "oddly fatigued and heavy" and sometimes "burny" in her right leg and right arm. She said that these symptoms were terrifying because her cousin had been diagnosed with MS and was now a complete invalid. The onset of these symptoms first began with her right little finger; she described a "robotically twitching" movement "like a metronome" three to four years before the right-sided symptoms began. When this neuralgia began it also had an upward movement pattern, like her heart symptoms. That is, she first felt heaviness in her right leg, and a week later it moved up into her right arm, accompanied by some tingling in her right face. Over time this right-sided numbness, tingling, heaviness, and burning occurred more and more frequently, with her right hip being particularly inflamed and painful, which caused her at times to be uncoordinated, to be "wobbly" on her feet, and to limp while walking.

Marilyn's third symptom was anxiety, with a tendency toward panic attacks. These attacks were especially severe in 1993 after a relationship ended; she would feel tingling in the back of her thighs and then a rush of electricity up to her heart, making it race. Everything felt "out of control" at that time and she was prescribed Xanax to reduce these anxiety symptoms.

There was a common experience among all of these symptoms—that of an upward rush or a rising sensation. This "whoosh" or "upward rush" experience was correlated to a homeopathic remedy with a similar sensation known as Aqua fida vetusta, sourced from the Yellowstone Geyser in Montana. As strange as it may sound, a geyser that has a rush of water spewing out of the ground and moving rapidly upward clearly matched Marilyn's symptoms of heart arrhythmia, elevated blood pressure, and tingling in her right arm and leg. In fact, this geyser remedy perhaps exemplifies the true nature of homeopathy as an incredible energy medicine that works at a quantum level of healing. On 10/14/09 Marilyn was prescribed Aqua fida vetusta 1M to be taken every two weeks over a six-week period, with a weekly "booster" dose of 30C.

Follow-up Appointment, Three Weeks Later

At a follow-up appointment three weeks later, Marilyn reported that her heart symptoms went away completely for most of the three weeks, and only came back mildly a few times toward the end. Additionally, the upward rush and what she described as "flooding"* feelings were a lot milder and not nearly as intense as they were before. She also reported that she felt more grounded and a lot less anxious—even in situations that would normally cause her to feel anxious. Marilyn said, however, that she was still experiencing her right-sided numbness and tingling under stress, although these symptoms were also better.

During this appointment a suspected right-sided scar interference field from her breast lumpectomy performed at age thirty-five tested positive. The scar was treated during this office visit by rubbing it with Notatum 4X drops, which were then photophoretically driven in deeper through a 100-milliwatt, 830-nanometer therapeutic infrared laser beam for thirty seconds. Marilyn rented this laser for the next week so that she could continue to rub the Notatum 4X into the breast scar along with thirty seconds of laser treatment, several times a day. She was additionally prescribed a low dose (2 drops each per day) of two plant stem cell herbal remedies: Olive, to help break down scar tissue, and Rosemary, which has been shown in several studies to treat staphylococcus bacteria.

Follow-up, 1/20/10

Marilyn again reported that her premature heartbeats were very infrequent, and that she rarely had sensations of an upward rushing feeling now. She also reported that her anxiety had been significantly reduced since taking the homeopathic remedy.

During this appointment a mild dairy allergy displayed, and Marilyn was given information on the elimination-challenge test. However, since this patient was a lacto-ovo vegetarian, it was suggested that she try to do more of a variety and rotation protocol since removing dairy from her diet would significantly reduce her protein intake. She was also given resource information on where to obtain raw dairy products through the Weston A. Price Foundation. Marilyn was additionally prescribed Quinton isotonic seawater to help remineralize her body and alkalinize acidic tissues. She was advised to continue on the Olive and Rosemary remedies five

*It is interesting to note that Marilyn described her "flooding" feelings despite being unaware of her remedy's connection to water.

days a week for another month. Her breast scar tested as neutral this visit, and her blood pressure was 124/86.

Follow-up, 3/26/10

Marilyn reported that she had been able to stop her Bacillin shots for three months now and was also off her blood pressure medication. She said she felt great, with no neuropathy, no arrhythmia, and much rarer episodes of anxiety—both milder and lasting for a much shorter duration than had been typical.

During this visit specific dairy products were tested individually for their degree of allergenicity. We then discussed the variety and rotation protocols of diversifying products as much as possible as well as trying to completely avoid the dairy foods that tested most positive.

Follow-up, 11/17/10

Marilyn missed a May appointment and then did not reschedule until November. She reported that she had a relapse during October and that her neurological symptoms returned. She injected herself with Bacillin a few times and had a terrible Herxheimer reaction from it for weeks. She later remembered to take her homeopathic remedy a couple of times and began to feel better.

After more inquiry it was revealed that both Marilyn and her daughter had severe sinus infections once in August and then again in September, and she had taken a ten-day round of antibiotics both times. Although not all drugs antidote the constitutional remedy, antibiotics are particularly notorious for this. Additionally, by injecting Bacillin again, Marilyn most probably antidoted the remedy's effects even more. This was explained to Marilyn and she was advised to call me if this ever happened again. Further, she was given the "emergency dose" instructions for taking a homeopathic remedy (a liquid dose that can be taken several times a day for a few days), which is the typical protocol patients (who are on their remedy) follow with the first signs of feeling sick.

During this period Marilyn also had an MRI and a cerebrospinal fluid analysis for MS, and she was re-tested for Lyme by IGeneX—all the results came back negative.

Follow-up, 1/24/11

Marilyn reported that she had been feeling great and "totally normal." She said that her neuropathy symptoms were clear and she was on no medications—just the nutritional supplements that her holistic M.D.s had earlier prescribed.

During this visit we took the time to test these supplements; none tested well except the fish oil (ProEPA). Additionally, Marilyn tested positive for the Fermented Cod Liver Oil as well as ghee—to be taken at the same time (based on Dr. Weston Price's recommendation). She further tested for high-quality probiotics (Original Formula), Pure Radiance C, and to continue the Quinton isotonic marine sea plasma vials for mineral supplementation. Finally Marilyn was put on a gentler (liquid dose) of her remedy Aqua fida vetusta 1M with a more steady dosage schedule (to be taken once every ten days for four months).

Marilyn also reported that she was on a wait list to start receiving raw milk products from a local dairy.

Discussion

This case is an excellent example of how constitutional homeopathy according to the Sankaran system can cure even serious Lyme symptoms. It also shows how essential it is for patients to contact their homeopath anytime symptoms return, as well as to be aware of the importance of re-dosing their remedy as soon as possible during times of significant stress. It further exemplifies the strong antidoting action of two rounds of antibiotics, and how that can cause a severe setback in patients on their constitutional homeopathic remedy. It is not clear why antibiotics can have such a strong antidoting effect, since other medications—for sleep, anxiety, hypertension, etc.—typically do not. But I have witnessed many times how a strong dose of antibiotics given for a ten-day period can antidote—that is, erase the effects of—a patient's homeopathic remedy.

5. TOURETTE'S (PANDAS) SECONDARY TO A TONSIL FOCUS AND MALOCCLUSION

Allopathic Diagnosis: Tourette's syndrome
Holistic Diagnosis: PANDAS (pediatric autoimmune neuropsychiatric disorders associated with streptococcus infections)
Treatment: Weston A. Price diet, avoiding dairy, treating the tonsil focus, clearing the malocclusion, and plant stem cell remedies

Symptoms

Robert N., an eleven-year-old boy, was brought in by his mother on 1/20/10 with symptoms of Tourette's consisting of various tics including intermittently furrowing his brow, head-jerking movements to the right, and kicking out his right foot when walking. These twitchlike movements had begun at age six and would typically increase under stress, but they could also occur during relatively stress-free quiet periods. Robert could somewhat disguise these embarrassing tics by making various volitional movements, but this had become a problem at school, where his teachers complained about his disruptive behavior during class.

Significant History

Robert had an unremarkable drug-free vaginal birth and was breast-fed for six months. He had three bouts of tonsillitis and four ear infections between the ages of two and six, with full courses of antibiotics given each time. He had also fallen and cut open his chin at age five, which required stitches. Robert demonstrated a sweet nature and was eager to please and cooperative during the appointment.

Significant Exam Findings

Robert's craniofacial tics were clearly apparent: brow furrowing every four to five seconds followed by a 15- to 20-degree quick head-jerking movement to the right. His tonsils were enlarged bilaterally but not touching. Robert also exhibited a Class II, type 1 dental malocclusion, or overbite. He had four dental fillings, but these were made up of composite material.

Energetic Testing

Using Matrix Reflex Testing (MRT), Robert presented with a right short leg and left short arm (Lesser Yin pattern in the six-channel system), and he was oscillating level 1 to the left (neurological disorganization). Kinesiologically, the supraspinatus muscle, generally associated with brain and nervous system functioning, tested weak bilaterally.

Treatment

Initial Visit, 1/20/10

Robert tested for a primary dairy allergy and a related tonsil focus, as well as a malocclusion (muscle weakening upon clenching teeth). His mother was given instructions on avoiding dairy and the elimination-challenge home test. Additionally, it was explained to her that although it was good that the family shopped at Whole Foods and tried to eat organically, she should also incorporate the principles of the Weston A. Price diet (bone broths, fermented vegetables, soaking the phytotoxins out of nuts, and so forth). Robert's tonsil focus was treated with Notatum 4X drops rubbed on externally bilaterally with an infrared laser (100 mw) applied to both sites for twenty seconds each. Robert's mother was instructed to continue rubbing a couple of drops on his external throat area overlying the tonsils every night before bed for the next month. We also discussed the fact that Robert's tics were more likely due to PANDAS (pediatric autoimmune neuropsychiatric disorders associated with streptococcus infections) from his history of tonsillitis and ear infections.

Robert was also prescribed 3 drops of the Linden Tree (double strength) plant stem cell remedy daily, an anti-anxiety and anti-spasmodic herbal to help reduce his tics. He was also referred to a holistic dentist specializing in treating malocclusions.

Second Visit, 4/7/10

Robert and his mother returned a few months later reporting that his tics were much improved. Robert's brow and head movements had significantly reduced after a week and remained that way until recently. Robert's mother reported that his tics had returned for the past few weeks, although they weren't as strong or as frequent as before. She further reported that she had embraced the Weston A. Price principles wholeheartedly and her whole family was enjoying this healthier diet. She also explained that they decided not to even challenge dairy since Robert's frequent clearing of his throat—a symptom they didn't initially mention—completely cleared up when he avoided dairy products. They had completed the course of rubbing the Notatum 4X drops over the tonsil sites and were still using the Linden Tree, which seemed to make a significant difference in reducing Robert's tics. For financial reasons they had not yet consulted the holistic dentist.

Although Robert's tics appeared to be reduced in intensity and frequency, they were apparent when he lay still on the exam table. Using the MRT diagnostic method, Robert presented with even legs and arms and no oscillation, and his previous weak supraspinatus muscle now tested strong bilaterally. His tonsils had reduced in size bilaterally and were almost normal for his age. However, he still tested weak to the kinesiological challenge of clenching his teeth together, indicating a primary dental malocclusion. Therefore, his mother was again urged to consult with a holistic dentist for treatment of this significant overbite that was affecting Robert's neurological functioning. Additionally, Robert was prescribed Fermented Skate Liver Oil, at a dose of 2 capsules a day, for its higher DHA content than cod liver in supporting brain functioning, as well as for the fat-soluble vitamins A and D in this supplement.

Third Visit, 6/3/10

Robert presented on 6/3/10 wearing upper and lower expansion appliances that had been made for him by his holistic orthopedic dentist in early May. His mother reported that within days of wearing the appliance his tics had virtually disappeared. Robert also noted that if he took his appliances out, after an hour or two he would begin to feel the "energy" of the tic movements again, but that this would disappear after he placed them back in his mouth.

Upon examination, Robert again presented with even arms and legs and no oscillation. His appliances tested well and no treatment was needed this visit. He and his mother were told to continue the Fermented Skate Liver Oil capsules at 2 a day taken with meals, but to see if they could begin reducing the Linden Tree drops to 1 to 2 drops, taken only during the school week. Robert tested for a probiotic during this visit and was prescribed Original Formula at a dose of ½ teaspoon daily. It was also suggested that he might be able to tolerate yogurt and kefir, eaten on a rotation basis at this point.

Fourth Visit, 10/13/10

Robert and his mother reported that he was doing great. His tics had cleared completely for months now and he was making better grades and no longer disrupting class. His mother said that he had become more confident and socially adept and just seemed happier. She further reported that he seemed fine (with no throat clearing) eating yogurt every few days, and even seemed to be able to eat raw goat or sheep cheese on a rotation basis. Robert no longer needed his Linden Tree remedy to reduce his tics and anxiety and hadn't taken regular doses for approximately six weeks.

My exam found that Robert's bite had expanded and his overbite was much reduced. His mother explained that the holistic dentist had told them that he would be wearing the appliances approximately six to eight more months and then would require braces to complete the finishing work of creating a harmonious bite. With MRT testing he again presented with even arms and legs, and no oscillation. His bite tested strong on challenge (strong indicator muscle remained strong when he clenched his teeth together, that is, bit down on his appliances).

Robert tested as needing to continue taking his Fermented Skate Liver Oil capsules at 1 daily and the Original Formula at ½ teaspoon five days a week. At this point his mother was told to bring him in as needed, but that he did not need to be rescheduled for a specific appointment.

Discussion

As discussed in chapter 12, this case clearly demonstrates that Tourette's is often caused by streptococcus infections typically from tonsillitis or otitis media (ear) infections in children. The obsessive-compulsive mental disorders and movement disorders such as tics from these childhood bacterial infections have been termed PANDAS (pediatric autoimmune neuropsychiatric disorders associated with streptococcus infections). Unfortunately, the conventional allopathic treatment for PANDAS is antibiotics, which actually implant the tonsil focus even deeper through their autoimmune effect on the system.

Robert's case also demonstrates the importance of treating both the tonsil focus and the dental malocclusion—two areas of dysfunction commonly seen in Tourette's, or PANDAS. By treating the tonsil focus, the chronic generation of streptococcus bacteria and its effect on the basal ganglia and other movement-regulating centers of the brain is reduced. By expanding the bite—and therefore the cranium—Robert's basal ganglia and other parts of his central nervous system were able to function and develop in a more balanced way. Parents should never neglect expansion of the bite through orthopedic appliances when it is needed for their children, especially since malocclusions have become so pandemic from inadequate nutrition during pregnancy, infancy, and early childhood.

Finally, this case exemplifies that sometimes even in a child, after significant dysbiotic damage from multiple rounds of antibiotics, it is often wise not to prescribe probiotics immediately, but to wait until the intestinal terrain is ready to receive and implant beneficial flora. This is often the case in adults, in whom, after decades of dysbiosis, probiotics actually make many patients feel worse—a key symptom of SIBO (small intestine bacterial overgrowth)—until the pathogenic microbes have been significantly reduced.

6. ALLERGIES AND ANXIETY CLEARED WITH AMALGAM REMOVAL AND CONSTITUTIONAL HOMEOPATHY

Allopathic Diagnosis: Patient does not see allopaths
Holistic Diagnosis: Atopic diathesis (allergy tendency) secondary to erethism (emotional dysfunction from mercury toxicity) and homeopathic constitution
Treatment: Mercury amalgam removal and detoxification, scar interference field protocol, constitutional homeopathy, nutritional supplementation, avoidance of primary dairy allergen, and isopathic remedies for a mild dental focus

Symptoms

Patty E., a forty-three-year-old female, presented on 7/14/07 with the following symptoms:

1. Chronic intermittent anxiety with a sense of breathlessness
2. Chronic sinus congestion
3. Rashes and itching

Significant History

When Patty came to me, she had been eating according to the Weston A. Price diet for the past five years, which had cleared the migraine headaches that she had suffered from for years. She was aware that she was mildly allergic to dairy, so she rotated the raw cheese and butter, kefir, and yogurt that she ate. However, this diet had not alleviated her rashes, sinus congestion and sneezing, and generalized anxiety symptoms. In her twenties, Patty had taken tetracycline for acne for almost a decade and noted that her rashes and itching began during this time. She had been on birth control pills for almost twenty years (until three years ago) but reported that eating a high-fat Weston A. Price diet had regulated her menstrual period over the last couple of years.

Patty said she had had lots of colds as a child and the flu almost every year. She had a tonsillectomy at age five and stitches from injuries in her left big toe at age three and her chin at age nine. She had six amalgam fillings placed as a child and all four wisdom teeth pulled at age twenty under general anesthesia. She said that the right lower socket (#32) was slow in healing and had never felt quite right.

Significant Exam Findings

Patty demonstrated a positive ankle clonus test bilaterally and hyperreactive deep tendon reflexes—both correlated with heavy metal toxicity. Her tonsil surgery sites had significant scarring on both sides. On Matrix Reflex Testing (MRT) she was oscillating level 1 (neurological disorganization), and her muscles tested in sympathicotonia (hypertonic).

Treatment

Initial Visit, 7/14/07

Patty tested positive for toxic metals, specifically mercury from her amalgam fillings. She was prescribed several nutritional products (Alginate Plus, Pure Synergy, etc.) to begin detoxification of these heavy metals. Since her blood tests were normal and her history and exam indicated that she was at a level of health where she could appropriately excrete, she was referred to a holistic dentist to have her amalgam fillings replaced. She was told to double the doses of her remedies during the Five Dental Detox Days after each quadrant was removed.

Second Visit, 4/9/08

Patty did not return until the following year, but on this visit she reported that she had had her amalgams removed in August of the previous year and that her sinus congestion was much improved, as was her skin, with only rare intermittent flare-ups. On this visit she presented in Greater Yang (left short leg and arm) and her liver was testing positive. She was prescribed herbal plant stem cell remedies (Black Poplar, Juniper, and Fig) to further the detoxification of heavy metals and to support her liver functioning. Additionally, her scars tested positive and she was prescribed Aspergillus 4X to treat them at home daily for three weeks.

Third Visit, 6/25/08

Patty reported that a mole over her liver had become red and swollen and then "blew up" and was now gone. She said it felt like the mole "was on fire" for a week and then it "blew up like a volcano" and then cleared. On examination this area of skin over the liver was indeed completely clear with no evidence of a previous mole there or any discoloration.

On this visit we did the constitutional homeopathic interview according to the Sankaran system, since Patty's anxiety—although improved after amalgam filling removal and implementing a nutrient-dense diet—was still present intermittently under stress. During the interview she described this anxiety as the "fear of not having enough air, that you don't breathe deep enough." She said that it felt like a heavy weight centered on her chest—"like an anchor of sadness"—and that this connected her to a sense of shame and not being valued or feeling good enough. When queried further she explained that when she experienced this shame she felt like she couldn't breathe and that she couldn't lift her head up, as if she were "collapsing inward." She further described that this felt like "contracting into yourself and a shutting down—the opposite of opening up and taking things in and being joyful." As the interview progressed, Patty continued to reiterate this same pattern—a distinct feeling of being hunched over and contracted and wanting to turn off feeling as opposed to the sense of "opening up, wide open, with the chest open and trusting in the world." During her childhood Patty said she would often "freeze in her tracks" and "suck in—you don't exist for a minute or so," during the times when she would "instantly get screamed at" by her father. She described these episodes as being scary and shocking, since they would often come out of nowhere and she would feel this "wrath of anger hitting you instantly." Patty said that for years she suffered from significant anxiety ("it was just part of my being—I didn't even realize I could be separate from it"), but now, after meeting her husband ten years ago, being on the Weston A. Price diet for five years, and detoxifying the mercury, she was better. However, she could still experience fear and anxiety several times a week, when "out of the blue" something would put her in that state of collapse and the "feeling of being squashed down" would come over her.

Upon analysis, according to the Sankaran system, Patty was expressing the sensation of the Cactaceae family (a feeling of being contracted, shrunk, heavy, and collapsed in contrast to the sense of expansion and being open) and the malarial miasm (the feeling of being intermittently attacked, with a sense of fear and anxiety alternating with feeling stuck, ashamed, and resigned to a restricted life), so she was prescribed the remedy Cactus grandiflorus 200C, to be taken every ten days for two months.

Fourth Visit, 9/9/08

Patty reported that since being on the homeopathic remedy she had been doing great. She had good energy and more motivation, was much more confident, and had no skin issues at all for the first time in her life—"the clearest skin since I was a kid!" She said that the Cactus remedy had given her a sense of buoyancy—like a "rubber balloon filled with air." However, on a recent business trip the feeling of being "kind of small" had come over her and she hadn't wanted to talk to anyone. She felt a lack of confidence, loneliness, and "brain fuzziness" on this trip, which was a problem since it was an important meeting where she needed to interact assertively with her colleagues. However, she stated that she hadn't had any episodes of completely "collapsing" since she had taken her remedy.

When further queried, Patty mentioned that on this trip she had been put in the Ion Mobility Spectrometer or IMS chamber at the airport during security screening. Realizing that the strong input from this machine (I myself had experienced the shocklike "whoosh" from this air being blown in at you before) had clearly antidoted her remedy, I had her re-dose her Cactus 200C in the office. After a few minutes she reported that she felt better—like the room had gotten "lighter and brighter" and that she felt more like herself.

During the MRT analysis it was determined that Patty should move to a stronger potency, Cactus grandiflorus 1M, taken two times over the next month, and then as needed thereafter.

Fifth Visit, 6/24/09

Again, Patty did not return for a year, but on this visit she reported that she had been doing "great with the Cactus!" She described that this feeling she had always had of "why bother, what's the point?"—a sense located in her solar plexus—was completely gone. She said that it felt like she could no longer collapse in this area even if she tried. Her skin was perfect and her sinus congestion was "almost nothing" (only occurring slightly when she traveled and ate poorly). She stated that she "got to a point this last fall and winter where I forgot I even needed the remedy." When asked about breathing she replied that her "lungs feel large now, more expansive—or I just don't even notice them because they are simply functioning normally when I exercise."

On MRT testing she tested with even arms and legs and a strong energetic field. She was again instructed to only re-dose the Cactus grandiflorus 1M as needed if she felt she had antidoted the remedy.

Sixth Visit, 3/11/10

Patty came in for one more check-up before moving out of state. She reported that she was still doing great and rarely needed to take her remedy. Sometimes she would have some sinus congestion in the morning and "hack up some stuff," but this was rare. Again she tested completely clear during the MRT exam. However, the need for High ORAC—an antioxidant and probiotic formula—did come up positive at a dosage of 2 capsules daily.

Phone Call, 12/7/10

Patty reported that lately she had experienced some joint pain, especially in her right elbow, which she overused quite a bit with her work. Since joint pain is so closely associated with a food allergy—especially to milk products—I inquired if she was still ingesting dairy on a rotation basis. She explained that since she was now living on a dairy ranch she was consuming raw milk on a daily basis. It was therefore suggested that she do the two-week elimination-challenge protocol with dairy products, as well as to do re-dose her Cactus grandiflorus 1M remedy in water (emergency dose protocol) for two to three days. Additionally, since she had never felt that her #32 wisdom tooth extraction site had fully healed and this potential dental focal infection (although negative on X-ray) could definitely cause ipsilateral (same-sided) joint pain, I wondered if that was affecting her now. She was therefore also sent Notatum 4X (anti-inflammatory) and Aspergillus 4X (soft-tissue healing) to drop on this extraction site, alternating with one in the morning and one in the evening, for approximately three weeks.

Phone Call, 1/7/11

Patty reported that after she gave up dairy and re-dosed her remedy her joint pain reduced greatly. She also felt that the isopathic drops (Notatum and Aspergillus) helped more fully heal her lower right socket and said that for the past month her right elbow had not bothered her. Patty was told to contact me if that right elbow pain (disturbed field) ever returned; in that case cavitation surgery with a biological dentist might be necessary. But since the X-ray of that site was negative (indicating possibly no significant bone lesion), I determined that this mild dental focus might heal on its own with the help of the isopathic drops, avoiding dairy, and taking her constitutional remedy. I advised Patty that as long as she felt well she could begin to eat fermented dairy products such as yogurt and kefir on a rotation basis again and possibly raw milk once a week if her joint and other symptoms did not reappear with this dietary protocol. Because of her almost ten years of tetracycline, High ORAC at 2 capsules a day was again prescribed. Patty was told to re-dose her Cactus remedy only as needed at this point (1M for major emotional/mental issues and 30C for more physical complaints) and to contact me in the future if any of her symptoms returned.

Discussion

First it is important to note how much the Weston A. Price diet had helped this patient before she even presented in my office. After a serious allopathic drug history—almost twenty years on birth control pills and ten years on tetracycline as well as a childhood history of antibiotics—it was very heartening to see how well she was doing during the initial visit. In many patients with a medication history that was this significantly damaging, I would not have immediately referred them for amalgam removal, but this nutrient-dense diet had allowed Patty a level of health where she was able to excrete these heavy metals adequately with support from additional supplementation.

Second, this case demonstrates the deep healing of the correct constitutional remedy. This patient's anxiety and fears, imprinted since childhood—although reduced from the Weston A. Price diet and the removal of mercury—could not be fully cleared without the homeopathic remedy. It also demonstrated a new antidoting agent to add to our list—the IMS chamber at airport security, where air is blown on you in order to detect if you have been in contact with illegal drugs, explosives, or chemical warfare agents. For many of us who are sensitive, this is a very strong—almost shocking—input, and can definitely antidote a constitutional remedy.

Third, this case demonstrates the seriousness of a primary food allergy and that, even with good detoxification and treatment, a major dairy allergy cannot be fully cleared (at least not in a patient with severe dysbiosis from excessive antibiotics). Although it will be interesting to see over the next few years if someday she can eat dairy products with impunity, for now she must continue to ingest them only on a rotation basis.

Finally, this case shows that a mild dental focus can emerge later in one's treatment, and that isopathic drops (in conjunction with homeopathy and avoiding primary allergens) can help heal this site (#32 extraction area) as well as its disturbed field (right elbow).

7. HEADACHES CLEARED WITH THE SANKARAN SYSTEM

Allopathic Diagnosis: Tension headaches
Holistic Diagnosis: Tension headaches secondary to a constitutional tendency
Treatment: Constitutional homeopathic remedy

Symptoms

Gail B., a forty-eight-year-old female, said she had headaches that often lasted three days or more and were aggravated by stress and weather changes. She said that they typically emanated from her right neck tension and then moved up to the top of her head. These headaches were so intense that she couldn't think straight and couldn't concentrate at all. She had had these headaches all her life.

Significant History

This patient was a European colleague who had attended my seminars in the 1990s, when I used to lecture in Europe twice a year. Her mercury amalgams were already removed and detoxified, she used only clean nontoxic personal care products, her foci had all been treated, she had greatly reduced her intake of her primary food allergen (wheat), and she had done a significant amount of psychological work. A previous MRI of her head and brain revealed no abnormalities.

Treatment

Initial Phone Appointment, 7/26/09

Gail's homeopathic appointment was done by phone since she lived in Europe. During the interview she described her headaches as being very painful, like a "boom, boom, boom" feeling in her head, almost like a sense that her head was "banging against a wooden door." She said her whole head felt pressed in, like there was not enough room for the brain. She also reported that her neck got very stiff and tense and she felt nerve pain like "lightning embedded in a continuous pressure feeling." Gail described a sense that her "head is too small and narrow—like being imprisoned" during these painful headache episodes. She said that she would feel like she was in a "dark black hole pulling me in a spiral form—like a sense of losing existence." She would feel "lost in this hole and get deeper and deeper in it" and "would feel this black nothingness, like a big black mouth—big animal—eating me." Gail further explained that it was a feeling that if she came too near the black hole that she "would be extinguished—that's the end of me."

Emotionally, she said she often felt that she was "not getting it right and not being good enough, and would be punished." However, nobody would notice when she felt this way. On the outside she would appear perfectly normal, but on the inside there was all this "inner chaos" and the feeling that there was something wrong with her but that she shouldn't show it. She also described that in this state she would feel very separate from other people, like a "little mini planet on its own totally—with no lights and no voices."

As a child Gail had a recurring dream that everywhere she walked and put her foot down on the earth it became a hole. There was no place she could put her foot without the earth breaking down and becoming a deep hole. During these dreams she would feel that she couldn't move because everywhere she went it was like she was "falling down into a hole and would be then gone forever." She said this childhood dream reminded her of her headaches, where "the feeling of the black hole is the same."

Gail was prescribed a newer remedy, Black Hole 1M, to be taken one time only, and then as needed if headaches arose.

Second Phone Appointment, 12/20/09

Gail reported that she had received the (intentionally unlabeled) remedy in the mail on a day when she had a headache and was "astonished that her headache dissolved almost immediately" after she took it. She noticed over time that she had fewer and fewer headaches and that when she felt one coming on, re-dosing her remedy would soon clear the pain.

She further reported that some sinus issues she hadn't mentioned in her last appointment were clearing. She said she had a two-day healing crisis with bad memories of her tonsillectomy combined with a sore rough throat, and then all of it resolved. Gail also said that her worried feelings about her son, which often made her heart feel "in pieces" and like she was "in a small dark hole away from the world and everything is black and I'm not connected to myself," were no longer there either. She still had some worried feelings but no longer felt "so completely gone" about it, like she had in the past. She said she felt more grounded and more secure, and that it is "fine to be alive and fine to be in a body now!"

Gail was told that she did not need to re-dose the remedy at this point, but that she could certainly re-dose it anytime she felt the symptoms of a headache returning.

Third Phone Appointment, 3/21/10

During this phone call Gail reported that she had had rare headaches and as soon as she took her remedy the pain would start diminishing. She felt more confident in herself and much more relaxed at home and at work, even during stressful times.

Since the remedy was clearly correct, she was told the name of it during this appointment, and it was explained to her why Black Hole fit her symptoms so well.

Fourth Phone Appointment, 9/19/10

Gail said that she had had no headaches for months now. Recently, when she had felt some pressure in her head, she simply relaxed for a few minutes and no headache occurred. She further reported that she was thrilled with the changes the remedy had made in her life—both physically and psychologically.

Discussion

Readers may wonder how this Black Hole remedy was made. I first learned about it in May 2008 from my teachers in India who specialize in the Sankaran system, Drs. Bhawisha and Shachindra Joshi. They explained that in response to an American patient of theirs whom they believed needed this remedy, they had asked an astronomer in Santa Fe, New Mexico, to make it for them. On December 3, 2007, this astronomer, along with a homeopath, taped a bottle of grain alcohol to the eyepiece of his telescope and then tracked the Cygnus XI binary star coordinates until its companion black hole transited the sky. The grain alcohol was left on the telescope aperture for eighty minutes in order to receive the information from this black hole. Since learning about this seemingly obscure remedy, I have been surprised to recognize its characteristics during several patient interviews and have successfully prescribed it five times since then.

Gail's symptoms perfectly fit this remedy. Although she never said "sucked in"—a common description of this homeopathic state—she described the feeling of falling into a hole during her painful headaches as well as in her childhood dream. Additionally, she experienced head pain and pressure—like that of being squeezed in the terrible pressure created by a black hole. She further expressed, like other patients who need this remedy, concomitant emotional symptoms of not feeling that she exists at times and having symptoms of low self-esteem and self-worth. The amazing thing about the correct constitutional remedy is that it works on every level—physically, mentally, emotionally, and even spiritually—to remove the particular distortion pattern a patient is suffering from. It then allows the human soul—less and less encumbered as this distortion pattern diminishes over time—to most fully develop. This was clearly seen in this exciting and satisfying case.

Appendix 3

ENERGETIC TESTING EXPLAINED

Any sufficiently advanced technology is indistinguishable from magic.
ARTHUR C. CLARKE, *PROFILES OF THE FUTURE*

Energetic testing is an umbrella term used to describe various techniques that interpret the body's various signals—muscle strength, arm and leg lengths, acupressure points, and energy fields—to arrive at a precise diagnosis and effective treatment. These methods have the benefit of directly testing a patient's body in present time, as opposed to attempting to interpret often days-, weeks-, or months-old radiographs and laboratory tests. In vivo* energetic testing can greatly augment these static tests, as well as the standard diagnostic office procedures (a thorough history and exam), thereby helping the doctor or practitioner arrive at a more specific and personalized treatment.

For example, through effective energetic testing measurements, it can be determined exactly which nutritional supplements a patient needs—in what particular form and which brand, how many per day, at what time of day (breakfast, lunch, dinner, or between meals), and for how long. In other cases, energetic testing can help in determining important dental referrals—when it is appropriate to remove mercury amalgam fillings, whether to replace a suspected toxic crown, and when to suggest the need for cavitation surgery.

ANCIENT SYSTEMS

India's Ayurvedic medicine (over 5,000 years old) and traditional Chinese medicine (over 2,000 years old) can be considered the first recorded systems of energetic testing. Through various methods of evaluating the patient's body—pulse and tongue diagnosis; reading the eyes, lips, face; and so forth—early Ayurvedic and Chinese doctors realized they could better determine the primary cause of the patient's symptoms. These assessments would then indicate the most appropriate treatments, such as a change of diet, herbal medicines, breathing exercises, essential oils, massage, acupuncture, and others. The Chinese, Indian Hindus, Egyptians, Persians, Medes, Etruscans, Greeks, and Romans also used the ancient science and art of dowsing to aid in their diagnosis of the ill.[1]* Furthermore, there have been countless other civilizations and indigenous tribes existing in various parts of the ancient world—including other parts of Asia and Europe, Africa, and South America—that had their own unique (but often not recorded or written) systems of divining treatments for disease.

*As opposed to *in vitro,* which means "within a glass or observable in a test tube," *in vivo* means "within the living body."

*Although dowsing is still not accepted as a science in the United States, it has considerably more respect in France, Germany, and other parts of the world. The practice of dowsing for water has been widely propagated, as well as being the most convincing form of energetic testing to skeptics. For example, in the early twentieth century, Henry Gross, probably the most celebrated American dowser, while sitting at his kitchen table in Maine, accurately pinpointed on a map of Bermuda (where no source of water had been yet found) the exact spots to drill to locate underground water (P. Tompkins and C. Bird, *The Secret Life of Plants* [New York: Avon Books, 1973], 310). For further information on the ancient art of dowsing, read Lloyd Youngblood's article, "Dowsing: Ancient Art," at www.neholistic.com/articles/0008.htm.

TWENTIETH CENTURY

However, as the centuries passed, the steady rise of industrialization and scientific materialism greatly contributed to the loss of these traditional forms of physical examination, as medicine became more and more tailored to a strictly pathological model. In fact, the majority of orthopedic, neurological, and physiological tests that students currently learn in (holistic and allopathic) medical schools are primarily indicators of serious disease *already present*—with few tests sensitive enough to reveal the more subtle signs indicative of future disease and dysfunction. Thus, not only does modern allopathic medicine fail individuals with the prescription of toxic medications, but it also often gives patients a false sense of security through a "clean bill of health" derived from a physical exam that is unable to detect anything other than present-time gross pathology. This trend is well illustrated by a warning—largely unheeded over the next century—from a physician in an article titled "The Sin of Treating Symptoms," published in a 1918 edition of the *Journal of the American Medical Association:*

> The clinician must not allow the laboratory or the specialist to make his diagnosis; if so, his days of usefulness are gone. These factors are only aids. One cannot always delay until the pathognomonic symptom appears. . . . We should, however, remember the plea to view the whole patient as a diagnostic problem.[2]

Fortunately, the second half of the twentieth century saw the birth of new and extremely innovative energetic testing methods, along with a revival in popularity and respect for systems of medicine from ancient cultures. With their precise and unique testing methods, these recently developed systems can greatly supplement the deficiencies found in modern orthodox physical examinations. Because they produce personalized diagnoses and more precise treatments, these newer methods can greatly help prevent the future onset of serious disease.

The renaissance of energetic testing systems that began evolving in the middle of the twentieth century continues to the present day. These systems primarily originated through the innovation of holistic medical doctors in Germany and France and chiropractic physicians in the United States.

Electroacupuncture

In 1955, the German physician Reinhold Voll originated electroacupuncture, a diagnostic method that combined the ancient principles of Chinese acupuncture with modern electronics.[3] Known as EAV (Electroacupuncture According to Voll), Voll's electroacupuncture method utilized what he termed a Dermatron instrument, consisting of four main components attached together in an electrical circuit: a diagnostic probe, an ohmmeter, an ampule container, and a cylindrical electrode. To operate, the patient holds the cylindrical electrode while the EAV practitioner tests his or her acupuncture points (beginning and end points on the distal fingers and toes) and observes the reading of the ohmmeter (or current detector).

For example, a patient suffering from acute abdominal pain and diarrhea might have his large intestine meridian point test positive with an increased conductivity reading on the ohmmeter (over 50 using a 1 to 100 range). The EAV practitioner can then place different diagnostic ampules in the ampule container (or honeycomb) to see which ones balance the ohmmeter (to a reading of 50). For example, if the patient recently returned from a trip with acute food poisoning, a homeopathic salmonella ampule may balance the ohmmeter. This patient's most appropriate treatment can then be ascertained through testing likely remedies in the ampule container, such as Arsenicum album 30C or Podyphyllum peltatum 30C.

A few years later, German physician Helmut Schimmel developed a similar instrument to Voll's Dermatron, which he called the Vega tester. In contrast to Voll's technique, Schimmel primarily utilized only one acupressure point on the foot or hand and measured this point over and over again while challenging different diagnostic and therapeutic ampules in the ampule container. Eventually, many other electroacupuncture instruments were generated throughout the world, including the United States, England, Hungary, and Russia.[4]

The primary benefit of these electronic instruments—similar to all quality energetic testing tools—is that they can often detect underlying pathophysiological processes that escape the standard diagnostic examination and laboratory tests.

However, electroacupuncture instruments have been criticized for two major reasons:

1. The ohmmeter or current detector can be influenced by the amount of pressure the examiner applies to the diagnostic probe (or point detector). Therefore, it is imperative that electroacupuncture practitioners become skilled at applying a consistent amount of pressure at all times on each point to arrive at the most objective and unbiased readings.
2. Electroacupuncture instruments induce low voltage into patients' acupressure points, as well as to the examiner, who is also part of the electrical circuit of energy, throughout testing. This causes two problems:

   Distortion in acupressure point readings. According to Dr. Van Benschoten, an Oriental medicine doctor in Southern California, *any* voltage introduced into the body over 180 millivolts causes neurological disturbance (nerves fire at around 60 millivolts) and disruption of the even-more-subtle acupuncture meridian energy flow of chi (qi).[5] For example, Voll's Dermatron instrument imparts 900 millivolts, and Schimmel's Vegatest imparts 1,500 millivolts into the patient's body. Therefore, although there is no danger of these voltages shocking the patient, Benschoten found that they were high enough to disrupt acupuncture meridian energy flow.

   Through this electrically induced distortion, Benschoten asserted, many of the locations of Voll's newly discovered acupuncture meridians, as well as the classic Chinese meridians for which Voll had discerned new locations, were actually in error. For example, without electrical interference, Benschoten found that the lung meridian corresponded to the same location where the ancient Chinese had determined it to be, and not on the other side of the thumb where Voll had later measured it. However, despite these voltage stresses and distortions, many electroacupuncture practitioners do good work. According to Benschoten's "working hypothesis," the reason is that examiners override the electromagnetic disturbance patterns of the instruments by "unconsciously varying the pressure" on the diagnostic probe to arrive at diagnostic conclusions consistent with their intuition and their years of clinical experience in treating patients.[6*]

   Electromagnetic stress induced in the patient and examiner. These low electrical currents cause mild to moderate stress in sensitive patients, as well as the examining doctor or practitioner—especially during lengthier visits. Dr. Schimmel recognized this problem, especially in the form of examiner fatigue, and tried to reduce this stress by placing magnets on the diagnostic probe or having the examiner wear a magnetic belt. However, over time these and other methods have proven limited in mitigating the electromagnetic stress to the nervous system, the subtle flow of acupuncture meridian chi, and the energy fields of the body. Thus far, no new electroacupuncture-type devices that conform to Benschoten's recommendations (180 millivolts of DC current or less) have been developed.

► For more information on electroacupuncture, go to www.vegatest.de for the VegaTest or www.biomeridian.com for Voll's Dermatron instrument.

Kinesiology

In 1964, a Michigan chiropractor named George Goodheart originated the technique of Applied Kinesiology (AK). This unique method of energetic testing uses the body's muscle tone as a feedback system to assess dysfunction in patients and to determine the most appropriate treatment. For example, in the presence of a major toxin, a previously strong muscle can test quite weak. The kinesiologist can then determine the needed treatment by challenging specific remedies to see which one causes the weakened muscle to strengthen (known as a "2-point"). Many readers may be vaguely familiar with

*Thus, what electroacupuncture practitioners are often criticized for—varying the pressure on the probe—is also the primary methodology intuitive practitioners often use unconsciously to arrive at diagnoses less affected by electromagnetic distortion.

muscle testing from observing someone demonstrating how refined sugar or other toxic foods adversely affect the body through the weakening of a previously strong muscle. Although these types of demonstrations can be dramatic and instructive, kinesiology is an art and a science best utilized by trained and experienced practitioners. For example, to become a diplomate in Applied Kinesiology a doctor must have practiced AK a minimum of three years, attended at least 300 hours of instruction given by a certified AK teacher, submitted two original papers, and passed both a written and a practical exam.

Goodheart and his colleagues introduced a host of original contributions in AK, including the diagnostic correlation of specific muscles to specific organs and tissues, the concept of a therapy localization (TL), and the phenomenon of a "2-point" (e.g., a weak muscle going to strength with a positive challenge). Other innovative treatments include numerous treatments for each muscle group, such as the use of neurovascular and neurolymphatic reflexes, acupuncture points, nutritional supplementation for the correlating organ, and related cranial and spinal adjustments. Due to the clinical success of these and other techniques experienced by more and more physicians, the International College of Applied Kinesiology (ICAK) was formed in 1973 to oversee the growing field of AK and to administer examinations for doctors wishing to become diplomates in the technique.

▶ For more information on becoming an AK diplomate, contact ICAK at (913) 384-5336 or e-mail ICAK@DCI-KansasCity.com.

Applied Kinesiology has been a collaborative effort since its inception. Through the innovative contributions of Walter Schmitt, D.C.; David Walther, D.C.; David Leaf, D.C.; Phillip Maffetone, D.C.; Michael Lebowitz, D.C.; Sheldon Deal, D.C.; John Bandy, D.C.; Robert Blaich, D.C.; and many more, the field of Applied Kinesiology has grown in sophistication and numbers. Through the efforts of these leading instructors—especially over the past two decades—AK doctors currently not only are taught the principles and skills involved in accurate muscle testing but also learn the neurological, physiological, immunological, and biochemical concepts and pathways underlying the particular dysfunction or disease they are diagnosing and treating.

The uniqueness and effectiveness of AK has inspired the development of other schools of kinesiology. In 1974, John Thie, D.C, an AK diplomate who was on the original AK board of directors, founded the Touch for Health Foundation (TFH), which has taught thousands of practitioners as well as the lay public all over the world the basic principles of muscle testing. Later, a psychiatrist, John Diamond, M.D., introduced another offshoot of AK—Behavioral Kinesiology (BK), which utilizes muscle testing principles to treat mental and emotional disturbances in patients. Another AK practitioner and clinical psychologist, Roger Callahan, Ph.D., has developed a system to address psychological issues called Thought Field Therapy (TFT). And in 1998, Scott Walker, D.C., another long-term AK physician, introduced Neuro Emotional Technique (NET), which has its own unique methodology and techniques to help assess and treat the emotional aspects of disease and dysfunction.

In 1978, another protégé of Goodheart, Alan Beardall, D.C., introduced his own form of advanced muscle testing called Clinical Kinesiology (CK). Through extensive clinical research on hundreds of patients, Beardall expanded Goodheart's original 54 muscle relationships to more than 250.[7] Additionally, Beardall introduced the use of specific finger positions known as hand modes to further augment the specificity of diagnosis in muscle testing. After Beardall's untimely death in a car accident in 1987, several of his students continued to teach as well as develop new concepts and hand modes in CK, including Gary Klepper, D.C.; Richard Holding, D.O.; Solihin Thom, D.O.; Rene Espy, D.C.; Nancy McBride, D.C.; Robert Shane; and myself.

In 1993, Dietrich Klinghardt, Ph.D., M.D., and I codeveloped Neural Kinesiology (NK), an offshoot of AK and CK that emphasizes the primacy of the autonomic nervous system in muscle responsiveness. Klinghardt and I used many European principles in NK, including blocked regulation (disturbed homeostasis) and the specific diagnosis and treatment through neural therapy (with and without needles) of dominant foci and toxic ganglia. Additionally, NK emphasizes the essential importance of appropriate detoxification of heavy metals and petroleum chemicals, as well as primary food allergies. Dr. Klinghardt continues to teach this style of muscle testing today through his Autonomic Response Testing (ART) method.

The primary criticism leveled at kinesiologists is that muscle testing can be too subjective. This is indeed a valid criticism because with muscle testing the practitioner's body *is* the primary unit of instrumentation. Although this obviates electromagnetic stress coming from a machine, it is imperative that the practitioner be as clear as possible. Skillful kinesiologists are aware of this situation and detoxify their heavy metals, use petroleum-free personal care and cleaning products, have their dominant foci treated, and so forth to allow them to conduct more authentic testing and therefore have less biased results. Furthermore, like all knowledgeable and experienced energetic testers, kinesiologists recognize that they must correlate their diagnostic findings with other information, including a thorough history, physical exam, and appropriate X-rays and laboratory tests.

▶ For more information on Applied Kinesiology, contact ICAK at (913) 384-5336 or go to www.icakusa.com. For information on Clinical Kinesiology, contact Dr. Christopher Beardall at (503) 982-6925 or beardall@hotmail.com, or Robert Shane at shanebob@msn.com. For information on Touch for Health seminars, call (310) 589-5269 or go to http://touch4health.com. For information on Dr. Klinghardt's ART seminars, go to www.klinghardtacademy.com.

Auriculomedicine

While electroacupuncture and kinesiology were being developed in Germany and the United States, Paul Nogier, M.D., was simultaneously researching his own form of energetic testing in France. After originating auriculotherapy in 1951, Dr. Nogier discovered in 1966

LAB TESTING AND BIOCHEMICAL INDIVIDUALITY

Because of each individual's unique biochemical makeup, laboratory tests should not be viewed as pillars of accuracy and objectivity. For example, through his innovative study of blood, urine, and other laboratory tests, world-renowned biochemist Roger Williams concluded that these supposedly objective tests are not free from error or misinterpretation. In Dr. Williams's landmark book, *Biochemical Individuality*—a must-read for all health practitioners—he cites the *wide* variations in individual biochemistry that can result in erroneous conclusions by doctors who are used to interpreting laboratory tests through the lens of "average ranges" laid down by orthodox medicine. For example, Dr. Williams cites "incontrovertible" and "substantial intra-individual variation" in glucose values, alkaline phosphatase, amino acids, and other factors in blood and urine tests in *healthy* individuals.[8] Additionally, he and his colleagues not only found "extremely variable" shapes, sizes, and locations of organs such as the thyroid gland (from 8 to 50 grams, some connected by an isthmus and others not, and some located at the base of the tongue), but also a "wide variation in thyroid activity" (from 2.5 to 11.5 micrograms of protein-bound iodine in the blood, and a tenfold variation in TSH) in *normal* individuals.[9] Williams further noted that when these average ranges were originally tabulated, a number of errors were made including the use of small samples (50, 20, 10, 5, or even fewer subjects tested), the throwing out of a substantial percentage of "abnormal" variations among healthy subjects, not repeating some tests, and failure to take into account diurnal, lunar, or seasonal variations.[10] In his book, originally published in 1956, Williams apologizes for the paucity of tests on this controversial subject. However, this lack of valid research on the variations of laboratory norms is *still* grossly inadequate, as dramatically evidenced today by the current popularity of the highly profitable statin drugs, based on the high cholesterol scare primarily propagated by pharmaceutical companies and their allopathic colleagues. In fact, in contrast to the ever-lowering bar pharmaceutical companies and medical doctors have assigned to "healthy" cholesterol levels (currently 170), a review of the scientific literature reveals that cholesterol levels ranging up to 400 and higher have been correlated *not* to atherosclerosis or cardiovascular disease but, in fact, with *increased* longevity.*

*For more information on cholesterol and statin drugs, see appendix 4, "How Scientific is Allopathic Medicine?" Furthermore, the two articles "The Benefits of High Cholesterol" and "The Dangers of Statin Drugs," in the Spring 2004 *Wise Traditions* journal, vol, 5, no. 1, have a wealth of well-documented information on this subject. Call (202) 333-HEAL or e-mail WestonAPrice@msn.com to obtain this issue.

that the radial pulse could be used to measure the state of health, or lack of it, through the body's electromagnetic field. He named this method Auriculomedicine, since he noticed changes in the radial (wrist) pulse or "vascular signal"—an intrinsic aspect of the technique—while stimulating the ear.[11]

> **Auriculomedicine/auriculotherapy:** *Auriculomedicine* is a diagnostic testing method, while *auriculotherapy* is a treatment method. Nogier underlined the fact that these two techniques are "totally different" and should not be confused with each other because of the similar-sounding names.[12]

In Auriculomedicine, the examiner challenges the patient's electromagnetic field (EMF) by waving a special three-phase filter (red, blue, and green Wratten color gels) beside the patient's ear, where the body's EMF is most apparent, while simultaneously monitoring the radial pulse (vascular autonomic signal, or VAS). A toxic challenge causes the EMF—which normally closely surrounds the body in an energetic protective manner (as measured by esoteric healers as well as through Kirlian photography)—to move out several feet. However, when an appropriate remedy is challenged, the EMF returns to a healthy and protective position in close proximity to the body's surface (less than approximately 3 to 4 millimeters away). During Dr. Nogier's life (1908–1996), as well as after his death, Auriculomedicine continued to be expanded and further refined. The most important contributors to this method include Raphaël Nogier, M.D., and Rene Bourdiol, M.D., in France; Frank Bahr, M.D., in Germany; and Mikhael Adams, N.D., in Canada.

▶ For more information on Auriculomedicine in North America, contact Dr. Adams at (905) 878-9994, Dr. Bryan Frank at www.auriculartherapy.com, Dr. Nader Soliman at www.alternativemedicineseminars.com, or the Auriculotherapy Certification Institute (ACI) at www.auriculotherapy.com. In Europe, contact Dr. Frank Bahr at www.akupunktur-arzt.de/dr.bahr or Dr. Beate Strittmatter at www.akupunktur-arzt.de/dr.strittmatter.

Arm and Leg Length Measurements

For over a century, chiropractic physicians have used leg measurement—for example, a patient presenting with a short right or left leg—as an indicator of the presence of spinal subluxations (misalignments). (Ninety-eight percent of the time the patient's leg length is not permanently short—except in the case of previous multiple leg fractures, surgical implants, congenital defects, and so forth—but simply temporarily appearing as short on one side as the result of a compensatory pelvic torque. This pelvic compensation is typically secondary to all the concepts described in this book—a chronic dominant focus, toxic metals and chemicals, dysbiosis, food allergy, and so forth.) Many specialized methods can assess this apparent signal of an osseous misalignment, most notably DNFT (Directional Non-Force Technique, originated and taught by Richard Van Rumpt, D.C.) and SOT (Sacro Occipital Technique, originated and taught by Major Bertrand DeJarnette, D.C.). In the 1970s, Dr. Alan Beardall included the arm length measurement—for example, diagnosing whether a patient was presenting with a short right or left arm—as another indicator of dysfunction in the body.

In the early 1990s, an Austrian osteopathic physician and renowned craniopath, Raphael van Assche, originated a variation of the arm length test he termed the arm length reflex (AR) test, also referred to as the reflex arm length (RAL) test. Dr. van Assche, a student of Beardall, was further inspired by the osteopathic research of Gordon Zink, D.O., who taught that the difference in muscle tone on the right and left sides of the body is regulated through the corpus callosum (the structure that separates the two hemispheres in the brain) and is compensated primarily by various fascial (soft tissue) patterns in the region of the chest. Through his clinical research, van Assche discovered that the AR test could measure this abnormal fascial disturbance initiated and regulated through the central nervous system (brain and spinal cord). Furthermore, by monitoring the change in arm length to various challenges—similar to a weak muscle going strong in kinesiology—the AR examiner can determine more accurate diagnoses as well as more specific treatments. The AR test has the benefit of being easier to learn and is slightly more sensitive than kinesiology testing. Furthermore, because no electrical apparatus is needed, it is electromagnetic-stress-free.

In 1998, I introduced the Arm Measurement–Field Measurement (AM-FM) technique, later renamed Matrix Reflex Testing (MRT), to better reflect that this method primarily assesses the state of the highly electromagnetically sensitive gel-like "matrix" tissue (also known as the "basic tissue" or "ground substance"). This method was originally inspired by van Assche's AR test and the assessment of the body's electromagnetic field (EMF) originated by Nogier. However, in the MRT method, the EMF is determined through a therapy localization of the ulnar bone, as a microrepresention of the body's energy field. The MRT technique also includes Dr. Beardall's hand modes for further specificity in diagnosis and emphasizes several sine qua non therapies described in *Radical Medicine,* including auriculotherapy and neural therapy in the treatment of chronic foci, their disturbed fields, and toxic ganglia; the appropriate removal and detoxification of amalgam fillings and petroleum chemicals; constitutional homeopathy according to the Sankaran system; and the use of drainage remedies.

The reflex arm length aspect of the test recognizes that there *is* a difference in a right versus a left short arm response, based on the six-channel adaptation patterns used in Chinese medicine. Dr. Alan Beardall originally correlated short arm and leg length to specific six-channel adaptation patterns. In the MRT method, these patterns demonstrate the patient's underlying adaptation—that is, why the pelvis (short leg) and shoulder girdle (short arm) compensated and misaligned (twist or torque). Over the years, extensive clinical research has shown that *any* dysfunction in the body—a congested liver, a tonsil focus, or a toxic celiac ganglion—can cause the structure to adapt, which then initiates a compensatory uneven arm and leg length pattern.

▶ For more information on the AR test, go to www.wso.at or contact Dr. van Assche at raphael.van.assche@wso.at. For more information on the MRT method, go to www.radicalmedicine.com, call (415) 460-1968, or e-mail info@radicalmedicine.com.

CONCLUSION

Energetic testing is just that—the testing of the energetic influence of a suspected diagnostic or therapeutic challenge, and the subsequent reading (positive or negative response) of the body's various signals (acupoints, muscle tone, pulse, electromagnetic field, and arm and leg lengths) to that challenge. Experienced practitioners are aware that no human endeavor is perfect. However, although energetic testing methods are not foolproof, they are an extremely valuable tool to help assess actual or potential disease and determine appropriate treatment protocols. Knowledgeable practitioners also incorporate in their decision-making process the data from laboratory tests and X-rays, the information from a thorough history and exam, and their years of clinical experience.

Because most of these methods just recently emerged during the mid-twentieth century, the renaissance period of the development of energetic testing is still in full bloom, and there is much work and additional research to do. Furthermore, although practitioners in different schools may argue about specific methodology and various techniques, they all agree about the primary principle underlying energetic testing: in vivo communication with the body's innate wisdom through the accurate interpretation of its signals can greatly augment diagnoses and help determine the most specific, appropriate, and effective treatments.

NOTES

1. P. Tompkins and C. Bird, *The Secret Life of Plants* (New York: Avon Books, 1973), 307.
2. H. Ward, "The Sin of Treating Symptoms," *Journal of the American Medical Association* 71 (July–December 1918): 9, 10.
3. P. Bellavite and A. Signorini, *The Emerging Science of Homeopathy* (Berkeley, Calif.: North Atlantic Books, 2002), 277.
4. H. Larsen, "New Technology Boosts Energy Medicine," www.yourhealthbase.com/energy_medicine.htm.
5. V. Benschoten, "A Critical Investigation of Electrodiagnostic Instrumentation Using Omera's Bidigital O-Ring Test," *American Journal of Acupuncture* 19, no. 3 (1991): 237–40.
6. Ibid., 239–40.
7. S. Levy and C. Lehr, *Your Body Can Talk* (Prescott, Ariz.: Hohm Press, 1996), 5.
8. R. Williams, *Biochemical Individuality* (Columbus, Ohio: McGraw-Hill, 1998), 57, 60–61, 78.
9. Ibid., 90–93.
10. Ibid., 61–64.
11. P. Nogier, *From Auriculotherapy to Auriculomedicine* (Sainte-Ruffine, France: Maisonneuve, 1983), 67.
12. Ibid.

Appendix 4

HOW SCIENTIFIC IS ALLOPATHIC MEDICINE?

I took so much medicine I was sick a long time after I got well.

CARL SANDBURG, *THE PEOPLE, YES*

Two primary falsehoods in medicine have been disseminated to the public:

1. Allopathic medicine is scientifically based.
2. Holistic medicine is not.

The following references can help dispel this massive prevarication propagated by the medical-pharmaceutical industrial complex and the media.

MORE THAN HALF OF ALL ALLOPATHIC TREATMENTS NEVER SCIENTIFICALLY VALIDATED

The general public has been led to believe that prescription drugs and surgical procedures—the primary therapeutic tools of allopathic medicine—undergo rigorous scientific testing. In the words of one respected doctor on the clinical faculty of Harvard Medical School, "Nothing could be further from the truth."[1] In a study published in the prestigious British medical journal *Lancet,* researchers discovered that more than 50 percent of all medical treatments (drugs and surgery)—and perhaps as much as 85 percent—have never been validated by scientific clinical trials.[2] In fact, an earlier study by the U.S. Congress found that "only 10 to 20 percent of all procedures currently used in a medical practice have been shown to be efficacious by controlled trial."[3] This surprising dearth of scientific protocol in conventional medicine was further evidenced by the National Institutes of Health (NIH) evaluation of more than 31,000 clinical trials conducted in the single discipline of gastroenterology. In this lengthy review it was found that *only 1 percent* of these gastrointestinal studies were properly randomized, and even more astounding, absolutely *none* satisfied the scientific requirements needed for objective research.[4]

PHARMACEUTICAL COMPANIES HAVE "NEARLY LIMITLESS" INFLUENCE

A recent book written by the former editor-in-chief of the *New England Journal of Medicine* and a current Harvard professor, Marcia Angell, M.D., reveals how drug companies routinely rig clinical trials to make their products look more effective than they actually are and have "nearly limitless influence over medical research, education, and how doctors do their jobs."[5] In the vastly profitable world of drug companies—and Dr. Angell points out that the pharmaceutical industry has been the *most profitable* of all businesses in the United States for over two decades—it is understandable how scientific objectivity is often overshadowed by bottom-line profits.[6] This lack of corporate integrity particularly flourishes in the capitalism-at-any-cost climate currently predominant in twenty-first-century America. However, in the world of health care, profit-driven allopathic medicine does not fall into the category of *minimal* harm from the shortcuts taken in other mass-produced consumer goods such as panty hose that run, poorly fitting shoes, or unreliable alarm clocks. Unfortunately, it falls into the arena of *maximum* consumer harm—that is, in the most serious category of all: that of causing morbidity (illness) and mortality (death).

THE HORMONE REPLACEMENT THERAPY DEBACLE

HRT Actually Increases the Risk for Heart Disease

The harm that can befall unwitting consumers of allopathic prescription drugs was exemplified by the spate of front-page headlines in 2002 that alerted millions of menopausal women to the significant danger incurred from taking hormone replacement therapy (HRT). In fact, a government study in July 2002 found that long-term use of estrogen and progesterone hormone replacement drugs not only does not help prevent heart disease but actually *increases* a healthy woman's risk of a heart attack (29 percent), stroke (41 percent), and breast cancer (26 percent).[7]

HRT Also Fails to Improve One's Sex Life

In 2003, a related federally sponsored study further found that contrary to popular belief, hormone replacement drugs also fail to improve the memory, sleep, and sex lives of older women.[8] As one *Newsweek* columnist commented, by deciding to "willy-nilly" prescribe hormones to every female menopausal patient, "doctors were doing just what was easiest," and by selling medication through "overstating its benefits and understating its risks, pharmaceutical companies were just doing what was most profitable."[9]

THE HYPE OVER CHOLESTEROL

But the hormone replacement therapy debacle is just one example of allopathic medicine's malfeasance through emphasizing quick fixes in the form of a pill over the more time-consuming process of searching for the underlying cause of each patient's unique symptoms and prescribing a personalized treatment protocol. (In one study, the time that patients spend face to face with their medical doctors averaged 1.7 minutes per visit.)[10]

The Serious Side Effects of Statin Drugs

In early 2004, Sally Fallon and Mary Enig, authors of the book *Nourishing Traditions,* presented scientific evidence to "demolish the hype" surrounding the use of popular statin drugs.[11] In a well-documented article about these cholesterol-lowering drugs purportedly prescribed to treat heart disease, Fallon and Enig referenced a host of significant side effects from ingesting statin drugs (Lipitor, Zocor, Crestor, Mevacor, Pravachol, etc.) sourced from prestigious medical journals such as the *Journal of the American Medical Association, New England Journal of Medicine,* and *Lancet.* These deleterious effects include muscle pain and weakness (rhabdomyolysis); pain and tingling in the extremities and difficulty walking (polyneuropathy); cognitive impairment including memory loss and slurred speech; depression and severe fatigue; pancreatitis; and cancer. In fact, in every single animal study (rodents) to date, statin drugs have caused cancer. Perhaps most mind-boggling of all, heart failure—one of the primary conditions statin drugs are prescribed to protect against—has been documented as one of the leading side effects of statin drugs, primarily through their action of blocking (along with cholesterol) the production of Co-Q10, which the heart muscle requires in high levels to function properly.[12] In fact, although statins were first approved for sale in 1987 and entered the market soon thereafter, deaths from heart failure more than doubled from 1989 to 1997.

The Benefits of High Cholesterol

In a related article, Uffe Ravnskov, M.D., Ph.D., a leading authority on lipids (fats) and their function in the body, further called into question the wisdom of prescribing statin drugs by citing the findings of numerous studies that chronic heart failure is actually *inversely* correlated with cholesterol, LDL-cholesterol, and triglyceride levels.

► For more information on Dr. Ravnskov's research findings, read his book *The Cholesterol Myths,* published by NewTrends Publishing in 2000.

That is, individuals with *high* lipid values (including the so-called bad LDL-cholesterol) actually live much longer than those with low levels, making high cholesterol a marker of longevity—and not mortality—in senior citizens. In fact, more than 200 articles and reviews of the scientific literature have pointed *not* to cholesterol as the underlying culprit of atherosclerosis and cardiovascular disease but to bacterial infections. Furthermore, these bacterial endotoxins—such as those produced from chronic dental and tonsil focal infections—have been *highly* correlated to death from heart failure. Based on the enormity of these numerous research findings—that high cholesterol is not the primary cause of heart disease and that infection is the most likely culprit—Dr. Ravnskov has made an astounding conclusion: the reason why high cholesterol levels are so strongly correlated with longevity is that they actually *protect* arterial walls from the damaging effects of microorganisms, and therefore also *protect* individuals from dying of heart disease—which most of us succumb to over the age of sixty.[13] Thus, the "problem" of high cholesterol is not a problem at all, and moreover, hypercholesterolemia can actually protect the body from future cardiovascular disease.*

> **hypercholesterolemia:** *Hypercholesterolemia* is the medical term for excess cholesterol levels in the blood. In the 1970s to early 1980s, the medical profession set this level at 240. In 1984, the level not to be exceeded was changed to 200. Recently this number has been further reduced to 170.[14]

ANTIBIOTICS FOR HEART DISEASE?

Based on their research correlating infection with atherosclerosis and heart failure, several studies have investigated the efficacy of treating cardiovascular disease with antibiotics. However, in four out of six trials—and one of these four trials included more than 7,000 patients—antibiotics consistently failed to prevent or successfully treat "cardiovascular events" or decrease the progression of atherosclerosis.[15] The reason is probably due to the high level of antibiotic resistance many individuals presently have resulting from excessive use of this drug previously, as well as the toxic effects of this medication.

*Conversely, low cholesterol is typically seen in very ill patients, such as those with cancer, AIDS, and chronic fatigue. In fact, cancer patients often succumb to death with a serum cholesterol between 100 and 150. Thus, as Dr. Tom Cowan states, "It is as though, in the wasting process, as all the fat is 'burned,' so too is the cholesterol." (T. Cowan, "Low Cholesterol," *Wise Traditions,* Spring 2005, 39.)

Harvard Physician Reveals Statistical "Insignificance" of Statin Drug

Despite overwhelming evidence linking statins with serious side effects, as well as the benefits of *not reducing* cholesterol levels, misleading studies purporting the effectiveness of these drugs continue to be published in prestigious medical journals. John Abramson, M.D., realized this fact when he took a closer look at an August 2000 study in which the statistics had been intentionally manipulated to make a statin drug, Pravachol, appear effective in reducing the risk of strokes among post–heart attack patients. After Dr. Abramson analyzed the data underlying this claim in more detail, he found that if 1,000 post–heart attack patients took Pravachol for one year, there would be only *one* less stroke occurring annually.[16]* This was indeed not a major finding at all, and certainly not statistically significant, as the authors of this study appearing in the *New England Journal of Medicine* (*NEJM*) had claimed. In fact, when one compares two other statistics—that simply eating fish once a week results in a 22 percent reduction in the chance of having a future stroke, and two hours of moderate exercise weekly results in a 60 percent reduction—it calls into question the wisdom as well as the integrity of the *NEJM* medical board that approved the publication of this misleading and deceptive article in the first place.[17] Even more alarming, Dr. Abramson, a family practitioner currently on the clinical faculty of Harvard Medical School, further realized after rectifying the data that for patients in this study who were older than seventy, Pravachol actually *increased* the rate of stroke by 21 percent.[18]

*Dr. Abramson determined the cost of the Pravachol drug that would be utilized by these sample 1,000 patients—a whopping $1.2 million. Furthermore, this figure does not include the cost of extra blood tests and physician visits that would be required to monitor the potentially dangerous side effects of this medication. (J. Abramson, *Overdosed America* [New York: HarperCollins Publishers Inc., 2004], 15.)

MODERN LONGEVITY EXPLAINED

In the minds of many readers, the question of longevity may come up here. That is, if these toxic drugs are so damaging, why are we living so much longer than our ancestors? The answer to this question is five-fold. First, many of our ancestors actually lived a lot longer than we do now. For example, the inhabitants of Soviet Georgia who ate liberally of pork and whole milk, yogurt, and cheese often lived to be over 100, with a significant percentage living to the rather astounding age of up to 130 years old in the nineteenth and twentieth centuries.[19] Great longevity was also reported by Arctic explorers in the earlier Eskimos, as well as among the Australian Aborigines, the Vilcabamba in Ecuador, and the Hunza in Pakistan.[20]

Second, no study has yet included the differences in sanitation that have had an enormous effect on longevity. With indoor toilets and showers, we can now bathe daily and therefore cleanse the dirt and microbes off our bodies before they trigger illness. This is in dramatic contrast to many of our European ancestors, who suffered from chronic skin diseases and infection from their terrible hygienic habits. For example, leaves and corncobs were most commonly used before the invention of toilet paper in 1890, and the Spanish Queen Isabella, who underwrote Christopher Columbus's voyages, boasted that she had only two baths in her life—at birth and prior to her wedding. In actuality, the importance of personal hygiene is still a relatively new concept that was rediscovered only in the late nineteenth century, having been popular almost two thousand years before (in the Western world) in ancient Greece and Rome.[21] Personal hygiene has also been a primary factor in reducing puerperal fever, the major cause of past infant mortality. In 1900, nearly 15 percent of American infants died before their first birthday, as compared with only 1 percent today. This improvement can be attributed in great part to Dr. Ignaz Semmelweis (1818–1865), who originated the practice of hand washing in obstetrics clinics, although this practice was not accepted until the late nineteenth century, after his death. Additionally, the contagious childhood diseases responsible for the deaths of many infants and children were greatly on the wane as a result of modern sanitation methods even before the widespread use of vaccines introduced in the mid-twentieth century.

Third, freedom from the drudgery of backbreaking work combined with modern-day comforts has also greatly supported the current longevity levels. That is, we no longer need to confront large and dangerous animals as in the Ice Age, try to survive fierce winters as the American colonials did, work all day under the searing sun in the fields, or clean and cook twelve or more hours daily as our earlier agrarian ancestors had to before the population shifted to the cities in the twentieth century, and before the inventions of the many modern time-saving appliances we now take for granted.[22]

Fourth, a 2006 study led by a Harvard School of Public Health researcher discovered a thirty-three-year disparity in longevity among Americans. At one extreme are the long-living Asian-American women in Bergen County, New Jersey, who had an average life expectancy of ninety-one years, while at the other end of the spectrum were the American Indians in South Dakota, who live on average only fifty-eight years. In fact, the life span disparities were so severe throughout the country that the researchers concluded that there were in actuality "eight Americas," with their specific groupings of race, geography, income, and life expectancy. Thus, the current average age of death of seventy-eight years varies so widely among the divergent cultures in the United States that it cannot be reliably used as a marker for the entire population.[23]

Finally, when one compares the pictures in chapter 16 that Dr. Price and his wife took of cultures before and after the introduction of toxic and refined foods, it further points out the question of the quality, not just quantity, of the years remaining. That is, although many of our ancestors dropped dead from the exhaustion of backbreaking work in their fields, factories, or homes, they often led much more robust lives than their present-day progeny. And when one considers the toll on mental, emotional, and physical health that poor diets and polypharmacy (taking two or more prescription drugs) have wrought on the average American, living longer must also be weighed with the quality of life of those years. Thus, the debate over longevity must include the fact that with all the benefits of labor-saving machines and modern sanitation, why are we not living even longer, and for a significant percentage of American seniors, not any richer?

FALSE CLAIMS REGARDING ARTHRITIS DRUGS VIOXX AND CELEBREX

Shocked that one of his profession's most highly respected journals had published this article, Abramson delved further into the literature on lipid levels and cardiovascular disease and discovered what Sally Fallon has been teaching for decades—that there is actually no scientific correlation between high cholesterol and heart disease.[24] In his subsequent book, *Overdosed America: The Broken Promise of American Medicine,* Abramson recounted his disillusionment with his profession and revealed other "false and misleading" claims made by the pharmaceutical companies that have been propagated through the seeming collusion of prestigious medical journals and the dearth of FDA regulatory action. These included the omission of six months of data in a study on the drug Celebrex that was published in the *Journal of the American Medical Association* and the manipulation of research statistics on the drug Vioxx from a study published in the *New England Journal of Medicine.* Through his extensive investigation, Abramson realized that when all of the data about these arthritis drugs was carefully analyzed, Celebrex was *not* significantly safer than NSAIDs such as Motrin and Advil and actually caused 11 percent more serious complications in the body than these much cheaper older anti-inflammatory drugs. He also discovered that the use of Vioxx did *not* result in "significantly fewer clinically important upper gastrointestinal events" but actually caused 21 percent more "serious adverse effects"* in study subjects than the cheaper anti-inflammatory drug to which it compared itself: naproxen.[25†]

*"Serious adverse effects" encompass gastrointestinal, cardiovascular, and other complications that lead to hospitalization or death.

†Vioxx costs $100 to $134 a month, compared with $18.19 to $7.50 per month for naproxen. In October 2004, Merck withdrew Vioxx from the market—one of the most widely used drugs ever to be withdrawn (in 2003 Merck received $2.5 billion in sales revenue from Vioxx). By March 2006, more than 10,000 cases and 190 class action suits had been filed against Merck over adverse cardiovascular events associated with Vioxx (www.druglibrary.org/library/vioxx2.html). Several lawsuits have now been won by the plaintiffs, including an August 17, 2006, ruling by a New Orleans jury that awarded a former FBI agent $50 million because Merck "knowingly represented or failed to disclose" important safety information on Vioxx (www.vioxx-lawsuit.ca).

INCREASED "EMOTIONAL LABILITY" FROM ANTIDEPRESSANTS

Dr. Abramson also recounted in his book what is perhaps the most reprehensible of all pharmaceutical deceptions—the marketing of SSRI antidepressant drugs to children. For example, he found that when the manufacturers of Paxil conducted nine clinical studies on the efficacy of their drug, they chose to publish only *one* of these studies, which showed beneficial results when adolescents took Paxil for depression. Why not publish the others? Because the other eight studies had shown that Paxil actually *increased* "emotional lability" in adolescents, which could potentially lead to suicidal thoughts as well as suicidal attempts.* This "mother of all sleight of hand" by drug companies that prey on our children is perhaps the most heartbreaking of all.[26]

BONE FRACTURE RISK INCREASED WITH OSTEOPOROSIS DRUG

Because it is such an excellent book, I'll mention one more subject covered extensively by Dr. John Abramson in *Overdosed America,* and that is the serious consequences of taking osteoporosis medications. Abramson writes that despite drug companies' aggressive marketing campaigns, bisphosphonate drugs such as Fosamax (alendronate) and Actonel (residronate) have little to no effect on preventing hip fractures, and in fact, in several studies they actually *increased* the risk of hip as well as wrist fractures. For example, in a 1998 *JAMA* study on osteopenia (bone thinning, which is less serious than osteoporosis), Fosamax actually increased the risk of wrist fractures by 50 percent and hip fractures by 84 percent in women.[27]

How could this be? The reason is that osteoporosis drugs strengthen the outer layer of bone, referred to as cortical bone, which makes up about 80 percent of the body's bone mass. However, these drugs have little effect on the other 20 percent, the lacelike internal bone structure called trabecular bone, which is essential for

*Increased suicide ideations as well as actual suicides have also been linked with other SSRI (selective serotonin reuptake inhibitors) drugs such as Prozac and Zoloft. (R. Degrandpre, "Bad Medicine," *Pacific Sun,* December 18–23, 2002, 11–14.)

providing extra strength to areas most vulnerable to fractures such as the hips, wrists, and vertebrae. And clearly, hip fractures are the most serious consequences of osteopenia and osteoporosis. The National Osteoporosis Foundation has reported that 24 percent of those who suffer a hip fracture die within one year, and 25 percent who previously had been living independently require long-term care.[28] It's unfortunate that osteoporosis drugs have little effect on this internal bone in these fracture-prone areas, since it's this trabecular bone that most rapidly reduces with age and therefore needs the most support.

Many allopathic doctors prescribe bisphosphonate drugs to their patients based on results of a bone mineral density (BMD) test that is used to measure osteoporosis. However, these BMD tests are not accurate indicators of the risk for hip fractures. In fact, a Netherlands study found that, for women between the ages of sixty and eighty, bone mineral density tests can determine the risk of fracturing a hip only one-sixth of the time. Other indicators need to be considered, such as muscle weakness, general frailty, activity level, a past history of cigarette smoking, and the side effects of past and present medications. As Abramson notes, "Routine BMD testing may not be the best way to help women prevent hip fractures, but it is an excellent way to sell more drugs."[29]

Equally disturbing is the serious "side effect" to jaws and teeth from these bisphosphonate drugs. Despite Sally Field's glowing endorsement and bright smile, Fosamax and other purported osteoporosis medications actually cause jawbone death. Although most cases occur in cancer patients who have received intravenous bisphosphonates (Zometa or Aredia), dentists are seeing jawbone degeneration from oral medications (Fosamax, Actonel, etc.) as well.[30]

Dr. Jacques Imbeau, a New Zealand dental physician, has reported in the *New Zealand Charter Journal* that this jawbone death, or jaw osteonecrosis, is usually detected from a lack of healing after a dental extraction but can also be seen in patients who present in dentists' offices displaying spontaneous cortical exposure through the gingival—that is, the jawbone begins to show through the gums. The mandible (lower jawbone) is affected more (by a 2:1 ratio) than the maxilla (upper jawbone), and the most culpable drugs linked with this jawbone ischemia (lack of blood supply) and eventual bone death are the nitrogen-containing bisphosphonates, including Fosamax (alendronate), Aredia (pamidronate), Zometa (zoledronate), Actonel (risedronate), and Boniva (ibandronate).[31]

Perhaps even more alarming, these bisphosphonate drugs remain in bone *indefinitely*. Therefore, if you are now taking—or have ever taken—any of these medications, it's important that you disclose this to your dentist and make sure that she is well aware of the serious consequences to the jawbone from these dangerous osteoporosis drugs.

ALLOPATHY CURRENTLY THE THIRD LEADING CAUSE OF DEATH

These examples of the significant harm that prescription drugs can do sheds light on the rather unbelievable statistic cited in the introduction to this book—that the combined effects of medical errors, adverse reactions to prescription drugs, and hospital infections are currently (at least) the *third* leading cause of death in the United States.[32] In light of this appalling statistic, no amount of explanation can legitimize, or excuse, the high levels of morbidity and mortality that allopathic medical practices continue to generate.

HOLISTIC MEDICINE VALIDATED BY THOUSANDS OF SCIENTIFIC STUDIES

First they ignore you,
then they laugh at you,
then they fight you,
then you win.

Mohandas "Mahatma" Gandhi (1869–1948)

Those who claim that there is no valid evidence for the efficacy of nutritional supplementation, botanical medicine, homeopathy, and other fields intrinsic to holistic medicine have simply not reviewed the scientific literature. In the *Textbook of Natural Medicine* alone, there are more than 10,000 citations from peer-reviewed research studies on the efficacy of various procedures and remedies used in natural medicine.[33]

Natural Medicine Often More Effective than Allopathic Drugs

Treating Memory Loss, Impotency, and Atherosclerosis

In fact, using the example of one botanical medicine alone that is commonly used by naturopathic physicians—*Ginkgo biloba* (ginkgo tree)—underscores this point even more dramatically. To date there have been more than 450 published articles on the efficacy of this botanical medicine prescribed primarily for memory loss and vascular insufficiency (in cases of stroke recovery, impotency, and arteriosclerosis), with 250 of these articles attesting to ginkgo's clinical potency (on satisfied patients). Furthermore, in nine double-blind randomized clinical trials, *Ginkgo biloba* extract proved to be "far superior" to the standard medications prescribed for the syndrome of intermittent claudication—pain and difficulty in walking from arterial obstruction or narrowing (atherosclerosis) in the legs.[34]

Treating Ulcers, Infection, Arthritis, and Hypertension

Numerous other natural medicines have also been proven in scientific studies (appropriately randomized and single- or double-blind controlled) to be far more efficacious (and less dangerous) than their much more widely publicized and costly allopathic prescription drug counterparts. These treatments include the use of licorice root (*Glycyrrhiza glabra*), fish oils (omega-3 fatty acids), vitamins A and C, and zinc as compared with cimetidine (Tagamet), ranitidine (Zantac), or antacids in the treatment of peptic ulcers; garlic (*Allium sativum*) in the inhibition of bacteria (staphylococcus, streptococcus, bacillus, brucella, and vibrio species) as compared with antibiotics (penicillin, streptomycin, chloramphenicol, erythromycin, and tetracyclines); glucosamine sulfate as compared with NSAIDs in the treatment of osteoarthritis; and celery, hawthorn extract, antioxidants (alpha lipoic acid, coenzyme Q10, vitamin E, L-carnitine, and omega-3 fatty acids), and minerals (potassium, magnesium, and calcium) in the treatment of hypertension.[35]

Holistic Principles Guide Physicians in Practice

Besides the use of natural and nontoxic medicines, holistic physicians have a further advantage in their practice by being thoroughly trained in the prevailing principles of natural medicine. These tenets, so integral to an effective holistic medical practice, are drilled into students from their first day as freshmen all the way through to their graduation (N.D. and D.C.), as well as annually thereafter in required postgraduate continuing education courses. Holistic doctors are further bound by oath to uphold the principles first elucidated by Hippocrates, many of which stand in stark contrast to the dangerous realities of modern allopathic medicine:

- First, *Primum non nocere* or "Do no harm"—that is, use therapies and interventions that are effective *and* safe;
- Second, *Vis medicatrix naturae* or "The healing power of nature," meaning the physician should primarily help support and facilitate the body's own inherent and innate power of healing;
- Third, *Tolle causam* or "Identify and treat the cause"—that is, treat the underlying cause of disease rather than simply suppressing the symptoms;
- Fourth, *Tolle totum* or "Treat the whole person," which points out that disease is multifaceted and must be diagnosed and treated according to all the possible causative factors in a patient's life—physical, mental, emotional, and spiritual;
- Fifth, *Docere* or "The physician as teacher," meaning that the major role of the holistic physician is to educate, motivate, and empower patients to take responsibility for their health;
- Sixth, *Prevention is optimum*—that is, prevention of future disease before it has fully manifested physically through insightful diagnosis and effective treatment is the highest form of medicine;
- And seventh, *The Law of Biogenesis* or "Only life can beget life," which asserts that only natural substances heal, and that synthetic or toxic medications can never be truly curative.[36]

Although holistic physicians are fallible human beings and can fall short of such lofty aims, these guiding principles stand as a continual reminder and incentive for them to always strive to serve their patients as safely and effectively as possible.

THE ALLOPATHIC INFLUENCE ON CONSUMERS

The scientific malfeasance of the medical-pharmaceutical industrial complex is so extensive that it's difficult to avoid sounding shrill when enumerating the overt (reports on "lifesaving" new drugs almost nightly on the six o'clock news) and covert (the glorification of allopathic medical doctors and the vilification of "alternative" treatments) means that have been used in propagating this present standard of medical care in the United States. Furthermore, when well-conducted studies have actually proven that certain natural medicines—botanicals, homeopathics, and nutritional supplements—are actually more effective and essentially *always* safer than prescription drugs, the iron grip that allopathic medicine has on the majority of consumers—over 50 percent of all Americans are taking at least one prescription drug—is all the more disheartening.[37]

The "Law of the Few"

However, the solution is not—and never can be—simply counterattacking the establishment or (vainly) attempting to influence the national media, which is already quite married to allopathic medical concepts ("find a drug to kill the bug"), as well as the advertising revenue it receives from its pharmaceutical company benefactors. Nor, and quite surprisingly so, are attempts to instigate change through communicating to large masses of people effective. In fact, radical change in a culture has been most effectively accomplished through the efforts of a surprisingly small number of people. As discussed in the conclusion of chapter 15,* Malcolm Gladwell explains in his book *The Tipping Point* that disease epidemics as well as social epidemics are actually initiated by a small but highly motivated minority; he refers to this phenomenon as the "Law of the Few."[38] That is, small but powerful word-of-mouth epidemics can be spread through the connections, energy, and enthusiasm of a small but exceptional group of people—such as the satisfied patients of skillful holistic practitioners.[39]*

*In chapter 15, this phenomenon was described citing the holistic communities in Oregon and other parts of the country where a majority of parents are now refusing to vaccinate their children.

Scales Almost "Tipped" at 40 Percent

Indeed, this law has already been demonstrated over the past two decades in augmenting significant changes in the American public's choice of medicine. Many readers are familiar with Dr. David Eisenberg's landmark study published in the 1993 *New England Journal of Medicine* revealing that 34 percent of Americans had had at least one "unconventional" therapy in 1992, even though 75 percent of these treatments were not covered by insurance and therefore paid for out of pocket. Furthermore, as evidenced by Eisenberg's subsequent study reported in a 1997 *Journal of the American Medical Association (JAMA)* article, this percentage actually increased to over 40 percent within just four years.[40] This word-of-mouth "epidemic" has been found to be especially contagious among cancer patients; it was reported in a 2000 study in the *Journal of Clinical Oncology* that the great majority—83 percent—had utilized at least one "alternative" therapy in conjunction with their allopathic treatments.[41]

Allopathic Medicine—The New "Alternative"?

This growing influence of the few is moving toward a critical mass in which a seismic shift in healthcare orientation can occur. At that crucial tipping point, it is foreseeable that the majority of Americans will finally begin to move away from the highly dangerous and

*Gladwell cites the number 150 as being the most significant to influence others and effect lasting change. This "rule of 150," as it is known to social scientists, has been known to initiate such a contagious milieu that the nature of thought and understanding can be radically changed overnight in a community. The rule of 150 also underscores an interesting analogy in the nature of epidemics: Just as major flu epidemics begin with small groups of individuals getting sick in scattered parts of the country, in order to create one contagious and powerful movement it is often necessary to create many small movements first. This "magical" number of 150 may be important for progressive leaders to keep in mind when they are in the process of organizing groups to help initiate change. It should be noted that the mystic and spiritual teacher G. I. Gurdjieff cited the number 200 for this context; he believed that if just 200 people existed and "if they found it necessary and legitimate, [they] could change the whole of life on the earth." (P. D. Ouspensky, *In Search of the Miraculous* [Boston: Houghton Mifflin Harcourt, 2001], 310.)

dubious treatments inherent in allopathic medicine and turn toward the safer and curative methods embodied in natural medicine. Through this more conservative portal-of-care paradigm, holistic physicians would be consulted first (except in the case of acute emergencies that necessitate emergency room visits), and the use of allopathic drugs and surgery would be considered only when initial conservative means fail. This trend would greatly reduce healthcare costs as well as the incidence of future chronic disease when, as a leading naturopathic physician most eloquently puts it, "the germinating weed of illness is pulled from the garden before it becomes a flaming bush."[42] In fact, this conservative care protocol is already the case for millions of satisfied patients who have been successfully treated by natural medicine and always choose to consult with their holistic physician first, before considering the allopathic alternatives of drugs and surgery.

EMERGENCY ROOM NATURAL MEDICINE

Even in the emergency room, the use of natural medicine could greatly benefit healing. For example, homeopathic Symphytum officinale heals broken bones so quickly that a compound fracture (bone sticking out of the skin) must first be set before the patient is given this remedy or it could begin healing the fracture in this abnormal position. Arnica montana is so effective in healing trauma in all its forms—wounds, head trauma, bruising, inflammation, and shock—that it should be stocked in every emergency room and considered after every accident or injury. And the use of glutamine—an amino acid with antioxidant effects that also helps reduce the permeability of a leaky gut—has already been reported to help patients in intensive care units recover so much faster that it has reduced medical care expenses by approximately $30,000 per patient.[43]

NOTES

1. J. Abramson, *Overdosed America* (New York: HarperCollins Publishers, 2004), 241.
2. M. Millenson, "What Your Doctor Doesn't Know, or Doesn't Practice, Can Harm Your Health," *Pacific Sun,* February 24–March 2, 1999, 12.
3. U.S. Congress, Office of Technology Assessment, *Assessing the Safety and Efficacy of Medical Technologies* (Washington, D.C.: USGPO, 1978), 7.
4. NIH, "Proceedings of the National Conference on Clinical Trials Methodology: Clinical Pharmacology and Therapeutics," *National Institutes for Health* 25 (1979): 630–31.
5. Ibid., xi–xx and cover flap.
6. M. Angell, *The Truth About Drug Companies* (New York: Random House, 2004), xv.
7. Associated Press, "Hormone Therapy Raises Cancer Risk," *Marin Independent Journal,* July 9, 2002, A-1.
8. Associated Press, "Hormone Pills Don't Improve Memory," *Marin Independent Journal,* August 18, 2003, A-1.
9. A. Quindlen, "And Now for a Hot Flash," *Newsweek,* July 29, 2002, 64.
10. J. Goldberg, *Deceits of the Mind* (Piscataway, N.J.: Transaction Publishers, 1991), 86.
11. S. Fallon and M. Enig, "Dangers of Statin Drugs," *Wise Traditions* 5, no. 1 (Spring 2004): 14–28.
12. Ibid., 18–21.
13. U. Ravnskov, "The Benefits of High Cholesterol," *Wise Traditions* 5, no. 1 (Spring 2004): 30, 31, 35, 36, 38.
14. S. Fallon and M. Enig, "Dangers of Statin Drugs," *Wise Traditions* 5, no. 1 (Spring 2004): 15.
15. U. Ravnskov, "The Benefits of High Cholesterol," *Wise Traditions* 5, no. 1 (Spring 2004): 36.
16. J. Abramson, *Overdosed America* (New York: HarperCollins Publishers, 2004), 13–16.
17. Ibid., 17.
18. J. Kramer, "Overprescribed Drugs," *Pacific Sun,* February 16–22, 2005, 14.
19. G. Pitskhelauri, *The Long Living of Soviet Georgia* (New York: Human Sciences Press, 1982), 37.
20. S. Fallon, "Nasty, Brutish and Short?" *The Ecologist* 29, no. 1 (January/February 1999): 26.
21. B. Wolf, "Great Moments in Toilet Paper History," http://abcnews.go.com/sections/us/WolfFiles/wolffiles156.html.
22. R. Halweil, "Is It Still Possible?" *Health and Healing Wisdom* 28, no. 2 (2006): 4.
23. T. Maugh II, "Lifespans in U.S. Disparate," *Press Democrat,* September 12, 2006, A6.
24. J. Kramer, "Overprescribed Drugs," *Pacific Sun,* February 16–22, 2005, 14.
25. J. Abramson, *Overdosed America* (New York: HarperCollins Publishers, 2004), 23, 30, 31, 32, 33, 34, 35.
26. Ibid., 242, 243.

27. Ibid., 213–15.
28. Ibid., 211.
29. Ibid., 214–15.
30. R. Rubin, "Drug Linked to Death of Jawbone," *USA Today,* www.usatoday.com/news/health/2005-03-13-jawbone-deaths_x.htm.
31. J. Imbeau, "Osteoporosis and Osteonecrosis of the Jaws: An Underestimated Problem with Multiple Ramifications," *New Zealand Charter Journal,* Summer 2007, 14, 15.
32. B. Starfield, "Is U.S. Health Really the Best in the World?" *Journal of the American Medical Association* 284, no. 4 (July 26, 2000): 483, 484.
33. J. Pizzorno and M. Murray, *Textbook of Natural Medicine,* vol. 1 (New York: Churchill Livingstone, 1999), 1.
34. Ibid., 757.
35. American Academy of Nurse Practitioners (AANP), *Naturopathic Medicine: Primary Care for the 21st Century* (Washington, D.C.: AANP), 22–29; J. Pizzorno and M. Murray, *Textbook of Natural Medicine,* vols. 1 and 2 (New York: Churchill Livingstone, 1999), 572, 771, 1444–45.
36. N. Calvino, "Integrative Medicine in Colon Cancer," *Townsend Letter for Doctors and Patients,* February/March 2004, 107; J. Boice, *Pocket Guide of Naturopathic Medicine* (Freedom, Calif.: The Crossing Press, 1996), 10–16.
37. HHS Secretary Tommy G. Thompson, "Almost Half of Americans Use at Least One Prescription Drug," *Health, United States 2004* (CDC), www.newsrx.com/newsletters/Science-Letter/2004-1228/122820043335525L.html (December 28, 2004); E. Wilcox, "Pharmacist Organization Unveils Snapshot of Medication Use in U.S.," www.ashp.org/news/ShowArticle.cfm?id=1998 (January 16, 2001).
38. M. Gladwell, *The Tipping Point* (New York: Little, Brown and Company, 2000), 18–19.
39. Ibid., 19–22, 88.
40. D. Eisenberg et al., "Trends in Alternative Medicine Use in the United States, 1990–1997," *Journal of the American Medical Association* 280 (1998): 1569.
41. K. Kohen et al., "Complementary/Alternative Medicine Use: Responsibilities and Implications for Pharmacy Services," *P & T* 27, no. 9: 440.
42. A. Vasquez, "Who Does the Healing? Who Should Do the Treating?" *Naturopathy Digest* 1, no. 9 (September 2006): 5.
43. Ibid., 4.

GLOSSARY

acute: A term describing a condition or disease that is usually brief in duration and self-limiting, such as a cold, flu, tonsillitis, or bladder infection that comes on suddenly and lasts for a short period of time.

aggravation: The homeopathic term for a healing crisis, when symptoms worsen for a brief period after the correct remedy (simillimum) triggers the release of toxins.

allopathy: The treatment of a disease by using medicines antagonistic and suppressive to the disease's symptoms, including *anti*histamines, *anti*biotics, and *anti*-inflammatories, or through the surgical removal (-ectomy) of diseased tissues, such as in append*ectomies*, hyster*ectomies,* and tonsill*ectomies*. Medical and osteopathic physicians are presently taught allopathic principles and practices in their medical schools.

amalgam: From the Greek word *malagma,* meaning soft mass, this term denotes any mixture or combination, typically an alloy of two or more metals. The term is most typically used to describe the amalgam filling that is a mixture of mercury (49–54%), silver (~35%), tin (~12%), copper (~ 3%), and zinc (~1%).

anamnesis: The taking of a careful and thorough history. Many physicians consider this history to be the most important key in accurate diagnosis and subsequent appropriate treatment.

antidote: This term can be used as a noun or a verb. It refers to a substance or procedure (essential oils, dental drilling, X-rays, etc.) that neutralizes or counteracts the effects of a homeopathic remedy.

Auriculomedicine: A term coined by Paul Nogier, M.D., to describe his energetic testing method in which he diagnosed patients' dysfunction and determined appropriate treatments through the measurement of their electromagnetic field (EMF) by monitoring their radial pulse or vascular autonomic signal (VAS).

auriculotherapy: The field of holistic medicine originated by Paul Nogier, M.D., that treats dysfunction and disease in the body through the stimulation of ear points. Auriculotherapy treats anatomical reflex points clinically correlated to specific areas of the body, in contrast to Chinese acupuncture ear charts (produced after Nogier's auriculotherapy was propagated worldwide) that are based on different points (reflex relationships).

autohemotherapy: The treatment practice wherein patients receive their own blood in a particular therapeutic manner. This treatment can be through a homeopathic remedy made from a drop of the patient's own blood and taken orally, or through the injection of the blood, which is often mixed first with a homeopathic remedy or treated with ozone (aka auto-sanguis or autosanguinous therapy).

Avogadro's number: The number of atoms or molecules contained in one mole (molecular weight in grams) of a substance was observed in 1811 by physicist Amedeo Avogadro (1776–1856) to be 6.023×10^{23}. In homeopathy, potencies diluted beyond Avogadro's number—that is, over 24X, 12C, and LM 3—contain no actual remaining physical molecules of the original plant, animal, or mineral from which they were made. These higher, "nonphysical" potencies of homeopathic remedies, however, have been proven in numerous research studies to have very real physical effects.

axonal transport: The capacity of nerves to conduct not only electrical nerve impulses but also chemicals along their axons. Nutrients as well as toxins (chemicals, heavy metals, and pathogenic microbes) can be transported along nerve axons.

bilateral: When both sides of the body are affected, as opposed to one side (unilateral or ipsilateral). For example, when there are multiple focal infections located on both sides of the mouth, such as in the case of both lower third molar (wisdom) teeth, *bilateral* symptoms in the body (from the disturbed fields) are commonly experienced.

blocked regulation: Employed most frequently in Europe, this term refers to the blockage of normal maintenance and control—that is, healthy regulation or homeostasis—in the body. The most typical factors that block regulation are steroids and other drugs, mercury and other toxic metals, toxic chemicals, chronic foci, continual ingestion of a primary food allergen, a major malocclusion, chronic geopathic or electromagnetic stress, and significant psychological stress.

bruxism: The rhythmic or spasmodic grinding of the teeth, especially when occurring at night during one's sleep. Bruxism is most commonly caused by dental malocclusions (bad bites) and emotional stress.

calomel: A mercury salt (mercurous chloride) that was used for centuries in skin creams and tooth powders has caused countless cases of mercury poisoning. It was banned for use in the 1950s.

cavitation: (1) The hole, or cavity, that can manifest in the maxillary or mandibular jawbone due to a focal infection. (2) The appropriate surgical methods required to remove the infected tissue in and around this hole, or cavitation area, in the bone. Cavitation surgery typically encompasses the removal of all infected soft tissue that may remain behind after simple extraction of a focal tooth (e.g., the periodontal ligament), as well as all infected gangrenous and necrotic (dead) jawbone areas. When this dead bone is thoroughly drilled out, new bone can then grow into the area as the site heals.

chi: This term in Chinese medicine, referred to as *prana* in Hinduism, as well as *vital force* or *vital principle,* is the power, force, or energy that has been said since ancient times to reside in and enliven every being. It is also spelled *qi.*

Class I, II, and III: The three classifications for various malocclusions ("bad bites") of the teeth. Class I refers to crowded and rotated teeth. Class II describes an overbite, or "buckteeth" appearance. Class III refers to an underbite malocclusion, or "bulldog" appearance. The *type* of class further defines the malocclusion. For example, a Class II, *type 1* malocclusion is an overjet of the maxillary teeth (upper jaw) over the mandibular teeth (lower jaw); whereas a Class II, *type 2* malocclusion is the trapping of mandibular teeth by the posterior-tipped (backward-tipped) maxillary teeth.

CNS: The acronym for the *central nervous system,* which includes the brain and the spinal cord.

constitutional homeopathy: A field of holistic medicine that uses a single remedy composed of potentized minute amounts (or just the energetic memory) of a plant, animal, or mineral that resonates with this same plant, animal, or mineral distortion pattern in an individual and subsequently heals related mental, emotional, and physical illness secondary to this chronic nonhuman pattern.

contralateral: In medicine, a condition wherein something is being affected on the opposite side of the body. For example, scar interference fields can cause disturbance (disturbed fields) on the ipsilateral (same) or contralateral (opposite) sides of the body.

counteracting relationship: A relationship that occurs when after years of "sharing the stress" with a disturbed field, a tooth may further compensate by disturbing other teeth. The counteractive pattern is one of three major patterns seen in Chinese five-element theory acupuncture. The other two are the *ko* destructive pattern and the *mother-son* promoting pattern.

craniopathy: The gentle and indirect treatment of restrictions of movement in the bones and fascia that surround either end of the central nervous system—the cranium (skull bones) and the sacroiliac (pelvis). Also known as *craniosacral therapy* or *craniosacral manipulation.*

craniosacral rhythm: The subtle motion of the cerebrospinal fluid (CSF) that circulates within the brain and spinal cord continuously from the head to the "tail," or sacrum. Typically, the craniosacral rhythm is about eight to twelve cycles per minute.

cutaneosomatic reflex: The reflex relationship between a scar interference field (cutaneo-) and the tissue in which it causes a disturbed field (-somatic). For example, chronic tension headaches (-somatic) can be triggered by a nearby scar, such as a surgical face-lift scar, but also from an interference field distal to the head, such as an appendix or episiotomy scar (cutaneo-).

cutaneovisceral: The reflex relationship between a scar interference field (cutaneo-) and an organ (*viscus,* singular; *viscera,* plural). For example, a hernia scar interference field that chronically irritates the large intestine (viscus) and triggers intermittent diarrhea is referred to as a cutaneovisceral reflex.

diathesis: See **miasm.**

disturbed field: Also known as a *burdened field,* the area that is secondarily disturbed by a focus. For example, right neck and shoulder pain is a typical disturbed field secondary to an ipsilateral—that is, on the right side of the mouth—dental focal infection.

dominant focus: An area of chronic disturbance—infected, inflamed, or fibrotic (scar tissue)—that is frequently asymptomatic but causes symptoms distally (in a disturbed field) in other parts of the body. The most common dominant foci are the teeth, tonsils, and scars. Synonyms include *focal infection, significant focus,* and *interference field.*

drainage: Drainage remedies (or techniques) stimulate the body's organs and tissues to release toxins at their own unique pace and within their own metabolic limits. As opposed to aggressive and non-personalized broad detoxification protocols that often trigger strong healing reactions, toxins are drained and released much more gently, naturally, and efficiently.

dysbiosis: From a Greek word meaning an "abnormal or bad way of living," this term refers to the overgrowth of pathogenic flora (primarily bacteria and fungi) throughout the body, but especially in the intestines. Dysbiosis is most commonly caused by the ingestion of sugar and other refined foods and the excessive intake of antibiotic drugs.

elective localization: See **selective affinity.**

electroacupuncture: A diagnostic method that combines the ancient principles of Chinese acupuncture with modern computer electronics. The two primary electroacupuncture systems originated in Germany, from Dr. Reinhold Voll, through a technique he termed EAV (Electroacupuncture According to Voll), and from Dr. Helmut Schimmel, who originated the Vega method.

emunctory: Derived from the Latin word *emungere,* meaning "to cleanse," this term is most commonly used to describe the organs and tissues that excrete toxins in the body. The primary emunctories in the body are the major excretory organs—the liver through bile, the kidneys through urine, and the intestines through feces. Other emunctories include the lungs, due to their removal of carbon dioxide and other gases through exhalation, and the skin, by the removal of waste via perspiration.

energetic testing: An umbrella term to describe the techniques that are utilized to interpret the body's various signals—muscle strength, arm and leg length, acupressure points, and energy fields. Energetic testing methods supplement standard history, exam, X-ray, and laboratory findings to arrive at a more precise diagnosis and help determine the most effective therapeutic intervention. Energetic testing techniques have an advantage over many diagnostic tests in that they assess the patient's state in vivo—that is, in present time—and directly on the patient's body. For more information, see appendix 3.

engram: The strong memory pattern that becomes embedded in the central nervous system (brain and spinal cord) after a major acute (e.g., earthquake) or chronic (e.g., child abuse) trauma.

enneagram: This term refers to both the ancient nine-pointed symbol and the system of nine personality fixation patterns that through self-observation and increased self-understanding can aid spiritual aspirants in differentiating their acquired and egoic personality tendencies from their true essential nature.

ephapse: As opposed to a *synapse*—the normal gap between two nerve fibers in which an impulse is transmitted from one neuron to the other—this condition refers to nerve impulses *not* being transmitted across a synapse properly. An ephapse is typically caused by faulty healing from a scar interference field, thereby causing the nerve impulse to no longer transmit across the neuronal gap properly.

episiotomy: A surgical incision commonly given during childbirth to avoid excessive stretching and tearing of the perineum and vagina just before the baby is delivered. Episiotomies commonly cause scar interference fields. Research since the 1980s has revealed that episiotomies do more harm than good and should be discontinued as a common delivery procedure.

equilibration: The grinding of an interfering surface on a single tooth, or on many teeth, in order to achieve a harmonious occlusion or bite.

erethism: The neurological and psychic disturbance most

typically seen in chronic mercury poisoning, which is characterized by irritability, emotional instability, anxiety, depression, shyness, fatigue, and, in advanced cases, hallucinations, loss of memory, and intellectual deterioration. Erethism due to mercury poisoning is also known as *erethismus mercurialis* or *micromercurialism*.

ergotropic: The "housecleaning" and body maintenance functions of the autonomic nervous system, such as the moment-to-moment adjustments that the autonomic nerves must make in the visceral (organs), circulatory (blood and lymph), and metabolic (thyroid, liver, etc.) systems. The chaotic and "noisy" sympathetic nerve activity in a scar interference field, for example, disrupts normal ergotropic (homeostatic or self-regulating) functioning.

false TMD syndrome: The effect on the temporomandibular joint (TMJ or jaw joint) from the pull of congested and contracted muscles and fascia due to a toxic neighboring vagal ganglion. This subtle but chronically disturbing pulling and pressure on the jaw joint, which can mimic primary temporomandibular joint dysfunction (TMD), is often caused by intestinal dysbiosis, mercury amalgam fillings, or a dental focal infection in which toxic microbes or metals are axonally transported along the vagus nerve and then stored in the vagal ganglion.

Flexner report: Written by educator Abraham Flexner, with the aid of Nathan Colwell of the American Medical Association (AMA), this study and subsequent report greatly favored the allopathic approach in medicine over the homeopathic. It became the final "death knell" in the mid-twentieth century for homeopathic colleges, as well as the widespread practice of homeopathy itself, in the United States. Based on the 1910 Flexner report, which was largely funded by the philanthropists Carnegie and Rockefeller, of the twenty-two homeopathic colleges operating in 1900, only two were still teaching homeopathy by 1923, and by 1950 not a single school was left.

focal chains: This expression refers to the fact that foci generate other foci. For example, a first molar dental focal infection that is causing a disturbed field in the pancreas, after enough years, can result in the pancreas itself eventually acting as a self-generating focus. After enough time, this pancreatic focus will trigger its own disturbed field, which in turn can become a focus itself at some point. This focal chain pattern—without significant therapeutic intervention such as auriculotherapy or neural therapy—will continue until enough tissue degeneration occurs that serious disease ensues, and eventually death.

focalsomatic referral: The musculoskeletal pain or dysfunction that can occur secondary to a primary focal infection or scar interference field. For example, a patient can experience chronic neck pain (aka "disturbed field") secondary to an undiagnosed tonsil or dental focus.

frozen regulation or **regulation paralysis:** The condition of the body being so inundated and overwhelmed with aberrant autonomic nerve signals emitting from numerous foci that homeostasis (normal functioning) is lost.

galvanism: The flow of an electric current produced by two or more dissimilar metals. *Dental galvanism,* or *electrogalvanism,* commonly occurs when gold, having a high positive charge, augments the rate of corrosion of the negatively charged mercury found in amalgam fillings, and thus the release of this latter toxic metal into the body is greatly potentiated.

ganglia: The clusters of autonomic nerve cells in the peripheral nervous system that act as "little brains" throughout the body to regulate local functioning. Ganglia secondarily function as adaptive storage centers by downloading and storing toxic metals, chemicals, and microbes from congested neighboring areas.

gangliosomatic referral: The pain or dysfunction in the body (-somatic) that occurs secondary to a toxic and congested ganglion. For example, painful and tense jaw muscles can be due to neighboring toxic vagal ganglia (see **false TMD syndrome**).

gemmotherapy: This potent form of drainage, also known as *plant stem cell therapy, blastotherapy,* or *embryophytotherapy,* involves the use of herbal remedies made of freshly harvested embryonic plant parts (buds, shoots, rootlets, etc.), which contain the strong active life essence and numerous growth factors inherent in young plants.

gnosis: Deriving from the Greek word meaning "knowledge" or "to know," this term refers to the special knowledge of spiritual and divine understanding that all individuals at times are privy to, but that is especially experienced by sages, saints, and other realized beings regularly.

gutta percha: This sticky substance from a rubber tree is the most common root canal filling material. However, only a minor portion of the gutta percha filling is made up of natural rubber. The rest is composed of zinc oxide, barium (15% to make it show up on an X-ray), and traces of heavy metals such as lead and cadmium (up to 0.6%).

healing crisis: Also known as *healing reaction, retracing of symptoms,* and, in homeopathy, *aggravation,* this term refers to a patient experiencing an increased intensity of symptoms during treatment while on the correct remedy or treatment regimen before feeling better.

Hering's law: Initially described in 1845 by Dr. Constantine Hering, this classic homeopathic principle describes the various responses seen when healing is proceeding appropriately: cure proceeds from above downward (head to toe), from inside out (from the most important organs to least important organs), and in the reverse order of the appearance of symptoms.

Hippocrates: A Greek physician (460–370 BCE) known as the father of medicine. His "like cures like" belief inspired Hahnemann (who was able to read his original Greek manuscripts) through quotes such as the following: "Disease is born of things, and by the attack of like things people are healed."

homeostasis: The state of healthy functioning that occurs when normal maintenance and control of the body is properly maintained. Homeostasis is the tendency for stability in the internal environment of the body—that is, a state of physiological equilibrium produced by a balance of the body's chemicals and nervous system, which can adapt to environmental stress.

homunculus: From the Latin word meaning "little man," this term refers to the microrepresentation, or small map, of the body that is represented neurologically in the brain's cortex. Other homunculi, or microsystems of nerve innervation in the body, are located in the thalamus (pain recognition and response), the cerebellum (regulation of posture), and the ear.

Huneke phenomenon: The instantaneous and often dramatic relief of a patient's disturbed field (i.e., pain or dysfunction) upon a neural therapy injection of local anesthetic into a focal infection or scar interference field. It is also known as the *seconds phenomenon* or the *lightning reaction*.

iatrogenic: A term describing any adverse state or condition produced by a doctor due to poor treatment.

idiopathic: The description for a disease or dysfunction that is of unknown origin.

ipsilateral: A reference to something being "on the same side." Dental focal infections often cause disturbance ("disturbed fields") ipsilaterally (on the same side of the body).

isopathy: A subset of homeopathy that is based on the principle of *sameness,* rather than on *similarity*. That is, the exact same microbe that caused the disease or condition (e.g., the tubercular bacillus) makes up the remedy (e.g., Tuberculinum). Isopathic remedies include those made from pathogenic microbes and other toxins (nosodes), as well as those made from harmless, and even beneficial, microbes (e.g., *Penicillium notatum*).

"K" potencies: Potencies made according to the Russian homeopath Korsakoff by using the same vial throughout the remedy preparation, whereas with Hahnemann's method (*C* or *CH* potency), the vial is discarded after making each particular potency level (1C, 2C, 3C, etc.).

kinesiology: A form of energetic testing that uses the body's muscle tone as a feedback system to assess dysfunction in patients and determine the most appropriate treatment. Applied Kinesiology (AK), originated in 1964 by Dr. George Goodheart, was the first school of kinesiology developed.

laser: The acronym for "light amplification by stimulated emission of radiation." The "radiation" aspect of this acronym refers simply to the expression of energy transmission by light, not harmful ionizing radiation.

"LM" potencies: Potencies diluted at a ratio of 1 (plant, animal, or mineral substance) to 50,000 (alcohol and water) at each step during the potentizing process. At the end of his life, Hahnemann highly recommended LM, also known as "Q" or "fifty-millesimal," potencies, which can be given more often than the "C" potencies. Purportedly, LM potencies often have a more profound impact on the patient and cause fewer healing aggravations.

luetic: The most pathogenic of the four primary miasms. It is characterized by ulceration, sclerosis (scar tissue formation), metastasis, and other forms of necrosis (tissue destruction). Chronic insomnia, stomach and duodenal ulcers, MS, ALS, Parkinson's, Alzheimer's disease, and cancer are characteristic of the luetic miasm.

malocclusion: The manner in which upper and lower teeth fit together. Often referred to as a *bad bite,* a malocclusion occurs when the teeth don't *occlude* or fit together properly upon closing.

materia medica: An encyclopedia-like book of homeopathic remedies that lists and describes in detail all of the remedies and the particular symptoms that they can potentially cure.

matrix tissue: The gel-like connective tissue, also referred to as the *ground substance* or *basic tissue,* that surrounds every cell in the body and through which nerves and blood vessels are able to communicate to organs and tissues. This highly sensitive semiliquid substance reacts to minute changes in the environment. A scar interference field can cause electrical chaos in the matrix tissue by disrupting normal conductivity and communication, and a chronic focal infection can cause this connective tissue to become congested with bacteria and their toxic by-products.

methylmercury: When metallic, or inorganic, mercury in mercury amalgam fillings comes in contact with bacteria, from a dental focal infection, gum disease, or intestinal dysbiosis, it becomes *methylated* to form one of the most potent poisons existing on the planet—organic, or methyl, mercury.

miasm: Also known as *diathesis* or *reaction mode,* the inherited or environmentally caused predisposition to chronic disease and the susceptibility to succumbing to that disease under stress.

morphogenetic field: The energetic or electromagnetic field that surrounds everything and encodes the basic pattern of that object or living being. First introduced by Paul Weiss in the 1930s, this concept was later developed and expanded by Rupert Sheldrake.

MRT (Matrix Reflex Testing): Energetic testing technique originated by the author of this book that utilizes the reflex arm length measurement and the body's electromagnetic field (EMF) to assist in the diagnosis of dysfunction in the body and to help determine the most appropriate treatments.

neural therapy: Classically, neural therapy is the treatment wherein local anesthetic is injected in and around a focus or its ganglion to temporarily block the abnormal neuronal signals emitting from this pathologically disturbed tissue. "Neural therapy without needles"—that is, through stimulation of the disturbed nerves and tissues of the focus with massage (isopathic drops, creams, or oils) or laser—was also recognized by Peter Dosch (the renowned German neural therapist and author) and has been proven effective for almost a century.

night guards: Hard plastic appliances that fit over both the upper and lower teeth and hold them rigidly in position to reduce nocturnal bruxism (grinding and clenching). These rigid appliances often disrupt rhythmic motion of the cranium, however, and impede the micromovement in the maxillary suture.

nosocomial: This term describes any hospital-related disturbance, such as infection acquired from bacteria (e.g., MRSA, or methicillin-resistant *Staphylococcus aureus*), that occurs in a patient while in the hospital.

nosode: A homeopathic remedy made from a microbe or diseased product designed to stimulate an immune system response to protect the body from succumbing to that particular microbe or disease. (For example, the Tuberculinum remedy is a nosode because it is made from the tubercular bacillus.)

odonton: This term refers to all aspects of the tooth—that is, the tooth itself, the pulp inside, the periodontal ligament, the nerves, and the jawbone.

odontosomatic: The reflex relationship a dental focus (odonto-) can have on the organs and tissues (-somatic) in the body (also called *focalsomatic*).

Organon: A reference to the book *Organon of the Medical Art,* which was written by the founder of homeopathy, Samuel Hahnemann, M.D. It is still considered to be the "bible" in guiding diagnosis and treatment by practitioners of constitutional homeopathy.

orthopedic dentists: As opposed to orthodontists, who typically pay little regard to the effect of retainers and braces on the rest of the patient's body, biological or holistic orthopedic dentists take into account the functioning of their patient's whole body—structurally, biochemically, and psychologically.

PANDAS: An acronym for "pediatric autoimmune neuropsychiatric disorders associated with streptococcal infections" that describes a wide spectrum of neurological and psychological disorders that can arise in children after a bout of strep throat. The two hallmark manifestations of PANDAS—tics or choreic-like movements and obsessive-compulsive disorders (OCD)—are also seen in Tourette's syndrome, as well as more subtly in patients with chronic tonsil focal infections.

Paracelsus: The Swiss physician (1493–1541) who advocated the "like cures like" principle as well as a belief in "the minimal dose" by stating that a poisonous substance that causes disease could also cure the disease if given in small enough dosages. Paracelsus succinctly characterized this law of minimum dose through the phrase *Dosis sola facit venenum*—that is, "only the dose makes the poison."

pathogenesis: The cellular events and organ and tissue dysfunction that lead to the development of disease.

pathognomonic: When a sign or symptom is so typical of a disease that a diagnosis can be confidently made from this single characteristic.

periodicity: A reference to the intermittent nature of symptoms, which is typical of the confounding nature of a disturbed field's waxing and waning symptoms and renders the underlying culpable focus difficult to locate, diagnose, and treat.

photophoresis: The effect of driving remedies, creams, or essential oils that have been rubbed into the skin deeper into the tissues through the cellular photon-stimulating effect of laser light.

phytotoxin: The natural—but toxic—substances found in some plants (e.g., alfalfa). Phytotoxins found in many nuts can be neutralized by soaking them before eating.

plant stem cells: When prescribed correctly, these primal, undifferentiated stem cells of embryonic plant parts (buds, shoots, rootlets, etc.) have the ability to repair and regenerate tissues and organs in the body. See also **gemmotherapy.**

pleomorphism: This controversial theory that microorganisms can be modified through their environment includes intraspecies metamorphoses such as streptococcus bacteria biologically transforming into pneumococcus bacteria, as well as interspecies changes such as a bacteria transforming into a virus.

PNS: The commonly used acronym for the "peripheral nervous system"—that is, the nerves in the body that lie outside of the central nervous system (or CNS, the brain and spinal cord).

polarity: A state of imbalanced or blocked life energy currents in the body. A pattern of obvious or even subtle right- or left-sided symptoms, such as muscle weakness, intermittent pain or numbness, or simply just a heightened awareness, causes what is referred to as "right-" or "left-sided polarity" in the body. From more current neurological understanding, these ipsilateral patterns are a sign of sympathetic nerve dysfunction expressed by thermatomal patterns.

potency: The power, vitality, or strength of a homeopathic remedy, based on the amount of dilution and succussion (shaking) the remedy undergoes. A low potency such as 6C has more of a physical effect in the body than a higher potency such as 1M, which acts more on the mental and emotional planes.

probiotics: Defined as "promoting or healthful to life," this term also refers to supplements such as *Lactobacillus acidophilus* and *Bifidus* bacteria, when they are used to replenish healthy intestinal flora.

proving: Uncharacteristic symptoms arising after taking a homeopathic remedy indicate that the remedy is not correct; this is called "proving the remedy."

psoric: The least pathogenic miasm or reaction mode, characterized by functional disorders that are reversible. Psorics are typically strong enough to eliminate toxins, and these eliminations do not exhaust them. Psoric manifestations primarily affect the skin, gastrointestinal, and respiratory systems.

psychogalvanic reflex: The traumatic emotions subconsciously associated with a chronic focus that are often the deepest factors underlying the focus's initial development as well as perpetuating its continued existence. The increased electrical current of the sympathetic nerves overlying a scar interference field, or *galvanism,* can be directly measured through autonomic instruments called dermometers.

psychosomatic referral: The secondary musculoskeletal pain or dysfunction (-somatic) referred from primary psychological stress (psycho-).

psychospiritual: Therapies, schools, or paths that meld modern Western psychology with Eastern spiritual traditions. In this way, individuals can potentially transcend their egoic patterns in the process of becoming fully human, through the realization of their deeper spiritual nature. Psychospiritual practice is synonymous with the field of psychology known as *transpersonal psychology.*

qi: See **chi**.

quack: A term that the holistic American Society of Dental Surgeons called the dentists in the American Dental Association (ADA) when they began to utilize and advocate the use of mercury amalgam in dental fillings in the late nineteenth century. The word *quack* derives from the German word *quecksilber,* which translates in English to "quicksilver"—another name for mercury.

reaction mode: See **miasm.**

rebirthing: Also known as *conscious breathing* or *breathwork,* the therapeutic process of breathing in a conscious and connected way that oxygenates and enlivens areas of suppressed emotions in the body and initiates the removal of painful psychological contraction patterns.

reflex arm length: The energetic testing method originated by Raphael van Assche, D.O., also known as the arm length reflex test (AR test), that measures changes in arm length to assess dysfunction in patients as well as to determine the most appropriate treatments. It is one of the primary methods for measurement in the Matrix Reflex Testing (MRT) technique.

repertory: This homeopathic book categorizes the numerous symptoms a patient may express according to the primary area of the body—mind, head, throat, abdomen, extremities, skin, and so forth—where the symptom is experienced.

retromolar space: Also referred to as the *trigone* region, it is the area just behind the wisdom teeth. When the retromolar space is crowded by malpositioned impacted wisdom teeth, it can have an adverse effect on brain function. Treatment can include orthopedic functional appliances (if caught early enough) or extraction and cavitation surgery of the wisdom teeth.

rheumatic disturbed fields: The disturbed fields created from streptococcus and staphylococcus bacterial focal infections, usually emanating from the teeth or the tonsils. The five most common rheumatic disturbed fields are the brain, the joints, the heart, the kidneys, and the stomach and intestine.

second intention: Healing by "first intention" or by "primary union" occurs when the edges of the tissue around the wound are very close together, there is no infection present, and a minimum of scar tissue is formed. Healing by "second intention" or by "secondary union" occurs in larger wounds or wounds complicated by infection, and the healing process is delayed and greater scarring results. Scars healed by second intention by definition will develop into chronic scar interference fields.

selective affinity: Also known as *elective localization,* this term refers to Edward C. Rosenow's theory that bacteria, especially streptococci, have a specific pathogenic affinity for certain tissues. Rosenow and other researchers, such as Weston Price, observed in numerous studies that bacteria taken from patients would replicate in animals the exact same eye infections, kidney disease, peptic ulcers, heart disease, and arthritis that the patients were suffering from.

sequelae: Any remaining disease or dysfunction that occurs after an illness. Thus, if an area heals "with no sequelae," it has resolved completely with no remaining symptoms (pain, numbness, tension, etc.) or signs (infection, inflammation, tissue contraction, and scarring, etc.).

silver filling: This is another term for the amalgam filling. However, this term is quite misleading, because silver makes up only around 35 percent of the amalgam filling, whereas mercury makes up from 49 to 54 percent. The rest is made up of tin at approximately 12 percent, copper at 0.5 to 3 percent, and zinc at around 1 percent.

simillimum: The most perfectly fitting constitutional homeopathic remedy based on the "like cures like" (*similia similibus curentur*) principle, in contrast to the principle of "opposite cures" (*contraria contraries*) employed by allopathic medicine.

somatesthesia: The perception or consciousness of having a body. A dominant focus negatively alters this body-consciousness, which further strengthens the self-perpetuating aspect of the focal engram in the brain's cortex.

somato-odonton: The description of how a focus in the body (somato-) can cause a dental disturbed field (odonton). For example, a toxic stomach (somato-) focus can cause decay and degeneration in a first molar tooth (-odonton) over time through this chronic somato-odonton reflex relationship.

somatovisceral: Structural dysfunction (joints and muscles) adversely affecting visceral organs.

stomatognathic system: This term refers to the mouth and jaws.

stomatognathicsomatic referral: Musculoskeletal disturbances in the body primarily initiated by jaw (TMD) and bite dysfunction (malocclusion).

succussion: The act of shaking a diluted homeopathic remedy against an immovable object (e.g., a book or one's palm) in the process of making a particular potency (e.g., 30C, 200K, etc.).

sycotic: This miasm is called the *pathology of adaptation* diathesis because instead of purging toxins it retains and adapts around them. In contrast to psora's strong but overreactive system, the sycotic, or second reaction mode, is one of progressive weakening and underreaction. Deeper skin conditions (warts, lipomas, skin tags, cystic acne, psoriasis, etc.), joint problems (tendonitis, bursitis, and arthritis), and digestive dysfunction (dysbiosis, gas, bloating, fatigue, constipation, diarrhea, liver congestion, enzyme deficiencies, hypoglycemia, diabetes, etc.) are classic sycotic symptoms.

syncytium: A group of nerve cells that are so closely allied that they function as a single unit, such as in the heart or the autonomic nervous system (neurovegetative system).

systemic: This term denotes when the entire body is affected as a whole. For example, a focus not only negatively affects a specific area (disturbed field) but also is chronically debilitating systemically.

tautopathy: A form of isopathy that uses a homeopathic medication made from an allopathic drug to treat the ill effects of that drug. The classic example of tautopathy is in the treatment of vaccinosis, for example, giving a child homeopathic MMR or DPT vaccine to treat the damaging effects of these measles/mumps/rubella or diphtheria/pertussis/tetanus immunizations.

therapy localization: A kinesiological term that describes a practitioner firmly touching an area of skin such as a suspected scar interference field while simultaneously challenging a strong muscle. If this previously strong muscle weakens with this therapy localization challenge, it is a positive "TL," and the scar is considered to be an active interference field.

thermatomes: Areas of skin innervated by sympathetic sensory nerves that reflect the cutaneous distribution of blood vessels, and thus the resulting skin temperature.

thermography: An imaging instrument that evaluates sympathetic nerve pathology, such as in the case of the tissues overlying a chronic focal area, through skin temperature.

thimerosal: In 1929, Eli Lilly repackaged its popular Merthiolate—the reddish orange antiseptic containing mercury—as thimerosal, for use as a preservative in injectible vaccines.

TMD: An acronym for "temporomandibular joint dysfunction," which occurs when the mandible (lower jawbone) shifts into an adapted and compensatory position and pulls the jaw joint, or temporomandibular joint (TMJ), out of its normal position or alignment.

transpersonal psychology: This field utilizes the insights of Western psychology to help individuals recognize their chronic negative egoic patterns concurrently with the wisdom inherent in Eastern religions to assist in releasing and transcending these patterns. It is a form of psychospiritual work.

trigger factor: Also referred to as *second insult,* this term describes when a particular stimulus activates a dormant focus, such as a previously asymptomatic root-canalled tooth becoming inflamed after getting one's teeth cleaned.

tropism: From a Greek root meaning "to turn to," this word refers to the affinity plants have for certain tissues. For example, Juniper, or *Juniperus communis,* the gemmotherapy remedy made from the young shoots of the evergreen shrub, has a natural tropism for the liver and is the primary drainage remedy for this organ.

tuberculinic: The tuberculinic miasm, or third reaction mode, is primarily characterized by a significantly weakened immune system that is susceptible to viruses (hepatitis, meningitis, herpes, influenza, HIV, etc.), chronic respiratory illnesses (colds, flu, bronchitis, pneumonia, tuberculosis, etc.), autoimmune syndromes, allergies, asthma, and disturbances in mineralization (rickets, scoliosis, osteomyelitis, rheumatoid arthritis, knock knees, bow legs, etc.).

vaccinosis: The adverse sequelae (aftereffects) following vaccinations, which can include acute and chronic illnesses.

viscerosomatic referral: These reflexes, also referred to as "Head's zones" in Europe, and simply "areas of referred pain" in the United States, describe somatic (skin, muscle, tendon, ligament, bursa, etc.) pain or dysfunction caused by a viscus (plural is viscera)—that is, an organ. An example of a classic viscerosomatic reflex is the left shoulder, arm, and central chest pain (angina) that often signals heart damage and an impending heart attack.

Waldeyer's ring: The five lymphatic tonsillar tissues: the paired palatine tonsils located in the back of the throat most typically called "the tonsils"; the pharyngeal tonsil, or adenoids, located in the nasopharynx in the roof of the mouth; the lingual tonsil located at the base of the tongue; the laryngeal tonsil located near the vocal cords in the larynx; and the bilateral tubal tonsils located inside the Eustachian tubes. These tissues are arranged in a ringlike formation in the throat (at the junction of the oral cavity and the pharynx).

xenobiotics: Alien and foreign chemicals; the term is commonly used to describe the toxic petroleum chemicals that are pandemic in our modern-day environment.

RECOMMENDED READING

The Adventure of Self-Discovery by Stanislav Grof (Albany: State University of New York Press, 1988). An incredible book on breath therapy by this innovative and renowned psychiatrist, who is not afraid to explore the furthest frontiers of human consciousness.

Affect Regulation and the Origin of the Self by Allan N. Schore (London: Psychology Press, 1999). Excellent neuropsychological text that helps explain how the brain integrates, records, and regulates emotions.

The Allergy Bible by Linda Gamlin (London: Quadrille Publishing, 2005). Very well-written book that covers all aspects of food allergies.

Alternative Approach to Allergies by Theron Randolph and Ralph Moss (New York: Harper Perennial, 1990). Excellent resource on the diagnosis and treatment of food and environmental allergies by the father of clinical ecology, Theron Randolph, and the science writer who helped expose the financially lucrative practice of allopathic oncology, Ralph Moss.

Alternative Medicine edited by John Anderson and Larry Trivieri, with an introduction by Burton Goldberg (Berkeley, Calif.: Celestial Arts, 2002). Excellent compendium of numerous holistic approaches by the editors of *Alternative Medicine* magazine

The Antibiotic Paradox by Stuart Levy (Cambridge, Mass.: Da Capo Press, 2002). Excellent book on the serious health consequences of cavalier antibiotic misuse by a leading international expert.

Applied Kinesiology: Synopsis by David Walther (Pueblo, Colo.: Systems DC, 1988). The most comprehensive text on this complex field of manual muscle testing covering the history, research, and many diagnostic and therapeutic methods used in AK.

Applied Kinesiology, volume 2 by David Walther (Pueblo, Colo.: Systems DC, 1981). Excellent text by a leading AK physician on the subject of TMD and malocclusions, including diagnosis of associated cranial faults and muscle weakness in the head and neck.

The Assault on Medical Freedom by P. Joseph Lisa (Newburyport, Mass.: Hampton Roads Publishing Company, 1994). A must-read for all D.C.s, N.D.s, D.O.s, acupuncturists, and other holistic practitioners from the intrepid researcher who infiltrated the AMA and exposed the covert tactics and conspiracy to destroy all other professions in competition with M.D.s.

Auricular Therapy: A Comprehensive Text by Bryan L. Frank, M.D., and Nader E. Soliman, M.D. (Bloomington, Ind.: AuthorHouse, 2006). The first definitive American text on this important healing method from France; well written with excellent illustrations.

Autohemotherapy Reference Manual by S. Hale Shakman (Seattle: CreateSpace, 1998). Incredibly thorough synopsis of all aspects on this form of serum therapy—a must-read for all holistic physicians who do homeopathic and isopathic injections.

Babies Remember Birth by David Chamberlain (New York: Ballantine Books, 1989). Extraordinary book on the very clear birth memories people recount under hypnosis and the importance of good prenatal and perinatal care for the health of the child. Also includes a section on the subject of abortion with conclusions similar to Dr. Helen Wambach's in her book *Life Before Life.*

Beyond Amalgam by Susan Stockton (Eustis, Fla.: Power of One Publishing, 2000). Concise booklet on the serious health consequences of chronic dental focal infections.

Biochemical Individuality by Roger J. Williams (New York: McGraw-Hill, 1998). A classic text with a timeless message: we are all genetically and biochemically unique and nutrition and lifestyle directly influence the functional expression (phenotype) of our genes (genotype).

Bioenergetics by Alexander Lowen (New York: Penguin/Arkana, 1994). One of the first books on the body-mind approach to liberating suppressed mental, emotional, and physical trauma hidden in the body's neuromusculoskeletal memory by the Reichian-influenced founder of the field of bioenergetics.

Birth without Violence by Frédérick Leboyer (Healing Arts Press, 2009). A beautiful book full of all kinds of essential truths about childbirth—a must-read for all parents-to-be.

Botanical Medicine: A European Professional Perspective by Dan Kenner and Yves Requena (Taos, N.Mex.: Paradigm Publications, 2001). Important information on the terrain, oligotherapy, gemmotherapy, and the correlation of herbal remedies to the five-element model.

Brain Allergies by William Philpott and Dwight Kalita (New York: McGraw-Hill, 2000). Philpott was one of the original pioneers to sound the alarm on the seriously deleterious effects food allergies can render on mental and emotional functioning in both susceptible children and adults.

Breath and Spirit by Gunnel Minett (New York: HarperCollins, 1994). Along with Grof's *The Adventure of Self-Discovery,* the best book ever written describing the process of rebirthing.

A Brief History of Everything by Ken Wilber (Boston: Shambhala, 2001). This book explains Wilber's very original and brilliant paradigm of the four "quadrants" of human development.

Care of the Soul by Thomas Moore (New York: HarperPerennial, 1994). Excellent book by a renowned theologian who reveals the various ways our lives have lost meaning and how to feel and experience the richness of our souls in our everyday life.

Chemical Deception by Marc Lappe (San Francisco: Sierra Club Books, 1992). Excellent book on the dangers to our health and environment from toxic chemicals.

Chemical Exposure and Human Health by Cynthia Wilson (Jefferson, N.C.: McFarland, 1993). Good resource book on the names of the most common toxic chemicals and the illnesses and syndromes they most typically cause.

Chemical Sensitivity by Bonnye L. Matthews (Jefferson, N.C.: McFarland, 2008). Detailed charts and descriptions of the various levels of the immune, endocrine, and nervous system response to toxic chemicals.

Chemical Sensitivity, volume 1 by William Rea (Boca Raton, Fla.: CRC Press, 1992). Good book for doctors and practitioners on the diagnosis and treatment of chemical sensitivity by this renowned clinical ecologist and his Dallas-based Environmental Health Center.

Chop Wood, Carry Water by Rick Fields (Los Angeles: Tarcher, 1984). This classic book from the early 1980s still holds up as an excellent guide to deepening one's inner journey through the wisdom gained from the world's great spiritual teachers.

Chronic Pain by Hooshang Hooshmand (Boca Raton, Fla.: CRC Press, 1993). A book that should be studied by every holistic physician and practitioner. Includes information on the ephapses created by unhealed scars as well as many other mechanisms of the autonomic nervous system.

Clinical Ecology by Iris Bell (Bolinas, Calif.: Common Knowledge, 1982). Concise book on the field of clinical ecology and the common foods and chemicals that trigger the wide range of physical, mental, and emotional disorders in susceptible individuals.

The Clinical Management of Basic Maxillofacial Orthopedic Appliances, volume 1, *Mechanics* by John W. Witzig and Terrance J. Spahl (Littleton, Mass.: PSG Publishing Company, 1987). Excellent comprehensive text by two renowned orthopedically oriented holistic dentists on the treatment of TMD and malocclusions through functional appliances.

Clinical Management of Head, Neck and TMJ Pain and Dysfunction by Harold Gelb (St. Louis, Mo.: Medico Dental Media International, 1991). A classic text that should be in the library of all physicians (dental and holistic medical) and practitioners who want to be able to assess and refer patients to orthopedically oriented dentists for treatment of TMD and malocclusions.

The Collected Papers of Irvin M. Korr (Colorado Springs: American Academy of Osteopathy, 1979). A compendium of the brilliant work of Dr. Korr, exploring his innovative research and contributions to osteopathic medicine and the deeper understanding of the functioning of the autonomic nervous system.

The Coming Plague by Laurie Garrett (New York: Penguin, 1995). Well-written book on the consequences of the excessive use of antibiotics, unpurified drinking water, and other factors in the emergence of new viruses and the need for worldwide medical as well as political solutions.

The Conscious Ear by Alfred A. Tomatis (Barrytown, N.Y.: Station Hill Press, 1992). Incredible autobiography by this brilliant scientist and educator on treating dyslexia, stuttering, lack of coordination, and other maladies associated with imbalanced listening.

A Consumer's Dictionary of Cosmetic Ingredients by Ruth Winter (New York: Three Rivers Press, 2009). A comprehensive guide to the harmful toxic chemicals in soaps and cosmetics.

Coping with Food Intolerances by Dick Thom (New York: Sterling, 2002). Good book on food allergies with an especially comprehensive section describing the various grains.

Craniosacral Therapy by John E. Upledger and Jon Vredevoogd (Seattle: Eastland Press, 1983). Classic, well-written, and well-illustrated text on the diagnosis of cranial distortion patterns and their treatment.

The Cure for All Cancers by Hulda Clark (Chula Vista, Calif.: New Century Press, 1993). Although the promise of this provocative title doesn't always hold true in clinical practice, Clark was one of the first to sound the alarm against isopropyl alcohol and other toxic chemicals.

The Curse of Louis Pasteur by Nancy Appleton (Santa Monica, Calif.: Choice, 1999). Never one to mince words, this courageous nutritionist explains the true cause of disease and shows how Pasteur's germ theory paradigm has utterly failed.

Death and Dentistry by Martin H. Fischer (Springfield, Ill.: Charles C. Thomas, 1940). A classic 1940s text on the very real and lethal effects of dental focal infections by the holistic physician who later inspired another holistic medical icon, Dr. Henry Bieler, author of *Food Is Your Best Medicine.*

Deceits of the Mind and Their Effects on the Body by Jane Goldberg (Piscataway, N.J.: Transaction Publishers, 1991). One of the best books ever written on mind-body interaction; an essential read for all medical and psychological professionals.

The Defective Delinquent and Insane: The Relation of Focal Infections to Their Causation, Treatment and Prevention by Henry A. Cotton (n.p.: reprinted General Books, 2010 [orig. pub. 1921]). Landmark 1921 book on the effect of focal infections on mental health and the amazing recoveries of various forms of "insanity" after the removal of infected teeth or tonsils.

Dental Caries as a Cause of Nervous Disorders by Patrick Störtebecker (Orlando, Fla.: Bio-Probe, 1986). Written by a brilliant researcher and original thinker, a text on how root-canalled teeth and other dental focal infections can potentiate multiple sclerosis, brain cancer, schizophrenia, epilepsy, and other neurological disease.

Dental Infections: Oral and Systemic, volumes 1 and 2 by Weston A. Price (Cleveland: The Penton Publishing Company, 1923). This classic two-volume set contains the brilliant research and knowledge gained from this father of holistic dentistry on the serious consequences to every system in the body from chronic dental focal infections.

The Dental Physician by Aelred C. Fonder (Rock Falls, Ill.: Medical-Dental Arts, 1985). A profoundly important text, recommended by the great Hans Selye, that should be studied by all biological dentists as well as every holistic physician who understands the importance of diagnosis and referral for the treatment of dental malocclusions in their patients.

Dentistry without Mercury by Sam Ziff and Michael Ziff (Orlando, Fla.: Bio-Probe, 2000). A classic and concise text by the Ziff brothers on the toxicity of mercury amalgam fillings.

Desktop Guide to Keynotes and Confirmatory Symptoms by Roger Morrison (Albany, Calif.: Hahnemann Clinic Pub, 1993). Very concise summary of the most common homeopathic remedies; recommended for every new homeopathic student. Morrison's other text, *Desktop Companion to Physical Pathology,* serves as an excellent resource for acute homeopathic treatment for both homeopathic physicians and parents.

The Diamond Approach by John Davis (Boston: Shambhala, 1999). One of the best overviews of the Diamond Heart psychospiritual approach, by one of the senior Ridhwan teachers.

Diamond Heart, book 1 by A. H. Almaas (Boston: Shambhala, 2000). An excellent introductory book explaining the Diamond Heart psychospiritual approach by the founder of this Ridhwan school.

Digestive Wellness by Elizabeth Lipski (New York: McGraw-Hill, 2004). Exceptionally clear and comprehensive; one of the best books written on the functioning of the digestive system as well as how it typically dysfunctions through dysbiosis and leaky gut syndrome.

Divided Legacy by Harris Coulter (Berkeley, Calif.: North Atlantic Books, 1994). This history of the chasm between homeopathic and allopathic medicine by one of our best science writers is a must-read for all homeopaths and their patients.

The DOs by Norman Gevitz (Baltimore: The Johns Hopkins University Press, 1991). The best historical account of the struggle of osteopathic physicians to become recognized despite the efforts of the medical profession, as well as the amalgamation of the California D.O.s in the early 1960s.

Dr. Pitcairn's New Complete Guide to Natural Health for Dogs and Cats by Richard H. Pitcairn and Susan Hubble Pitcairn (Emmaus, Pa.: Rodale Books, 2005). The leading American holistic veterinarian describes the problems with pet vaccinations as well as guidelines for raising healthy animals.

Dr. Schuessler's Biochemistry by J. B. Chapman (n.p.: Merchant Books, 2008). Practical guide to using cell salts in clinical practice.

Drop-Dead Gorgeous by Kim Erickson (New York: McGraw-Hill, 2002). Excellent book on the serious dangers of chemical-laden cosmetics and soaps, with many natural home alternatives.

E. C. Rosenow and Associates: A Reference Manual by S. H. Shakman (Santa Monica, Calif.: Institute of Science, 1998). In his inimitable precise and detailed way, S. H. Shakman details the life and research of one of the most brilliant physicians, Dr. Edward C. Rosenow, who researched the focal infection theory and had amazing therapeutic results in the early twentieth century.

The E.I. Syndrome by Sherry A. Rogers (Sarasota, Fla.: SK Publishing, 1995). Excellent and practical book on all aspects of environmental sensitivity by this leading holistic physician who knows the suffering of this illness firsthand.

Electromagnetic Fields by B. Blake Levitt (Orlando, Fla.: Harcourt, Brace & Co., 2007). One of the rare resource books on the hazards of electromagnetic fields (EMFs) and their link to modern illnesses such as cancer, chronic fatigue, and learning disabilities.

The Emerging Science of Homeopathy, second edition, by Paolo Bellavite and Andrea Signorini (Berkeley, Calif.: North Atlantic Books, 2002). The best book to date covering the history, principles, and scientific research underlying homeopathy.

The Enneagram by Helen Palmer (New York: HarperOne, 1991). This classic book has held up over time as an excellent introduction to the enneagram.

The Enneagram of Passions and Virtues by Sandra Maitri (New York: Tarcher, 2009). Unique and in-depth book written on two aspects of the enneagram rarely explained: the ego-driven and emotional passions that are transformed through effective psychospiritual work into the associated virtues of inner realization of each enneatype.

Essence by A. H. Almaas (Newburyport, Mass.: Red Wheel Weiser, 1986). Clearly describes the state of what Gurdjieff described as "self-remembering," or essence, and the mental and emotional blocks to deeply experiencing our true essential nature.

Evidence of Harm by David Kirby (New York: St. Martin's Griffin, 2006). This masterful book reads like a modern Watergate detective novel, describing the mysterious rider inserted into the 2002 Homeland Security Bill that shields Eli Lilly from billions of dollars in potential thimerosal litigation by parents who have witnessed the onset of autism clearly linked to their children's vaccinations with products containing this mercury preservative.

Facets of Unity by A. H. Almaas (Boston: Shambhala, 2000). Almaas's masterful book on the Holy Ideas of each psychological type on the enneagram.

Fatal Harvest: The Tragedy of Industrial Agriculture edited by Andrew Kimbrell (Sausalito, Calif.: Foundation for Deep Ecology, 2002). A beautiful book with stunning photographs of the serious environmental and health effects from agribusiness farming, and the hope from organic farming and a "new agrarian consciousness."

Fats That Heal, Fats That Kill by Udo Erasmus (Burnaby, B.C.: Alive Books, 1993). The classic text on all aspects of these essential components of our diet—their various forms, our bodies' ability to digest and assimilate them, the history of margarine versus butter, and much more.

Fiber Menace by Konstantin Monastyrsky (n.p.: Ageless Press, 2005). A must-read for all holistic advocates. This book describes both the constipating effects of fiber and the fallacy of drinking eight glasses of water a day.

The Field by Lynne McTaggart (New York: Harper Paperbacks, 2008). The clearest explanation on the subject of quantum physics ever written.

Focal Infection by Frank Billings (Charleston, S.C.: Nabu Press, 2010). A concise text on the theory of focal infections by one of the originators of this discovery; should be read and studied by all physicians interested in diagnosing and treating foci.

From Auriculotherapy to Auriculomedicine by Paul Nogier (Moulins-les-Metz, France: Maisonneuve, 1983). An essential read for all physicians and practitioners who want to utilize auriculotherapy and/or Auriculomedicine in their practice.

Genetically Engineered Food by Ronnie Cummins and Ben Lilliston (Cambridge, Mass.: Da Capo Press, 2004). Describes the serious health risks of eating GE foods, and how to identify these foods if you still dare to shop in conventional grocery stores.

Germs, Biological Warfare, Vaccinations by Gary Null with James Feast (New York: Seven Stories Press, 2003). Packed with information on the health hazards of vaccines and antibiotics and natural ways to boost the functioning of your immune system as well as "anti-biowarfare regimens."

Headaches Aren't Forever by Gerald Smith (Langhorne, Pa.: International Center for Nutritional Research, 1987). Dr. Smith was the first to alert the holistic community about the health problems, including headaches and musculoskeletal pain in the body, that can arise from crossing the maxillary midline with appliances or bridges.

Heal Yourself with Natural Foods by Nancy Appleton (New York: Sterling, 2000). Another excellent and concise book by this renowned nutritionist on how diet affects every aspect of our lives and the importance of eating a healthy diet.

Healthy Mouth, Healthy Body by Victor Zeines (New York: Kensington, 2000). Loaded with information on holistic dentistry and remedies for patients.

Healthy Teeth for Kids by Jerome and Beverly Mittelman and Jean Barilla (New York: Kensington, 2001). Excellent guide on how to grow strong teeth and fully developed jaw and cranial bones in children.

Holistic Herbal, fourth edition, by David Hoffmann (London: Thorsons, 2003). Comprehensive illustrated guide to the use of botanical medicine in healing from this renowned herbalist.

Homoeopathic Alternatives to Immunisation by Susan Curtis (Kent, U.K.: Winter Press, 1994). Well-written and concise book for travelers and parents on the use of homeopathy as an alternative to vaccines.

Homeopathic Care for Cats and Dogs by Don Hamilton (Berkeley, Calif.: North Atlantic Books, 1999). A convincing book on the dangers of vaccines that will have you searching for an alternative to allopathically oriented veterinarians.

Homeopathic Cell Salt Remedies by Nigey Lennon and Lionel Rolfe (Garden City Park, N.Y.: Square One Publishers, 2004). An excellent guide to choosing cell (tissue) salts.

Homeopathic Remedy Guide by Robin Murphy (Blacksburg, Va.: H.A.N.A. Press, 2000). The best guide to the most common homeopathic remedies outside of homeopathic software; excellent reference for the beginning homeopath.

Homeopathic Science and Modern Medicine by Harris Coulter (Berkeley, Calif.: North Atlantic Books, 1981). This outstanding writer on holistic medicine clearly explains the scientific basis underlying homeopathy.

Homeopathy in Epidemic Diseases by Dorothy Shepherd (London: Random House UK, 2004). The amazing effects of homeopathic remedies on diphtheria, measles, mumps, influenza, pertussis, chicken pox, and other infectious diseases when the early symptoms are treated promptly.

Hormone Deception by D. Lindsey Berkson (New York: McGraw-Hill, 2001). Frightening and thorough book on how toxic chemicals in our environment are mimicking our sex hormones and causing chaos in humans and animals, resulting in infertility, menstrual dysfunction, behavior and learning disabilities, and cancer.

How to Save Your Teeth by David Kennedy (Delaware, Ohio: Health Action Press, 1996). Clear description of levels of gum disease as well as the dangers from mercury amalgam fillings and fluoride.

Identifying and Treating Blockages to Healing by Beate Strittmatter (New York: Thieme, 2004). One of the few books on the treatment of foci by auriculotherapy diagnosed through Auriculomedicine energetic testing methods.

In Search of the Miraculous by P. D. Ouspensky (Boston: Mariner Books, 2001). One of the best books ever written on the teachings of the brilliant spiritual teacher G. I. Gurdjieff.

An Insight into Plants, volumes 1 and 2 by Rajan Sankaran (Mumbai, India: Homeopathic Medical Publishers, 2004). This two-volume set is a must for homeopaths who want to utilize the Sankaran system in their practice.

Integral Psychology by Ken Wilber (Boston: Shambhala, 2000). One of the best works on the integration of Western psychology with Eastern spiritual traditions by this original and brilliant thinker.

Interrelations of Odontons and Tonsils to Organs, Fields of Disturbance, and Tissue Systems by Reinhold Voll, translated by Hartwig Schuldt (Hamburg, Germany: Missing Link Verlag, 1978). One of the few books available in English from this master of energetic testing.

Is It "Just a Phase"? by Susan Anderson Swedo and Henrietta L. Leonard (New York: Broadway Books, 1999). The first book describing the ramifications of PANDAS by the two pediatricians who originated the acronym after years of observing children with obsessive-compulsive disorders.

It's All in Your Head by Hal A. Huggins (New York: Avery Publishing, 1993). Classic book on the health hazards of mercury amalgam fillings written by the holistic dentist who alerted millions to this problem.

Job's Body by Deanne Juhan (Barrytown, N.Y.: Barrytown Limited, 1998). One of the few—and quite possibly the best—books written on the connective tissue. This book should be read and studied by all body workers, D.C.s, and D.O.s.

Know Your Fats by Mary Enig (Silver Spring, Md.: Bethesda Press, 2000). Sally Fallon's coauthor and colleague presents the most comprehensive text on fats ever written, which includes the importance of cholesterol for optimal brain functioning, the need for saturated fats in our diets, and the dangers of trans-fats.

Leaving My Father's House by Marion Woodman (Boston: Shambhala, 1992). Important book on the need to bring "conscious femininity" into a (still) patriarchal world.

Let the Tooth Be Known by Dawn Ewing (Spring, Tex.: Holistic Health Alternatives, 2002). Excellent, very readable overview of all aspects of holistic dentistry.

Lick the Sugar Habit by Nancy Appleton (New York: Avery Trade, 1988). This exceptionally well-written book clearly delineates the very destructive damage sugar does to our immune system and body chemistry, often aided by sugar's "little helpers" such as antibiotics, mercury, steroids, and toxic oils and fats.

Living Downstream by Sandra Steingraber (Cambridge, Mass.: Da Capo Press, 2010). Well-written and comprehensive book by this ecologist that clearly links the growth of cancer in our society to environmental contamination.

Love and Awakening by John Welwood (New York: Harper Paperbacks, 1997). Excellent book by this leading transpersonal psychologist on conscious relationships through an integrated psychospiritual approach.

The Man in the Ear by Paul Nogier and Raphaël Nogier (Moulins-les-Metz, France: Maisonneuve, 1985). A classic text on the origins of auriculotherapy and Auriculomedicine.

Manual of Neural Therapy According to Huneke by Peter Dosch and Mathias Dosch (New York: Thieme, 2007). The original "bible" on the treatment of dominant foci through neural therapy. A must-read for all physicians and practitioners interested in diagnosing and treating scar interference fields and chronic teeth and tonsil focal infections.

Matrix and Matrix Regulation by Alfred Pischinger (Portland, Ore.: Medicina Biologica, 1991). Not an easy read, but this book is a classic from the Austrian master of neural therapy research.

The MD Emperor Has No Clothes by Peter Glidden (self-published, www.drglidden.com, 2010). An excellent exposé on allopathic medical care in this country and the benefits of naturopathic medicine.

Mental Deficiency by Alfred Frank Tredgold (Charleston, S.C.: Nabu Press, 2010). An early-twentieth-century writer referenced by Dr. Price on the association between narrow palates and mental deficiency.

Mental Health and Chiropractic edited by Herman C. Schwartz (New Hyde Park, N.Y.: Sessions Publishers, 1973). This book describes the amazing effects of chiropractic care on psychiatric patients in the mid-nineteenth century—a must-read for all holistic D.C.s.

The Mercury in Your Mouth by Quicksilver Associates (New York: Quicksilver Press, 1997). Excellent book that details the many research studies proving the serious toxicity of mercury amalgam fillings.

Mercury Poisoning from Dental Amalgam—a Hazard to the Human Brain by Patrick Störtebecker (Orlando, Fla.: Bio-Probe, 1986). This short book is packed with valuable information such as Störtebecker's research proving axonal transport of toxins along nerves, the storage of these toxins in various ganglia, and the importance of the valveless venous system in the brain and spine.

The Micro-Organisms of the Human Mouth by Willoughby D. Miller (Birmingham, Ala.: The Classics of Dentistry Library, 1980). First published in 1889 by this father of the focal infection theory, this book should be read by all physicians interested in the history of the field of focal infections, as well as diagnosing and treating them.

The Milk Book by William Campbell Douglass (Panama: Rhino Publishing, 2004). Excellent book on how pasteurization and, even worse, homogenization have destroyed nature's "perfect food."

The Missing Link by Michael Ziff and Sam Ziff (Orlando, Fla.: Bio-Probe, 1991). This concise book details the substantial number of research studies clearly establishing the link between mercury amalgam fillings and chronic cardiovascular disease.

More from the Gluten-Free Gourmet by Bette Hagman (New York: Holt Paperbacks, 2000). Excellent cookbook of gluten-free recipes, including delicious gluten-free bread.

Natural Detoxification by Jacqueline Krohn and Frances Taylor (Seattle: Hartley and Marks Publishers, 2000). Well-written book on various methods for detoxification of toxic metals, chemicals, foods, and drugs.

Natural Healing with Cell Salts by Skye Weintraub (Salt Lake City, Utah: Woodland Publishing, 1996). Probably the best book written on cell salts, with a very easy-to-use guide for their various uses in healing.

Nature Doctors by Friedhelm Kirchfeld and Wade Boyle (Portland, Ore.: NCNM Press, 1994). Excellent book on the life and work of Priessnitz (originator of the water cure), Kneipp and the Lusts (founders of naturopathy), Carroll (founder of constitutional hydrotherapy), and other colorful and amazing healers from the nineteenth and twentieth centuries; should be read by all holistic physicians and practitioners.

Nature's Open Secret by Rudolf Steiner (Great Barrington, Mass.: Anthroposophic Press, 2010). Includes a description of Goethe's discovery of the premaxilla bone as well as a deeper understanding of the nature of plants, animals, and human beings through the brilliant lens of these two geniuses.

Neural Therapy: Applied Neurophysiology and Other Topics by Robert F. Kidd (self-published, www.neuraltherapybook.com, 2005). This Canadian physician has written an excellent reference book for physicians that details neural therapy treatment of various foci and their related ganglia—one of the rare books written on these subjects.

The Neurodynamics of the Vertebral Subluxation by A. E. Homewood (St. Petersburg, Fla.: Valkyrie Press, 1979). A classic chiropractic text that not only describes the neurology of the somatovisceral and other reflexes but also includes tidbits like D. D. Palmer's abhorrence of toxic food and water, as well as "the outrageous practice of the M.D. who injects vaccine poison into a healthy person."

Neurology for Barefoot Doctors in All Countries by Patrick Störtebecker (Stockholm, Sweden: Störtebecker Foundation for Research, 1988). Another incredible book by this brilliant researcher; this text is an essential read for all holistic practitioners.

A New Model for Health and Disease by George Vithoulkas (Berkeley, Calif.: North Atlantic Books, 1995). Excellent summary of how modern medicine has failed in curing disease from this world-renowned homeopath.

No Milk by Daniel A. Twogood (Victorville, Calif.: Wilhelmina Books, 1992). California chiropractor clearly links back pain and headaches with an allergy to dairy, a connection often seen in holistic practices.

Nontoxic, Natural and Earthwise by Debra Lynn Dadd (Los Angeles: Tarcher, 1990). Excellent book by this internationally recognized consumer advocate on the safest products for our homes and the environment.

Nourishing Traditions by Sally Fallon (Winona Lake, Ind.: NewTrends Publishing, 1999). This combination cookbook and nutritional book that teaches ancestral dietary wisdom has become a classic and is a must-read for every holistically minded individual.

Nutrition and Physical Degeneration by Weston A. Price (Lemon Grove, Calif.: Price Pottenger Nutrition, 2008). As A. C. Fonder said, this book is the most important book ever written and essential for everyone in the healing profession.

Operative Dentistry by G. V. Black (Chicago: Medico-Dental Publishing Co., 1936). This classic four-volume text by the father of operative dentistry has an excellent chapter on focal infections (volume 4) as well as other timeless information on appropriate cavitation surgery.

Optimal Wellness by Ralph Golan (New York: Wellspring/Ballantine, 1995). Excellent compendium of holistic treatments for common chronic disorders by a holistic Seattle physician.

Organon of the Medical Art by Samuel Hahnemann, edited by Wenda Brewster O'Reilly (Palo Alto, Calif.: Birdcage Books, 1996). The *Organon* is the "bible" of every homeopath, and it has never been clearer in explaining the art and science of homeopathy than in this edition edited by O'Reilly.

Other Healers: Unorthodox Medicine in America by Norman Gevitz (Baltimore: The Johns Hopkins University Press, 1988). Well-written perspective on "unorthodox healers"—D.O.s, D.C.s, homeopaths, and others—in their struggle to receive acceptance despite pressure and outright persecution by the medical profession.

The Other Song, by Rajan Sankaran (Mumbai, India: Homeopathic Medical Publishers, 2008). An excellent description of how the new sensation method works, for homeopathic patients and practitioners alike.

Our Stolen Future by Theo Colborn, Dianne Dumanoski, and John Peterson Myers (New York: Plume, 1997). A landmark book on the widespread birth defects and sexual abnormalities seen in wildlife around the world as a result of endocrine-disrupting synthetic chemicals, as well as their effects on human sexuality and reproduction.

Overdosed America: The Broken Promise of American Medicine by John Abramson (New York: Harper Perennial, 2008). A must-read book for both physicians and patients by a Harvard physician whose statistical acumen allowed him to expose the specious research propagated by pharmaceutical companies.

The Pearl Beyond Price by A. H. Almaas (Boston: Shambhala, 2000). Extraordinary psychospiritual text describing the process of becoming truly human by this brilliant author and founder of the Ridhwan school.

The Point of Existence by A. H. Almaas (Boston: Shambhala, 2000). This classic text by the leader of the Ridhwan school reveals how the various levels of narcissism are simply incomplete stages of development that block self-understanding and our essential nature from emerging.

Pottenger's Cats by Francis Pottenger (Lemon Grove, Calif.: Price Pottenger Nutrition, 1995). Short text on the brilliant research conducted by Dr. Pottenger where he determined raw milk and other nontoxic foods were essential to adequate bone and brain development in cats and humans.

Principles of Holistic Therapy with Herbal Essences by Dietrich Gümbel (Portland, Ore.: Medicina Biologica, 1993). One of the best and most scientific treatises on the effects of essential oils on the nervous, circulatory, and endocrine systems, and an excellent anatomy and physiology review with insights that all holistic physicians will enjoy.

Probiotics: Nature's Internal Healers by Natasha Trenev (New York: Avery, 1998). Explains the importance of healthy intestinal flora with a comprehensive guide to discerning quality (live) cultured dairy products and acidophilus supplements.

Psychotherapy East and West by Alan Watts (New York: Vintage, 1975). One of the early classics in the field of transpersonal psychology by this brilliant expert on Eastern spiritual traditions and Western psychology.

Reclaiming Our Health by John Robbins (Tiburon, Calif.: H. J. Kramer, 1998). Excellent "whistle-blowing" book on the many serious health consequences of allopathic medicine.

Root Canal Cover-Up by George E. Meinig (Lemon Grove, Calif.: Price Pottenger Nutrition, 2008). This book by a past founding member of the American Association of Endodontists details the damage done from root canals and also describes much of the history of the focal infection theory.

The Roots of Disease by Robert Kulacz and Thomas E. Levy (Bloomington, Ind.: Xlibris, 2002). Details the detrimental health effects of root canals.

The Sanctity of Human Blood by Tim O'Shea, thirteenth edition (www.thedoctorwithin.com, 2009). One of the most well-documented books on the toxicity of vaccines.

The Science of Homeopathy by George Vithoulkas (New York: Grove Press, 1980). A book about not just homeopathy but also the cause and treatment of disease. A must-read for all holistic practitioners.

The Second Brain by Michael Gershon (New York: Harper Paperbacks, 1999). One of the most important and illuminating books on the digestive system, filled with incredible facts (e.g., 95 percent of the neurotransmitter serotonin is manufactured and contained in the gut, which, when deficient, can trigger both constipation and depression).

The Secret Life of the Unborn Child by Thomas Verny with John Kelly (New York: Dell, 1982). A pioneering work on the importance of prenatal care and evidence of the parental and environmental memories and patterns imprinted on the fetus before birth.

The Sensation in Homeopathy by Rajan Sankaran (Mumbai, India: Homeopathic Medical Publishers, 2004). This is the most comprehensive text written so far on the "vital sensation" that underlies each remedy pattern. The Sankaran system is incredibly effective in determining a patient's deepest constitutional homeopathic remedy, and this book is a must-read for all interested homeopaths willing to put the time and energy into studying and learning this revolutionary new method.

A Shot in the Dark by Harris Coulter and Barbara Loe Fisher (New York: Avery Trade, 1991). A "chilling account" of how dangerous the pertussis vaccine (DPT) is to children's health.

Silent Spring by Rachel Carson (Boston: Houghton Mifflin, 1994). The landmark book that forced the banning of DDT, now with an introduction by Al Gore.

Silver Dental Fillings: The Toxic Time Bomb by Sam Ziff (Santa Fe, N.Mex.: Aurora Press, 1986). Another excellent book on the scientific evidence of the damaging health effects of mercury from amalgam fillings as well as from dental galvanism.

Somatovisceral Aspects of Chiropractic by Charles S. Masarsky and Marion Todres-Masarsky (New York: Churchill Livingstone, 2001). One of the rare modern-day books written on the important somatovisceral (spinal-organ) aspects of chiropractic care.

The Soul of Remedies by Rajan Sankaran (Mumbai, India: Homeopathic Medical Publishers, 1997). One of Dr. Sankaran's earlier books that describes the basic delusion, miasm, and symptoms that underlie the most common homeopathic remedies—an important resource for all homeopaths.

Soul Without Shame by Byron Brown (Boston: Shambhala, 1998). This book by a senior Ridhwan teacher helps readers identify the insidious and relentless "inner critic" (superego) inside and through awareness and presence move away from these debilitating judgmental thoughts and beliefs.

Spacecruiser Inquiry by A. H. Almaas (Boston: Shambhala, 2002). One of Almaas's best books. Describes the various lataif—the centers of perception and essential states—in more detail than any other of this texts.

The Spirit of Homoeopathy by Rajan Sankaran (Berkeley, Calif.: Homeopathic Educational Services, 1999). Excellent book for homeopaths to read about the "central disturbance" and other philosophies that describe Sankaran's understanding of disease as delusion.

The Spiritual Dimension of the Enneagram by Sandra Maitri (New York: Tarcher, 2001). Very well-written book that explains in depth each of the nine enneatypes' personality distortion tendencies resulting from the loss of a particular enlightened perspective, or Holy Idea.

Sri Aurobindo or the Adventure of Consciousness by Satprem (Mysore, India: Mira Aditi Centre, 2000). One of the best books written on the life of Aurobindo, one of the few Eastern gurus who understood the essential need for psychological self-understanding in concert with spiritual work.

Staying Well in a Toxic World by Lynn Lawson (Chicago: Noble Press, 1993). Classic and valuable text on the devastating effects of toxic chemicals in our homes, schools, and workplaces.

The Stress of Life by Hans Selye (New York: McGraw-Hill, 1978). This brilliant researcher describes the debilitating effects psychological and physical stress exerts on the adrenals, thymus, and entire body; a classic text that should be read and studied by all holistic practitioners.

The Substance of Homoeopathy by Rajan Sankaran (Berkeley, Calif.: Homeopathic Educational Services, 1999). Important book for all homeopaths on the theory of miasms, detailed and expanded through the original thinking of this brilliant teacher.

Textbook of Natural Medicine, third edition, volumes 1 and 2 by Joseph E. Pizzorno Jr. and Michael T. Murray (New York: Churchill Livingstone, 2005). The "bible" of holistic medicine with over 10,000 research literature references; this has become the standard text internationally for science-based naturopathic medicine.

The Tipping Point by Malcolm Gladwell (New York: Back Bay Books, 2002). This very entertaining read will change the way you think about how to effect changes in your life as well as in the world.

Tooth Truth by Frank J. Jerome (Chula Vista, Calif.: New Century Press, 2000). Excellent book on holistic dentistry with a clear description of the procedure of placing crowns and the more conservative options of inlays and onlays.

Toward a Psychology of Awakening by John Welwood (Boston: Shambhala, 2002). Excellent book by this renowned transpersonal psychologist exploring spiritual, psychological, and interpersonal transformation.

Toxic Deception by Dan Fagin, Marianne Lavelle, and the Center for Public Integrity (Monroe, Maine: Common Courage Press, 1999). Describes how chemical companies, in collusion with the EPA, are deceptive regarding the toxicity of their products.

Toxic Metal Syndrome by H. Richard Casdorph and Morton Walker (New York: Avery, 1994). Clearly describes the neurotoxicity of aluminum, mercury, cadmium, and lead and the beneficial detoxifying effects of chelation therapy.

Transpersonal Psychologies edited by Charles T. Tart (New York: HarperCollins, 1992). Rare book on this important field of modern psychospiritual approaches with a fascinating chapter on the original enneagram training in Arica, Chile, that was coauthored by the renowned John C. Lilly.

The Trials of Homeopathy by Michael Emmans Dean (Essen, Germany: KVC Verlag, 2004). Reveals the long history (since 1821) of scientifically conducted clinical trials homeopathic remedies have been subjected to and the effectiveness of this form of natural medicine.

The Truth About the Drug Companies by Marcia Angell (New York: Random House Trade Paperbacks, 2005). Excellent and well-referenced indictment of the lies pharmaceutical companies tell in order to sell their drugs and the modern reversed trend of promoting diseases to fit an existing drug in the name of corporate profit.

Vaccination? A Review of Risks and Alternatives, fifth edition by Isaac Golden (Canberra, Australia: National Library, 1998). This book presents the pros and cons on routine immunizations and the effectiveness of homeopathic alternatives to vaccination.

Vaccination, Social Violence, and Criminality by Harris Coulter (Berkeley, Calif.: North Atlantic Books, 1993). A disturbing exposé by this excellent science writer. Considered by Dr. Harold Buttram, a leader in this field, to be a "masterpiece" and one of the most important works on childhood vaccination programs and subsequent violence in our society.

Vaccinations and Immune Malfunction by Harold E. Buttram and John Chriss Hoffman (Quakerstown, Pa.: The Randolph Society, 1985). Excellent booklet on the damage done by compulsory mass medication with vaccines and the resulting vaccine-induced immune dysfunction.

Vaccine Guide for Dogs and Cats by Catherine J. M. Diodati (Santa Fe, N.Mex.: New Atlantean Press, 2003). Describes the debilitating and sometimes fatal consequences of annual pet vaccinations and their link to chronic autoimmune and neurological disorders.

Vaccines: Are They Really Safe and Effective? by Neil Z. Miller (Santa Fe, N.Mex.: New Atlantean Press, 2008). A revised edition of the classic and most comprehensive and concise book on the damage done to our immune, endocrine, and nervous systems from toxic vaccinations.

Vaccines, Autism and Childhood Disorders by Neil Z. Miller (Santa Fe, N.Mex.: New Atlantean Press, 2003). This second book by the leading writer on the serious health consequences of vaccines is a must-read for all parents considering immunizations for their children.

Vitalism: The History of Herbalism, Homeopathy, and Flower Essences by Matthew Wood (Berkeley, Calif.: North Atlantic Books, 2000). Includes fascinating biographies of Paracelsus, Hahnemann, Bach, and the other brilliant forefathers of holistic medicine.

What Every Parent Should Know About Childhood Immunization by Jamie Murphy (Boston: Earth Healing Products, 1993). Excellent and concise book on the adverse reactions to vaccines, the "witch's brew" of toxic chemicals contained in them, and the "myth of vaccine immunity."

When Antibiotics Fail by Marc Lappe (Berkeley, Calif.: North Atlantic Books, 1995). Older book but still holds up well in explaining the inappropriate use of antibiotics and how these drugs have caused widespread bacterial resistance.

Whiplash and Temporomandibular Disorders by Dennis Steigerwald et al. (Encinitas, Calif.: Keiser Publishing, 1992). Well-researched book on the traumatic onset of TMD and the multidisciplinary chiropractic-dental integrated approach to treatment.

Whole-Body Dentistry by Mark A. Breiner (Fairfield, Conn.: Quantum Health Press, 1999). Excellent comprehensive book on all aspects of holistic dentistry.

The Whole Food Bible by Chris Kilham (Rochester, Vt.: Healing Arts Press, 1996). Comprehensive guide to eating safe and organically. Discusses the dangers of toxic preservatives, pesticides, bovine growth hormones, chlorine-dipped fish, and bioengineering.

Whole Food Facts by Evelyn Roehl (Rochester, Vt.: Healing Arts Press, 1996). Good reference on the source, nutritional value, storage, and preparation of foods, from adzuki beans to zahidi dates.

Women and Autoimmune Disease by Robert G. Lahita (New York: Harper Paperbacks, 2005). A clear description of the most common autoimmune diseases including the little-known PANDAS.

Yasgur's Homeopathic Dictionary and Holistic Health Reference by Jay Yasgur (El Paso, Tex.: Van Hoy, 2004). An essential book for all homeopaths full of definitions of obscure homeopathic medical terminology as well as more modern terms.

Your Body Can Talk by Susan L. Levy and Carol Lehr (Prescott, Ariz.: Hohm Press, 1996). An explanation of how muscle testing works based on AK and CK principles; suitable for all readers.

Your Jaws, Your Life by David C. Page (Baltimore: Smilepage Pub, 2003). Excellent book on the deleterious effects of TMD syndrome and dental malocclusions; flawed only by this author's stance on the "safety" of mercury amalgam fillings.

RESOURCES

AURICULOTHERAPY PRODUCTS FOR PRACTITIONERS

CEPES-Laser: Contact Med Servi-Systems in Canada at (800) 267-6868 or go to the website of Advanced Medical Systems at www.magnetotherapy.de.

Needles: Order ML1-2215 AcuGlide needles from Helio Medical Supplies, Inc., at (800) 672-2726 or go to www.heliomed.com.

Pointer Plus: Contact Lhasa OMS at (800) 722-8775 or go to www. lhasaoms.com. (Suggested for diagnosis only.)

Pointoselect DT: Contact Schwa-Medico in Germany at zentrale@schwa-medico.de or go to www.schwa-medico.de. (For diagnosis and treatment.)

CAVITATION SURGERY SUPPORT

Dr. Jerry Bouquot at the University of Texas Health Science Center: Dentists and oral surgeons can order biopsy kits to utilize after cavitation surgery by calling (713) 500-4420 or e-mailing Dr. Bouquot at jerry.bouquot@uth.tmc.edu.

HOMEOPATHIC COMPANIES

Hahnemann Laboratories: Call (888) 427-6422 or go to www.hahnemannlabs.com.

Helios: Call (in London) 01892 536393 or go to www.helios.co.uk.

JOURNALS

PPNF *Health and Healing Wisdom* Journal: The Price-Pottenger Nutrition Foundation, dedicated to propagating the benefits of whole foods and ancestral wisdom researched by Francis Pottenger, M.D., and Weston Price, D.D.S., publishes this excellent quarterly journal. Contact PPNF at (800) FOODS-4-U (366-3748), e-mail them at info@ price-pottenger.org, or go to www.ppnf.org.

Wise Traditions: Get well-referenced and cutting-edge information on nutrient-dense whole foods, the soy controversy, vaccinations and autism, breast-feeding and alternatives, statin drugs, and much more from this valuable quarterly journal that teaches the traditional dietary wisdom articulated by Weston Price, D.D.S. Contact the Weston A. Price Foundation at (202) 333-HEAL (4325) or (202) 363-4394, e-mail them at info@westonaprice.org, or go to www.westonaprice.org.

LABORATORIES TO TEST FOR HEAVY METALS AND TOXIC CHEMICALS

Doctor's Data: Practitioners may call (800) 323-2784, or go to www.doctorsdata.com, to order the Fecal Heavy Metal test as well as other diagnostic tests.

MELISA: Call (888) 342-7272 or go to www.neuroscienceinc.com. This test does not require provocation and can differentiate between metallic mercury from dental amalgams and ethyl mercury (thimerosal) used in vaccines.

Pacific Toxicology Laboratories: Call (800) 538-6942 or go to www.pactox.com.

LASERS

"Canadian" Laser: Contact Rick McKay at (250) 474-3514 or e-mail him at jarek.mfg@shaw.ca.

LOCAL ANESTHETIC

ApothéCure: Physicians, call (800) 969-6601 or go to www.apothecure.com to order epinephrine-free, preservative-free bupivacaine, the least toxic local anesthetic presently available.

NEURAL THERAPY WITHOUT NEEDLES PRODUCTS

BioResource Isopathic Drops: Practitioners, call (800) 203-3775 or go to www.bioresourceinc.com to order Notatum 4X, Aspergillus 4X, and Kombination 4X drops.

Laser: Practitioners, see "Canadian" Laser information above.

Organic Essence Pure Organic Shea Butter: Call (707) 465-8955 or go to www.orgess.com to order shea butter to rub into scar interference fields.

NUTRITIONAL PRODUCT COMPANIES

BioImmersion: Healthcare professionals, call (425) 451-3112 or go to www.bioimmersion.com to order probiotic and antioxidant formulas including High ORAC, Original Formula, Triple Berry, Wild Blueberry Extract, and more.

BioResource: Practitioners, call (800) 203-3775 or go to www.bioresourceinc.com to order Notatum 4X drops or capsules, Aspergillus 4X drops, Kombination 4X drops, and essential oils (e.g., Niaouli for chronic tonsil foci).

Biotics: Healthcare practitioners, call (800) 231-5777 or go to www.bioticsresearch.com to order organic virgin sesame seed oil for use in Dr. Karach's oil pulling treatment.

Dragon Herbs: Call (888) 558-6642 or go to www.dragonherbs.com to order Jing and other Chinese herbal medicines.

Enzymes, Inc.: Healthcare practitioners, call (800) 637-7893 or go to www.enzymesinc.com to order Gastric Comfort (#601) for those with a sensitive stomach and gut.

Gaia Herbs: Call (888) 917-8269 or go to www.gaiaherbs.com to order Sweetish Bitters, to help stimulate hydrochloric acid (HCL) and enzyme release during meals.

Gemmos LLC: Healthcare professionals, call (877) 417-6298 or go to www.gemmos-usa.com to order gemmotherapy herbal remedies.

Green Pasture: Call (402) 858-4818 or go to www.greenpasture.org to order Blue Ice Fermented Cod Liver Oil and Blue Ice Fermented Skate Liver Oil.

Mary Cordaro: Go to www.marycordaro.com to order reverse osmosis water filters or for more information on creating healthy, nontoxic homes.

Nordic Naturals: Call (800) 662-2544 or go to www.nordicnaturals.com to order ProDHA or other quality fish oils.

Original Quinton: Call (888) 278-4686 or go to www.originalquinton.com to order the very assimilable marine plasma supplements.

PC NetwoRx, Inc.: Call (800) 453-7516 or go to www.msm-msm.com to order the crystal form of MSM (sulfur).

Protocol for Life Balance: Pracitioners, call (877) 776-8610 or go to www.protocolforlife.com to order ubiquinol, the antioxidant form of coenzyme Q10.

PSC Distribution: Call (631) 477-6696 or go to www.epsce.com to order herbal gemmotherapy (plant stem cell) remedies.

Pure Indian Foods: Call (877) 588-4433 or go to www.pureindianfoods.com to order organic ghee with high X factor (vitamin K_2) and other fat-soluble vitamins.

Radiant Life Company: Call (888) 593-9595 or go to www.radiantlifecatalog.com to order the book *Nourishing Traditions* by Sally Fallon and for water filtration systems (designed by Dennis Higgins, M.D.), extra virgin coconut oil, cod liver oil, fermenting crocks, slow-speed grain mills, and much more.

Seroyal: Physicians, call (888) 737-6925 or go to www.seroyal.com to order Schuessler cell salts.

The Synergy Company: Call (800) 723-0277 or go to www.thesynergycompany.com to order Pure Radiance C, a natural form of vitamin C.

Thorne: Practitioners, call (800) 228-1966 or go to www.thorne.com to order Herbal Bulk, Magnesium Citramate, Calcium-Magnesium Citramate, Formula SF734, Dipan 9, Bio-Gest, B.P.P., Artecin, and a multitude of other excellent nutritional products.

PSYCHOSPIRITUAL SCHOOLS OR PATHS

Breathwork: To locate a holotropic-certified practitioner based on Dr. Stanislav Grof's teaching, call (415) 383-8779 or go to www.holotropic.com. To locate a Reichian-oriented therapist, go to the Radix Institute website at www.radix.org. For rebirthers utilizing the Orr method, consult the www.rebirthingbreathwork.com website.

Ridhwan or **Diamond Heart School:** For more information on the school, call (510) 841-1283, e-mail them at office@dhat.org, or go to www.ridhwan.org.

Transpersonal Psychology: Contact the Association for Transpersonal Psychology at (650) 424-8764, or visit their website at www.atpweb.org. For those who would like to train in transpersonal psychology, the Institute of Transpersonal Psychology (ITP) in Palo Alto (650-493-4430 or www.itp.edu) and the California Institute of Integral Studies (CIIS) in San Francisco (415-575-6150 or www.ciis.edu) are both excellent and internationally renowned. Dr. John Welwood, who is on the CIIS faculty, also holds workshops and trainings in transpersonal psychology, and he can be reached at (415) 381-6077. To study the work and teachings of Ken Wilber, contact the Integral Institute at (866) 483-0168, or go to www.integralinstitute.org.

SEMINARS AND PRACTITIONERS: AURICULOTHERAPY

Dr. Bryan Frank and Dr. Nader Soliman: Contact Dr. Bryan Frank for upcoming seminars, referrals to practitioners trained in auriculotherapy, or an excellent auricular wall chart and atlas at (405) 623-7667, or go to www.auriculartherapy.com. Contact Dr. Nader Soliman by going to www.alternativemedicineseminars.com. These two doctors have also written an excellent book together titled *Auricular Therapy: A Comprehensive Text.*

Dr. Louisa Williams: Go to www.radicalmedicine.com, e-mail info@radicalmedicine.com, or call (415) 460-1968 for information on Dr. Williams's upcoming seminars or for referrals to practitioners trained in auriculotherapy.

Dr. Mikhael Adams: Call (905) 878-9994 or go to www.integralhealth.ca for information on upcoming seminars or for referrals to practitioners trained in auriculotherapy.

SEMINARS AND PRACTITIONERS: HOLISTIC DENTISTRY

For information on continuing education seminars or to locate a holistically oriented or "biological" dentist, contact one of the following organizations:

Consumers for Dental Choice at (202) 822-6307 or www.toxicteeth.org

Dental Amalgam Mercury Solutions (DAMS) at (800) 311-6265, (651) 644-4572, or dams@usfamily.net

Dental Wellness Institute at (800) 335-7755 or www.dentalwellness4u.com

Holistic Dental Association (HDA) at (305) 356-7338 or www.holisticdental.org

International Academy of Biological Dentistry and Medicine (IABDM) at (281) 651-1745 or www.iabdm.org

International Academy of Oral Medicine and Toxicology (IAOMT) at (863) 420-6373 or www.iaomt.org

SEMINARS AND PRACTITIONERS: ORTHOPEDIC DENTISTRY

For information on continuing education seminars or to locate holistic dentists trained in treating TMD and malocclusions, contact one of the following organizations:

American Academy of Craniofacial Pain (AACP) at (800) 322-8651 or www.aacfp.org

American Academy of Gnathologic Orthopedics (AAGO) at (800) 510-AAGO or www.aago.com

American Association for Functional Orthodontics (AAFO) at (800) 441-3850 or www.aafo.org

International Association of Facial Growth Guidance (IAFGG) (Biobloc appliances) at (888) 404-3223 or www.orthotropics.com

OrthoSmile Inc. (Homeoblock appliances) at (518) 943-7703 or www.facialdevelopment.com

(Dentists in the previous "Holistic Dentistry" list may also have referrals to orthopedically trained dentists.)

SEMINARS AND PRACTITIONERS: DRAINAGE

Dr. Louisa Williams: Call (415) 460-1968 or go to www.radicalmedicine.com for information on upcoming seminars that include gemmotherapy drainage remedies.

Dr. Mikhael Adams: Call (905) 878-9994 or go to www.integralhealth.ca for information on upcoming seminars and practitioners trained in the use of drainage remedies.

Gemmos LLC: Call (877) 417-6298 or go to www.gemmos-usa.com for information on upcoming seminars on gemmotherapy.

Seroyal: Call (888) 737-6925 or go to www.seroyal.com for information on upcoming courses.

SEMINARS AND PRACTITIONERS: ENERGETIC TESTING

Applied Kinesiology (AK): Contact the International College of Applied Kinesiology (ICAK) at (913) 384-5336 or go to www.icakusa.com.

Autonomic Response Testing (ART): Go to www.klinghardtacademy.com for information on Dr. Dietrich Klinghardt's ART method.

Clinical Kinesiology (CK): E-mail Dr. Chris Beardall at beardall@hotmail.com or call him at (503) 982-6925, or contact Robert Shane at shanebob@msn.com, for more information.

Matrix Reflex Testing (MRT): Go to www.radicalmedicine.com, e-mail info@radicalmedicine.com, or call (415) 460-1968 for information on Dr. Louisa Williams's MRT technique.

Touch for Health: Contact the foundation at (310) 589-5269 or go to http://touch4health.com for information on Touch for Health courses.

SEMINARS AND PRACTITIONERS: HOMEOPATHY

There are many great homeopathic teachers and methods. However, the most accurate and profound technique today is that taught by Dr. Rajan Sankaran and his Mumbai colleagues, referred to as the Sankaran system. To learn about their next seminar in the United States, to find a Sankaran-trained homeopath near you, or to study at the **California Center for Homeopathic Education (CCHE)**, call (760) 466-7581 or go to www.cchomeopathic.com.

For information on Dr. Sankaran's seminars worldwide, go to **Homeopathic Medical Publishers** at www.rajansankaran.com.

For information on other excellent seminars by Sankaran-trained Mumbai practitioners, go to **Dr. Joshis' Homeopathic Care** website at www.drjoshisclinic.com.

Dr. Betty Wood also maintains a calendar of homeopathy courses in North America, many of them taught by Sankaran-trained homeopaths. To subscribe, e-mail her at bw@bettywoodmd.com.

SEMINARS AND PRACTITIONERS: TREATING FOCI AND DETOXIFYING HEAVY METALS AND CHEMICALS

There is no one group at this point that addresses all the different aspects of healing described in this book. For example, it is very difficult to find a holistic practitioner who both specializes in constitutional homeopathy according to the Sankaran system and *also* is knowledgeable in detoxifying mercury amalgam fillings, using herbal drainage remedies, treating focal infections and scar interference fields, and so forth. Therefore, in most cases, individuals should plan on seeing at least two physicians or practitioners, as well as a holistic dentist, for both their constitutional remedy and the diagnosis and appropriate treatment of their suspected toxic fillings and crowns, foci, and scars. However, the following contacts can help direct you to training courses as well as practitioners who have studied all, or at least a great majority, of these concepts:

Klinghardt Academy: Go to www.klinghardtacademy.com for a referral to practitioners who have learned Dr. Dietrich Klinghardt's ART (Autonomic Response Testing) technique and for information on upcoming seminars on the diagnosis and treatment of foci and their disturbed fields and ganglia, toxic metals and chemicals, food allergies, dental malocclusions (TMD), and geopathic and electromagnetic stress. Treatments taught include neural therapy, isopathy, nosodes, complex homeopathy, nutritional supplementation, microcurrent therapy, and psycho-neurobiology.

Dr. Louisa Williams: Go to www.radicalmedicine.com, e-mail info@radicalmedicine.com, or call (415) 460-1968 for referral to practitioners who have learned Dr. Louisa Williams's MRT (Matrix Reflex Testing) energetic testing method and for information on upcoming seminars on the diagnosis and treatment of foci and their disturbed fields and ganglia, toxic metals and chemicals, dental malocclusions (TMD), food allergies, and geopathic and electromagnetic stress. Treatments taught include the use of gemmotherapy drainage remedies, auriculotherapy, neural therapy, Schuessler cell salts, isopathy, nosodes, and nutritional supplementation, and here you can also find information on the Sankaran system of constitutional homeopathy and referral to schools and teachers who teach this method.

INDEX

Page numbers in *italics* indicate photographs and illustrations.